THE HUMAN BRAIN AND SPINAL CORD

The Human Brain
and
Spinal Cord

A HISTORICAL STUDY ILLUSTRATED

BY WRITINGS FROM ANTIQUITY

TO THE TWENTIETH CENTURY

Edwin Clarke and C. D. O'Malley

1968

UNIVERSITY OF CALIFORNIA PRESS

Berkeley and Los Angeles

University of California Press   Berkeley and Los Angeles, California
Cambridge University Press   London, England
© 1968 by the regents of the university of california
library of congress catalog card number: 68–11275
designed by david pauly
printed in the united states of america

PREFACE

DURING recent years there has been a considerable increase in the publication of collections of readings or so-called source books to illustrate the historical development of different areas of medicine, and it is hoped that this further contribution to this category of books will be found of value to those interested in the historical development of knowledge of the brain and nervous system.

It seems appropriate here to describe the principle guiding the selection of material for inclusion. First of all, a decision was made, on the basis of inherent importance, as to what material ought properly be included, and then, wherever necessary, it was translated into English. In consequence the present work contains a considerable number of selections hitherto not available except in their original language. Such translations as were available for the most part were not used because of faults of translation or misleading omissions, antiquated terminology, or a hackneyed quality resulting from repeated use in the past. Finally, it may be added that some of the classic works were astonishingly rare and difficult to find even in their original languages, as, for example, one of Haller's, those of Mistichelli and of Pourfour du Petit, and several of the papers of Ramón y Cajal.

In line with the principle of desirability rather than availability, the selections illustrating the evolution of knowledge of neuroanatomy and neurophysiology have been arranged under broad headings representing the main anatomical structures such as the spinal cord and the cerebellum, and basic physiological principles such as those of cerebral localization and the reflex. However, the vastness of the total subject is such that certain omissions had to be made, and in consequence material on the basal ganglia, thalamus, hypothalamus, pituitary, cranial nerves, meninges, the embryology of the nervous system, the autonomic nervous system, the physiology of the special senses, and sensory modalities, among other subjects, has not been included.

Within the chapters illustrating the chief divisions the selections have been arranged in chronological order, each preceded by a brief biographical account of the contributor and some attempt to relate his contributions to those of other investigators. Occasionally, however, two or more contemporary themes have been considered in sequence rather than in strict chronological order for the sake of clarity. In this way we have attempted to present a connected story of historical development. We are well aware that a full textual commentary might occasionally have been desirable, but limitations of space precluded any such effort.

Whenever translation was necessary it was kept as close to the original text as possible so that on many occasions style has been sacrificed to accuracy. It has been our primary intention to reproduce the individual's ideas or data as faithfully as possible. References and footnotes that appeared in the original texts have been mostly excluded since those who need them will in any case consult the original text for which a full citation has been provided with the selection. These citations have been repeated in the Bibliography where the secondary works referred to throughout the book will also be found. Titles of journals have been abbreviated to conform as much as possible with the practice followed in the *World List of Scientific Periodicals*. Despite a general disregard of existing translations, they have nevertheless been indicated in the Bibliography for the use of those who may wish to pursue a topic more extensively than our selections permit. The inclusion of such translations carries no recommendation of them but merely recognizes their existence. Omissions within texts have been indicated in the customary way, and material within brackets is invariably of editorial origin and intended to elucidate the text.

Although illustrations referred to within the text have been included, occasionally one not cited but essential to a full comprehension of some passage has been added. As a general rule portraits of individuals have been sacrificed in favor of text illustrations if a choice had to be made. This is merely an application of our guiding principle of placing emphasis on the concept rather than on the man *per se*.

We are very well aware of the potential dangers of this type of book. Essentially it is a compromise between all the sources at one end of the scale and a condensed history of neuroanatomy and neurophysiology at the other. For a historical presentation certain main pathways can usually be followed and minute detail is not always essential, but an anthology such as the present one demands precise selection from the onset. As soon as the main themes have been determined those individuals considered important must be selected. Next a selection has to be made within the individual's works, in many instances voluminous, and finally a choice of parts of the preferred texts. At each stage individual preferences are likely to intervene and hence criticism courted.

In some instances we have brought our material nearer to the present day than is perhaps wise, but only to illustrate general principles that we judge will continue to be influential into the future. We have preferred to run the risk of being proved incorrect in our choices among current materials in order to connect the more distant past with the present and with the future. After all, the main role of a book of this sort is not only to indicate the birth of modern concepts, but also to trace forwards the lines of progress from their most distant roots.

ACKNOWLEDGMENTS

WE are very appreciative of the kindness of the authors, editors of journals, and publishers who have permitted us to reproduce selections from the texts and illustrations of a number of papers and books indicated here by authors and the chapters of the present work in which their writings are cited. Further bibliographical information will be found in the chapters, and it is repeated as well in the Bibliography where, in the instance of books, the publishers' names are also given. We wish therefore to express our thanks to the Editor of the *Journal of the American Medical Association* for Lashley, IX, Larsell, XI, Dandy, XII; to the Editor of *The American Journal of the Medical Sciences,* and the publishers Lea & Febiger, Philadelphia, for Loewi, III; to the Editor of *The American Journal of Pathology* for Weed, XII; to The American Physiological Society for papers of Forbes and Gregg, Erlanger and Gasser, III, Lashley, IX, Dusser de Barenne, X, Weed, XII, Snider and Magoun, XI, that appeared in the *American Journal of Physiology*, the *Physiological Reviews,* and the *Journal of Neurophysiology*; to the Editor of *The Anatomical Record* and the Wister Institute of Anatomy and Biology, Philadelphia, for Harrison, II; to the J. B. Lippincott Company of Philadelphia for papers of Weed, XII, that appeared in the *Annals of Surgery*; to the Trustees of The Association for Research in Nervous and Mental Disease and to the authors H. S. Forbes and S. Cobb for an article, XIII, in the *Transactions*; to the Editor of *Brain* for Lewis, VIII, Munk, Henschen, Bianchi, IX, Jackson, Holmes, XI, Beevor, XII; to the British Association for the Advancement of Science for an article of Sherrington, VI, that appeared in the *Transactions*; to the Editor of the *British Medical Journal* for Pavlov, VI, Holmes, IX; to the Cambridge University Press for Galen, IV, V, IX; to J. & A. Churchill, Ltd., London, for Hill, XIII; to the Clarendon Press, Oxford, for Adrian, III, Aristotle, I, III, VI, and Sherrington, VI; to The Company of Biologists, Ltd., Cambridge, for Lashley, IX; to the Elsevier Publishing Company, Amsterdam, for Erlanger, Dale, III; to the Federation of American Societies for Experimental Biology for articles of Snider and Magoun, XI and of Schmidt, XIII, that appeared in the *Proceedings*; to the Hafner Publishing Company, New York, for Ramón y Cajal, II; to the Editor of *The Journal of Physiology* for Lucas, Adrian, Elliott, Dale, III, Sherrington, V, VI, Löwenthal, XI, Roy and Sherrington, XIII; to the Editor of *The Lancet* for Flechsig, IX; to the Liverpool University Press and to A. L. Hodgkin for Hodgkin, III; to Luzac & Company, Ltd., London, for Avicenna, I, IX; to the Editor of *The Journal of the Mount Sinae Hospital* for Dale, III; to the Editor of *Nature* for Hodgkin, III; to the Editor of the *Quarterly Journal of Experimental Physiology* for Grünbaum and Sherrington, IX; to Dr. F. Rahman for Avicenna, IX; to the Oxford University Press, London, for Ramón y Cajal, II;

to Routledge & Kegan Paul, Ltd., London, for Plato, I; to the Council of the Royal Society, London, for papers by Leeuwenhoek, Waller, Kühne, II, Müller, Lucas, Hodgkin, Loewi, III, Sherrington, V, VI, Lewis and Clarke, Campbell, VIII, Grünbaum and Sherrington, Schäfer and Brown, IX, Löwenthal, Magnus, XI, Beevor, XII, that appeared in the *Philosophical Transactions* and the *Proceedings*; to the SCM Press, Ltd., London, and the Westminster Press, Philadelphia, for Nemesius, IX; to the Springer-Verlag, Heidelberg, for Loewi, III, Magnus, Kleijn and Magnus, XI, appearing in *Pflügers Archiv für die gesamte Physiologie des Menschen und der Tiere* and Pfeifer, XIII; to the Georg Thieme Verlag, Stuttgart, for Flechsig, IX; to Charles C Thomas, Publisher, Springfield, Illinois, for Magoun, XI, and Schmidt, XIII; to the University of Chicago Press for selections from the Edwin Smith Surgical Papyrus, VII; to the University of Pennsylvania Press for Adrian, III; to the Year Book Medical Publishers, Inc., Chicago, for Kety, XIII; to The Williams & Wilkins Co., Baltimore, for Dale, III, appearing in the *Journal of Pharmacology*; to the Yale University Press for Sherrington, III, VI, XI; and to W. H. Freeman and Co., for Snider, XI.

CONTENTS

ix

CHAPTER I

ANTIQUITY AND THE MEDIEVAL PERIOD

Introduction

Because of the rapid advances made in science during the last hundred years and because of its present-day complexity and sophistication, there is a tendency to neglect the most distant past. The ancient Greeks seem to be so far away in thought, as well as in time, that we tend to forget that their ideas, some of which now appear to be archaic and curious, were in many instances the origins of concepts that today are held to be of the greatest importance. This is certainly true in respect to the history of neuroanatomy and neurophysiology, and, in this work, in order to emphasize the direct links of modern beliefs with those of antiquity, the latter have been included with each theme or chapter, whenever appropriate, rather than collected in a single chapter. Nevertheless, there are several reasons that favor the inclusion of an additional, introductory chapter dealing primarily with certain aspects of the neurological knowledge of antiquity.

The first reason is the most important and has for the most part determined the choice of the material presented below. Although the overall objective of this book is to discuss only ideas that have survived into the present era, there is one exception to this rule. Throughout antiquity, and to some extent up to the end of the eighteenth century, there was controversy on the question of which organ was the seat of the soul, the intellect, the passions, and the guiding force in the control of the motor and sensory phenomena of the body. The problem is one that no doubt engaged man's attention from a very early period, but it does not become apparent to us in any detail until the time of the pre-Socratic philosophers of ancient Greece (6th century B.C.). Thereafter it became a major issue, and the field was divided between those who selected the brain and those who preferred the heart. As with any controversy, this one stimulated men to ponder and to seek evidence in support of one side or the other, and thus indirectly it centered interest upon the brain and also, of course, upon the heart. This then is the main theme of the first chapter: the cephalocentric versus the cardiocentric soul.

Although earlier Western civilizations such as those of the ancient Egyptians, the Mesopotamians, and the Hebrews had selected the heart as the central organ, the Greeks were divided on this matter. Thus Empedocles, Democritus, Aristotle, Diocles, Praxagoras, the Stoics, and the Epicureans favored the heart, whereas Alcmaeon, Pythagoras, one of the Hippocratic Writers, Plato, Herophilus, Erasistratus, Rufus, and Galen chose the brain. In view of the fact that we today belong to the second group, selections will be taken mainly from its representatives. There are, however, remnants of the contrary opinion still with us, preserved in the many expressions that refer to the heart and are probably chiefly Hebrew in origin.

The second reason for the inclusion of this first chapter arises from a fundamentally important concept that matured in antiquity. This was the notion of the nervous system as an anatomical and functional unit. Although the contributions to it were few, they could only be included in a chapter dealing with antiquity in general.

A further reason lies in the fact that a few authors, such as Rufus of Ephesus, gave brief yet outstanding accounts of the nervous system that could not conveniently be split up into their component sentences and distributed among the various chapters; hence almost all of Rufus's account has been reproduced here and will be referred to from the appropriate, later chapters.

In this first chapter, the writings of philosophers such as Plato and Aristotle must come under consideration. We are well aware of the hazards involved in removing portions of them from the general context of their authors' philosophy and considering them in isolation; and since it is difficult within restricted limits to set the selected passages in their correct perspective, authorities have been cited to whom the reader may refer for further assistance in this matter.

Finally, two writers from the medieval period have been included, not because of any original contribution but because of their wide influence in the maintenance and furtherance of classical ideas. These are Avicenna, one of the most outstanding representatives of Moslem medicine, and Mondino, the most important anatomist of the late medieval and early Renaissance period. In the instance of the former, his opinions regarding the heart–brain controversy have been illustrated, and in that of the latter, his description of the brain.

ALCMAEON
(fl. c. 500 B.C.)

Although there are occasional references to parts of the nervous system in the fragmentary remains of Ancient Egyptian (see p. 383) and Mesopotamian writings available to us today, we can discern in them no clear opinions concerning its function. Such opinions did not appear until the pre-Socratic philosophers of the sixth and fifth centuries B.C., the earliest ancient Greeks to be interested in natural phenomena, began their studies. One of them, Alcmaeon of Croton, is of special importance in the history of knowledge of the brain.

Very little is known about Alcmaeon and even his *floruit* is still debated. He seems to have belonged to the earliest Greek school of physicians at Croton in southern Italy, but he was not closely associated with Pythagoras (*c.* 580–500 B.C.) as is sometimes claimed. Unfortunately only a few fragments of his writings have survived, and later writers must be relied upon for his opinions, so that exposure to possible errors and misrepresentations is unavoidable. Nevertheless he has been acclaimed by some as the founder of empirical psychology (Beare, 1906), and his theory of opposites formed an important part of Hippocratic medicine. Alcmaeon appears to have dissected animals and to have discussed nerves. One of his most striking contributions was the recognition of the brain as the central organ of sensation and thought, and this, as well as other perceptive observations, was included in a book on nature that may have been written between 480 and 440 B.C. but, which apart from a few sentences, has been lost (see Kayserling, 1901; Guthrie, 1962, pp. 341–359; Freeman, 1959, pp. 135–139; Schumacher, 1963, pp. 66–81; Diels, 1964, I, 210–216).

The following passage has been taken from the works of Theophrastus (372/369–288/285 B.C.), the peripatetic philosopher who was a pupil of Aristotle and succeeded to the direction of his master's school in Athens. His treatise, *On sense perceptions* (*Theophrasti Eresii opera, quae supersunt, omnia*, edita Fridericus Wimmer [Paris, 1866]) presents Alcmaeon's opinions of the mechanism of the special sense organs connected to the brain, and these ideas are known to have influenced later writers such as Plato (pp. 6–7).

EXCERPT P. 326

IV. (25) Among those who have decided that perception is not accomplished through similarity, Alcmaeon was the first to define the difference between man and animals, saying that man differs from the latter in the fact that he alone has the power of understanding. The others perceive but do not understand since to understand is different from perceiving and not, as Empedocles believed, the same thing. Then [Alcmaeon] discussed the separate senses. He tells us that we hear by means of the ears and that sound is heard because of the empty space in them; he says that the [internal] air resounds by means of that hollow space. [He asserts that] we smell by means of the nostrils when in respiration the air has been carried to the brain; that we distinguish flavors by the tongue, for since it is warm and soft it melts [substances] by its heat, and because of its yielding fineness it receives and passes on [the flavors]. (26) The eyes see through the surrounding water that obviously contains fire because it flashes out in those that have been struck a blow. Vision occurs when that shining, translucent quality [in the eye] reflects, and the more so the greater its purity. All the senses are related in some way to the brain so that if it is moved or if it changes its position, they are blunted because the passages by which sensation occurs are blocked. He did not define touch, nor how or by what organs it occurs. Such then are Alcmaeon's opinions about these matters.

The Hippocratic Writers
(c. 430–350 b.c.)

Alcmaeon's belief that the brain was the body's dominant organ is also to be found in the writings of the Hippocratic physicians. Although there is no doubt that Hippocrates of Cos existed (*c.* 460–*c.* 379 b.c.), it seems certain that the eminence accorded him today was acquired some time after his death. Moreover, the writings attributed to him were clearly the work of a group of physicians, and it is thus more accurate to speak of the "Hippocratic Writers" rather than of "Hippocrates."

It is clear from their writings that the Hippocratic physicians were keen observers of the human body in health and in disease, even though their knowledge of anatomy was slight. They based their interpretations upon the theory of the four elements (air, water, earth, fire) and of the four humors (blood, phlegm, yellow bile, black bile), and in therapy their aim was to assist and not to impede nature's own healing powers. By so doing they broke with the supernatural, magicoreligious concepts of disease that had dominated previous civilizations (see Heidel, 1941; Sigerist, 1961, pp. 260–295; Schumacher, 1963, pp. 177–211).

The clearest expression of this rational approach to disease occurs in a book on epilepsy, *The sacred disease* (Littré [1839–1861], VI, 350–397), written perhaps by a younger contemporary of Socrates (470–399 b.c.). The author declared epilepsy to be a disturbance of the brain and then described that organ's functions in health and disease. Abnormalities were due to changes in the elements, and the brain functioned by having contact with the inspired air, presumably through the cribriform plate, and thus with the extracorporeal world. The distribution of the air from the brain to different parts of the body may be described as a very crude form of what we today call nervous transmission (see p. 140). The role of the brain as the seat of mental processes was here clearly accepted, probably for the first time. The following excerpts have been translated from chapters 14 (pp. 387–389) and 16 (pp. 391–393).

14. One ought to know that on the one hand pleasure, joy, laughter, and games, and on the other, grief, sorrow, discontent, and dissatisfaction arise only from [the brain]. It is especially by it that we think, comprehend, see, and hear, that we distinguish the ugly from the beautiful, the bad from the good, the agreeable from the disagreeable, whether we distinguish these things through custom and use, or whether we recognize them by the benefit they gain us and through this very same benefit experience pleasure or displeasure; or, according to the occasion, the same things may not be pleasing to us. Furthermore, it is by [the brain] that we are mad, that we rave, that fears and terrors assail us—be it by night or by day—dreams,

untimely errors, groundless anxiety, blunders, awkwardness, want of experience. We are affected by all these things when the brain is not healthy, that is, when it is too hot or too cold, too moist or too dry, or when it has experienced some other unnatural injury to which it is not accustomed. Madness results from its moistness; in fact, having become too moist, it is set in motion, and during motion neither sight nor hearing is trustworthy; the patient sees and hears sometimes one thing, sometimes another, and the tongue expresses what he sees and what he hears. But all the time that the brain is at rest, man has understanding.

15. . . . .

16. For these reasons I consider the brain to be the most powerful organ of man's body, for when it is healthy it is our interpreter of the impressions produced by the air; now, the air gives it intelligence. The eyes, the ears, the tongue, the hands, the feet, act according to the brain's understanding; in fact, the whole body participates in the intelligence in proportion to its participation in the air; now, the brain is the messenger for the intelligence. When man draws breath into himself, this breath first arrives at the brain, and it is in this way that the air disperses itself through the rest of the body, leaving in the brain its most active part, the part that has intelligence and understanding. If the air were to proceed first of all into the body, and from there to the brain, it would leave the intelligence in the flesh and veins, and this would reach the brain overheated, not pure but mixed with the humors originated from the flesh and blood, so that it would no longer have its perfect qualities.

PLATO

(*c. 429–347* B.C.)

The renowned Athenian philosopher Plato also believed that the brain was the most important organ of the body. Plato came of an aristocratic family and studied under Socrates, by whom he was greatly influenced. In 387, or thereabouts, he began teaching at Athens in what was later known as the Academy. For the remaining forty years of his life this was his principal occupation, and by his writings, which have been mostly preserved, he contributed probably more than any other philosopher to the moral and intellectual culture of mankind. This fact can be attributed to his remarkable intellect, his outstanding philosophical views, and to his poetic power and attractive style of writing (see Field, 1930; King, 1954; Taylor, 1956; Schumacher, 1963, pp. 212–250).

Although Plato had no firsthand knowledge of biology, it was necessary for his philosophical considerations that he should be familiar with the form and functions of the human body. He therefore acquired this information from others, and particularly, it seems, from the physicians of Sicily and southern Italy. His most extensive reference to the nervous system occurs in the *Timaeus,* a dialogue written towards the end of his life, which is a survey of natural science and of the creation of the world by the gods. In it Plato dealt with man's perceptions, the composition of his soul, his body, his diseases, and his health. He believed that a dualism existed between body and soul, mind and senses. The soul was made up of three parts, and the most important part, the rational, was assigned to the head and presumably to the brain; the other parts were in the heart and in the upper abdomen.

Although he added no new data to the knowledge of the anatomy and physiology of the nervous system, nevertheless Plato supported the concept of a cephalocentric organism, which is our idea today. His comments were vague, obscure, and archaic, reminiscent of the cult of the head that seems to have been popular in some earlier civilizations. The approximation of the head and the brain to the perfect figure, the sphere, had also influenced Pythagoras in his acceptance of the brain as the most important organ and as the seat of the mental processes.

The following passages have been taken from the translation of the *Timaeus* by F. M. Cornford (*Plato's cosmology. The Timaeus,* translated with a running commentary [London, 1937]), in which Plato described the creation of the human body, in which the head was supreme, and compared and contrasted it with the universe. It is felt that these statements are worthy of reproduction here, especially in view of the widespread influence of the *Timaeus* during the Middle Ages.

EXCERPT 44*d* (P. 150)

Copying the round shape of the universe, they [the gods] confined the two divine revolutions [orbits] in a spherical body—the head, as we now call it—which is the divinest part of us and lord over all the rest.

He discussed the three parts of the soul. The most important was in the head and therefore this must be the chief bodily part.

EXCERPT 89*e*–90*b* (P. 353)

As we have said more than once, there dwell in us three distinct forms of soul, each having its own motions . . . .

As concerning the most sovereign form of soul in us we must conceive that heaven has given it to each man as a guiding genius—that part which we say dwells in the summit of our body and lifts us from earth towards our celestial affinity, like a plant whose roots are not in earth, but in the heavens. And this is most true, for it is to the heavens, whence the soul first came to birth, that the divine part attaches the head or root of us and keeps the whole body upright.

The following passage is obscure, but in it Plato was probably relating the creation of the brain and bone marrow, and perhaps of the spinal cord, from a life substance, marrow, of which the seed was a part. The similarity between brain substance, bone marrow, and semen is frequently encountered in early Greek scientific writings, and may relate simply to a similarity in appearance.

EXCERPT 73c–73d (PP. 293–294)

Next he implanted [universal seed] and made fast therein the several kinds of souls; also from the first, in his original distribution, he divided the marrow into shapes corresponding in number and fashion to those which the several kinds were destined to wear. And he moulded into spherical shape the ploughland, as it were, that was to contain the divine seed [semen]; and this part of the marrow he named 'brain,' signifying that, when each living creature was completed, the vessel containing this should be the head. That part, on the other hand, which was to retain the remaining, mortal, kind of soul he divided into shapes at once round and elongated, naming them all 'marrow.' From these, as if from anchors, he put forth bonds to fasten all the soul; and now began to fashion our whole body round this thing, first framing round the whole of it a solid shield of bone.

Alcmaeon's concept of the special senses seems to have influenced Plato who stated in the dialogue, *Phaedo*, 96 (Jowett [1892], II, 242), that "the brain may be the originating power of the perceptions of hearing and sight and smell, and memory and opinion may come from them, and science may be based on memory and opinion." This is one of the first references to a belief that became universal in the Middle Ages whereby mental activity was thought to take place by means of a threefold sequence: accumulation of sensations, reasoning, and memory, in this order (p. 459).

Concerning the faculty of hearing, Plato made the following statement that may have originated with Diogenes (*fl.* 440 or 430 B.C.) or with Anaxagoras (*c.* 500–*c.* 428 B.C.).

EXCERPT 67b (P. 275)

. . . Sound we may define in general terms as the stroke inflicted by air on the brain and blood through the ears and passed onto the soul.

ARISTOTLE

(384–322 B.C.)

Consideration has thus far been given to the minority opinion of those who held that the brain was the body's primary organ. The opposing, cardiocentric view, notably supported by the physicians of the Sicilian and southern Italian schools, will be illustrated here by the writings of its most distinguished advocate, the great Greek philosopher and biologist Aristotle.

Aristotle was born at Stagirus in Chalcidice. He studied in Plato's Academy where he remained for about twenty years, until the death of Plato. Thereafter he moved from place to place, but in each he lost no opportunity to observe the local fauna and flora. He spent two years as tutor to the future Alexander the Great (343/2–340), and in 335 he established a research and teaching institution outside Athens, the Lyceum, from which he retired in 323.

Only a part of Aristotle's very numerous writings have survived, but they are sufficient to show us that he was probably the most outstanding thinker of all time. Aristotle did not accept Plato's idea of a central role for mathematics in philosophy, and this may be a reason for the remarkable quality of his biological studies. His interests and energies were, however, very widespread and covered most of contemporary knowledge. Furthermore, he possessed notable common sense and a passion for orderliness. As his opinions matured, he became more interested in biology, although there was no decline in his philosophical prowess (see Lewes, 1864; Geoffroy, 1878; Volprecht, 1895; Lones, 1912; Ross, 1923; Jaeger, 1934; Randall, 1960; Clarke, 1963).

Aristotle argued that the heart was the chief organ of the body and the center for thought and the appreciation of sensation. The brain, an important structure, was secondary to it and functioned only as a means of cooling the heart's heat. The special sense organs grouped around the brain were in direct communication by vascular channels with the heart and not with the brain. Of all the proponents of a cardiocentric arrangement, Aristotle was the most active and eloquent, and his influence can be followed to the seventeenth century when William Harvey, for example, still showed traces of it. Praxagoras of Cos (*fl.* 300 b.c.), the teacher of Herophilus, took over Aristotle's teachings on this matter and developed them to the extent of stating that all nerves arose from the heart (see pp. 142–143).

One of the reasons for selecting passages from the writings of Aristotle is the fact that in them we find the first account in any detail of structures of the nervous system. Admittedly this is vague and in some instances puzzling, and, moreover, we know that Aristotle dissected only animals and projected their anatomy to man. Nevertheless his influence in subsequent centuries was immense.

The following passages have been taken from the Oxford translations (*The works of Aristotle*, edited by J. A. Smith and W. D. Ross) by permission of the Clarendon Press. The first selection is from *The account of animals*, I, 16 (*Historia animalium*, [translated] by D'Arcy W. Thompson [Oxford, 1910]). The curious statement that the brain lies in the front part of the cranium has been variously interpreted (see Clarke and Stannard, 1963).

EXCERPT 494*b*:25—495*a*:17

In the first place then, the brain lies in the front part of the head. And this holds alike with all animals possessed of a brain; and all blooded animals are possessed thereof, and, by the way, molluscs as well. But, taking size for size of animal, the largest brain, and the moistest, is that of man. Two membranes enclose it: the stronger one nearer the bone of the skull [dura mater]; the inner one [pia mater], round the brain itself, is finer. The brain in all cases is bilateral. Behind this, right at the back, comes what is termed the 'cerebellum,' differing in form from the brain as we may both feel and see.

. . . .

The brain in all animals is bloodless, devoid of veins, and naturally cold to the touch; in the great majority of animals it has a small hollow in its centre [ventricles]. The brain-caul around it is reticulated with veins; and this brain-caul is that skin-like membrane which closely surrounds the brain [pia mater]. Above the brain is the thinnest and weakest bone of the head, which is termed 'bregma' or 'sinciput.'

From the eye there go three ducts to the brain [? cranial nerves]: the largest and the medium-sized to the cerebellum, the least to the brain itself; and the least is the one situated nearest to the nostril. The two largest ones, then, run side by side and do not meet; the medium-sized ones meet—and this is particularly visible in fishes—for they lie nearer than the large ones to the brain; the smallest pair are the most widely separate from one another, and do not meet.

The following selections have been taken from *The parts of animals*, II, 7 (*De partibus animalium*, translated by William Ogle [Oxford, 1911]). In them Aristotle dealt mainly with the cooling properties of the brain, but it is important to note that their purpose was "the preservation of the whole body." This indicates that despite its secondary status in Aristotle's schema, the brain was nevertheless an important organ.

EXCERPT 652*a*:24—653*a*:31

From the [bone] marrow we pass on in natural sequence to the brain. For there are many who think that the brain itself consists of marrow [cf. Plato, p. 7], and that it forms the commencement of that substance, because they see that the spinal marrow [cord] is continuous with it. In reality the two may be said to be utterly opposite to each other in character. For of all the parts of the body there is none so cold as the brain; whereas the marrow is of a hot nature, as is plainly shown by its fat and unctuous character . . . . The coldness of the brain is also manifest enough. For in the first place it is cold even to the touch; and, secondly, of all the fluid parts of the body it is the driest and the one that has the least blood; for in fact it has no blood at all in its proper substance. This brain is not residual matter, nor yet is it one of the parts which are anatomically continuous with each other; but it has a character peculiar to itself, as might indeed be expected. That it has no continuity with the organs of sense is plain from simple inspection, and is still more clearly shown by the fact, that, when it is touched, no sensation is produced; in which respect it resembles the blood of animals and their excrement. The purpose of its presence in animals is no less than the preservation of the whole body . . . . But as all influences require to be counterbalanced, so that they may be reduced to moderation and brought to the mean (for in the mean, and not in either extreme, lies the true and rational position), nature has contrived the brain as a counterpoise to the region of the heart with its contained heat, and has given it to animals to moderate the latter, combining in it the properties of earth and water. For this reason it is, that every sanguineous animal has a brain; whereas no bloodless creature has such an organ, unless indeed it be, as the Poulp, by analogy. For where there is no blood, there in consequence there is but little heat. The brain, then, tempers the heat and seething of the heart. In order, however, that it may not itself be absolutely without heat. but may have a moderate amount, branches run from both blood-vessels, that is to say, from the great vessel and from what is called the aorta, and end in the membrane which surrounds the brain [pia mater]; while at the same time, in order to prevent any injury from the heat, these encompassing vessels, instead of being few and large, are numerous and small, and their blood scanty and clear, instead of being abundant and thick . . . . We must suppose, to compare small things with great, that the like happens here as occurs in the production of showers. For when vapour steams up from the earth and is carried by the heat into the upper regions, so soon as it reaches the cold air that is above the earth, it condenses again into water owing to the refrigeration, and falls back to the earth as rain . . . .

. . . .

That the brain is a compound of earth and water is shown by what occurs when it is boiled. For, when so treated, it turns hard and solid, inasmuch as the water is evaporated by the heat, and leaves the earthy part behind . . . .

Of all animals, man has the largest brain in proportion to his size; and it is larger in men than in women. This is because the region of the heart and of the lung is hotter and richer in blood in man than in any other animal; and in men than in women.

HEROPHILUS   ERASISTRATUS

(*fl. c. 300* B.C.)   (*fl. c. 260* B.C.)

The city of Alexandria was founded by Alexander the Great in 332 B.C., and it was there that the most famous medical school of antiquity was founded. Its two best known physicians were Herophilus and Erasistratus who were especially re-nowned for their knowledge of anatomy; unfortunately, however, all their own writings have perished and what limited information is available about these two men must be gathered from fragments of their works imbedded in those of other authors, notably in the writings of Galen more than four centuries later. Nevertheless, there appears to be no doubt that both Herophilus and Erasistratus possessed an extensive understanding of the anatomy of the nervous system; this resulted from the fact that in Alexandria, for the first and only time in antiquity, data on the structure of the human body could be derived directly from dissection of the body rather than indirectly from analogy based upon animal dissection.

Herophilus and Erasistratus considered the brain as the organ of the soul, and, in addition, they made a number of important contributions to knowledge of the nervous system which were influential upon the thought of succeeding times. For this reason they have been included here and will also be referred to in several of the subsequent chapters.

Herophilus was born at Chalcedon, on the shores of the Bosphorus, and as a member of the Hippocratic school he was a Dogmatist. He was a practising physician and, like his teacher, Praxagoras (see p. 142), was famous for his study of the pulse, in which he used the clepsydra and so was an important pioneer in the use of quantitation in medicine. However, his most important work was on human anatomy, and the terms *duodenum, prostate,* and others to be mentioned hereafter were derived from his writings. He was particularly interested in the brain, and his contributions to neuroanatomy will be discussed in later chapters. He placed the soul in the ventricles, of which he considered the fourth as the most important (p. 713), and the animal spirits in the cerebrum. He described and gave their names to the *rete mirabile* (see p. 757), the *calamus scriptorius* (see p. 713), the *torcular* (p. 762), and the *choroid.* Herophilus also distinguished between motor and sensory nerves (p. 146). Although we know something of his studies from the writings of others, nevertheless there are no suitable portions of such fragments that can be presented here (see Marx, 1838; Finlayson, 1893; Dobson, 1925).

Erasistratus was born on the island of Chios in the Aegean Sea and worked in the Alexandrian School together with, and after, Herophilus. He practised medicine and carried out scientific research that today we should term physiological. His solidist explanation for bodily function and disease opposed that of the Hippocratics, and Galen denounced him repeatedly on this account. Again we are dependent upon later writers, especially Galen and Rufus, for our knowledge of his work, but there seems to be no doubt that he greatly influenced medical thought up to the time of Galen. We know a little about his ideas on digestion, respiration, metabolism, and the cardiovascular system, as well as his contributions to pathology, treatment, surgery, and hygiene; like Herophilus he used quantitation, in this instance for metabolic studies. On the whole, more is known of Erasistratus than of Herophilus, mainly because Galen often cited his theories, or those of his followers, before attacking them (see Finlayson, 1893; Dobson, 1927).

The work of Erasistratus will be referred to in other chapters but, in addition, a statement made apparently by Erasistratus and reproduced by Galen, *On the opinions of Hippocrates and Plato,* VII, 3 (Kühn [1821–1833], V), is given in translation immediately below. Erasistratus's general knowledge of the nervous system is reviewed, but Galen's comments on it are, as usual, derogatory.

EXCERPT PP. 602–604

Erasistratus, for such a long time seeing only the external part of the nerve which advances from the dural membrane, believed that the whole arose there. He has several large books in which he says that the nerves arise from the membrane surrounding the brain. But when he was an old man and free to devote himself solely to investigation of the art, he attempted more exact dissections. He learned how the medulla of the nerves originates from the brain. These are his words: "I investigated the nature of the brain; and the brain [in man] was indeed bipartite as in other animals. It had a ventricle placed longitudinally on each side, and these were pierced through into [another] one at the junction of the [two] parts [foramen of Monro]. This [third] one extended to the so-called cerebellum, where there was another, smaller ventricle [fourth], each side walled off by membranes; for the cerebellum was set off by itself, as well as the cerebrum, and was like the jejunum and very much folded. The cerebrum was constructed from even more and differing foldings. From this the observer may learn that as in those animals that surpass the others in speed of running, such as the stag and hare, well constructed with muscles and nerves useful for this, so also, since man greatly surpasses other beings in intelligence, his brain was greatly convoluted. All the processes of the nerves were from the cerebrum; and, in brief, the brain appeared to be the origin of the nerves of the body; for the sensation which comes from the nostrils reaches this opening (*foramen* [? olfactory plates]), likewise [in regard to that] coming from the ears. Processes were also carried from the brain to the tongue and the eyes."

Here Erasistratus states what was first unknown to him, and then that he clearly saw single nerves proceeding from the brain. He writes exactly of the four ventricles that he had not seen even the year before. If he had made the experiment in live animals, which I have made not once or twice but many times, he would have had a firm understanding of the hard and thick membrane which was formed for containing the brain, and for its sake also the soft and thin; in addition, that they may gather together all the vessels, that is, arteries and veins, of the brain.

Rufus of Ephesus
(*fl.* A.D. *98–117*)

Another important medical school in antiquity was at Ephesus on the western coast of Asia Minor. Rufus, a physician who practised there, is especially noteworthy for his important work on anatomy and for the considerable authority he exercised as a teacher and writer. Little is known of him, but we are aware that he had studied at Alexandria and that he considered anatomy necessary for the understanding of disease. His books are also a valuable source of opinions of individuals such as Herophilus and Erasistratus (*Œuvres de Rufus d'Éphèse*, translated by C. Daremberg and C. E. Ruelle [Paris, 1879], 2 vols. For biographical details, see I, ii–x).

Because of the fragmentary state of their writings it is impossible to determine if Herophilus or Erasistratus considered the brain, spinal cord, and nerves as a connected system and whether they ever described them in that way. Although they may have done so, the first definite presentation of the matter that has come down to us is that of Rufus. He was clearly aware of the brain, cranial nerves, spinal cord, and nerves as an anatomical entity, although he had little to say about function. Admittedly and obviously much of his knowledge was derived from the earlier anatomists of Alexandria, but some of the observations were probably his own, and, in any case, his contribution as an influential teacher is worthy of recognition.

In his book, *On the names of the parts of the human body* (I, 133–167), Rufus described for a student the bodily structures of a monkey. The following excerpt, in which the relationships between the marrow of the cranium (brain), of the spine (spinal cord), and of bone (medulla) are mentioned, has been translated from sentences 147 to 152, and 217.

EXCERPT PP. 153–154

The brain is located inside the skull; it is covered by meninges; one, denser and more resistant, is attached to the bone [dura mater]; the other, thinner but also resistant, although to a lesser extent, stretches over the brain [pia mater]. The upper surface of the brain is called varicose [convoluted], its inner and posterior surface is called the base; the extension from the base is the parencephalon [cerebellum]; the cavities of the brain have been designated hollows [ventricles]. The membrane which lines the ventricles is called the choroid membrane. Herophilus also calls it the choroid meninges. The processes springing from the brain are the sensory and the motor nerves with the help of which we are able to feel and to move voluntarily and which are responsible for all activities of the body. There are also those nerves which issue from the spinal marrow, and from the meninges which surround it. One may designate indifferently all of the marrow which descends through the vertebrae either as dorsal or spinal.

EXCERPT P. 164

The marrow contained in the spine is called spinal marrow, and at the back, dorsal marrow; the meninges clothing it are called dorsal meninges; the marrow enclosed in the cranial bone is called brain but that of the other bones has received the name of bony marrow, found, for example, in the large cavities of the [bones of the] thigh and the arm, or in the small cavities of the ribs and the clavicle.

The second excerpt has been translated from Rufus's *Anatomy of the parts of the body* ([1879], I, 168–185) and comprises sentences 3 to 9.

EXCERPT PP. 169–170

The brain, with the meninges covering it, is enclosed in the head between the walls of the cranium and it is more voluminous in man in proportion to his body than in other animals; it is a pulpy and viscous concretion; it is ash gray [colored]; the part situated below at the occiput is called the parencephalon [cerebellum]. Of the two meninges, one is moulded on the bones of the cranium [dura mater]; it has a movement in time with that of the pulse; the other [pia mater], following the sinuosities of the brain, holds it together and preserves its fragile substance from disintegration. These two envelopes are nervous [i.e., fibrous] and membranous; they have an undoubted sensitivity and manifest an interlacing of vessels. The inner membrane is lacking in movement; the thicker, outer membrane moves freely. The marrow [spinal cord] arises from the brain and escapes through the hole of the cranium at the occiput [foramen magnum] and descends as far as the base of the spine through all the vertebrae; it is not a special substance but an extension from the brain; it is called the marrow of the back. Nervous channels [nerves] which are distributed to the senses arise and emerge from the brain: for example, to the ears, to the nose, and to the other sensory parts.

One of these processes comes off in front from the base of the brain, is divided into two branches [optic nerves], and inclines towards each of the eyes in the part called the basin or cavity of vision, in the form of a fossa, and which is found on each side of the nose.

GALEN OF PERGAMUM
(A.D. 129–199)

The most voluminous body of medical writings of antiquity available to us is that of Galen of Pergamum, and in these writings are to be found extended arguments directed against such investigators as Aristotle, who maintained that the brain was secondary to the heart. In addition, Galen wrote at length on the form and function of the nervous system, and reference will be made to this data in many of the subsequent chapters.

Galen was born in Pergamum, north of Ephesus and near the western coast of

Asia Minor. He studied medicine at Smyrna, Corinth, and Alexandria. In A.D. 157 he was appointed surgeon to the gladiators at Pergamum and five years later began practice in Rome, but returned to his home town after four years. During his second visit to Rome, *c*. 169–*c*. 193, he became medical attendant to a succession of emperors and was considered the leading physician of his day, as, indeed, he was of all antiquity. It is clear from his writings, however, that he was possessed of a strong and, indeed, prickly personality. His final several years until his death were passed in the more peaceful surroundings of his native land.

As an eclectic Galen selected those ideas best suited to the trend of his own thought and work, but in particular leaned towards the medicine of the Hippocratic physicians and the biology of Aristotle. To the experiences of others he added his own, especially his knowledge acquired from surgery as well as from dissection—which latter although extensive was limited to that of animals—and from numerous experiments aimed at the investigation of function. This knowledge he then attempted to apply to disease and its treatment. Probably his most outstanding contributions to medicine, which underlay much of his work, were his insistence upon the importance of experimental studies and upon the necessity of relating form to function.

Galen's reasoning and his experiments cannot fail to evoke respect even today, and various attempts by historians to minimize his contributions are unjustified. His teachings became universal dogmata throughout the Middle Ages and later; some were, in fact, still accepted in a modified form in the first few decades of the nineteenth century (see Thorndike, 1943, I, 117–181; Sarton, 1954, a good source of factual information).

If, as has been indicated, Aristotle was the foremost proponent of the cardiocentric theory (p. 8), then Galen was his most vocal opponent. He marshaled an imposing array of arguments and made use of experiment, reasoning, and analogy to demolish the ancient belief and to establish his own—and ours—that the seat of intelligence, motion, and sensation is the brain, not the heart. That the cardiocentric idea was still a widely held opinion in the second century A.D., is reflected in the fact that Galen took so much trouble over its refutation. The following passage has been translated from his book, *On the opinions of Hippocrates and Plato*, II, 8 (Kühn [1821–1833], V). Despite Galen's forceful denial of Aristotle's cardiocentric opinions, he had much respect for the great philosopher's teachings as a whole.

EXCERPT PP. 278–279

. . . . Therefore we shall agree with Plato and Hippocrates, and contrary to Aristotle and Chrysippus [? of Cnidus, *fl*. 350 B.C.], that the brain is the source of voluntary motion and the heart of another involuntary motion, and these propositions were satisfactorily demonstrated . . . . Aristotle's assumption relates to what I considered at the end of the first book; it is derived from those things residing in the heart, for, he says, a supply of nerves is observed in it [cf. Praxagoras, p. 142]. I pointed out that there are nervous bodies in the heart but no nerves; likewise, that the parts of the nervous bodies correspond to nerves only in appearance but not in action and use . . . . We shall turn our attention to something else which is mentioned by almost all who believe the heart of animate beings to be the source of all the faculties. They assert that the being's faculty of reasoning is located at the being's source of nourishment; that the source of nourishment of animate beings is in the heart, and therefore that the power of reason and intelligence is located in it. They are deceived in each assumption, for I do not grant that the source of nourishment in beings is in the heart.

Whenever possible Galen had recourse to experiment to support his arguments, and in the following extract from the same work he gave experimental evidence that favored the ascendancy of the brain. It occurred in the course of another dispute, on this occasion directed against Erasistratus's belief that arteries contained air or spirit, a much older tradition from which our terms *aorta* and *artery*, or air-containing structures, derived. Galen demonstrated that whereas pressure on the heart did not render an animal senseless and immobile, pressure on the brain did. Thus the most important spirits were in the brain and not in the heart.

EXCERPT PP. 185–187

. . . . If you press so much upon a [cerebral] ventricle that you wound it, immediately the living being will be without movement and sensation, without spirit and voice, not otherwise than is seen to happen in men whose heads have been pierced. For when the bones have been broken, we cut away what are called the guardians of the membranes [meninges]—we are compelled to add for the sake of protecting the brain—lest if we press the brain a little too much, the victim is rendered without sensation and without all voluntary movement; this does not happen if we press the naked heart. I recall that once I permitted a certain person to grasp it with blacksmith's tongs since otherwise, when it moved, beating very strongly, it slipped from the hands; but not even thus was the animal injured in its sensation or voluntary movement, only it cried out greatly, breathed incessantly, and all its limbs shook violently. For with the heart grasped that way only the movement of the arteries is impaired; the animal suffers nothing else, but as long as it lives it moves all its limbs and breathes. However, if you compress the brain in the same way you will see everything to happen quite contrarily.

Galen's most telling repudiation of Aristotle's notion occurred in his book, *The use of parts*, VIII, 2, 3 (Daremberg [1854–1856], I). He first of all employed a technique reminiscent of Aristotle, the comparative anatomical approach. One cannot avoid admiring the way in which Galen attacked his opponent, and after reading the following excerpts it is difficult to understand why the Aristotelian theory survived the onslaught. Its authority in the medieval period and later was probably owing to the greater availability of Aristotle's works.

EXCERPT PP. 527–530

The head seems to many persons to have been created for the brain, and consequently to enclose all the senses as the servitors and satellites of the great king [the brain]. However, crabs and other crustacea do not have a head. The part that directs the senses and the voluntary movements is placed in the thorax, and all the organs of the senses are to be found there. Thus that which in us is the brain, in these animals is that part which refers to movements and sensations. Now if it is not the brain but the heart that is the origin of all these phenomena, it is with reason that among the acephalous the organs of the senses have been fixed in the chest, for in this way they are directed towards the heart which is situated near them; and it is, on the contrary, incorrect that in some they have been attached to the brain. Those who hold this opinion must find the head all the more superfluous since they are unable to indicate a use for the brain, nor to lodge around it the organs of the senses. Indeed, to imagine that the brain was created because of the natural heat of the heart, to refresh it and moderate its temperature, is wholly absurd. Presumably nature, instead of placing it so far from the heart, either would have provided it as a covering for the heart, as she did the lung, or at least she would have placed it in the thorax; but she would not have placed the origins of all the senses in the brain.

Even though she pushed negligence to the point of putting the brain distant from the heart, at least she had no need to attach the senses to it; but she ought not to have separated these two organs by two coverings so solid and so thick, in covering the one with the cranium and the other with the thorax. Even though she had neglected these matters she should certainly not have established the neck between the two organs, a neck so long in the hottest-blooded animals, which take their name from their sharp teeth [i.e., carnivores], a neck still longer in birds, so that in them the brain is as distant from the heart as are the feet. In my opinion it is just as sensible to say that the heel was created for the heart. Do not believe that I speak thus in jest, since an attentive examination will show you that refrigeration reaches the heart more promptly from the heel than from the brain.

. . . . Under all conditions one finds the brain to be much warmer than the air, whether one places his hand on a fracture of the cranium, whether in the course of experiment one takes some animal, and lifting a part of the cranium, incises the membranes and touches the brain. Furthermore, everyone is aware that [in the case of fracture] we always use the greatest care in removing the bone of the head so that the brain may not be chilled; and if it is chilled, that is the most dangerous happening for the patient . . . .

. . . . Perhaps someone will say the evil arises not from the brain but from the chilling of the membranes, especially the thin membrane [pia mater] that encloses the very numerous veins and arteries, and which pulsates constantly through all its extent and has no part that does not produce a bubbling heat. You simple men, with the idea that the thin membrane is hot, you dare again to declare that the brain is cold, when the membrane penetrates its tissue on all sides [via sulci] so that one finds no part of the brain that is lacking it! Or indeed, ignore this fact and think that the brain is only covered by it but not traversed and enfolded in every way. Besides, if it were confined to covering it, the brain would be unable to cool the heart from which it is so distant, from which it is separated by a double barrier of bone [skull and thorax]; and ought it not, besides, be heated by the membrane with which it is in constant contact; at least were a cold part to cool regions so distant, would not a hot part heat neighboring regions? For, such are necessarily the frivolous reasons of those who are less anxious to defend the truth than their own opinions, who not only do not trust their senses and logical deductions, but rashly turn to contradictions.

EXCERPT PP. 532–535

. . . . Why is the brain capable of cooling the heart and why is the heart not rather capable of heating the brain which is placed above it, since all heat tends to rise? And why does the brain send to the heart only an imperceptible nerve while all the sensory organs draw a large part of their substance from the brain?

Again, how to explain that the brain, destined to cool the heart, is of a quite different use for the organs of the senses? Indeed, an organ created to cool the heart must necessarily, I think, have in it a source of refrigeration and communicate that to all the neighboring bodies. Also, the brain, alone among all the organs, would then be a marvel if it could, through the numerous interposed bodies, cool distant parts warmer than itself, but be incapable of exercising the same action on the less warm, very close bodies that it touches.

But, said Aristotle, all the organs of the senses do not abut on the brain. What is this language? I blush even today to cite this statement. Does not a considerable nerve enter into one and the other ear with the membranes? Does not a part of the brain descend to each side of the nose [olfactory nerves], even more important than that which goes to the ears? Does not each of the eyes receive a soft [sensory] and a hard [motor] nerve, the one inserting at its root, the other on the moving muscles? Do not four of them go to the tongue, two soft ones penetrating by the palate [? hypoglossal, ? lingual], two other hard ones descending through the ear [? chorda tympani]? Thus, if one must put faith in one's eyes and touch, all the senses are in relationship with the brain. Shall I announce the other parts that enter into the structure of the brain? Shall I say what use is provided by the meninges, the reticular plexus [*rete mirabile*], the pineal gland, the pituitary body, the infundibulum, the lyre [fornix], the vermiform eminence [vermis], the multiplicity of the ventricles, the openings by which they communicate with one another and the variety of configurations, the two meninges, the processes that go to the spinal marrow, the roots of the nerves that abut not only on the organs of the senses but also on the pharynx, on the larynx, the oesophagus, the stomach, and all the viscera and all the intestines, and go to all parts of the face?

Aristotle did not attempt to explain the use of any of these parts, no more than that of the nerves of the heart; but the brain is the source of all the nerves. If it were destined only for refrigeration, the brain would have to be a useless and shapeless sponge, having no skillfully produced structure; and the heart, if it be not the origin of the arteries or of the innate heat, ought not have a complicated configuration, or even exist.

These admirable goals, marked in the two organs by a consummate wisdom, are again proved, especially by this circumstance, that the followers of Aristotle not only did not believe that the brain is the origin of the nerves and the heart the origin of the arteries, but they avowed even that one of the two organs lacked all usefulness; some declaring it loudly, as Philotimus [pupil of Praxagoras of Cos: ". . . Philotimus placed the governing principle in the heart. For whence joy and grief take their beginning, there reason evidently originates," Steckerl, 1958, p. 108], the others in an indirect fashion, as Aristotle himself. Indeed, in recognizing the brain as only a useless property, and imagining that it has no other purpose, evidently he condemned it to complete uselessness although he did not dare acknowledge it openly. But this is not the place to speak of functions. That which we said at the beginning of the whole work becomes evident by the fact that it is impossible to reveal suitably the usefulness of any part without understanding the function of the whole organ.

Galen also attacked the followers of Aristotle such as Praxagoras of Cos (pp. 18–19), who extended the heart versus brain controversy. In respect to nomenclature, Galen discussed the terms for the cerebellum and the cerebral hemispheres when dealing with the anatomy of the former structure (pp. 630–631).

Another matter of general significance was the vital concept of the nervous system as a functional unit. As noted, it is possible that the Alexandrian anatomists envisaged a continuity between brain, cord, and nerves, and that Rufus had a clear idea of it. However, there is no doubt that Galen's concept of a system composed of brain, cord, and nerves was the same as ours but, as he stated, it was by no means universally accepted in the second century A.D. The following comment is from *On the dissection of nerves*, I (Kühn [1821–1833], II, 831); a second is to be found in his argument against Praxagoras (p. 142).

It is agreed by all physicians that none of the parts of the animal possesses either what we term voluntary motion or sensation without a nerve; and that, if the nerve should be cut, the part immediately becomes motionless and insensitive. But it is not yet realized by all that the brain is the beginning of the nerves, just as it is of the spinal cord; and that some of them originate from the brain itself, others from the spinal cord; and yet in dissections the fact is thus.

AVICENNA
(980–1037)

After Galen's death in A.D. 199, little new was added to the corpus of knowledge he had assembled until the sixteenth century. His works were carefully transmitted and became eventually a body of dogmata for the medical world, comparable in sanctity to the Bible. Consequently his ideas and those of other writers he had accepted can be detected throughout the medieval period and later. In addition, the teachings of the Hippocratic Writers, Plato, Aristotle, and other ancients are found in amounts determined, as in the case of Galen, by the availability of their books.

During the medieval period the Moslems were active in preserving and, in some instances, extending the Greek medical learning. One of the most outstanding was the Persian Ibn Sina or Avicenna. He was born near Bukhara in central Asia, not far from Samarkand. His intellectual precocity was remarkable and he seems to have mastered all branches of learning at an early age. His activities were, however, devoted mainly to medicine, philosophy, and politics. His most important medical work was a system of medicine or *Canon* which is a huge digest of Greek anatomy and physiology, materia medica, diseases, and therapy. This work had a profound and widespread influence, and it is said to be used even today in parts of the East and Middle East. No man, except Aristotle and Galen, had such absolute authority in science during the medieval period. Yet his work was mainly a compilation of Greek learning and especially from these two authors (see Wickens, 1952; Afnan, 1958).

In view of Avicenna's universal influence it is appropriate to select a small portion of his writings for inclusion here. But his anatomy, like that of 'Ali Abbas (Wiberg, 1914), was mainly Galenic in origin, and repetition is unnecessary. A translation of Avicenna's account of the anatomy of the nervous system is to be found in Koning (1903), taken from Book III of the *Canon*. The portion, "Concerning the brain" (pp. 646–660), deals mainly with the meninges and ventricles, reflecting Galen's predominant interest in these structures (pp. 461–462).

Although Avicenna's anatomical knowledge was limited to the findings of others, he could express an opinion with greater authority on the partially philosophical controversy of the heart versus the brain. On the whole he sided with Aristotle, as is clear from the following passages taken from Book I of the *Canon* (O. C. Gruner, *A treatise on the Canon of Medicine of Avicenna incorporating a translation of the first book* [London, 1930]).

EXCERPT PP. 110–111

138. Many philosophers, and all physicians who follow Galen, consider that each faculty has its own principal member, which forms its storehouse, and from which its functions emerge. On this view the rational faculty resides in the brain, and its functions proceed from the brain.

139. . . . .

140. The *vital faculty* preserves the integrity of the breath [*pneuma* or spirit], and is the vehicle of sensation and movement, and makes the breath able to receive these impressions (of sensation and movement), and, having reached the brain, makes it capable of imparting life, and then spreads in every direction. The seat of this faculty is the heart, and its function proceeds from this.

141. Now the great philosopher Aristotle believes that the heart is the source of all these functions, though they are manifested in the several principal organs. But physicians still keep to the opinion that the brain is the chief seat of sentient life, and that each sense has its own distinct member whereby it manifests function. But if physicians thought over the whole matter as thoroughly as they should, they would take Aristotle's view instead. They would find that they have been only regarding appearances instead of realities, taking non-essentials for essentials. The establishment of this truth is for the philosopher and natural scientist, and not for the doctor as doctor. But the latter, looking on members as being initiators of the faculties instead of as their manifestation—thus despising or ignoring philosophy—fails to see which things are prior, and accordingly overlooks the proper basis for the treatment of diseases, and for the remedying of bodily defects.

Avicenna, repeating Aristotle, thought the first organ to develop in the embryo was the heart and that it influenced the growth of other organs, including the brain.

EXCERPT P. 124

172. The foundation or beginning of all these faculties [of sensation, movement, nutrition, growth, and generation] is traceable [in the embryo]

to the heart, as is agreed upon even by those philosophers who think that
the source of visual, auditory, and gustatory power lies in the brain.

Mondino de' Luzzi
(c. 1270–1326)

Avicenna's knowledge of anatomy came from the books of Greek writers, for in
common with other Moslem physicians he had no practical experience of, at least,
human dissection. Not until the close of the thirteenth century, after a hiatus of
about fifteen hundred years, was human dissection undertaken again. One of those
who played a principal role in restoring anatomy to its rightful place in medicine
was Mondino. Admittedly his work was very considerably based on the writings of
Galen, but a portion of it is included here mainly because of the extremely wide
authority it achieved and because of the few minor contributions he made to the
anatomy of the brain. His writing also summarized, albeit somewhat inadequately,
the knowledge of the anatomy of the brain current before the advent of the great
anatomists of the Renaissance.

Mondino was born at Bologna where he studied at the University; he completed
his medical studies about 1290, and in 1306 he joined the faculty of medicine.
Mondino distinguished himself by his systematic work in anatomy and by the fact
that he carried out the dissections himself rather than allowing someone else to do
them for him as was to become the usual practice. On the whole, he followed
Moslem authorities who in their turn had followed the Greeks, and in consequence
Mondino showed little originality. Nevertheless, his anatomical treatise, the *Anath-
omia*, written in 1316, is a landmark in the history of anatomy. In content it is akin
to our modern manuals of dissection, and it became the most popular anatomical
treatise of the fourteenth, fifteenth, and early sixteenth centuries; it passed through
about thirty printed editions and was still in use even after the works of the
Renaissance anatomists began to appear (see Singer, 1925, pp. 74–86; Singer's
introduction to Mondino, 1925; Mondino, 1930, pp. 1–22; Kudlien, 1964).

The following passages have been translated from Mondino's text as incorporated with one of the most famous commentaries upon it, that of Berengario da
Carpi (1521). Mondino clearly drew upon the teachings of Aristotle, Galen, and
Avicenna, and the large amount of space he allotted to the ventricular system was a
reflection of Galen's extended discussions of it (pp. 711–714). His account of the
thalami was better than that of Galen who connected them with the eyes; the
cooling properties of the brain (p. 23) were also mentioned. The localization of
psychological functions in the ventricles of the brain will be dealt with later (p.
463).

EXCERPT FOLS. CCCCXXVIIr–CCCCXXVIIIv

The anatomy of the cerebral marrow and of those things contained in it.
When the membranes have been seen, the brain will appear, larger in

quantity in man than in any other animal of the same size because he has a hotter brain than they, and because he requires more animal spirit for the operation of his intellect.

This brain has two parts, anterior and posterior, and the anterior part [cerebrum] is divided into right and left; this division appears clearly in the substance of the brain and consequently in the ventricles. Its substance is a cold and humid marrow, different from other marrows; it is not contained to nourish the cranium but rather the cranium is nourished that it may contain the brain of which the purpose is to temper by its complexion the vital spirit [from the heart] so that it may become animal spirit.

Then cut lightly through the middle until you reach the greater anterior [lateral] ventricle. Before you reach the depth of the lacuna [infundibulum] note that the ventricle is divided into right and left, as I said; also that there are walls on this side descending as far as the base, dividing right from left; then you will immediately see the size of each ventricle. Phantasy, which retains the appearances received by particular senses, is located in the anterior angle. Imagination, which apprehends those appearances received by phantasy, is in the posterior angle; it apprehends them by composing and dividing, not by perceiving that this thing is this [see pp. 463–465].

In the middle is the *sensus communis* which apprehends appearances carried from the particular senses, and so, as you will see, the sensitive parts end at this place like rivers in a fountain. All these things are in accordance with the opinion of Avicenna, *De virtutibus animalibus*, although as I declared elsewhere, according to the opinion of Aristotle and Galen there is only the *sensus communis* which is variously called phantasy and imagination.

. . . .
. . . .
. . . .
. . . .

If it is wholly obstructing either it obstructs ventricles and substance at the same time, or only the ventricles. If the ventricles and substance, it is apoplexy, if only the ventricles it is epilepsy. Although this obstruction may block the other ventricles, not as much as the anterior. It can also suffer a bad complexion, as melancholy and the like.

Before you proceed to the middle [third] ventricle, give consideration to that which intervenes between anterior and middle ventricles; there are three things, that is, *anchae* [thalami], which are a kind of base of this anterior ventricle on the right and left [floor of lateral ventricles], and they are of the substance of the brain in the shape of buttocks. At the side of each *ancha*, between the aforesaid ventricles, there is a blood red substance formed like a long worm such as an earthworm [choroid plexus], attached by ligaments and nervules on each side; by lengthening it constricts and closes the *anchae* and the way or passage from the anterior to the middle [ventricle], and the reverse. When a man wishes to cease cogitation, and again in consideration, he raises the walls and dilates the *anchae* so that the spirit may pass from one ventricle to the others; it is called a worm because it resembles an earthworm in substance and form, and also in its contractive and extensive movement.

After this, investigate lower, little by little, and first you will meet with the *lacuna* [infundibulum] which is a round and long concavity in the middle of which is a foramen extending downwards diagonally [through the sella turcica] to the palate and running directly to it; it descends directly from the middle ventricle to the *colatorium* [cribriform plate], and this *lacuna* [infundibulum] has around it large, round eminences formed for sustaining the ascending veins and arteries from the *rete mirabile* to the aforesaid ventricles of the brain; its base is glandular, rising near the *rete mirabile* [see p. 763], and through this *lacuna* the anterior ventricles and the middle part of the brain purge their superfluities, but as much of the brain as is in the anterior parts purges its superfluities [directly] through the cribriform plate [see pp. 709–710].

When these things have been investigated, the middle ventricle will appear to you, which is a kind of way and passage from the anterior to the posterior [fourth ventricle]; the cogitative power is placed in it, and deservedly, because this power works by composing phantasy and memory so that from what has been perceived it may draw forth what has not been perceived. Likewise, because it is the ruling power of the whole animal. The system of the whole animal consists in comprehension of the present, memory of things passed, and prognostication of the future; hence cogitation ought to be in the middle of the powers of apprehension and memory; also it is in the middle of these ventricles so that its power may be in direct line with the heart, because the power of the heart is immediately subservient to the intellect, so that cogitation ought to be in the middle ventricle and in the middle of the aforesaid powers.

Continuing onwards from this ventricle, you will see the posterior [fourth] ventricle, which is situated and located in the posterior brain [cerebellum], and this brain is veiled and separated from the anterior brain [cerebrum] by the two membranes already mentioned, because the former, that is the anterior, is soft, and the posterior hard.

This brain is placed posteriorly because it is the source of the spinal marrow, and because it is the origin of many of the motor nerves. Movement occurs through motor nerves which are the stronger the harder they are.

This brain has the shape of a pyramid because the ventricle placed in it also has the shape of a pyramid, and the reason that this posterior ventricle is of this shape is that it must receive through its lower part, which is its base, and so it must have breadth; but it must retain through its upper part, and so, sharp and restricted, it must have a point in order to retain what is received, because appearances are held better in a narrow space than in a wide one; hence its shape.

From these things it is apparent what are the operations or uses of this posterior brain; one is that it may be the source of the motor nerves and spinal marrow, another that it may be the instrument of the power of memory. From this it appears that its own affliction is injury to the memory, and also to the power of movement, just as when the cogitation is injured it is a special affliction of the middle ventricle, and when the imagination is injured it is an affliction of the anterior ventricle. When an affliction is communicated to the whole brain, all the forces and operations of all these powers are injured.

But you will ask what is the reason that the middle ventricle does not have a distinct middle brain like the other ventricles; it must be replied that the reason is because that ventricle is the way and passage of those other two, and so it ought not be distinct from them as regards the brain. So much for the anatomy of the brain.

Conclusion

Throughout the medieval period there was to be continued controversy over the relative merits of the heart or the brain as the central organ of the body. Although all Aristotle's original arguments, which had been dealt with so brilliantly by Galen, were not invoked, nevertheless, many individuals felt that there was sufficient evidence to support the argument in favor of the cardiocentric theory. The experimental data provided by Galen were not considered necessary by the medieval philosopher, who was content to solve the problem by disputation alone. In his eyes this was a more worthy and reliable method of tackling a controversial issue.

Such polemics were a feature of the Middle Ages; nor were they immediately dispelled by the new learning of the scientific revolution of the sixteenth and seventeenth centuries. The University of Padua was one of the strongholds of Aristotelian teaching, and its influence can be seen in the work of Harvey and his contemporaries. Andrea Cesalpino (1519–1603), a rigid Aristotelian, still believed in 1588 that nerves originated from the heart and stated that "the heart is not only the origin of all the veins but also of the nerves" (*Tractationum philosophicarum tomus unus. . . . Quaestionum peripateticarum libri* V [Geneva, 1588], col. 516). Descartes, writing in 1649 (p. 471), noted that some would place the seat of the soul in the heart, and such opinion can be traced well into the eighteenth century.

It is clear from the foregoing that a large body of ideas about the anatomy and function of the nervous system was assembled in Greco-Roman antiquity, some of which resulted from the heart versus brain controversy. Further details about this knowledge will be included in most of the subsequent chapters, and when brought together they reveal the remarkable legacy of achievement bequeathed to the neurological sciences by antiquity.

CHAPTER II

THE NEURON

Introduction

This first chapter to deal with a special topic is concerned with the fundamental constituent of the nervous system, the nerve cell or neuron. The term *neuron*, which was not introduced until 1891, can be defined as the nerve cell body and all its processes; the account by Barker (1899) and his well-known illustration (fig. 38) represent our present-day concept of the neuron in its simplest form.

It need hardly be mentioned that the neuron is one of the most complex and important cells of the body, and that one of the greatest advances in the neurological sciences during the last century and a half has been the gradual elucidation of its structure and function and the application of that knowledge to the problems of morbid anatomy. This has proved to be the most difficult task in the whole field of histology, and even today with the help of new and more powerful methods of investigation such as the electron microscope and physical and chemical intracellular techniques, investigators are still only at the edge of the problem.

It follows that the body of literature produced by those who have worked in this field is of very considerable dimensions, and even to find one's way through the part that concerns morphological characteristics is a daunting endeavor. The chronological sequence of events has therefore been divided into four sections.

The evolution of the microscope was vital to them and to some extent determined their boundaries. The microscope was first applied to biological problems in the middle of the seventeenth century and at that time was either simple with one lens or compound with more than one. It was crude in structure and difficult to use but nevertheless Robert Hooke was able to identify plant cells in 1665 and Leeuwenhoek, the red blood cell in 1674. Thereafter there were no important improvements in the instrument until the achromatic compound microscope was introduced in the 1820's. It then became possible to observe plant and animal structures without the troublesome chromatic and spherical aberrations which had confused earlier workers. The staining of animal tissues was not introduced until the middle of the nineteenth century and since then the development of it and of other essential histological techniques and of the microscope itself have largely determined the growth of knowledge of the neuron.

The first section of the present chapter deals with the early observations of nervous tissue by the classic microscopists in the latter half of the seventeenth century. These were continued sporadically through the eighteenth century and into the 1830's culminating in the enunciation of the cell theory of animal tissue by Schwann in 1839. Until then observers had only seen the nerve cell and the nerve fibre separately, and although a connection had been occasionally assumed, it had not yet been demonstrated irrefutably. That advancement is represented in the second section. In the third are descriptions of certain important morphological characteristics of the cell body and fibre; here will be found an account of the neuroglia of Virchow, the only other component of nervous tissue, in addition to the neuron, to be included. The fourth and final group of selections deals with attempts to solve the problem of neuronal individuality. On the one hand, the neuronists considered the nerve cell and its processes to be an independent unit in contact but not in continuity with its neighbors. On the other, there were those who favored the concept of a diffuse network connecting the cells and made up of their processes. The former group has so far prevailed, and the neuron doctrine enunciated in 1891 has not been displaced. The most modern work, which began about two decades ago with the invention of the electron microscope, has so far produced only support for it.

It is of particular interest to note that most of the work in this field of the neurological sciences was carried out in Germany. The arduous and painstaking tasks imposed by the study of the nerve cell may have appealed to the German temperament, and, furthermore, they were acceptable to the materialistic German scientist of the nineteenth century who was dissociating himself from the *Naturphilosophie* of earlier decades. Other factors such as the excellent German lens grinding and the microscope workshops of Berlin, Vienna, and Munich, as well as the German dyestuffs industry were also of no little significance.

There are four useful sources of information for the history of neurohistology: (1) Barker (1899) whose first two chapters give a good account of the neuron theory because the author surveyed the complex literature with precise and critical discernment; (2) Andreoli (1961), whose account covers the periods outlined above, is a less reliable source of information; (3) Stieda (1899), who deals with the period from about 1790 to 1865, although in parts less reliable than Barker or Andreoli, offers more detail than either; and (4) Rasmussen (1947) who devotes one chapter to "The microscopic structure of nervous tissue and the development of the central nervous system" (pp. 51–53). These chapters contain much accurate information, but, unfortunately, the author gives no references. The general history of cytology is to be found in two excellent works: Hughes (1959) and Baker (1948–1953).

Early Accounts of Nerve Cell and Fibre

The history of attempts to elucidate the morphological appearance of the ultimate structure of nervous tissue, the nerve cell, is obviously a part of the development of knowledge concerning the cell in general and must be considered against this background. This is especially true of the first period which represents, in fact, an important aspect of the early history of cytology. In dealing with this early period there are three dangerous pitfalls that occasionally engulf the unwary.

First of all, the word *fibre* must be considered with care whenever it is found in literature before the end of the eighteenth century. The nerve fibre, as we know it today, was first identified by Fontana in 1781 (pp. 36–38). Before that time the word *fibre*, considered as a synonym for *thread, filament,* and the like, in many instances was used to refer to a bundle of axons visible to the naked eye; Vesalius, for example, mentions how one may recognize the threadlike composition of nerves in cooked meat (p. 155). Occasionally, the individual axon may have been seen but not recognized, as was probably true in the instance of Leeuwenhoek (pp. 32–34). In addition, early authors sometimes used *fibre* to describe an elementary but hypothetical unit of plant and animal tissue in much the same way that atoms, which were thought to make up the fibre, were theoretical, fundamental units of matter. Thus the fibres discussed by Glisson (pp. 167–169) were of the theoretical variety, and when Descartes spoke of threads inside the nerve (p. 156 and fig. 42), he may have been referring to these rather than to the individual nerve fibres or axons that his diagram certainly suggests. An excellent review of the fibre has been published by Alexander Berg (1942).

Second, there is the problem of the structures described by early microscopists such as the cortical "glands" of Malpighi (pp. 417–418) and the "globuls" of Leeuwenhoek and others. It is easy to accept them as nerve cell bodies, but it is almost certain that they were not. As Baker observed (1948–1953, 89:114–121), the "globule theory" preceded the cell theory of 1839, and the lack of a critical evaluation of early descriptions of so-called nerve cells has deceived many historians of the subject. Others, in addition to Leeuwenhoek, made similar observations and some found globules associated with peripheral nerve fibres: Procháska in 1779; Fontana in 1781; J. and C. Wenzel in 1812; Treviranus in 1816; Milne Edwards in 1823 (Baker, *loc. cit.*; Della Torre, 1776). In each instance the globules seen and described were almost certainly not nerve cells, and may have been fat cells or fat globules. But it seems likely that more often they were optical artifacts owing to aberrations produced by the primitive microscopes then in use; particles smaller than cells were thereby surrounded by haloes and given a globular appearance; and, no doubt, products of degeneration also produced confusion. Care must also be taken in interpreting the term "cellular tissue," or its foreign equivalent, used before the enunciation of the cell theory in 1839. Early authors using it usually meant connective tissue, what we today call areolar connective tissue.

Third, it is essential to realize that up to the middle of the nineteenth century there were no methods of fixing or staining tissues and that most investigators used only aqueous preparations. Obviously this not only limited their examination of histological material but it also meant that water could enter the cell or fibre by osmosis to produce distortions such as the varicosity of the nerve fibre described by Ehrenberg (pp. 41–42) and perhaps, in some cases, the "globules" just mentioned.

Thus accounts of nerve cell bodies and fibres recorded before the introduction in the 1820's of the achromatic compound microscope (which reduced the distorting influence of aberration) and before the development of histological techniques in the middle of the nineteenth century must be accepted with caution. Some have been included below because of their widespread influence on subsequent investigators; Malpighi's account of the gray matter "glands" was the first and one of the most influential (see pp. 417–418); that of Leeuwenhoek is of equal importance and is to be found in the present chapter.

As soon as the achromatic microscope became freely available, the globule theory was quickly displaced by the first accurate descriptions of nerve cells, and these led to the cell theory of Schwann in 1839. One of the papers that marked this vital transition from a world of shadows to one of precise cytological structures was that of Hodgkin and Lister who employed the new achromatic microscope perfected by the latter, the father of Joseph, Lord Lister ("Notice of some microscopic observations of the blood and animal tissues," *Phil. Mag.*, 1827, ii:130–138). In it they referred (p. 137) to brain tissue as follows:

> Our examination of it has yet been but slight; but we have noticed that when a portion of it, however fresh, is sufficiently extended to allow of its being viewed in the microscope, one sees instead of globules a multitude of very small particles, which are most irregular in shape and size.

With the preachromatic instrument, these "very small particles" would no doubt have been seen as "globules."

Almost immediately, detailed studies of the nerve cell were carried out by young German and Czech microscopists, and their findings, which mostly antedate the cell theory of Schwann, support the claims of those who question his absolute priority (see Studnička, 1931–1932; Florian, 1932; Studnička's claims for Purkyně have, however, a nationalistic flavor, and he failed in some instances to assess correctly the findings of the pre-Schwann investigators). The way was now open to more accurate and detailed descriptions of the nerve cell.

The nerve fibre, on the other hand, caused less deception, and the majority of the authors mentioned above were examining and describing it as well as the cell. The continuity between the two had not yet been verified, however, although strongly suspected by Remak and Purkyně.

It has been thought preferable to include some of the first accounts of the cerebral cortical cells and white matter fibres in the chapters dealing with the history of these structures (Chapters VIII and X respectively), and they should be read in conjunction with the material offered in the present chapter.

Antony van Leeuwenhoek
(*24 October 1632—26 August 1723*)

The nerve fibre was discovered before the nerve cell body was, and this was probably due to the fact that the fibre was more readily available in peripheral nerves and that it was more robust than the cell and easier to examine in the unstained state by means of a primitive microscope.

The theory of nerve function current in the seventeenth and eighteenth centuries was very similar to that of Greek antiquity (pp. 144–153); it was believed that a spiritous substance passed along the nerve which was thought to be hollow. The early investigators of the nerve's structure were therefore looking for passages that would act as pathways. Some, like Leeuwenhoek, believed that they had found them when they encountered the myelinated fibre, since they thought the central axon was a tubular space.

One of the earliest suggestions concerning the contents of the nerve was that of Descartes; it was mostly speculative (p. 157) but of considerable importance because of its influence on others. Also in the seventeenth century, Thomas Willis of Oxford and London made reference to nerve fibres (p. 161), but it seems that like Marcello Malpighi of Bologna, who compared the cerebral white matter to a mass of fibres or tubes (p. 580), he was using a microscope. However, the first important account of the peripheral nerve and its fibre, the axon, was that of the great Dutch microscopist Leeuwenhoek in 1717.

Leeuwenhoek was born in Delft, the son of a prosperous basket-maker, and died there in his ninetieth year. By trade he was a clothier and haberdasher, and he was active in local politics. However, after 1670 his interest turned more and more to the new science of microscopy, mainly because of his great skill in lens grinding and in the production of simple microscopes and possibly because of his very acute visual powers. He examined a great variety of substances, both living and non-living, and many of his results were published in the form of letters to the Royal Society of London. He was distinguished from contemporary microscopists by his attempts to measure the objects he observed. Unfortunately, however, he did not make public the details of his instruments, and, in many instances, it is impossible to deduce the exact magnification he used in individual experiments (see Dobell, 1932; Schierbeek, 1959; Cole, 1937; this last work includes a bibliography and analytical index of Leeuwenhoek's writings).

In 1674, and therefore early in his career as a microscopist, Leeuwenhoek reported his examination of the optic nerve of the cow ("More observations from Mr. Leewenhook, in a letter of Sept. 7. 1674. sent to the Publisher," *Phil. Trans. R. Soc.*, 1674, 9:178–182). He was primarily concerned with proving or disproving the old theory of hollow nerves, especially in regard to the optic nerves. He concluded as follows:

> . . . but I could find no hollowness in them; I only took notice, that they were made up of many filamentous particles, of a very soft substance, as if they only consisted of the corpuscles of the Brain joined together, the threds were so very soft and loose: They were composed of conjoined globuls, and wound about again with particles consisting of other transparent globuls [p. 180].

Although on this occasion Leeuwenhoek did not find the nerve hollow as the ancient theory demanded, the selection given below describes how Leeuwenhoek discovered an apparent hollowness of the fibres which make up a nerve. He published further observations on this problem in the following year ("Microscopical observations of Mr. Leewenhoeck, concerning the optic nerve . . . ," *Phil. Trans. R. Soc.*, 1675, 10:378–380) and again in 1677, 1685, and 1693. In these papers he became increasingly obsessed with "globuls" but, as suggested already, these may have been fat cells or globules, optical artifacts, or products of degeneration. His paper on cerebral cortical "globuls" should also be consulted (see pp. 418–420).

More than forty years later, Leeuwenhoek wrote a letter to Abraham van Bleiswyk of Delft, 2 March 1717, providing in it an account of the peripheral nerve fibre and spinal cord (*Epistolae physiologicae super compluribus naturae arcanis* [Delft, 1719], Epistola XXXII, pp. 310–317. See also Letters XXXIV [6 March 1717] and XXXVI [26 May 1717]). One of the most interesting features relating to the letter of 2 March 1717 is the accompanying illustration (fig. 2, fig. 2), for it is probably the first attempt to represent the cross section of a peripheral nerve. Individual nerve fibres can be seen, and the central stroke contained in each is meant to indicate the collapsed central tube, which he assumed was present; or, as we should put it today, the axis cylinder surrounded by the myelin sheath. It seems likely therefore that Leeuwenhoek observed the myelinated nerve fibre although his interpretation was incorrect; and having discovered no cavities in the nerve itself, he found in the individual fibres the hollowness that the then current theory of nerve function demanded. The thin sections of the nerves which he cut were probably the first ever.

The penultimate paragraph of the selection translated below has also been used to support the claim that Leeuwenhoek described the myelin sheath (see, for example, Schierbeek, 1959, p. 121). He stated that the fibres increase in size and take on a new tunic as they pass from the spinal cord out through the meninges. The acquired covering may, however, have been from the latter, and the description does not necessarily refer to the change from a non-myelinated to a myelinated fibre.

EXCERPT PP. 310–315

Delft, 2 March 1717

A few days ago I arranged to have the spinal marrow of three cows and a sheep brought to my home so that I might dissect out the nerves. Often, and not without pleasure, I have observed the structure of the nerves to be composed of very slender vessels of an indescribable fineness, running lengthwise to form the nerve. The diameter of the vessels is such that if you compare it with its canal, it is a third larger than the canal [i.e., the lumen is two-thirds the total diameter].

I regret that in this matter I have been unable to display these visible canals to anyone, for no sooner did I move them to my eyes for examination than almost immediately, in less than a minute, they dried out and contracted so that this astonishing sight wholly vanished beyond recall. I not only saw the circumference of those vessels—up to several hundreds seem to join together to form a nerve—but also I very distinctly recognized the canals in some of them; just as if we were to perforate a piece of paper in certain places with a very fine needle and look at the sun shining through those holes. And even though that space [the lumen] was so small, yet I have seen live animalcules swimming in water that were able to move and swim freely through it. In brief, the minuteness of certain things seems to surpass all belief.

Thereafter I cut a nerve into slices or round sections, not any or little thicker than the hair of a man's chin. I placed those round slices, previously moistened, on a glass plate to dry. When I looked at them when dried, I saw many little hills raised on them, which it seemed to me required explanation. A nervule of that sort is composed of many little vessels which, when contracted through the drying out of the nervule, what humor was in them is driven out and rises up like little hills.

It frequently happened that when I moistened a small slice of dried-out nervule with clean water and looked at it so moistened through the microscope, I noticed a large number of small particles swimming and floating in the water [probably fat globules and/or tissue debris]. I believe that these particles had issued from the vessels, for the little knife which I employed for cutting was so sharp that it could be used for shaving.

. . . .

A few weeks ago, despite my advanced years [he was eighty-four years of age], I was encouraged by a worthy gentleman to continue my studies since fruits that ripen in the autumn are by their nature the more lasting.

Therefore, here are the things I have observed in my old age, not without great effort. Indeed, it is no easy task to pursue investigations into all those [very minute] divisions, and it can scarcely be understood how the most minute nerve can be divided into so many little branches.

Although I am unable to provide a drawing of a nerve cut transversely, as it appeared to my eyes [but see fig. 2, fig. 2], nevertheless I can offer one in longitudinal extension. Thus a portion of such a slender nerve is reproduced in Fig. 1 [fig. 2] at $ABCDEFG$, where the main portion is denoted $ABCDEF$ and the part designated AGF is only a branch extending from the larger nerve.

In this portion of the nerve, not only was I able to recognize the fibres that compose the nerve and which serve in place of vessels, but also I saw that the single nerves, as far as they extended lengthwise, were hollow or pervious like a kind of channel. Furthermore, it seemed to me that I could visibly distinguish the very particles contained in the aforesaid vessels [? products of degeneration or osmosis].

I cut those little nerves transversely and as accurately as possible several times, and I moistened the sections so that not only might the artist observe those parts or vessels, but, furthermore, that we might see the course of the little longitudinal lines from which, as I advised, the nerve is composed; which, in fact, was nothing except that hollow but compressed passage of the vessel [nerve fibre]. We find this to occur in blood vessels when the flesh has dried out.

In illustration 2 [fig. 2] the nervule is indicated by $BCDEF$, of which the many vessels have been dissected transversely, in which the individual little lines indicate the cavity of individual vessels. Five other nerves, designated in the same illustration by $GGGGG$, partly surround this nerve. I have had delineated only their outline and the tunics enveloping them which protect the enclosed vessels.

In the same illustration 2, in four places, that is, BNG, $GHID$, $EKLF$, and AFN, the fatty parts are indicated. Sometimes I observed a nervule of that sort to be completely surrounded by fatty parts. However, I believe that the nerves are contiguous to one another in a lean animal so that they are separated only by their little membranes [perineurium]. Whence it follows that the juices distributed through the body, and thickened into fat, have the ability to separate the nerves from one another. Through a certain portion of the same nerve, not wider than several hairs, I saw seven extended nervules, all lacking fat.

After this I dissected the spinal marrow [cord] so that I might be able to discover the parts extending through it longitudinally; I delineated a small portion of this marrow, insofar as I was able to imitate nature, and it is represented in illustration 3 at $MNOP$.

I also made numerous transverse sections of the spinal marrow, and finally, with singular pleasure, I discovered that its parts were arranged in the very same order represented in Fig. 2, except that I saw them a little larger. Furthermore, in many places I was able to distinguish the light of the sun piercing transversely through the hollow passages of the vessels, and pointed it out to the artist. Since everything agreed with Fig. 2, I decided that it would be unnecessary to present a new drawing.

While I was separating from the spinal marrow the strong tunic that surrounds it [spinal meninges], I saw numerous small nervules extending here and there from the spinal marrow; some of these were so minute that very often what I believed to be a simple nervule turned out to be at least five, and each of those five nervules was as small as that which is designated by GAF in Fig. 1. It astonished me that as soon as those nervules had issued from the spinal marrow they were inserted into part of the hard (*cornea*) tunic which I have said surrounded it, and were, so to speak, united with it. But when they again emerged from that hard part, they seemed to be increased in size and to have acquired a new tunic. I found the nerves which I had severed near their origin here to be so covered with fat and invested with such strong membranes that I was unable to separate them.

. . . .

. . . . What the material is that was enclosed in them [spinal cord fibres or tubes] I was never able to determine with certainty, although I believe that it was a very fluid humor which passed off as vapor.

FELICE GASPAR FERDINAND FONTANA
(*15 April 1730—9 March 1805*)

There was no important improvement in the fundamental structure of the microscope during the eighteenth century, and on the whole the instrument fell into disrepute for investigation of animal and human biology because of the frequent artifacts that misled those who used it. It was for this very reason that Alexander Monro II (1783, pp. 67–73), having attempted a study of the microscopical features of nerve fibres, abandoned further work on the problem. Gall and Spurzheim (pp. 598–602) likewise preferred macroscopic studies. Others did, however, examine nervous tissue microscopically, but their conclusions were not outstanding (see Stieda, 1899, p. 313; Baker, 1948–1953, 89:114–121). There was only one noteworthy contribution made after Leeuwenhoek's observations of 1717 and before the invention of the achromatic, compound microscope. That was the investigation of nerve fibres carried out by Fontana in 1779 and published in 1781.

Fontana was born at Pomarole in the Austrian Alps and received his education in Italy, at Verona, Parma, Padua, and Bologna. He was appointed to the chair of logic at Pisa in 1765, but soon accepted the directorship of the Museum of Physics and Natural Sciences in Florence, where he remained for the rest of his life. His scientific interests were very wide, but he is best known for his work on the venom of vipers, *Ricerche fisiche sopra il veleno della vipera*, Lucca, 1767 (see Earles, 1960; and on irritability, Marchand and Hoff, 1955). Fontana also described the refractory period of the heart (Hoff, 1942). For further aspects of Fontana's work, see Garrison (1935) and Brazier (1963).

Fontana's observations on the nerve fibre were stimulated by Monro's preliminary communication (1779), and are to be found in a section added to a later edition of his work on viper venom (*Traité sur le vénin de la vipère* [Florence, 1781], 2 vols., "Observations sur la structure des nerfs faites à Londres en 1779," Vol. II, 187–208). He summarized contemporary opinion regarding the nervous system in the first paragraph (p. 187):

Of all the organic parts of which the living animal is formed, in my opinion, there is none of which the structure is less well known and at the same time deserves the greatest understanding, than the brain, together with the nerves derived from it.

The following selection has been translated from Fontana's revised Florentine edition of 1781, in which he identified the nerve fibre as the ultimate structure of nerves and termed it "the primitive nerve cylinder." It has been claimed by Zanobio (1959) and Brazier (1963) that Fontana described the axis cylinder and the enveloping myelin sheath; however, it is difficult to be certain that this was so. The vital portions of his description are confusing, and it is possible that all he was describing was the nerve fibre as a whole and its sheath of endoneurium. This is similar to the conclusion of Remak, who gave the first accurate description of the axon and the myelin sheath (pp. 46–52) in a careful analysis of Fontana's findings (Remak, 1844, pp. 463–472). It has also been claimed (Hoff, 1959) that Fontana (1784) observed the fluidity of the axoplasm; and he certainly described a material issuing from a nerve fibre just as J. Z. Young (1935) did in his classic account. But Fontana had no idea of its precise origin nor of its function, for he naturally interpreted it in terms of the then current concept of animal spirits. Nevertheless, his report on the nerve fibre is worthy of notice, unlike the portion of his book that dealt with the microscopical structure of the brain and retina (Vol. II, 209–221) but did not advance beyond previous descriptions. He made no direct reference to Leeuwenhoek.

EXCERPT PP. 203–206

. . . . The problem was to appreciate the elementary structure of the nerve; that is, whether it is composed of channels or of simple threads; whether it consists only of globules or whether it contains a non-organic, irregular, spongy substance. This investigation is as important as it is difficult, since it is no less than the establishment, once and for all, of anatomists' ideas on the nature of the nerves; that is, of the structure of the organ of motion and sensation in animals. There has been dispute concerning this for more than three thousand years, from Hippocrates to Albinus, from the Greeks to the moderns, and it seems as if all that has been achieved is the multiplication of doubts and hypotheses.

. . . .

I began my observations on a very small nerve from which I had stripped the areolar connection tissue (*tissu cellulaire* [see p. 37; this does not mean cellular tissue as we think of it today]). With a very strong lens I observed the winding fibres [circular fibres of collagen in the epineurium] very clearly, and I determined their size. This done, I cut the nerve lengthwise and, with a very sharp needle, I divided the parts or threads and separated them from each other. I immersed the nerve in water and the threads floated in it. After many fruitless attempts and after several observations, either suspect or inconsistent, I finally succeeded in finding several very small, more or less transparent cylinders which seemed to possess a pellicle and to be partly filled with a transparent, gelatinous fluid and small globules or bodies of unequal size. Fig. III, Plate IV [fig. 3] illustrates three of these tubes which I shall call primitive nerve cylinders, because they are the structures which constitute the nerve or its medullary [central] part. Fig. V represents another of these cylinders.

I examined a large number of these primitive nerve cylinders with a lens which magnified five hundred times, so that I could recognize their structure and shape better. Fig. I depicts one that appeared to have some fragments of winding threads here and there on its walls and some spheroidal corpuscles in the inner part of the cylinder [? effect of water transuding into nerve fibre]. In Fig. II is to be seen another which appeared to contain very small, scattered globular corpuscles submerged in a transparent, jelly-like fluid. I have seen others which could be considered to be filled with a jelly-like substance, interrupted here and there and divided into various fragments so that one might consider the jelly of the cylinders as interrupted or divided into large, transparent and irregular masses [? products of degeneration and/or osmosis in a water-mounted preparation].

However, all the efforts which I made to convince myself of the reality and nature of these irregular corpuscles belonging to the primitive cylinders were not sufficient to let me make a precise judgment. It seemed to me sometimes that these were spots or irregularities in the exterior coats; but I did not dare to decide, and my doubts multiplied proportionately with my observations. I used the strongest lens with a magnification of 700 diameters, and, after several unsuccessful attempts, I finally succeeded in satisfying myself that the walls of the primitive nerve cylinders were uneven and full of irregularities. Fig. IV represents four of these cylinders (*ac, om, rs, ne*) in which the irregularities are clear in two (*ac, rs*). When I finally convinced myself of this new truth, it remained for me to learn better the true nature of the irregularities of these cylinders and to find out if they contained globules or corpuscles of varying shapes.

In order to succeed in such a difficult study I began by separating the primitive cylinders of several nerves with the point of a needle.

The nerves or their ends were placed in water, and I ran the point of the needle along the length of the nerve to break the cylinders or to deprive them somehow of their irregularities, and I was able finally to see one of them which had the shape depicted in Fig. VI; approximately half of this cylinder (*ac*) was made of a transparent and uniform thread, and the other half (*ma*) was almost twice as thick, less transparent, irregular, and rough. I suspected therefore that the primitive nerve cylinder was made of a transparent, smaller, and more uniform cylinder and covered by another substance, perhaps connective [again, the term *cellulaire* means *connective* rather than *cellular*] in nature [? neurilemma].

The observations which I have since made have always confirmed this hypothesis, which finally became an established fact. On many occasions I have seen these two parts of which the primitive nerve cylinder is composed. One of them is completely exterior, uneven, and rough, the other a cylinder which appears to be formed of a special transparent, homogeneous membrane filled with a gelatinous fluid of a definite constituency.

As already mentioned, Fig. IV represents a group of these primitive nerve cylinders which I saw when examining a rabbit's nerve. One of them, that is (*om*), was completely stripped from the external, rough membrane and appeared in the shape of a uniform, transparent cylinder. A second likewise was completely exposed except for the extremity (*ne*) which seemed covered and surrounded by a rough, outer membrane. A third (*ac*) was almost entirely covered by the rough membrane and was only partly exposed. The fourth (*rs*) was completely covered with the rough membrane.

EXCERPT PP. 207–208

The basic structure of nerves is as follows: a nerve is formed of a large number of transparent, homogeneous, uniform, and simple cylinders. These cylinders seem to be fashioned like a very thin, uniform wall or tunic which is filled, as far as one can see, with a transparent, gelatinous fluid insoluble in water. Each of these cylinders receives a cover in the form of an outer sheath which is composed of an immense number of winding threads [? confusion with neurofibrils of axon or with artifacts of preparation]. A very large number of transparent cylinders together can form a nerve so small that it is barely visible but which shows the white bands [winding threads] on the outside [i.e., in the epineurium]. Several of these nerves together form the larger nerves which are thicker than those seen in animals.

I was fully convinced by my own observations, which I repeated many times with the same result, that the cylinders I have described are the simple and first organic elements of nerves, for I never succeeded in dividing them further, no matter what investigations I carried out with the help of the sharpest and finest needles. I could easily tear and break them here and there; but they always remained indivisible. I could strip them off their sheaths and separate the winding cylinders of which they were formed, although they were very small [perhaps a reference to the perineurium of a bundle of fibres]. The primitive nerve cylinder then appeared transparent, homogeneous, and of equal diameter everywhere. Thus one may see how much even the greatest anatomists were wrong in maintaining that the nerves divide and subdivide endlessly, and that there was no hope of ever being able to understand this or to see the primary threads or the primary organic elements.

CHRISTIAN GOTTFRIED EHRENBERG
(*19 April 1795—27 June 1876*)

Fontana's findings were widely known, owing to the wide distribution of his book, and for the time being they were universally accepted, even by Remak who later, however, changed his mind. But there was no advance beyond them until the appearance of achromatic microscopes.

One of the first to employ the new tool in a special study of nervous tissue was Ehrenberg. He was born at Delitizsch, near Leipzig, and studied medicine and science at the Universities of Leipzig and Berlin. After extensive travels in Asia, he was made professor *extraordinarius* of medicine in Berlin in 1826 and *ordinarius* in 1847. He became secretary to the Berlin Academy of Science but devoted most of his time to microscopy. His most famous publication was the mammoth *Die Infusionsthierchen als volkommene Organismen* (Leipzig, 1838), but although this work on the morphological characteristics and classification of bacteria is important, his idea that each was a "complete organism" with all the organs and systems of higher animals led him into scientific obscurity (see Hanstein, 1877; Hofmeier, 1963).

Ehrenberg's remarkable paper on the microscopic structure of the nerve cell and fibre appeared in 1833, "Nothwendigkeit einer feineren mechanischen Zerlegung des Gehirns und der Nerven vor der chemischen, dargestellt aus Beobachtungen von C. G. Ehrenberg" ([Poggendorffs] *Annln. Phys.*, 1833, 28:449–473). It should be noted that he examined several parts of the nervous system and that he was working with unstained material, probably mounted only in water.

The selections given below in translation deal with the cerebral white matter, peripheral nerves, and ganglion cells; a further portion of the paper, in which the microscopic appearances of the cerebral cortex were described, appears on pages 421 to 422. Although the cerebral and peripheral fibres had each been described independently previously and their connections usually assumed, Ehrenberg demonstrated that this was so. The fibres of the brain, which could be compared with a capillary vascular system, were asserted to be continuous with those of the spinal cord that they formed. These are what he called "varicose or articulated tubes," and he declared them to be in direct connection with the "cylindrical fibres" of the peripheral nerves. It is difficult to avoid the conclusion that they were the nonmyelinated and myelinated fibres respectively, although Ehrenberg's account is not always easy to follow. He also described the myelin that he could express from the myelinated fibres like toothpaste from a tube.

To amplify and elucidate the text, figure 11 of Plate VI has been reproduced (fig. 4). It represents a part of the frog's femoral nerve at the origin of one of its roots from the spinal cord and shows how the varicose fibres on the left at *a'*, change into the cylindrical fibres at *x*; the myelin content of the latter is shown extruded at ρ. Remak was to show later (p. 48) that this strict differentiation into a central and a peripheral fibre was not constant because, as we now know, myelinated fibres may be found in the brain or cord. The varicosity exclusive to central nerve fibres was also described by Remak (p. 48 and fig. 7, *c*) and was probably owing to the passage of water into the nerve fibre; Hannover was able to prevent this with his fixation technique (p. 833). It perhaps corresponds to the *unduloids* of Young (1945, especially pp. 88–90) which also appear only in central tissues; Young gives a modern physicochemical explanation for this phenomenon.

Ehrenberg also described the nerve cell of the cerebral cortex (pp. 421–422) and of the ganglion cell for the first time. There is no doubt that he was observing the cell and not an artifact of preparation or of his microscope. He can thus be considered one of the first to examine an animal cell in anything approaching an intact state other than the red blood cell. His interpretation, however, often did not match his powers of observation.

EXCERPT PP. 451–452

. . . . In the vicinity of the white matter, the fibre content of the cortical substance becomes increasingly evident, and, in the same proportion, the blood vessels become rarer. The white or medullary substance exhibits much more prominent brain fibres as continuations of the finer cortical ones. They began especially at certain crests, that is, linear or bandlike places of origin on the surface of the brain, located in the longitudinal direction of the lateral cerebral convolutions which run towards the base [of the brain]. These are not simple, cylindrical fibres; rather they resemble strings of pearls, of which the pearls do not touch each other but are separated by a thread (narrow interspace), or they resemble [nodular] vesicular tubes [fig. 4]. They are always straight, mostly parallel, and sometimes crossing; only very rarely did I see individual fibres split in two, for otherwise they never anastomose. In the vicinity of the base of the brain one always finds individual fibres, much thicker than the rest, between these nodular fasciculi. These have the distinct appearance of an outer and an inner boundary of the wall, which makes it perfectly obvious that they are hollow inside. Therefore one cannot designate these nodular, linear elements of the brain as either fibres or filaments, but they are *alternatingly swollen* (that is, *varicose* or *articulated* [*gegliederte* used in the sense of a joining together of sections as, for example, a string of beads]) *tubes* or *channels* [fig. 4].

EXCERPT PP. 453–456

THE [PERIPHERAL] NERVES

The optic, auditory, and olfactory nerves, that is, the three most vital sensory nerves, as had already been accurately deduced in part from other phenomena, are also, according to microscopic findings, direct extensions of the unchanged, varicose, tubular medullary substance; all the remaining nerves, with the exception of the sympathetic in the middle of its course, are essentially distinguishable from the brain substance; they contain the latter which has an altered form and a different function.

All nerves, except for the three named above and the sympathetic, consist of cylindrical fibres which run parallel to one another and never anastomose; they are approximately $\frac{1}{120}$ of a line * thick and are collected in bundles which in turn form larger bundles called nerve fasciculi. Each individual fasciculus and the entire tracts are surrounded by a very sinewy sheath, rich in vessels (pia mater, neurilemma [perineurium]). Frequently different nerve bundles unite by false anastomosis, in that the tubes [fibres] issuing from a fasciculus continue into one another without the individual tubes fusing; these are the plexuses which the nerve roots resemble mostly, one of which partially forms the retina. I shall discuss the ganglia separately. In the divided roots of most nerves, where they emerge from the surface of the brain or spinal cord, I have recognized almost equally stout varicose (articulated) fibres between the cylindrical tubes [fig. 4] . . . . In the sympathetic I clearly saw articulated tubes, everywhere mixed with stouter cylindrical ones.

The cylindrical, simple nerve fibres, however, demonstrate an essential difference from the articulated brain fibres, for they have a much larger internal cavity, and enclosed in it there is a very noticeable, less transparent content which has been recognized for a long time. This content of the simple nerve fibres appears also in fresh nerves as a medullary, almost coalescent substance consisting of small, rounded, regular particles; at times the mass appears reticular or striated, and when divided up, can, upon light pressure, be expelled from the fibres [fig. 4, ρ]. In the cross section of each nerve it is pushed out of the individual fibres by the contraction of the fibrous sheath and forms the resultant thickening at the end of the nerve. Its color is white . . . .

Now I followed very carefully each cylindrical fibre of the motor nerves as far as the brain substance and convinced myself that they are direct extensions of the varicose (articulated) brain fibres. When leaving the brain or the spinal cord they slowly lose their varicose shape, because the connecting parts between the spherical or oval pieces become thicker and the whole ultimately becomes an increasingly uniform cylinder. I found it difficult to be convinced of this, but I finally discovered ready proof of it. In the [proximal] roots of the nerves, outside the brain substance, individual,

---

* Before the universal acceptance of the metric system the *line* was employed as a unit of measure, especially when describing microscopic appearances. In most instances the French *ligne* was referred to and this seems to have been an eleventh or a twelfth part of an inch and equivalent to the English barley corn. The following quotation is from the translator's preface to Kölliker (1853, I, viii): ". . . the Paris line, equal to about $\frac{1}{11}$ (0.0888138) of an English inch (and now very generally adopted on the continent), is taken as the unit . . . the signs ‴ for 'of a line,' and ″ for 'of an inch.'" The Paris line is therefore equivalent to about 2.00 mm.

articulated filaments very similar to the brain fibres are found in the process of transition into the cylindrical state. Evidence of this formation was important because it shows that the clear nerve medulla [myelin sheath] contained in the nerve fibres appears only after the nerve fibres have left the cerebral or spinal medulla; however, so long as the same fibre containing medulla remains part of the brain and is articulated (varicose), it exhibits a perfectly transparent, clear interior when free of medulla. Consequently the gelatinous, milky, granular content of the nerve fibres is not the cerebral substance enveloped by a neurilemmal fibre (as Treviranus asserts in his report which, by the way, is excellent as are all his works), but is a peculiar nerve medulla, which is either completely absent in the cerebrum, of which the finer fibres are water-clear, or is present in it in the form of a much more transparent, quite different matter, as a vapor or a sticky, non-discharging, homogeneous juice. According to this the cerebrum can obviously be compared to a *capillary vascular system for the nerve fibres.*

EXCERPT PP. 458–459

GANGLIA

The nerve nodules or ganglia differ in their structure. Almost all of them have this in common, that they consist of agglomerations of articulated cerebral fibres which either alone form the ganglion, as in the optic chiasma, or, as in all sympathetic ganglia which I have examined, are mixed with stouter, cylindrical nerve fibres. The latter are enclosed in a delicate, dense, vascular net, and in its larger meshes those large granules which cover the retina and belong to the cerebral nerve endings again appear. However, in the ganglion of the spinal nerves in birds, I saw only nerve fibres and very large, almost spherical (approximately $\frac{1}{48}$ of a line thick [see p. 41]), irregular bodies [cells] which produce the actual swelling [of the ganglion] and give more the appearance of a glandular substance . . . . When following their course, I could see very distinctly the articulated cerebral fibres of the ganglionic nerves gradually becoming thicker and almost equal in size to the nerve fibres; however, as far as I followed them, they always demonstrated a peculiar structure, a more or less prominent arrangement, and they never attained the diameter of the other cylindrical nerve fibres. An understanding of their structure favors the idea that the ganglia are comparable to small brains. However, the universally accepted theory that they are comparable to the cortical substance of the cerebrum must be corrected since, although their color is similar, the cortical substance consists of a mixture of vessels and very delicate, articulating (varicose) fibres that can scarcely be differentiated [apparently finely granular medullary substance]; genuine cortical substance has an overwhelming number of stout, articulating fibres and is therefore genuine medullary substance. This cerebral substance is deposited around cylindrical nerve fibres which do not change but are reinforced by mixing with articulating fibres in their bundles.

GABRIEL GUSTAV VALENTIN

(8 July 1810—24 May 1883)

Knowledge of the microscopic characteristics of nervous tissue was now growing rapidly, and Ehrenberg's primitive observations on nerve cells were supplemented three years later by a more detailed study carried out by Valentin.

Valentin, a German who was described by Julius Pagel (1895) as "one of the most eminent physiologists of the nineteenth century," was born in Breslau and studied medicine there from 1828 to 1832. Among his teachers and friends was the famous Czech biologist Purkyně (p. 53). In 1836 Valentin went to Berne as professor of physiology and zootomy and remained there for more than forty-five years. His researches were in the fields of embryology, histology, physiology, biochemistry, parasitology, and teratology (see Kisch, 1954, pp. 139–317; Hintzsche, 1953, 1963; Freund and Berg, 1963–1964, II, 413–422).

In 1836 Valentin published a classic paper, "Über den Verlauf und die letzten Ende der Nerven" (*Nova Acta phys.-med. Acad. caes. Leopold.-Carol. Nat. Curiosorum, Breslau*, 18 [i]:51–240), described by the great Swiss histologist Koelliker, who was himself no mean contributor to our knowledge of neurohistology (pp. 61–62), as "the epoch-making and first good description of the nervous system elements." It dealt with the microscopic morphology of several parts of the nervous system in both vertebrates and invertebrates, but a very important contribution was the account of the nerve cell. Valentin identified its parenchyma, a term he introduced into cytology, as well as the nucleus and nucleolus, and his illustration (fig. 5) is the first of its kind in biological literature. It is important to realize when reading this report that the cell theory of Schwann (pp. 56–57) was not to be enunciated until three years later, in 1839, thus showing that considerable knowledge of the nerve cell, at least, had already been acquired.

The passages from Valentin's paper of 1836 presented below contain an account of the ganglion "globules," and those of the cerebellum and cerebrum (for the description of the cortical cell, see pp. 422–423). Finally, a section contains his perceptive comments on the two ultimate elements of the nervous system, the nerve cell (*Kugel*) and the nerve fibre (*Primitivfaser*), with a comparison of the central and peripheral nervous systems; this is his most outstanding contribution to neurohistology. He did not believe, however, that the cell and fibre were connected but thought them to be merely juxtaposed. Thus Valentin was led into a bitter controversy with Remak (pp. 46–52) which retarded the advance of knowledge in this field.

EXCERPT PP. 138–139

The globules proper [*Kugeln* = nerve cells] demonstrate the most marked differences as well as generally the most interesting peculiarities. Their chief or parenchymatous substance (*Parenchymmasse*) is mostly a gray-reddish, finely granular material which is saturated with fluid and held together by a clear, transparent, slightly viscous mass (*Blastem*) which not infrequently contains filaments. In the fish this parenchyma is extremely transparent and clear as water, and it contains small, dispersed, separate, round particles. In this way there is a direct transition into a form which we shall see again below as a common feature in invertebrate animals.

Concerning the structure of this parenchymatous substance, each globule, either inside the intact ganglion or still enclosed or surrounded by its primary fibres, has a circular border throughout. This is not so, however, as soon as it [the globule] is isolated and freed from its environment. Not infrequently it then has an oblong shape. Often one end is slightly pointed, often even elongated into a small, tail-like appendix. In particular, the latter configuration could well lead us to assume that this elongation continues as an individual, organic nerve fibre. Apart merely from the great differences between the content of the primary fibres and the parenchyma of the globules, the fact alone that one occasionally finds such a tailed globule completely enclosed by its sheath of cellular tissue must bring to naught this assumption which hitherto was based only upon the doctrine of neurophysics (*Nervenphysik*).

More or less in the center of the parenchyma of such a globule one notes a round, clear nucleus, and in its center a circular corpuscle [nucleolus (fig. 5)]. If, however, one looks at these [two] objects with aplanatic glasses or with lenses of short focal distance, it becomes apparent that they do not by any means lie in the same plane. The large nucleus is sunk into the depth of the parenchyma whereas the small corpuscle which seems to be inside it, is completely on the surface. This evidence is even better confirmed as soon as one succeeds in turning the globule, which is always somewhat flat, in such manner that the corpuscle [nucleolus] lies on one side. Whatever the nature of the parenchyma may be, both *nuclei* [i.e., nucleus and nucleolus] are always clear and transparent, and when subjected to continuous crushing they are easily destroyed. The large one [nucleus] consists of an enveloping membrane and an enclosed, clear liquid. The smaller one [nucleolus] appears to be solid throughout.

EXCERPT PP. 152–153

Wherever the grayish-red [gray matter] and the white matter are in direct contact, all parts of the globules, as has already been pointed out, can be better distinguished. Provided that a moderate section, neither too thin nor too thick, has been made from the yellow substance at the junction of the cortical and medullary substances of the cerebellar hemispheres, individual globules in the fluid, and at times also in the margin, rounded at one side but furnished with a tail-like ending on the other, can be observed (Pl. VII, fig. 54 [fig. 5]). This observation was first made by Purkyně in sheep, and I succeeded later in finding the same structure in man, the calf, the sheep, the pig, and the horse, at this site as well as in the yellow substance of the cerebral hemispheres. One recognizes at a glance the identical shape which we have described above in the ganglia. Under exactly the same conditions we find an inner, clearer nucleus and a small nucleus [nucleolus] at the external surface of the nucleus. I should merely repeat literally [what I have already said] if I were going to describe the parenchymatous mass as well as the nuclei, since what I stated in the case of the ganglia fully applies here, too.

EXCERPT PP. 157–158

From this description of the finer structure of the nervous systems in man and vertebrates, the following may be stated when we take the entire picture into consideration. This picture has an admirable simplicity such as the human mind could hardly understand until now. Two principal propositions are paramount for the complete comparison:

1. The entire nervous system is made up of two elementary basic substances, namely the isolated globules of the covering substance [cortex] and the isolated, continuous primitive fibres. The former probably represent the creative, active, higher principle, the latter the receptive, passive, lower principle. Each is surrounded by a sheath of connective tissue, the strength of which is defined precisely for each small part. It [the sheath] effects the degree of influence of each heterogeneous part upon the other. These are the genuine and distinctive structures of the nervous system . . . .

2. The central and peripheral nervous systems in their smallest details are extraordinarily similar to each other, a similarity hitherto unknown for other opposing portions of a system of the body. Apart from the fact that in theory it is possible that centralization is manifested in the central nervous system, whereas possibly dissemination is manifested in the peripheral system, they differ from each other only in the thickness of the sheaths of their two components, that is, of the primary fibres and the globules. If one now imagines the complete system of primary fibres, central as well as peripheral, as an aggregate of many elipses because of their absolutely continuous course from one end to the other, and because of their retroverted loops (*Endumbiegungsschlingen*) at each end, one half of the curve

is found in the central nervous system whereas the other half is in the peripheral system.

Robert Remak
(30 July 1815—29 August 1865)

It seems likely that both Leeuwenhoek and Fontana had seen the myelinated fibre but without recognizing its significance. Treviranus of Bremen (Gottfried Reinhold Treviranus. *Vermischte Schriften. Anatomischen und physiologischen Inhalts*, Bd. I [Göttingen, 1816], II. Vermischts Abhandlungen. "4. Ueber die organischen Elemente des Thierischen Körps," pp. 117–144, especially p. 128), who used the terms "nerve medulla" (*Nervenmark*) and "nerve tube" (*Nervenröhr*), likewise had seen it and produced the first clear illustration of it; others, such as Ehrenberg and Valentin, had also recorded their observations. It was, however, Remak who gave the first accurate and detailed account of the myelinated and non-myelinated nerve fibre.

Remak was born in Posnan, Poland, of a Jewish family and studied medicine at the University of Berlin, where he remained for the rest of his life. There he was one of the first pupils of, and was greatly influenced by, Johannes Müller, the great German physiologist (p. 203). He was graduated in 1838, and after a variety of appointments eventually became professor *extraordinarius* in the University of Berlin in 1859 but was never promoted to a higher position. His work was in the histology and embryology of the nervous system, including important studies on the intrinsic cardiac ganglia, galvanotherapy, and clinical neurology. Remak met with opposition and adversity throughout his life, probably because of his Jewish origin, and of his personality. As a result, his brilliant work is even today less well appreciated than it should be (see Kisch, 1954, pp. 227–296; Haymaker, 1953, pp. 80–83). Like other young physicians in the 1830's, such as Purkyně, Müller, Valentin, Schwann, and Henle, Remak soon realized the importance of the microscope in the study of anatomy. He was allowed to use Müller's instrument and also that of Ehrenberg, who was another of his teachers. The results of his studies were of great significance to neurohistology, his three most important contributions being:

1) Identification and description of the central core of the myelinated fibre, the axon, which he called "the primitive band"—soon to be known as "the band of Remak"—and the whole fibre, "the primitive tube";

2) Discovery of the non-myelinated, sympathetic fibre which he called "the organic fibre" or "primitive fibre," which became known as "the fibre of Remak," a term still used today;

3) Suggestion that the nerve cell and nerve fibre were in direct communication with one another.

In his first paper, written as a prize essay—for which he was awarded second prize—Remak described the various fibres he could identify in the embryonic tissues of the rabbit ("Verläufige Mittheilung microscopischer Beobachtungen über den innern Bau der Cerebrospinalnerven und über die Entwickelung ihrer Formelemente," *Arch. Anat. Physiol.*, 1836, pp. 145–161). In the portion from it translated below he described briefly the myelinated fibre with its central "band of Remak," or axon, and gave passing mention to the non-myelinated fibre or "fibre of Remak." He also identified the varicose and cylindrical fibres, previously reported by Ehrenberg, and these are seen in the figure which accompanied the article; however, their description has not been included in the selection below. In his illustration Remak depicted the constriction of a fibre (fig. 7, *b*), and this may have been a node of Ranvier (see p. 79) or a Schmidt-Lantermann incisure, the significance of which is still unknown.

EXCERPT PP. 148–149

During the fourth and fifth weeks the following conditions were seen in the rabbit:

The cerebrospinal nerves contain:

(1) Stout cylindrical fibres (medullary fibres, 0.0025–0.0060 Engl. line in diameter [see p. 41]), which occasionally are clear and transparent but for the most part are filled with a medulla which is not very transparent [fig. 7, *f*]. They appear to be outlined now by straight, now by irregularly sinuous, markedly notched margins, on the inside of which a parallel, finer line can be distinguished. The narrow space between the thicker and the finer boundary lines often appears opaque, especially in those areas that do not contain any medulla. Upon squeezing it, I have seen the medulla flow out, and I have thus observed the phenomenon as Ehrenberg demonstrated it [see fig. 4]. However, in fibres torn off [and viewed] transversely I have also frequently seen the lumen of the outer wall as a double circle [myelin sheath], as Valentin noted in the varicose variety; but these cases were always of the kind in which there was no sure guarantee against deception.

(2) Finer cylindrical fibres of 0.0008 to approximately 0.0025 Engl. line [see p. 41] that are always without medulla (*marklos*) and transparent. They are provided with straight, rarely slightly sinuous, margins which are never notched, and in the inner partition of which no double border can be distinguished [fig. 7, *e*].

(3) Fibres varicose throughout.

This publication of 1836 was a preliminary communication, for in the following year Remak reported the characteristics of the myelinated and the non-myelinated fibres in greater detail ("Weitere microscopische Beobachtungen über die Primitivfasern des Nervensystem der Wirbelthiere," [Froriep's] *Neue Notizen*, 1837, 3:cols. 35–40).

However, Remak's most famous publication on this subject was his graduation dissertation of 1838, *Observationes anatomicae et microscopicae de systematis nervosi structura* (Berlin, 1838). In it he discussed the myelinated fibre, or "primitive tube," and in so doing corrected some of Ehrenberg's errors. He also cast doubt on the claim that Fontana had first described the myelinated fibre, and six years later he was to refute it (p. 49). Figure 8 (Tab. I, 6) shows the myelinated and non-myelinated nerve fibres. The following excerpt has been translated from the first section, "On the parts of the peripheral nervous system," Chapter I, "On the tubules and primitive fibres of the cerebrospinal nerves."

EXCERPT PP. 1–4

1. It is not our purpose in any way to review those various and often contrary things that have been said in recent years about the primitive nerve fibres. It suffices to call to mind that the tubular structure of the fibres was distinctly described by the eminent Ehrenberg [pp. 41–42], but what is contained in them was so explained by everyone that to an observer many things yet remain in doubt about the structure of the tubules. In that particular matter, moreover, all recent investigators have erred, because they believe that the rough condition of the fibres is produced by something irregular contained within.

2. After I had accepted this error for many years, my later investigation taught me very clearly that the content of the primitive tubules, both in the nerves and in the central parts [of the nervous system], was by no means either an oily or globular or generally amorphous mass, but solid *fibre* [see p. 49], flat, very pellucid, with straight, parallel margins, an even surface only slightly rough, and of remarkably strong texture so that it is torn with much more difficulty than the sheath. The latter, however, is now thinner, now thicker, and closely surrounds the fibre; in the nerves of freshly killed animals it displays a pellucid membrane [neurilemma], wholly smooth without any roughness or irregularity, but, according to various physicians, after some time it finally contracts, now more easily now with more difficulty, according to the different ages of the animals, so that, especially in the tubules of the nerves, it produces that rough condition and appearance of some conglomerate substance placed within; also it sometimes seems to produce in the tubules of the central parts of the nerves that varicose form which, after the eminent Ehrenberg detected it [see pp. 40–42] and believed it to be peculiar to certain parts of the nervous system, I found in all the nerves of animals of whatever age, so that according to those conditions

by which the supply and thickness of varicose tubules in various nerves is harmful, certain distinctions may be drawn between the motor and sensory nerves.

3. Now even if very recently the force of water pressure was considered especially to produce the varicose forms, nevertheless wherever I observed them under such contrary conditions, although I hold them as a modification of the contractions of the sheath, yet I believe that there is some not yet recognized internal cause; under wholly equal conditions regular contractures of the sheath affect some tubules, irregular ones others. Finally, what may be the shape of the various tubules [sheath + contents = *tubule*; contents only = *fibre*] in the live animals, whether or not it undergoes some change in the animal, remains for investigation.

4. It will scarcely be doubted that the structure of the nerve tubules that I have now represented was first learned by me very recently [1836]. When reading Fontana's observations on the nerves a few days ago, I was greatly astonished to discover that almost sixty years ago that investigator had seen the primitive fibre which I described, but he described it so vaguely that it could not be intelligible to anyone before the true structure of the tubules was finally uncovered and clearly described. Nevertheless he did not recognize correctly either our primitive nerve fibre [axon] or the structure of the sheath [neurilemma], for the latter is tubular and filled with a gelatinous humor which he considered to be composed of certain twisted cylinders. In the first place, according to our observations, the primitive fibre [axon] is by no means hollow, but wholly solid and flat; therefore those twisted cylinders can have been nothing except the turnings and folds of the sheath produced by its irregular contraction; in very fresh nerves they are completely lacking.

This account of the myelinated fibre or "primitive tube" may be supplemented by a passage from a later paper, "Neurologische Erläuterungen" (*Arch. Anat. Physiol.*, 1844, pp. 463–472). It is of special importance because we find here the first reference to the "granular fibres" or neurofibrils, in this instance in the cell and axon of the freshwater crab. As is frequently the case with early accounts of morphology, the illustration (fig. 9) is easier to comprehend than the textual description.

EXCERPT PP. 468–469

Fig. 8, magnified × 250, illustrates a primitive tube [or cylinder] from the umbilical cord of the river crab with the fasciculus (*m*) in its natural position. At the point of exit (*n*) disintegration of the fibres is indicated by a punctiform area. Although I may have expressed doubts concerning the identity of this bundle with the axis cylinder (the primitive cord, the pale central fibres) of vertebrates, it seems to me that an observation which I made repeatedly and which I have represented schematically in Fig. 9 speaks for the identity. Where, for instance, a finer *tube* (*p*), in which one can distinguish only a punctate and non-fibre content, runs to a ganglion cell, one sometimes recognizes in this cell (*r*) very delicate granular fibres which circulate around the nucleus to form the substance of the cell. They collect at the site of transition from cell to tube to form a continuation of the latter's punctate content. This makes the assumption more probable that finer lumens, too, have a fibrous content which, owing to their greater fragility, disintegrate more easily into a granular substance. If, by the way, Henle and Koelliker emphasize the lack of similarity of the central bundle with the axis cylinder of the higher animals, I feel compelled to recall the striated condition of the axis cylinder which I described (*Anat. Observ.*, p. 2 [p. 48]).

The following passages, also taken from the *Observationes* of 1838, amplify Remak's preliminary account of the non-myelinated or "organic fibre" or "primitive fibre," as he called it ("the fibre of Remak"). It is described in the first paragraph (see fig. 8, 6, *a*), and in the second there is a discussion of the sympathetic nerves and ganglia where the organic fibres are found. He refers to the neurofibrils, and probably to the cells of Schwann, as well as to the connection of cell and nerve (see p. 56), and he notes that sympathetic nerves are gray because of the non-myelinated fibres they contain.

EXCERPT P. 5

6. . . . . . They are not tubular, that is, surrounded by a sheath, but naked, being transparent, almost gelatinous, and much finer than most of the primitive tubes [myelinated fibres]. Almost invariably they have longitudinal lines upon their surface and they readily divide into very small fibres [neurofibrils]. In their course they are frequently provided with oval nodules, and they are covered with certain small, oval or rounded, but more rarely irregular, corpuscles [cells of Schwann] with one or more nuclei which are about the same size as the nuclei of the ganglion globules [nerve cells].

EXCERPT PP. 10–11

15. Now since the same organic [non-myelinated] fibres constitute the larger part of the sympathetic nerves and originate from the nucleated globules, which together make up the ganglia, the *sympathetic ganglia must be considered as the true centers of the organic* [autonomic] *nervous*

system. The only difference between the sympathetic and the spinal ganglia is in the supply of fibres which arise from them; otherwise there is no difference in the number of nuclei, and the *spinal ganglia seem to relate to the organic nervous system,* although the reason why the origins of the organic fibres are joined to the posterior roots rather than to the anterior remains as yet unexplained. First it must be noted that very important organic processes exist in the skin to which the posterior roots are especially directed. Long ago, moreover, I frequently observed in the rabbit that when those cutaneous nerves pierced the muscles they appeared on each side of the vertebral column and, corresponding very closely in number and site to the spinal ganglia and displaying a certain analogy with the first branch of the trigeminal nerve, they extended from those ganglia. For this reason I suspect that the spinal ganglia were specially constructed to receive the necessary organic fibres from the sympathetic ganglia by way of the posterior and largely sensory spinal nerve roots. In addition, numerous organic fibres are observed in the spinal nerves (also in the trigeminal nerve) after they have formed ganglia and before they have received anything from the sympathetic nerve, but only a few occur in the roots; and the communicating branch, according to the distinguished *Müller* and my own observations, often displays a distinctly gray color [gray ramus], which, as I have learned with the aid of the microscope, is produced by the great number of organic [non-myelinated] fibres in it.

As well as describing different kinds of nerve fibres, Remak also reported the morphological features of the nerve cell. His account of cerebral cortical cells is on pages 428 to 430, and in the *Observationes* of 1838 he described a variety of cells (fig. 8, at 7, 11, 17, 31). However, his greatest and most original contribution to the anatomy of the nervous system was his suggestion that the nerve fibre and nerve cell, which had been described separately by a number of observers, were in fact joined together. Hitherto no one had considered this, and Valentin (pp. 43–46) had even denied the possibility. Nevertheless, more than one investigator claimed the discovery for himself; Kisch (1954, pp. 245–250) has discussed in detail the development of the idea of the cell fibre connection and has established beyond doubt Remak's priority. In the following passage from the *Observationes* of 1838, Remak discusses the relationship between the "organic" fibres and cells in the sympathetic ganglion. It is taken from the second section, "The central parts of the nervous system," Chapter I, "The sympathetic and spinal ganglia, or the centers of the organic nervous system."

EXCERPT PP. 8–10

11. The distinguished *Purkyně* and the celebrated *Valentin* were the first to bring a little light to our understanding of the structure of the

ganglia. The former [pp. 53–56] observed that the primitive tubules [nerve fibres] so traverse the ganglia that, partly forming a plexus, they continue their passage directly (continuous fibres), partly, and especially in the exterior part of the ganglion, they encompass the nucleated globules [nerve cells] on all sides (woven fibres); in addition, the ganglionic globules [nerve cells], often covered with pigment and containing the nucleus, and in its circumference the nucleolus, are, according to the latter [Valentin, pp. 41–46], surrounded by a kind of connective sheath and are *contiguous only* with the nerve [fibre] elements.

12. I am able to confirm only the smaller and less significant part of these observations. First, according to my observations, partly confirmed by Valentin's illustrations, there is no significant difference between those *traversing* and *encompassing* tubules [continuous and woven fibres mentioned above] except that the tubules, especially in the middle of the ganglia, form bundles. These, a little distant from one another, have small globules placed between them, and they pass directly through the ganglion; but in the exterior part the individual tubules, following a somewhat twisted course, hold several globules in wider spaces. That traverse of the tubules seems to be explained by the fact that in the particles of ganglia torn and spread out with a needle, convoluted loops of tubules in the form of intestines are often found in individual globules, as I have described elsewhere.

13. But that investigator [Valentin] did not understand, nor could he understand a thing undoubtedly of very great importance for the comprehension of the nature of the ganglia. *The organic* [non-myelinated] *fibres originate from the very substance of the nucleated globules* [nerve cells], and this observation, although it is very difficult and requires great skill in preparation and observation, is nevertheless so clear that it cannot be doubted.

Now from the very substance of those globules arise either bundles, varying in thickness but sometimes equal to the primitive tubules, exceedingly clear, much like the *primitive fibres* [non-myelinated fibre of Remak], but with this difference that they appear to be composed distinctly of very thin, non-tubular threads, into which they readily divide, and that then in their passage the organic fibres, into which they pass, display similar nodules and similar nucleated corpuscles [fig. 8]; or very thin fibres are extended from several parts of the globule, usually nodulated in the place of origin and passing distinctly into the organic fibres of the nerve itself.

14. . . . . . Finally, I could not find any special connective sheath of the globules, and it seems likely to me that the celebrated *Valentin* mistook for that sheath some nervous part, especially the organic fibres by which the globules are covered, altered by too much pressure.

Jan Evangelista Purkyně
(17 December 1787—28 July 1869)

In the last two decades the electron microscope has revealed a wealth of morphological detail, and this was also the case after the introduction of the achromatic
light microscope, for observers were presented with a complexity of histological
appearances. One of the most outstanding exponents of the new technique was the
Czech biologist Purkyně, whose name is still associated with one of his many
discoveries, the Purkyně cell of the cerebellum.

He was born in Libochovice in Bohemia and studied philosophy and medicine in
Prague from 1813 to 1818. Five years later he was appointed to the chair of
physiology and pathology in the Prussian University of Breslau (now Wroclaw)
where he remained for twenty-seven years. When the opportunity arose in 1850, he
returned to Prague as professor of physiology and spent the rest of his life in this
post. His studies were mainly in the fields of physiology, histology, and embryology;
these included his study of the cardiac nerves that were named after him. In
addition, he was an outstanding Czech patriot and a close friend of Goethe (see
Studnička, 1936; Purkyně Society, 1937, especially pp. 15–18, 66–75; Haymaker,
1953, pp. 70–74; John, 1959; Kruta, 1962, 1964; Freund and Berg, 1963–1964, II,
299–309).

Purkyně acquired an achromatic compound microscope in 1832 and at once
began to study a variety of materials. One of them was nervous tissue, and although
he described the myelinated and non-myelinated fibres three months after Remak,
his account nevertheless deserves to be recorded here. Moreover, he was the first to
describe accurately nerve cells other than those of the cerebral cortex and of
ganglia, spinal and sympathetic; he had been stimulated to do so after reading
Ehrenberg's account of his "globules" or nerve cells (pp. 40–43); Purkyně's best
known description is that of the cerebellar "cell of Purkyně."

The two passages presented below in translation are from the report of a paper
he read at a meeting of German scientists and physicians in Prague on 23 September 1837 (*Bericht über die Versammlung deutscher Naturforscher und Ärzte in
Prag im September,* 1837 [Prague, 1838], pt. 3, sec. 5, A. Anatomisch-physiologische
Verhandlungen, pp. 177–180), and deal with the fibres and then with the cerebellar cell. His comments in the final paragraph on the role of the cell are especially
pertinent, for they indicate that Purkyně played a larger part in the formation of
the cell theory than he is usually credited with. Like others in the early nineteenth
century, he was overshadowed by Schwann (Studnička, 1927–1928). Of equal
importance was Purkyně's suggestion that the cell may be connected with the fibre.

EXCERPT PP. 177–178

. . . . With the help of very thin, transparent, transverse sections of the
nerve bundles of a fresh nerve he [Purkyně] succeeded in visualizing the

lumens of the elementary nerve fibres. A double, circular line was noted at
the outer periphery which corresponded to the enveloping membrane of
the nerve cylinder, which, like a vessel, contains the nerve medulla
[myelin]; towards the center there was a thicker circle, the heart of the
medullary nerve, and in the center a completely transparent spot, for the
most part polyangular, which could be considered to be the inner canal of
the medullary nerve [axon]. However, as successful sections like these are
entirely dependent upon a rare and fortunate chance, he used hardened
nerves for his investigations with which the finest and most transparent
tranverse sections can always be produced with great certainty. Here, too,
the lumen of every nerve fibre exhibited exactly the same feature (Fig. 9
[fig. 11]) . . . .

If a thin, longitudinal section of the fixed nerve was examined, a thin,
more transparent strip right in the middle of the medullary nerve was
observed. Something similar [myelin] was noted in the cylindrical medullary fibres which, when squeezed, protruded from the tubes of the elementary fibres (Fig. 10). Again, Purkyně doubted the *constancy* of these differences in the medullary nerve; he therefore examined fresh nerves, after
Burdach's method, in lukewarm water, and he saw that the inner substance
of the elementary nerve filament [axon] was very limpid and without a
trace of an inner canaliculus. Nevertheless, these observations pointed to an
organic structure inside the medulla of the elementary nerve cylinders; it
can hardly be presumed that these morphological features were due to the
process of fixation. Furthermore, Purkyně discussed the continuation of the
sympathetic nerve [unmyelinated fibres] onto the cerebral arteries. These
nerves had been seen already by Lancisi, Wrisberg, Soemmerring, and
others. In part one can follow them from the intervertebral arteries, in part
from the ophthalmic artery to the large arteries at the base of the brain,
and, with the help of magnification, to the second branching of the arteries
of the Sylvian fossa and the corpus callosum. In this investigation, however,
one must be extremely careful not to confuse these delicate nerve plexuses
with the fibres of the arachnoid which everywhere proceed from the inside
towards the pia mater and which profusely envelop the larger arteries in
particular. Considering the minuteness and fragility of these nerve fibres, it
is not a little difficult to be certain of their nerve character by means of the
microscope. The elementary cylinders which are almost naked, lie on the
surface, and lack the firm neurilemma [perineurium] which surrounds the
bundles of other nerves. Fig. 11 is a slightly enlarged illustration of such a
nerve plexus which enmeshes the pontine arteries; Fig. 12, a portion of a
small branch of this plexus with its elementary cylinders and its own blood
vessels.

EXCERPT PP. 179–180

a) The essential characteristics of a ganglion corpuscle (*Körperchen*) in the nerve ganglion as well as in the brain are: a granular, partly spherical, partly round-edged shape, with or without processes. The substance is hardish, transparent, and consists of a free mass of circumscribed substance (*Punktmasse*) which is probably neural. It resists pressure and chemical *reagents* longer than other nerve substance. The ganglion granule is, in comparison with other microscopic structures, large, $\frac{8-30}{800}$ of a Vienna line [see p. 41]. Inside, it contains a round, somewhat transparent nucleus, enclosed by a large, spherical covering, the size of which corresponds to the dimensions of the whole ganglion granule; these granules [nerve cells] have their own connective tissue or even fibrous coverings in the nerve ganglions, from which they will emerge only upon extreme pressure; such coverings cannot be seen on the ganglionic corpuscles of the brain. Pigmented spots of various shades of brown and of different distribution are seen in many ganglion granules in the brain and in the nervous system; for the most part they leave a free, clear area laterally or in their center, through which shines the central nucleus; as elsewhere, the pigment itself consists of very fine corpuscles which demonstrate Brownian movement.

b) Nothing definite could be ascertained about the connection between the ganglionic corpuscles and the elementary nerve and brain fibres.

c) Now, the topography of the ganglionic corpuscles in the brain and the spinal cord is as follows: they are most noticeable in the substantia nigra of the cerebral peduncles, in the rust-colored substance [? red nucleus], and in the anterior angle of the fourth ventricle. There they have many processes which exhibit the most extravagant shapes (see Fig. 16); their pigment is dark brown and in some individuals very dense, but in others, especially the younger, rather sparse. In the fourth ventricle the corpuscles are roundish, they rarely show distinct processes, and their pigment is lighter and reddish-brown. In addition, ganglionic corpuscles can be found in different sites in the substance of the thalamus and the geniculate bodies. Here, they are mostly very soft, roundish, and their pigmentary granules are of a lighter brown and relatively large (Fig. 17). Moreover, small, tetrahedral, ganglionic corpuscles with processes and weakly pigmented areas are seen in a specific gray layer of the spiral lamina of Ammon's horn. In the posterior lobe of the cerebrum, in the vicinity of the yellow substance [junction between gray and white matter] and in the white matter, ganglionic, longitudinal, figlike corpuscles with processes at their thin end are found together. Similar corpuscles surrounding the yellow substance in large numbers, are seen everywhere in rows in the laminae of the cerebellum [Purkyně cells]. Each of these corpuscles faces the inside [of the organ], with the blunt, roundish endings towards the yellow substance, and it displays distinctly in its body the central nucleus together with its corona; the tail-like ending faces the outside and, by means of two processes, mostly disappears into the gray matter which extends close to the outer surface which is surrounded by the pia mater (Fig. 18). The gray-brown substance is similarly constituted and surrounds the olivary body of the medulla oblongata, like a shell (Fig. 19). Finally, the brain nodule, or pons, also has the characteristics of a ganglion, owing to the large number of roundish ganglionic corpuscles covered with gray pigment which are interspersed through the alternating fibre layers of its gray mass.

d) Apart from these ganglionic corpuscles, there are others in the brain which do not contain a central nucleus and which are of an entirely different type. Thus there are large, gray-white granules, consisting of a circumscribed mass of substance (*Punktmasse*) found all over the gray matter of the cerebral convolutions. In addition, there is a special arrangement of clear, transparent, round or roundish, angular corpuscles, similar to starch granules and of a waxlike consistency (Fig. 20) which are frequently found in the lamina cribrosa in front of the optic chiasma and in the stria cornea on both sides of the thalami [corpora amylacae]. Another type of small, very uniform corpuscle constitutes, together with elementary brain fibres, the yellow central substance of the cerebellum [? deep nuclei].

e) With reference to the importance of the ganglionic corpuscles, it could be suggested that they are probably central structures. This fact is likely because of their whole organization in three concentric circles [i.e., periphery of cell, nuclear membrane, and confines of the nucleolus] which may be related to the elementary brain and nerve fibres in the same way as centers of force are related to the conduction pathways of force, or like the ganglia to the nerves of the ganglion, or like the brain substance to the spinal cord and cranial nerves. This means that they would be collectors, generators, and distributors of the neural organ.

THEODOR SCHWANN
(7 December 1810—11 January 1882)

Much has been learned about the nerve fibre since the pioneer work of the 1830's, and recently it has been shown by means of electron microscopy that one of its most important component parts is the covering that invests the myelinated fibre. It plays a vital role in the development of the fibre and also in the processes of myelination, regeneration, and neoplasia. This is the sheath or membrane of Schwann and the nucleus of Schwann (see fig. 13). It seems that today "sheath of Schwann," "membrane of Schwann," and "neurilemma" are synonymous terms and that "cell of Schwann" should be restricted to the Schwann cell nucleus and its immediately surrounding protoplasm (Causey, 1960).

Schwann was born at Neuss, near Düsseldorf, and attended the Universities of Bonn, Würzburg, and Berlin where he studied medicine, natural science, mathematics, and philosophy. He came into contact with Johannes Müller in both Bonn and Berlin and in the latter was Müller's favorite assistant. He received the M.D. degree from the University of Berlin in 1834 and worked there on the physiology of muscle and the problem of fermentation. He also discovered pepsin, and his work on the cell theory of animal life began at this time. In 1839 Schwann left Berlin to take the chair of anatomy at the University of Louvain, and in 1848 accepted the same post at Liège, from which he retired in 1880 (see Münzer, 1939; Florkin, 1960; Watermann, 1960*a*, 1960*b*).

As indicated above (p. 53), much was already known about the animal cell before Schwann enunciated the cell theory in 1839; but although he may in some respects have been anticipated by a number of investigators, nevertheless his contribution to the concept was greater than that of any one of them. The book in which he published his observations and the theory based upon them also contains his account of the nerve fibre structures which bear his name (*Mikroskopische Untersuchungen über die Übereinstimmung in der Struktur und dem Wachsthum der Thiere und Pflanzen* [Berlin, 1839]). The main enunciation of the cell theory is on page 196 and states "that there is one common principle of development for the most diverse elementary parts of the organism, and that this principle is the formation of cells."

Schwann also discussed the varicosity of nerve fibres which had appeared so frequently in the reports of earlier workers (Ehrenberg and Remak in particular) and concluded that they were artifacts owing to the passage of water through the cell membrane (pp. 176–177). As noted above (p. 50), Remak had already seen cells associated with the non-myelinated fibre. The following extract describes the sheath and cell of Schwann.

EXCERPT PP. 174–175

. . . . The conclusion that I have reached concerning these few observations is that the latter view, namely, that the white substance [myelin] is a secondary deposit on the inner surface of the cell membrane, seems to me to be the most probable. The white substance of each nerve is surrounded externally by a structureless and peculiar membrane which appears to be finely granular. This membrane appears as a narrow, clear border which is clearly differentiated from the darker contours of the white substance. It seems that this membrane has hitherto been included with the neurilemma or with the connective tissue which surrounds the nerve fibre. Although in the frog's nerve this membrane is more sharply defined externally, it would

be more difficult to arrive at a conclusion when examining the intact
mammalian nerve fibre if there were no opportunity of seeing the membrane in an isolated state. Plate IV, Fig. 9, *a* [fig. 13] provides such a
preparation which is the vagus nerve from the cranial cavity of a calf. In
one place the continuity of the white substance of the nerve has been
broken during preparation. But where it still exists, the double contours,
and hence the thickness of the white substance, can be distinguished
clearly. But the nerve still exists where the white substance is removed, and
it is sharply defined externally, although with only pale contours. This pale
contour does not change into the outer dark contour of the white substance, but is placed externally as a thin border parallel to both contours of
the white substance. The white substance of the nerve is, therefore, surrounded externally by a thin, pale membrane which is sharply defined
externally. If the membrane is very thin, it cannot be recognized as a pale
border around the nerve fibre; but it is still seen clearly in places where the
white substance is destroyed: see Fig. 9, *b* [fig. 13]. The distinct external
boundary certainly is evidence against this membrane having a connective
tissue structure; it is apparent from the isolated piece of the membrane that
it does not have a fibrous structure; it merely appears to be somewhat finely
granular. If this is correct, the membrane cannot be anything else than the
cell membrane of the nerve fibre or of a secondary deposit on its surface.
The position of the cell nucleus is also evidence for this view. Most of the
cell nuclei which are found in the youngest and as yet pale nerve fibres,
disappear during the formation of the white substance, which is often the
case with most other cells. Some, however, seem to last for a longer time.
Occasionally, although not often, a cell nucleus is seen here and developed;
it lies in the pale boundary which surrounds the white substance externally.
Fig. 9, *c*, *d* [fig. 13] show such a fibre from the vagus nerve of the same calf.
In the fibre *c*, the white substance corresponding to the nucleus even makes
a small indentation in the cavity of the fibre. This cell nucleus seems
actually to belong to the fibre and to be lying on the inner surface of the
cell membrane, while the white substance is so deposited that the nucleus
remains lying external to it. The band discovered by Remak [axon] would
then be the true cell contents.

Continuity between Nerve Cell and Fibre

By 1840 the nerve cell in various parts of the nervous system had been recognized
and described as far as the available primitive techniques would permit. The two

types of nerve fibre, the myelinated and non-myelinated, had also been identified. The next step was to establish the connection between the cell body and the fibre, the existence of which had been suggested vaguely by Purkyně and with certainty by Remak. This took about twenty years, and the individuals selected here for consideration are representative of the large number of investigators who helped to verify Remak's discovery (Kisch, 1954, pp. 245–250).

ADOLPH HANNOVER
(24 November 1814—7 July 1894)

Full confirmation of the pioneer work of Purkyně and Remak came from the studies of a Dane, Adolph Hannover, who worked in the Berlin laboratory of Johannes Müller from 1839 to 1840 and used Müller's microscope.

He was born in Copenhagen where he received his medical license in 1839. After studying with Müller, he practised medicine in Copenhagen, but continued his histological investigations as a Privatdocent. He is usually considered to have been the first outstanding Danish microscopist, and he directed his attention to both normal and abnormal tissues. With regard to the latter, he is remembered for his work on malignancies, and his name is still occasionally associated with the term "epithelioma." His studies also included teratology, parasitology, medical statistics, and hygiene (see Salomonsen, 1915; Johnsson, 1915).

While working in Berlin, Hannover became friendly with Remak who described him (1841, p. 506) as "this scholar whose exactness I esteem very highly." It may, in fact, have been Remak who encouraged him in his examination of the microscopic structure of the nervous system. In 1840 Hannover wrote a letter to Professor Jacobson of Copenhagen in which he reported a new technique for treating nervous tissue with chromic acid to facilitate its inspection under the microscope; his description of this is on page 833. This was one of the first fixation techniques used in histology, and Hannover illustrated its results by giving an account of the myelinated fibre. In particular he confirmed Remak's findings concerning the central band or axon which at this time had not been fully accepted.

Of equal, if not greater, importance was Hannover's substantiation of Remak's opinion that nerve fibres originated from nerve cells. He was the first to observe this in the brain, although he worked only with vertebrates; the same observation was made by Helmholtz in invertebrates two years later (*De fabrica systematis nervosi evertebratorum*, Berlin, 1842). Hannover's letter was published by Müller in his journal ("Die Chromsäure, ein verzügliches Mittel beim mikroskopischen Untersuchungen," *Arch. Anat. Physiol.*, 1840, pp. 549–558), and the following selections have been translated from it. In 1844 he published a more detailed work (*Recherches microscopiques sur le système nerveux*, Copenhagen) that included illustrations.

EXCERPT PP. 552–556

In the *cerebrospinal* [myelinated] *nerve fibres* the liquid medullary sheath, which is transparent in the fresh state, coagulates after some time. That is, such a fibre consists of a connective tissue sheath and a primitive band [band of Remak = axon] which is also visible before any coagulation occurs; between it and the connective tissue sheath lies the liquid medulla [myelin]. When this has been coagulated with acid, it can be easily removed by light pressure. One then sees only the primitive band, surrounded by the connective tissue sheath, in the middle of the fibre as well as at its cut end. I have convinced myself of the existence of this very tough band, because I saw it, more than a line [see p. 41] long and hanging freely out of the open end of a fibre [see fig. 7]. I was also aware of it because if only a portion of the connective tissue of the nerve fibre with the coagulated medulla was broken, while the tough band remained intact and both ends of it (the one free, the other still connected to the rest of the fibre) were visible, the band was surrounded by the tube formed by the mentioned parts; its lumen was recognized at both ends of the tube. As concerns the band itself, it is not round but either flat or, still more likely, a hollow tube. . . . One can see the primitive band of the nerve best in the [spinal] nerve roots of mammals, especially in the posterior ones; the band is often seen as a light or dark stripe lying in the coagulated medulla (according to the variation of focus).

In all vertebrates, the primitive band of the brain fibres [axon] is seen best in the thick fibres that line the floor of the fourth ventricle and run down from there into the spinal cord; here I have seen it surrounded by a piece torn loose from the coagulated medulla and the connective tissue sheath as in the primitive nerve fibres. These fibres are as thick as nerve fibres and are very similar in appearance. With the help of chromic acid, I have convinced myself that the band does not participate in the varicosities of the brain fibre [see Ehrenberg, pp. 40–43]. Incidentally, brain fibres, except for the staining which takes place, remain unchanged even after many months of preservation in the solution and rarely become varicose . . . . When examining the brain one always sees a larger number of [free] nuclei than of nuclei lying in their cells . . . . Apart from these small cells [molecular layer of cerebellar cortex], there are very large cells in the cerebellum, with a large nucleus and one or two nuclear bodies [Purkyně cells]; these large cells also occur in the spinal cord [anterior horn cells] but are lacking in the cerebrum . . . .

. . . . I shall report that by using the chromic acid method I noticed transverse fibres, running individually as well as in bundles, in the spinal cord of birds, frogs, and fish (as yet I have not explored this in mammals), and that it now seems to me more than probable that the brain fibres originate from the brain cells and retain a lifelong, permanent connection with these central structures; I have made this observation so many times that I personally have hardly any doubt as to the truth of this interesting phenomenon. For those who would like to investigate the subject, I should like to report two errors into which one may easily fall: first, one must be careful not to mistake a floating varicosity attached to a thread for a brain cell with its brain fibre; second, one must not consider the granular and often very long processes and tails of the cell as fibres. The fibre that originates in the cell must appear as a fibre (the best criterion is its intermittent varicosity), and the cells must contain a definite and distinct nucleus. I have found the cerebrum as well as the cerebellum of all vertebrates equally useful for this observation, but there exists a class of cells from which no fibres originate. In general, however, two fibres emerge from one cell.

Rudolf Albert von Koelliker
(6 July 1817—2 November 1905)

Despite the assertions of Purkyně, Remak, Hannover, and others that nerve fibres arose from nerve cells, this had not been proved conclusively and opposition to it still existed in 1849. It could be agreed that no one had yet demonstrated the origin of genuine and undoubted nerve fibres from a cell, and this was the argument put forward at this time by Koelliker, the great Swiss histologist. His investigations, however, showed with brilliant clarity that the earlier workers had been correct, although their evidence had not warranted their dogmatic statements.

Koelliker was born in Zürich where he studied zoology, anatomy, and botany. In 1839 he encountered Johannes Müller in Berlin and was no doubt influenced by him to devote his time to histology, which he did as soon as he was graduated in medicine at Zürich. After spending four further years in Zürich, Koelliker was called to Würzburg as professor of physiology and microscopic and comparative anatomy; he held this post for fifty-five years and became one of the foremost histologists and biologists of his time. His books, *Mikroskopische Anatomie* (Leipzig, 1850–1854, 3 vols.) and *Handbuch der Gewebelehre des Menschen* (Leipzig, 1852), were the first of their kind, and the latter was one of the first textbooks to apply the cell theory to descriptive embryology. Koelliker made numerous discoveries in the field of histology and with them helped to reinforce the cell theory of animal life; he was also interested in comparative embryology, toxicology, protozoology, and evolution (see Weldon, 1898; Koelliker, 1899; Ehlers, 1906; Cameron, 1955; Haymaker, 1963, pp. 52–54; Freund and Berg, 1963–1964, II, 201–213; Buess, 1964).

In his classic paper, "Neurologische Bemerkungen" (Z. *wiss.* *Zool.*, 1849, 1:135–163), Koelliker showed that myelinated, or "dark-bordered," fibres originate from nerve cells and that this takes place in the central nervous system as well as in peripheral ganglia. Now as only nerve fibres have a myelin sheath, it can be said that he was the first to demonstrate the indisputable connection between cell and fibre. His conclusion, furthermore, that there are no nerve fibres that are not connected with nerve cells was a distinct step towards the concept of the independent neuron, the establishment of which forms the fourth section of this chapter. When the fibre, or axon, arises from the cell it is at first pale, that is unmyelinated, and then receives its myelin covering. He compared the sympathetic non-myelinated fibre with similar fibres in the central nervous system and showed the latter to be continuous with the myelinated fibres of the peripheral nerve. Furthermore, he found that sympathetic fibres arise from the spinal cord.

In view of the vital significance of Koelliker's observations, it is unfortunate that he gave no acknowledgement to Remak who had first insisted upon a cell fibre connection. In fact, he made only one brief reference to Remak in the paper (p. 142), and in the introduction to it he discussed his own priority as follows (p. 135):

> As far as the origin of nerve fibres is concerned, it is well known that in 1845 I was the first to reveal the connection of genuine nerve fibres with the pale process of the ganglion globule in vertebrates.

Koelliker's account of the histology of each type of nervous tissue can be read in his *Handbuch* (Leipzig, 1852, pp. 28–71, 262–339). Here he introduced further evidence to support the connection between cell and fibre but admitted that he had been unable to establish its presence between cerebral cortical cells and white matter fibres; his account of the cortex is on pages 430 to 432.

In his *Handbuch* (p. 70) he also made a brief reference to the problem of the relationships between the fibres of one cell and those of others. As we shall see, this was to engage his attention and that of many others later in the century. He stated:

> How these ultimate [fibre] processes finally end, whether freely or in connection with nerve fibres, or whether they anastomose with similar processes, is not yet known, although it seems not at all improbable that the three possibilities mentioned according to the location may be found.

The following excerpts have been translated from the paper of 1849 mentioned above, "Neurologische Bemerkungen."

EXCERPT PP. 142–146

Investigation of the origin of the nerve fibres in the brain and spinal cord is far from easy, and it is made still more difficult by the contradictory reports of the latest investigators. I consider the following as certain and established: (1) that nerve cells with one or two processes exist in these areas; (2) that some of the former are definitely continuous with dark-bordered [myelinated] fibres; (3) that there are also nerve cells with more than two processes which are definitely not continuous with peripheral nerves.

Concerning (1), it must be noted that nerve cells with a single process occur very frequently in the brain and spinal cord in all vertebrates and have been adequately described by Hannover as well as by others (Figs. I, 2; VIII, 2; X, 2, 3 [fig. 15]). Likewise cells with two processes are not at all rare in certain areas (Figs. V, 3, 4; VIII, 3). . . . . It should be noted that nerve cells with more than two processes can also be recognized (Fig. V, 5) . . . . in addition, the processes are frequently very long, very delicately branched, and sharply outlined, from which we may conclude that these cells are normal structures.

. . . .

As for (2), regarding the origin of the dark [myelinated] nerve fibres in the brain and cord, I have already reported the first, sound and definite fact in my paper on the sympathetic nerve. That is to say, from the small ganglion cells of the frog's cord, single or double, pale processes originate which, in the latter case, lie either on the same or on opposite sides [of the cell]. It is easy to follow these processes for considerable distances. They appear pale, slightly granular, sharply outlined, and without branches; it is very rare to see them become dark and assume the characteristics of genuine, fine nerve fibre, and this is invariably at some distance from the cell (Fig. VII). In those cases in which I was successful, it was a cell with a single process; but it should be said, therefore, that those with two could not for their part also be continuous with genuine nerve fibres . . . .

If we review the above statements, it will undoubtedly be apparent how much those who base their conclusion upon the observation that two nerve fibres originate from one ganglion cell, and have assumed that this is the only mode of origin, are deceived. I consider that the occurrence of single fibres originating from ganglia and from the cord, as I first described it, is an absolutely established fact. It is far from being discredited by more recent experiments and to some extent has been further strengthened by them . . . .

The question of the origin of nerve fibres is now joined closely to the questions whether or not there are also nerve cells which do not give off fibres, and what the relation of the other cells is to the fibres which originate in them. Concerning the first point, I have already designated ganglion cells with processes, from which fibres originate, as so-called free or independent ganglion cells, and as component parts of the ganglions . . . . *They are not only very frequent in the actual central organs, brain*

and cord, but they occur so constantly and frequently in the ganglia of the sympathetic and of the cerebrospinal nerves that the question for me is whether there exists a ganglion in which they are completely lacking . . . .
. . . .

When I discovered the connection between nerve cell and fibre, I designated the relationship of the cells to the fibres as simply *the origin of the fibres from the cells in such a way that the pale process of a ganglion cell, because of an alteration in its appearance, changes into a dark-bordered* [myelinated] *nerve fibre and is continuous with it* . . . .

. . . . I have stated that the ganglion cells are connected with the nerve fibres by their processes and that these two are continuous with one another; I did not interpret this otherwise *than that (1) the sheath of the ganglion cell continues as that of the primary nerve fibre, and (2) that the content of the ganglion cell and its pale process are continuous with the content of the primary fibre.*

EXCERPT PP. 151–156

. . . . A second, still questionable point is the relationship between the contents of the ganglion cells and the nerve fibres. I consider it proved that in this respect two somewhat different circumstances exist. In one instance, which appears to be of frequent occurrence in ganglion cells of fish, the nerve fibre, starting at the point where it leaves the ganglion cell, has the characteristic, homogeneous, darkly outlined, viscous content; or, in the second, some of the fibre is filled for a longer or shorter distance with a pale, granular substance or, less frequently, with the contents of the ganglion cell (Fig. III, 2). This behavior in the spinal cord and brain is the only event which is standard in the ganglion cells of all animals, beginning with the amphibia. Until now the pale parts of the nerve fibres were designated as "processes of the ganglion spheres." However, since most of the nerve fibres of the invertebrates are of a similar quality, since, moreover, all embryonic nerve fibres appear equally pale and granular, and since, finally, in adult animals also (Pacinian corpuscles, terminal ramifications in the retina, in the olfactory organ, in the cornea, and in the electric organ of the torpedo) the same pale, granular fibres are present, one may say without question that the so-called processes of the ganglion cells are to some extent nerve fibres of embryonic character. Even if it should turn out that these pale portions of the fibres are constantly formed by growth from the ganglion cells, I should nevertheless attribute to them this meaning without wishing to replace the expression "process of ganglion cells" . . . . The dark medulla of the nerve fibres and the granular light substance meet in all cases. Under normal conditions, that is, if no pressure occurred, this is probably always without sharp demarcation, regardless of whether it does or does not extend beyond the actual ganglion cell into the nerve fibre [Figs. IV, 1, 2; VI].

. . . .

. . . .

1) *The fine fibres of the sympathetic nerves and the thick fibres of the cerebrospinal nerves do not differ from each other in their essential character* . . . .

2) *Apart from the sympathetic nerves there are fine nerve fibres in other areas, such as the brain and special sensory nerves, which do not differ from their fine elements by any specific characteristics.* Volkmann and Purkyně, too, seem inclined to consider these further fine nerve fibres as a special, third type of fibres because of their striking propensity to form varicosities and because of their extraordinary capability of being torn; however, I should like to point out that in many areas the fine fibres of the central nervous system are connected continuously with those of the peripheral nerves, as, for example, those of the spinal cord with those of the spinal nerve roots; this clearly proves that both these sorts of fibres must not be separated from each other. They are rather related to one another in the same way as the thick fibres of the peripheral nerves are to certain thick, brain and cord fibres. Like these latter, as soon as they enter into the cord they receive more delicate sheaths and therefore become varicose and disintegrate more easily, as also the former . . . .

3) *In many areas even the thick nerve fibres are continuous with fine* [non-medullated] *fibres which cannot be differentiated from those of the sympathetic nerve by any anatomical criterion.* Here we must differentiate two features. One, which I have mentioned already in an earlier work, is *that thick nerve fibres prior to and during the terminal ramifications rejuvenate so much that they become very similar to the fine fibres of the sympathetic* . . . . I myself note now that one may express a general law, at least for mammals, that all thick nerves without exception, sensory as well as motor, appear in their terminal ramifications as fine fibres which in essence are not different in any way from those of the sympathetic nerves . . . . Second, what the latest investigations have taught us that the endings of nerves must be considered carefully. For wherever nerve fibres divide one observes as a frequent phenomenon *that thick fibres give off branches that are fine fibres that have all the characteristics of the so-called sympathetic fibres* . . . . Like everyone who knows these relations, I, too, at this point can confirm from my own observations that thick primitive fibres of 0.004 to 0.006''' divide into small branches that do not measure more than 0.002 to 0.003''' and in their last ramifications are always below

0.001‴. All fibres below 0.003‴ have simple outlines and are identical in appearance with sympathetic fibres.

. . . .

. . . . Concerning the spinal cord, although we cannot report definitely that fibres of the sympathetic originate in it, nevertheless it seems permissible to assume so, considering that (1) the roots of the cerebrospinal nerves contain fine fibres (in mammals a considerable number which enter, at least partly, into the sympathetic by the communicating branches), and (2) that I have observed directly the origin of fine fibres in the nerve cells of the spinal cord of frogs.

OTTO FRIEDRICH KARL DEITERS
(15 November 1834—5 December 1863)

The early investigators were greatly limited in their observations by the paucity of methods to fix and stain tissues, but by the middle of the nineteenth century several of these techniques had been introduced. Tissue fixation had begun with Reil who used alcohol in 1809 (p. 830); Hannover introduced chromic acid in 1840 (p. 833), and other methods were soon developed. Carmine as a stain was first used on animal material in 1858 by Gerlach (pp. 840–841), and his application of it to nervous tissue had very important results. Indigo was used in 1859, and aniline dyes in 1862. In consequence, more and more of the complexities of the nerve cell and fibre were revealed, and one of the most important advances, made by Deiters in 1865, resulted from these new histological methods. He not only gave an excellent description of the nerve cell body and its processes, but also presented further evidence for its union with the nerve fibre.

Deiters was born in Bonn and attended medical school there. He later worked in Berlin under Virchow and then returned to Bonn where he carried out his neurohistological work. Unfortunately he died of typhus at the early age of thirty, and as a result, his study of the microscopic appearance of nervous tissue was published posthumously by the great German histologist Max Schultze (*Untersuchungen über Gehirn und Rückenmark des Menschen und der Säugethiere* [Braunschweig, 1865]). The fact that the book was edited posthumously from notes is reflected in the translation below, where, in certain instances, obscurities could not be avoided (see Diepgen, 1960, pp. 24–28; Nieschlag, 1965).

Concerning the nerve cell body, Deiters differentiated two kinds of processes: (1) *protoplasmic*, or, according to modern terminology, *dendrites*, and (2) *nervous*, our *axon* or *axis cylinder*. He also explored the problem of contact between cells, which was soon to become the most important issue in the history of nervous tissue and will be considered in the fourth section of the present chapter. The appearances of the cell processes at their terminations were, in fact, a preliminary step towards the creation of Gerlach's nerve net theory (see pp. 88–90). The lateral vestibular nucleus, which still retains Deiters' name, was also described in his book.

EXCERPT PP. 55–57

I am not premising a definition of the ganglion cell by which it may be distinguished from similar structures; I do not know if there is an exact one; however, I shall designate as such every cell *which is connected with definite nerve fibres* . . . .

With few exceptions, the central ganglion cell is an irregularly shaped mass of granular protoplasm which is either wax-soft and malleable, or, as in most cases, brittle and fragile; at times it is markedly flat and thin, but for the most part it appears bulky and drawn out on all sides; it is demarcated from its surroundings by either a rather smooth outline or a somewhat ragged border, and carries in its interior a large, rounded, bubble-like nucleus with enclosed granular bodies; it is not separated from its environment by an external, insulated covering, the so-called cell membrane [see fig. 16]. The body of the cell is continuous uninterruptedly with a more or less large number of processes which branch frequently but have long [unbranched] stretches in between. The granular, frequently even pigmented, protoplasm can be followed into them readily, and it consequently appears directly in the processes. These ultimately become immeasurably thin and lose themselves in the spongy ground substance which can always be recognized close to these extremely fine, ragged processes. These processes which, even in their ultimate, invariable branches, must not be considered as the source of axis cylinders, or as having a nerve fibre growing from them, for the sake of convenience, will hereafter be called *protoplasmic processes* [dendrites]. A prominent, single process which originates either in the body of the cell or in one of the largest *protoplasmic processes*, immediately at its origin from the cell, is distinguishable from these at a glance [fig. 16, *a*]. However, at its point of origin, we can still recognize in this single *nerve fibre* or *axis cylinder*, the granules of the protoplasm in which [the base of the process] loses itself, for there is no easily recognizable break. But, as soon as it leaves the cell it appears at once as a rigid, hyaline mass, much more resistant to reagents, and on the whole with a different reaction to them; and, from the start, it does not branch. *Shortly after leaving the cell this process becomes thinner* [fig. 16, *a*], *and as a rule it simultaneously snaps off because of the angle which usually occurs here.* But such torn-off pieces are also characteristic and easily and distinctly recognizable among the small cells in well-preserved areas. They are sufficiently characteristic for a cell to be identified as a nerve cell. They are sufficient for anyone who does not wish to take the time to explore the direct transition [of a cell] into a dark-bordered nerve fibre which is found only by chance, but is always a possibility, as will be asserted in the subsequent discussion. This characteristic is not peculiar merely to the large motor cells in which Remak has already partly recognized it, *but also to the sensory ones, to those of the olive, the pons, and, on the whole, to all which could so far be examined thoroughly; indeed, if I am not mistaken, it is also peculiar to the cells of the cerebrum.*

If one checks the various protoplasmic processes [dendrites], one becomes aware of a second, important circumstance analogous to the above. One notices in many processes of the larger, as well as of the smaller cells, that, in a variation from the usual branching, a number of very fine, easily destroyed fibres proceed from them, which do not appear as simple branches since, for the most part, they rest laterally on a triangular base [fig. 16, *b, b*]. These processes are very delicate and can be preserved intact only in certain solutions; they show no marked difference from the axis cylinder of the finest nerve fibres with which they share a somewhat irregular appearance [because of] slight varicosity and the same physicochemical behavior. [In fact, Deiters calls them "axis cylinders" in the legend to the figure.] Sometimes they branch. I very rarely succeeded in identifying a dark-bordered outline in any of these processes, and I do not hesitate to consider them as a second system of efferent axis cylinders which seem to be altogether different from the large ones just mentioned.

Thus the ganglion cells which I have examined so far appear to be central points for two systems of genuine nerve fibres; a system of mostly large, always simple, and undivided fibres, and a second extensive system of the smallest fibres, which are attached to the protoplasmic processes.

EXCERPT PP. 58–59

While I am entering into a discussion of the individual characteristics of the ganglion cell, I should like to touch upon only the points which are of basic importance and for which we have well-founded observations. First of all, the protoplasm is a slightly granular substance with a dull finish, in which a characteristic pigmentation is demonstrable in many cells. In some parts, particularly in large cells with broad processes, it also takes on a slightly striated appearance [? neurofibrils], a characteristic which I have thus far been unable to trace back to definite, finer formative elements. In the fresh state the cells can be easily destroyed; they are soft and firmly fixed to their surroundings, and therefore difficult to isolate. It is not easy to establish what degree of consistency ought to be attributed to their various layers during life. In large, pigmented ganglion cells the fine, pigmented granules seem to be able to change position upon pressure, but it is hardly possible to decide whether the differentiation between the fluid nucleus and the solid cortex ought to be attributed to death or to the influence of various reagents. In addition, the protoplasm has the quality of easily precipitating the dissolved contents of weak solutions, as for example, the pigment of carmine and probably also chromic acid in weak dilutions. By means of stronger reagents, such as alkalis and acids, if they exert their influence in the fresh state, the cells are soon destroyed, otherwise they coagulate with only slow change; but the behavior in different areas is extremely variable. Such effects are very rare but well tolerated also in the fresh state, especially if they are of only short duration and then are terminated completely. Chromic acid solutions of strong concentration coagulate the substance and make it resistant and, later on, very suitable for the penetration of dye; however, this is usually accompanied by a high degree of brittleness and friability. The use of weak chromic acid and potassium chromate solutions, by which one can isolate the parts and preserve them completely and thus present all the essential characteristics, with the help of an especially suitable mixture of early coagulation and maceration, is here of great importance. It is important less for the establishment of absolute chemical characteristics than for the detection of differential physicochemical criteria in different ganglion cells.

EXCERPT PP. 99–100

For the time being only very few clues are available regarding the local physiological layout in the individual ganglion cell. If, according to reported experiences, the cell, as a central point, appears to be of different significance for two fibre systems, such a fact gives rise to a variety of possible questions. As has been mentioned, the two systems are not similar; one of them is represented by one fibre [axon, fig. 16, *a*], the other by many [dendrites, fig. 16, *b, b*]. In this way one can think of the area of influence (*Strömgebiet*) of the nerve tract as either simple or complicated; one can imagine the establishment of connections to opposite points. For the time being, it is hardly possible to arrive at definitive conclusions regarding such assumptions, simply because further exploration of the two systems is not feasible. Only this much seems certain to me, that in the motor ganglion cell the efferent nerve trunk belongs to the *emerging* [anterior] *nerve root*. But even here it is proper to ask if all ganglion cells must follow the same principle. It is certainly not only possible but also probable that in this connection even ganglion cells, which otherwise have the same appearance, function completely differently. If at present, investigation of structures which are relatively easy to distinguish [axons] occasionally exceeds the limits of anatomical methods, this is the case to a much greater degree with the second system of fibres which occur in large numbers [dendrites]. Theory demands a connection between tracts of different functions, and it demands the influence of different organs upon one point; as is known, the reflex phenomena particularly demand such an arrangement. Since cells are not connected by means of the protoplasmic processes, and since a simple union of different fibres without the intervention of cells is hardly sufficient for the theory, it follows that one necessarily falls back upon the fine nerve fibres [axons; presumably Deiters meant the terminal branches of the axis cylinder proper, although some have thought that he referred to the terminal dendritic branches (fig. 16, *b*) which he also called axis cylinders] which ramify and therefore may well unite. One is not only justified but, it seems to me, one has the duty of considering such possibilities because, if the arrangement does not take place in the assumed manner, we are dealing with a fact which in all likelihood will always exceed the limits of anatomical research.

Miscellaneous Morphological Features of the Nerve Cell and Fibre

The next significant advancement in knowledge of the nerve cells was the result of the investigation of the relationship between them. But before dealing with this important matter, the discovery of certain morphological characteristics must be considered, some of them still known by the names of their discoverers. These discoveries were made and described concurrently with the events considered in the previous section and those to be considered next, but they are more conveniently dealt with separately: Wallerian degeneration, Kühne's muscle end plates, the node of Ranvier, the granules of Nissl, and, finally, Virchow's account of the neuroglia.

Augustus Volney Waller
(21 December 1816—18 September 1870)

One of the most difficult problems besetting the student of neurohistology is the process of degeneration and its reverse, regeneration. From the earliest studies of the nerve fibre, degeneration hampered observations, and, in retrospect, it seems clear that some early investigators mistook the products of degeneration in nerve fibres for normal structures. Thus some of the "globules" and other findings in the first reports may have been of this origin. Inadequate techniques, as well as inadequate experience, were also responsible for erroneous conclusions; hence Burdach (1837, p. 42) stated that ligating a nerve had no effect upon it. No further advancement could be made, moreover, until the relationship between the fibre and the nerve cell had been firmly established (see Kennedy, 1897–1898; Ramón y Cajal, 1959, I, 3–26).

Today we know that the nerve cell body is a trophic center and that a detached process will disintegrate and die. The studies that have led to this concept began with the work of Waller. His experiments on the frog's tongue showed that after section of its nerve, degeneration took place throughout the distal segment, and this process is still known as Wallerian or secondary degeneration.

Waller was born at Faversham, Kent, and received the M.D. degree from the University of Paris in 1840. After practising medicine in London for ten years, during which time he carried out many investigations, in addition to the one mentioned here, he joined the ophthalmologist J. L. Budge in Bonn. During the five years Waller spent there important investigations were carried out on the autonomic nervous system. He was able to elucidate Horner's syndrome in experimental animals, and he carried out fundamental studies of the vasomotor system. He then worked in Paris, Birmingham, and Bruges, but, due to continued ill health, did little more scientific work. He eventually took up medical practice in Geneva where he died at the age of fifty-four (see Power, 1899; Haymaker, 1953, pp. 95–98; Gertler-Samuel, 1965).

Waller's first paper on secondary degeneration represented work done in 1849 and first reported to the Royal Society on 21 February 1850 ("Experiments on the section of the glossopharyngeal and hypoglossal nerves of the frog, and observations of the alterations produced thereby in the structure of their primitive fibres," *Phil. Trans. R. Soc.*, 1850, 140 (i):423–429). His belief that although the distal portion of the severed nerve degenerated, the proximal part and the cell did not, has since been modified through the use of better staining methods, especially that of Nissl (pp. 850–851). However, Waller's paper gave further evidence for the connection between fibre and nerve cell. Moreover, his work formed the basis of a very important method of tracing nerve fibres in the nervous system (see Gudden, pp. 854–857), and the findings of Forel, which helped to establish the neuron theory, were dependent upon it. Further discussion of degeneration is to be found in Forel's paper (pp. 104–109).

EXCERPT PP. 425–427

During the first two or three days after section, no alteration in the texture and transparency of the tubes of the papillary nerves [of the tongue] can be detected. Generally, at the end of the third and fourth day, we detect the first alteration by a slightly turbid or coagulated appearance of the medulla, which no longer appears completely to fill the tubular membrane, which does not appear to be affected. These alterations of the medulla are best seen in a fragment to which a little distilled water has been added to render it more transparent. When examined twenty-four hours after death, the difference between these and the nerves on the healthy side is still more evident. Commencing decomposition on the healthy side causes the nerve-tubes to swell considerably, so as to attain nearly double their ordinary size. On the divided side the disorganized nerve retains nearly the same size and appearance as when fresh. Caustic potash, which dissolves all the tissues except the nerves, renders the altered nerves more transparent, and consequently the morphological changes are

less apparent. Nevertheless, by comparative experiments made simultaneously, we may still detect a difference between the nerves of the two
sides. In some cases, in about three or four days after section, I have traced
the turbid state of the nerve from the fungiform papillae into branches
containing forty or fifty tubes, where it did not appear to terminate, but
where the opacity of the nerve prevented my observing it any further.
About five or six days after section, the alteration of the nerve-tubes in the
papillae has become much more distinct, by a kind of coagulation or
curdling of the medulla into separate particles of various sizes. Sometimes
the coagulated particles have an uneven spongy appearance, as if the component parts of the medulla, i.e., the white substance and the axis cylinder,
were mixed together. Often they appear merely like separated particles of
the medulla, such as are frequently effused from the ends of a divided
nerve, and present the double contour and the central nucleus characteristic of the nervous medulla. In some cases the coagulated particles are very
uniform in size and appearance, averaging $\frac{1}{7000}$th of an inch. In others,
the limits between the maximum and minimum dimensions are far greater,
namely, from $\frac{1}{2500}$th to $\frac{1}{12,500}$th of an inch. The diameter of the altered
tubes, examined in the ordinary manner in water, is about a fourth smaller
than that of the sound ones, and in many instances the tubular cylinders
appear wanting, and the medullary particles to have escaped from the
cylinder, and to be merely held together by the neurilema [sic] which
surrounds the whole nerve. After the application of potash, the diameter of
the altered and unaltered nerves is as nearly as possible the same. This
equalization of the two is produced almost entirely by a decrease in the size
of the sound tubes, which swell considerably in water, and afterwards
contract by the application of the alkali. It is therefore probable that the
difference of size at this stage between the altered and unaltered nerves
arises from the former not absorbing so much within them as the latter.
Whether this arises from a ruptured state of the membrane or from a
chemical change of the medulla, is not evident. After the surrounding
tissues have been removed by potash, the tubular membrane offers no signs
of rupture, and the medulla appears less disorganized than before the
denudation. The disjointed condition of the medulla is greatest towards the
extremities. A portion of each nerve-tube is frequently so disorganized as to
be carried away among the tissues dissolved by the alkali. The circular rim
so frequently presented by the extremity of the tubes is absent. We often
observe around the healthy nervous branches, and the papillary nerve in
particular, a common sheath or neurilema [sic] fitting closely to the nerve.
After a disorganization has attained this degree, it appears to form a kind of
loose pouch around the nerve and separated from it by an interval of
$\frac{1}{5000}$th of an inch. This pouch appears to form the sole investment of the

curdled medullary particles, which, as we have stated, previous to the action of the alkali, appear void of any tubular investment. As we ascend towards the brain the disorganization appears to decrease, the coagulated medulla is more apt to assume the oval form, and at some places it presents its double contour apparently unaffected. The effect of decomposition in the unaltered and altered nerve is similar to that in the former stage. In consequence of the above changes the disorganized nerve is more opake than the unaltered one . . . .

. . . .

. . . .

On the seventh, eighth and ninth days the disorganization of the nervous structure continues to progress. In the papillae the curdled particles of medulla become still more disconnected, and in parts are removed by absorption. The tubular sheath also is ruptured and disorganized near the extremities of the tubes. In the other ramifications of the glossopharyngeal, the medulla becomes more and more disjointed and collected into oval or circular coagulated masses.

On the tenth day and upwards we perceive another morphological state of the medulla. The coagulated particles lose their amorphous structure and assume a granulated texture. The granules, retained together by slight cohesion, are dark by transmitted light, but of a light white colour by reflexion, and average $1/20,000$th of an inch.

About the twentieth day the medullary particles are completely reduced to a granular state. The condition of the papillary nerve is represented in Plate XXXI. fig. 2 [fig. 17], where we find the presence of the nervous element merely indicated by numerous black granules, generally arranged in a row like the beads of a necklace. In their arrangement it is easy to detect the wavy direction characteristic of the nerves. They are still contained in the tubular membrane, which is but very faintly distinguished, probably from the loss of the medulla and from atrophy of its tissue. The resistance of these granular bodies to chemical agents is most remarkable, for they remain unaffected by acids, alkalies and the ethers, which have so great an influence over the nervous medulla. These granules may be detected within the papillary nerves for a considerable period of time. I have seen them apparently unaltered in the papillae upwards of five months after division of the nerve, reunion not having taken place.

EXCERPT P. 428

At present we have restricted our observations to the alterations which take place in the ramifications originating from two trunks [ninth and twelfth cranial nerves], but we cannot suppose that this is a local phenomenon, and that other nerves do not participate in similar alterations, and that the brain itself, composed in great part of tubular fibres, must be excluded. Experiments on other nerves already enable me to affirm that such is not the case, and that they are to be found on [*sic*] other nerves, such as the sciatic, &c., and, moreover, that they are as extensive as the nervous system itself. It is impossible not to anticipate important results from the application of this inquiry to the different nerves of the animal system. But it is particularly with reference to nervous diseases that it will be most desirable to extend these researches.

An important result of Waller's work was the idea of the cell body as a nutritional and trophic center and of the law of dependence of the nerve fibre upon it; this was not, however, fully accepted until long after his time. His subsequent papers, which reported further evidence for the concept, as far as the peripheral nervous system was concerned, were published in Müller's *Archiv* or in the proceedings of the Académie des Sciences of Paris. The three following extracts come from the latter, and they vaguely foreshadowed the neuron theory. The first, "Examen des altérations qui ont lieu dans les filets d'origine du nerf pneumogastrique et des nerfs rachidiens, par suite de la section de ces nerfs au-dessus de leurs ganglions" (*C. r. hebd. Acad. Sci., Paris*, 1852, 34:842–847), is concerned with posterior spinal root ganglion cells.

EXCERPT P. 847

According to the interpretation of my researches, each of the fibres which is attached to one of the two poles of these cells finds in it the center of its nutritive life. If the cell is disorganized, so likewise the fibre, as we have seen in the instance of the inferior ganglion of the vagus nerve [ganglion nodosum]. If by cutting the fibres their connections with the corpuscles [nerve cells] are interrupted, they are disorganized and consequently lose their functions which are easily reestablished by the development of new fibres which arise from the cut fibres of the ganglion.

The second extract, from "Septième mémoire sur le système nerveux" (*ibid.*, 1852, 35:301–306), is concerned with the spinal cord and its roots.

EXCERPT P. 301

. . . . I have arrived at the conclusion that the central nutrition of the sensory spinal fibres is to be found in the vertebral [posterior root] ganglia, while that of the motor fibres is in the spinal cord.

The third extract, from "Huitième mémoire sur le système nerveux" (*ibid.*, 1852, 35:561–564), includes Waller's concept of the vital forces inherent in the cell.

EXCERPT P. 563

. . . . the animal body, as all physiologists admit, is composed of parts which are being destroyed and renewed ceaselessly. If we need direct assurance of this fact, it can be found in the equilibrium which exists between these two contrary processes. As long as the influence of the ganglion on the nerve fibre is in force, the equilibrium is maintained; but as soon as the connection between the ganglion corpuscle [cell] and the nerve fibre is destroyed, the peripheral end of the latter remains in the tissues like a foreign body, and destructive forces are brought to bear upon it so that, according to the degree of their activity, it is eliminated more or less quickly. The decentralized nerve fibre can thus serve as an index of the activity of vital forces, be it by structural changes, be it by the loss of motor qualities, if it is a motor nerve. I have no doublt that anything that has an influence on vital activity will also affect the speed with which the alteration of structure and the loss of functional properties is brought about.

Willy Kühne
(28 March 1837—10 June 1900)

Not only was attention being paid to the nerve fibre itself and to its attached cell, but its endings in the periphery of the body were also being examined, since once the fibre's origin from the cell had been established it was natural to investigate its extremity. Some of the first to be described were the sensory receptors such as the Pacinian corpuscle (Henle and Koelliker, 1844), Meissner's corpuscle in 1852, and Krause's end bulb in 1860; others were discovered later in the century (Merkel's tactile corpuscle in 1880, and the corpuscle of Ruffini in 1893). Meantime, however, the effector organ, or the ending of the nerve in muscle, was also being studied, and Willy Kühne of Heidelberg was the most active investigator in this field.

Kühne was born in Hamburg and had the good fortune to be able to study and work under Wöhler, R. Wagner, Weber, Henle, Lehmann, Virchow, Claude Bernard, Ludwig, Brücke, and du Bois-Reymond. After having been assistant in chemistry at the Institute of Pathology in Berlin and professor of physiology in Amsterdam, in 1871 he was appointed professor of physiology and director of the Institute of Physiology at Heidelberg as successor to Helmholtz. His work lay in three main areas: the physiology of muscle, the physiology of the retina, and the chemistry of the digestion of proteins. In particular he demonstrated the axon reflex and the fluidity of the sarcoplasm (see Voit, 1900).

His first detailed account of the nerve endings in muscles was published in 1862 (*Über die peripherischen Endorgane der motorischen Nerven* [Leipzig, 1862]), and the following selection has been translated from it.

EXCERPT PP. 17–18

We shall now consider the end apparatus of the motor nerves. As already noted, the terminal nerve bulbs appear to be very intimately associated with the axis cylinder, or with whatever one wishes to call the intramuscular continuation of the nerve. Its firm attachment, as well as the termination of the short axis cylinder with a single terminal bulb set on it [see figs. 18 and 19, *a*], speak adequately for this. For reasons that have already been mentioned, there can be no question of confusion here with the well-known muscle nuclei, the more so if one subjects the behavior of these [two] structures to further scrutiny. The muscle nuclei are such durable structures that almost no reagent can make them disappear completely, while the terminal nerve bulbs, when subjected to strong acids, disappear almost instantaneously and leave behind a crumpled, coagulated substance. This is also the reason why it was just as difficult to recognize them as to recognize the intramuscular axis cylinders, other than by their remnants in muscle fibres, isolated with nitric acid and potassium chlorate. Furthermore, the varying behavior of the terminal end bulbs to sodium hydroxide solution is much less than that of the muscle nuclei so that they always disappear first. However, a strong concentration of sodium hydroxide does not get rid of the muscle nuclei at all, while the terminal end bulbs immediately become invisible. Just as their chemical behavior is different, so the terminal bulbs are also clearly distinguished by their shape. The peculiar shape, pointed at one end, the markedly granular appearance, the constant absence of a nucleolus, and the complete lack of a membrane, are very specific characteristics. Not infrequently one also observes a "brush-like" disintegration [see Fig. VI in fig. 18, *b*], especially after too strong maceration of the muscle; this permits the conclusion that they have a characteristic fine structure. However, although these observations may serve to protect against objections regarding the existence of these structures, which are to be newly introduced into histology, so, too, I do not wish to omit examination of them under still more advantageous circumstances, that is, to recognize them in an isolated state. Surely this was not possible when we pulled the nerves, so to speak, out of the sarcolemma, but only by taking the muscle substance from the sarcolemma and leaving the nerves in it. For this purpose one selects a muscle fibre which exhibits as clearly as possible the nerve ending formation and treats it in a beaker with 0.1% hydrochloric acid. In order that as much as possible of the contents of the transversely striated muscle fibre may be removed, this procedure ought to be continued for a considerable time—for the best results, several days—with frequent shaking and storage in a cool place. With this technique the muscle fibre becomes almost twice as long and so transparent that it is difficult to find and remove it from the acid. Then place the long, delicate thread very carefully under the microscope and look for the place where the nerve enters. The contractile contents have completely disappeared, and the entire tube is filled with a slightly opaque liquid which can be put in motion by pushing the cover slip down gently. Thus the ending of the nerve can now be identified; it is completely isolated in the interior of the sarcolemma, so that when the liquid is shaken, the entire organ, which during the treatment becomes only slightly paler, moves to and fro in it like threads in water. One can observe the same picture as was described above, recognize the axis cylinder with its swellings and the marginal buds, and, with great distinctness, the pointed endings of the longer processes [figs. 18, 19].

In his chapter contributed to Stricker's textbook of histology, "Nerv und Muskel-faser" (*Handbuch der Lehre von den Geweben des Menschen und der Thiere*, Vol. I [Leipzig, 1869], 147–169), Kühne dealt with the terminations of motor nerves in the muscles of a wide variety of animals. He admitted that:

. . . the appearances of the motor nerve endings are so various that it is difficult today to construct a scheme which conforms faithfully to reality and which reproduces the end-apparatus in accordance with its physiological and morphological significance in all animals [p. 162].

However, he summarized the state of knowledge in 1871 in the passage which follows. Figure 20, which illustrates it, has been reproduced many times in textbooks of anatomy. The terms used by Kühne, such as, for example, "nerve end plate," "nerve end bulbs," and "nerve end apparatus," are now universally employed.

EXCERPT P. 165

In all striated muscle the nerve ends beneath the sarcolemma with which the sheath of Schwann is continuous [fig. 20]. The medullary sheath accompanies the axis cylinder up to this spot. The end of the axis cylinder always spreads out over a considerably enlarged area which invariably forms a flat, spread-out ramification. This nerve end plate (*Nervenendplatte*) is at times comparable to a membrane and at others, to a system of fibres. In most cases the plate rests on a substratum of nuclei and finely granular protoplasm, but in other cases this residue is absent and the nerve plates then have so-called nerve end bulbs (*Nervenendknospen*). The nerve ending never penetrates into the interior of the contractile cylinder, nor does it surround its whole periphery. Short muscle fibres accommodate only one nerve ending, but long fibres have more.

Seventeen years later Kühne delivered a Croonian Lecture to the Royal Society on 28 May 1888, and one can see from it that little new histological information had been added during the intervening years ("On the origin and the causation of vital movement," *Proc. R. Soc.*, 1888, 44:427–447).

EXCERPT P. 441

Nerves end blindly in the muscles; as a rule they are not even finely pointed, and still less do they spread out diffusely in such a way as might make the true ending difficult to find. They end quite distinctly. But the ends always lie beneath the sarcolemma in such a way that no foreign tissue intrudes between them and the muscle, so that what is fluid in the muscle can directly moisten the nerve. The sublemmal nerve is clothed with nothing else than the axolemma. The nerve never penetrates into the depths of the muscle substance; on the contrary, it remains confined to the sublemmal surface of the contractile cylinder or prism. Each nerve end consists of several branches, like antlers, arising by division, which together form the terminal nerve-branch. Apart from the form of the antlers, this short description is exhaustive for many animals, since neither in the sublemmal nerve need any special additional structures occur, such as nuclei, nor any kind of modification of the muscle substance in the field of innervation. There is much to indicate that the nerve-fibre proper, or axis-cylinder, does not change its constitution in passing through the sarcolemma; still it is to be remarked that the twigs of the terminal branches, although as long as they live often apparently longitudinally striated, have not yet, even in the most favourable strainings, been found to present the general fibrillar structure of nerves.

According to these results of morphological research, it appears that contact of the muscle substance with the non-medullated nerve suffices to allow the transfer of the excitation from the latter to the former.

Louis-Antoine Ranvier
(2 October 1835—22 March 1922)

It is always difficult to understand why obvious anatomical structures were not recognized and described earlier. There seems little doubt that in many cases they were in fact observed but their significance was not understood or it was misinterpreted, and at times the primitive nature of the investigations was responsible for such failure. A case in point is the node of Ranvier. We have seen that Remak observed a break in the myelin sheath (fig. 7, *b*; this could, however, have been a Schmidt-Lantermann incisure), and Koelliker, Dalton, and Todd had seen it, too, and had, like Remak, figured it in their illustrations (Stirling, 1881). It was, however, thought to be an artifact, an understandable interpretation when one recalls the primitive techniques of the early microscopists. In this instance the delay in recognition was due to the absence of an adequate staining technique. Thus it was not until 1871 that Ranvier, using a new silver impregnation method, which gave him the certainty that had been denied his predecessors, provided a detailed account of the structure which is still known by his name.

Ranvier was born at Lyons where he was graduated in medicine in 1865. In Paris he first worked as an assistant to Claude Bernard, and in 1872 became director of the histological laboratory of the Collège de France in Paris. Three years later he was appointed professor of histology in the same institution. He spent his professional career studying the microscopical appearances of normal and pathological tissues and was considered by his countrymen to be continuing the French histological tradition of Xavier Bichat, the founder of histology, who had not, however, used the microscope (see Nageotte, 1922; Jolly, 1923).

Ranvier's first account of the nerve fibre constriction, or node of Ranvier, appeared in 1871 ("Contributions à l'histologie et à la physiologie des nerfs periphériques," *C. r. hebd. Acad. Sci., Paris,* 1871, 73:1168–1171). He was also the first to describe in detail the perineurium of the nerve, but this account has not been included in the following selection.

EXCERPT PP. 1169–1171

In the mouse we find extremely small thoracic nerve filaments which are over two centimeters long. When one of these nerves has been placed for one hour in a solution of silver nitrate, 1 in 300, washed in distilled water, preserved in glycerine, and then subjected to light, it shows a remarkable structure which so far has escaped the attention of histologists. On the outside of the nerve [fibre] one will notice a layer of connective tissue containing adipose cells [endoneurium]; below that layer a continuous epithelial covering formed by large, flat, and polygonal cells [neurilemma], and then the mass of nervous tissue. In this mass, in the center of which one may distinguish a longitudinal fibrillation [neurofibrils] which corresponds to the nerve tube [axon], small, black, transverse lines of remarkable clarity, arranged like the rungs of a ladder, appear at different points. In order to give an exact idea of the distribution of these little lines an illustration would be necessary [none provided. Fig. 21 is from a later article]. A large number of these small transverse lines are cut perpendicularly near their center by a black line [axon], and the preparation also appears to be covered with small Latin crosses. This preliminary observation, which was made with a magnification of 150 diameters, is insufficient; the study must be pursued with much greater magnification, when one will then be convinced that the black, transverse lines are placed on the nerve tubes to produce a smaller diameter than in the other parts of their length, and that the longitudinal lines occupy the center of the nerve tubes and correspond to the axis cylinder.

The isolation of large nerves, the sciatic nerve of the rabbit, for example, in a solution of silver nitrate, 1 in 300, provides a preparation in which the black, transverse line can be seen to correspond to a ring which constricts the nerve tube, and that the longitudinal line is the axis cylinder which has been stained with silver at the base of the ring and in a small part of its length on each side of the ring, proving that the silver solution penetrated the nerve tube at this point only.

If one employs a different method, the action of neutral, 1 in 100, ammonium picrocarminate upon isolated nerve tubes, straightaway one will notice under the microscope the penetration of the staining substance at the base of the ring. Wherever it occurs, the axis cylinder is clearly outlined, but beyond, it escapes observation. This method also permits a more exact analysis of the ring itself. The study of the ring-shaped constriction with stronger magnification will show that this is not an artifact of preparation but that the observation which was first carried out in the thoracic nerves of the mouse, subjected to the effect of silver nitrate, has unquestionably established its physiological reality. Indeed, with a magnification of 800 diameters the constriction of the nerve tube at the majority of the points where it occurred, seemed to be owing to a narrow, convex ring which, when the object is adjusted, coincides with Schwann's membrane; it is brilliant when one moves the object away, and darker when it is brought closer, which are positive characteristics as reported by Dujardin for refractive and convex bodies. I shall call this ring the *constriction ring of the nerve tube*.

In the following year, in the paper from which figure 21 is reproduced ("Recherches sur l'histologie et la physiologie des nerfs," *Archs. Physiol. norm. path.*, 1872, 4:129–149), Ranvier summarized his account of the constriction.

EXCERPT PP. 145–146

The various methods that I have applied to the study of the annular constrictions of the nerve tubes give us fairly precise ideas about their condition, structure, and morphological significance. These ideas can be formulated in a few words.

A. The annular constrictions are almost equally distant from one another in the same nerve tube. They are a little closer together in the thin than in the thick tubes.

B. The segments of a nerve tube between two constrictions show only a single nucleus of the membrane of Schwann, situated almost in the middle of the segment, that is, at an equal distance from the two neighboring constrictions. A mass of protoplasm surrounds this nucleus and extends on to the inner surface of the membrane of Schwann as can be observed clearly in young animals. These facts lead to the following hypothesis regarding the morphological development of the nerve tube: each segment represents a cell joined to its neighbors at the corresponding constrictions. Staining the ring with silver nitrate confirms this hypothesis, for it is known that intercellular cements are always the first parts of tissues to be impregnated with silver.

C. The myelin sheath of a nerve tube is interrupted completely by the ring of constriction, and the crystalloid material that bathes the nerve tube reaches the axis cylinder by way of the colloid medium of the ring.

D. The study of the nerves of animals during the course of growth establishes the fact that the interannular segments of the nerve tubes, once formed, increase in size.

Franz Nissl

(*9 September 1860—11 August 1919*)

The delineation of the processes of the cell body proved to be a difficult yet vital task. But while it was advancing, attention was also directed towards the problem of the contents of the nerve cell. One of the individuals who in the last decade of the nineteenth century made the greatest progress in this area was Nissl, whose name is still applied to the Nissl bodies or material of the cell, and to a staining technique.

Nissl was born in Frankenthal in Bavaria and was educated at Munich where he was graduated in medicine in 1885. He worked first at the Munich Kreisirrenanstalt, and after spending twenty-three years at Heidelberg, where he was professor of psychiatry and director of the Psychiatric Clinic, he returned to Munich to work in Kraepelin's Deutsche Forschungsanstalt für Psychiatrie. He was widely active in the fields of neurohistology and neuropathology as well as in psychiatry (see McGill, 1936, pp. 107–113; Haymaker, 1953, pp. 195–198; Farrar, 1954; Cerletti, 1959; Kolle, 1956–1963, II, 13–31).

His method of staining (see pp. 850–851), which employed basic aniline dyes, allowed him to stain the cell contents selectively. On the basis of which parts of the cell took up the dyes and which did not, and their relationships, Nissl was able to evolve an elaborate classification of normal cells. He could also detect pathological changes in the cell by means of his technique which revealed, for instance, that contrary to Waller's claim (p. 71) the ganglion cell can be affected by peripheral axonal injury; this Nissl described for the first time and called it "primary irritation" or chromatolysis as we should call it today.

Nissl's first detailed account of the nerve cell contents appeared in 1894 (Über die sogenannten Granula der Nervenzellen," *Neurol. Zbl.*, 1894, 13:676–685, 781–789, 810–814). This is a long, rambling paper which is principally a reply to criticism made by Heinrich Rosin (1863–1934) of Berlin ("Entgegnung auf Nissl's Bemerkungen: Über Rosin's neue Färbemethode des gesammten Nervensystems und dessen Bemerkungen über Ganglienzellen," *Neurol. Zbl.*, 1894, 13:210–214). Nissl's style is awkward and long-winded so that some editing of his text has been necessary.

The following extracts describe the varieties of cellular constituents. The related problems of nomenclature are discussed in an excellent review of the nerve cell written by Robertson (1899) which conveniently summarizes, in the form of a critical digest, the data on neurocytology available at the turn of the century.

Nissl also discussed the interpretation of the results of staining and believed that the chemical state of the granules could not necessarily be predicted by their response to the dyes employed, as Rosin had claimed when he stated that "the staining of the (acid) granule with the (basic) pigment granule is a chemical process" and that "the granule of the nerve cell is more a chemical than a morphological concept." In reply Nissl made an important statement concerning the relations between morphological and tinctorial phenomena in histology.

EXCERPT PP. 676–677

Therefore, although Rosin believes that he can demonstrate substances in the granules, which he claims possess basic pigments related to acid properties, I maintain a purely descriptive viewpoint and consider these structures in a more morphological sense. For me, the question is that of fragments, i.e., the stainable or visible, formed part of the nerve cell body and fragments which are not even morphologically homogeneous. With the exception of chromophilic cells, which are in a class by themselves and therefore will not be discussed at this point, the body of all nerve cells consists of a formed portion which can be stained and one that cannot be stained. Besides, some nerve cells contain a disorganized substance, a pigment which, as a rule is deposited in the form of granules in the unstained portion of the cell body. The stainable portion shows a variety of different forms: at times we find small and large granules of regular or irregular shape, groups of granules, rows of granules, and granular fibres; at other times we find smooth or coarse threads of varying thickness which differ in their course and length; or we find larger formations of regular or irregular shape. These last have either characteristic shapes, such as spindles or wedges (*Versweigungskeln*), or they sit like a skullcap on the nucleus (*Kernkappen*) (Fig. 5 [fig. 22]) and are either all of the same kind or are in combinations; or they appear in a form which is difficult to define for they are variously shaped yet homogeneous bodies; or they prove to be composite, and their process-like outgrowth is frequently not dissimilar from a starlike or ray-shaped body (Figs. 2 and 4 [fig. 22]). Because of this variability in structure shown by the stainable portion of the cell substance, the latter, owing to a certain mode of arrangement of the stainable substance of the cell body, can appear in many forms. The unstainable portion fills in the remaining part. According to the site of origin of a nerve cell, the arrangement of the stainable substance of the cell body may differ considerably. In some of the cells it presents a continuous network, the meshes of which are filled with the unstainable part (Figs. 2 and 4 [fig. 22]). In others, the stainable portion of the cell body substance apparently does not form a connected mass; single spindles or differently shaped portions of the substance, filaments, granules, and series of granules, arrange themselves in the unstainable part of the cell body in such a way that they give it a sort of parallel-striped design (Figs. 1, 5, and 3). In still other cells, the netlike arrangement combines with the parallel-striped variety (Fig. 6), etc. However, as soon as it is firmly established that nerve cells are divided into a series of well-defined morphological types and, furthermore, that the individual type of cell also has a cell nucleus with a very definite, morphological and substantial behavior, i.e., specific cell nuclei, and, finally, that a legitimate, recurring association exists in animals between the individual types of nerve cells and their sites of origin, then the classification of nerve cells follows automatically and naturally. With these assumptions, we are not dealing with a subjective classification determined by one investigator; this plan is entirely the result of the actual conditions which have been encountered. If, with regard to the classification of nerve cells, I recognize an analogue in the concept of the gland cell, the following ratio may be established: a pancreas cell compares to a liver cell as a nerve cell with a parallel-striped arrangement compares to one with a netlike configuration.

EXCERPT P. 681

. . . . I am, however, of the opinion that we have the right to speak of substance in the chemical sense only when we have proved it. As long as we cannot do this, the nerve cell body must remain for us an object of morphological investigation. If, in such research we first of all use selective stains, we may, however, draw *a posteriori* conclusions from the cell's differential ability to be stained owing to the considerable diversity of these parts. Important as these [stains] are for the evaluation of cell bodies *per se*, they are, however, in a chemical sense and according to their general nature, not immediately useful for the recognition of the actual state of the individual cell's substance. Because of this, the goal of tinctorial analysis need not be always a chemical one. It is often simply morphological, for when stained the cell body can be broken down into different substances, the shapes of which can be determined.

EXCERPT P. 814

We can characterize one element of the nerve cell body as visible, formed, or stainable, and the second as invisible, unformed, or unstainable. We can term the individual, elementary shapes, i.e., the components of the stainable parts, according to their shape: "granules," "granular fibres," "-series," "-groups," and, in addition, "fibres" of this or that constituency; finally, the larger portions of the substances we can term "corpuscles," attributing specific names to the typical ones, such as "spindles," "nuclear caps," or "ramified cones." We thus have a completely adequate terminology for the formed elements of the nerve cell body which is acceptable and which says no more, but also no less, of one portion of the cell body than what we know of it.

Rudolf Virchow
(13 October 1821—5 September 1902)

Although neurohistological investigations during the nineteenth century were centered mainly on the elucidation of the nerve cell and its processes, it was also recognized that there were other constituents of nervous tissue. Here consideration will be given only to the neuroglia and only to the first description of it.

With the aid of tissue culture techniques, neurochemistry, and electron microscopy, modern investigation has led to the belief that the neuroglia represents a dynamic, functional system (Glees, 1955). But the opinion universally accepted until very recently that it was a static, interstitial, supporting tissue was the concept of those who first described it. The original accounts are by no means clear, because the investigators were confronted with a complexity of cells and fibres that could not be stained adequately by the techniques then available. It is usually agreed that Virchow, the great German pathologist, was the first to describe the neuroglia, and it is known that he supplied its name.

Virchow was born in the small Pomeranian town of Schivelbein and studied medicine in Berlin until 1844. He worked in the autopsy room of the Charité Hospital for the next four years, after which he took up the position of professor of pathological anatomy at Würzburg. His early and brilliant researches were on thrombosis, embolism, leukemia, coagulation, cretinism, and other topics. His microscopical investigations culminated in the cellular theory of life and cellular pathology, which is basically the modern explanation of disease. In 1856 he returned to Berlin as professor of pathology, but after 1870 his main interests were anthropology, archeology, and ethnology. Throughout his life Virchow was involved in politics and local government and at one time was leader of the liberal party. He was not only the foremost pathologist of his day but as well one of the most outstanding and versatile medical scientists of the nineteenth century, whose work helped in no small measure to establish contemporary medicine (see Ackerknecht, 1953).

While devoting himself to the study of normal and abnormal histology, Virchow called attention in 1846 to a layer of tissue beneath the ependyma of the cerebral ventricles ("Über das granulirte Ansehen der Wanderungen der Gehirnventrikel," *Allg. Z. Psychiat.*, 1846, 3:242–250). This was the first reference to what he thought was a special kind of connective tissue, which he mentions towards the end of the following selection. Some of the appearances, however, may have been due to the inflammatory process present in the material he was examining. The ependyma is also described here and in subsequent passages.

EXCERPT PP. 247–248

. . . The epithelial cells [ependyma], in which I must confess that I have never been able to recognize the cilia in human cadavers although their presence in thick layers can be easily verified, are located on an almost completely structureless membrane that often appears to be composed of rather regular, very thin and pale fibrils which lie parallel to each other; these fibrils can be very easily distinguished at the border of the area where they are usually ravelled, and, when treated with acetic acid, they occasionally demonstrate longitudinal-oval, very tiny, granular nuclei which in most instances, however, are lacking [spongioblasts]. The presence of such membrane is particularly demonstrable in those areas where the nerve fibres run parallel to it and where the finely granular cortical layer, which is mixed with clear vesicles, is missing; the most suitable for this might be the floor of the fourth ventricle. In the normal state this membrane forms thickenings in some places and is folded in others . . . .

The described elevations consist of the same connective substance as the ependyma proper; only it is tighter, denser, and tougher, so that it gives the microscopic appearance of being distinctly fibrous; in it, too, the nuclei can rarely be verified. The small nodules in particular consist of a tissue that exhibits more or less concentric fibres, similar to Pacchionian granulations; above and around them is a similar substance in which I have recognized large numbers of longitudinal-oval nuclei. Otherwise they do not contain any trace of cell formation.

Some years later, in an article dealing with corpora amylacea found in the brain and spinal cord ("Über eine im Gehirn und Rückenmark des Menschen aufgefundene Substanz mit der chemischen Reaction der Cellulose," *Virchows Arch. path. Anat. Physiol.*, 1854, 6:135–138), Virchow again referred to a material like connective tissue associated with the ependyma of the cerebral ventricles.

EXCERPT P. 136

As for the cerebral ventricles, I have already declared many times that I have found them lined everywhere with a connective tissue type of membrane upon which the epithelium lies. This membrane in turn contains very fine cellular elements, and a stroma which at times is compact and at times soft, and which is continued centrally without any special boundary between it and the nerve elements.

This paper was dated 4 September 1853, but a supplement was added with the date 25 September 1853 (p. 138). In the latter Virchow again discussed the curious tissue.

EXCERPT P. 138

Since recording the above, I have repeated and confirmed my observations.

. . . .

Although I have already mentioned above that the ependyma continues among the nerve elements without special boundaries, I can now assert that there is a continuous spreading out of a similar substance inside the special sense nerves. From a series of pathological observations, I accept the fact that a soft stroma, which is a kind of connective tissue substance, pervades and holds together the central nervous system elements everywhere, and that the ependyma is only an expansion of it on the surface of the nerve elements. The assertion that the epithelium of the cerebral ventricles lies immediately on nerve elements seems to be owing to a confusion of this interstitial substance (*Zwischensubstanz*) with the nerve substance proper.

In 1856 Virchow gave the name "neuroglia" to this tissue (*Gesammelte Abhandlungen zur wissenschaftlichen Medizin* [Frankfurt am Main, 1856]).

EXCERPT P. 890

. . . . According to my investigations, the ependyma consists not only of an epithelium, but essentially of a layer of connective tissue covered with epithelium. Although it can be separated without difficulty from the surface, yet it does not constitute an isolated membrane in the narrowest sense of the word but only a layer of an interstitial connective tissue of the brain substance which is prominent on the surface (Virchow, *Arch. path. Anat.*, VI, 138 [p. 86]). This connective substance, which is in the brain, the spinal cord, and the special sense nerves, is a kind of glue (*neuroglia*) in which the nervous elements are planted and which is the main site of the corpora amylacea (the bright vesicles mentioned in the text). If one investigates it in the fresh state, a fine-grained, very plentiful substance with longish, oval and fairly large nuclei can be found which was earlier mistaken for a special kind of nerve substance. The nuclei are, however, contained in very soft and fragile cells, as can be seen at times in fresh material and even more clearly in that which has been artificially hardened.

The neuroglia is of particular importance in pathological states of the nervous tissue. It can for example provide scavenger cells such as the microglia, although some would argue that these cells should not be classified as neuroglial elements. Nevertheless, Virchow noted the phagocytic behavior of certain nerve cells and described it in a paper published in 1867 ("Zur pathologischen Anatomie des Gehirns. I. Congenitale Encephalitis und Myelitis," *Virchows Arch. path. Anat. Physiol.*, 1867, 38:129–142). It is interesting to compare this work with that of his pupil Julius Cohnheim (1839–1884) who at this time was laying down the general principles of inflammation.

EXCERPT PP. 131–132

To wit, the principal change consists in a metamorphosis of fat in the neuroglial cells . . . . The neuroglial cells increase in size considerably during this metamorphosis; they are filled more and more with fine, fat granules, and after a time they represent large, round, granular cells in which the nucleus is at first still distinguishable but later is not. If the metamorphosis reaches an advanced stage, the globule loses its continuity and all that is seen is a small circular accumulation of fat granules without membrane and proper ground substance.

These granular cells and accumulations of granules are located predominantly in the white matter, and the gray matter remains almost entirely free of them or is involved only secondarily. The main sites are the *cerebral hemispheres* and the *tracts of the spinal cord*. In marked cases, the majority of the neuroglial cells of these areas take part in the change, and then the microscopic picture seen at certain intervals shows, with the utmost regularity, the tissue infiltrated by the fatty accumulations . . . .

Subsequent elucidation of the neuroglia had to await the development of more subtle staining methods. Although Deiters' contribution (1865) was important, Golgi demonstrated its precise histological characteristics in 1886, Weigert discovered the fibrillae in 1895 and, most important of all, Ramón y Cajal's investigations with a gold sublimate stain revealed the complete picture. But studies of the form and especially the function of the neuroglia continue today (see Rand, 1953).

The Neuron versus Nerve Net Controversy

One of the steps in the establishment of the animal cell theory was the elucidation of the connective strands between cells (Baker, 1948–1953, 93:168–177). In the instance of the nerve cell this proved to be a very difficult task and one that was to engage investigators up to the present.

When the more obvious morphological characteristics of the nerve cell body and its processes had been identified and the relationships between the two had been universally accepted, the next problem was to determine how they made contact with their neighbors. Although this had interested investigators for some time, no certain advance could be made until a method of staining the cell and all its prolongations, or at least most of them, had been devised. When this had been accomplished, however, two opposing groups of neurohistologists arose. On the one hand there were those who believed that the nerve cells and their processes, like the

trees of a forest, constituted independent units in contiguity with other units but
not in continuity. They developed the concept of what was later known as the
neuron and the *neuron theory,* and they are usually called *neuronists.* Their
opponents, on the other hand, who used much the same techniques, considered the
cells and fibres to be in direct continuity with one another by way of a network to
which the fibres contributed; these were the *reticularists.* The ensuing conflict
stimulated a great deal of excellent work that advanced the histology of the nervous
tissue considerably rather than slowing it down as might have been feared. For the
rest of the nineteenth century and well into the twentieth the controversy continued and some few would say that the debate has not yet been concluded. It can,
however, be observed that up to the present time no certain evidence to disprove
the concept of independent cells has been brought forward. In view of this,
although we shall trace the establishment of both theories, only three representatives of the reticularists have been selected; the remainder are neuronists.

Joseph von Gerlach
(3 April 1820—17 December 1896)

In 1855 Franz von Leydig identified in the central nervous organs of the spider a
Punktsubstanz consisting of innumerable interlacing fibrils (Freund and Berg,
1963–1964, II, 215–220), and in 1872 Gerlach found what he took to be an
essentially similar material in the central nervous system of vertebrates. In this way
the nerve net or reticular theory of nervous tissue came into being.

Gerlach was born at Mainz and studied at Würzburg, Munich, and Berlin. He
received the M.D. degree from the University of Würzburg in 1841 and then
practised medicine in Mainz, but continued his study of histology. In 1850 he was
appointed professor of anatomy at Erlangen, and it was there that he carried out
his most important histological studies. He has been considered to be among the
most outstanding anatomists of the second half of the nineteenth century (Freund
and Berg, 1963–1964, II, 97–100).

Gerlach was greatly interested in the techniques of staining tissues and was
responsible for the widespread use of carmine as a stain (see pp. 840–841). The
so-called nerve net which he described resulted from this technique and from his
experiments on the effect of gold chloride on nerve cells and their processes. His
hypothesis stated that the ultimate divisions of Deiters' protoplasmic processes, or
dendrites, formed a fine-fibred, diffuse plexus that connected together all cells, and
that from it axons arose to form a second, much coarser network. Although Golgi,
the greatest proponent of the net theory, subsequently demonstrated that the
dendritic net did not exist and that only the one formed by axons could be
substantiated (pp. 92–96), Gerlach must nevertheless be considered the originator of the net theory of nervous tissue. In fact, they were both wrong.

The following selections have been taken from Gerlach's famous paper dated 19 April 1872 ("Über die Structur der grauern Substanz des menschlichen Grosshirns. Vorläufige Mittheilung," *Zbl. med. Wiss.*, 1872, 10:273–275). One of the editors of the journal, J. Rosenthal, stated that he had examined Gerlach's preparations and confirmed the presence of the two networks, one produced by dendrites and the other by axons.

EXCERPT PP. 274–275

1) In addition to the long-recognized medullary [myelinated] nerve fibres that enter the [cerebral] gray matter from the white and radiate in bundles to near the surface of the cerebrum, there are innumerable nerve fibres that are also medullary but which extend horizontally. These are particularly distinct in the interstices between the bundles of the radiating fibres, where we also find the main location of the ganglion cells which enter into connection with each other as well as with the radiating fibres. The result is a wide-meshed network of medullary fibres visible at sixty magnifications.

2) In the interstices of this coarse network of medullary fibres, and close to the nerve cells, lies a second extremely fine-meshed network of the finest fibres that are no longer medullated; these, as well as the network proper, can only be seen by means of a powerful immersion system. Participating in the formation of this second network are, on the one hand, the most delicate fibres of the protoplasmic processes [dendrites] of the nerve cells; on the other hand, large nerve fibres [axons] which are soon enveloped by myelin, originate from this network and subsequently enter the wide-meshed network of medullary fibres first mentioned. Although Rindfleish believes that a finely granular substance is inserted between the origins of the second, more delicate network and the terminations of the protoplasmic processes of the nerve cells, with the help of the gold method I succeeded in demonstrating the continuity of the network with protoplasmic processes of the nerve cells [fig. 24].

3) Deiters' nerve process [axon] is found at the nerve cell itself. Without branching, it at once becomes the axis cylinder of a medullary tube [myelinated fibre] which subsequently joins a bundle of radiating fibres. Whether all cortical nerve cells have been provided with a nerve process [axon] must be left undecided. To date I have seen obvious nerve processes on only a few occasions and these only in large nerve cells which send a wide and frequently very long, branching protoplasmic process towards the cerebral surface, and numerous finer ones also towards the outside. The nerve process is always found among the latter.

4) Consequently, there exists in the gray matter of the convolutions of

the human cerebrum two sites of origin for medullary nerve fibres, directly from the cells, or from the network.

As I proved earlier, we also find two types of origin in the spinal cord; the two fibre groups are differentiated into those which proceed directly from the cells and leave the spinal cord through the anterior [motor] roots, and those which originate from the network and leave the cord through the posterior [sensory] roots. I hardly need call attention to the importance of this explanation of the double origin of nerve fibres in the gray substance of the cortex.

In the same year that the above paper was published, 1872, Gerlach's chapter on the spinal cord, "Von dem Rückenmark," appeared in Stricker's textbook of histology (1869–1872, II, 665–693). The following passage which describes the nerve net in the spinal cord has been taken from it.

EXCERPT PP. 683–684

Regarding the second of the questions in hand, which concerns the further relations of the protoplasmic processes [dendrites], Deiters' observation [pp. 66–70] must not be ignored. The finest branches of these processes are occasionally surrounded by a dark-edged, double contour, and in a few instances they are seen to divide into further portions. Supported by these observations, Deiters thinks that these ultimate endings of the protoplasmic processes do not differ from the axis cylinders of the finest nerve fibrils and that they form a system of nerve pathways connected with the ganglion cells. If Deiters had taken a step further, he would have discovered the fine nerve fibre plexus; but as he did not use ammonium carminate in his preparations, and as the gold [chloride] method was unknown to him, the nerve fibre plexus remained hidden from him. I can confirm those observations of Deiters that have been cited, but, in addition, the finest branches of the protoplasmic processes ultimately take part in the formation of the fine nerve fibre network which I consider to be an essential constituent of the gray matter of the spinal cord (see Fig. 223 [fig. 24]). The finest divisions of the protoplasmic processes which are surrounded by a dark-edged, double contour are none other than the beginning of this nerve fibre net. The cells of the gray matter, which are provided with nerve processes [axons] and protoplasmic processes, are therefore *doubly* connected with the nerve fibre elements of the spinal cord: on the one hand *by means of the nerve process which becomes the axis fibre of the tubules of the anterior roots, and on the other through the finest branches of the protoplasmic processes which become a part of the fine nerve fibre net of the gray matter.*

CAMILLO GOLGI

(7 July 1843—21 February 1926)

Gerlach's use of the carmine and gold stains permitted him to make observations denied to his predecessors such as Deiters, even though the conclusions he drew were incorrect. Nevertheless, there was still no available technique which could render the cell and its processes adequately visible in their entirety. As soon as one did become available, a new era in the tracing of nerve fibres and the elucidation of their relationships began. The technique which opened up this new field was the silver staining method of the renowned Italian histologist Golgi, first described in 1873; there is an account of it on pages 842 to 845. It was incomparably better than any of its forerunners, and by means of it Golgi was able to make beautiful preparations in which the nerve elements were silhouetted against a white or yellow background. He discovered structures which had hitherto remained invisible and he established a new theory of nerve connections. These observations led him to become the most ardent and influential proponent of the nerve net.

Golgi was born in Corteno, in the province of Brescia, and he was graduated in medicine at the University of Pavia in 1865. Soon thereafter he decided to study the microscopic structure of nervous tissue and did so in Pavia under very primitive conditions. In 1875 he was appointed professor of histology in the University where he spent the rest of his active career, retiring in 1918. As well as his neurohistological investigations, his work included outstanding contributions to malarial research (see Da Fano, 1926; McGill, 1936, pp. 141–150; Haymaker, 1953, pp. 41–44; Kolle, 1956–1963, II, 3–12; Freund and Berg, 1963–1964, II, 101–116; Zanobio, 1963; Golgi, 1903).

In 1883 Golgi published a classic paper which is remarkable for its clarity and orderly presentation, "Recherches sur l'histologie des centres nerveux" (*Archs. ital. Biol.*, 1883, 3:285–317; 1884, 4:92–123; an edited version of this paper was published in the same journal, 1959, 97:279–299, whence the following excerpts have been taken). Golgi used the terms *nerve extension* for the axon and *protoplasmic extension* for the dendrite, thus slightly modifying Deiters' nomenclature. After summarizing the work of his predecessors, he dismissed the dendritic network of Gerlach and others. In the remainder of the paper he reported his three important contributions to the morphology of the nerve cell and its processes: the silver-staining method, the recognition of two basic types of central cells, and the discovery of the right-angled branches of the axon. However, the main purpose of the paper was to present evidence supporting the existence of an axonic net which replaced Gerlach's plexus. When Golgi's work became known to German histologists three years later, the neuron versus net controversy received an important stimulus; the argument dominated this field of study for the rest of the nineteenth century.

EXCERPT PP. 289–290

If a method of preparation capable of demonstrating the anastomoses of different cells [i.e., between the dendrites of different cells] exists, it must be that of black [Golgi] staining, obtained by the combined action of potassium bichromate and silver nitrate [pp. 842–845]. Thanks to this reagent one notes not only the cell body with its primary extension [axon] clearly revealed, but, in addition, the most delicate ramifications. The use of the black dye can be limited to a small number of cells or to more extensive groups; occasionally one may even obtain a comprehensive view of an entire area of the central nervous system.

Now, I have never succeeded in discovering a single [dendritic] anastomosis in these preparations (although I have examined several hundreds of them with the greatest care), either among the large extensions or their branches.

It is true that very often one believes that one sees two extensions approaching each other and fusing, especially when this observation is made with low magnifications; but a more careful examination with the help of powerful objectives leads easily to the discovery that this is merely an appearance produced by simple contact.

EXCERPT PP. 294–295

In summarizing, I consider myself justified in declaring that the protoplasmic extensions [dendrites] take no part in the formation of nerve fibres [axons], that they are not in direct connection with them, and that, on the contrary, they enter into relation with connective cells [neuroglia] and with the walls of [blood] vessels.

Consequently, it can be suggested that they must have a nutritional function and that their essential role is to carry nutritive plasma from the blood vessels and connective cells to the nerve elements.

If nerve fibres [axons] proceed neither directly nor indirectly from the protoplasmic extensions, and if there is no communication between the different groups of cells of the nervous system, either by way of anastomoses or by the diffuse network, what then is the mode of origin of the nerve fibre in the gray matter? How then is a functional relationship, which one is forced to admit *a priori*, established between the various cells of different parts of the nervous system?

In the next selection Golgi first of all described the axon (nerve extension) of the cerebral cortical cell. He agreed with Deiters that peripheral nerve fibres and those of the cerebral white matter originated from axons, but, in addition, he described lateral branches of the axon for the first time. In his opinion, fibres entering the cortex connected with outgoing elements by way of an anastomotic network and not by synapse as we today know to be the case. This nerve net, unlike the diffuse nerve net substance of Leydig and the dendritic net of Gerlach, was formed by the axons of two types of cells which Golgi identified as Type I, with a long axon, and Type II, with a short axon (figs. 25 and 26). Thus the net was made up from the union of afferent terminals with the complicated subdivisions of the terminals of Type II cell axons and the collateral fibrils of axons of Type I cells. It is perhaps significant that Golgi did not figure the network he proposed.

EXCERPT PP. 297–299

In submitting the cortical substance to the preparation already mentioned, one ascertains first of all that for the majority of the ganglion cells, the manner in which this nerve extension [axon] acts does not agree with Deiters' description or with those of the authors who followed him.

Sometimes it leaves the cell body itself, most often on the side nearest the white matter (base of the pyramidal cells), and sometimes it takes origin from the base of a large protoplasmic extension which emanates from the cell; it then proceeds by gradually thinning for 20 or 30 microns from the point of its emergence, and constitutes a simple, smooth, rectilinear, unbranched filament; commencing at the indicated distance [20 to 30 microns], it winds slightly and then most often starts to branch at once and to give off lateral branches at very regular intervals as far as one can follow it with the help of the black reagent. Preserving its smooth and simple appearance, it follows a slightly tortuous course (perhaps caused by the drying up of the tissue), and not infrequently it is observed to traverse in this way the entire thickness of the cerebral cortex, and to plunge into the nerve fibre layer. In several cases I was able to follow it up to a distance of 600 and 800 microns. The thickness varies within very considerable limits; sometimes the extension preserves almost the same diameter from the first tortuosity and reaches the fibre layer as a clearly defined filament; more often it gradually becomes thinner as it gives off branches, until it is extremely thin.

I have stated that throughout its entire course the nerve extension from time to time gives off lateral filaments very regularly; as a rule these emerge at a right angle, and they in turn send out lateral branches which continue to divide into still thinner branches of the third, fourth, and even fifth order. The mass of these ramifications forms an inextricable plexus of fibres throughout the entire thickness of the gray matter. It is probable that these innumerable subdivisions anastomose among one another and thus form a genuine plexus, but the extreme complexity of this network does not permit me to make any positive statement on the subject. It is important to note that several of these nerve extensions reach their greatest thinness midway, well before they arrive at the fibre layer, and at that moment they divide into three, four, or five filaments which in their turn branch and mingle with the diffuse network mentioned above.

Finally, let us note that in a certain number of nerve cells, especially those belonging to the deep cortical layer, the nerve extension originates at the extremity of the cell which is towards the white matter, but subsequently proceeds towards the opposite side to subdivide into branches of the second, third, and fourth order and to become lost in the network, as with the preceding ones.

In summary, two types of ganglion cells can be distinguished in the cerebral cortex, and probably in the gray matter of the nerve centers in general, to wit:

(1) Ganglion cells, the nerve extensions of which give off only a small number of lateral filaments and change directly into the axis cylinder of a myelinated nerve fibre [Type I cell; Plate IV: fig. 25].

(2) Ganglion cells, the nerve extensions of which subdivide in a complicated manner, lose their identity and participate *in toto* in the formation of a nerve network which traverses all layers of the gray matter [Type II cell; Pl. III: fig. 26].

In this connection it is not without value to call attention to the manner in which certain nerve fibres which penetrate the gray matter behave.

In examining the preparations obtained by the method already described, one often notes, in addition to the bundles of nerve extensions which are directed towards the white matter, other bundles of axis cylinders, also stained black, of identical appearance, branching in the same manner, but nevertheless behaving differently. Some of these accompany the main bundles of nerve extensions and mingle with them so thoroughly that it becomes difficult to distinguish them; but others, by contrast, give off a considerable number of secondary filaments which end by becoming extremely thin fibrils, and then are lost in the gray matter network in the same way as those which we described earlier. Just as we have distinguished two types of nerve cells by following the way in which the nerve extensions behave, so we may establish two categories of nerve fibres which correspond to them exactly.

(1) Nerve fibres which, while giving off secondary fibrils (of which the ramifications get lost in the diffuse network) preserve their own identity, however, and proceed in direct connection with the ganglion cells of the first type by continuing with the nerve extension.

(2) Nerve fibres which subdivide in a complicated manner, lose their identity and participate *in toto* in the formation of the diffuse network of the gray matter.

Here then are the elements which participate in the formation of the network:

(1) Fibrils which emanate from nerve extensions of cells of the first type.

(2) All the nerve extensions of cells of the second type.

(3) The secondary branches of axis cylinders belonging to the nerve fibres of the first category.

(4) Certain axis cylinders *in toto* which break down into ever more tenuous filaments and end by losing themselves in the network and by losing their identity (nerve fibres of the second category).

The following excerpt deals with the relationships of cells and fibres as well as with their function. As pointed out by Fuortes (1959), there is here a very important reference to the principle of convergence and divergence which was basic to Sherrington's concept of the nervous system.

EXCERPT P. 303

The nerve fibre as an organ of centripetal and centrifugal transmission is found in the majority of cases in connection with numerous groups of cells; each cell is inversely related to a certain number of fibres having a different destination and probably a different function. This point deserves to be illustrated by an example.

During my recent studies of the olfactory lobes I stated that each cell is in connection with at least three kinds of nerve fibres; for example, a cell of the first type, by means of its nerve extension, is connected with (1) the fibres of the [olfactory] tract; (2) the fibres of the anterior commissure; and (3) the fibres of the corona radiata. In all cases, the connection is an indirect one. Similarly each cell of the second type is in connection with the same three types of fibres, with this difference that, in this case, the connection is a direct one with the fibres of the tract and probably also with those of the commissure.

I have observed similar things in the spinal medulla.

In conclusion, we see that in the majority of nerve centers isolated and individual connection with the fibres and cells does not occur at all, but, on the contrary, there is an arrangement evidently destined to permit the greatest variety and complexity in their mutual connections, this not only for the central elements or groups of elements but also for the entire areas.

The following excerpt comes from the excellent summary in which Golgi again defined his two types of cells and speculated on their possible functions.

EXCERPT PP. 305–306

I. Cells whose nerve extension is in direct continuity with a fibre without losing its identity, despite the lateral branches which it distributes [Type I cell].

II. Cells of which the nerve extension does not enter into direct connection with the fibres at all and loses itself in the diffuse network [Type II cell].

The distribution of these two types of cells seems to indicate that those of the first type are motor or psychomotor cells, and those of the second, sensory or psychosensory cells.

(9) These two types of cells are found *brought together and mixed in all the areas* of the nerve centers; they are not specific to any one. This is the more so if, in some zones, one distinguishes the prevalence of one or the other type, or clearly, in the same zone, a separate group of the two types.

Golgi concluded his summary by judging contemporary physiological work on the basis of his axonic net. Thus, if nerve cells were connected by way of a diffuse network, their communication would naturally be complex and they could not act in isolation, nor would a strict localization of cerebral functions be possible. As may be seen in Chapter VIII, the latter conclusion has been proved correct, but today it seems certain that Golgi's idea of continuity of nerve cells as opposed to contiguity was quite erroneous. Nevertheless, his staining method and some of his ideas proved to be a very important stimulus for neurohistology, as was eventually acknowledged by the award of the Nobel Prize for Physiology and Medicine in 1906. He shared this with his contemporary and adversary Ramón y Cajal (pp. 127–129). Despite the mounting evidence against him, Golgi had not entirely abandoned his original ideas in 1906, as is evident in his Nobel Prize oration, although by 1891 he had modified his views concerning the net. Even though he did not emphasize the postulated network in 1906, he upheld its consequences which supported the idea that the nervous system acts as a whole and not as a group of isolated centers, a concept that would be received with sympathy today. The following excerpt has been taken from Golgi's Nobel Prize oration ("La doctrine du neurone," *Les Prix Nobel en 1906*, Stockholm, 1908).

EXCERPT P. 30

. . . . As we have said with respect to the functional mechanism, far from being willing to admit the idea of individuality and of functional independence of each nerve element, I have never had cause even now to abandon the idea which I have always insisted upon, and to know that the nerve cells display an individual action. They act together so that it is necessary to consider that several groups of elements exert a cumulative action on the peripheral organs by the mediation of entire bundles of fibres . . . . I cannot abandon the idea of a unitarian action of the nervous system without being uneasy that by so doing I shall become reconciled to the old beliefs.

PAUL EHRLICH
(14 March 1854—20 August 1915)

At first, Golgi's "black stain" (pp. 842–845) was the only method that outlined the nerve cell and all its processes, but, revolutionary as this was, the investigator often had difficulty in fully tracing fibres with it. Thus the technique of staining nervous tissue *intra vitam* with methylene blue, described by Ehrlich in 1886 ("Über die Methylenblaureaction der lebenden Nervensubstanz," *Dt. med. Wschr.*, 1886, 12:49–52), was a notable advancement, for by means of it a more certain and complete delineation of structures became possible. In particular, it stained well the nerve endings and myelinated nerve fibres.

Ehrlich was born in Strehlen in Upper Silesia. He studied medicine at Breslau (now Wroclaw) and was graduated at Leipzig in 1878. He did clinical work in Berlin under Frerichs and later worked there at the Institute for Infectious Diseases with Koch and Behring. In 1891 Ehrlich was created professor *extraordinarius* and five years later director of the Institute of Serum Research and Control at Steiglitz, Berlin, whence he became director of a new institute for experimental therapy at Frankfurt am Main, which was opened in 1899. Ehrlich is remembered especially for his discovery of the basic principles of chemotherapy and immunology (see Marquandt, 1949; Freund and Berg, 1963–1964, II, 79–89).

The introduction of Ehrlich's *intra vitam* methylene blue staining technique was an important event in the history of the study of nervous tissue, since it played a significant role in the foundation of the neuron theory. In addition, his method suggested an experimental biochemical and pharmacological approach to the nerve cell and its processes which could perhaps reveal exact information regarding the properties of the living cells (cf. Nissl, pp. 850–851). Although some of his arguments on morphology are no longer tenable, Ehrlich may be considered to have been a pioneer of neurocytochemistry. It was from his studies of vital staining that Ehrlich developed his revolutionary ideas of chemotherapy and antigen-antibody relationships.

EXCERPT P. 49

During the course of my investigations I discovered that methylene blue has an extraordinary affinity for the finest branches of the axis cylinder, and that it is therefore possible to follow certain nerve endings in the living state with a clarity that cannot be achieved with any other method. For some time, as you know, we have had, for the preparation of nerve endings, only the gold impregnation method discovered by Cohnheim, to which we are indebted for all progress in this field. Nevertheless, there has existed for a long time an urgent need for another method for the preparation of nerve endings, above all for the following reason: on the one hand gold impregnation often fails completely, and on the other, artifacts are by no means out of the question when powerful reagents are used.

The advantage of the biological methylene blue staining over the gold method lies in the fact that first, we can distinguish the terminal apparatus in its perfectly natural state; second, that it often shows nerve endings which could not be obtained in any other way. Of course the methylene blue staining also has its definite disadvantages, of which I should like to emphasize at this time only the instability of the preparations and the limitations imposed by certain areas of the nervous system.

Ehrlich concluded as follows. He seems to have confused axon and dendrite but he made an important statement supporting what was soon to be known as the neuron doctrine.

EXCERPT P. 50

What conclusions can now be drawn from these findings? The fact that I discovered that the straight process (*der gerade Fortsatz* [axon]) does not have the slightest affinity for methylene blue points on principle to a difference of function; such an assumption is in complete agreement with the observation of Axel Key and Retzius, that only the encircling fibre (*die umwundene Faser* [dendrite]) surrounds itself with a myelin sheath [?]. In my experience, the difference in staining supports the fact that the encircling fibre serves centripetal conduction, and the straight fibre, the centrifugal type. Anyone who has once seen such illustrations will be involuntarily prompted to assume that the ending which is applied to the surface of a cell finds its analogue in the nerve ending in the transversely striated muscle fibre and that it differs from this arrangement only by having a special arrangement. We therefore arrive at the concept that stimuli are conducted by the encircling fibres which project very regularly upon the surface of the cell by means of terminal ramifications. Whereas the muscle fibre responds to this discharge by contraction, the ganglion cell reacts in its own specific way by a process of stimulation which propagates itself outwards in the straight fibre. I should like to mention that I have several times seen pictures that enabled me to recognize yet another analogy between the muscle fibre and the ganglion cell. That is, I found variations in the ganglion cell itself in that the voluminous central part which included the nucleus and was in continuity with the straight process, contrasted, with the help of blue dye, with the homogeneous peripheral part, on the surface of which was the darkly stained terminal ramification. In such a cell it is easy to compare [first] the terminal ramification with the muscle terminal arborization or antler, [second] the light peripheral zone with the substance of the sole [motor end plate], [and third] the blue stained center with the muscle fibre proper. I believe that these facts will be of importance to physiology and pharmacology since it is very probable that this terminal ramification, as with methylene blue, will localize other [toxic] substances in it and thus, like the muscle terminal plate, can be paralysed in isolation.

It is certainly astonishing that the axis cylinders do not fuse uniformly with the substance of the cell, but terminate on it in sharp contrast, almost as on a foreign, heterogeneous substance; with this, the old assumption that the processes of the ganglion cell are promiscuous and directly connecting, is definitely ended. Considering the importance of this principle, it seemed appropriate for me to examine still another kind of ganglion cell with this in mind. I selected the spinal ganglion of the frog as a subject of study. As you know, it consists of large ganglion cells that hang like pears from stalks, and from a thick process that divides at its distal end like a fork [i.e., like a letter T]. I found through my methylene-blue experiments that the bodies of the cells proper usually remained colorless while the nerve fibre stained intensively. The transition of the nerve fibre into the ganglion cell took place with the help of a short, intermediate part that consists of blue fibrils [neurofibrils] that end as soon as they enter the cell.

WILHELM HIS
(9 July 1831—1 May 1904)

Opposed to Golgi's nerve net theory was the concept that later became known as the neuron doctrine. According to this concept it was argued that terminal, afferent nerve fibres, instead of ending in an anastomotic plexus, extended close to other cells or processes but did not unite with them. This remains the present-day doctrine, and, even if in the future it may be modified in the light of improved modes of examination, it is unlikely that it will be wholly displaced. Although it did not originate with them, there is no doubt that the Swiss embryologist Wilhelm His and the Swiss psychiatrist August Forel produced the first irrefutable evidence for this concept.

His, a native of Basel, was educated there and at Berne, and at Berlin, where he was influenced by Johannes Müller and Robert Remak, at Würzburg, where Virchow was teaching, and in Paris, where he did postgraduate work with Brown-Séquard and Claude Bernard. After having begun his professional career in Basel, in 1872 he accepted the chair of anatomy in the University of Leipzig and remained there for the rest of his life. His work was mainly in the fields of developmental anatomy, especially that of the nervous system, in histology and in anthropology. The bundle of His was named for his son, Wilhelm His, Jr., who described it in 1893 (see Mall, 1905; Haymaker, 1953, pp. 49–52; His's own summary of his life's work, 1894, pp. 35–41, 51; His [Jr.], 1931; Buess, 1964).

One of the methods of determining whether a nerve cell and its processes remain isolated or whether they anastomose with their neighbors is to observe their growth. This was the approach employed by His, using hematoxylin stains and human material, and he showed that in the beginning the nervous system was a mass of essentially independent cells (neuropiles) from which the nerve cells and their fibres developed; at the early stages of growth it was easy to establish the individuality of the units. Thus he was able to conclude that every nerve fibre arose from a single nerve cell and that this cell was the nutritive and functional center of the fibre, and that, furthermore, all other connections of the fibre were either indirect or arose secondarily. Hence the axon of the peripheral afferent fibre, the spinal ganglion cell, and the axon in the posterior columns of the spinal cord represented parts of one and the same cell. His work can be compared with Harrison's (pp. 132–136).

The paper in which His first reported his findings on this matter appeared in 1887 ("Zur Geschichte des menschlichen Rückenmarkes und der Nervenwurzeln," *Abh. k. sächs. Ges. Wiss.*, Math.-Phys. Classe, 1887, 13:477–514), and in the selection from it presented below His discusses the components of the embryonic spinal cord.

EXCERPT PP. 509–513

THE DEVELOPMENT OF THE NERVE FIBRE AND THE SEQUEL

The results reported in previous sections have shown that some of the cells of the spinal cord participate in the formation of stroma, and the others in nerve fibres . . . .

Of the nerve fibres which appear first in the spinal cord, some pass into the motor roots, others into the anterior commissure, or into the anterior and anterolateral columns. Not more than one nerve fibre appears to arise from any one spinal cord cell. The branching processes of the motor cells [dendrites] develop later than the axis cylinder, and they, too, probably spread out very slowly. Two fibres grow out from each of the cells of the spinal root ganglion, one of which enters the spinal cord and the other extends to the periphery [of the body]. Wherever fibres occur, there are at first few of them, and they increase [in number] only gradually. This can be said of the anterior root bundles, of the anterior and anterolateral columns, of the anterior commissure, and of the oval posterior column fasciculus [Interfascicular fasciculus or comma tract of Schultze].

The fibres which grow out from the nerve cells advance by growing into existing interstitial spaces between other tissue elements. In the spinal cord and in the brain, the medullary stroma already formed, provides pathways for expansion and its structure undoubtedly determines the course of the process of extension . . . . (Cf. Harrison.)

. . . .

Now, if fibres originate in the whole nerve as processes of ganglion cells and spread out gradually to their central or peripheral terminations, the necessary conclusion with respect to the union with the parent cell is that any other connections, if they exist, are only secondary. In the past, one has been very liberal with these central and peripheral nerve connections. According to the opinion of Schröder van der Kolk, the connections of nerve cells among each other have long since been recognized as illusions, but most of us still tacitly imagine that the central nerve fibres serve in some manner as a common connector of cells, and, in the case of the peripheral areas, their ending in so-called sensory cells has become the prevalent dogma, at least for the sensory nerves, since Max Schultze's reports.

The possibility that nerve fibres which penetrate into epithelial layers can also reach the inside of cells cannot be denied *a priori*. However, the nerve endings which were discovered by Hensen in the tail of the frog larvae and which, with respect to their position, are indeed not indisputable, are perhaps applicable in this connection. But, on the other hand, we know of an overwhelmingly large number of terminal fibrils in the corneal epithelium, and in the epidermis, the endings in Pacini's corpuscles and Krause's end bulbs, the plate in the tactile corpuscles of the duck's bill, the ramifications of the motor end plate, etc. A soft mass can accumulate around the end of the respective fibres, as in motor end plates, or it may, if the nerves project into the connective tissue, form a more or less complicated system of capsules which lends a somatic character to the end-apparatus. The example of the end apparatus provided with connective tissue capsules (Pacini's corpuscles, end bulbs, tactile corpuscles, touch spherules, etc.) is therefore of particular interest because it demonstrates that a kind of stimulus is exercised on the part of the nerves, upon the environment at the terminal site, and this causes the accumulation of special cell layers. In the special sense organs, in the retina, and in the auditory, gustatory, and olfactory organs, according to the more recent observations by G. Retzius, Schwalbe *et al.*, we do not get beyond the projection of the nerve fibrils in the vicinity of the so-called sensory cells, and we must ultimately resign ourselves to consider the possibility of a transmitted stimulus to these organs without direct continuity.

The motor end plates are an unquestionable example of a stimulus transmitted without continuity of substance between it and the centrifugally conducting nerves. It can even be shown that Kühne's end plate (*Sohle* [see p. 77]) is inserted here as a separating, intermediate layer, between the endings of the axis cylinders which terminate in stumps, and the muscle.

I believe that one can also arrive at simple concepts regarding the nervous system if one abandons the idea that nerve fibres, in order to affect a part, must necessarily be in continuity with each other. For the development of a fibre, the law of insulated conduction is incontestable; however, if a fibre ends, because it is stopped short, new conditions for transmitting the stimulus prevail at the stump. The multiplicity of stumps, as shown by Kühne's motor end plate ramifications, gains special significance from this point of view. However, if the concept of the importance of the stimulus transmitted by a nerve stump is justified, the continuity between two tracts is not mandatory for the explanation of the influence of one fibre system upon another; it suffices that both end stumps project into the same medullary area and that an intermediate substance which can transmit the stimulus [synapse] be inserted between. If we select as an example the fibres of the pyramidal tracts, their influence upon [spinal root and peripheral nerve] motor fibres remains understandable if we can prove that they end in the vicinity of the motor [anterior horn] cells as simple or branching stumps, and that they appear to move close to the terminations of the branching processes of the cell. Each of the bilateral tract systems is complete until its ending; but between the two ends the medullary stroma, along with its interstices, is inserted as an open area, and here the spread, for instance, of chemical processes can occur in very different directions.

Gerlach, with whose concepts I concur on several points, postulates a nerve plexus within the gray substance as an intermediate structure between fibres and cells [see p. 89]. However, proof for such a plexus cannot be obtained, either from his own observations or from those of others, since what can be positively seen and what Gerlach also shows in illustrations [see fig. 24] is always a richly branching plexus of cell processes only, without actual anastomosis of the decussating branches. If a generally conducting, intermediate mass is now inserted in one or another between the nerve tracts which end separately, the conclusion follows that, within a certain area, the stimulus which is transmitted by a neighboring tract can be communicated to various adjacent pathways. On the basis of this same presumption, it is likewise conceivable that, with an inhibition of conduction in nearer tracts, the more distantly located ones may take over the conduction. The physiological experiences concerning the transmitting status of the spinal cord are not at all favorable to a strict application of the principle of isolated transmission and, at least within the gray substance, the potential radius of transmission is so large that it is hardly possible to succeed with the concept of completely separate tracts.

The comments expressed above which partly agree with the assumptions of Golgi, based on histological investigations, in no way pretend to pass summary judgment on the overall problem of central and peripheral nerve endings, but I believe that I am justified in reviving the discussion with a new series of questions. In consequence I defend the following postulate as an indisputable principle: *that each nerve fibre originates as a process from a single cell. This is its genetic, nutritive, and functional center; all other connections of the fibre are either indirect or secondary.*

On the 21st of May of the following year, His read an important paper ("Über die embryonale Entwickelung der Nervenbahnen," *Anat. Anz.* 1888, 3:499–506) to a meeting of the Anatomical Society at Würzburg. In it he summarized his findings in thirteen succinct points, and the main statements of ten of them have been translated below. He considered the microscopic structure of the nervous system and its development in terms of his concept of independent nerve cell bodies and fibre units.

EXCERPT PP. 501–504

(1) There is a period in embryonic life when no nerve fibres exist, either central or peripheral.

(2) The motor cells [*sic. Zellen*, presumably *fibres*] originate as processes from specific cells of the spinal cord and brain.

(3) The axis cylinder processes [axons] appear as primary processes of the motor cells; the branching processes [dendrites] are formed considerably later.

(4) From an early time, the motor cells display a fibrillary, striped body and the streaking is continued into the relatively broad axis cylinder [neurofibrils].

(5) The motor cells of both the spinal cord and brain are situated in a quite specific part of the medullary tube [i.e., brain and spinal cord].

(6) All motor nerve roots [i.e., fibres] arise from mantle cells [anterior horn cells] in the ventral part of the tube, but not all the cells of that part send their axons into the motor roots.

(7) . . . .

(8) The cells of the spinal ganglia at first do not have long processes [axons]. A stage follows when the cell is bipolar, and later it is characterized by two fibrillary axis cylinder processes which leave the cell in different directions. The cell is in a position eccentric to them.

(8 [*sic*]) The central processes of the spinal ganglion cells grow towards the medullary tube [spinal cord] and remain mainly near its surface in the form of a longitudinal tract.

(9) The sensory roots [i.e., fibres] which grow into the spinal cord make up the primary posterior column. In the brain the so-called ascending

roots [pneumogastric, glossopharyngeal, etc.] are equivalent to the posterior column formation of the cord.

(10) Not all sensory root fibres of the medullary tube grow simultaneously.

August-Henri Forel
(1 September 1848—27 July 1931)

Almost immediately, within two months in fact, Wilhelm His's histogenic studies, which gave proof of the independence of the nerve cell and its processes, were corroborated by independent observations that had employed an entirely different approach. These were made by a fellow Swiss, August Forel.

Forel was born near Morges, on the shore of Lake Geneva. He studied medicine at Zürich and was greatly influenced by the writings of the neuroanatomist and psychiatrist, Bernhard von Gudden (pp. 606–611). After having been graduated in 1871, Forel studied with Meynert in Vienna (p. 433) and then with Gudden in Munich. In 1879 he was appointed professor of psychiatry in the University of Zürich and director of the Burgholzli Asylum where he remained until his retirement in 1898. His work covered many problems of neuroanatomy and psychiatry as well as philosophy, biology, temperance, pacificism, and socialism (see Forel, 1935, 1937; Haymaker, 1953, pp. 35–38; Buess, 1964.

Forel's paper "Einige hirnanatomische Betrachtungen und Ergebnisse" (*Arch. Psychiat. NervKrankh.*, 1887, 18:162–198) was based upon observations made with Golgi's method of staining and with the technique of retrograde degeneration, first used by his teacher Gudden. It was the utilization of the latter technique that made Forel's contribution important, although his accurate and critical analysis of other investigators' findings was of equal importance. His remarkable keenness of perception allowed him to separate the facts from the hypotheses, of which there were many. He admitted that his paper was fragmentary and incomplete and that he wished only "to emphasize certain opinions which seem to me to point in the right direction" rather than to enunciate "conclusive theories which for the most part always turn out to be erroneous as soon as our knowledge becomes expanded" (p. 195). It is not easy, however, to abstract or to select representative passages from this paper. The following are the principles established in it, although Forel did not summarize them himself:

1) A nerve network does not exist, and each nerve cell is in contact with, but not in continuity with, its neighbor. This has been called the Contact Theory of Forel.

2) Nerve fibres originate only from cells.

3) In view of this, a fibre will degenerate if the cell is damaged, and, contrary to Waller's conclusions (pp. 71–75), the reverse may also take place.

In other words, both actions are governed by the general laws of cell vitality. The various types of degeneration produced by animal experiment are thus accounted for; if a fibre termination in the central nervous system is cut where regeneration is impossible, the whole cell will atrophy slowly and, in the case of the newborn at least, it will degenerate and disappear. But Forel's primary evidence for independent nerve units was found in the fact that the process of degeneration was restricted to the unit that had been directly damaged. In a way, therefore, this was the reverse of the evidence of His who had declared that nerve cells and fibres grew as a unit; now Forel could demonstrate that this was also true for degeneration. These two Swiss anatomists, whose work was remarkably complementary, can thus be considered as the originators of what Waldeyer (pp. 113–117) in 1891 called the *neuron theory*. It was the first important challenge to Golgi's network theory.

After having fully reviewed Golgi's work, Forel then argued against the existence of the nerve network. He pointed out that even Golgi was not completely certain of its occurrence and, as already mentioned, nowhere did Golgi figure the plexus he postulated.

EXCERPT PP. 165–166

Now, where do we stand in relation to the *a priori* assumptions which still exist in the most recent textbooks and reports, that the ganglion cells represent, so to speak, nodal points (*Knotenpunkte*) between fibre systems? Although for the most part, one no longer thinks of Schroeder's naive illustrations in this connection, nevertheless, one hears again and again discussion of the interruption of a fibre system by a gray nucleus; and most workers tacitly assume that apparently each ganglion cell is associated with at least two nerve fibres; that these, if not directly, yet indirectly are in direct *continuity* with nerve fibres by means of a fibre net, despite the fact that no certain evidence exists on this matter. One might point out, however, the so-called T-shaped division of the process of the spinal ganglion cells. But if it does exist, it must in any case be interpreted quite differently, because of Veja's experimental work which he did under von Gudden's direction; and there can no longer be any doubt concerning the transition into a nerve fibre of the branch which is directed towards the spinal cord. He asserts that he has recently observed in the embryo that the sensory fibres grow from the spinal ganglion towards the spinal cord. However, this may be just as well explained by the fact that they simply pass through the ganglion rather than that they originate in its cells.

If however we pay more heed to comparative histology and embryology, we must arrive at quite different viewpoints. The nervous system which, as is well known, originates in epiplastic cells, is present in the lowest animals, first in the shape of isolated ganglia and neuroepithelial cells. The nerves are merely outgrowths of epithelial cells. To the best of my knowledge, no one has yet seen, in the development of the nerve elements of vertebrates, any reliable anastomotic processes between the outgrowths of the ganglion cells, the fibres [axons], or the protoplasmic processes [dendrites] of one element, with those of others. Even the manner in which the nerve attaches itself to the muscle fibre, the so-called nerve ending in the transversely striated muscle, is a kind of cementing and does not represent a direct continuity.

But now the fibre plexus. One ordinarily imagines it to be a true network, the most delicate branches of which are in direct continuity among themselves, but even Golgi's method cannot establish this point definitively, and Golgi expresses himself with extreme caution in this matter. The most delicate little branches of the nerve fibre are, after all, much too thin for it to be certain whether they can be seen lying on top of each other or anastomosing with one another, when the branches of some of the elements meet. However, when such enormous ramifications of the elements, which Golgi's method exhibits, meet, they must, of necessity, anastomose with each other in such manner that a dreadful feltlike maze must result, even if they do not form a genuine plexus of fibres. This felt could thus be a *phantom net*. And, indeed, how could we possibly imagine such a process in which these very delicate and innumerable cell processes, which originally were not connected with each other, should all meet exactly with their free endings in order to coalesce into a continuous network? Such an idea becomes even more improbable if we consider that this plexus of fibres must develop still further during the years of development, and this, after all, would not be easy to imagine in the case of a true anastomosis.

Gradually, I can see less and less reason why an actual, continuous union of the finest little branches of the nervous elements ought to be a physiological postulate. If the branches of the trees of the various nerve elements interlock in the manner they actually do, this is quite sufficient for the transmission of stimuli. Electricity gives us such innumerable examples of similar transmissions without direct continuity that it could well be the same in the nervous system.

I like to assume that all fibre systems and the so-called fibre net of the nervous system are nothing else than mere nerve processes, each of an individual ganglion cell. The nerve process proceeds from its base in the cell. It then branches in various ways and gives off fibrils at different points. Some are not far away [from the cell] (cells of the second [Golgi] category), some are both close to it and at a greater distance, but they remain temporarily united as medullary fibres. Ultimately [the branching] always takes the shape of extensively ramified, interlocked trees, but anastomosing [is found] nowhere.

In the following passage, Forel pointed out that the optic pathway is made up of two parts. The first carried the retinal cell fibres via the optic nerve, chiasma, and tract to the lateral geniculate body, and here the second part took over and the fibres of cells, which began among the ramifications of the retinal cell axons, ran via the optic radiation to the visual cortex. This basic arrangement of the visual system was vital evidence in favor of cell and fibre units in contiguity, not continuity, with each other.

EXCERPT PP. 170–171

As is well known, von Monakow demonstrated that a principal center of the optic system, the external geniculate body, can be made to atrophy by [lesions of] the eye (as von Gudden demonstrated) as well as by [lesions of] a specific area of the cerebral cortex. Earlier, von Gudden emphasized the occurrence of atrophy following removal of the entire hemisphere. But, according to von Monakow, it atrophies differently in each case. With the extirpation of the cortex, *all its cells are destroyed;* with the removal of the eye, in the main only the *gelatinous ground substance* is destroyed, especially in the so-called dorsal nucleus [of the external geniculate body], so that the cells lie closer together. Certainly the assumption therefore becomes obvious that visual fibres terminate as processes of the ganglion cells of the retina with treelike branching in the external geniculate body. A second fibre system would then proceed from the cells of the external geniculate body to the cortex of the visual [cortical] area (*Sehsphäre*), that is, the cuneus as Seguin has established (the so-called optic radiation), and it probably terminates there, too, in treelike ramifications. The atrophy starting at the cortex, when all cells and their processes are destroyed, is in any case by far the more severe. According to von Monakow, the external geniculate body atrophies almost to the size of a pinpoint, stains dark with carmine, and exhibits the remains of the atrophied elements. This speaks in favor of its cells belonging to his first category. I have carried out this experiment, too, in a rat, although slightly incomplete, and I have confirmed the results mentioned. Thus, the treelike branchings of the optic [retinal] fibres would probably transmit the optic stimuli to the cell system of the external geniculate body and through it to the visual cortex, probably by intimate contiguity, but without direct continuity according to our assumption, provided it is correct.

Forel's work was based upon the phenomenon of nerve degeneration, and his findings advanced the relatively simple concepts of Waller (pp. 71–75). For example, it was fundamental to Forel's work that cell atrophy followed axonal injury; the slow cellulipetal degeneration had been discovered by his teacher Gudden, and is sometimes known as Gudden's Law (pp. 608–609). The following are some of Forel's general statements on the matter, concluded by further applications of them to fibre pathways and nuclei. He thus provided additional evidence for neuronal units, rather than an interlocked plexus.

EXCERPT PP. 181–184

It seems to me that all these processes can be easily explained if we consider the nerve such as it is, a process of the ganglion cell. If one excises a small piece from a lower organism, it regenerates. Even the fingers of tritons and the tail of the lizard regenerate. However, if the part which has grown again and regenerated can no longer function, it gradually shrivels up, and this is probably the case with the regeneration of motor nerves. If a fibre, because of section (as in our case), is prevented from reaching the muscle again, or if the muscle has been removed, the entire element, the entire nerve cell, loses its function, and it disintegrates gradually like the muscle proper, albeit very slowly. However, if in a lower organism, too large a part of the body is severed, the entire organism dies as well as the extirpated part. It seems to me that this latter process is very similar to the one which occurs in the nucleus, the root, and in the peripheral part of the extirpated nerve. If these operations are carried out in the newborn animal, the products of death resorb very rapidly and completely because of the extremely active adjacent life. On principle, this is probably the only difference. Lastly, if a fibre is cut close to its peripheral end, the extirpated portion constitutes a small fragment of the element which, despite deficient function, can remain alive much more easily.

. . . . I presume, to put it very simply, that the cell of origin of the degenerated fibre is found on that side which does not degenerate, and even, perhaps, at a greater distance from the severed area, so that the fibre can stay alive. However, such maintenance of life is best explained when the sectioned fibre does not contain almost all of the fibrils of the nerve process but when a large portion of these ramifications has still other destinations which are capable of maintaining the cell, partially or completely, alive. There also seem to be differences depending on whether the process takes place in the newborn or in the adult. Owing to the rapid resorption, a rapid atrophy is produced in the former, with or without minute residuals only, whereas in the adult these residuals cause the so-called "secondary" degeneration [Wallerian]. In addition, in the newborn, too, the cells of the surface of the fibre sometimes seem to atrophy jointly with the cell proper, which does not happen in the adult under the same circumstances. However, in this respect I have become very suspicious and am convinced that comparable experiments are of prime necessity. I presume that in those cases in which this degeneration of the element takes place in the newborn, it would, for the most part, be the same in the adult, as seen by experiment. And now I also believe that this destruction of the cell does not always take place in the newborn . . . .

It is well known that the pyramidal tract degenerates downwards only.

Evidently it therefore originates in ganglion cells of the first type [Golgi] of the cerebral cortex, as is also evident from von Gudden's experiments and those of von Monakow . . . .

If one excises the superior peduncle of the cerebellum, as Laufer and I have demonstrated, a partial atrophy of the opposite red nucleus of the tegmentum begins. One sees here again shrinkage of ganglion cells, owing perhaps to the fact that they are only partially dependent on the fibre, for the cells do not stain paler, they are simply smaller. In this respect, too, it seems very important to explore the size of the pyramid and its fibres long after the pyramidal tract has been severed in the spinal cord.

The fact is that atrophies which are undoubtedly entirely central and which von Gudden produced by intervention in the newly born animal also occur in the adult following destructions, if only in a less marked form. Thus, I have convinced myself above all that each of the more extensive lesions of the cerebral hemisphere in man, when it has existed for any length of time, is followed, according to its location, by a marked atrophy of this or that portion of the thalamus. This is confirmed by von Gudden's and von Monakow's findings in the newly born animal [pp. 608–609].

An interesting illustration of my assumption is seen in the relation of the nucleus of the Funiculus gracilis (so-called Goll's tract) to the fibres which lead to it . . . . I conclude from these facts that the cells of origin of the Funiculus gracilis lie probably caudal in the spinal cord and that its fibres in its so-called nucleus probably have treelike branchings only; and, finally, that the cells of this so-called nucleus dispatch the main branch of their nerve process through the cortical lemniscus to the cerebral cortex. In any event I should like to note that, according to Spitzka, the cortical lemniscus degenerates downwards (perhaps also upwards), while the Funiculus gracilis is destroyed cephalad only.

Santiago Ramón y Cajal
(1 May 1852—17 October 1934)

While His and Forel were developing their ideas concerning the individuality of nerve cells, unknown to them a Spanish histologist, Ramón y Cajal, using Golgi's staining method and modifications of it, was working on the same problem. When Cajal published his important paper, "Estructura de los centros nerviosos de los aves" (*Rev. trimest. Histol. norm. patol.*, 1888, 1:305–315), he had not read the work of his Swiss contemporaries but was making an independent attack on Golgi's net theory; nevertheless, his purely histological findings amply confirmed the results of the Swiss investigators. The concept of the independence of nerve units had thus been examined by three quite different techniques and the answer was the same in each case: there seemed to be no evidence for Golgi's net.

Ramón y Cajal, son of a surgeon of modest means, was born in the small village of Petilla de Aragon in the province of Navarre, northeastern Spain. In 1873 he was graduated in medicine from the University of Zaragoza where in 1877 he was appointed temporarily as professor of anatomy. His interests soon turned to histology, however, and during the period 1884 to 1892 he passed from Zaragoza to Valencia, from Valencia to Barcelona, and from Barcelona to Madrid. It was in Barcelona, and particularly in Madrid, that his outstanding studies of the nervous system were carried out. Cajal's work was not known to the rest of Europe until 1889, but thereafter he became one of the acknowledged masters of neurohistology and founded a school at the Laboratorio de Investigaciones Biológicas of the University of Madrid. Among many awards, in 1906 he shared with Golgi the Nobel Prize for Medicine and Physiology (see Ramón y Cajal, 1923, 1937; Sherrington, 1935; Cannon, 1949; Haymaker, 1953, pp. 74–77; Kolle, 1956–1963, I, 27–38; Freund and Berg, 1963–1964, II, 311–325).

The ingenuity, the acuity of observation, the tireless energy, and the immense patience of Ramón y Cajal allowed him to carry out remarkably extensive investigations of the morphology of the nerve cell and its processes, of degeneration and regeneration, and of the neuroglia. By means of his work he established more certainly than ever before the independence of nerve units. The first occasion on which he emphatically supported this theory and effectively attacked the nerve net concept of Golgi was in the paper of 1888 cited above. There he described the cortical cells of the cerebellum and, in particular, observed that the cells of the molecular layer which formed "baskets" around the Purkyně cells were in contiguity with them but not in continuity. This was in fact the first direct evidence of actual contact between nerve cells and of the manner in which an adult axon terminates. It was also in this paper that he demonstrated that the afferent, so-called climbing fibres were in intimate contact with the dendrites of the Purkyně cells, thus refuting Golgi's suggestion that the latter were for nutritional purposes only. This evidence and that concerning the contact between cells and fibres formed the foundation of Cajal's later theory of dynamic polarization of the nerve cell. His later (1894) and more detailed account of the cerebellar cortex will be found on pages 122 to 124.

The first excerpt presented below is from the article of 1888, already mentioned, and the second, in which the author discussed his findings, has been taken from a paper which appeared on the 15th of August of the same year ("Estructura del cerebelo," *Gac. méd. Catalana*, 1888, 11:449–457), the contents of which are very similar to the earlier publication.

EXCERPT PP. 309–310

2. *Starlike cells* [basket cells of the molecular layer of the cerebellar cortex]. They are small, globular, and irregular, situated at different levels in the thickness of the molecular layer, and supplied with numerous protoplasmic prolongations [dendrites]. The special character of these cells is the

striking arrangement of their nerve filament [cylinder or axon], which arises from the cell body but also very often from any thick, protoplasmic expansion [dendrite]. It immediately adopts a horizontal position, runs for a considerable distance through the molecular layer, and is supplied with numerous branches, some ascending and others descending. The ascending ones are delicate, and after various ramifications they end in the molecular layer in a manner as yet unknown, but perhaps by terminating freely since we have been unable to find anastomoses between these fibres and the branches of the *cylinders* [axons] of more superficial cells. The small descending branches are always given off at a certain [right] angle along the length of the nerve prolongations (pl. 1, fig. 1, *L* [fig. 31]); they descend, growing visibly in size, and branching at acute angles, and they terminate in tufts of short, varicose fibres [the baskets] that completely envelope the bodies of the Purkyně cells [pl. 1, fig. 1, *A*]. On account of their abundance and thickness, these fringes [baskets] form a true layer in the transitional zone between the molecular and granular layers. The fibres that form them do not anastomose among themselves and, as it appears, end freely [pointing] downwards after they have become considerably thickened and varicose (pl. 1, fig. 1, *C*).

In numerous preparations we have never been able to find the prolongation of one of these varicose fibres of the fringes extending deeper than the granular layer [pl. 1, fig. 1, *B*]. With regard to the termination of the [horizontal] *cylinder* [axon], it appears to take place through a descending fringe somewhat stouter than the others, but without any new features. This singular way in which the *cylinder* ends and these same arrangements of descending fringes or tassels are found in man. But in man the fringes contain fewer fibres (two or three somewhat larger and uneven), and the arcs formed by the *cylinder* in its horizontal direction are much more delicate or incomplete. We are not astonished that Golgi has not mentioned these features, since we ourselves learned to see them in mammals only after having discovered them in birds. For the sake of completeness we may describe a very frequent arrangement of the *cylinder*. Immediately after its origin, it carries out a complete and horizontal circle around the cell; sometimes it is a semicircle so that the fibre goes in the opposite direction; finally, on some occasions these circles, or more or less extended arcs, occur at the termination of the *cylinder* (pl. 1, fig. 1, *O*).

EXCERPT PP. 455–457

3. *Connections of the cerebellar elements*. This is a difficult question and the solution is impossible since only limited and extremely incomplete data are available. The technique of Golgi, which is so excellent for staining the protoplasmic extensions [dendrites] of the nerve cells, is very inconstant

in the case of the nerve prolongations [axons] because almost invariably they appear to be cut off. An opinion concerning the course and connections of this fibre cannot be made without a comparative study of a large number of good preparations.

The first result that we obtained in the preparations of the cerebellum of the bird was the same as in mammals; the nerve cells do not anastomose directly, that is, by means of their protoplasmic expansions. This phenomenon [anastomosis], which is so much against our physiological and anatomical theories concerning the connections of the nerve centers, has not escaped Golgi, who in some way or other finds an explanation and establishes in the substance of the gray matter of the centers [brain and cord], a network of axis cylinders (the small branches of the prolongations of Deiters [terminal branches of dendrites]) and of the nerve fibres [axons] which is called the *diffuse net* through which the cells can be directly joined together. We have made careful investigations of the course and connections of nerve fibres in the cerebral and cerebellar convolutions of man, monkey, dog, etc., and we have never seen an anastomosis between the ramifications of two different protoplasmic expansions, nor have we observed them between the filaments emanating from the expansions of Deiters [i.e., from axons]; the fibres intermingle in a very complex manner, producing a thick and intricate plexus but never a net. The observations which we have just explained, concerning the structure of the avian cerebellum, also support this viewpoint; it could be said that each element is an absolutely autonomous physiological canton. This is not to deny indirect anastomosis (by branches of the filaments of Deiters) but to affirm simply that never having seen them, we dismiss them from our opinion.

A problem no less difficult and closely related to the previous question is the investigation of the connections that Deiters' prolongations [dendrites] which have lost their individuality, make with the fibres of the white matter. It is well known that in the cerebellum there are cells of the motor type (those of Purkyně), of which the cylinder [axon] preserves its identity as far as the white matter [pl. 1, fig. 1, B]; and the cells in which it is not preserved (the little starlike cells, large starlike cells, and dwarf corpuscles [granule cells]) are the ones, if we accept Golgi's hypothesis, that can be considered as sensory. But when are the descending fringes [baskets] continuous with the fibres of the white matter, and which of the infinite fibres into which the cylinder [axon] of the large starlike cells [basket cells] is divided, are continuous with a nerve fibre? This is what we have been unable to determine. Undoubtedly many of the varicose and branching fibres of the descending fringes [baskets] are terminal arborizations, since they constantly present the same appearances as the discontinuous globules

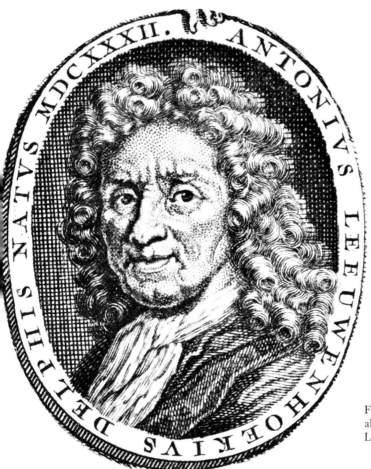

Fig. 1. Antony van Leeuwenhoek at about 85 years. From frontispiece to Leeuwenhoek (1719).

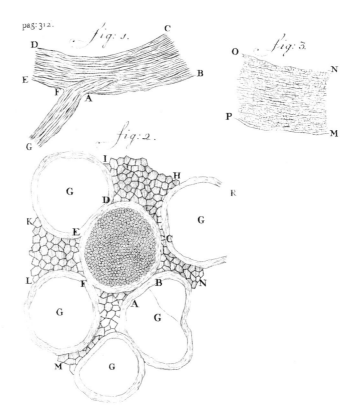

Fig. 2. Leeuwenhoek (1719, facing p. 312). 1, longitudinal section of peripheral nerve; 2, transverse section of same; 3, longitudinal section of spinal cord. For explanation see text (p. 33).

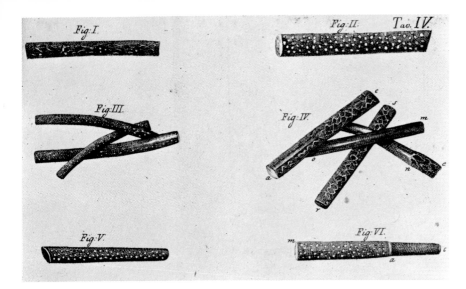

FIG. 3. Fontana (1781, Plate IV, figs. 1–6). For explanation see text (p. 37).

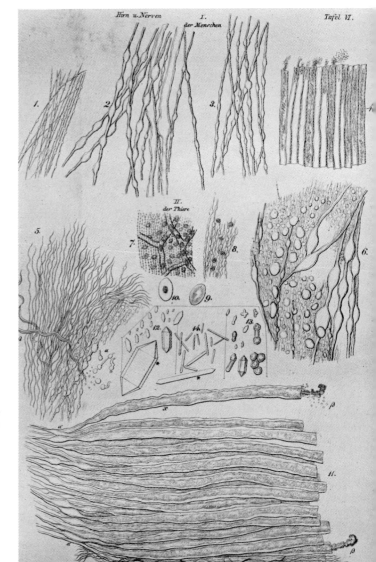

FIG. 4. Ehrenberg (1833, Plate VI, fig. 11). For explanation see text (p. 39).

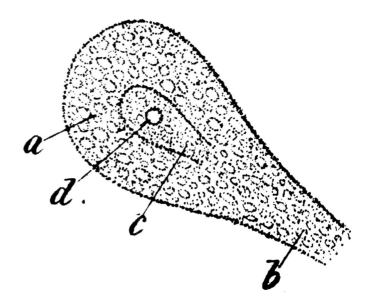

Fig. 5. Valentin (1836, Plate VII, fig. 54). Cell from human cerebellar cortex: *a*, parenchyma; *b*, tail-like appendage; *c*, nucleus; *d*, small corpuscle (nucleolus).

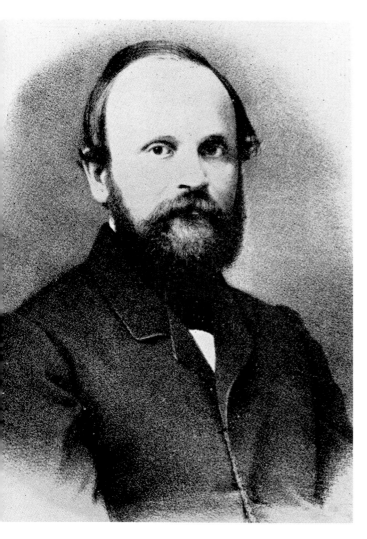

Fig. 6. Robert Remak, later than 1859. From *Naissance et déviation de la théorie cellulaire dans l'oeuvre de Théodore Schwann*, by M. Florkin, Paris & Liège, 1960, p. 70. Courtesy of Professor Florkin.

FIG. 7. Remak (1836, Plate IV, fig. 5). Cutaneous nerve, four-week-old rabbit, X 300: *a*, site of accidental damage; *b*, constriction, often seen on fibres; *c*, varicose fibres; *d*, crossing fibres; *e*, fibre without medulla (fibre of Remak); *f*, myelinated fibre.

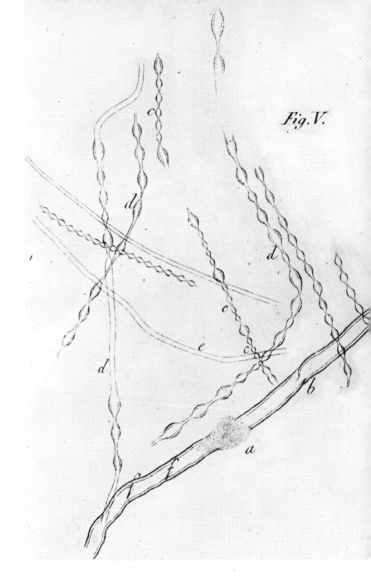

Fig. V.

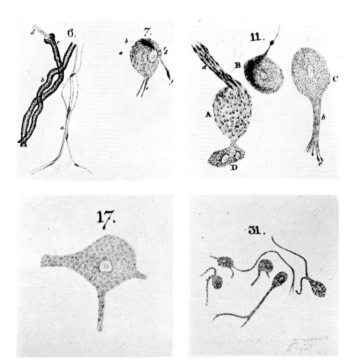

FIG. 8. Remak (1838, Plate I, figs. 6–7, 11; Plate II, figs. 17, 31). Fig. 6, from posterior lumbar root of sheep, X c. 200: *a*, organic fibre, *b, c*, primitive tube, *d*, extruded myelin; fig. 7, globule from sympathetic ganglion of ox: *a*, parenchyma, *b*, pigment spots, *c*, nucleus, *d*, nucleolus, *e, f*, organic fibres leaving cell; fig. 11, globules from spinal ganglion of calf with originating organic fibres *a*, and *b*, X c. 200; fig. 17, globule from *substantia spongiosa* of pigeon cord with originating fibre, X c. 200; fig. 31, globules from yellow substance of ox with branching fibres, X c. 75.

Fig. 9. Remak (1844, Plate XII, figs. 8–9). For explanation see text (p. 49).

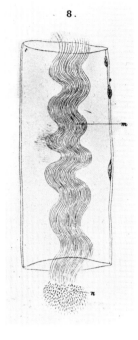

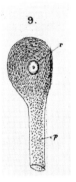

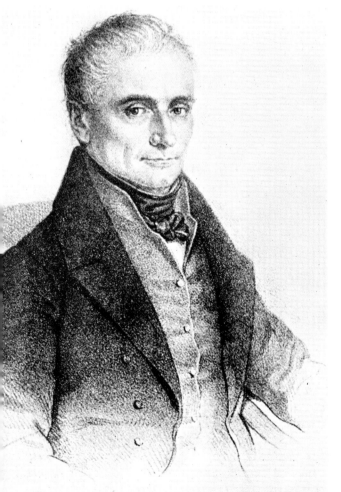

Fig. 10. Jan Evangelista Purkyně. By permission, National Library of Medicine.

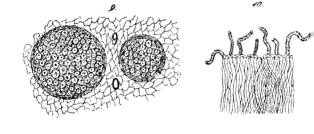

Fig. 11. Purkyně (1837, facing p. 174). For explanation see text (p. 54).

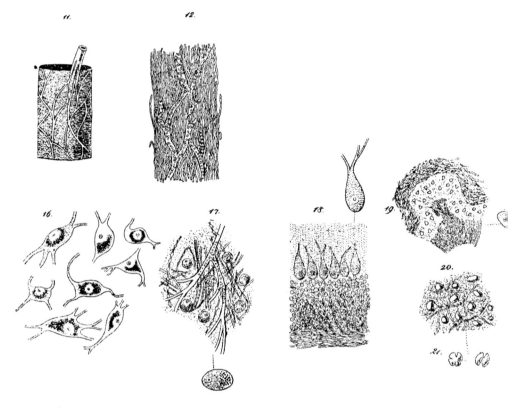

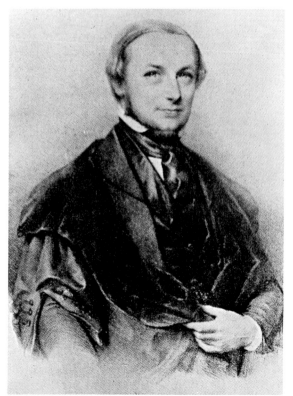

Fig. 12. Theodor Schwann in 1846. From same source as fig. 6. Courtesy of Professor Florkin.

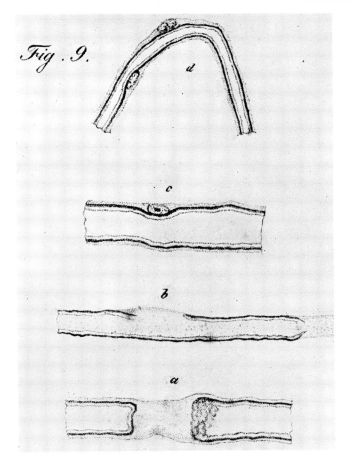

FIG. 13. Schwann (1839, Plate IV, fig. 9). For explanation see text (p. 58).

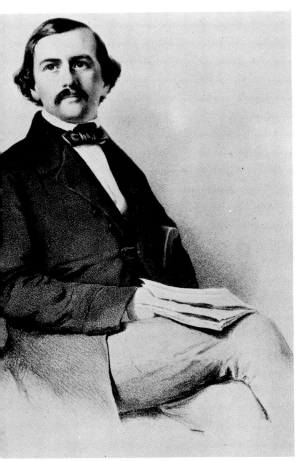

FIG. 14. Rudolf Albert von Koelliker. From *Recherches, découvertes et inventions de médecins suisses*, Bâle, Ciba SA, 1946, p. 67. By permission.

Fig. 15. Koelliker (1849, Plate XI). All figures X 350 and of animal origin: *a*, membrane of cells; *b*, contents; *c*, granular process; *d*, dark-bordered nerve tubes into which *c* extends; *e*, boundary of cell and fibre (neurilemmal sheath of Schwann).

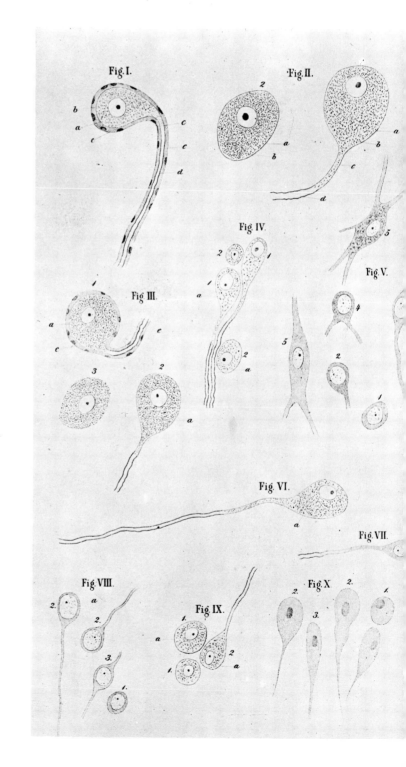

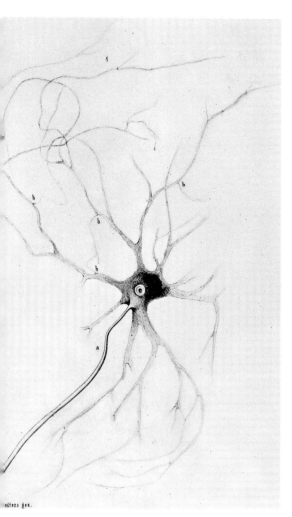

Fɪɢ. 16. Deiters (1865, Plate I, fig. 1).
Anterior horn cell: *a*, main axis cylinder; *b*, fine axis cylinders arising from
protoplasmic processes; dark yellow pigment in cell.

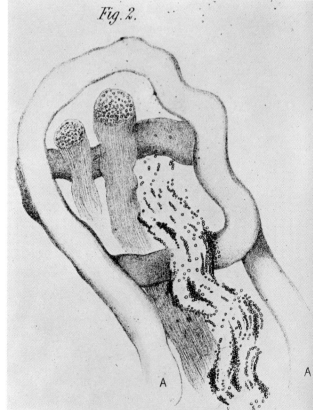

Fɪɢ. 17. Waller (1850, Plate XXXI,
fig. 2). Papillary nerve of frog after
section; muscle fibres inside capillary
coil at summit of fungiform papilla.
For explanation see text (p. 73).

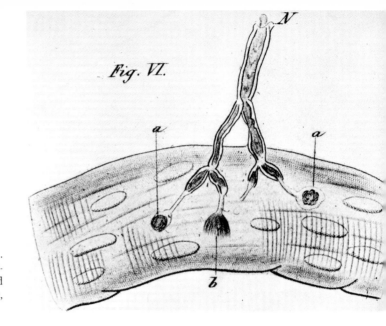

FIG. 18. Kühne (1862, Plate I, fig. 6).
Frog muscle fibre with marked alteration of substance. Nerve branches end
in single end bulb, *a, a*; *b*, brushlike,
disintegrated bulb.

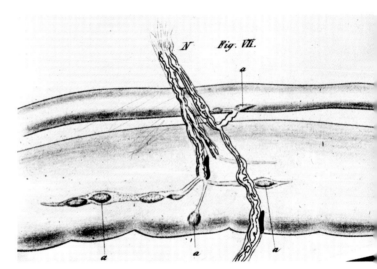

FIG. 19. Kühne (1862, Plate II, fig.
7). Two muscle fibres from frog's sartorius treated as described in text (p.
76). End bulbs of nerve *a, a*, float
free in fluid fibre contents; remains of
its nucleus omitted.

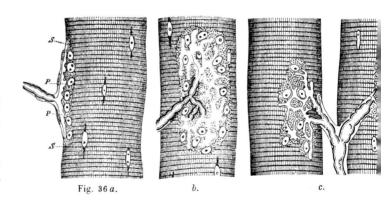

FIG. 20. Kühne (1871, p. 159, fig.
36). Muscle fibres with nerve endings
from *Lacerta viridis*: *a*, profile; *pp*, end
plate; *ss*, base (sole) of plate consisting of granular mass and nuclei; *b*,
fresh muscle fibre, probably still excitable; contours of branched plate not
shown; *c*, after death of nerve end—
two hours after giving curare.

Fig. 21. Ranvier (1872). Large sciatic nerve fibres of adult rabbit one hour after removal from 1:100 ammonium picrocarminate solution: *a*, annular constriction; *m*, myelin that has become granular; *cy*, stained axon now visible; at X 600 double boundary [axolemma] seen.

Fig. 22. Nissl (1894, pp. 678–683, figs. 1–6). Normal, adult rabbit cells, Nissl's stain. X Zeiss 2.0, Homog. Immers. Apert, 1.30. Fig. 1, anterior horn cell; fig. 2, enarkyochrome cell from dorsal nucleus of proximal medulla; fig. 3, cervical spinal ganglion cell; fig. 4, arkyochrome olfactory bulb cell; fig. 5, Ammon's horn cell; fig. 6, Purkyně cell. (Footnote, pp. 678–679, Nissl details inaccuracies: cell boundaries too clear-cut; too much contrast of unstained parts, stained parts too sharply outlined, nuclei poorly seen because of inadequate staining.)

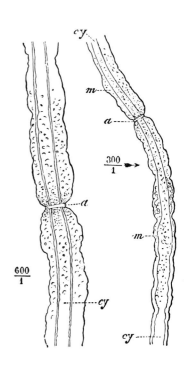

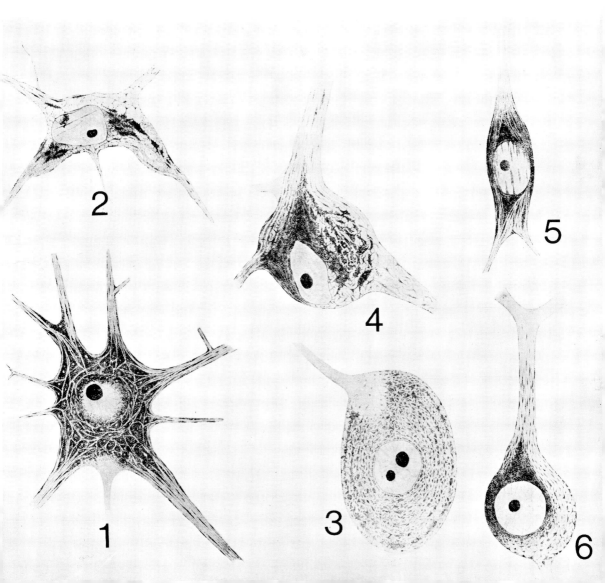

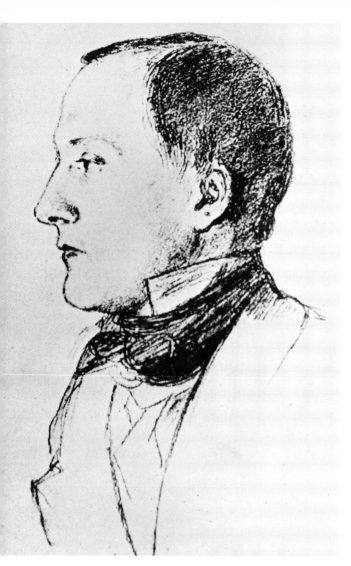

Fig. 23. Rudolf Virchow, 2 February 1849. Courtesy of Prof. Dr. R. Rabl, grandson of Virchow.

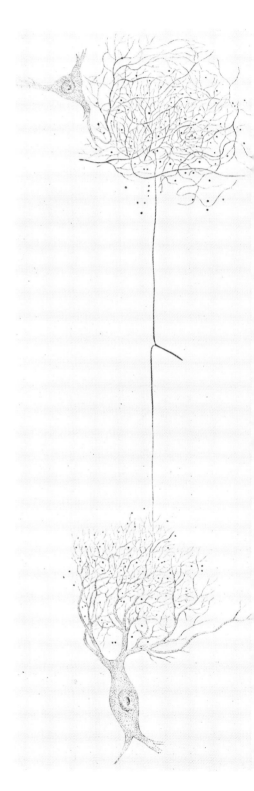

Fig. 24. Gerlach, in Stricker (1872, p. 679, fig. 223). Spinal cord fibre of ox divides into two branches and this communicates with fibre plexuses of two cell bodies. Ammonium carminate, X 150.

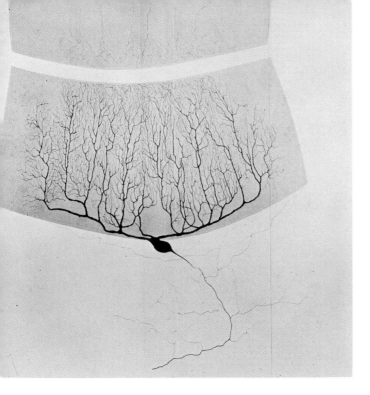

FIG. 25. Golgi (1883, Plate IV, Type I cell). Human Purkyně cell: dendritic branches subdivide continually and many reach limits of molecular layer. Axon provides many secondary fibrils, but maintains individuality; can be followed as thread of constant diameter to layer of axons (medullary fibres).

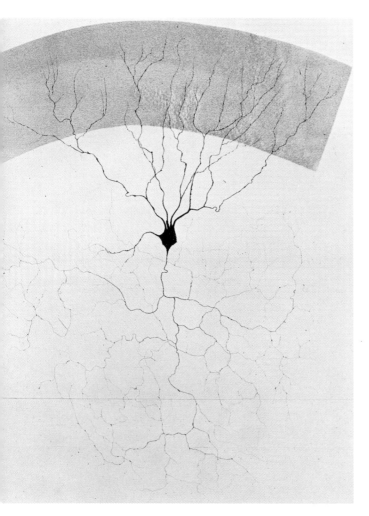

FIG. 26. Golgi (1883, Plate III, Type II cell). Cerebellar cortex, granular layer, newborn kitten: dendritic branches reach only to upper part of molecular layer; plentiful axonal branches form complex network filling all granular layer and horizontally it mingles closely with networks of other cells.

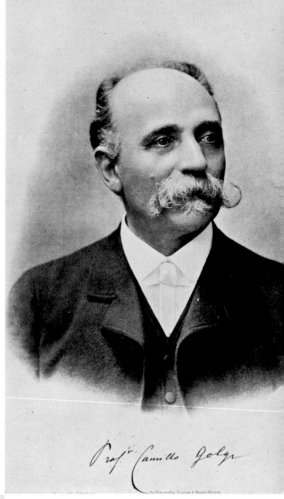

Fig. 27. Camillo Golgi. By permission of the Wellcome Trustees.

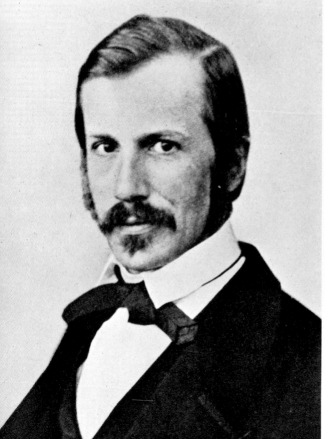

Fig. 28. Wilhelm His, Senior. From W. Kolb, *Geschichte des anatomischen Unterrichtes an der Universität zu Basel 1460–1900*, Basel, Schwabe, 1951, facing p. 116. By permission.

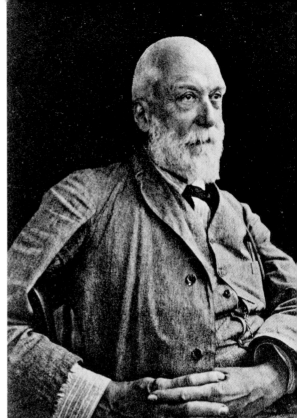

Fig. 29. August-Henri Forel.

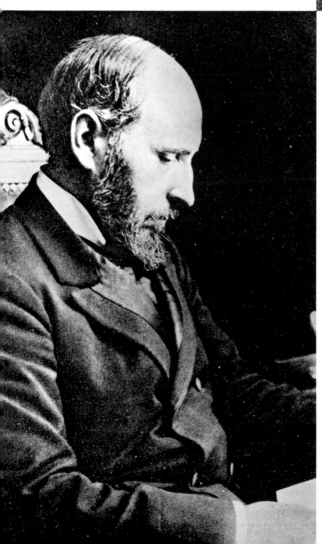

Fig. 30. Santiago Ramón y Cajal. From *Obit. Not. R. Soc.*, 1935, no. 4, facing p. 425. By permission of the Royal Society.

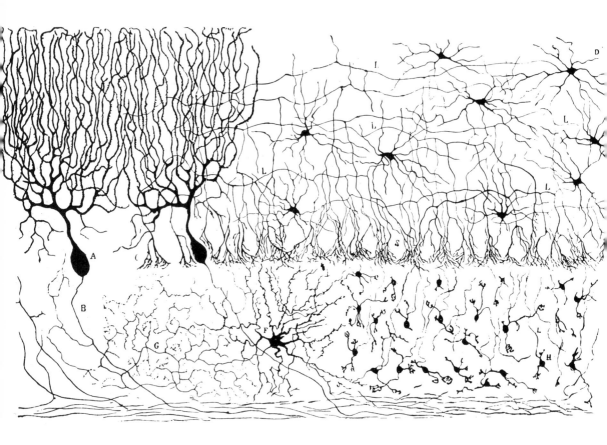

Fig. 31. Ramón y Cajal (1888, Plate I, fig. 1). Vertical section of cerebellar convolution of hen; Golgi method. A, molecular layer, B, granular layer, C, white matter. A, body of Purkyně cell, B, its axon, C, descending branch ending in arborization [basket], S, space made by this for Purkyně cell, H, dwarf cell of granular layer with cylinder, L, directed upwards. F, large star-shaped cell in the granular layer, G, its repeatedly branching axon.

which are peculiar to nerve endings; also it is certain that almost all the varicose and arcuate expansions that provide the lateral filaments of the nerve extension [axons] of the large starlike cells [basket cells] display a terminal arborization (analogous to that presented by the feet of the bipolar cells of the retina), but Golgi's method never reveals extension beyond this. There are one or two hypotheses here: either Golgi's method is insufficient to demonstrate the unifying bridges these fibres have with those of the white matter, or the connection between these and the axis cylinders is possible, and the transmission of the nerve action, like electrical currents from the inductor filaments upon the induced, is verified.

The fact that the descending branches of the axis cylinders of the starlike cells of the molecular layer approach the bodies of the Purkyně cells lends support to this latter hypothesis. The contacts between these [cells] and the aforesaid fibres (descending fringes [baskets]) are such and they are so numerous that it is possible to say that each of the Purkyně cells lies on a cushion of ramifications of the cylinder. Now then, could not these very extensive and intimate connections be the means which nature provides to allow the nerve current to pass from one cell to the other; for example, from the starlike [basket] cells that have hitherto been considered sensory, to those of Purkyně which have been supposed to be motor? Would it not be possible likewise to determine, as with the procedure of indirect contiguity, that those innumerable arcuate endings of the branches of the cylinder of the plump or starlike little bodies of the granular layer [pl. 1, fig. 1, F], that are never without them, stimulate the surface of the granular or dwarf cells? [pl. 1, fig. 1, H].

Although anatomy does not prove the existence of direct connections, this hypothesis of the transmission by contact appears as likely as any other, and has the advantage of harmonizing better with the discoveries that have been made in the structure of the central nervous system through the use of Golgi's black stain.

[HEINRICH] WILHELM [GOTTFRIED VON] WALDEYER [-HARTZ]
(6 October 1836—23 January 1921)

By 1891 the literature dealing with the morphology of the nerve cell and its processes had assumed formidable proportions. On the one hand there were those who carried on the work of His and Forel and maintained the independence of nerve units, the most ardent and active supporter being Ramón y Cajal. On the other there were the "reticularists" led by Golgi and his followers who upheld the existence of a nerve net. The time had now come for someone to analyze the evidence critically and from it to decide in favor of one or the other theory. It was Waldeyer, the German anatomist, who undertook this task, and although he made no individual contribution to the data already available, he was able to enunciate general laws. He concluded that the evidence favored the independent nerve unit, to which he applied the term *neuron*. This fundamental concept of the structure of nervous tissue thus became known as the *neuron doctrine*. Waldeyer had done little more than summarize a mass of data and provide a name. Nevertheless, the latter alone was an important advance, because once an anatomical structure has an appropriate and universally accepted name it is more readily acceptable as a conceptual entity. Furthermore, his famous article ("Über einige neuere Forschungen im Gebiete der Anatomie des Centralnervensystems," *Dt. med. Wschr.*, 1891, 17:1213–1218, 1244–1246, 1267–1269, 1287–1289, 1331–1332, and 1352–1356) probably did more than any other single publication to popularize the doctrine of the individuality of nerve elements in the nervous system. Thereafter the neuron doctrine received increasing acceptance. There were many, however, who felt that Waldeyer did not deserve the credit he later received; today one still reads of "the neuron theory of Waldeyer" (e.g., Gray's *Anatomy*, 32d ed. [London, 1958], p. 916). He should perhaps be considered as a persuasive promoter rather than as the originator of a theory. Ramón y Cajal, whose work more than that of anyone else paved the way for the acceptance of the theory, looked back with some bitterness and remarked that "all Waldeyer did was to publish in a weekly newspaper a résumé of my research and to invent the term 'neuron.' "

Waldeyer was born in Hehlen a.d. Weser in Braunschweig and studied at Göttingen and Berlin (1856–1862). He had already decided to devote himself to anatomy and so worked with Wittich at Königsberg and with Heidenhain at Breslau (now Wroclaw). In 1872 he became professor of normal anatomy and director of the Anatomical Institute at Strassburg and eleven years later moved to Berlin as director of the University's Anatomical Institute, which he completely reorganized. He had wide interests in anatomy and his numerous books and papers cover many areas of the field. He retired in 1917 at the age of eighty. As well as introducing the term "neuron," he also created the terms "chromosome" and "plasma cell" (see Waldeyer-Hartz, 1920; Fick, 1921; Sobotta, 1922; Freund and Berg, 1963–1964, II, 455–461).

The following selections have been taken from his paper of 1891, which was serialized between October and December of that year; they are from the final instalment, entitled "Summary and physiological observations."

EXCERPT PP. 1352–1354

I. The axis cylinders of all nerve fibres (motor, secretory, sensitive, and sensory, conducting centrifugally or centripetally) have been proved to proceed directly from the cells. A connection with a fibre network, or an origin from such a network, does not take place . . . .

II. *All these nerve fibres terminate freely with "end arborizations"* (*Kölliker*) *without network or anastomotic formation.*

Examples: The end branches of the motor fibres in the muscle fibres, the end branches of the pyramidal fibres in the spinal cord, the endings of the sensory fibres at the periphery (free nerve endings in the cornea, free nerve endings in the end corpuscles of nerves of the skin—Schwalbe, G. Retzius *et al.*—the exposed tactile disc of Grandry's corpuscles), as well as in the central organs (end branches of the sensory collaterals). Transmission therefore does not take place, as one might say, continuously, but, at the most, contiguously, by way of contact or by spreading from one free end to another . . . .

Regarding sentences one and two [*I* and *II* above] there are still certain difficulties regarding the sensory nerves if one wishes to enter into a more precise definition of the concept of "origin" and "end" of a nerve. In this connection, three distinct factors could prevail: *a*) physiological; *b*) topographic-anatomical; *c*) genetic. Physiologically, the origin of a nerve is evidently the location where the process of conduction, which normally takes its course in the nerve, originates; the end of a nerve is that place where it terminates when proceeding in this direction. Topographical, as well as descriptive anatomy, transfers the origin to the central organs, the end to the periphery. The genetic factor refers to the place from which a nerve fibre develops, the origin; the place where it stops in its further development, its end. For the motor and psychomotor fibres, all is now simple and clear since all three combine here . . . .

. . . . Let us set aside once and for all the varying concepts of "origin" and "end"; then all those investigators who do not assume a reticular connection of the nerve fibres within the central organs (Ramón y Cajal, Kölliker, His, Nansen, Lenhossek, Retzius) can easily consolidate sentences one and two [I and II above] into a general, concise and fundamental law of extreme importance. This would read as follows:

"The nervous system consists of numerous nerve units (neurons) connected with one another neither anatomically nor genetically. Each nerve unit is composed of three parts: the nerve cell, the nerve fibre, and the terminal arborizations. The physiological process of conduction can take place in the direction from cell to end arborizations, as well as in the reverse direction. Motor conduction takes place only in the direction from cell to terminal arborization, sensory conduction runs now in one, now in the other direction."

If we now look at the condition of the tracts which lead from the seat of conscious perception and conscious will to the periphery, we always find, as far as we are now aware, several neurons, at least two in these tracts. For example, only two should exist for the pyramidal tract: the one nerve unit after decussating, extends from a ganglion cell of the cerebral cortex, to the end arborizations in the gray matter of the spinal cord [upper motor neuron], the second from the motor cell of the anterior horn to the end arborizations in a muscle fibre [lower motor neuron]. (See Fig. 9, tracts 15–17–18–19–20–21–23 [fig. 32].) Probably all sensory nerve conduction pathways consist of more than two neurons. These ratios can be easily illustrated in Kölliker's diagrams (Fig. 4, A.B.C. [fig. 32]) and in the one which I designed (Figs. 9 and 10). In Kölliker's schemata (Fig. 4), A represents the conduction through the pyramidal tracts and the anterior roots: (1), illustrates the direct pyramidal tract, (2), the lateral [crossed] pyramidal tract, with its various decussations, the repeated decussations in the anterior commissure for (1), and the large single crossing in the decussation of the pyramid for (2). The longitudinal, pyramidal fibres either turn altogether into the gray substance or they send out collaterals. The latter, as well as the whole fibres, terminate in end branches (1*a* and 2*a*) from which the stimulus is transmitted to the ganglionic cells of the anterior horn, including their processes, the anterior motor root fibres (3). The tract with two neurons has been shown in more detail in my schematic illustration (Fig. 9). (15), represents a pyramidal cell of the cerebral cortex where the pyramidal fibres presumably originate. As is known, the course of the pyramidal fibres is uninterrupted and decussated (Figs. 9, 17–18). The circle (18), indicates the bending of the fibre into the longitudinal direction of the anterior column (here we take as an example the direct pyramidal tract); at this point the collateral supplied with end arborizations originates (19), and passes to the gray matter in the vicinity of an anterior [horn] ganglion cell (20), transfers in it the psychomotor stimulus, which extends along the nerve fibre (21), to the motor end arborizations (23), in the muscle fibre. (22), illustrates a collateral of the motor nerve fibre, as Golgi [see p. 93] and Ramón y Cajal have demonstrated in some animals. As we have seen, it is questionable (Kölliker) whether they are present everywhere. (22*a*) [not marked], indicates the branching to which the motor fibres are repeatedly subjected in their course.

The diagram of a sensory reflex-conducting pathway represented in Kölliker's Fig. 4, B: 1, the spinal ganglion cell, 2, the conducting fibre originating at the periphery, 3, the root fibre gravitating towards the brain; it separates into an ascending and descending branch (4, 4); from here depart the collaterals (5, 5), with their end branches which in turn transmit the stimulus to the anterior horn (6, 6, etc.). We are dealing here with three neurons: the first one from the periphery to the spinal ganglion cell; the second one from the latter to the sensory end branches; and the third one from the motor ganglion cell to the muscle fibre.

Fig. 9 illustrates this reflex arc in more detail . . . . [1–2–5–6–7–7$_1$–9–20–21–23].

. . . .

. . . . In Kölliker's diagram, Fig. 4, C, we have the illustration of a long extended reflex conduction. The sensory conduction, 2, 1, 3, 4, 5, acts upon a tract cell 7, the latter upon both longitudinal fibres which are T-shaped, and through their numerous collaterals, simultaneously, upon many motor fibres [6].

These concepts of the course of conduction are, however, based upon the assumption that in reality there are no anastomotic nerve plexuses, but that only a nerve felt (Neuropile of His) occurs. If we assume, with Golgi and B. Haller, the existence of nerve networks, the concept is somewhat modified, yet we may retain the nerve units. The boundaries between two nerve units would then always lie in a system of nerve networks and, anatomically at least, could not be accurately defined with our present methods of investigation.

Regarding the question of the dendritic plexus or nerve [axonal] plexus, it may be pointed out briefly that the majority of the investigators who more recently devoted considerable attention to this subject, denied the nerve plexus. Indeed, Kölliker, at the Anatomical Congress at Munich [May 1891], gave the important and surprising report that Golgi, in a written and oral communication, had informed him that he had been misunderstood if the assumption of a true, anastomotic nerve plexus had been ascribed to him. In any event, Golgi would then have had to change his opinion, for his publications in the *Anatomischer Anzeiger* are, as I understand it, definitive, and so are the reports of his disciple, L. Sala, which were published only a few months ago. That Golgi no longer strictly emphasizes a nerve plexus is also evident from his most recent paper. As matters stand today one may be permitted to assert that the evidence of an anastomotic nerve net has not been proved as yet, and that most investigators express themselves in favor of a "Neuropile."

EXCERPT P. 1356

If we review the principal benefit that we have derived from the anatomical investigations we have discussed, in my opinion this is above all the more exact outline of the anatomical and functional elements of the nervous system which has been made possible. According to this we must consider the nerve units (neurons) as well as the discovery of the axon collaterals with their end branchings by Golgi and S. Ramón y Cajal. These matters enable us to understand isolated conduction—although it must remain questionable whether this does in fact take place—as well as the diffusion of conduction over long stretches.

HANS HELD

(*8 August 1866–1942*)

It might be thought that the data produced by His, Forel, and Ramón y Cajal, which was then distilled by Waldeyer into the neuron doctrine, would have been sufficient to rout the reticularists. But this was not so and the controversy between neuronists and reticularists proceeded unabated, with attention being paid almost exclusively to histological evidence. The key problem was that of whether the terminal axons, or telochondria, made simple contact with the nerve cells and dendrites or whether they became continuous with them. As staining techniques increased in number and in versatility, each side brought forward new evidence to support its respective contention.

In view of the fact that today the neuron theory is the more acceptable, we have selected almost exclusively from the writings of those who made this possible. Their opponents, however, although their basic premise was incorrect, contributed to the **morphology** of the neuron. The most important reticularists, in addition to Golgi, were Apáthy of Hungary, Bethé of Strassburg, and von Lenhossék. Opposition to the neuron theory was also offered by Hans Held, who is especially important for his work on the general structure of the neuron.

Held was born at Neukloster in Mecklenburg and studied at the Universities of Rostock and Leipzig. At the latter he came into contact with two men who influenced his future career, Paul Flechsig and Wilhelm His. Owing to their stimulus he devoted the rest of his life to the histology of the nervous system. In 1891 he was appointed assistant, and then *Prosektor* in anatomy at Leipzig. He was promoted to professor *ordinarius* of anatomy and director of the anatomical institute in 1917 and retired in 1935. His major publications were only forty-nine but they were important contributions to the histology of the nervous system and the inner ear (see Stieve, 1936).

First of all, Held discovered that whereas in the embryo a terminal axon in contact with another nerve cell body was separated from it by a line of demarcation, this was not present in the adult and a growing together or "concrescence" had taken place. Furthermore, he first discovered in 1891, that the terminal axons surrounding the cells of the trapezoid nucleus in the pons, for example, broke up into a basket formation (*Endkörb* of Koelliker or *chalice* of Ramón y Cajal, fig. 31), and at times he could see their thick rodlike fibres entering the cell body itself. These results were reported in a paper of 1897 ("Beiträge zur Structur der Nervenzellen und ihrer Fortsätze. Zweite Abhandlung," *Arch. Anat. Physiol.* (Anat. Abt.), 1897, pp. 204–294), and figure 34 illustrates some of them. The following passages are from this report. He employed either iron-hematoxylin or erythrosin-methylene blue stains.

EXCERPT PP. 259–262

1. In the newborn animal, and still in the two-day old, the body of the trapezoid nucleus cell is already more or less extensively surrounded by end fibres. In most cases the end fibres spread into the enveloping basket-like area directly at the cell body surface. (Figs. 2 and 6, pl. XII [fig. 37].) This splitting up occurs partly at some distance from the cell, although a minimal distance. (Fig. 11, Pl. IX, Fig. 7, Pl. XII in the adult animal [figs. 35, 37].) Despite the relative smallness of the structures (as compared with the size in the fully grown animal) the end fibres, as well as the end areas, show distinctly the uniform, longitudinal vacuolization characteristic of the axis cylinders, and the very small-sized neurosomes which are arranged densely in the network. There can be no possibility of it being an axis cylinder arising from the cell, first, because the characteristic basal protuberance [axon hillock] is missing, and, second, the basket-like spreading process which approaches and encloses the cell is much too voluminous for its respective size. That these distinguishing features are real is demonstrated by observations in which the cross section of the cell shows its outgoing axis cylinder at the same time as the terminating one [from another cell] (Fig. 2, Pl. XII). At the place where the terminating axis cylinder approaches the protoplasm of the cell a line of differentiation is noted along the whole area of contact, not unlike the membrane of a nucleus; like the nucleus, it stains intensely red with an erythrosin-methylene blue double stain (Fig. 6, Pl. X shows the same as Fig. 2, Pl. XII but in a nine-day-old dog). I cannot say whether this homogeneous boundary line belongs to the ectoplasm of the nerve [cell] as a differentiated product of it, or to the axis cylinder protoplasm. After many detailed observations I am of the opinion that the former is correct, because the axis cylinder protoplasm exhibits an extraordinarily fine and delicate axospongium, whereas the cytospongium of the cell shows a much more compact and coarser meshwork which can thus be stained much more intensively with erythrosin. Now, whether this marginal membrane represents a gluelike substance, that is, a nerve glue, seems to me improbable for additional reasons: (1) it extends into the protoplasm of the enveloped cell, disintegrating very gradually, and (2) at a later age not only is it no longer formed and developed but it may disappear completely. However, its presence shows with certainty that the actual protoplasm of the axis cylinder at this stage of development does not directly border that of the cell, because this membrane-like line can be distinguished in the whole area of investment; consequently, the designation "nerve contact" (*Nervencontact*) seems significant and appropriate. This layer, which appears as a surface differentiation of the nerve-cell protoplasm, I regard as

produced by the contact of the end of the axis cylinder which grows and
spreads around the involved cell. As for the shape of this terminal part of
the axis cylinder, Cajal's designation "terminal cup" (*Endkelch*) is incorrect, insofar as one does not observe cross sections in which a completely
annular outline of this structure invariably appears; one always observes
cross sections in which only a more or less irregular basket of small and
independent branches of axis cylinders encloses the cell. These forms,
regarding which my earlier nomenclature of *fibre basket* (*Faserkorb*) is
perfectly appropriate, become increasingly distinct and pronounced in all
further stages of growth, as in the young and the newborn animal.

2. It can be noted that in the nine-day-old animal, apart from the
increased proportions owing to growth and thus more distinct observation
with respect to all these structures, an essential difference from the earlier
stage exists, because the line of differentiation already described can no
longer be observed everywhere as distinctly as before. Distinctly and
markedly pronounced in many trapezoid nucleus cells, it can no longer be
seen in others, so that it becomes difficult, if not impossible in a few cases,
to verify where the axospongium ends and the cytospongium of the trapezoid nucleus cells begins.

3. . . . . If one now examines in the thinnest sections, of one μ, the
relation of the ramifications of the axis cylinders to the protoplasm of the
entwined cell with regard to their structure, one is unable in many instances
and many fibres to prove a *pericellularly located boundary zone between
the axo- and cytospongium; rather, one and the same thinnest plasma mass
appears as the separating line between rows of meshes or, as a separating
wall between two rows of vacuoles of which one seems to belong to the axis
cylinder, the other to the cellular ground substance proper* . . . .

This mode of *association of the terminal surfaces of the axis cylinder
with the ground substance of the entwined nerve cells,* just described, no
longer appears to me to be commensurate with the concept of mere contact, but rather to demonstrate a more intimate association between nerve
cells than that which the contact theory has had reason to assume until
now. I do not conceal the fact with the delicacy of the relations discussed
here—be the sections ever so fine and brilliantly stained—that sources of
error are inherent in the limitation of the optical efficiency even of the best
lenses, so that it is justifiable to assume that the very dense, thinnest parts
of protoplasm are fused together. For a long time I was therefore not at all
sure whether the connection is really such an extraordinarily close one; but
by a repeated series of investigations I have observed the same and often
still more convincing evidence.

I must therefore designate all those cases in which the conditions described in the trapezoid nucleus of the adult animal are distinctly present

between the end of the axis cylinder and the cell protoplasm, *as pericellular concrescence*, in order to signify that a union of two neurons exceeding mere contact has occurred, and that this has taken place in the parts of the ground substance of the nerve cell which are located on the surface. (Figs. 1–4, Pl. XII [only fig. 2 is seen in fig. 37].)

EXCERPT PP. 265–266

If I summarize the preceding observations which have been briefly reported, the important conclusion is as follows. *The connections of neurons in the trapezoid nucleus cells of the adult, as distinct from the newborn animal and that only a few days old, become more intimate and closer* if the more delicate histological *relationships between the axis cylinder ending and the protoplasm of the enveloped nerve cell are considered.*

Held also described the terminal feet or *Endfüsse* of axonal filaments in contact with another nerve cell. He believed, however, that direct continuity occurred between the protoplasm of the axon and that of the cell body or dendrite, but later thought this was owing to the neurofibrils of the axon connecting directly with the intracellular reticulum. Thus he supported the doctrine of continuity, also upheld by Apáthy and Bethé. Subsequent studies, especially those of Ramón y Cajal (1952 for an excellent survey of his and those of others), verified the presence of the *Endkörben* and the *Endfüsse* but denied the existence of direct continuity by way of the latter. Likewise the evidence brought forward by other reticularists was eventually shown to be false, and this was owing in great measure to the patient work of the Spanish school of histology and its followers. The following account of the *Endfüsse* is from another paper published by Held in 1897 ("Beiträge zur Structur der Nervenzellen und ihrer Fortsätze. Dritte Abhandlung," *Arch. Anat. Physiol.* (Anat. Abt.), 1897, pp. 273–312).

EXCERPT PP. 283–285

. . . . Concerning the method of connection between the protoplasm of the end surface of the axis cylinder in central nerve cells and that of the cell body, according to new observations in agreement with my earlier assertions, one can with certainty assume a firm union of these two parts of the protoplasm of different nerve cells in adult animals. The illustrations 1 to 5 in Plate XII [fig. 34; fig. 3 only is reproduced, X, continuity between protoplasms of cell and axon] show this in multipolar, anterior horn cells of the lumbar spinal cord of dogs . . . . [Some axons are closely connected with the cell membrane.] The other attached axis cylinders do not give any certain indication regarding the way in which they are connected with the cell or with one of the dendrites. Because of this I do not dare to distinguish whether this is a case of closest contact or concrescence that already exists. There are layers of both protoplasmic parts lying on top of one another according to whether they have been cut transversely or horizontally; hence a definite decision as to whether they lie side by side or in continuity is impossible. In the decision concerning continuity between the axis cylinder protoplasm and the dendrites, such sources of error can be easily removed by comparing longitudinal and transverse sections. From each, one can deduce that the protoplasm of the terminal axis cylinder is connected with the dendrite protoplasm *per continuitatem* . . . .

I designate as *endfeet* the axis cylinder terminal surfaces of such axis cylinders, coming from the nervous membrane of nerve cells and firmly connected with the protoplasm of the cell itself. I do this in order to recall Deiters' description of the small-fibred axis cylinders of his second system that came out from the cell protoplasm with "footlike, small expansions." I have observed such axis cylinder endfeet on dendrites, on the cell body, and on the loosely formed axon hillock of the axis cylinder process.

. . . . On the dendrite the endfoot appears markedly concave, as can be seen in the illustration of the transverse section, so that in this way the cylindrical   protoplasmic   formation   of   the   dendrite   is   almost surrounded . . . .

In agreement with His's neuroblast teaching, a short time ago I called such endfeet in central nerve cells, *sites of concrescence between different nerve cells situated at a distance from one another.* This was because I was able to convince myself of such continuity in the adult nervous system but not in the undeveloped (mature fetuses of rabbit, newborn cats and dogs or those a few days old). I do not yet fully understand to what degree one must take into account the factors related to the relative fineness and thinness of the protoplasm of the axis cylinder terminal surface.

SANTIAGO RAMÓN Y CAJAL
(See p. 109)

(See p. 109)

Six years after his paper of 1888 in which he had presented preliminary evidence in favor of the neuron theory, Ramón y Cajal was in a position to make even more precise statements in support of it. During a visit to England (see Sherrington, 1935), he delivered the Croonian Lecture to the Royal Society on 8 March 1894 ("La fine structure des centres nerveux," *Proc. R. Soc.,* 1894, 55:444–468). In it he summarized his extensive studies which refuted Golgi's theory and replaced it with the doctrine of the neuron. He also referred to the function of the neuron.

EXCERPT PP. 446–447

The studies which we have carried out during these past five years on the structure of almost all the nerve centers, cerebellum, spinal cord, brain, olfactory bulb, sympathetic ganglia, optic centers, retina, etc., if they have permitted us to confirm in large part the facts reported by Golgi, at the same time they have led us to substitute the following propositions which we consider fully demonstrated for the three anatomicophysiological hypotheses of the Italian scientist; the existence of an interstitial nerve plexus, the differentiations of the cells into sensory and motor, and the nutritive role of the protoplasmic extensions [dendrites].

The axis cylinders, as well as the protoplasmic expansions, terminate in the thickness of the gray matter by absolutely independent branches.

The protoplasmic extensions, as well as the body of the nerve cells, can serve for the conduction of nerve currents.

The two physiological types of nerve cells recognized by Golgi [p. 93] do not have a precise physiological or functional reality. Their morphological reality is, on the contrary, beyond doubt. In fact, in the gray matter, next to the elements which we have called cells with short axis cylinders [Golgi Type II cell], of which the axis cylindrical extensions break up into a terminal arborization around the adjacent cells, one encounters others that we call cells with long axis cylinders [Golgi Type I cell], of which the functional extension is continued with a fibre of the white substance. But these latter, the cells with a long axis cylinder, are abundant in organs that are essentially and undoubtedly sensory, such as the retina and the olfactory bulb; hence the conclusion that they do not necessarily and exclusively perform a motor role.

The same circumstance and reasoning apply to the cells with a short axis cylinder; they cannot really be considered as sensory cells since they are found indistinctly in all nerve centers, such as the cerebrum, cerebellum, corpus striatum, retina, olfactory bulb, etc.

The connections established between the fibres and the nerve cells take place by means of contact, that is, with the help of a genuine articulation between the varicose arborizations of the axis cylinders on the one hand and the body and the protoplasmic extensions on the other. Also, one is led to imagine the cerebrospinal axis as a structure composed of superimposed nerve entities, of *neurons* to use Waldeyer's expression.

EXCERPT PP. 464–465

In a synthetic manner one can say that the whole nerve center is the result of the association of the four following parts: the nerve cells with short axis cylinders, that is, branching in the very thickness of the gray matter; the terminal nerve fibres which come from other centers or from distant regions of the same center; nerve cells with a long axis cylinder, that is, extending as far as the white matter; the collaterals which originate either during the passage of the axis cylinder extensions of the cells with long nerve processes [axons] across the gray matter, or during the course of the tubes of the white matter. In certain organs, such as the retina, the olfactory bulb, and the first cerebral [cortical] layer, one must add a fifth structural factor; this is the elements characterized by the absence of differentiation into nerve and protoplasmic expansions [axons and dendrites]. This is reminiscent of the cerebellar granules, the spongioblasts of the retina, and the special cells of the cerebral cortex.

Each nerve fibre is the continuation of the functional expansion of a nerve cell. This law also holds in the case of ganglia of the great sympathetic, the elements of which, according to our observations, confirmed by Retzius, van Gehuchten, L. Sala, and von Lenhossék, offer two kinds of extensions: branching or protoplasmic appendices which terminate freely in the ganglion proper, and an axis cylinder extension which is continuous with Remak's fibre [non-medullated fibre].

The nerve cells constitute entities, the *neurons* of Waldeyer, of which the reciprocal relations consist of genuine articulations. The features of each contact are, on the one hand, the body and the protoplasmic expansions of the cells, and on the other the terminal arborizations of nerve fibres [axons].

In organs where the origin of excitation has been well established one recognizes that the cells are polarized, that is, that the nerve current always enters by way of the protoplasmic apparatus of the cellular body, and that it leaves by the axis cylinder which transmits it to a new protoplasmic apparatus.

RUDOLPH ALBERT VON KOELLIKER

(See p. 61)

It was only natural that as more and more morphological and physiological characteristics of the neuron were discovered, attempts should be made to provide general correlations between the two groups of findings. Koelliker, who has already been cited as one of the outstanding early investigators of the nerve cell and its processes, discussed this problem in the 1896 edition of his famous textbook, *Handbuch der Gewebelehre des Menschen* (6th ed., Vol. II [Leipzig, 1896], "Vom Nervensysteme"). He had accepted the neuron theory and when discussing the function of neurons, he declared that they all had the same basic structure and function which varied, however, with their location. This has been described as "an epitome of his belief" (Haymaker, 1953, p. 53) and is an application of the law of specific nerve energy of Helmholtz (pp. 207–209). In fact Deiters had already remarked (p. 69) that nerve cells may look the same but may act quite differently.

EXCERPT PP. 809–810

Therefore, although among the pyramidal cells of the cerebrum, too, no important differences are known, it is still possible that more specific distinctions may exist between these and the motor cells of the medulla and the cerebral motor nuclei, and, furthermore, between these two varieties and the sensory ganglion cells, and other cells. If this be so, one would have to confess that anatomy is unable to establish and prove the anatomical characteristics of such differences. On the other hand, it is conceivable that *all the nerve cells present essentially the same function and that their respective performance depends upon the different relations of the cells to their environment.* A nerve cell which is in communication only with a sound-producing apparatus would be unable to transmit smells, and centrifugal axons which are not connected with muscle fibres would not produce movements! Such a concept seems at first sight to be too general and therefore unacceptable. However, if one considers the gradual development of the functions of the nervous system and the organs serving it in the animal kingdom, it is found to contain a grain of truth. With what simple means does a *protozoon* feel and move? Little by little, simple nerve cells develop and join into ever more complicated organs; in addition, peripheral sensory cells develop and are gradually transformed into an entire series of simple and higher sensory organs. The same applies to the motor apparatus. If one considers all this carefully and keeps in mind that along with the ever higher development of functions the formation of the elementary anatomical apparatus also goes hand in hand, one is eventually forcefully convinced *that all nerve cells originally possess essentially the same function and that their coming into existence depends exclusively upon the manifold external influences or stimuli by which they are affected, and upon the many possible ways of reacting to these stimuli.*

LEWELLYS FRANKLIN BARKER

(16 September 1867—13 July 1943)

At the end of the nineteenth century the weight of evidence favored the neuron theory, although the neuron versus net controversy was by no means over. One of the most ardent neuronists was the American anatomist and clinician Lewellys F. Barker.

He was born at Milldale, Ontario, Canada, but spent his adult life in the United States. After having been graduated in medicine at the University of Toronto in 1890, he was attracted to Baltimore by the presence there of William Osler, a fellow Canadian. After a succession of posts in anatomy, pathology, and clinical medicine in Johns Hopkins University, he went to Rush Medical College, Chicago, as professor of medicine but returned to Baltimore in 1905 to succeed Osler. In 1921 he became professor emeritus of medicine. His work covered many areas of anatomy and clinical medicine, and his neurohistological investigations resulted from a visit to Germany in 1895, where he studied under His, Wundt, Flechsig, and Frey (see Austrian, 1943; Barker, 1942).

Barker made no outstanding practical contribution to the neuron doctrine but his importance is due to the articulate support he gave it. He did for the English-speaking countries what Waldeyer had done for the German-speaking. In his book, *The nervous system and its constituent neurones* (New York, 1899), he brought together the important data which favored or opposed the doctrines and presented them with critical analysis and balanced judgment. These personal qualities, together with thoroughness, clarity, and excellent illustrations, made the book a useful source of nineteenth century concepts, as well as an important medium for the popularization of the neuron doctrine.

The following passage from his book gives a succinct summary of the theory. Figure 38 accompanied it, and it has since appeared in many textbooks to illustrate the prototype neuron. Also in a footnote on page 40 is a discussion of the term *neuron* not included below.

EXCERPT PP. 40–42

Enough has been said, I hope, to make clear what is meant by the "neurone concept" of the nervous system. To sum it up in a few words: The nervous system, aside from its neuroglia, ependymal cells, blood-vessels, and lymphatics, consists of an enormous number of individual elements or neurones. Each neurone in its entirety represents a single body cell. These units are at first *entirely* (if protoplasmic bridges be excepted) and continue throughout life *relatively* to be morphologically, and in part, at least, physiologically, independent of one another.

There is no evidence of the existence of a diffuse nerve network either in the sense in which von Gerlach or in that in which Golgi used the term, though should it be forthcoming, it would not, and Waldeyer stated this in his article, interfere with the neurone conception. The axis cylinder of every nerve fibre, just as much as every protoplasmic process, is an integral part of a neurone, and has an organic connection somewhere with a nerve cell. Nerve conduction paths may, and probably usually do, in higher animals at least, involve more than one neurone, the neurones being, as it were, superimposed upon one another to make simple or more complex neurone chains or chains of neurone groups, one individual neurone through its various processes being in a position to be affected by and in turn to affect several or many other neurones. Notwithstanding almost infinite minor variations in form, the neurones in the most different parts of the nervous system present surprisingly similar general external morphological characteristics. The nerve life of the individual, including all his reflex, instinctive, and volitional activities, is the sum total of the life of his milliard of neurones.

Santiago Ramón y Cajal

(*See p. 109*)

Adequate recognition of Ramón y Cajal's contributions to the histology of nervous tissue was received in 1906 when he shared the Nobel Prize for Medicine and Physiology with his opponent Golgi, the leader of the reticularists (p. 91). On 12 December 1906 he gave his address ("Structure et connexions des neurones," *Les Prix Nobel en 1906* [Stockholm, 1908]), in which he summarized his many observations on the neuron, and declared it to be an independent unit that does not anastomose. He also discussed the function of the neuron and, like Koelliker (pp. 61–66), he was struck by its basic uniformity. He considered further the concept of neuronal transmission of the nerve impulse which involved dendrite, cell body, and axon.

EXCERPT PP. 1–2

From my collected researches there emerges a general concept that comprises the following propositions:

1. The nerve cells are morphologic entities or, to use Professor Waldeyer's term, neurons [pp. 114–117]. This property has already been demonstrated by my illustrious colleague Professor Golgi in regard to the dendritic or protoplasmic prolongations of the nerve cells [pp. 94–95]; but as regards the arrangement of the most peripheral branchings of the axons and their collaterals, there were, at the beginning of our researches, only conjectures that might or might not be sustained. With the aid of Golgi's method, I believe that our observations, first on the cerebellum [pp. 110–113], and thereafter on the spinal cord, the cerebrum, the olfactory bulb, the optic lobe, the retina, etc., revealed the ultimate arrangement of the nerve fibres. These branch several times and are always carried towards the neuronal body or towards the protoplasmic expansions around which arise very compact, abundant plexuses or nerve nests. The pericellular baskets (*Endkörben*), the climbing plexuses, and other morphological arrangements, of which the form varies according to the nerve centers studied, attest that the nerve elements possess reciprocal relationships of *contiguity* and not of *continuity*; and that these relationships of more or less intimate contact are always established, not only between nerve arborizations but between these

branches on the one hand and the cell body and the protoplasmic prolongations on the other. A granular cement or special conducting substance serves to keep the neuronal surfaces in very intimate contact.

EXCERPT PP. 17–18

From the entire collection of these facts an inevitable postulate emerges; this is the neuronal doctrine of His and Forel, accepted by a large number of neurologists and physiologists. Nevertheless, it must be said that some of the physiological deductions drawn from observations made during these past twenty years by means of selective methods, have been attacked and naturally, therefore, they cannot be considered as infallible dogmata. Despite the solid foundation of its inferences, present day science has no right to foretell the future. Our assertions should not go beyond the revelations of contemporary methods. Perhaps technology will in time discover some staining procedure capable of revealing new and more intimate connections between neurons which we suppose to be in contact. One cannot reject a priori the possibility that the tangled forest of the brain, of which we imagine that we have discovered the last branches and leaves, may still possess some bewildering system of filaments binding together the neuronal mass as lianas bind the trees of tropical forests. That idea, presenting itself to us with the attraction of unity and simplicity, has always exercised and continues to exercise a powerful influence even upon the most placid minds. From the analytic point of view it would be very convenient and economical if all the nerve centers formed a continuous network intermediate between motor nerves and sensitive and sensory nerves. Unfortunately, nature seems to ignore our intellectual need for convenience and unity, and is very often pleased with complexity and diversity.

Besides, we believe that we have no reason to be skeptical if while awaiting the work of the future we remain quietly confident in the future of our work. We recall that these terminal arrangements that modern neurology has discovered in the axons were established through the concordance of several methods, and if the science of the future reserves some great surprises and astonishing conquests for us, one must believe that it will complete and develop our knowledge infinitely, all in keeping with the actual facts.

The irresistible suggestion of the reticular concept, of which I have spoken to you (the formula of which changes every five or six years), has persuaded some physiologists and zoologists to raise objections to the doctrine of the propagation of nerve currents by contact or at a distance. All their allegations are based upon the revelations of incomplete methods infinitely less demonstrable than those that have served to construct the imposing edifice of the neuron concept. Some of these arguments belong to the morphologic, others to the histogenic category.

With regard to the morphologic objections (of which we no longer hear so much since the discovery of Donaggio's method and our own), I shall declare only that despite the efforts I have made to observe the supposed intercellular anastomoses in preparations made with various staining procedures (those of Bethé, Simarro, Donaggio, ours, that of Bielschowsky, etc.), I have never succeeded in finding any incontestable examples of them (that is, displaying themselves as clearly and distinctly as the free terminations), neither in the pericellular nerve plexuses, nor in the *boutons* of Held-Auerbach, nor between the neurofibrils belonging to the different neurons. (Such wise and experienced neurologists as His, Koelliker, Retzius, v. Lenhossék, Duval, van Gehuchten, Lugaro, Schiefferdecker, Dejerine, etc., are of the same opinion.) If the aforementioned intercellular unions are not illusory, they represent fortuitous arrangements, perhaps anomalies of almost no value in contrast to the almost infinite quantity of clearly observed facts concerning the free termination.

As to the histogenic arguments which the adversaries of the neuron doctrine have strongly advocated in recent times, considering them as the most weighty and decisive evidence possible against the neuron concept, I shall reply that my recent researches, as well as those of Perroncito, Marinesco, Lugaro, and Nageotte, made with the assistance of a more positive procedure than those employed by the antineuronists, demonstrate conclusively the lack of foundation for the hypothesis of discontinued development of nerve fibres. Purpura, a student of my illustrious colleague, C. Golgi, analyzing the regenerative process of sectioned nerves by means of the silver chromate procedure, and very recently Krassin of St. Petersburg, using Ehrlich's method [pp. 97–99] for the same purpose, both arrived at the same conclusions.

Another field of neurohistology in which Ramón y Cajal predominated was that of the degeneration and regeneration of nervous tissue. He favored the ideas of Waller regarding degeneration (pp. 71–75), and this phenomenon together with the reverse, regeneration, gave support to the monogenist doctrine to which he subscribed; this doctrine that was soon to receive further support from Harrison's tissue culture experiments (pp. 132–136), recognized fibre growth only from the central end of a cut nerve. Ramón y Cajal considered that his own studies refuted the tenets of his opponents, the polygenists, who held that the distal portion of a cut nerve could regenerate without the help of its cell body, in short, the doctrine of autogenous regeneration. In 1913 he published his evidence in a book entitled *Estudios sobre la degeneración y regeneración del sistema nervioso* (2 vols., Madrid, 1913–1914), which, however, remained almost unknown in much of Europe and in

North America until it appeared in English translation in 1928 (*Degeneration and regeneration of the nervous system,* translated by R. M. May, 2 vols., London). The following passage from Volume I summarizes Ramón y Cajal's conclusions concerning regeneration.

EXCERPT PP. 17–19

1. When the sciatic nerve of a young animal is cut and the animal is killed at a longer or shorter interval after the operation, one notes in impregnated preparations that a great number of the axons of the central stump are actively in the process of sprouting. This sprouting is effected in two ways: (*a*) The new fibre or fibres are terminal, and are budded from the enlarged tip of the old axon. (*b*) The new fibres are collateral, and arise at right or acute angles to the old axon. In both cases the newly-formed shoots have no medullated sheaths, invade the exudate that is present between the two nervous stumps, ramify as they proceed, and, finally, end freely in a terminal club or bud, a kind of battering-ram, which is used to push aside the mesodermal cells and to form a path across the future cicatricial substance.

The discovery of this terminal excrescence, later confirmed by the investigations of Perroncito, Marinesco, Nageotte, Sala, Tello, Dustin, Rossi, etc., assumes a certain importance for the resolution of the debated question, since with such a terminal protoplasmic bud one can tell in the sections not only the level which the regenerative process has reached, but also the origin and orientation of newly-formed axons.

2. During their initial phases the newly-formed nerve fibres, as well as their terminal buds, lack nuclei or cells of Schwann. From the third or fourth day on, embryonic connective cells are attracted, and around the naked axons and clubs appear marginal nuclei. This important observation of the formative precedence of the regenerated axons over the cells of Schwann singularly compromises the polygenist theory, since it shows that during the first phases of the evolution of the fibres there are absolutely no cellular chains.

3. If one studies the growth of the newly-formed fibres during the first six days after section of the nerve one can easily see that the terminal clubs grow indeterminately along the paths of least resistance. A great many take a reverse direction, in the central stump, where they go back very far, as well as in perinervous tissues. Other fibres, disorientated and wandering, stop before obstacles, follow complicated paths, and lose themselves definitely, as far as the nervous reunion of the peripheral stump is concerned. Such diverted axons, abundantly found where pieces of nerve are taken out or where the two stumps are intentionally pulled apart, are characterized by

gigantic encapsulated clubs or spheres, often in process of degeneration. These spheres are nothing else than the so-called *nerve cells*, shown some time ago by S. Mayer of Prague, in the substance of regenerating nerves, and described by Ranvier as enigmatic monstrous formations, situated in the paths of central fibres.

4. After ten or twelve days in adult animals, and six or seven in animals a few weeks old, the young fibres that have not lost their way, wandering in the intercalary cicatricial tissue, approach the sheaths of the peripheral stump, grow into them, and push from their path the remnants of the myelin that are as yet unabsorbed. Before obstacles the new fibres subdivide minutely, and the shoots go forward flexibly and indifferently either through the bands of Büngner or in their interstices.

5. If one repeats the experiment of Vulpian, Brown-Sequard, Bethe, etc., by putting obstacles between the two stumps of a cut nerve, so as to keep them from immediately uniting, one often notes, after two or three months, a well-advanced regeneration of the distal segment. When this is examined by means of our method of staining one can see in its interior numerous young axons which always end, at different levels, with small buds of growth.

An examination of the varied and extensive scar which unites the stumps reveals, not the absence of uniting fibres, as the polygenists arbitrarily claimed, but a complex nerve plexus, formed by small bundles of unmyelinated nerve fibres, which extends uninterruptedly from the central to the peripheral segments.

6. The newly-formed nerve fibres repeatedly subdivide in the scar, especially at the edge of the peripheral stump, where, very often, a large axon reduces itself to a *bouquet* of fine terminal twigs. The branches of a single axon do not go to one old nerve tube, but they distribute themselves to several empty sheaths. From this it follows that a group which is relatively poor in afferent axons can still innervate a good portion of the regenerated nerve. It is to be noted that such branches, always oriented towards the periphery, as well as their free end-clubs, are observed facts irreconcilable with the polygenist theory.

7. When the obstacles to reunion of the nervous fragments are insuperable (suture of the peripheral stump to the skin, insertion of the central segment in the abdominal cavity, etc.), the peripheral segment shows absolutely no regeneration, even months after the operation, and no matter what the age of the animal.

8. The multiplication of the cells of Schwann of the peripheral stump does not occur for the purpose of producing chains of elements which can be transformed by autogeneration, as Büngner and Bethe claimed, but its

object is to segregate stimulating substances which are able to attract and direct to the motor and sensory nerve endings the young nerve fibres that are wandering in the scar.

Ross Granville Harrison
(13 January 1870—30 September 1959)

So far the vast majority of data supporting the neuron doctrine had come from the painstaking labors of the neurohistologists. But clearly, one of the ways by which the neuron could be adequately examined would be to grow and maintain it outside the body. By this technique its form and development could be studied fully. This was a prerequisite for the elucidation of any type of cell structure, but in the case of the neuron the evidence derived would be vital to the neuron–net controversy. Admittedly, by the early twentieth century the majority of investigators were in favor of the neuron theory, and although their opponents were not necessarily thinking in terms of either Gerlach's or Golgi's original concept, they nevertheless felt that some form of close connection occurred between cells.

Many attempts at tissue culture, or the growth of cells *in vitro*, had been made, but the first successful one, and the one that opened up a new field of general cytological research, was that of the American biologist Ross G. Harrison. It was, furthermore, a decisive confirmation and demonstration of the neuron doctrine and of His's work (pp. 98–104).

Harrison was born in Germantown, Pennsylvania, received a Ph.D. degree from the Johns Hopkins University in 1894, and the M.D. from the University of Bonn in 1899. He devoted himself chiefly to embryology, tissue culture, and transplantation. After holding appointments in the department of anatomy of the Johns Hopkins University, in 1907, the year in which his first paper on tissue culture was published, he went to Yale University as professor of comparative anatomy and director of the department of zoology. Harrison spent the rest of his academic career at Yale, retiring in 1938 from the chair of biology which he had occupied since 1927. He retained widespread contacts with the biological sciences during his retirement, and his eminence in the field was acknowledged by his many awards and honors (see Abercrombie, 1961; Freund and Berg, 1963–1964, II, 117–126; Rook, 1964, pp. 158–163, where the 1907 article is reproduced in full; Oppenheimer, 1966).

Harrison's classic paper in which he described his tissue culture methods appeared in 1907 ("Observations on the living developing nerve fiber," *Anat. Rec.*, 1907, 1:116–118), a model of clarity and brevity. It was read before the Society of Experimental Biology and Medicine in New York on 22 May 1907, and is reproduced in its entirety below.

The immediate object of the following experiments was to obtain a method by which the end of a growing nerve could be brought under direct observation while alive, in order that a correct conception might be had regarding what takes place as the fiber extends during embryonic development from the nerve center out to the periphery.

The method employed was to isolate pieces of embryonic tissue, known to give rise to nerve fibers, as for example, the whole or fragments of the medullary tube, or ectoderm from the branchial region, and to observe their further development. The pieces were taken from frog embryos about 3 mm. long at which stage, i.e., shortly after the closure of the medullary folds, there is no visible differentiation of the nerve elements. After carefully dissecting it out, the piece of tissue is removed by a fine pipette to a cover slip upon which is a drop of lymph freshly drawn from one of the lymph-sacs of an adult frog. The lymph clots very quickly, holding the tissue in a fixed position. The cover slip is then inverted over a hollow slide and the rim sealed with paraffine. When reasonable aseptic precautions are taken, tissues will live under these conditions for a week and in some cases specimens have been kept alive for nearly four weeks. Such specimens may be readily observed from day to day under highly magnifying powers.

While the cell aggregates, which make up the different organs and organ complexes of the embryo, do not undergo normal transformation in form, owing, no doubt, in part, to the abnormal conditions of mechanical tension to which they are subjected; nevertheless, the individual tissue elements do differentiate characteristically. Groups of epidermis cells round themselves off into little spheres or stretch out into long bands, their cilia remain active for a week or more and a typical cuticular border develops. Masses of cells taken from the myotomes differentiate into muscle fibers showing fibrillae with typical striations. When portions of myotomes are left attached to a piece of the medullary cord the muscle fibers which develop will, after two or three days, exhibit frequent contractions. In pieces of nervous tissue numerous fibers are formed, though, owing to the fact that they are developed largely within the mass of transplanted tissue itself, their mode of development cannot always be followed. However, in a large number of cases fibers were observed which left the mass of nerve tissue and extended out into the surrounding lymph-clot. It is these structures which concern us at the present time.

In the majority of cases the fibers were not observed until they had almost completed their development, having been found usually two, occasionally three, and once or twice four days after isolation of the tissue. They consist of an almost hyaline protoplasm, entirely devoid of the yolk granules, with which the cell-bodies are gorged. Within this protoplasm there is no definiteness of structure; though a faint fibrillation may sometimes be observed and faintly-defined granules are discernible. The fibers are about 1.5–3 μ thick and their contours show here and there irregular varicosities.

The most remarkable feature of the fiber is its enlarged end, from which extend numerous fine simple or branched filaments. The end swelling bears a resemblance to certain rhizopods and close observation reveals a continual change in form, especially as regards the origin and branching of the filaments. In fact, the changes are so rapid that it is difficult to draw the details accurately. It is clear we have before us a mass of protoplasm undergoing amoeboid movements. If we examine sections of young normal embryos shortly after the first nerves have developed, we find exactly similar structures at the end of the developing nerve fibers. This is especially so in the case of the fibers which are connected with the giant cells described by Rohon and Beard.

Still more instructive are the cases in which the fiber is brought under observation before it has completed its growth. Then it is found that the end is very active and that its movement results in the drawing out and lengthening of the fiber to which it is attached. One fiber was observed to lengthen almost 20 μ in 25 minutes, another over 25 μ in 50 minutes. The longest fibers observed were 0.2 mm. in length.

When the placodal thickenings of the branchial region are isolated, similar fibers are formed and in several of these cases they have been seen to arise from individual cells. On the other hand, other tissues of the embryo, such as myotomes, yolk endoderm, notochord, and indifferent ectoderm from the abdominal region do not give rise to structures of this kind. There can, therefore, be no doubt that we are dealing with a specific characteristic of nervous tissue.

It has not as yet been found possible to make permanent specimens which show the isolated nerve fibers completely intact. The structures are so delicate that the mere immersion in the preserving fluid is sufficient to cause violent tearing and this very frequently results in the tearing away of the tissue in its entirety from the clot. Nevertheless, sections have been cut of some of the specimens and nerves have been traced from the walls of the medullary tube but they were in all cases broken off short.

In view of this difficulty an effort, which resulted successfully, was made to obtain permanent specimens in a somewhat different way. A piece of medullary cord about four or five segments long was excised from an embryo and this was replaced by a cylindrical clot of proper length and caliber which was obtained by allowing blood or lymph of an adult frog to clot in a capillary tube. No difficulty was experienced in healing [sic] the clot into the embryo in proper position. After two, three, or four days the specimens were preserved and examined in serial sections. It was found that the funicular fibers from the brain and anterior part of the cord, consisting of naked axones without sheath cells, had grown for a considerable distance into the clot.

These observations show beyond question that the nerve fiber develops by the outflowing of protoplasm from the central cells. This protoplasm retains its amoeboid activity at its distal end, the result being that it is drawn out into a long thread which becomes the axis cylinder. No other cells or living structures take part in this process.

The development of the nerve fiber is thus brought about by means of one of the very primitive properties of living protoplasm, amoeboid movement, which, though probably common to some extent to all the cells of the embryo, is especially accentuated in the nerve cells at this period of development.

The possibility becomes apparent of applying the above method to the study of the influences which act upon a growing nerve. While at present it seems certain that the mere outgrowth of the fibers is largely independent of external stimuli, it is, of course, probable that in the body of the embryo there are many influences which guide the moving end and bring about contact with the proper end structure. The method here employed may be of value in analyzing these factors.

A year later Harrison published another paper dealing with the same subject ("Embryonic transplantation and development of the nervous system," *Anat. Rec.,* 1908, 2:385–410). Its concluding remarks follow.

EXCERPT PP. 409–410

The foregoing observations show beyond question that the nerve fiber begins as an outflow of hyaline protoplasm from cells situated within the central nervous system. The protoplasm is very actively amoeboid, and as a result of this activity, it extends farther and farther from its cell of origin [see fig. 39]. Retaining its pseudopodia at its distal end, the protoplasm is drawn out into a thread, which becomes the axis-cylinder of a nerve fiber. The early development of this structure is thus but a manifestation in a marked degree of one of the primitive properties of protoplasm, amoeboid activity. We have in the foregoing a positive proof of the hypothesis first put forward by Ramón y Cajal [1893] and von Lenhossék [1895], who based it upon the consideration of the cones of growth found by the Golgi method at the end of the growing fiber.

. . . .

As regards the theories of nerve development that have been the subject of the foregoing argument, I need scarcely point out that the experiments now place the outgrowth theory of His upon the firmest possible basis— that of direct observation. The attractive idea of Hensen [protoplasmic bridges are left everywhere between dividing cells of the embryo and these form nerve fibres] must be abandoned as untenable. The embryological basis of the neurone concept thus becomes more firmly established than ever.

Santiago Ramón y Cajal
(See p. 109)

Although opposition to the neuron theory declined rapidly as the twentieth century progressed, Ramón y Cajal in 1933 felt impelled to reevaluate the evidence for and against it, "Neuronismo o reticularismo? Las pruebas objectivas de la unidad anatómica, de las células nerviosas" (*Archos. Neurobiol.*, 1933, 13:217–291, 579–646). This was his last important publication, and in view of his unwavering support of the theory and the overwhelming amount of histological data with which he had helped to establish it, it is appropriate that his statement should be included here. In this essay Ramón y Cajal looked back over his many investigations and those of others and reevaluated the evidence for the neuron theory. The conclusion reached was the same as the one he had pronounced about forty-five years earlier, in 1888 (pp. 110–113). The following two selections have been translated from the opening and closing sections of the 1933 paper.

EXCERPT PP. 217–218

Notwithstanding the innumerable objective proofs offered in support of the discontinuity of the component elements of the gray matter, from time to time we notice the reappearance of the reticular theory, especially since Apathy's apparent demonstration of the existence of a net, as it seems, continuous between the neurofibrils of the *Püncksubstanz* [*sic*; see Purkyně, p. 54, and Gerlach, p. 90]. Today we likewise encounter a resurrection of the hypothesis of continuity, thanks to the indefatigable activity of Held [pp. 118–122] and his followers.

We do not wonder at this return to the old tradition of Gerlach's nets. It is necessary to realize that for certain minds the reticular theory offers an extraordinarily seductive and convenient explanation. Among other physical advantages, it offers the invaluable one of readily understanding the propagation of the nerve impulse from one neuron to another and its diffusion in a multitude of directions within the gray matter.

However, it is not just a question of examining closely the theoretical simplicity and convenience (more apparent than real) of a concept, but rather to appraise how it conforms to the known and easily demonstrable facts.

The present paper will be a concise exposition of observations contrary to the concepts of Bethe and Held, rather than a polemical attack, which is almost always sterile. I propose to describe briefly *what I have seen* during fifty years of work and what any observer who is free from the prejudice of a doctrine can easily verify, not by [relying on] this or that nerve cell, perhaps badly fixed or of an abnormal type, but instead on millions of neurons deeply stained by different methods of impregnation.

We are impelled moreover by an eagerness for clarity. The reticular theory, although defended by its more authoritative and brilliant champions, always appears to be nebulous and contradictory. Each antineuronist obstinately defends a personal profession of faith which has few points of contact with that sustained by his companions. And what is more serious, all of these have little in common with the positive data derived from the physiology, pathology, ontogeny, and phylogeny of the nervous system. On the contrary, the basis of the neuron theory is invigorated and extended by the influence of neurogeny, nerve regeneration, physio-pathology, etc.

It is clear that the techniques of the future may bring a new and [unsuspected] argument in favor of the reticular theory or of other concepts. A little improvement in the output of a method or a histological discovery of a general nature may oblige us to modify our conclusions. But at the present, this revision seems neither near nor probable. We can then still adopt without reservation the genial doctrine of His, Forel, and Kölliker because it rests upon innumerable concordant facts drawn from the nervous system of vertebrates and invertebrates.

EXCERPT PP. 645–646

We believe that we have cited numerous and conclusive proofs of the neuron doctrine. To provide details on all of them would have required a book. [This article was, in fact, published subsequently in book form.] For us, as for the observers of the first epoch (Kölliker, Retzius, van Gehuchten, Athias, Duval, Marinesco, etc.), it is not the case of a more or less probable theory but of a positive fact. What about doubtful appearances observed in some cases and by means of certain techniques? We do not deny them. But the neurologist has the inevitable duty—common to all scientific investigators—of distinguishing the apparent from the real, the fortuitous technical fact from the preexisting and general fact. And at the hour of judgment, we must depersonalize ourselves, forget seductive prejudices, those both of ourselves and of others, and see things, as Gracián says, as if they were contemplated for the first time. And let us not fear future technical inventions, because if the facts have been well observed, they will last although the interpretations may change.

We are neither exclusive nor dogmatic. We have to take pride in conserving a mental flexibility which is not ashamed of corrections. Neuronal discontinuity, which is evident in innumerable examples, could suffer exceptions. We ourselves have referred to some of them, for example: those probably existing in glands, vessels, and intestines (our *interstitial neurons*). Recently, Lawrentjew has confirmed [the presence of] anastomoses in the latter type of cell. Nor should we be surprised at the existence of these unions by continuity in the coelenterata, although recently Bozler has denied their existence in preparations made by Ehrlich's method. (This point demands an investigation with modern methods.)

Let us not fear, then, that by the impetuous attacks of the reticularists, the old and genial cellular theory of Virchow will suffer grave damage. The normal organism, so much an association of relatively autonomous cells, always contains, in the manner of a populous city, defective, deformed, monstrous, and even gravely sick, as well as healthy elements. For this reason, which we have moreover indicated previously and now insist upon, when dealing with the morphology and neuronal connections, we should rely on the law of large numbers, that is to say, on a rigorously statistical criterion.

Conclusion

In this chapter excerpts have been presented which have dealt almost exclusively with the morphological characteristics of the neuron. Throughout the period covered, however, concurrent investigations that attempted to correlate this structural data with function were taking place, and the two groups of information must be considered together. The function of the nerve is the subject of Chapter III.

During the last few decades, new techniques have accelerated this process of correlation, and in the last twenty-five years in particular, the electron microscope, together with increasingly sophisticated chemical and physical intracellular techniques, have helped to relate the basic histological findings of the nineteenth century to the cellular physiology of the twentieth (see Eccles, 1957). No attempt has been made to enter this current era of research, thought of perhaps as a fifth period of development, since an adequate evaluation of its themes will not be possible for several decades. At that time, it will be necessary to review the work that has been chosen here to illustrate the history of the neuron.

NERVE FUNCTION

Introduction

In Chapter II attention was directed to the steady accumulation of knowledge regarding the nerve's microscopical structure; now the history of its function requires consideration. As already mentioned, the two must be thought of together, although for the present purpose it has been found necessary to separate them.

Chapter III covers a much longer historical period than the previous chapter, since it includes all the more important attempts made by man to explain how the central organ controls movements and appreciates incoming sensory stimuli. As soon as the nerve was found to be responsible for these functions, the question arose as to how messages travelled through or along it. It was first asked by the pre-Socratic philosophers (*c.* 500 B.C.) and is still being asked today. The search for an answer, as described in this chapter and illustrated by the writings of some of the important contributors, began therefore in antiquity; present-day investigations, although proceeding at a greater rate than ever before, are as yet far from solving the problem. In modern terms the nerve message may be regarded as an electrochemical disturbance travelling like a wave along the surface of a neuron from the point of stimulation to the point where the neuron passes the stimulus to another neuron or to an effector organ.

Earlier authors, especially those of antiquity, did not make a strict division between structure and function so that their discussions invariably contained accounts of both. Hence the selections chosen from authors up to the seventeenth century, although concerned mainly with the function of the nerve, may also deal with its anatomy.

To facilitate an appreciation of the major concepts of nerve function, the selections have been grouped according to their main themes. The first group also represents a historical period because it includes all of antiquity and contains the ideas that were to dominate thought for many centuries; just as the ancient concept of the hollow nerve existed until the 1830's, so the Greek idea of a subtle agent that caused the nerve to function was likewise viable early in the nineteenth century. The second section of the chapter covers the seventeenth and eighteenth centuries when new physical and chemical notions and data were applied to biological problems. But more important, they also witnessed the origin of the theory of irritability. The third and fourth sections had their beginnings in the nineteenth century and deal with matters that are still current. Thus the two major present-day approaches to the problem of the nerve impulse are physical and chemical or pharmacological, and each has its roots in the last century. The electrophysiological investigators have always acknowledged Galvani as their progenitor, and it is this group that is considered in the third section. The physiological chemist or the pharmacologist, working on the problem of the chemical transmission of nerve impulses, claims the chemist and pharmacologist of the nineteenth and the early decades of the present century as the instigator of his line of thought; their investigations and ideas are included in section four. It seems that the future elucidation of nervous transmission lies in the hands of these latter two groups.

So far there has been no adequate history of the evolution of knowledge of the nerve impulse although parts of that story can be discovered in a variety of publications referred to either here or later in the chapter (see Rothschuh, 1958; Brazier, 1959).

Antiquity

The problem of how the special sense organs, such as the eyes and ears, perceive information reaching them from the outside world was frequently discussed by the early Greeks (Beare, 1906). The next step, the transmission of these sensory messages to the central organ of perception, whether brain or heart, was of importance to the philosopher as well as to the physician. Likewise other forms of sensation, such as touch and pain, were of interest, and the related enigma of how the central organ initiated and controlled movements of the body was a frequent topic of discussion. Some of this material has already been presented (pp. 10–20), and attention was called to one of the earliest concepts of message transmission through the body (pp. 13–14).

The early history of the notion that channels carry the various kinds of messages has been examined closely by Solmsen (1961) who deals with the pre-Socratic philosophers, Plato, Aristotle, the post-Aristotelian doctrines and, finally, with Herophilus and Erasistratus. It is to the last two that the origin of our present-day concept of nerve function can be traced with any certainty.

The Hippocratic Writers
(See p. 4)

Although the pre-Socratic Alcmaeon (pp. 2–3) concluded that the brain was the sensory center of the body and that all special sensations were carried to it, we have no reliable information on how he thought they were conveyed. Some have argued that he had identified the optic nerves and that he considered them as channels; if this was so, he was anterior by two hundred years to Herophilus who had the same idea (p. 10). Diogenes (*fl.* 440–430 B.C.) thought that air was responsible for the movements of the limbs and that it probably found its way to them by means of blood vessels.

Such a view was reflected in the fact that the Hippocratic Writers considered the nerves to have no special function, and that in the Hippocratic writings, as in other contemporaneous works, there was invariably confusion among nerve, tendon, ligament, and vein; the word *neuron* was used interchangeably for all of them. It is interesting to note that some of this confusion is reflected today in the Dutch word *zenuw* that can mean either nerve or tendon. The several references in the various Hippocratic books to so-called nerves are in fact to ligaments or sinews, as can be readily detected in each instance from the context (Littré [1839–1861], X, 701). The other use of the word "nerve" was to describe channels that carried sperm to the testes and were cut during the operation of castration (*On generation*, 2, Littré [1839–1861], VII, 470–473). Nowhere in the writings are the true nerves described except in a doubtful passage (*Second book of epidemics*, IV, 2, Littré [1839–1861], V, 124–126) where the author may have been referring to the vagus nerve and the sympathetic trunk. The only section of the writings (*Articulations*, 45, Littré [1839–1861], II, 118, n. 2) that Galen accepted as a description of the spinal cord and nerves is clearly not this; the author was describing vertebral ligaments. In the following passage (*On the different parts of man*, 5, Littré [1839–1861], VI, 284–285) the term *neuron* obviously means tendon, but the reference to "hollow nerves" is of great importance in view of subsequent developments:

> . . . . The neurons surround the joints and are spread throughout the whole length of the body. They are particularly strong and always largest where there is the least flesh. The entire body is full of neurons; however, on the face and on the head there are no neurons, but some fibres that are more slender and solid and that are located between bone and flesh resemble neurons; some of them are hollow neurons.

ARISTOTLE
(*See p. 7*)

Plato had little knowledge of physiology except for that acquired from other writers, and therefore he experienced their difficulty in accounting for the transmission of sensory impressions. On the whole he favored blood as the conveying agent.

Aristotle, on the other hand, favored a spirit or "pneuma" for this task. It controlled sense perception and voluntary movements but was not necessarily contained within channels. The concept of *pneuma* is complex and not readily comprehensible today. As with the Hippocratic Writers and others, Aristotle applied the word *neuron* to tendons and ligaments as well as to nerves, if in fact he ever considered this last structure. The resultant confusion is evident from the following translation of *The account of animals*, III, 5 (*Historia animalium*, [translated] by D'Arcy Thompson [1910], 515*b*:20).

> A feeling of numbness is incidental only to parts of the frame where sinew is situated.

Presumably Aristotle was referring to nerves, although he used the term *neuron*. Apart from a few possible references to cranial nerves (p. 9) he ignored the nerves; this is to be expected since his belief that the heart and not the brain was the central and controlling organ of the body made the nerves superfluous. In fact, if he ever recognized them, they were probably an embarrassment to him and to his followers, a situation that Galen was quick to detect in the case of Praxagoras, one of those who accepted Aristotle's cardiocentric system.

PRAXAGORAS
(*fl. 300* B.C.)

Among the generation that followed Aristotle there were some who accepted his doctrine of the supremacy of the heart over the brain as the central and controlling organ of the body (pp. 8–10). Of these Praxagoras is especially noteworthy because of his differentiation of vein from artery and his suggestion that the latter might function as a channel for the *pneuma*.

Praxagoras, son of the physician Nicharchus, was a native of Cos, and in antiquity he was considered one of the most famous representatives of the Hippocratic or Dogmatic school. He was an authority on medicine and appears to have been an outstanding teacher; among his pupils was the great Herophilus. The influence of Praxagoras on Greek medicine was therefore widespread (see Steckerl, 1958, pp. 1–6; Baumann, 1937).

Praxagoras followed Aristotle when he argued that since the heart was the central organ of the body, not only blood vessels, but also the nerves should arise from it. He therefore suggested that blood vessels passing out from the heart gradually lost their lumen and became solid nerves as they proceeded to the periphery of the body. All we know of Praxagoras's doctrines is contained in the writings of others, and recently these fragmentary remains were collected by Fritz Steckerl (*The fragments of Praxagoras of Cos and his school* [Leiden, 1958]). The following passage has, however, been translated directly from Galen's book, *On the opinions of Hippocrates and Plato*, I (Kühn [1821–1833], V, 187–200; cf. Steckerl, pp. 49–53). In the presentation of his argument, Galen gives his own ideas on the origin of nerves, and these correspond to ours of today; they will be given amplification later (pp. 147–153).

EXCERPT PP. 187–200

. . . . You may rightly censure Aristotle and Praxagoras since they assert, contrary to the facts, that the heart is the origin of the nerves. However, one may learn from their extant writings that they did observe carefully many other things pertaining to anatomy, but either they were entirely blind or talked with blind men when they wrote of the origin of the nerves. There is no reason why I should discuss the matter further; hence, allow me to hasten on to what is perceptible. As I demonstrated before, some nerves clearly arise from the brain, some from the spinal marrow, and the spinal marrow itself from the brain. Therefore it was better not to say simply, as Aristotle, nor with deliberate slyness, as Praxagoras, that the heart is the origin of the nerves. For although the latter saw no nerve arisen from the heart, he argued against Hippocrates, and when he sought to convince that the brain is not at all the origin of the nerves, he was not ashamed to deceive, saying that when in their course the arteries have been divided into many branches, becoming narrower and more slender, they are finally changed into nerves. Since their body is sinewy and hollow, after they have been much and variously divided and distributed in the body of the animal, their cavities are rendered so small and narrow that the covering parts collapse together. He says that when this first happens the nerve appears in place of the artery. Erasistratus decided that the opinion of Praxagoras was based upon impudent audacity and was not even worthy of refutation.

CHAPTER VII

. . . . We do not hesitate to say that if anyone were to accept as correct what Praxagoras considers to be the case, that the heart is the origin of the nerves, it would have to be apparent from anatomy. But such is not the case, as we have demonstrated thousands of times to those who desired to know the truth . . . . Therefore let us consider the arteries that are outside the thorax. Of these the first pair are those that are carried upwards to the scapulae, from which a sizeable pair [vertebral] creep internally to the spinal marrow and are distributed in the muscles of the neck; but it is the second pair, which extend to the arms [subclavian] that seem to me to be those in particular that Praxagoras wished to indicate as ending in nerves. As these are larger than those in the thorax, so they can be observed more clearly as they extend throughout the whole arm as far as the fingers. But none of them is seen to become a nerve. Those in the wrist that are felt for the sake of determining fevers, and those that are located between the thumb and index finger are very slender but do not become nerves, and even without dissection are clearly felt to pulsate. Regarding these matters, perhaps Praxagoras ought not be too strongly censured, but rather pardoned if he did not see the small arteries, although when he said that the arteries are transformed into nerves, it ought to be noted that he did not wish to plead blunted vision but that he saw very acutely. I wish to call to the attention of those who so strongly support Praxagoras, the fact that the axillary arteries (for there is one in each arm), since they are large, they have around them four pairs of large nerves. No artery has begun to divide in these parts, and the nerves are so large that even were one blind they would not at all lie hidden from his touch. Therefore, it is proper that Praxagoras say whence they arise and from which arteries they extend. Such being the case, I challenge Praxagoras to explain this . . . . And so it has been demonstrated that all the arteries arise from the heart, and none of them is changed into nerve since the origin of all the nerves is in the brain.

HEROPHILUS AND ERASISTRATUS
(*See p.* 10)

As noted above, it was owing to Herophilus and especially to Erasistratus, his younger contemporary at Alexandria, that the structure which transmits messages throughout the body was discovered. Furthermore, Herophilus seems to have differentiated between motor and sensory nerves (see Rufus, p. 146) and thus resolved generations of controversy. Most important of all, he suggested that the nerves originating from the brain and cord were hollow (Galen, *The use of parts*, X, 12, Daremberg [1854–1856], I, 637): ". . . for the sensory nerves that descend to the eyes from the brain, and which Herophilus called conduits, because they alone display visible channels for the passage of the [animal] spirit." Hence Herophilus, according to Galen, considered the nerves to contain a spirit or *pneuma*.

The idea of a hollow nerve transmitting a subtle substance, either fluid or gaseous, was to dominate all theories of nerve function until the late eighteenth century. As demonstrated in Chapter II, it was for this reason that investigators studying the morphological features of the nerve, such as Leeuwenhoek, felt impelled to discover a hollowness, if not in the nerve bundle then in the nerve fibre, in order to satisfy the theory of function originated by Herophilus.

The exact opinions of Herophilus are no longer available, and his arguments must be reconstructed from a few references made to them by other authors. This is also true of the slightly later Erasistratus, except that in his case the material is somewhat more plentiful, owing to the fact that he was a frequent target, about four centuries later, for the scorn and criticism of Galen who usually presented his opponents' opinions while attacking them.

In his book, *On the natural faculties*, II, 6 (Kühn, 1821–1833, II), Galen, while discussing "nutrition," first mentioned the nutrition of veins from their contents and then went on to consider how nerves were nourished. The nerve was hollow and contained *psychic pneuma*, or the Latin equivalent, *animal spirit*. This was to be the basis of Galen's theory of nerve action.

EXCERPT PP. 96–97

. . . . But how are the nerves nourished since they do not contain blood? The obvious answer is that they draw nourishment from the veins, but [Erasistratus] will not agree to this. What then does he propose? He says that the nerve has within itself veins and arteries, like a cord woven from three different strands. He believed that through this hypothesis he could avoid the argument of attraction; for if a large nerve were to have a blood vessel within itself, it would not require other blood flowing outside from the neighboring true vein, but there would be sufficient nourishment supplied by that fictitious vessel which his scheme recognizes. But here again he faces another problem. For could this slender little vessel nourish itself, it would be unable to nourish that simple nerve or artery that lies adjacent unless he were to grant to them some innate force for attracting nourishment. How could that simple nerve attract nourishment in that way in which the composite do by a refilling of what is emptied? Although, according to [Erasistratus] it contains a cavity, that cavity is full of animal spirit, not blood. We must consider that nourishment to be introduced not into this cavity but into the vessel that contains it whether it be required only for nourishment or for growth. Therefore in what way should we consider it to be introduced? For that simple vessel is so slender, like each of the other two, that if you puncture any part of it, even with the finest needle, you will at once tear the three of them. And so it cannot be that there is a perceptible, wholly empty space in it. A theoretical empty space cannot compel the associated [fluid] to enter and fill it.

Another fundamental idea originating from Erasistratus' work concerned the contraction of muscle. When the *psychic pneuma* reached the muscle from the motor nerve, the muscle was ballooned (*The sites of diseases*, VI, 5, Daremberg [1854–1856], II, 693): "Erasistratus has said that if the muscles are filled with spirit and increased in breadth, they are decreased in length and therefore that they are shortened." Muscle contraction was still explained on the basis of this statement in the seventeenth century.

Like Herophilus, Erasistratus traced the nerves to the brain, although at first he thought they arose from its meninges, and he described both motor and sensory types (see Rufus, p. 146). He also considered the role of the nerves in disease, and, in keeping with then current ideas, thought that the blocking of them by a humor was a pathogenic process. He discussed this in the following statement (Galen, *The black bile*, V, Kühn [1821–1833], V) and made the very important comment that nerves mediate voluntary movements.

EXCERPT P. 125

. . . . It was demonstrated by us elsewhere that humor also arises in serious illnesses, since Erasistratus himself granted that certain diseases originate from a humor of that sort. However much he may have sought to ascribe the cause to perverse humors, nevertheless he declared the sticky and thick humors to be the causes of the weakness of the nerves, writing: And so the disease arises from obstruction by the humors in the vessels [i.e., channels] of the spirit, which are in the nerves, by which the voluntary motions are performed. And a little later he says: There is obstruction of the aliment by which the nerves are nourished; it [the humor] is sticky and tractile, and it can be separated out with difficulty. Yet he did not say that a humor of this sort is the cause of apoplexy, lethargy, epilepsy, or of many other affections.

RUFUS OF EPHESUS
(See p. 12)

The anatomical descriptions given by Rufus are of outstanding significance, although their value is diminished by the difficulty of dating them accurately (c. A.D. 100?); nevertheless they supplement the accounts given by others of the lost writings of Herophilus and Erasistratus. Reference has already been made to the nerve as described in Rufus's writings (see p. 14), and in the following passage from *The anatomy of the parts of the body*, 71–75 (*Œuvres*, 1879) the nerves are again described; it will be noted that the confusion over the word *neuron* continues. Rufus's statements concerning the Alexandrian anatomists must be correlated with those of Galen on the same topic.

EXCERPT PP. 184–185

The nerve is a simple and dense body; it is the source of voluntary movement; but it lacks sensitivity when it has been cut. According to Erasistratus and Herophilus, there are nerves of sensation; but according to Asclepius, there is none of this sort. Thus Erasistratus declares that there are two kinds of nerves, those of movement and those of sensation; these latter are hollow and their origin is on the meninges; the others arise from the cerebrum and cerebellum. If one believes Herophilus about them, there are nerves of voluntary movement that arise from the brain and the spinal cord, others that insert themselves, some from one bone to another [ligaments], some from a muscle to another muscle [aponeuroses], and, finally, others that bind articulations [tendons].

The second excerpt is from *The names of the parts of the body*, 211–212.

EXCERPT PP. 163–164

Among the nerves that issue from the brain and from the spinal marrow, the motor or sensory ones are called voluntary and tensor; the others that are around the articulations are called ligaments. The thick fascia that extends from the nape of the neck [nuchal ligament] and that which passes from the muscle into the heel [tendo Achillis] are called tendons.

GALEN

(See p. 14)

Galen was the coordinator of Greek medicine, and in his writings we find included many of his predecessors' theories which he was attempting to fuse into a complete system with his own. Concerning nerve function, he relied heavily upon Herophilus and Erasistratus despite his frequent castigation of the latter. In his discussion of their ideas of nerve action (pp. 144–145 and 145–146) and those of Praxagoras (pp. 143–144), some of Galen's beliefs can be deduced from his accompanying comments. He accepted and incorporated into his system the doctrine of the hollow nerve which either transmitted *psychic pneuma* from the brain to the muscle, which it ballooned, or was used to carry sensory impressions. His explanations of how the *pneuma* travelled through the nerves varied; for example, when thinking of the more solid nerves he said it passed through them like "the rays of the sun through air and water" (*The causes of symptoms*, I, 5, Kühn [1821–1833], VII, 110).

His view of the importance of the nerve in the nervous system has already been cited (p. 18); and his basic concept of nerve function is to be found in his book, *The sites of diseases*, IV (Daremberg [1854–1856], II, 583ff.). In summary form it may be stated as follows: There are nerves destined for the muscles and others for the skin. When the first kind has been affected, movement is abolished, and when the second, sensation.

Galen's writings are notoriously difficult to handle for illustration of his concepts. They are long-winded, circuitous, repetitive, and occasionally contradictory. He discusses some topics in several different works, and it is rare to find a succinct summary of his ideas. We must therefore select a number of separate passages.

His extensive experience of dissection taught him much about the anatomy of nerves that had escaped earlier investigators. The problem of differentiating nerves from structures of similar appearance still existed, but Galen's division of nerves into hard and soft was to persist for many centuries. In the following passage he included a third variety, midway between hard and soft (*Commentaries on Hippocrates' book on nourishment*, III, 1 [Kühn (1821–1833), XV, 257]).

. . . . There are three kinds of "nerves." [1] Some, which we call voluntary, originate from the brain and spinal marrow; [2] some, which, so to speak, we call ligaments, from bones; and [3] some, which we call tendons, from muscles. Some are hard and some soft, and the origin of all the hard is from the spinal marrow. The lower extremity of the latter is the source of the hard, but the brain is the source of all the soft nerves; the middle of its anterior parts is asserted to be for the very soft. The origin of the substance of the middle nerves is where the brain and spinal marrow are joined. Aristotle, however, did not know this, he who in other respects was a distinguished ornament of science but was not especially skilled in dissection of bodies.

According to Galen, the hard and soft nerves came from parts of the central nervous system of like consistency, and as this implies a functional division of the brain, one may think of it as the first suggestion of brain localization (see p. 147). Concerning the texture of nerves, he asserted that their substance was like that of the brain but that in the case of the optic nerves canals were present (see Leeuwenhoek, p. 33), and in his book, *The dissection of the nerves*, 2 (Kühn [1821–1833], II, 833), he stated this even more clearly.

> . . . . But in these nerves alone, before they enter the eye, there is a clearly perceptible canal or passage, whence some anatomists have called them canals, not nerves; and some term them optic (*visorii*) nerves, bestowing the name from the function.

The division of the brain into hard and soft can be understood if one considers the relative firmness of the cerebellum and the softer consistency of the cerebrum in a fresh, unfixed brain. It is more difficult to comprehend the hard nerves coming from the anterior, soft brain, but both varieties of nerves from this part may represent a reference to motor and sensory cranial nerves. The following passage has been taken from *The use of parts*, VIII, 6 (Daremberg [1854–1856], I, 541–543).

> . . . . This [brain], then, is very similar in substance to the nerves, of which it was destined to be the origin except insofar as it is softer than they. I emphasize this, for it befits that which receives all sensations into itself, and also imagines all phantasies, and conceives all concepts and ideas. It is the most easily modified in all such functions and the most suitable for experiences, as a softer substance is always more easily modified than a harder. It is for this reason that the brain is softer than the nerves. Because of their need to be dual in nature, as was also said previously, the brain itself was likewise created dual, softer in front, and the rest, which the anatomists call the cerebellum, harder. And therefore, too, it is walled off by a double dura mater [tentorium cerebelli], and is connected only at the passage lying under the crown of the head and the bodies surrounding it [tentorial opening]. Since it was necessary that the front be softer, since it was destined to be the source of the soft nerves extended for sensations, and harder behind as the source of the hard nerves distributed to the entire body, and since contact of the soft with the hard would not be safe, therefore nature separated one from the other by placing between them the dura mater [tentorium cerebelli], which was also required to contain, invest, and surround the entire brain consisting of the aforesaid parts. Furthermore, those parts of the anterior brain itself [cerebral cortex] which touch this covering that is called the dura mater or pachymeninges, are also

made sensibly harder, and those parts surrounded in the middle by these, softer. For it was necessary to make the external parts harder for protection and for the production of the harder nerves, but the parts in the middle have protection from their position itself and so were a suitable source for the soft nerves. From the posterior brain not a single soft nerve is produced, but it was necessary that some of the hard nerves should spring from the anterior brain, like those I consider to have been provided to move the eyes. Although these are near the soft nerves, yet nature did not give them origin from the [soft] deep parts from which soft nerves arise, but from the superficial [hard] parts. Hence all the nerves are harder than brain sub-stance, not as being another altogether different kind of substance, but as being of the same nature though differing from the brain in dryness and density. The sensory nerves going to the eyes are altogether denser than brain, but do not appear altogether harder; but it will seem to you that these, of all nerves, were created of, as it were, condensed but not dried brain substance. Then, too, these alone appear to contain perceptible pores, wherefore many anatomists call them porous or perforate, saying that two such passages [hyaloid canals] grow from the brain into the roots of the eyes, one in each of them; and when these break up, broaden, and flatten out, the retinal tunic is formed; furthermore, they say that nerves pass into their muscles.

Galen returned to this problem in the next book of the *Use of parts*, IX, 14 (Daremberg [1854–1856], I, 597–598) and made more precise statements concern-ing the motor and sensory nerves. His intermediate group perhaps reflected his uncertainty over a strict division of nerves into hard and soft, or the need for a mixed motor and sensory nerve.

EXCERPT PP. 597–598

. . . . So understand that there are two kinds of nerves, one hardest of all those in the body and the other softest. And again understand that there is a third kind between these two, proportionally an exactly equal distance from each of the extremes. Those, therefore, between the median and the hardest are all called hard; and those remaining, relative to the softest, soft. The hard are to be considered best adapted for motion and the most unsuited for sensation; on the contrary, the soft have good constitution for accuracy of sensation, but weakness for strength of motion.

Those that are absolutely soft are not motor at all, and those less soft than these may be considered as approaching the mean; these are motor also, but they fall far short of the function of the hard nerves. Consider, therefore, that the source of all the hard nerves is the spinal cord, and its lower extremity is the source of the extremely hard ones; the source of all the soft nerves is the brain, and the parts between its anterior lobes are the source of the softest; this is the source of the substance of the intermediate nerves [mixed, motor, and sensory] where both brain and spinal cord join.

In his book, *The movement of muscles*, I, 1 (Daremberg [1854–1856], II, 323), Galen differentiated the nerve from the ligament and then the nerve from bone marrow; evidence of the early confusion with the last is still found in several modern European languages. He went on to account for the muscle's motive force which reaches it by way of the nerve. His realization that damage to a nerve had certain specific sequelae was a vital factor in his considerations on nerve disease as well as on function.

EXCERPT P. 323

All the muscles have very important relationships with the brain and the spinal marrow, for they need to receive from the brain or from the spinal marrow a nerve which is small to our sight, but the force of which is far from slight. You will recognize this fact from injuries to this nerve. Indeed, incision, compression, contusion, ligation, hardening, or gangrene of the nerve takes away all movement and sensation from the muscle . . . . There exists then in the nerves a considerable force that runs down from above, from the great principle, for this power is not innate in the muscles and does not originate in them. You will understand this best by the following fact: if you choose to cut certain nerves or, indeed, the spinal cord, all that part situated above the incision that remains in relationship with the brain will still preserve the forces that come from this principle, but all that part below will no longer be able to communicate sensation or movement to any organ.

The nerves which in consequence enjoy the role of conduits, carry to the muscles the forces that they draw from the brain as from a source; from the instant that the nerves enter into contact with them they are variously divided through several successive bifurcations, being at the end completely distributed into thin membranous fibres; these bifurcations form a network for the body of the muscle.

In the muscle itself, the nerve was considered to be joined to the tendon and thus to the elementary fibres which were not thought of as muscle fibres (see p. 141) but as derived from the tendon, for according to Galen's concept, these alone contracted; the muscle substance or flesh was only packing material. This was to be the accepted doctrine until refuted by Steno, Charleton, and others in the seventeenth century (Bastholm, 1950, ch. 5). Galen described the nerve ending in the muscle as follows (*The movement of muscles*, I, 2; Daremberg [1854–1856], II, 326).

EXCERPT P. 326

. . . . The nerve that comes to [the muscle] from the brain is a route for the motive force; its goal is to communicate this force. It is also extended at the side of the ligament and mixed with it; in this way the tendon is formed from these two organs.

Galen's fame rested in large degree on his efforts to correlate anatomy, physiology, and medicine, and in this regard his careful dissections of animals were especially noteworthy. He had a great deal to say about the distribution of cranial and peripheral nerves.

We have chosen for presentation a passage from his account of the recurrent laryngeal nerve, for which he provided the name that we use today. The following account, given in full, has been taken from *The use of parts*, VII, 14–15 (Daremberg [1854–1856], I, 504–508). It illustrates well Galen's methods of anatomical description and argumentation, and, in addition, his style of writing. His analogies are appropriate, his teleology is apparent; his desire to praise the handiwork of the Creator, which was his frequent reaction to the wonders of the animal body, later proved to be an important reason for the universal acceptance of his writings in the East and in the West.

EXCERPT PP. 504–508

Listen very carefully to this discourse in which an attempt will be made to explain an incredible fact that is very difficult to demonstrate. You must have indulgence for those anatomists who have preceded me if a fact so difficult to discover escaped them.

In the passage of the nerves across the thorax a branch reascends on each side by the same pathway which it took before in descending; thus it accomplishes a double course. Please remember the return route which I have just mentioned, resembling the course of those runners who cover a double distance. Both courses represent the one direction of the nerves; as for the return route, although the origin of these nerves is derived from the brain, when the will desires the muscles of the larynx to be stretched as if by cords, that route emanating from the origin of the nerves is directed from the top downwards; and, descending across the neck to a somewhat distant part of the thorax, it reascends from there to the larynx where the nerves insert themselves into the muscles in question; each of these six muscles is drawn downwards as if by the hands. It is the same as in that instrument made for the leg [glossocomion]; there the origin of the movement arises from our hands around the axis and carries along the motion of the principal springs to the pulleys; and from these the motion returns from the top downwards from the pulleys towards the part of the leg which is in the course of being stretched. The nerves of the larynx behave in the same way; the bundle of nerves issuing from the brain is like the axis, the origin of the motion. The part of the thorax whence the nerves commence to retrace their course is like the pulley [on the right the nerve turns around the subclavian artery; to the left around the arch of the aorta]. In comparing passage of the nerves with the double course of the stadium you will find that this part does not at all represent the pulley but what is called the point of reflexion; the runners who run a double course circle it, then retracing their steps, begin to run the same course again.

The reason why the nerve does not retrace its previous route, although it has run through such a long passage across the neck and a considerable part of the thorax, is that there is no part of the thorax which could take over the function of boundary or pulley. Such a part would have to be firm and smooth in order to provide a means for the return movement without injury to itself or to the nerve. In that interval [from the brain to the thorax] there is only the clavicle or the first rib which, being lined with a membranous sheathing, might offer its convexity to the nerve so that it could turn as on a pulley; but in this event the nerve would be almost flush with the skin, exposed to all kinds of lesions. Nevertheless, it would not have been wise thus to bring back to the larynx without reflexion, a small nerve detached from a large one. It would run the risk of breaking if it were not wrapped around, and since such protection was necessary, no expedient offered itself except for the nerve to approach the heart. With good reason, since it was bound to return and run through a considerable distance, nature did not hesitate to extend it. This detour did not take strength away from the nerve. On the contrary, all the nerves are soft at their origin and resemble the brain itself, but in advancing they become harder and harder. Consequently these nerves attain a remarkable strength through the length of their passage and, after their reflexion, cover a distance which is almost as long as that of their descent.

CHAPTER XV

Now it is time to discuss this admirable part which you may call the pulley, the boundary or point of reflexion of the nerves of the larynx. However, we are not concerned at present with a search for beauty of names, nor a waste of time in matters of such slight and frivolous interest, when we find such a magnificent and imposing beauty in nature's work. Surely it exists in this area of veins and large arteries which arise from the heart and cross the neck, some following a perpendicular, others a diagonal pathway; none of them exhibits the horizontal direction required for the reflexion of the nerves. The perpendicular would not permit this reflexion to the descending nerves since the vessels and nerves go in opposite directions; in the case of the diagonal, the bending around would be possible to a certain degree, but deprived of stability and firmness, especially if the diagonal were to deviate much from the horizontal and approach the perpendicular. As far as I am concerned, I cannot praise sufficiently the wisdom and power of him who created the animals. Such beautiful works are above, I shall not say merely eulogies, but even hymns. Before seeing them we are convinced that their existence is impossible, but when we have seen them we realize that our judgment was poor, especially when the craftsman, without elaborate equipment and using only a single, small medium, reveals from every angle an irreproachable and accomplished masterpiece, such as one sees in the reflexion of these nerves.

Indeed, in extending the left branch a long distance, nature did not hesitate to make it turn around the large artery [arch of the aorta]; it chose the point where, upon emerging from the heart, the artery [aorta] turns towards the spine. The nerve, therefore, had everything that it needed, horizontal position, smooth, circular flexion, very strong and very solid support. As for the right branch, not finding similar support on this side of the thorax, it was compelled to turn around the artery which exists on this side, an artery which reascends diagonally from the heart towards the right axilla [right subclavian artery]. Nature compensated for this inferiority of means of diagonal reflexion [on the right], compared to the means of horizontal reflexion [on the left], by the multitude of ramifications issuing from the two sides of the nerve and by the strength of the ligaments. Indeed, all the nerves which she had to send to the right side of the thorax she produced in quantity in this region [posterior pulmonary plexus] and inserted them into the organs for which they were destined, giving roots to the nerves as to vegetables planted in the ground. Thus she established this nerve of the larynx in the center of all these roots so that they might protect it on the two sides, and she attached it by membranous ligaments to the artery and adjacent bodies in order that, maintained, so to speak, within these limits, it could safely accomplish its reflexion around the artery, wrapping itself around it as around the neck of a pulley.

Since these nerves reascend immediately after their reflexion, the large nerve extends a ramification like a hand by means of which it straightens and lifts them. From there, both advance to the head of the trachea, repassing along the route previously followed, but no longer distributing the smallest nerve filaments to any muscle, since none needs to receive the principle of motion from the inferior parts [i.e., ascending]; both divide again symmetrically and equally, each into the series of muscles of the larynx that relates to it, the one into the muscles located on the right, the other into the three muscles located on the left, both nerves limiting themselves to the six muscles which open and close the larynx.

ANDREAS VESALIUS
(31 December 1514—October 1564)

After the death of Galen in A.D. 199, little was added to his account of the nerves and their function. Even as late as the appearance of Vesalius's famous anatomical treatise, *De humani corporis fabrica* (Basel, 1543), there had been no significant change. Vesalius has therefore been included with the authors of classical antiquity but forms a bridge to the next group of investigators. Although his anatomy belonged to the Renaissance, much of his physiology stemmed from the classical period.

Vesalius was born in Brussels and studied first at Louvain, then at Paris with Guinter of Andernach and Sylvius, and returned to Louvain to complete his studies for the M.B. At the close of 1537 he received his M.D. at Padua where he was appointed professor of surgery and anatomy. Having realized that Galen had dissected and described only animals and that all those after him had made the error of thinking these descriptions applied to the human body, Vesalius was inspired to write the *Fabrica* which greatly supplemented the relatively insignificant efforts of his predecessors to found modern anatomy. Thereafter he became a court physician and died at the early age of fifty (O'Malley, 1964). The following passage has been taken from the *Fabrica* (1543) Book VII, Chapter I, "A brief enumeration of the functions and parts of the brain."

EXCERPT P. 632

. . . . [The brain] prepares the very finely attenuated animal spirit that it employs partly for the divine operations of the principal soul [in the brain] and partly for continuous distribution through the nerves, as through little cords, to the instruments of sensation and movement. The organs that are considered the chief authors of those functioning instruments, the liver and heart, never lack spirit, and—so long as man is healthy—leave no parts of the body that require them without their materials, even if they are not always distributed in the same quality and quantity. As we indicated in the fourth book, the nerves which take origin from the brain have that relationship to the brain that the aorta has to the heart and the vena cava to the liver. The nerves may be considered as the diligent servants and messengers of the brain as they deliver the spirit prepared by the brain to those instruments to which it must be sent.

Galen had taught that the vital spirit was generated in the heart and that the animal spirit was elaborated from it in the brain (see p. 759). After having described this, Vesalius then mentioned the role of the animal spirit in the nerves, noting, however, that variant theories existed.

EXCERPT P. 633

. . . . A considerable portion of animal spirit is distributed from this [fourth] ventricle into the dorsal marrow [spinal cord] and into the nerves arising from it. I believe that the spirit is dispensed from the other [lateral and third] ventricles into the nerves taking origin near them, and so into the organs of sensation and movement. I have no desire to go into the question of whether that very refined spirit is transmitted through passages in the nerves, like the vital spirit through the arteries, whether it is transmitted along the sides of the nerve's body like light along a column, or whether the power of the brain extends to the parts merely by the continuity of [the substance of] the nerves.

Vesalius's refusal to discuss the question of how the spirit was transmitted by way of the nerves arose from the fact that although compelled to accept the neurophysiology of his time, through personal observation of the human structure he had come to doubt at least some aspects of neuroanatomy. Thus, contrary to the belief then current, he denied that the nerves were hollow. In Book IV, Chapter I, of the *Fabrica* (p. 315) he declared the nerves to be ". . . long, rounded structures without any apparent internal cavity, slipping from the skull or dorsal vertebrae and carrying down animal spirit from the brain to produce the animal faculty for the parts of the body." Later on he was more emphatic (p. 317): "I scarcely dare to deny the hollowness of the nerve although I have never seen a channel even in the optic nerve; this despite the fact that the nerves, like the veins and arteries, are called vessels and that I am aware that professors of anatomy declare the optic nerves to be hollow."

On the same page he stated that the nerves can be identified in cooked meat: "You will see the end of the nerve to resemble a thick cord, twisted from many threads, and as if it had been cut across with a blunt knife."

Vesalius was, therefore, refuting the ancient concept of the hollow nerve, and his mention of "threads" in the nerve may have been the first reference to the internal structure and it indicates that he had seen bundles of primitive fibres there. However, he was in agreement with Galen's general theory of nerve action.

New Theories of Nerve Function

RENÉ DESCARTES
(31 *March* 1596—11 *February* 1650)

The basic features of Galen's concept of nerve function were still alive a hundred years after the publication of Vesalius's *Fabrica*, but thereafter they were subjected to modifications out of which present-day beliefs subsequently developed. One of the most interesting modifications of the Galenic concept of nerve function was that of the great French philosopher Descartes.

Descartes was born in La Haye, Touraine, and was educated at the Jesuit College of La Flèche in Anjou. Thereafter he renounced all he had learned and would admit nothing that could not bear the test of reason. He travelled widely in Europe, served briefly in the Bavarian army, studied, and meditated. His books on mathematics, pure and applied, and on philosophy were the product of an independent genius whose influence was widespread in the seventeenth century. Descartes aroused in the philosophy of mind the same revolution that Bacon had aroused in the natural sciences. He died in Sweden where he had been invited by Queen Christina, reputedly from the rigors of the winter and the equally rigorous intellectual demands of the queen (see Baillet, 1691; Saint-Germain, 1869; Mahaffy, 1880; Adam, 1910, 1937; Haldane, 1913; Souques, 1938).

Descartes' dualistic philosophy separated the mind from the body, the latter, according to his belief, constructed like a machine. Messages to and from the brain, in which the rational soul was situated in the pineal body, travelled by way of the nerves; his explanation of the functioning of the nerves was based upon mechanical phenomena. This aspect of Descartes' work was therefore characteristic of the efforts of the iatrophysicists of the seventeenth century who attempted to explain biological phenomena on the basis of physical laws.

The following brief summary of Descartes' concept of nerve function occurs in his celebrated discourse on the method of reasoning (*Discours de la méthode pour bien conduire sa raison, & chercher la verité dans les sciences. Plus la dioptriques* . . . [Leiden, 1637], "The senses in general, Fourth discourse").

EXCERPT P. 31

. . . . it is necessary to believe that the [animal] spirits, flowing through the nerves into the muscles, and inflating them sometimes more and sometimes less, now some, now others according to the different ways in which the brain distributes them, cause the movements of all the limbs; and that the little threads of which the internal substance of the nerves is composed serve the senses.

Descartes' anatomy and physiology were based upon that of Galen, but they also included his own ideas which helped to explain his preconceived theory. The next passage has been taken from a book which, although probably written in 1634, was not published until 1662 when it appeared in a Latin translation (*De homine*, Leiden, 1662); Descartes' original French text, *L'homme* (Paris, 1664), was not published until two years later. It contains the classical theory of animal spirits manufactured in the brain, stored in the ventricles, and passed into the hollow nerves to initiate muscular movements. The most interesting part of his description concerned the nerve's fine threads, already mentioned, which allowed sensation to be appreciated. The origin of this idea is unknown, and it is tempting to suggest that the threads may have been nerve fibres or small bundles of them. It is much more likely, however, that Descartes was referring to the elemental "fibre" (p. 29); he argued that the fibre common to other animal and plant tissues should also be in the brain (p. 158). Figure 42 appears in *L'homme* of 1664, whereas in *De homine* of 1662 the same text is illustrated by figure 42 with the addition of a drawing of the brain and optic nerves (p. 20; not illustrated here). Descartes' account of his system in action is found in his discussion of the reflex (pp. 329–333). The following selection has been taken from Part II, "How the Bodily

Machine Moves," Article 15, "That the Animal Spirits are the Great Force which moves this Machine."

EXCERPT PP. 12–15

Now as these spirits thus enter into the cavity of the brain, so they pass from there into the pores of its substance, and from these pores into the nerves; where, as they enter, or, indeed, where they only advance to enter, now into some, now into other pores, they have the power to change the shape of the muscles in which the nerves are inserted, and by this means to cause motion in all the parts. Just as you may have seen that the power of moving water, travelling from its source, is alone sufficient to move the different machines in the grottos and fountains in our kings' gardens, according to the various arrangements of the pipes conducting it, even causing those machines to play several instruments or to pronounce several words.

ART. 16

ACCURATE COMPARISON MADE WITH THE ARTIFICIAL MACHINES

In fact, one can readily compare the nerves of the [human] machine that I am describing to you to the pipes of the machines of these fountains; its muscles and tendons to various other engines and springs that serve the movements; its animal spirits, of which the heart is the source, to the water that moves them, and the cavities of the brain to reservoirs. Furthermore, respiration and other such natural and ordinary actions which depend upon the flow of the spirits are like the movements of a clock or a mill rendered continuous by the normal flow of water. The external objects that by their presence alone act upon the sensory organs, and that by this means cause [the human machine] to move itself in many different ways, according to the disposition of its brain, are like strangers who, entering into one of the grottos of these fountains, without giving thought to the movements that are performed there in their presence, in fact, themselves cause them; for they cannot enter except by walking on certain tiles so placed that, for example, if they approach a bathing Diana they will cause her to hide in the rushes; and if they go further in pursuit of her, they will cause Neptune to approach menacingly with his trident; or if they go to one side, they will cause a sea monster to appear and spew water in their faces, or similar things according to the whim of the engineers who made them. Finally, there is a *reasoning soul* in this machine; it has its principal site in the brain where it is like the fountaineer who must be at the reservoir, whither all the pipes of these machines are extended, when he wishes to start, stop, or in some way alter their actions.

ART. 17 . . . .

ART. 18

WHAT IS THE STRUCTURE OF THE NERVES?

Here, then, observe, for example, the nerve A [fig. 42] of which the outer membrane is like a great pipe containing many other, smaller pipes, *b, c, k, l*, etc., composed of a thinner outer membrane; and these two membranes are continuous with the two, *K, L*, that envelope the brain *M, N, o*.

Observe, too, that in each of these smaller pipes there is a kind of marrow composed of many very fine threads that come from the substance of the brain itself, *N*, of which the extremities terminate at one end at the internal surface that faces the cavity, and at the other, at the membranes and fleshes against which the containing pipe terminates. But because this marrow does not at all serve for the movement of the parts, it suffices for the present that you know that it does not fill the little pipes containing it in such a way that the animal spirits cannot find enough room to run easily from the brain into the muscles, into which these little pipes, that must here be considered as little nerves, extend.

Descartes' writings resemble those of Galen in that he repeated himself frequently and no one statement is adequate. Thus, in regard to the nerves and their threads we find more details in the first section of his work *Les passions de l'ame* ([Amsterdam], 1649), Article XII.

EXCERPT PP. 19–20

. . . . I shall repeat here that there are three things to be considered in the nerves: to know that their medulla or internal substance is extended in the form of little threads from the brain, from which they take their origin, to the extremities of the lobes where they are attached; then, that the membranes which surround them and which are continuous with the one that envelopes the brain are composed of little tubes in which these fine threads are enclosed; and, finally, that the animal spirits that are carried in these same tubes from the brain to the muscles, explain why the threads are quite free and so plentiful, so that the least thing which moves the part of the body or extremity to which one of them is attached, in the same way causes movement in the part of the brain from which it comes; just as when one end of a cord is pulled the other end moves.

THOMAS WILLIS
(27 January 1621—11 November 1675)

Whereas Descartes and others after him—for example, Borelli—attempted to apply the laws of the physical sciences to the functioning of animal and human nerves, another group of investigators preferred to relate chemical data to the problem. These were the iatrochemists, and one of the most important of them was Thomas Willis of Oxford and London.

Willis was born at Great Bedwyn in Wiltshire and educated at Oxford where he eventually became professor of natural philosophy. He also practised medicine and, although very successful, nevertheless in 1666 moved to London where he also gained a high reputation as a practitioner. Despite Michael Foster's denigration of him (Foster, 1901, pp. 269–279), it is clear that Willis's contribution to the anatomy and physiology of the nervous system was an important one, and that his clinical work was likewise worthy of note. His name is still associated with the arterial circle at the base of the brain (see Munk, 1878, I, 338–342; Dow, 1940; Hierons and Meyer, 1962, 1964; Dewhurst, 1964).

Willis's important book, *Cerebri anatome* (London, 1664), contains his theory of nerve function which is basically Galenic. Characteristically he indulged in considerable speculation beyond the observable facts, and his account of how a muscle is invoked to contract was a mixture of chemical and physical analogies. The basis of nerve function was a chemical process; and the substance that passed to the muscle there met the vital spirits from the blood, and the resultant reaction produced contraction. Willis frequently spoke of fibres and in some instances may have been referring to the elemental "fibre" (p. 29). But as he made mention of the microscope, perhaps the first reference to it in relationship to the study of the nerve, some of his "fibres" could have been small bundles of true nerve fibres. The following passages have been translated from Chapter XIX, "On the nervous system in general." Although the translation by Pordage (*Dr. Willis's practice of physick . . . new* translated by Samuel Pordage, London, 1684) has a quaint and vigorous style, it has been thought preferable to retranslate the selections below, as well as those included in other chapters.

EXCERPT PP. 125–128

We revealed above that the animal spirits are created only in *the brain* and *cerebellum*, and running continuously thence they inflate and fill the medullary trunk [spinal cord] that is like the organ's box which receives the air to be blown into all the pipes. Carried thence into *the nerves* those spirits fully inflate them as if they were so many pipes hanging from the medullary trunk, and actuate them. Then those which overflow from the nerves enter the fibres dispersed throughout the membranes, muscles, and other parts, and so they communicate *motor and sensory force* into those bodies in which the nerve fibres are interwoven . . . .

Indeed, *the animal spirits* flowing within *the nerves* are like a river from a lively, bubbling and perennial source; they are in nowise stagnant nor remain still, but flowing down with a continual current are ever newly supplied by an inflow from the source. Meanwhile, *the remaining nervous spirits*, especially abundant in the membranes and muscular fibres, are like ponds and lakes of waters widely flooded beyond their river beds, of which the standing waters are not much moved of their own accord but rather by things cast into them or are agitated by the blowing of winds and so produce various sorts of waves.

But since there is considerable difference between the movements and lack of them of the spirits and waters, perhaps the matter would be better illustrated if each kind of *spirit*, the inflowing and the implanted, were compared to *the beams* of different rays of light. When illumination is let into a dark room and instantly lights up the whole of it, one must conceive of those so swiftly diffused particles of light as *of two kinds*, that is, *some* are little bodies sent from the light itself and diffused everywhere into an orb: in addition, there are *other* luminous particles, little ethereal bodies already existing within the pores of the air. When the latter particles are agitated by the former and, so to speak, set alight, a very tenuous, quasi flammy texture is produced in the whole transparent extent. In like manner the animal spirits running from the medullary substance [white matter] into the nerves are like the rays diffused from the light itself, and the other spirits, abundant throughout the fibres, are like the lucid particles enclosed and implanted in the air which are activated and aroused into movement by the former particles, and thus the acts of the sensory and motor faculties are performed.

. . ˙. .

. . . .

The passages *of the nerves* are not hollowed out like those of the arteries and veins, because their substance is not only impervious to any stylus, but the use of a lens or microscope confirms that there is no cavity present in them. As regards the olfactory tubules, they seem to be so made, not for the passage of animal spirits but in order that certain serosities may slip out by that route; but the spirits are carried in the sides and not in the cavity of each tubule [cf. Vesalius, p. 155]. The other nerves are clearly formed of a compact and firm substance so that the subtle humor, which is the vehicle of the spirits, may pass through their structures not otherwise than spirits of wine through the tensed cords of a lute, only by slowly creeping through. Hence it may be argued that the animal spirits require no manifest cavity within the nerves for their expansion . . . .

. . . . *The nerves* themselves, as may be detected with the aid of a microscope, are formed throughout with pores and passages like so many holes densely packed one next to another [cf. Leeuwenhoek, p. 33]; thus their tubelike substance, similar to sugarcane, is porous and pervious throughout. Within these little spaces the animal spirits, or very subtle corpuscles, by their nature always ready for movement, are in gentle agitation. A *watery liquid* of very subtle parts is added to them as both *a vehicle* and *a bridle*. This *humor*, by its *fluidity*, diffuses the spirits through the whole nervous system, and by its *viscosity* prevents their dissipation and retains them as in a kind of composed or uninterrupted series; for it seems that without such a humor the spirits would be unable to remain within the nervous fibres but would vanish into thin air. The same humor is no less required for the passage of sensory perceptions; indeed, we suppose that the animal spirits, like rays of light, are diffused through the whole nervous system, and those rays, unless the humid particles of the air are mixed with them, do not easily transmit the appearances or images of things, as is obvious in a painted scene that is obscured by too brilliant and strong sunshine. Likewise, we can readily display that by a *defect* or *lack of the nervous juice* a disarrangement of the animal spirits and often horrid cerebral and nervous affections arise.

That *nervous juice* that is directed from the brain and cerebellum into the medullary appendix [spinal cord], from there is carried in a gentle downward course through the whole nervous structure and irrigates the entire system . . . . meanwhile, however, as occasion arises, those spirits, like a breath moving over those waters, conceive of other and more rapid distribution. For just as waves are aroused in a river by winds and various things cast in, so the animal spirits aroused by objects for performing the functions of sensation and motion, move this way and that within the nervous structure and by other means are driven hither and thither.

EXCERPT PP. 130–131

The animal spirits that enter the ordered arrangement of *the fibres* [of the nerve] and, so to speak, fill their little compartments, flow thither through the nerve ducts; nevertheless *the spirits* that occupy *the fibres* woven together with *muscular fibres* receive *nourishment* and, as it were, *subsidiary supplies*, from *the arterial blood* flowing abundantly into the same place; by this the spirits acquire *a greater kind of elastic force for the performance of their movements*, so that their onset, aroused by a powerful urge, seems like *an explosion of gunpowder*; then those same spirits, more diffused within the muscles than is usual in the membranes and other parts, and continually nourished by their *sanguineous fodder*, are to a certain degree restored. Indeed, when *the arterial juice*, which is plentifully abundant within the sanguineous parts, approaches *the nervous juice*, it is permissible to believe that it also adds and affixes intimately to the spirits brought there certain quasi *nitrosulphurous particles*. Because of this highly *gaseous union*, suitable for rarefaction, those *spirits* then become more active so that in whatever their motive effort by which they suddenly inflate the muscle, it is as if *having been ignited they are exploded*. For this reason a swift *restoration* of *the spirits* exhausted by their strong effort is in some degree accomplished by *the blood*, that is, inasmuch as the *spiritous particles* remain after *the movement*, and at once there is a *new union* of that material suitable for explosion. It is not possible that the immense loss of spirits—if they are not completely dispersed—which happens in such great effort, could be restored in a short time by supplements received only through the nerves.

The final selection is from the *De motu musculari* of Willis, which first appeared in a volume entitled *Affectionum quae dicuntur hystericae & hypochondriacae*, London, 1670. It is of special interest because in it we find possibly the first reference to the fact that peripheral nerves need not always be in direct communication with the brain. Willis argued that muscles must have nerve connections between themselves in order to account for associated movements. This arrangement was also of basic importance in reflex action and underlay the phenomenon of "sympathy" (pp. 328–329). In the paragraph preceding the excerpt Willis described the nerves as being made up of "many hairlike nervules collected in the same bundle for the sake of better conduction" which could be traced "to the parts and members to which they are directed." These no doubt were small bundles of primary nerve fibres, rather than theoretical "fibres."

EXCERPT PP. 104–105

   Meanwhile, although it may be that many nerves are separate passages or channels of the animal spirits, yet some communicate variously with others through shoots and branches extended between them. This is required so that when many nerves are needed simultaneously for some motion of a muscle, all of them, because of the mutual relationships between them, take part in the same action. Hence in certain motions of the members, as in the plucking of a harp and other very complicated actions, several muscles cooperate with such astonishing speed that, although many may be involved at the same time, without any confusion each separately performs its service. Moreover, it is necessary for the nerves to communicate mutually with one another because of the consonant motions of certain members and parts; it is for no other reason that the nerve of the diaphragm is attached to the brachial branches, so that the activities of animals, especially in running and flying, may be proportionate to the state of respiration. Hence it also happens that in any passion, with the praecordia constricted or dilated, the appearance of the countenance and face, indeed, the gestures of the hands and members, reflect the emotions.

GIOVANNI ALFONSO BORELLI
(28 January 1608—31 December 1679)

One of the most ardent proponents of the iatrophysical explanation of biological phenomena was the Italian mathematician and physicist Borelli. He was born in

Naples and studied medicine and mathematics in Rome. After having held a professorship in the University of Messina, in 1656 he was appointed professor of mathematics at Pisa where he worked in close touch with Malpighi; but after spending twelve years there he returned to Messina in 1668. Six years later he went to Rome where, under the patronage of Queen Christina of Sweden, he was engaged upon his most outstanding work, *De motu animalium* (Rome, 1680–1681, 2 vols.), a study of the mechanics of animal movement. He died before it was published (see Foster, 1901, pp. 62–83, 281–285; Meier, 1937; Gaizo, 1904, 1908, 1909; Bastholm, 1950, pp. 163–175. There is also an unpublished dissertation by Wilson, 1955–1956).

One of the problems which Borelli tackled from the mechanical point of view was the transmission of messages through the nerves. His basic pattern was again the same as that of his predecessors except that he postulated a new vehicle to carry the messages. This was the *succus nerveus* which, although bearing a name substituted for the term animal spirit, was declared to have properties that adhered strictly to physical laws. However, when the *succus* reached the muscle, a chemical process took place, reminiscent of that postulated by Willis. It is important to note that some of Borelli's statements are vaguely and distantly in keeping with present-day ideas of nervous transmission. The following selections are from *De motu animalium. Pars altera*, 1681, chapters 3 and 11.

EXCERPT PP. 59–60

PROPOSITION XXIV

THE NERVOUS JUICE (*succus nerveus*) CAN BE VOLUNTARILY INSTILLED WITHIN THE MUSCLES

It seems impossible to deny that the animal spirit is a very subtle and pure fluid substance moving itself. . . .

Hence we perceive that when those cerebral juices or spirits have been agitated they move or pluck the origins of the fibres of some nerve either through a shaking motion or a penetrating sharpness by which perhaps they operate; and so they irritate and arouse. In their structure the nerves are of very delicate and sensitive balance, as is clear from experience, for if the inner part of the nostrils or the ears is touched lightly with a straw, the nerves are agitated so forcibly through their whole lengh that they arouse convulsive movements of sneezing and coughing. Therefore it is not astonishing that when a slight agitation or irritation of the nerves has occurred in the brain a convulsive agitation is produced through their whole length from which there then follows a forcing out and an outflowing of some drops of that juice by which they are swollen.

Because wherever the terminal orifices of those nerve fibres are dispersed through the mass of the muscle, even though they may be open, yet their spongy texture fulfills the function of valves, for we see that the suspended droplets of a moist sponge do not run forth. Hence it occurs that an agitating power is necessary to force them out.

Perhaps this is how the nervous juice is discharged into and instilled through the whole mass of the muscle at the command of the will.

EXCERPT PP. 321–324

PROPOSITION CLVII

EXPLANATION OF THE MECHANICAL ARTIFICE BY WHICH THE SPIRITOUS JUICE CAN BE MOVED OUTWARDS AND INWARDS THROUGH THE SAME NERVE DUCTS

We said that the spirits are moved through the nerves by a double motion. First is that by which local motions of the joints occur and sensations are communicated to the brain. Consideration ought to be given to these things first. From investigation of them it must be revealed that the nerve fibres are neither entirely solid, filled and impermeable, nor are they empty, tubular hollows similar to reeds, but are channels filled with a certain spongy substance, like the pith of the elder tree. This spongy pith of the fibres is easily moistened by the spiritous juice of the brain, to which they are directly attached, and can be saturated to the point of swelling, just as we observe sponges and filters to be saturated by water touching them.

Then I observe that the sheep's intestine may be rendered, so to speak, swollen if it is filled only with water and if also its cavity contains a spongy cord impregnated with the water. The intestine becomes swollen in each case, and if it is slightly compressed or struck at its swollen end, that blow will be simultaneously communicated as far as the other end. In the same way the tubes of the nerve fibres containing a spongy pith can be saturated and swollen by the spiritous juice of the brain, and then if one end is compressed, set in motion, struck, or twitched, the vibration, shaking, or surge must immediately be communicated to the other end; in that ordered arrangement, because of contiguity, the parts following, by impelling those ahead, communicate the blow and impulse to the farthest [part].

Hence it follows that from that slight movement of the spirits by which the acts of the controlling will are exercised, the fibres or spongy ducts of some of the nerves, swollen by the spiritous juice, may be shaken or twitched. Then because of the convulsive irritation shaking the whole length of the nerve, some spiritous droplets can be squeezed out from their terminal orifices into the corresponding muscle, whence a boiling up and dilatation follow and the muscle is thereby contracted and dilated.

On the other hand, when the extremities of the sensory nerves which end in the skin, tongue, nostrils, ears, and eyes are lightly compressed, struck, or tickled, at once a shaking, surging, and tickling of the spiritous juice contained within the tubules is of necessity spread through the whole length of that nerve until it reaches the part of the brain to which the nerve fibres are attached; the faculty of the sensitive soul is thus able to pronounce judgment of the object from the incarried [afferent] motion, from the place struck in the brain, and from the force and manner of the blow and the nature of the motion.

Thus it is easily established that irritation produced in one end of the nerve can, by the action of the farther end, in that same moment be spread and communicated in remote parts without their being touched, pricked, or twitched; because there are nerves of such nature that when one end has been pricked, the sensation of pain is perceived in another place remote from it, as is revealed by many experiments . . . .

. . . .

There remains only one point to be settled, that is, in what way two contrary vibrations can be carried simultaneously through the same nerve so that at the same time local motion and sensation can be exercised, as for example, in the tongue, when a piece of rhubarb is spit out of the mouth and a bitter taste is perceived; and when all the muscles perceive a piercing pain when they have been strongly contracted.

It seems to me that there are two possible explanations of this problem. First, that the aforesaid contrary vibrations do not occur through the same fibre ducts but through separate ones, so that the movement of the sensation of pain is not received through the same fibres by which the movement of the directing will is spread, but through different ones.

Second, and more likely, as the surge of the juice contained in the tube cannot be received without reciprocal movement impelling the extremities of the nerve backwards and forwards by two alternate strokes, not unlike what happens in a tremor. Therefore, those contrary vibrations do not occur at the same but at different times; because of frequency and brevity, they cannot be distinguished and so are concealed; it is thus that from time to time we are deceived in many interrupted sensations and motions.

FRANCIS GLISSON
(1597—14 or 16 October 1677)

In addition to the mechanical and chemical explanations of nerve and muscle function formulated in the seventeenth century, there was another which, although entirely speculative, proved to be of greater importance than many of those based upon a more practical approach. This was the concept of irritability, first put forward by the English physician, Glisson, and representative of the attitude of the vitalists who opposed the materialism of the iatrochemists and physicists.

Glisson was born at Rampisham in Dorset and educated at Cambridge where he first studied philosophy and became lecturer in Greek. He was graduated in medicine in 1634 and two years later was appointed Regius Professor of Physic, a post he held until his death. However, he spent most of his life in London where he both practised medicine and produced treatises on that subject. His name is still associated with the capsule of the liver, and his treatise on rickets, although not the first description of the disease as is often claimed, was a classic contribution to clinical medicine (see Munk, 1878, I, 218–221; Marion, 1882; Foster, 1901, pp. 286–288; Moore, 1908).

By creating his vitalistic doctrine, Glisson was opposing in particular Descartes' materialistic explanation of life. In so doing he stumbled upon a biological phenomenon which in the hands of Haller and others, came to be accepted as a fundamental property of living matter. His notion of the fibre was that already referred to (p. 29), and he discussed it at length in his book, *Tractatus de ventriculo et intestinis* ([London, 1677], pp. 138–143). Unlike our present-day interpretation, the fibre, like the atom of the Greek atomists, was essentially a theoretical concept and presumed to be a basic element of the animal body. However, the uniqueness of Glisson's approach lay in the fact that he included the body's vital force in it. One of the fibre's inherent properties (*robur insitus*) was "irritability," which Glisson first discussed in his book, *Anatomia hepatis* (London, 1654). In the following passage (from Chapter XLIV) Glisson stated that the gall bladder and its ducts were able to secrete bile because of their irritability which was itself dependent upon the nerve supply. The bile irritated the passages and they reacted to rid themselves of the irritant and therefore moved.

EXCERPT P. 396

IRRITATION OF THE BILE DUCTS

. . . . There is a small matter concerning merely the biliary duct and the gall bladder, which must be noted here; that is, how those vessels are irritated to cause abundant excretions at one time rather than at another.

No one doubts that from time to time the biliary ducts may be *irritated* because when cathartics or emetics have been taken, a large amount of this humor is ejected upwards or downwards or in both directions, and that within a very few hours, although otherwise in a period six times as long not even a quarter part of it may be evacuated. The reason for this difference cannot be adequately explained unless we give consideration to those parts of the nerves concerned with the actions and uses, and therefore we must consider here both at the same time.

Recently Temkin (1964) traced the origins of Glisson's idea and rectified several long-standing misconceptions; his paper is therefore an important introduction to any consideration of Glisson's work on irritability. Bastholm (1950, pp. 219–225) has also analyzed the theory clearly (see also Meyer, 1843; Singer, 1937).

Although published posthumously in the year of his death, 1677, Glisson's book, *Tractatus de ventriculo et intestinis*, was written probably as early as 1662. In it he gave a full account of his doctrine of irritability of living substance, which for complete comprehension must be considered as part of the system of natural philosophy that he built up in his book, *Tractatus de natura substantiae energetica* (London, 1672). This system was itself founded upon Aristotelian philosophy, and styled by Max Vervorn (1913, p. 3) as a "wilderness of scholastic phraseology." There is no present intention of delving deeply into it, and the selections below, translated from the *Tractatus de ventriculo et intestinis*, deal with some of the simpler and more readily comprehensible portions of the doctrine.

Glisson differentiated between *perception*, which was the ability to react to a stimulus, and *sensation* or feeling, which was dependent upon the intervention of nerves and brain. *Natural perception* was an unconscious, inherent property and a dynamic principle of the fibre; in modern terms it is the direct response to an artificial stimulus applied directly, and as it is independent of the nervous system it does not enter consciousness. This was the first of three ways in which the fibre could react. The second was by *sensory perception*, owing to an external stimulus which acted by way of the sensory nerves and thus reached consciousness, and the third was by means of *animal desire*, an internal stimulus from the brain. *External sensation* was that in which the impulse acted upon the fibre at the periphery. *Internal sensation*, however, acted centrally in the brain and on the soul (*phantasia*) and went by way of the nerves to produce movement of fibres; it was equivalent to the *vis nervosa* of Haller (p. 172), or to our *nerve impulse*. The movement owing to external sensation can therefore be thought of as reflex and that owing to internal as voluntary.

EXCERPT PP. 147–149

CHAPTER VII, THE IRRITABILITY OF THE FIBRES

1. *Irritability supposes perception.* Unless irritability existed, the motive capacity of the fibres would be either constantly in action or in continual disuse. Therefore the varieties and differences of their actions clearly demonstrate their irritability. However, this supposes perception and desire so that the fibre may be excited repeatedly. But perception having been granted, desire and motion are a natural consequence, so that the mere appearance of perception of the fibres suffices to cause their irritability.

The method of investigating it. Meanwhile, since frequently sensation, and in fact the sensation of desire, are involved with natural perception in this irritation of the fibres, it would be necessary that now natural perception alone, now with the conjoined sensation, now finally impelled by the sensation of desire, contribute to the movement of the fibres. In order that this may be done more easily, it has seemed best to divide [perception] into three kinds and to describe each separately, and so to examine the perception concerned with the movement of the fibres. And so we suppose that perception of irritation related to the fibres is threefold (we suppose it to be, whether it is so or not): natural, sensitive, and regulated by animal desire. First is the natural, that is, by which the fibre perceiving change carried to it, whether pleasing or displeasing, is excited to move itself either towards or away from it. Second, sensible is that by which the fibre by its sensible property [sensation], noting the change made in the external organ, is impelled to seek something and in consequence to move itself. Third, regulated by animal desire is that by which the brain from within moves the fibre of the muscles in order to seek that which it desires. A few things now about these matters in order.

2. *Whether natural perception is inherent in the fibres.* Some perhaps doubt whether there is a natural perception which irritates the fibres; but I, on the contrary, have asserted the existence of natural perception in general, and notably in my book *De vita naturae* [*Tractatus de natura substantiae energetica*, London, 1672], so that he who knows my book may grant that same thing much more readily to the fibres imbued with resident spirits and with those inflowing, vital spirits. One must not expect here a general proof of this, but whatever can be adduced from the structure, actions, and use of the fibres, and confirmed by experience, will be considered later. There is no doubt that the fibres are now at rest and now are moved, for during sleep all of them are relaxed (excepting only those that serve the circulation of the blood and respiration, and whichever of them in turn are now stretched, now relaxed); during wakefulness, again all of them are invigorated by a slight tonic movement so that in all movements of the members, the fibres of the opposed muscles spontaneously yield to one another so that if the adducting muscle is contracted, the abducting relaxes itself, and on the other hand, if the latter is stretched, the other relaxes. And so it is certain that sometimes the fibres are moved and sometimes they yield to rest. Therefore, since they are not the principal agents or indeed the source of decision, it is necessary that when they act anew, they be irritated from somewhere, for it is impossible for quiescent fibres to be put in motion again without an irritating cause; nor is it possible that they can be irritated if they do not perceive the irritation, just as if you were to speak to a deaf person or to attempt to arouse someone dead. You may say that the fibres are ["atomic"] particles equipped with sensibility which can be excited by reason of their capacity of sensation [feeling]. I confess that there are sensible parts and that they are able to indicate, through sensibility, some, but not all, of the causes irritating them. But whether the sensibility moves the fibres immediately, whether it extends directly to the brain and irritates the animal desire and similarly whether the animal desire immediately affects the motion of the fibres, and to what kind of perception this irritation ought properly and appropriately be ascribed, will be said below in order when we come to the explanation of sensible perception and then that directed by phantasy.

3. *It is asserted by the fibres.* Meanwhile let us remain in this area and show that natural perception can be underlying in cases where there is no trace of sensation. The pulsation of the heart neither acts nor is varied by any sensibility. The fibres of the heart by reason of the rapid motion of the vital blood contained in the ventricles, which in turn have been irritated, are excited to contract themselves and to cause pulsation; then with the irritation remitted they are relaxed and seek the natural position of their parts. It cannot be denied that as a result evident irritation of the fibres occurs here. The rhythm of pulsation is varied, as is clear from the differences of pulses in fevers and other diseases. It is not possible that sensibility of the fibres is the cause of this since this perception of irritation occurs in turn equally during sleep, at which time the senses are at rest, and during wakefulness when they are exercised. Therefore, they do not perceive the irritation of the vital blood in these parts by sensible perception, but they are excited both for contraction, and in turn for relaxation by natural perception. The same idea is corroborated by the violent movement of animals which sometimes persists when their heads have been cut off. Similarly, intestines as yet warm in an abdomen which has been opened recently, move and twist themselves in various ways. The fibres of muscles in dead animals contract when touched with sharp and stinging liquids. Likewise all muscles in the dead having been excited by exposure to cold, are strongly constricted by tonic motion and make the body rigid. The hearts of some animals having been removed, and indeed even dissected, continue to pulsate. What more is necessary? Hence it may be inferred with sufficient certainty that the fibres without the aid of sensation can perceive irritation and move themselves in conformity.

EXCERPT P. 152

6. . . . . I have no doubt that external sensation is inherent in the nervous parts of the outer organ [e.g., ear, eye, etc.], whence it may be inferred that it can adequately arouse the fibres of the organ to which it is intimately related, for desire and movement. For since sensation is carried through the nerves to the brain, it cannot be [otherwise than] that the nerves and all nervous parts which have fibres are connected to the brain. Therefore, just as sensation causes its subject to sense, so the same prepares it easily for the conformable [state of] desiring and moving. For perception of the subject is vain if it is unable to desire, and desire is useless if it is unable to move itself. Therefore external sensation is properly said to render the fibres irritable in action, that is, as often as an irritating cause is perceived by the sensation, for as often as it perceives not by the sensation but only by natural perception, this alone is what constitutes an irritable fibre.

ALBRECHT VON HALLER
(*16 October 1708—12 December 1777*)

Glisson's doctrine of irritability received little or no immediate acknowledgment. By the time it appeared in print its author was dead, and it was couched in terms of scholasticism that were no longer fully understood or tolerated in the late seventeenth and early eighteenth centuries. Furthermore, it had not been supported by experiment and so was unacceptable to the experimentalists of the period. Thus it lay dormant for about seventy years until it was resurrected by the renowned Swiss physiologist and anatomist Haller.

Haller was one of the most outstanding medical scientists of the eighteenth century. He was born at Berne and studied medicine at Leyden under Boerhaave, becoming his favorite pupil. In 1736 Haller was appointed professor of anatomy, botany, and medicine at the new University of Göttingen, and during the seventeen years he spent there he carried out a remarkable variety and number of scientific investigations. In 1753 he returned to Berne where he spent the rest of his life writing many books and taking part in municipal and state duties. His publications were voluminous (Lundsgaard-Hansen-von Fischer, 1959) and included literary and poetical compositions (Coffman, 1934). Unfortunately there is no adequate biography of Haller in English (see, however, Hemmeter, 1908; Klotz, 1936; d'Irsay [1930]. There are two recent studies by Rudolph, 1959, 1964).

Under Haller's influence anatomy became an experimental science, and his application of dynamic principles to physiological problems is well exemplified by his investigation of irritability. His handling of this phenomenon differed from that of Glisson in two important respects. First, whereas for Glisson, irritability was a property of all elements of the body, Haller restricted it exclusively to muscle. Second, unlike Glisson, Haller substantiated each statement with experimental evidence. Similarly, Glisson's universal sensibility became in Haller's hands restricted to nerves. Glisson and Haller thus illustrate respectively the medieval scholastic approach to a biological problem, and that of the new scientist of the Scientific Revolution. Each in his own way helped to establish a fundamental process of animal life.

Having made a number of preliminary references to the problem of irritability in earlier publications, Haller read his classic paper on the subject before the Royal Society of Sciences of Göttingen on 22 April and 6 May 1752 ("De partibus corporis humani sensibilibus et irritabilibus," *Comment. Soc. Reg. Sci. Göttingen.*, 1753, 2:114–158).

Haller gives full credit to Glisson for having first formulated the idea of irritability (pp. 154–155) and deals first with sensibility, which is invariably owing to the presence of nerves, and then with irritability or contractility, which belongs exclusively to muscles and is present with or without an intact nerve supply. On this basis he divides the body into parts with sensibility and parts with irritability. The study is essentially an experimental one, for Haller eschewed theory.

. . . . I do not even conjecture very much beyond the scalpel and microscope and readily abstain from teaching those things that I do not know, since it is pride of ignorance to present oneself as a guide for others when one sees nothing oneself [p. 115].

In the original printing of the essay there is a gap in the text between pages 136 and 137. Tissot, in his French translation (1755), completed the unfinished sentence, and the portion given below (p. 174) in brackets is our version of it. The sentence has also been completed in the English and Italian translations of 1755 since they were derived from that of Tissot. The passage in question is to be found originally and in its entirety in Friedrich Ortlob's *Nova anatomia ratiociniis illustrata* ([Württemberg, 1694], "Praefatio," fol. *b*3): "If the phrenic nerve is digitally compressed the diaphragm ceases to beat, but if now a more proximal part of the nerve is also compressed and the first compression released, the diaphragm will make a few movements and will then cease. In other words, the first compression prevents the animal spirits from reaching the muscle and thus prevents its contraction, but when the spirits in the portion of the nerve lying between the two sites of compression are allowed to flow distally, they induce transient contractions." This was refuted by Haller. The following selections have been translated from the essay of 1753.

EXCERPT P. 116

I say that the irritable part of the human body is that which by some external contact becomes shorter; very irritable if upon light contact it is impelled into brevity [i.e., contracts], less so, finally, if upon strong.

I call that a sensible part of the human body, in which the [impression of] contact is transmitted to the soul, and in brutes, in which the soul is not correspondingly evident, I call those parts of the animal sensible which upon being irritated, display clear indications of pain and discomfort; the insensible, on the other hand, is that which upon being burned, torn, pricked, or cut even to the point of destruction, arouses no indication of pain, convulsion, or change in the position of the whole body. For it is known that an animal in pain removes the affected part from the pain-producing cause, that it pulls away an injured leg, shakes the skin if it is pricked, and gives other indications from which you may perceive that it is in pain.

I observe that only through experiments can one define what part of the body is sensible or irritable, and what the physiologists and physicians have undertaken to explain about these qualities without experiment has been the cause and source of errors in this respect and in others.

EXCERPT P. 117

I sought to learn which of these parts are sensible by the following experiments.

In living animals of different kinds and different ages, I laid bare that part in which I was interested; I waited until the animal was quiet and ceased complaining, and with it silent and at rest, I irritated that part with a blast of air, heat, spirit of wine, the scalpel, *lapis infernalis* [caustic potash or potassium hydroxide], oil of vitriol, and butter of antimony. I noted whether the animal was aroused from its quiet and silence when the part was touched, torn, cut, burned, or lacerated, and whether it struggled or whether it pulled away the wounded limb, whether the limb was convulsed, or whether it experienced none of those things I have mentioned.

Haller then related his experiments on the sensitivity or lack of sensitivity of a wide variety of structures such as skin, tendons, ligaments, joint capsule, periosteum, meninges, blood vessels, viscera, glands, etc. He finally discussed the nerves and concluded that they were wholly responsible for the state of sensitivity.

EXCERPT PP. 133–139

Finally, as the nerve is the source of all sensibility so it is the site of the most acute sensitivity. For upon its having been touched, irritated, or even tied, it is astonishing to one without experience what disquiet and indications of pain the animals display. I have learned from experience that with only the larger nerves tied—not only a nerve of the eighth pair [ninth, tenth, eleventh cranial nerves] but even of their legs—after several days dogs have died. This made me even more fearful than before of tying those usual ones in amputation. But when a nerve has been cut and irritated below the section, it arouses no sensation of discomfort in the animal. It seems that sensation is not extended by anastomosis from one nerve into another.

We have seen that the sensible parts are the nerves, and hence the parts of the body which have the greatest abundance of nerves. When the nerve that communicates with that part has been compressed, tied, or cut, it loses sensation. Such experiments are known, as my commentaries on Boerhaave have sufficed to indicate. Therefore the nerve alone is sensitive, and in the nerve neither the dural membrane, nor the pia, but only the medullary structure that comes from the brain and is contained by coverings originating from the pia mater.

Next, he turned to the central theme of his discourse, irritability.

SECTION II
PRESENTED ON THE 6TH MAY

Now let us proceed to irritability, which so differs from sensibility that the most sensible parts lack all irritability and the irritable are without sensibility. I shall prove each conclusion by experiments and I shall demonstrate as well that irritability does not, as is commonly believed, arise from a nerve, but is innate in the fabric of the irritable part.

First, the nerve by which all sensation is carried to the soul, lacks all irritability. This will seem astonishing, but it is as true as it is astonishing. When a nerve has been irritated, each muscle to which that nerve is distributed through its branches is convulsed, and I know no example to the contrary. Very often I have seen the diaphragm and abdominal muscles (in the dormouse), and especially the fore and hind leg of a frog, convulsed in that way when the nerve was excited. Observe the like experiments of Swammerdam; in that observation I, like Georg Christian Oeder, found that when a nerve has been irritated it does not tremble or convulse muscles other than those which receive branches from that nerve itself.

I have also constantly seen that when the nerve has been irritated with a scalpel it causes a convulsion of the muscles, not in the same way as if it had been irritated by a corrosive.

But if the nerve fibres of a muscle have been irritated, the muscle is contracted; nothing similar occurs in the nerves . . . .

. . . .

These are new proofs which indicate that it would be contrary to the results of experiment to attribute an oscillating force to the nerve fibres.

Neither the skin, which is the seat of feeling, nor the nervous membranes of the stomach, intestines, or urethra are irritable . . . .

Nor are irritability and the acuteness of sensibility in the same proportion. The stomach is highly sensible, the intestines are rather less sensible; certainly the pain is less sharp, and yet I have found them to be more irritable. The heart, which is highly irritable, is of slight sensibility, and if touched in a living man, it induces unconsciousness rather than pain.

Therefore, a part of the body is not sensible because it is irritable. For when a nerve has been tied or cut, that part which is supplied from this nerve, does not therefore lack irritability; I have often repeated that celebrated experiment mentioned by Bellini, although the result was a little different from what is commonly described. I grasped and compressed the phrenic nerve of a live animal or one recently dead, for it makes no difference. By this irritating compression of the nerve, the diaphragm was convulsed. If I tied the nerve the same occurred. If I cut it and irritated the nerve below the cut, hence without any communication with the brain and without any sensation, the diaphragm, just as before, reacted and was convulsed. If in the same way I cut the crural nerve of the dog, the sensation perishes in the living beast, and the leg can everywhere be lacerated without indication of pain. But if the nerve is irritated, the same leg trembles; therefore although it becomes irritable, it is insensible.

I have found that too much has been said of this experiment of Bellini. It

is true that a constricted and irritated nerve causes a tremor in the diaphragm whether it be constricted proximally or distally; nor does distal
constriction produce anything different from proximal, nor is the diaphragm moved more if the nerve is constricted distally, nor is it quiescent if
proximally. Irritation of a tense nerve, however, produces its effect better
than irritation of a lax one, as I have learned by experience. If you compress
the nerve and then irritate it above the compression, or then compress it
distally, or very slightly, the diaphragm remains quiescent and therefore
what Friedrich Ortlob wrote is not true, that motion begins in the diaphragm when the nerve [is compressed distally and ceases upon the fingers
being slid towards the upper part of the thorax. [See p. 171].

Finally, in smaller animals I have tied the nerve trunks going to the limbs
so that the limb became paralyzed and insensible. Then I irritated the
exposed muscles with a scalpel and I saw their fibres tremble and palpitate
as much as before, although each muscle was no longer under the control of
the will.

. . . .

. . . .

. . . . Therefore, irritability does not depend upon the will or upon the
soul. These same experiments demonstrate that all the force of the muscles
does not depend upon the nerves since when these have been tied or cut,
the fibre is [still] irritable and contractile.

ALEXANDER MUNRO, SECUNDUS
(*10 March 1733—2 October 1817*)

Apart from introduction of the doctrine of irritability, it can be said that as late
as the end of the eighteenth century, knowledge concerning nerve action had not
greatly advanced beyond that of Galen in the second century, A.D. Admittedly
animal spirits were no longer held responsible, but the new theories had merely
introduced terms and concepts which, although based on known physical or chemical processes, had done little to elucidate the problem. There was available,
however, negative evidence which, for example, refuted the idea of a fluid being
responsible. Thus, Alexander Monro *primus* (1697–1767) writing in 1746 (*The
anatomy of the human bones and nerves* [etc.], 4th ed. [Edinburgh, 1746] discussed
some of this evidence.

39. . . . .

. . . . it is further urged that tho' we might not see the nervous Tubes or
the Liquors they contain, as they naturally flow; yet if such Liquors really
exist, they ought to discover themselves, either by a Nerve's swelling when

it is firmly tied; or that however subtile their Fluids are, they might be collected in some Drops at least, when the cut End of a Nerve of a living Animal is kept some Time in the exhausted Receiver of an Air-Pump. It is affirmed, that neither did the tied Nerve swell between the Brain and the Ligature, nor was there any Liquor collected in the Receiver of the Air-Pump; from which it is concluded that there is no Liquor in the nerves [p. 332].

At this time electricity had been demonstrated, and it was only natural that attempts should be made to apply the new force to the nerve which, after all, was not unlike a conducting wire. Stephen Hales (1732), Haller (1762), and others entertained the possibility, but most investigators agreed that there were more objections to it than supporting evidence. Monro in the same publication of 1746 (p. 339, par. 51) rejected it; the words in brackets in the excerpt below were added or changed in later editions (for example, 6th ed. [Edinburgh, 1758], p. 349, par. 52 and *The works of Alexander Monro M.D.*, published by his son Alexander Monro [*secundus*] [Edinburgh, 1781], p. 333, par. 52).

We are not sufficiently acquainted with the Properties of an Aether [or *electrical effluvia*] pervading every Thing, to apply it [them] justly in the animal Oeconomy, and it is as difficult to conceive how it [they] should be retained [or conducted] in a long nervous Cord as it is to have any Idea how it should act. These are Difficulties not to be surmounted.

Whytt (see p. 336) (Robert Whytt, *An essay on the vital and other involuntary motions of animals*, 2d ed. [Edinburgh, 1763]) dismissed all previous theories of muscle contraction thus:

. . . . Upon the whole then, we may fairly conclude that the contraction of an irritated muscle cannot be owing to any effervescence, explosion, ethereal oscillation, or electrical energy excited in its fibres or membranes, by the mechanical action of *stimuli* upon them [p. 265].

Later in the century, Alexander Monro *secundus* again summarized the position concerning nerve function and, like his father and others, argued against the electrical fluid.

Alexander Monro *secundus*, the second of the Monro dynasty, was born in Edinburgh. His father was professor of anatomy, and in 1754, one year before the younger Alexander received the M.D. degree, he joined his father as conjoint professor of anatomy. In 1777 he was appointed professor of medicine, anatomy, and surgery, and in 1808 his son, Alexander Monro *tertius*, took over his teaching duties entirely. Of the three, the second Alexander was probably the best anatomist, and his name is still associated with the interventricular foramen and with the Monro-Kellie doctrine. He is remembered in particular for his book on the anatomy of the nervous system (see Wright–St. Clair, 1964).

The following selection has been taken from Chapter XXIII of his book,

Observations on the structure and functions of the nervous system (Edinburgh, 1783), which is entitled "Of the nature of the energy of the nerves."

EXCERPT PP. 74–76

Most authors have supposed that the nerves are tubes or ducts conveying a fluid secreted in the brain, cerebellum, and spinal marrow. But, of late years, several ingenious physiologists have contended, that a secreted fluid was too inert for serving the offices performed by the nerves, and, therefore, supposed that they conducted a fluid the same as, or similar to, the electrical fluid.

Two arguments chiefly seem to have led them to this conclusion.

First, The nervous energy appeared to them to be moved with prodigious velocity. Thus, Dr. Haller observes how often a muscle of any part could act in a minute; and supposing that, previous to every contraction, the nervous fluid moved from the brain to that part, has attempted to calculate its velocity [footnote: . . . . not less than 9,000 feet in the first minute].

But if the nerves are constantly filled or charged with their fluid or energy, which, from our instantly perceiving injury done to every the most remote part, we have reason to suppose is the case, an impulse given to that fluid at the brain may be suddenly communicated to the most distant organ, although the velocity of the fluid be very small. Nay, in fact, we find, after cutting through the nerve of a muscle, that, by irritating the nerve, repeated motions can be performed; whereas, by Dr. Haller's theory of great velocity from end to end of the nerve, as the nerve now wants supply from the reservoir in the brain, the fluid should be exhausted by a single effort of the muscle. Such an argument as this no more proves that the nervous fluid moves with great velocity, than our letting out, in the space of a minute, a hundred successive drops of water from the end of a pipe, a mile distant from the reservoir which filled it, would prove that the water was moving in that pipe at the rate of a hundred miles every minute.

The other principal argument is more direct; and has been thought very conclusive, to wit, that some animals, as the torpedo and gymnotus electricus, have the power of giving an electrical shock, and that, on dissecting them, a piece of machinery, proper to them, is discovered, in which large and numerous nerves terminate.

But, perhaps, all we can conclude from these facts is, that the nerves enable this machinery to perform its proper office of collecting the electrical fluid, but without directly furnishing to it any of that fluid. Just as we, by rubbing a glass tube, excite electricity without there being any reason to suspect that the electrical matter is, in particular, derived from the nerves of our hand, since the electricity could be as readily excited by the hand of a dead man, as by that of a living, rubbed against the glass with the same force.

We seem, therefore, far from possessing positive arguments that the nerves operate by the medium of an electrical fluid, especially if we add, that, after cutting a nerve across, and again bringing its parts contiguous, its offices cannot be immediately restored . . . .

That the matter on which the energy depends is a secreted fluid, we are, indeed, far from being able to prove.

Electrophysiology

The report of Alexander Monro *secundus* has been chosen to represent the opinion of eighteenth century investigators who rejected all the available explanations for nerve action but could find nothing to take their place. It summarizes for us the situation towards the end of the eighteenth century when every effort to elucidate the nerve's ability to carry motor and sensory messages had failed. Clearly no further advance was possible unless some entirely new phenomenon or concept could be applied to the problem. As it happened these investigators were standing at the close of one era and at the beginning of another that will now be presented as the third section of this chapter.

As Monro was writing his book in 1780, the Italian, Galvani, was carrying out experiments that opened up an entirely new approach. Admittedly the electricity that Galvani and others were to find associated with muscle and nerve activity had been considered as an explanation for nerve transmission ever since Hales had referred to this possibility in 1732, and the properties of the electric fish had been known since antiquity (Kellaway, 1946). Nevertheless, no extensive experimental work had been carried out before Galvani devoted himself to the problem. The background against which his experiments were conducted and the data that were already available to him are discussed in detail by Hoff (1936) and by Walker (1937).

Galvani's work had two important results. It led eventually to universal acceptance of animal electricity as a biological phenomenon; thus the study of electrophysiology began with Galvani. An indirect but more immediate result came from the work of Alessandro Volta (1745–1827) of Pavia who, in opposing Galvani's contentions, developed the field of "metallic electricity" that led to the Voltaic pile and to the manifold technological applications of this new force, the use of which we enjoy today (Dibner, 1952). Hence Galvani's indirect influence in these fields must be remembered, for he had, after all, led Volta to bimetallic electricity. After Galvani's death in 1798, several of his countrymen carried on his investigations, but after the discovery of the pile by Volta in 1800, there was a lull until apparatus to detect and measure electricity was invented. Thereafter there was a revival of interest in the 1830's and 1840's, owing to the work of Nobili and Matteucci. In turn the Italians became less important, and in the 1840's the center of interest in experimental electrophysiology moved to Germany as its great schools of physiology began to take shape. Physiological materialism was fostered by du Bois-Reymond and Helmholtz, and the problems set by electrophysiology were largely responsible for its growth. Germany remained the center for study of the physiology of nerve conduction until the rise of the British school of physiology in the fourth quarter of the nineteenth century, followed by the rise of American centers. In the present century, most of the important work has taken place in Great Britain and in the United States.

The growth of electrical theories of nerve function gave rise to three important and productive controversies. The first, already mentioned, was that between Galvani and Volta in the 1790's. The second involved Matteucci and the great German physiologist du Bois-Reymond in the 1840's and 1850's, and the third developed between the latter and his pupil Hermann in the 1860's. All were beneficial to the subject for they stimulated widespread interest in experimental work.

Just as the development of the neuron concept was determined by advances made in microscopy and its auxiliary techniques, so the accumulation of data concerning the function of the cell and fibre was mainly dependent upon advances made in the physical and chemical sciences, and especially in the development of methods of detecting and recording minute and momentary electrical changes in biological materials. The mechanical ingenuity and the experimental skill of the electrophysiologist and the neuropharmacologist were directly equivalent to the earlier visual acuity and patient attention to detail of the histologist. Although in this section we are primarily interested in the function of the nerve, much must be said about the muscle, which is inseparable from its nerve supply. But it was early recognized that principles of muscular function could mostly be applied to the nerve.

This third period in the history of neurophysiology witnessed the beginning of an idea that is still in force, and its patient development by a number of investigators is illustrated below by some of the more outstanding contributions. Nevertheless, despite the considerable advances that have been made, only a small part of the enigma of nerve function has been resolved.

The electrical concept of nerve activity has been separated from the chemical for the sake of clarity, but they obviously have advanced, and will continue to advance, side by side. Similarly there is a close connection between the morphological data selected for Chapter II and the knowledge of function given in the selections below. The early history of electrophysiology is related by Brazier (1959) and by Pupilli and Fadiga (1963); the most complete account of the pre-1848 history is to be found in the first volume of du Bois-Reymond (1848–1884).

Luigi Galvani
(9 September 1737—4 December 1798)

Galvani did not discover animal electricity. It had been identified in 1772 in the electric fish by John Walsh (1774). Moreover, the name was already in use before

Galvani's time. Nor was he the first to stimulate muscles and nerves electrically since others before him had suggested electricity as a possible basis for the contraction of muscle, although no one had demonstrated its presence. In addition, the electrostatic charging of the human body had aroused much interest and curiosity. Galvani's work, therefore, although of the greatest importance—for he was the first to find electricity in an animal other than the electric fish—was not as original as is often maintained (Hoff, 1936*a*; Walker, 1937).

Galvani was born and died in Bologna where he was graduated in medicine and philosophy at the University in 1759. He held a number of positions in the University, including several in anatomy, and in the Institute of Sciences. Although his teaching and research were devoted mainly to anatomy, he also practised medicine and obstetrics and was professor of obstetrics in the Institute of Sciences. In the last year of his life he refused allegiance to the Cisalpine Republic created by Napoleon and in consequence was deprived of all his appointments. He died probably of pyloric stenosis (see Medici, 1845; Fulton and Cushing, 1936; Galvani, 1953*a*, pp. xvii–xx; Rothschuh, 1963; E. Benassi, 1963).

Galvani's discoveries were by no means the chance observations which one is led to infer from the accounts of his experiments that one finds in secondary sources. He must have been aware of at least some of the investigations that had been carried out already. Nevertheless, his enthusiasm, which at times admittedly carried him astray, and his painstaking deliberation resulted eventually in the demonstration that animal tissues possess electricity (pp. 184–185). His experiments probably began in or before 1780 but he did not publish them until 1791 ("De viribus electricitatis in motu musculari commentarius. Pars prima," *Bononien. Sci. Art. Instit. Acad.*, 1791, 7:363–418; this appeared separately with the same title and with the imprint, Bologna, Ex Typographia Instituti Scientiarum, 1791).

Galvani reported his findings in four sections. The first dealt with muscular contraction in the frog and other animals, resulting from exposure to electricity manufactured by the electric machine, the Leyden jar, or from other sources. The second discussed the effects of atmospheric electricity on the same preparations. The third and fourth parts are the most important, for in them Galvani described and discussed his demonstration of animal electricity which he claimed must surely represent the animal spirits of the ancients. In retrospect it is clear that his experiments demonstrated what we today would call the *current of injury*, which is set up between a healthy and injured part of a muscle.

However, his findings did not in themselves prove that animal electricity was present in the muscles, but merely that contact between two different metals could lead to a difference of potential which would then stimulate the muscle. None of the experiments in the *De viribus electricitatis* actually demonstrated animal electricity, although Galvani at first thought they did. The only experiment that did so is described on page 185.

C. H. Pfaff (1773–1852) of Kiel, who supported these findings, enumerated Galvani's findings in his book, *Über thierische Elektricität und Reizbarkeit. Ein Beytrag zu den neuesten Entdeckungen über diese Gegenstände* ([Leipzig, 1795], pp. 329–330):

I. Animals have an electricity peculiar to themselves to which the name *animal electricity* is given.

II. The organs in which animal electricity acts above all others, and by which it is distributed throughout the whole body, are the nerves, and the most important organ of secretion is the brain.

III. The inner substance of the nerve, especially the thinnest lymph, has the ability to conduct electricity and makes possible its free and swift passage through the nerve. But the outer, oily layer [the myelin sheath had not at this time been named] of the nerve prevents the dispersion of this electricity and permits its accumulation.

IV. The most excellent reservoirs of animal electricity are the muscles. They are like a Leyden jar and are negative on the external surface, but the inside where the electricity accumulates is, on the contrary, positive. The nerve is the conductor of the jar, which also provides the blood vessels of the muscles with electricity.

V. The mechanism of all movement is owing to the electrical fluid from the inside of the muscle migrating and being conducted by way of the nerve itself to the outside surface of the muscle. This discharge of the muscle–Leyden jar provides an electrical stimulus to the outer surface of the muscle and the irritable muscle fibres therefore contract.

For various reasons it was thought best to retranslate the selections given below from *De viribus electricitatis* (1791*b*) rather than to make use of existing translations.

EXCERPT PP. 17–20

Since from time to time I had seen the frog preparations, hung from brass hooks in their spinal cords along an iron fence surrounding our home's sunken garden, exhibit the usual contractions, not only during electrical storms but also with the sky quietly serene, I believed that those contractions were the result of the changes that occur during the day in the atmosphere's electricity. Hence it was not without hope that I began a careful study of the effects of these changes on such muscular movements, attempting a variety of procedures. At different times over a period of many days I observed the animals suitably arranged for the purpose, but there was scarcely any movement of their muscles. Finally, disappointed in this vain expectation I began to press and squeeze the brass hooks fixed into the spinal cord against the iron fence to see if muscular contractions might be aroused by this sort of procedure, and if they might display any difference or change relative to the changing state of the atmosphere and its electricity; I frequently did observe contractions, but they had no relation to the changing state of the atmosphere and its electricity.

However, since I had observed these contractions only outdoors and had not yet attempted to experiment elsewhere, I was on the point of deciding that such contractions arose from atmospheric electricity gradually introduced and accumulated in the animals and then rapidly discharged when the hook came in contact with the iron fence; it is easy to be deceived in one's investigations and to accept as seen and discovered what one wishes to see and discover.

But when I brought the animal into a closed room, placed it on an iron plate, and began to press the hook fixed in the spinal cord against the plate, behold, the same contractions and the same movements. I performed the same experiment over and over, using different metals, at different places, and at different hours and days, with the same result except that the contractions differed according to the metals used; that is, more violent with some, weaker with others. Then it occurred to me to employ for this same experiment other substances that were either weak conductors of electricity or not at all such as glass, gum, resin, stones, and dry wood. There was no like result, and no muscular contractions or movements could be observed. These results caused us great astonishment and led us to give some thought to inherent animal electricity itself. Both astonishment and suspicion were increased when by chance we noticed that when the phenomenon of contraction occurred the flow of very tenuous nervous fluid from nerves to muscles resembled the electrical flow that is discharged in a Leyden jar.

For while I held in one hand the hook fixed into the spinal cord of a prepared frog, and did this so that its feet rested on a silver box, with the other hand I touched the surface of the box on which the frog's feet or its side rested, with a metallic object, and beyond my expectations I saw the frog exhibit strong contractions as often as I repeated that same procedure.

. . . .

. . . .

. . . . [Galvani showed that the same effect could be produced with a human chain instead of one person, either by the clasping of hands or with a conducting body between the two experimenters.]

But in order to present the matter more clearly, I found it most suitable to have the frog placed on an insulating surface, that is, glass or resin; then to use now the conducting arc, now one either wholly or partly nonconducting, and to apply one end of it to the hook affixed to the spinal cord, the other to the muscles of the leg or to the feet. When the trial had been made, we saw that contractions occurred when the conducting arc was used, but were wholly lacking when the partly conducting, partly nonconducting arc Fig. 9, Plate III [fig. 44], was used, as in Fig. 10. The conducting arc was of iron wire and the hook of brass wire.

When these things had been observed, it seemed to us that the contractions that we said were made in frogs placed on a metal surface while the hook of the spinal cord was pressed against the same surface, must be ascribed to a like arc, of which the metal plate served as a substitute, so that, providing precisely the same procedures were used, the contraction would not be aroused in frogs placed on some insulating surface.

A suitable phenomenon, observed by chance, clearly confirmed our opinion; for if a frog is held in the fingers by one leg so that the hook fixed into the spinal cord touches some silver surface, and the other leg falls freely on the same surface, Fig. 11, Plate III, immediately this same leg touches the surface the muscles undergo a series of contractions, so that the leg rises and is carried upwards, then of its own accord relaxes and again falls to the surface; as soon as it makes that same contact, for the same reason it is carried upwards again, and so alternately it is raised and drops, so that, not without some astonishment and pleasure for the observer, the same leg seems to imitate an electrical pendulum.

EXCERPT PP. 34–36

From what has hitherto been learned and investigated I consider it sufficiently well established that there is an electricity in animals that we, with Bartholon [*sic*; Pierre Bertholon, abbé de St. Lazare] and others, may refer to by the general term "animal." If it is not contained in all parts of animals, yet it is to be found in many and displays itself most conspicuously in muscles and nerves. It seems to have the special, hitherto unrecognized quality of moving strongly from muscles to nerves, or rather from the latter to the former, and may then immediately enter either an arc or a human chain or any other conducting bodies that lead from nerves to muscles by the shortest and quickest route, and runs very swiftly through them from the one to the other.

From this, two things in particular seem evident, that is, that the electricity in these parts is of two kinds, one, as it seems, positive, the other negative, and that the one is by its nature completely distinct from the other; for were an equilibrium established, there would be no motion, no flow of electricity, no phenomenon of muscular contraction.

But in which of the aforesaid parts one electricity resides, in which the other, that is, whether there is one in muscle, the other in nerve, or both in one and the same muscle, and whence it flows, is very difficult to determine. Nevertheless, if I may have an opinion about such an obscure matter, I favor the location of both kinds of electricity in muscle . . . it seems a plausible conjecture that muscle is the proper seat of the electricity investigated by us, but that nerve performs the function of a conductor.

If these things be admitted, then perhaps that hypothesis and conjecture is neither absurd nor far from the truth that would compare a muscle fibre to a small Leyden jar, or to some other similar electrical body charged with two opposed kinds of electricity, with the nerve compared in some degree to the jar's conductor, and, therefore, the whole muscle as if it were composed of a collection of Leyden jars.

EXCERPT P. 42

So much for the nature and character of animal electricity. Now a few things about its source. I believe this is not unlike that which physiologists have hitherto selected for the animal spirits, that is, the brain. For although we have indicated that electricity is inherent in muscles, yet we do not hold with the opinion that it also emanates from them as from its own natural source.

For since all nerves, both those carried to the muscles and those to other parts of the body, seem to be entirely the same in appearance as well as in nature, who will rightfully deny that all carry fluid of the same sort? But we have already demonstrated above that electrical fluid is carried through the nerves of the muscles; therefore it will be carried through all of them; and so they draw from one common source, that is, the brain, the beginning and origin of all. Otherwise there would be as many sources as there are parts in which the nerves terminate; and although they are very unlike in nature and construction, they do not seem to be suited, as would be necessary, for the elaboration and secretion of one and the same fluid.

Therefore, we believe it most likely that the electrical fluid is prepared by the force of the brain, is extracted from the blood, that it enters the nerves, and that it runs through them internally whether they are hollow and empty, whether, as seems more probable, they carry a very tenuous lymph or another similar, special, very tenuous fluid, as it seems to many, secreted from the cortical substance of the brain. If this is so, the obscure and for so long vainly sought nature of the animal spirits will perhaps finally be explicable.

GIOVANNI ALDINI
(16 April 1762—17 January 1834)

Galvani's experiments were confirmed by many, but his conclusion that animals possessed a type of electricity peculiar to themselves was attacked almost immediately. His main opponent was the physicist Volta, and the controversy which resulted is one of the most famous in the history of science (see p. 177). As Volta repeated the experiments he became increasingly convinced that the electricity demonstrated by Galvani came not from the animal tissue but from the contact between dissimilar metals; this he termed *metallic electricity*. His first publication on the matter appeared in 1792 ("Memorie sull'elettricità animale," G. *fis.-med. L. Brugnatelli*, 1792, 1 [ii]:146–187, 241–270, 287–290), and the controversy continued until Galvani's death in 1798.

Clearly the only way to sustain the concept of animal electricity was to show that muscle contraction could take place in the absence of metals. The crucial experiment was first described in an anonymous publication of 1794 (*Dell'uso e dell'attività dell'arco conduttore nelle contrazioni dei muscoli* [with a supplement] [Bologna, 1794], pp. 3–10, 13–14). The manuscript, which was said to have been partly in Galvani's hand, is now missing, and although it seems certain that it was the work of Galvani, or inspired by him, we have preferred to rely upon the description given nine years later by Aldini, the nephew of Galvani and one of his most ardent supporters. A translation into English of the pertinent part of the 1794 tract is to be found in Galvani (1953*b*, p. 161) and in Pupilli (1963, pp. 568–569).

Aldini was born in Bologna and received the doctor of philosophy degree from the University there in 1782. After holding appointments in physics at the Institute of Sciences as well as in the University he was made professor of experimental physics in 1803 when the two chairs were combined, and he held this post until 1808. He travelled widely in Europe, lecturing on animal electricity and demonstrating its presence in animal and human preparations, the latter including an executed criminal at Newgate Prison, London. His reasons for supporting Galvani's work have been questioned and some have concluded that they were purely selfish and not primarily concerned with popularizing it.

The critical experiment was reported in a little-known book by Aldini, *An account of the late improvements in galvanism* [etc.] (London, 1803) which comprises lectures given at Guy's and St. Thomas's Hospitals in London and is on the whole a slender piece; a French translation (1804) was considerably enlarged. We must consider the experiment as an extension of Galvani's work and not as an original contribution by Aldini. Although Aldini's support for his uncle's beliefs may have been motivated by a desire for personal gain, it nevertheless contributed to the survival of the belief in animal electricity. This experiment gave conclusive evidence that electricity could be of purely animal origin and that it was not dependent upon the presence of metals or upon any other external factors. The response described is now known as the *current of injury*; in other words, the sciatic nerve of the frog was excited by the demarcation potential of another nerve.

A part of Proposition VI, entitled "Galvanism is excited in the animal machine without any intermediate body, and merely by the application of the nerves to the muscles," is given below.

EXCERPT PP. 14–17

Several philosophers have endeavoured to obtain this interesting result. Professor Volta, in a letter which he addressed to me, in Brugnatelli's Journal, observed, "that various parts of animals can excite Galvanism, independently of metals." Galvani, a short time before his death, proposed two ingenious methods of obtaining this result, and gave me a description of them. This, however, has not been able to destroy the incredulity of some philosophers, who hitherto have confounded Galvanism with metallic electricity, under an idea that all contractions proceed from irritation, produced by the action of metals. For this reason I have, with confidence, announced my method, which enables any one to observe this important result.

EXPERIMENT I

Having prepared a frog in the usual manner, I hold the spinal marrow in one hand (Pl. I, fig. 3 [fig. 47]), and with the other form an angle with the leg and foot, in such a manner that the muscles of the leg touch the crural nerves. On this contact strong contractions, forming a real electrico-animal alarum (*carillon*), which continue longer or shorter according to the degree of vitality, are produced in the extremity left to itself. In this experiment, as well as in the following, it is necessary that the frogs should be strong and full of vitality, and that the muscles should not be overcharged with blood.

EXPERIMENT II

By observing the directions already given, very strong convulsions will be obtained; but they must not be ascribed to the impulse produced by bringing the nerve into contact with the muscle. If the experiment be repeated, covering the muscle, at the place of contact, with a nonconducting substance, the contractions will entirely cease; but they will be re-produced as soon as the nerve is made to touch the muscular substance. In performing this experiment, in public, I obtained several times more than two hundred successive contractions; but this was never the case when I formed the same contact with the muscle by means of a conducting substance, and even with a plate of metal.

To ensure the success of this interesting experiment, the nerves must be prepared as speedily as possible, by disengaging them from every foreign substance. It will be proper also to apply the nerves not to one but to several points of the muscle, throughout its whole length. It is observed, that the contact of the nerves with the tendinous parts which communicate with the muscles, often serves to increase the muscular contractions.

CARLO MATTEUCCI

(*21 June 1811—24 June 1868*)

In the last decade of the eighteenth century there was widespread interest in Galvani's observations and theories, and in Volta's denial of them. Experiments on frogs were carried out all over Europe, but after Galvani's death in 1798 and after the invention of the Voltaic pile by Volta in 1800, during the subsequent thirty years less attention was paid to animal electricity, especially as there was as yet no accurate means of detecting its presence or strength. A method of doing this was provided by the Dane, Hans Christian Oersted (1777–1851), and by Johann Salomo Christoph Schweigger (1779–1857) who invented the galvanometer (Hoff and Geddes, 1957, pp. 213–217). The Italian physicist Leopoldo Nobili (1784–1835; see Pupilli, 1963, p. 587) improved on this to produce the astatic galvanometer in 1825 ("Über einen neuen Galvanometer"), and with this instrument he detected in the frog the *corrente della rana*, the "frog current" or *courant propre* for the first time. This current had been responsible for the findings of Galvani and Aldini, and we recognize it today as the "current of injury" or "demarcation potential" because it appears in an injured muscle and at the area of demarcation between healthy and injured tissue, or is found in frogs after the injury of decapitation. It was later recognized that the electrical activity of muscle and nerve were identical. Nobili was, however, unable to interpret his observations correctly, and his work was later taken up by another Italian physicist, Matteucci. Interest in animal electricity had by now returned, and Matteucci was one of the most active early members of the new group of investigators.

Matteucci was born in Forlì and studied mathematics and the physical sciences at Bologna and Paris. In 1834 he joined Nobili and G. B. Amici at the museum of physics and natural history in Florence. Here his work on electrophysiology began and he continued it at Forlì, Ravenna, and Paris. With Carl Ludwig he was one of the pioneers in the application of graphic recording to physiology. He was appointed professor of physics at the University of Pisa in 1840 where he also interested himself in the application of physics to telegraphy; after holding a number of government posts, he became minister of public instruction of the recently established Kingdom of Italy (see Moruzzi, 1963 and 1964; Pupilli, 1963).

Matteucci's studies of animal electricity began with an extensive investigation of the electric fishes and his next experiments led to the further elucidation of the muscle demarcation potential.

In an article published in 1842 ("Deuxième mémoire sur le courant électrique propre de la grenouille et sur celui des animaux à sang chaud," *Annls. Chim. Phys.*, 1842, 6 [3d ser.]:301–339), Matteucci reported several experiments on the *courant propre* or "frog current" of Nobili; he had begun his studies with the galvanometer in 1838. At the conclusion of the second chapter (pp. 307–327) which is entitled "On the *courant propre* of the frog," he gave a summary of his findings and the following is part of it.

EXCERPT P. 327

The experiments that I have reported are clearly sufficient to establish the common origin of the *courant propre* of the frog and of the phenomenon of contractions discovered by Galvani.

I shall limit myself to the following conclusions:

1. The frog current exists in the absence of the intact cerebrospinal nervous system.

2. When the nervous system is included in the experiment and one obtains indications of the *courant propre* on the galvanometer, it fulfills the same function as the muscle mass of the thigh.
3. The current in the frog becomes weaker when it has been seized by a kind of tetanic state, whatever the procedure by which this is aroused [see p. 191].

Matteucci then gave an account of further observations which, despite the work of Nobili, establish beyond doubt that Matteucci had given the first adequate demonstration of the demarcation potential or current of injury. By means of a galvanometer, he detected in mammals the invariable presence of an electric current when an injured portion of a striated muscle was connected with its intact surface. This, as will be seen, was a step towards the membrane theory of resting polarization of today [p. 214]. It was also a demonstration of the presence of a potential in an inactive muscle (resting potential) which is released when the muscle is injured. Neither of these concepts was otherwise to appear for several decades.

EXCERPT PP. 330–331

I have made another discovery in the living, warm-blooded animal which proves the existence of a phenomenon comparable to that found in the frog.

In an old and sturdy rabbit, I separated the two thighs and quickly prepared rather long portions of their nerves.

On lifting a nerve with a glass rod and then letting it fall on the muscle mass of the legs, I invariably saw that the whole thigh contracted strongly during the space of two or three minutes. I placed the thighs together, put the nerve of one on the muscle of the other, and when the circuit was closed by putting one of these nerves in contact with the muscles or the tendons of the other leg, the two thighs contracted strongly.

Pacinotti and Puccinotti have also observed that when one plate of a very sensitive galvanometer is introduced into the brain of a living animal and the other into a muscle, there are well-marked signs of an electric current which is always directed from the brain to the muscle in the animal, and consequently opposite to that of the frog. I have repeated the experiment of these natural philosophers [physicists] in rabbits and in pigeons, and I have obtained currents on my galvanometer which in several experiments have been up to 80 or 90 degrees on the first immersion. In all these experiments the direction of the current was, on the first immersion, always from brain to muscle in the animal. I found that this current was of the same intensity and in the same direction when one of the plates was immersed in the brain and the other merely placed on the surface of the muscle.

Furthermore, I have obtained a very distinct current of 20 to 30 degrees by making a wound in the chest or thigh of a living animal (pigeon, rabbit, sheep) and by placing in it one of the plates [of the galvanometer] while the other was placed on the exposed surface of the injured muscles. The current in the animal was invariably conducted from the inside of the wound to the exterior surface of the muscle. The constant direction of these currents and the quite distinct signs that I got on my galvanometer have assured me that they cannot be attributed to any flaw in the experiment.

During his many investigations, Matteucci perfected a number of useful devices, the most important of which were two preparations, of which he termed one "the galvanoscopic frog" and the other an electrophysiological pile comparable to Volta's electrophysical pile. The following description of the first is taken from his *Traité des phénomènes électro-physiologiques des animaux* ([Paris, 1844], Pt. I, Ch. II).

EXCERPT PP. 28–30

The suitably prepared frog gives us another instrument that can be employed to great advantage in electrophysiological research. For this purpose it is necessary to begin by selecting a very lively frog as Galvani did. Cut off about two-thirds of its body just below its front legs; throw away the head and all the entrails and strip off the skin from the two-thirds of the frog that remain. In this way there is a piece of the spinal cord with the pelvis and the two back legs. Then by introducing scissors between the lumbar nerves and the pelvis and cutting the latter in two places, you will have what is usually called the frog *prepared according to the method of Galvani* (Fig. 3 [fig. 48]). In order to use the frog for study of the electric current, it is necessary to pass the current into the single nerve filament of the frog. To this end cut in half the frog prepared according to the method of Galvani, and by a very simple procedure the thigh bone and thigh muscles of the half-frog can be removed with the nerve remaining intact. Now one has a frog's leg, composed of the lumbar portion of the pelvis and the crural part of the thigh to which a long nerve filament is attached. In order to produce an instrument very sensitive to the passage of an electric current, nothing remains to be done except to place this leg in a tube of varnished glass. To use this type of galvanoscope (Fig. 4), hold the glass tube by the end opposite to that into which the frog's leg was introduced, and touch the nerve filament that falls outside the tube, with the two points of the electromotor element that you wish to study [z and c in Fig. 4; see fig. 49]. If an electric current runs through the nerve filament, you will notice at once that the leg contracts. If it is feared that direct contact of the nerve with the points of the electromotor element may irritate the nerve, independently of the electric current, you need only join two strips of paper moistened with water to the two points of the electromotor element and then close the circuit by touching the two strips to the nerve filament. [Fig. 5; see fig. 49.]

The frog used in this way, which I shall henceforth call the *galvanoscopic frog*, is certainly the most sensitive apparatus at our disposal, provided one renews it from time to time. This instrument is still more accurate in its information if one is careful to strip the nerve well and to close the circuit with the nerve alone without including any part of the leg muscle. The galvanoscopic frog not only indicates the existence of an electric current, but more than that, it assists us in determining the direction of the current with a considerable degree of probability.

Matteucci then used this preparation to demonstrate the demarcation currents in muscle (Chapter V, "On the existence of the electric muscle current in living animals or in those recently killed").

EXCERPT PP. 51–52

There is an experiment which is very simple and very easy to carry out and which proves the existence of the electric current produced by bringing together, by means of a conducting body, different parts of a muscle mass of a living animal, or of one recently killed. For this a frog preparation which I have called the galvanoscopic frog (Fig. 4 [fig. 49]) is used. Then the muscle of a living animal is cut in any way whatsoever and the nerve of the galvanoscopic frog introduced into the wound. When only this has been done, it often happens that the [galvanoscopic] frog contracts. If the experiment is performed with care, it is readily seen that in order to succeed it is necessary to touch two different parts of the nerve filament. If as well as touching the depths of the wound with the end of the nerve of the galvanoscopic frog, another part of the same nerve touches the sides of the wound or the surface of the muscle, the frog invariably contracts. This obviously proves that it is indeed an electric current which moves in the nerve, since it is necessary to form an arc in which this same nerve is included. That this contraction of the frog is stimulated by an electric current owing to the different parts of the muscle of the living animal, is again well proved when it is seen that if two parts of the nerve are touched with liquid or with the conducting body, contractions are never produced.

Matteucci next described how it could be proved that the intrinsic muscle current was independent of all external factors introduced by the experiment. He used his second contrivance, the electrophysiological pile, comparable to a somewhat similar arrangement of "frog piles" made by Nobili (1828), to show that the demarcation potential could be increased if muscles were arranged in series or, as we would say today, the increased intensity of the current was owing to summation; as will be noted later, du Bois-Reymond's claim for priority in describing the muscle current is without foundation.

One prepares five or six frogs, or a still larger number if greater deviations are required. They are prepared after the manner of Galvani and are cut in half and then all the legs are removed by disarticulation carried out as carefully as possible so that the muscle mass is not damaged.

Finally the thighs are cut in half and thus a certain number of half-thighs are obtained (Fig. 13 [fig. 51]). It is now necessary to begin by placing on the board which I have described [a varnished board which has small cup-shaped depressions or cavities, Fig. 12 (fig. 51)], one of these half-thighs in such a way that it is lying at the edge of one of the little cavities hollowed out of the board. Then all the others are placed in series to the first half-thigh so that each half-thigh touches the one following and so that the cut surfaces obtained by bisecting the thighs face in the same direction. Thus at the end of this series, one half-thigh, like the first one, will be lying on the edge of another cavity in the board. The arrangement of this pile of half-thighs can be seen in Fig. 13 [fig. 51]. It can be seen that each point of contact of two neighboring half-thighs is the interior of one muscle and the surface of the other. Similarly, by this arrangement it happens that one of the extremities (B) of the pile is formed by the interior of the muscle and the other (A) is formed by the surface of a muscle. Water is let into the two cavities through a pipette; or better, a solution similar to that in which the two plates of a galvanometer are immersed. The two plates [of a galvanometer] are lifted out of the liquid and brought together without touching the liquid of one of the two cavities of the muscle pile. If after this manoeuvre the needle stands at zero, the two plates must be lifted out again and then at the same time reimmersed, one into each of the two cavities at the extremities of the pile, in such a way as to close the circuit. When the deviation of the needle takes place, it will soon be seen that it varies according to the number of half-thighs, that is the elements of the pile. Thus I obtain on my galvanometer 15°, 20°, 30°, 40°, 60° etc., according to the number of half-thighs, and providing the frogs are of equal liveliness; I obtain 3° or 4° with two elements, 6° to 8° with four elements, 10° to 12° with six elements, and so on.

The current [intrinsic current of muscle] is always directed in the pile from the internal part of the muscle to the surface.

Various modifications of this basic experiment were possible, and further refinements were also included in a description which appeared in Lecture IX, "Electric currents of muscles," in *Lectures on the physical phenomena of living beings* (translated by Jonathan Pereira [London, 1847], pp. 192–194).

Included in this lecture is a comment which indicates that Matteucci's interpretations of his findings in the late 1840's were no longer worthy of notice. He denied that electricity was present in the nervous system and believed that some other "nervous force" was responsible for its activity. This accounts in part for the dispute with du Bois-Reymond (see p. 194), but it does not diminish the worth of Matteucci's fundamental contributions to the electrophysiology of the nervous system.

Also a suggestion of the muscle action potential is to be found in Matteucci's writings. In the presence of muscle tetanus the intrinsic or muscle current, or *courant propre*, was diminished or disappeared; in other words, he demonstrated the negative deviation of the demarcation potential, which is the action potential. This experiment, that he says Galvani knew about but failed to interpret correctly, was described in several of Matteucci's works and has already been referred to briefly (p. 187). The following selection has been taken from a paper published originally in 1838 ("Sur le courant électrique ou propre de la grenouille," *Bibl. univ. Genève*, 1838, 7:156–168); reference, however, is to the reprint published in *Essai sur les phénomènes électriques des animaux* ([Paris, 1840], Ch. VI).

EXCERPT PP. 81–82

Another factor that greatly modifies the *courant propre* of the frog is a state of tetanus. This often happens in lively specimens that have been prepared quickly; they extend and stiffen their legs so that it is impossible to bend them. The tetanic convulsion can also be induced in a few seconds with a solution of strychnine or the extract of *nux vomica*. The influence of the tetanus is such that the *courant propre* is diminished when the frog is stimulated. There are no longer any contractions nor any galvanometric signs. If the animal has been killed by the poison, it is impossible to reestablish them. But, conversely, if the tetanus is produced by the stimulation of preparing the specimen, once the convulsions have stopped the signs of the *courant propre* reappear.

In his article of 1842 ("Deuxième mémoire . . .") Matteucci reported the phenomenon again.

EXCERPT P. 325

I have prepared frogs seized by convulsions produced by an extract of *nux vomica* introduced into their stomachs. In these frogs there are indications of a current on the galvanometer, but weaker than usual; the contractions themselves are likewise less frequent and more difficult to obtain.

These findings led Matteucci into confusion for he now had two opposing observations: an electric current had appeared with muscle contraction, but with tetanus it had disappeared. He did not understand the latter phenomenon and therefore rejected it later; his alternative explanation turned out to be incorrect. Du Bois-Reymond was to continue this work and to recognize its vital significance (p. 195).

Another basic contribution that Metteucci made to electrophysiology was his demonstration of the fact that the contraction of a muscle was always accompanied by an electrical change that could be detected by the secondary contraction of a rheoscopic frog. It was the first experimental demonstration of the existence of the action current. Although the report of his findings was read by Dumas to the Academy of Sciences in Paris on 24 October 1842 (*C. r. Acad. Sci., Paris*, 1842, 15:797–798), it had been written earlier and deposited with the Academy in a sealed package. The same experiment, but in more detail, appeared in "Sur un phénomène physiologique produit par les muscles en contraction" (*Annls. Chim. Phys.*, 1842, 6 [3d ser.]:339–343). The following selection has been translated from the *Comptes Rendus* of the Academy.

EXCERPT P. 797

Prepare quickly the thigh of a frog, leaving the nerve attached; place this nerve on the thighs of another frog prepared in the usual way [i.e., in the manner used by Galvani, see fig. 49]. If you make the muscles of the second frog contract, either by means of an electrical stimulus or by any other method, at the moment that the muscle contraction takes place, you will see the leg muscles of the first frog also contract.

Both the primary contraction in the second frog and the secondary, or induced, response in the first were produced and Dumas commented: ". . . it is the first time that the muscle contraction of an animal has exercised any influence on the nerves of another animal to bring about contraction." Although Matteucci correctly distinguished this phenomenon from the frog current, he unfortunately misinterpreted it. Du Bois-Reymond thought it was owing to excitation of the second nerve by the negative variations of the first muscle.

EMIL DU BOIS-REYMOND
(7 November 1818—26 December 1896)

The role of Matteucci as a pioneer of muscle-nerve electrophysiology cannot be denied, although it is often underestimated. Admittedly his writings are confusing on account of their volume and their contradictions, but it is difficult to understand why he incurred the persistent wrath and lifelong antagonism of the man who confirmed and extended his work, Emil du Bois-Reymond. The following is du Bois-Reymond's brief appraisal of Matteucci's work and of his own, taken from the preface to his *Untersuchungen über thierische Elektricität* (Vol. I [Berlin, 1848], xiv–xv).

There are, according to him [Matteucci], no electric currents in the nerve. The muscle current circulates in the muscles only if they are prepared in a certain manner, and has no relation to their contraction. The so-called nerve principle is to him [in later life] still a special, hypothetical entity which he likes to explain on the basis of ether vibrations, and he declares it to be distinguished from electricity under all conditions.

I shall now venture to defend the very opposite view. If I have not completely deluded myself, I have succeeded in restoring to life in full reality that hundred-year-old dream of the physicist and physiologist, the identity of the nerve principle with electricity.

In the spring of 1841, Johannes Müller of Berlin (see pp. 203–204) gave a copy of Matteucci's book, *Essai sur les phénomènes électriques des animaux* (Paris, 1840), to his twenty-two-year-old assistant, du Bois-Reymond, and suggested that he devote himself to the complex, yet important, field of muscle-nerve physiology. With remarkable singleness of purpose, du Bois-Reymond spent the next forty years of his professional life investigating this subject, and its development from an empirical to a rational study is due to him more than to anyone else. His pupil, L. Hermann, with whom he quarreled, described him (1884, p. 161) as "the creator of this rich field [electrophysiology], the discoverer of its methods, the man who helped to teach his contemporaries in medicine to think in accordance with physics."

Du Bois-Reymond was of Swiss-French extraction. He was born in Berlin and completed his medical education there in 1840. He worked with Müller until the latter's death in 1858 when he succeeded him in the chair of physiology in the University of Berlin. He was one of the group of German materialists which included Helmholtz (see pp. 206–207), Brücke, and Carl Ludwig, from the work and teaching of whom the influential school of German physiology developed. In 1877 a new institute of physiology was completed in the University of Berlin, and du Bois-Reymond was its active head for the next twenty years. Although his research was limited to a small area, he was a man of wide interests and culture and he combined the best of the German and French national characteristics (see Stirling, 1896–1897; Waller, 1905; Boruttau, 1922; Diepgen, 1927; Haymaker, 1953, pp. 116–119; Cranefield, 1957; Rothschuh, 1964).

Du Bois-Reymond was devoted to the new materialistic and mechanical physiology, and it was mainly his work which finally led to the break with the ancient theories of nerve function. He was also noted for his many ingenious inventions which made his experiments possible. Thus with a new and more sensitive galvanometer, he first of all verified Matteucci's finding of an electric current in the intact muscle itself as well as in the muscle when attached to its nerve. This he called the *muscle current* (*Muskelstrom*) and, like Matteucci, he considered it to be different from the *frog current* of Nobili. It was owing, he thought, to an attempt to preserve a resting difference of potential between the negative inner and the positive outer surface of the fibre; it seems likely that this was an early link with the membrane theory of today (Hoff and Geddes, 1957). He postulated a natural and artificial (that is, by cutting) cross section of the muscle, and although this produced many perplexities, it nonetheless led to the concept of the "resting" or "pre-existing" potential of muscle or nerve which was the source of electromotive power appearing with injury.

The most succinct account of du Bois-Reymond's muscle current is found in a letter sent to the English physician, Bence Jones, in 1853 (*On Signor Carlo Matteucci's letter to H. Bence Jones*, etc. [London, 1853]). In it du Bois-Reymond attacked Matteucci, at times without justification, and his claim for priority concerning the muscle current cannot be accepted. The following excerpt from Section VI appeared originally in his first paper which was published in 1843 ("Vorläufiger Abriss einer Untersuchung über den sogenannten Froschström und über die elektromotorischen Fische," [Poggendorffs] *Annln. Phys.*, 1843, 58:1–30).

EXCERPT PP. 16–19

1. Currents, in all respects similar to the so-called frog current, may be observed in any limb of any animal, whether cold or warm-blooded . . . .

2. . . . .

3. These currents are produced by the muscles. If any undissected muscle of any animal be brought into the circuit longitudinally, it generally exhibits an electro-motive action, the direction of which depends on the position of the muscle on the ends of the galvanometer circuit, according to the law which will immediately be stated. Thus, the current might be a downward one, or it might be an upward one [*sic*]. The current of the whole limb is nothing but the resultant of the partial currents which are engendered by each muscle of the limb; and the frog current as well as the similar currents observed in other animals, are thus simply reduced to a general *muscular current* [Muskelstrom]. *I therefore invented and first used this term, and it does not occur in Signor Matteucci's papers anterior to mine.*

4. To make the law, according to which this current may be regularly obtained, more easily understood, it will be useful to premise some definitions.

By *longitudinal section* of the muscle, I understand a surface formed only by the *sides* of the fibres of the muscles considered as prisms. By *transverse section* of the muscle I likewise understand a surface formed by the *base* of the fibres of the muscles again considered as prisms. Both the transverse and the longitudinal section may be either *artificial* or *natural*. In fig. 2 [fig. 52] which of course is an ideal one, a section of the muscle through *a b* would be an artificial transverse one; a section through *c d* an artificial longitudinal one. As to the natural transverse section, it is at each end of the muscle formed by the ends of all the fibres, and hidden beneath a coating of tendinous tissue, which is in connexion with the tendon itself, and, in an electric point of view, plays the part of an indifferent conducting body (*e f g h* in the diagram). Thus, the above-mentioned aponeurosis of the tendo-Achillis on the back of the gastrocnemius muscle covers the under natural transverse section [*sic*] of that muscle. Finally, the natural longitudinal section of the muscle is that part of its external surface which extends from one natural transverse section to the other, being free from the tendinous coating, and exhibiting the red colour peculiar to muscles (*fh, e g* in the diagram).

This being thus stated, the law of the muscular current may be shortly expressed as follows: *Any point of the natural or artificial longitudinal section of the muscle is positive in relation to any point of the natural or artificial transverse section.* (See the algebraic signs in fig. 2.)

5. . . . . Again, according to that law, every particle of a muscle, however minute, ought to produce a current in the same manner as the whole muscle, or as a larger piece of it. This consequence in my first paper [1843] is shown to be true even as regards shreds of muscle, consisting only of a few primary fibres, and such as, accordingly, admit of microscopical investigation, as shown in fig. 3 [fig. 53].

6. As to the nerves, I have stated in my paper that they are possessed of an electro-motive power, which acts according to the same law as the muscles.

Du Bois-Reymond confirmed Matteucci's observation that the muscle current in a tetanized muscle is reduced. This is the *negative variation* (*negative Schwankung*) of du Bois-Reymond, the discovery of which has been thought by some to mark the beginning of modern electrophysiology. It is known today as the *action current* of the muscle and is owing to the change in distribution of electrical charges on its surfaces. From this followed the concept of the *action potential* producing the action current and brought about by the potential difference between the region activated and any inactive part.

His experiments were reported in the paper of 1843, and more elaborately in the second volume of his *Untersuchungen über thierische Elektricität* ([Berlin, 1849], pp. 425–430). They appear in a more compact form in the letter to Bence Jones which was published ten years later. The selection offered below has been taken from Section IX of that letter, entitled "On the negative variation of the muscle current during contraction." It should be noted again that du Bois-Reymond's comments regarding Matteucci were unjustified. It is worth noting from the standpoint of later theories that du Bois-Reymond pointed out the fact that simple decrease of current was not the only possibility for negative variation but that reversal could also account for it.

EXCERPT PP. 27–28

Since the middle of the last century, innumerable attempts have been made to detect any electric phenomenon exhibited by the muscles during contraction. Signor Matteucci himself had made some random experiments on the subject [footnote: "Essai sur les Phénomènes électriques des Animaux" (Paris, 1840), p. 36]. They were all made in vain. [See pp. 191–192.]

In the summer, 1842, as soon as I had mastered the electric phenomena of muscles when at rest, by the discovery of the law of the muscular current, I also turned my attention to that most important problem, and, I am told, was fortunate enough to solve it satisfactorily.

I simply put a muscle into the circuit of the galvanometer, and waited until the needle took up its new position of equilibrium under the influence of the muscular current, whatever its direction in the muscle might be, in consequence of the position of the muscle on the ends of the galvanometer circuit, and in accordance with the law of the muscular current. I then proceeded to tetanize the muscle—that is, to make it contract powerfully and uninterruptedly as long as possible, in order to protract the action, and therefore to increase the effect exerted upon the needle by any change which the electric condition of the muscle might undergo during the contraction. In order to effect this the muscle was still attached to its motor nerve which, however, did not form part of the circuit of the galvanometer, and to which, therefore, any stimulus could be applied without endangering the equilibrium of the needle otherwise than by the very effect to be observed—namely, by any electro-motive action taking place during the contraction of the muscle.

The result was, that at the moment when the muscle was convulsed a sudden and considerable decrease of its action on the needle occurred. This decrease lasts as long as the tetanus itself, and cannot be accounted for by any change of the resistance of the circuit, for it is also obtained when there are two muscles in the circuit, the currents of which counter-balance each other; in this case no perturbation of the electric equilibrium can ever arise from any change of the resistance of the circuit.

Thus far my results on that subject were published in my paper of January 1843. It is well known that I have since extended those experiments successfully to the living body of the frog, of the rabbit, and even of man and that I have detected a negative variation * of a similar description which the nerve current undergoes while the nerve is conveying to the brain or to the muscle, those material changes which give rise to sensation and motion.

* Instead of "decrease" I usually say "negative variation" of the muscular current during the contraction, because as yet I have not been able to make out whether during contraction there is only a decrease in the intensity current, or whether the direction of the current is reversed. In the following remarks the phenomenon in question will, for the sake of brevity, be called simply —"The negative variation."

In 1848 the first volume of du Bois-Reymond's classic work, *Untersuchungen über thierische Elektricität* (Berlin, 1848), appeared; the second volume was published in 1849, and the second part of this volume, containing the eighth and last chapter, in 1860. It was in the second volume (Pt. II, ch. 2, Sec. II, 1) that du Bois-Reymond discussed the universal law of nerve stimulation by electric current, first reported to the Physics Society of Berlin on 8 August 1845. The current itself does not produce excitation; it is owing to the changes that accompany making or breaking the current or when it varies in strength. The following account is the author's general expression of the law.

EXCERPT PP. 258–259

We have just recalled the fact that a thigh tested with a current reacts with twitches only at the start and the cessation of the current but remains at rest while the current flows. Only if the nerve is subjected to excessively strong currents may one occasionally note the muscles supplied by it to be seized by a continuous series of twitchings despite the constant strength of the current. However, in such cases the twitches not infrequently continue after the opening of the circuit, but, if the latter remains closed for some time, calm is very soon restored and for good. One is therefore justified in concluding that under these circumstances the twitches are no longer the result of an ordinary type of stimulus by the electric current, but originate rather from its destructive effect, which is undoubtedly based upon electrolysis and has nothing to do with the law in question.

Contrary to this, one finds that twitchings occur freely in the nerve subsequent to the opening and closing of the circuit, as well as upon mere fluctuations in the density of the current, as long as these events proceed with sufficient speed. Indeed, one might also compare the start and the end of the current with a mere positive fluctuation in the first case and a negative one in the second, which starts at zero in the former and returns the current to zero in the latter. For the time being we can therefore establish the following hypothesis that should be adhered to as the basic and essential law for the whole immense field of experimental electrical stimulation: "It is not the absolute value of the current density * at any given moment to which the motor nerve responds by the contraction of its appropriate muscle, but the change of this value from one moment to the next. This means that the stimulation to move, which results from these changes, is the more powerful the more rapidly these changes of the same magnitude occur or the greater they are per unit of time."

The following passages have been translated from the second volume of *Untersuchungen über thierische Elektricität* ([1849], Pt. III, ch. 7, Sec. I, 1) and deal with

---

* Du Bois-Reymond means by the *density of the current* in any section of the circuit, the quotient of the intensity of the current divided by the area of cross section of the nerve.

the electrotonic state of the nerve. In them the author referred to several interesting and important findings.

1. Paragraph 1 refers to his idea of "electromotive particles" or molecules which were arranged on the surface of the muscle or nerve. A nerve was a chain of dipolar electromotor molecules, positive at their middle and negative at their two ends. Between the longitudinal surface and transverse cross section a resting current existed and this was decreased (the negative variation) during excitation of the nerve or muscle. The electrotonic state was represented by the molecules arranged with their negative poles towards the anode and their positive poles towards the cathode. This was later disproved by Hermann, but the basic idea is important for it was the earliest link with the theory of polarization which underlies modern concepts of nerve conduction. Du Bois-Reymond's state of electrotonus is identical with polarization in nerves. It is also important to note that he was differentiating between the process in the nerve (*nerve principle*) and its electrical accompaniment.

2. In paragraph 2 he is concerned with the vital question of *nerve principle* (nerve transmission).

3. In paragraphs 3 ff. he deals with the problem of nerve tetanization and is grappling with the problem of whether the nerve's negative variation in potential (i.e., current of action) was the same as the nerve principle (excitatory process or nerve impulse). This led later to attempts to measure the speed of the conduction rate of the nerve (see pp. 206–209).

4. The terms he gives in the last paragraphs allow us to understand his work better.

EXCERPT PP. 289–294

We now know that muscles and nerve tissues more than all others are distinguished by the possession of an excessively strong current; we know the law according to which they exercise this function; it is identical in both. We have seen that all phenomena which, under this law, participate in the resting nerve and muscle can be explained by the simple hypothesis that muscle and nerve are uniformly composed of molecules whose equatorial zone is positive, their polar zone negative, and whose axes thereby are all placed parallel to one another and to the direction of the primary bundles, or to that of the nerve fibres. In addition, we know that the electromotive activity [resting potential] which we attribute to these hypothetical molecules is associated essentially with a condition represented by certain functions and qualities characteristic for both tissues in the comparatively intact [undamaged] state; indeed, we have found that the electric current alters in a muscle with the manifestation of life the contraction which is peculiar to muscle tissue. Now, fortified by these promising hypotheses, we shall proceed with the investigation; how does the nerve current behave while the so-called nerve principle is in action, that is, while the nerve communicates the material changes which we perceive as motion, as sensation, to the muscle or to the central structures.

In the beginning, the investigation follows the same order here as that for the behavior of the electric current in muscle during contraction. It again is divided into experiments with the multiplier [the first name used for the galvanometer (Schweigger, 1826)] and into supplementary ones with the frog thigh which is tested with the current. With regard to the multiplier tests, exactly the same principles prevail which were determined above for the investigation of the electric current in muscle during contraction. With the rapid speed of nerve reactions and the low value of the current which must be assumed here, it is just as impossible, for reasons that we discussed above, to observe immediately the effect of a single impulse of the nerve principle upon the multiplier needle as it is with that of a single muscle twitch. If a change in the nerve current accompanies the process which transmits motion and sensation [i.e., the nerve principle] at all, the latter cannot be noted on the multiplier in any other way than if it were to occur either continuously or be constantly repetitive in the same manner during as short a time as possible. It may be noted that here, in contrast to the previous endeavors in this field, with the exception of those by Person, the objection may be raised again that this essential point has not been considered.

Therefore our goal must be directed towards establishing a procedure whereby we can reproduce in the nerve a condition which, with respect to its particular living characteristics, is the same as tetany of the muscle. Such a condition is for the nerve in motion evidently the same that causes tetany in the respective muscles; for the sensory nerve it is the condition in which sensations of any kind, but as lively as possible, occur either steadily or in individual bursts which are repeated in uninterrupted and close sequence. For the sake of brevity and convenience we shall continue to refer to the experimental procedure which produces such a state in the nerve by the expression "tetanize," regardless of whether it is of motor or sensory type.

One may already realize that the means at our disposal for reaching our goal must correspond for the most part to those which we reported when exploring muscle tissue, since in that case our aim was to produce sustained contraction by the nerve. We can choose between the electric current, strychnine poisoning, and mechanical, thermal, and chemical stimulations applied directly to the nerve. It can hardly elude us that here, too, a great preponderance of certainty, convenience, strength, and duration of the stimulus are all in favor of the electric current; we shall therefore start with it in our order of procedure . . . .

Furthermore, for the sake of simplicity and convenience, we shall use at first only single, dissected sections of nerve . . . .

The manner in which the electric current is applied here is absolutely identical with the one we investigated in the muscle. The question here is

merely to investigate which electromotive process takes place perhaps between the cross section and longitudinal section of the nerve pathway
which during tetanization of the muscle is located between it and the
platinum ends of the induction cylinder; in lieu of the muscle one now
places the end of the nerve itself, which was cut off above the former, on
the pad in the usual manner. Everything that has been said concerning the
contractions in the muscle, how they are produced, their alternating course,
etc., etc., remains fully valid; also everything that has been said from the
beginning and demonstrated in the schematic tests, so that the suspicion
may be removed that if, with the procedure applied, the stimulating current could pass directly into the multiplier circuit.

However, for the sake of greater certainty we shall once more carry out a
controlled experiment with respect to this latter point. This precautionary
measure proves to be of great significance. In order to bring this about, one
must not use induction stimuli but a direct current which, as may still be
remembered from the above discussion and which, as we believe to be the
case, does not affect the nerve principle at all provided it does not exceed a
certain strength. Although the insertion of a nerve between platinum electrodes renders the consistency of the current impossible, it is yet of advantage to use a pile of consistent voltage. In order to deflect the direction of
the current in the nerve easily, either a Poggendorff inverter or, since
stoppage by the spring on metal, or the exact motion of the wheel at a
certain fraction of its circumference cannot be carried out without definite
attention, a Pohl commutator is inserted into the loop of the nerve and the
pile.

It is self-evident that here, too, as in the corresponding experiments on
the current in muscle, the greatest care must be taken to avoid any direct
influence of the circuit upon the needle . . . .

Now it is found that at the moment when the circuit through the nerve
is closed, what must happen by the intervention of metals is that the
current is considerably changed in size, while the nerve lies there on top
and while the needle is kept in a position of constant deviation in one of
the mercury vessels of the commutator. And so the law which seems to
determine the height of the current is as follows:

If the current of the circuit in the nerve has the same direction as the
current in that of a length of nerve circuit which is part of the multiplier
circuit, we then have an increased nerve current; apparently, diminution of
the latter occurs if both currents in the nerve have the opposite direction.

See Figs. 99, 100, Plate II [fig. 54] where the arrows point in the
direction of the currents, the plus and minus signs respectively indicate
increase and decrease of currents. The sign of the change of the nerve

current has nothing to do with the ascending and descending course of the extrinsic electric current; indeed, the phenomenon is exactly the same, regardless of whether the central end of the nerve rests on the platinum plates, or the muscle end on the pads, or vice versa. The change of the current is of a steady nature; it lasts as long as the extrinsic current circulates through the other end. This is seen first, in a continuous increase or decrease in the constant deflection which, under favorable circumstances, is easily noticeable; second, in that by opening the circuit one produces a reduction in the current when the currents of the nerve and that in the circuit run in the same direction, and cause an increase in current when they run in opposite directions.

However, at first inspection of these phenomena, it is not easy to avoid the conclusion that they are simply based upon the flow of the extrinsic electric current into the multiplier circuit, and the reader may perhaps be astonished that one subjects him to the detailed description of such an insignificant point. But such is not the case; a brief observation and a few tests will suffice to demonstrate that such interpretation is out of the question and that we are dealing with nothing less than a new electromotive function of the nerves which they display under the influence of a constant electric current which makes contact with a fraction of their length at all its points. Just as welcome as this concept is to us, since it permits sudden recognition of the nerves as endowed apparently with other special electric functions, apart from their ordinary current, so just as little can we conceal the great difficulties which prevent the pursuit of the actual goal we envisaged; that is, to find out whether a noticeable change takes place in the nerve current at the moment when the nerve principle is functioning. As we know, because of previous reports (see above, Vol. I, p. 258 [p. 197]) this moment corresponds only with the beginning and ending of the stimulating current. By contrast, we now find that the electric conditions of the nerve are also changed by the continuation of the current at the same strength. Because of the function of the nerve principle this change is also going to interfere, in all probability, with the possible fluctuation of the current at the beginning and the ending of the current . . . .

We shall continue to designate the current which changes the electric conditions in the nerves by the already familiar name of *stimulating current*.

We propose to call the state of the change of its electromotive powers which are produced by the stimulating currents, the *electrotonic condition of the nerve* . . . .

We shall say of the portion of a nerve which is in an electrotonic state and which demonstrates an increase of its original current, that it is in a positive phase of this condition. We shall ascribe the *negative phase* to the portion which showed decrease in its original current.

We shall call the parts of the nerve which are resting on pads and from where the nerve current is conducted to the multiplier, the *conducting nerve section;* the one on the platinum plates of the current-conducting device which is subjected to the stimulating current will be called the *stimulated section.*

It is difficult to summarize even a portion of du Bois-Reymond's work because his reports of it are numerous and diffuse. However, one of his friends, Henry Bence Jones, in acquainting the English-reading world with them (*On animal electricity: being an abstract of the discoveries of Emil du Bois-Reymond* [London, 1852]) included a chapter of conclusions. Some of these are reproduced below, and they conveniently sum up the first ten years of du Bois-Reymond's labors.

EXCERPT PP. 210–212

1. The muscles and nerves, including the brain and the spinal cord, are endowed during life with an electromotive power.

2. This electromotive power acts according to a definite law, which is the same in the nerves and muscles, and may be briefly stated as the law of the antagonism of the longitudinal and transverse section. The longitudinal surface being positive, and the transverse section negative.

3. As the nerves have no natural transverse section, their electromotive power, when they are in a state of rest, cannot be made apparent unless they have previously been divided.

4. . . . .

5. Every minute particle of the nerves and muscles acts according to the same law as the whole nerve or muscle.

6. The currents which the nerves and muscles produce in circuits, of which they form part, must be considered only as derived portions of incomparably more intense currents circulating in the interior of the nerves and muscles around their ultimate particles.

7. The electromotive power lasts after death, or in dissected nerves and muscles after separation from the body of the animal, as long as the excitability of the nervous and muscular fibre; whether these fibres are permitted to die gradually from the cessation of the conditions necessary to the support of life, or whether they are suddenly deprived of their vital properties, by heat, chemical means, etc.

8. . . . .

9. . . . .

10. The current in muscles when in the act of contraction, and in nerves when conveying motion or sensation, undergoes a sudden and great negative variation of its intensity.

EXCERPT PP. 213–214

16. If any part of a nerve is submitted to the action of a permanent current, the nerve in its whole extent suddenly undergoes a material change in its internal constitution, which disappears on breaking the circuit, as suddenly as it came on. This change, which is called the electrotonic state, is evidenced by a new electromotive power, which every point of the whole length of the nerve acquires during the passage of the current, so as to produce, in addition to the usual current, a current in the direction of the extrinsic current. As regards this new mode of action, the nerve may be compared to a voltaic pile, and the transverse section loses its essential import. Hence the electric effects of the nerve, when in the electrotonic state, may also be observed in nerves without previously dividing them.

17. The electrotonic state of a nerve is the commencement of its electrolysis. The contraction of making the circuit is caused by the nerve passing into the electrotonic state, and that on breaking the circuit by the nerve passing out of this state.

18. In the muscles the electrotonic state does not manifest itself as it does in the nerves.

19. Approaching death and severe injuries of the muscular and nervous tissue cause other modifications of the electromotive power of the nerves and muscles, of which some are permanent, and connected with the total extinction of that power; others are only transitory.

20. The electric phenomena of motor and sensitive nerves are identical. Both classes of nerves transmit irritation in both directions.

JOHANNES MÜLLER
(14 July 1801—28 April 1858)

While the electrical phenomena of the nerve and its attached muscle were receiving widespread attention, other properties of nerves were also being studied. One of these concerned the behavior of sensory nerves and the basic observation that specific nerves transmit specific sensations. This led to the formulation of a law, the elements of which were provided by the famous German physiologist, Johannes Müller (see Boring, 1942, pp. 80–95).

He was born in Coblenz, the son of a cobbler, and studied medicine at the University of Bonn where he was graduated in 1822. Four years later he went to Berlin, and by 1833 was professor of anatomy and physiology and director of the anatomical theatre and museum. Müller was one of the most outstanding biologists of all time and his interests were widespread in medicine and biology. It is said that he produced, on an average, one scientific publication every seven weeks from the age of nineteen to his death. He worked on the physiology of motion, foetal life, nerves, and vision; the anatomy of invertebrates, embryology, histology, and comparative anatomy. His students formed a galaxy of famous men and included du Bois-Reymond, Virchow, Schwann, Helmholtz, and Koelliker. As a group they were responsible for the dominance of German physiology in the second half of the nineteenth century (see Platt, 1896; Haberling, 1924; Ebbecke, 1951; Steudel, 1964).

Riese and Arrington (1963) have traced the origins in Müller's writings of the so-called law of specific nerve energies although he did not formulate a law as such. These authors term it more correctly the doctrine of specific energies of the senses rather than of the nerves, a point already made by McKeag in 1902. Müller admitted that others had considered the problem; indeed, Robert Whytt of Edinburgh (p. 336) had made vague references to the phenomenon, and Charles Bell of London discussed it in 1823 ("Second paper on the nerves of the orbit," *Phil. Trans. R. Soc.*, 1823, 113 [i]:289–307). It is interesting to detect the remnants of Galenic beliefs in the following passage.

EXCERPT P. 304

This notion of a fluid moving backwards and forwards in the tubes of the nerves, equally adapted to produce motion and sensation, has perpetuated the error, that the different nerves of sensation are appropriated to their offices by the texture of their extremities, "that there exists a certain relation between the softness of the nervous extremities, and the nature of the bodies which produce an impression on them." On the contrary, every nerve of sense is limited in its exercise, and can minister to certain perceptions only. Whatever may be the nature of the impulse communicated to a nerve, pressure, vibration, heat, electricity, the perception excited in the mind will have reference to the organ exercised, not to the impression made upon it. Fire will not give the sensation of heat to any nerve but that appropriated to the surface. However delicate the retina be, it does not feel like the skin. The point which pricks the skin being thrust against the retina, will cause a spark of fire or a flash of light. The tongue enjoys two senses, touch and taste; but by selecting the extremity of a particular nerve, or what is the same thing, a particular papilla, we can exercise either the one or the other sense separately. If we press a needle against a nerve of touch, we shall feel the sharpness and recognize the part of the tongue in contact with the point; but if we touch a nerve of taste, we shall have no perception of form or of place, we shall experience a metallic taste.

The first full discussion of this matter, however, was published by Müller in 1826 (*Zur vergleichenden Physiologie des Gesichtssinnes des Menschen und der Thiere* [Leipzig, 1826]), but the final version of his Law appears in the second edition of his famous textbook of physiology (*Handbuch der Physiologie des Menschen für Vorlesungen* [Coblenz, 1835], Vol. I, bk. 3, sec. 4, "On the peculiar properties of individual nerves"). As the English translation by William Baly (1838) is inaccurate and incomplete, a new version of the appropriate section has been prepared.

To evaluate Müller's argument correctly we must recall that at this time external bodies were thought to give off vibrations that could travel as such through the sensory nerve to the sensorium. Müller's new idea was in part owing to an increasing interest in physics which dispelled the concept of vibrations; its survival was assured by Helmholtz who applied it to the problem of color vision. Although Müller's Law seems to state a fact which is very obvious to us, its elucidation still occupies investigators of sensory physiology as a central theme.

EXCERPT PP. 752–753

CHAPTER 1. THE SENSORY NERVES

The nerves have always been considered conductors for the mutual effect of the external world on our organs. Thus physicians have regarded the sensory nerves as mere conductors of the properties of external matter so that the nerves have been supposed to transmit the qualities of such bodies almost passively to the consciousness without any change in the impressions of these qualities. More recently some physiologists have begun to analyze these concepts of passive conduction by the nerves. If the nerves are merely passive conductors for the impression of light, of sound vibrations, and odors, how does it happen that the nerve that perceives odors is perceptive only of this kind of impression, and not of others, and that by contrast another nerve cannot perceive odors; that a nerve which is sensitive to light radiation or to its oscillations, cannot sense the oscillations of sound-producing bodies; that the auditory nerve is insensible to light, the gustatory to odors; that the sensory nerve does not sense the oscillations of bodies as sound, but as tremors. These considerations have led physiologists to attribute to the individual sensory nerves a specific sensibility for certain impressions by virtue of which they are supposed to be conductors of certain qualities only, but not of others.

However, a comparison of the facts with this explanation, which ten or twenty years ago was not doubted in the least, soon proved it to be unsatisfactory. For the same cause, such as electricity, can simultaneously affect all sensory organs, since they are all sensitive to it; and yet, every sensory nerve reacts to it differently; one nerve perceives it as light, another hears its sound, another one smells it; another tastes the electricity, and another one feels it as pain and shock. One nerve perceives a luminous picture through mechanical irritation, another one hears it as buzzing, another one senses it as pain. The increased stimulation of the blood produces spontaneous impressions of light in one organ, buzzing in another, tickling, pain, etc., in yet another one. He who feels compelled to consider the consequences of these facts cannot but realize that the specific sensibility of nerves for certain impressions is not enough, since all sensory nerves are sensitive to the same cause but react to the same cause in different ways. Consequently some have come to the realization that a sensory nerve is not a mere passive conductor, but that inherent in each particular sensory nerve are also certain special energies or qualities that are merely stimulated and brought out by exciting causes. *Therefore, sensation is not the conduction of a quality or state of external bodies to consciousness, but the conduction of a quality or a state of our nerves to consciousness, excited by an external cause.* We do not feel the knife that causes us pain, only the painful state of our nerves; the probable mechanical oscillation of light is not a sensation of light *per se*; even if it could reach into consciousness it would only be as the awareness of an oscillation; only because it affects the optic nerve as the mediator between cause and consciousness is it perceived as luminosity; the vibration of bodies *per se* is not sound, but sound originates only as a sensation through a quality of the auditory nerve; and the nerve of touch perceives this same vibration of the seemingly sonorous body as a sensation of tremor. Therefore, only by virtue of the conditions that are stimulated in our nerves by external influences do we communicate sensorily with the external world.

This truth, which is the result of a simple and impartial analysis of facts, not only leads us to a knowledge of the peculiar energies of the various sensory nerves, apart from their general distinction from the motor nerves, but it also points the way to banish once and for all from physiology a number of erroneous concepts regarding the ability of nerves to substitute for one another. It has long been known that blind men *cannot* recognize colors as colors with their fingers; but we now realize its impossibility from facts that are an explanation for many other facts. However much the feeling in the blind man's fingers may be increased by practice, it always remains a quality of the sensory nerves, touch. What educated physician would want to believe in such fairy tales as the sensation of light and vision with the fingers, or the so-called magnetism [i.e., animal magnetism or hypnosis] with the pit of the stomach?

Hermann Ludwig Ferdinand von Helmholtz
(31 August 1821—8 September 1894)

Ever since man first realized that the brain initiated movements of the limbs and interpreted sensations, he must have been astonished at the speed with which messages could be sent along the nerves. It was at first generally thought that it would never be possible to measure that speed, and even Johannes Müller agreed with this conclusion. However, one of his pupils, Helmholtz, achieved the seemingly impossible.

Helmholtz was born in Potsdam and studied at the Army Medical School in Berlin. Like others in the nineteenth century and earlier, Helmholtz, whose main interests lay in the basic sciences, qualified in medicine so as to acquire a respectable education, a position in society, and a source of income while carrying out purely scientific research. He was graduated in 1842 and then studied with Johannes Müller at the University of Berlin. He became professor of physiology in the University of Königsberg until 1856 and held the same post at Heidelberg until 1871 when he was appointed professor of physics in the University of Berlin. His work included the pronouncement of the law of conservation of energy (Livingston, 1947), invention of the ophthalmoscope, fundamental studies of the physiology of vision and hearing, and important work in physics. In modern terminology, he was a biophysicist and his influence on nineteenth century mechanistic physiology was immense (see M'Kendrick, 1899; Wood, 1902; Knapp, 1902; Hall, 1902; Randall, 1902; Goodspeed, 1902; Koenigsberger, 1902–1903, English translation 1906; Boring, 1942, pp. 297–315; Haymaker, 1953, pp. 135–138; Kolle, 1956–1963, II, 67–77; Sechenov, 1962, pp. 467–478; W. Blasius, 1964).

Helmholtz used two methods to measure the time that elapses between electrical stimulation of the nerve and contraction of the muscle. The first, as Hoff and Geddes (1960) have pointed out, was based upon analogy to the velocity of a bullet from a gun. He therefore applied the knowledge and techniques of ballistics to the problem and was completely successful. He measured the duration of an electric current sent through a galvanometer from the moment the nerve was stimulated to its interruption when the muscle contracted. The results of his experiments appeared first in the report of the Academy of Science in Berlin, January 1850. This preliminary announcement was published in Müller's *Archiv* in the same year ("Vorläufiger Bericht über die Fortpflanzungsgeschwindigkeit der Nervenreizung," *Arch. Anat. Physiol.*, 1850, pp. 71–73).

EXCERPT PP. 71–73

I have found that a measurable period of time elapses before the stimulus applied to the iliac plexus of the frog is transmitted to the insertion of the crural nerve into the gastrocnemius muscle by a brief electric current. In large frogs, in which the nerves were from 50–60 mm. in length, and which were preserved at a temperature of 2–6° C, although the temperature of the observation chamber was between 11° and 15° C, the elapsed time was 0.0014 to 0.0020 of a second.

The nerve was stimulated by a current induced in a coil by the interruption of the current in a second coil [a double galvanic induction coil]. At the very moment when the current in the induction coil was interrupted, a second current conducted through a multiplier [galvanometer] was closed by means of a special mechanical device. I convinced myself that the errors in the exact timing of the opening and closing were always less than $\frac{1}{10}$ of the time element in question. The current circulated through the multiplier until the contraction of the stimulated gastrocnemius muscle had increased sufficiently so that a certain weight suspended from a platinum point, and resting on a gilded base, was raised off this base, with the platinum point, and so interrupted the current conducted through these parts. Therefore, the duration of the current equals the lapse of time between the stimulation of the nerve and the beginning of the mechanical reaction of the muscle. The deflection produced by the current during its passage through the bar magnet of the multiplier is proportional to its duration and can be calculated from it, the more so if one knows the duration of oscillation of the magnet and the deflection that would have been elicited by the uninterrupted current. I measured the deflection with mirror and telescope. The essentials of the method correspond to those established by Pouillet [who invented the ballistic galvanometer and influenced Helmholtz in the planning of his experiments] for the measurement of short periods of time.

The results were as follows:

Following standard stimulation the time required by the muscle to reach the degree of contraction necessary to lift the attached weight was longer the heavier the weight.

With equal attached weights and changing intensity of stimulus or excitability of the muscle, the time became longer the lower the height to which the muscle raised the weight.

With stimulation of the upper end of the sciatic nerve, the height of elevation was usually, but not always, smaller than with stimulation of a part adjacent to the muscle; this agrees with the known facts regarding degeneration of the nerve when severed from its central portion. However, one can bring about similarity of elevation by reducing the induction currents in the stimulated area. The deflection of the magnet then demonstrates that the same mechanical effect occurs slightly earlier when the distal end of the nerve is stimulated rather than the proximal. This differentiation is constant in the same individual, regardless of the weights which have been attached. In a series of experiments with different specimens this alternated between 0.0014 and 0.0020 of a second; the higher values occurred on colder days. In experiments with smaller weights, the individual contractions were somewhat more irregular, and it was necessary to calculate the constant value of the difference from the averages of the test series, whereas with a load of from 100 to 180 grams, this was read off immediately by comparing the individual figures.

Helmholtz did not give the velocities of the nerve impulse in this paper, but they can be estimated at 25.00 to 42.50 meters per second (Hoff and Geddes, 1960, p. 143). Later that same year, 1850, he published figures and the range was 24.6 to 38.4 meters per second.

By 1852 he had developed his second technique, a graphic method of recording the times of nerve excitation and muscle contraction on a cylinder, from which he could calculate the speed of the impulse. The details appeared in one of a series of publications on this topic ("Messungen über Fortpflanzungsgeschwindigkeit der Reizung in den Nerven, zweite Reihe," *Arch. Anat. Physiol.*, 1852, pp. 199–216), and the following account represents his conclusion. The figures obtained corresponded well with those derived from the ballistic or electromagnetic method.

EXCERPT PP. 215–216

The great advantage of the method described lies in the fact that one can recognize immediately in each individual drawing of two correlated curves if the muscle is acting regularly or not in both cases, whereas with the electromagnetic method of measuring time this can only be established after a long series of separate experiments. With regard to absolute value of the speed of [nerve] transmission, the horizontal distances of the two curves cannot be measured very accurately; however, the values are found to be approximately as large as shown by the previous method. For example, *in Fig. 5* [fig. 58] the horizontal distance is approximately 1 mm., the size of the circumference of the cylinder approximately 85.7 mm., which corresponds to $\frac{1}{6}$ second; therefore, the length of the abscissa is 514.2 mm., for 1 second. 1 mm. corresponds to $\frac{1}{514.2}$ seconds. The length of the nerve circuit was 53 mm.: hence it follows that the speed of transmission [in the frog] is 27.25 meters per second. The most probable value from previous experiments was 26.4 meters [per second].

It might be thought that the repercussions of this fundamental discovery would be restricted to the field of physiology but, in fact, they were much wider. Helmholtz and Baxt were able to measure the conductivity rate in human motor nerves (30–35 m. per second), and from this it followed that man could now experiment upon the human mind and, with mathematical precision, measure the speed with which it sent messages along the nerves. The influence upon the development of experimental psychology was, therefore, of the greatest importance. Another momentous effect of Helmholtz's discovery that the velocity of nerve messages could be successfully measured was to provide important evidence that the conductivity of nerves could not be compared with electricity flowing along a wire. The process, whatever its nature, was slower, and Hermann's theory of nerve transmission was to derive support from this finding.

LUDIMAR HERMANN

(*21 October 1838—5 June 1914*)

Du Bois-Reymond's theories of nerve and muscle function dominated the field of electrophysiology until the 1860's when opposition to some of them began to develop. The simple concept which likened nerve and muscle currents to electricity flowing along a wire became untenable when evidence such as that provided by Helmholtz on the velocity of nerve conduction became available (pp. 207–209). As it happened, du Bois-Reymond's most effective critic was one of his own assistants working in his laboratories, Ludimar Hermann.

Hermann was born in Berlin and studied medicine there. After having been graduated, he worked in du Bois-Reymond's Institute of Physiology, but as his results did not agree with the latter's theories of nerve and muscle function, relations between the two became strained and in 1868 Hermann left to take up the post of professor of physiology in the University of Zürich. In 1884 he moved to Königsberg where he worked until his retirement. He published widely on topics concerning physiology, chemistry, and physics, and wrote a popular textbook of physiology, *Grundriss der Physiologie des Menschen* (1863), frequently re-published over the next few decades and translated into several foreign languages. His interests lay mainly in the field of muscle physiology where his work on the chemical, as well as the electrical, aspects of contraction was important, and in the physiology of voice and speech and of digestion.

Like his teacher du Bois-Reymond, Hermann had a remarkable ability for designing and producing the apparatus necessary for his experiments. Moreover, he was an example of the pure physiologist who appeared in Germany in the middle of the nineteenth century, who had little connection with medicine. Concerning his personality, his fortitude in opposing the opinions of his world-renowned master should not be overlooked (see Boruttau, 1914; Bayliss, 1920).

Contrary to du Bois-Reymond's concept of electromotive molecules producing a potential difference on the longitudinal surface of the uninjured muscle or nerve at rest, and thus accounting for muscle and nerve currents (p. 198), Hermann maintained that in normal muscle or nerve the whole surface was isoelectric or equipotential and, incorrectly, that resting potentials, or the current of rest, did not exist. Differences of potential occurred when cells under one electrode were injured, the "plane of demarcation," the current of injury or "demarcation potential" arose at the area between sound and injured tissue (1867). According to this "alteration theory," a fundamental discovery which paved the way for our present-day theory, cells which altered their chemical nature by injury or death became electronegative. Any active or injured area of a nerve or muscle was negative to a part at rest and intact; thus arose the idea that an active area was comparable to an injured area. Hermann's ideas, based on physicochemical data, eventually replaced the hypotheses of du Bois-Reymond.

The negative variation of du Bois-Reymond (p. 199) represented Hermann's "current of action," and he examined it with delicate and ingenious apparatus demonstrating it to be in the form of a wave of negative excitation which progressed along the structure from the point of stimulation although not like an electric current in a wire. In his view the wave was a self-propagating state carried from one section of the nerve to the next by a sequence of decreased excitability (*anelectrotonus*) in a resting region and increased excitability (*catalectrotonus*) in an active region; these terms had been introduced by E. F. N. Pflüger (*Untersuchungen über die Physiologie des Electrotonus* [Berlin, 1859], p. 456: "A given piece of nerve is stimulated by the appearance of catelectrotonus and the disappearance of anelectrotonus but not by the reverse"). The galvanometer represented this process as a diphasic variation, and any two points of the nerve in the same stage of activity were equipotential. There was thus a closed electrical circuit with the current flowing from the resting to the active region and returning to the negative interior of the fibre and then to a resting area, as in a cylindrical, electrically polarized membrane.

This action current was later shown to be the release of the resting potential, likened by Glees (1961, p. 115) to the pressure in water mains released through a hole. Hermann's denial of the resting electrical potential had been unwarranted; yet he was correct in opposing du Bois-Reymond's concept of surface potential differences, as he was also in stating that du Bois-Reymond's electrotonic currents were polarization effects owing to electrolysis. The spread of excitation was the result of the polarization effect of the action current.

The following selections have been translated from various editions of Hermann's *Grundriss*. The first, in which the author defined certain terms such as *electrotonus*, which is today used to describe the longitudinal spread of current in the nerve or the state of polarization, has been taken from the third edition (Berlin, 1870).

EXCERPT PP. 296–297

7. . . . . If a constant galvanic current is led through any section of a nerve, the condition of the whole length of the nerve changes (du Bois-Reymond), so that its state of excitation becomes modified (Eckhard, Pflüger). This state is called "electrotonic," or "electrotonus" (du Bois-Reymond); moreover, the state in the neighborhood of the positive electrode (anode) is called "anelectronic" and near the negative electrode (cathode) "catelectronic" (Pflüger); the constant current itself [which produces this change] is called "polarizing" or "electrotonizing." The boundary between the electrodes (in the "intrapolar region"), between anelectrotonus and catelectrotonus (the "indifferent point"), lies near the anode when the [polarizing] current is weak and moves towards the cathode as the current increases in strength. The influence of electrotonus is strongest in the neighborhood of the pole. The irritability *is increased in the catelectrotonic region and decreased in the anelectrotonic.* When the polarizing current ceases, the [state of] irritability gradually returns to normal after a reversal (positive for anelectrotonus, negative for catelectrotonus).

The second excerpt provides a brief explanation of Hermann's theory of the transmission of activity along the nerve and has been translated from the same edition.

EXCERPT P. 303

The simplest explanation for this behavior [transmission of the state of activity along nerve fibres] is that when the end organ is stimulated naturally the whole nerve does not go into an active state. Instead, the activity is transmitted from one cross section to the next and in this way it is transmitted throughout the whole length of the nerve. Furthermore, any stimulus applied to any portion of the nerve produces an active state at that point first, and in this way causes the same chain of transmission as with the natural stimulation of the end organ. The ability of the nerve to transmit the active state from one point to the next, and in this way to the end organ, is called the capacity for conduction [conductivity].

In the third excerpt, translated from the fifth edition (Berlin, 1874), Hermann referred to his concept of the nerve behaving like a core conductor with a membrane separating it from its conducting envelope.

EXCERPT PP. 308–309

The other theory (Hermann) explains the nerve current as analogous to the muscle current and thus owing to two effects of contact: nerve fibre contents that are dying or active are negative to the same contents that are living and at rest. The cause of the electrotonic phenomenon is the above-mentioned polarization at the boundary between the covering and the medullary substance of the nerve fibre.

In later editions the title of Hermann's text became *Lehrbuch der Physiologie,* and the next selection, from the thirteenth edition (Berlin, 1905) so entitled, presents a fuller account of his theory. The first paragraph gives a brief history of nerve conduction, and the diagram (fig. 59) has been reproduced on many occasions in the past.

EXCERPT PP. 242–243

The older theories that tried to explain the activity of nerves by the movement of fluids or some such substance, can be left out of our consideration completely. The idea that nerve activity consisted of electricity (Hausen 1743 [Hermann overlooked Hales, 1732, II, 58]) could not be developed into a usable theory even when the electric telegraph had been invented and it became a happy commonplace to compare the nervous system in some respects to the telegraphic system. The absence of closed-current circuits speaks against any close analogy with the telegraph; so likewise do the absence of a battery-like apparatus to produce currents, the absence of any galvanic insulation of the nerve fibres, the effect of ligation, and, above all, the slowness of nerve conduction. After the discovery of the nerve current (du Bois-Reymond, 1843) new possibilities for electric theories were opened up; especially as it was sometimes thought that the regularly arranged electromotive molecules in the nerves, which were assumed to explain the nerve current, at the same time caused the conduction by means of an electrodynamic effect of the molecules upon each other; however, neither has such a theory been developed in more detail, nor has the assumption of these molecules been found to be necessary or admissible.

Nowadays nerve conduction is nearly always understood in such a way that each segment of the fibre is stimulated by the neighboring segment, just as if by an external stimulation; that is, as a transmission of excitation from particle to particle. Against this simple view it is asserted that a stretch of nerve can conduct without being mechanically or chemically stimulated by an external stimulus (Schiff and others); but this can be explained by the very reasonable assumption that excitation by the stimulus of the neighboring particle finds more favorable conditions than by external stimulation which, after all, does not occur under completely normal circumstances. Moreover, because more excitable stretches of nerve (for instance, heated) increase the passing excitation (Grützner and others), conduction must be based upon excitation.

But what the changes of excitation consist of, and how it is transmitted to the neighboring segment or particle, is unknown. The only thing that is known for certain is that each change is closely connected with a negativity of the stimulated area. As the electric current is not only the most effective stimulus for the nerve but also influences the excitability greatly, it is true that action currents most probably play the main part during the conduction of excitation. Especially in favor of this is the latest finding that in the central nervous system and in the retina, excitation is not dependent upon continuity but flows between neighboring structures.

The conduction of excitation is probably secured by the fact that the action current runs in a neighboring area of the nerve in such a way that it places the stimulated area itself into anelectrotonus but the nearest neighboring area into catelectrotonus (Hermann). Fig. 114 [fig. 59] explains this: *KK* is the nucleus [axon], *HHHH* the covering of the nerve fibre, and *pqrs* a stimulated area of the nucleus; then the electromotor areas *ps* and *qr* of the action current produce the two little sketched currents which, it must be realized, are extremely strong because of the small resistance in microscopic dimensions; these form for the nucleus at *c, c* cathodes, with *a, a* anodes, which therefore have a quietening effect upon the stimulated area and an excitatory effect upon the neighboring area.

JULIUS BERNSTEIN
(*8 December 1839—6 February 1917*)

The source of the electromotive force manifested by the resting potential and the relationship between the resting potential and the action current had not yet been discovered. This was the work of Bernstein who adapted Hermann's idea of current flow in the nerve and developed his membrane theory of nerve conduction from the observation that all living animal tissues contain ions of salt solutions and that these are electrically charged. Is it not possible, he argued, that this is the source of the electrical charge in the nerve?

Bernstein was born in Berlin and studied there and at Breslau. In Berlin he came under the influence of du Bois-Reymond and was assistant to Helmholtz in Heidelberg. In 1871 he returned to Berlin briefly and then spent the remainder of his active career as successor to Goltz, professor of physiology at Halle. He retired in 1911, having worked especially in the fields of electrophysiology and the physiology of the cardiovascular and respiratory systems, as well as of the special senses. He was also interested in toxicology, medical education, physics, and mathematics. Bernstein was one of the second generation of German mechanistic physiologists, in succession to such men as du Bois-Reymond, Helmholtz, and Brücke (Tschermak, 1919).

The membrane theory was based upon the presence in the nerve fibre of a selectively permeable membrane which, in the resting, polarized state (it sustains a potential difference that corresponds to the resting or demarcation potential) separates the internal, potassium cations from the external, sodium cations. Excitation at one point increases the permeability of the membrane there and the negative ions inside the fibre pass through it to produce a state of depolarization. The small electric currents thus generated, stimulate adjacent parts and the process is repeated so that a self-propagating wave of negativity passes along the fibre.

Bernstein used the capillary electrometer, invented by Gabriel Lippmann in 1872, to confirm his earlier ideas, and he was able to detect these minute currents. He also invented an ingenious analyzing instrument, the rheotome (Hoff and Geddes, 1957), with which he proved that the electrical response of nerve or muscle to a stimulus (i.e., the negative variation in nerve potential) was a true index of the tissue's active state, the nerve impulse, and kept time with it. He was the first to plot the negative variation of nerve and to prove that it was propagated at the same velocity as the nerve impulse. Hence the nerve impulse and the negative variation are one and the same. Some of his conclusions were incorrect; nevertheless his theory has survived the searching analysis of modern electrophysiology and today is still acceptable although somewhat modified (see Hodgkin, pp. 234–237).

It is impossible to avoid a comparison, already barely touched on, between Bernstein's membrane theory and du Bois-Reymond's electromotive particles. Likewise, the current of injury of earlier investigators can be explained by the migration of electrically charged ions from the normal to the injured area with the creation of a potential difference. The action current is the electromotive disturbance induced by a temporary change in the permeability of the internal surface of the membrane, brought about by stimulation.

The following selection is the conclusion to Bernstein's article of 1902 ("Untersuchungen zur Thermodynamik der biolektrischen Ströme," *Pflügers Arch.*, 1902, 92:521–562) in which he sought to apply some of the recent advances in thermodynamics and electrochemistry to the problems posed by the electric currents of living organisms. His primary assumption that "these currents have a similar if not identical cause and that they occur with different energy and magnitude according to the prevailing conditions of the structure and of the chemical composition of the cells which constitute the organs" (p. 521) is still acceptable.

EXCERPT PP. 560–562

The resting currents of muscle and of nerve are considered to be current concentrations. Their circuits differ from the physical concentration circuits though the fact that their chemical composition depends inversely and within narrow limits upon temperature.

The origin of these current concentrations may be interpreted in two ways:

a) according to the alteration theory [Hermann, p. 210] by the formation of an organic electrolyte at the cross section, of which the ions have different mobilities and *Überführungszahlen* [the relation of the velocity of one ion to the sum of the velocities of both ions] in the fibre and the sheath.

b) according to the membrane theory, with the help of an electrolyte [potassium] preexisting in the fibre, which, for the most part, consists of inorganic salts, with the assumption that the living plasma membranes of fibres or fibrils are not easily, or not at all, permeable for one of two ions. Therefore this theory is at the same time a theory of preexistence.

Of course one may also combine the membrane theory with that of alteration, since on the whole a difference by degree only between the assumption of various, relative mobilities (*Überführungszahlen*) and semi-permeability of the membranes exists for the ions. Therefore the essential difference of the two theories lies on the one hand in the acceptance of the formation of an electrolyte coherently participating with the current at the cross section by alteration, and on the other the preexistence of this electrolyte in the living fibre or fibril. However, this theory of preexistence is based essentially on the membrane theory. It is obvious that the negative variation (i.e., action current) by stimulation can be equally well explained by either theory; according to the theory of alteration, by the formation and disappearance of the organic electrolyte in the living fibre; according to the membrane theory, by an increase of permeability for the retained ion owing to a chemical change in the plasma.

Experiments regarding the time of origin of the currents following the construction of a cross section can decide between these two theories only when such a time factor is actually proved. As I have argued, this is not the case according to Hermann's experiments, and the more recent studies by

S. Garten seem to me just as little convincing. However, this would still not be evidence for a theory of preexistence, because the alteration, too, might be a process of molecular velocity.

The molecular theory of E. du Bois-Reymond [p. 198] could not and, according to the author's own opinion, was not, supposed to be anything but a model for the distribution of electric potentials in muscle and nerve, transmitted as electromotive elements to the smallest part of the fibre. Du Bois-Reymond considered even these potentials as only expressions of physical and chemical energies which are active during life. However, this theory in its original form did not permit a further expansion based upon physics and chemistry, useful as it appeared at the start. On the other hand, on the basis of electrochemical data, I have tried to give it a different form by assuming the electromotive elements to be polarized or polarizable. This theory is not in such great contrast to the opinions of modern physical chemistry and electrochemistry as Oker-Bloom seems to surmise. On the contrary, it can be easily correlated with the membrane theory. It compares the molecules and molecular threads with metal particles and metal threads which, at their surface, are polarized towards the liquid, and the surface is polarized by currents conducted to it. But, according to the membrane theory, a fibre behaves to its surrounding fluid exactly as a metal thread, for the phenomena of polarization in semipermeable membranes are completely analogous to those of metal polarization.

ERNEST OVERTON

(25 February 1865—27 January 1933)

Although in his paper of 1902 Bernstein (pp. 215–216) did not discuss in detail the properties and activities of the sodium and potassium ions that were basic to his membrane theory, in the same volume of *Pflügers Archiv* that contained it there were two reports on this subject by Overton ("Beiträge zur allgemeinen Muskel- und Nervenphysiologie" 1902, 92:115–280, and "Beiträge zur allgemeinen Muskel- und Nervenphysiologie, II. Mittheilung. Über die Unentbehrlichkeit von Natrium- (oder Lithium-) Ionen für den Contractionsact des Muskel," 92:346–386). Of the second paper, a remarkable contribution to the subject of muscle contraction and nerve transmission, an excerpt has been given below. It complemented Bernstein's work perfectly for it gave information about sodium ions and their role in muscle and nerve function.

Ernest Overton was born in Stretton, England, but in 1882 moved to Zürich. In 1901 he was appointed assistant professor of physiology at Würzburg and in 1907 became the first occupant of the chair of pharmacology at Lund (1907–1933). He was trained initially as a botanist and his research work was in the field of cell osmosis and permeability which led to his lipid-cell membrane theory and his concept of the mechanism of narcosis (see Collander, 1933; Holmstedt and Liljestrand, 1963, pp. 150–154).

Overton demonstrated that sodium ions are necessary for muscle contraction and that in active muscle and nerve there is an exchange between potassium ions inside the fibres and sodium ions in the surrounding fluid.

EXCERPT PP. 384–386

1. If muscles and blood are put into isosmotic solutions of sucrose, or solutions of other non-electrolytes to which the muscle fibres are impermeable or only slowly permeable, after some time they lose their ability to contract and to transmit excitability.

2. The inexcitability of the muscles is owing to the exosmosis of sodium chloride from the intermuscular fluid, that is from the solution flowing around the single muscle fibres [extracellular fluid].

3. The nerve fibres do not lose their excitability by staying in pure sugar solutions, etc.; but it is possible that under these circumstances a solution of sodium chloride remains between the axis cylinder and the myelin sheath, insofar as a peri-axial space containing lymph exists around the axis cylinder.

4. The excitability of muscles which have become inexcitable by staying too long in sugar solutions, etc., slowly returns when small quantities of sodium chloride are added to the solutions in question.

5. The inexcitable state is not owing to the increase in the electrical resistance of the muscles produced by sodium chloride loss, because the muscles are just as insensitive to mechanical as to electrical stimulation. With the gradual reduction of sodium chloride in the fluid between the muscle, the muscle excitability at first decreases only a little (until the concentration of this salt has fallen to c. 0.12%). Yet when the reduction of sodium chloride is increased, the muscle excitability suffers an enormous decrease very quickly and is soon completely extinguished.

6. In 6% cane sugar solutions, etc., containing about 0.1–0.12% sodium chloride, the muscles remain excitable for about as long as in 0.6–0.7% sodium chloride solution.

7. The lowest content of sodium chloride in a solution, just sufficient to keep the muscles noticeably excitable, is $0.07 \pm 0.003\%$ (at a temperature of 16–22° C).

8. The sodium chloride can be replaced by any non-toxic sodium salt so that the lowest concentrations of any of these salts, just sufficient to preserve the excitability, are equivalent to about 0.70% sodium chloride. Thus the conservation of excitability of muscle depends, almost certainly,

only upon the sodium ions, while the anions (electrically neutral molecules) remain inactive.

9. Sodium salts can be replaced by those of lithium but not potassium, rubidium, caesium, or ammonium and similarly not magnesium, calcium, strontium, or barium salts. The lowest concentrations of the lithium salts which make contraction possible are the same as with the corresponding sodium salts, if one goes by molecular concentrations; but they are smaller if one is guided by the percentage weight.

10. The role played by sodium or lithium ions in the transmission of excitability and in the contraction of muscle has not yet been explained; perhaps during these processes a certain exchange takes place between the potassium ions of the muscle fibres and the sodium ions of the solution flowing around them [extracellular], but this assumption is associated with considerable difficulties.

KEITH LUCAS
(8 March 1879—5 October 1916)

By the end of the nineteenth century it was well established that a rapid wave, the nervous impulse, could be set up in the nerve by means of an electrical stimulus. Moreover, it seemed certain, although not yet proved, that natural transmission consisted of like impulses which travelled at the same rate and which could be detected by a change of potential, and accounted for by Bernstein's theory.

The "all or none" property which was later called, more correctly, the "all or nothing" law, had been demonstrated in the heart muscle by Bowditch in 1871: "an induction shock results in a contraction or fails to do so according to its strength; if it does so at all, it produces in the muscle at that time the maximal contraction that can result from stimuli of any strength." In 1902, Gotch of Oxford had hinted at the presence of the all-or-nothing law in nerve and had detected its effects, but it was Adrian who verified its presence (p. 225).

Striated muscle fibres, like nerve fibres, perhaps also manifested all-or-nothing behavior and it was Keith Lucas of Cambridge who was able to demonstrate this as well as to investigate another vital characteristic which became known as the refractory phase of nerve or muscle. The elucidation of these two phenomena has led to greater understanding of the nerve impulse, and the early work on them was carried out by the ill-fated Lucas.

Lucas was born in Greenwich, England, and studied science at Cambridge, where in 1911 he was appointed lecturer in natural sciences. He turned his attention to the physiology of the nerve and, as in the case of his distinguished predecessors in this field, his manual dexterity and engineering capacity allowed him to design and construct new scientific instruments and apparatus necessary for his experiments. His work was only on muscle and nerve physiology which he continued until the outbreak of World War I. Thereafter he worked at the Royal Aircraft Factory and after joining the Royal Flying Corps was killed in a flying accident (see Langley, 1916–1917; Bayliss, 1919).

In 1903 Lucas began a systematic study of muscle and nerve function which led him to his main theme, the nerve impulse, or, as he termed it, the propagated disturbance which he defined as: "A change of unknown nature travels along the nerve in both directions from the seat of stimulation; it is this change which I shall speak of as the propagated disturbance" ("Croonian Lecture: The process of excitation in nerves and muscles," *Proc. R. Soc.*, 1912, 85B:495–524, see p. 496).

To investigate the all-or-nothing property, he studied the cutaneous dorsal muscle of the frog because it has only eight or nine motor nerve fibres to it, and he found that it reacted to increasing stimuli by sudden steps, equal in number to the number of fibres. Thus skeletal muscle also obeyed the all-or-nothing law. This was the first direct evidence of the ungraded nature of the wave of excitation in excitable tissues, other than cardiac muscle, and the first work on individual nerve-muscle units. The following excerpt is from an article written in 1909 ("The 'all or none' contraction of the amphibian skeletal muscle fibre," *J. Physiol., London*, 1909, 38:113–133).

EXCERPT PP. 132–133

It is found that when a series of stimuli of increasing strength is sent into the nerve to the cutaneous dorsi the contraction of the muscle increases in a few definite steps. When once a step has been established further increase of the stimulus causes no further increase of the contraction until a new step is reached. Such continuous increase of contraction as is observed after any step has been reached appears to be due to the favourable effect of previous contractions, since it still follows the sequence of the contractions in time if the experiment is reversed so that each stimulus is weaker than the last.

Presumably each step in the increase of contraction means that another nerve-fibre (or group of nerve-fibres of like excitability) has been excited, and that the muscle-fibres to which that nerve-fibre runs have consequently contracted. It follows that in each muscle-fibre the contraction is always maximal regardless of the strength of stimulus which excites the nerve-fibre.

The skeletal striated muscle cell of amphibia therefore resembles the cardiac striated muscle cell in the property of "all or none" contraction. The difference which renders it possible to obtain 'submaximal' contractions from a whole skeletal muscle but not from a whole heart is not a difference in the functional capabilities of the two types of cell; it depends upon the fact that cardiac muscle cells are connected one with another, whereas skeletal muscle cells are isolated by their sarcolemma. The 'submaximal' contraction of a skeletal muscle is the maximal contraction of less than all its fibres.

In the Croonian Lecture of 1912 he referred to the refractory period as follows: ". . . . its recognition as a part of the process of propagation cannot fail to be a significant fact for any hypothesis of the propagated disturbance" [p. 510]. When a nerve is stimulated there is a redistribution of electrical potential in the nerve and this is the electrical response. It is found, however, that a second stimulus fails to produce like effects until a few thousandths of a second have passed; this momentary inactive period is the refractory state (for early history of the refractory period, see Hoff, 1942) that Lucas mentioned as follows in his Croonian Lecture (see p. 218).

EXCERPT P. 509

The sum of this evidence is that in all these phenomena of impaired activity we have expressions of a single process of recovery from some change which is associated with the propagated disturbance. From what change precisely the tissue is recovering we do not yet know. It seems very probable that in these phenomena we measure the actual return of the tissue to the equilibrium position after its disturbance by that change which is the basis of propagation.

In the year following Lucas's death, his book, *The conduction of the nervous impulse*, edited by his pupil E. D. Adrian, was published (London, 1917) and presented its author's important conclusions regarding the refractory period.

EXCERPT P. 44

We have seen that the passage of a nervous impulse leaves in its wake a period of depressed function known as the refractory phase. In the earlier stages the nerve is inexcitable to any stimuli and also quite unable to conduct impulses which have been set up in some region where the recovery was more advanced. The excitability of the nerve returns gradually during the relative refractory period and the power of conduction also returns gradually. The impairment in conduction is of a different kind from that brought about by a narcotic. The nerve does not conduct with a decrement, but it will not conduct impulses of the normal intensity. The intensity remains constant as the impulse travels down the nerve, but it is less than the normal because the impulse can be extinguished by compelling it to undergo a decrement which is not great enough to extinguish an impulse of the normal intensity. The intensity of the second impulse becomes gradually greater and greater as the interval between it and the first is increased.

So far the function of the nerve fibre had been studied almost exclusively in the peripheral nervous system because of the ease of using it in experiments. Nevertheless, as more was learned about the connections between the central nervous system and the periphery (Chapter II), investigators naturally wondered if functional as well as morphological likenesses existed. Lucas was one of them, and the following extracts have been taken from his posthumous book of 1917. The ideas expressed are those of Lucas but the words are mainly those of the editor. As Alexander Forbes noted (1939), this has had important repercussions.

EXCERPT PP. 101–102

All this may seem a laboured attempt to magnify the likeness between peripheral and central conduction beyond all reason. The likeness may be there, but why insist on it at such length? The answer is that it is very much easier to investigate a simple case than a complex. If we have reasonable ground for supposing that the process of conduction depends on much the same mechanism in the central nervous system as in the peripheral nerve, it will be worth while to analyse the mechanism of peripheral conduction as fully as possible in the hope that we may learn more of the workings of the central nervous system. If the central nervous system involves processes which are entirely unknown in peripheral nerve, then the analysis of peripheral conduction loses a great deal of its interest and the problem of central conduction becomes infinitely more formidable. Indeed the complex structure of the central nervous system would make it almost impossible to attempt more than the most superficial analysis, if all our information is to be drawn from the central nervous system alone. But if we can assume that the same laws govern the conduction of an impulse in the central nervous system and in a peripheral nerve, the problem becomes very much simpler. In a muscle-nerve preparation it is possible to control every important factor to a degree which would be quite out of the question in the central nervous system, and our analysis of peripheral conduction, though far from complete, is still advanced enough to allow us to predict what will happen in different circumstances with a fair degree of accuracy. On the basis of this analysis we have pictured the central nervous system as a network of conductors having different refractory periods, communicating through regions of decrement, easily fatigued and capable of setting up a train of impulses in answer to a single stimulus. Several difficulties have been mentioned already, and it would not be hard to find others. Whether they can be solved without introducing any new factors in central conduction is a question which must be left for future experiment to decide. In any case it will be worth while to continue the investigation on these lines until we find clear evidence of a mechanism of conduction in the central nervous system which differs fundamentally from that found in simple tissues such as muscle and nerve.

ALEXANDER FORBES

(*14 May 1882—27 March 1965*)

In the vast majority of the experimental work carried out thus far on the nerve and muscle, their characteristics had been studied through the application of artificial stimuli. Hence it was reasonable to inquire whether or not their responses might differ when they were subjected to natural stimulation. This problem was discussed by Forbes.

Forbes was born in Milton, Massachusetts, and received the M.D. degree from Harvard University in 1910. He worked exclusively in physiology, and apart from spending a year with Sherrington at Liverpool (1911–1912) and a period with Adrian in 1921, his career was spent at Harvard where he was professor from 1936 until he became Emeritus in 1948. However, he did not retire from neurophysiological work but continued in research in the Biological Laboratories at Harvard until his death (see Adrian, 1965; Davis, 1965).

Forbes studied the electrical phenomena of reflexes in mammals, and in a paper dealing with the flexion reflex, written with a medical student (Alan Gregg, later to become prominent in medical education), he considered the difference to be observed between the responses of nerves to artificial or direct stimulation and to naturally occurring excitation ("Electrical studies in mammalian reflexes. I. The flexion reflex," *Am. J. Physiol.*, 1915, 37:118–176). In this paper the term "propagated disturbance" was used, originally introduced by Keith Lucas as a noncommittal epithet for the nerve impulse (p. 219). Forbes was the first to show that the nature of nerve impulses was always the same, whether elicited by natural or by non-natural causes, a fact more directly proved in a later publication (A. Forbes, C. J. Campbell, and H. B. Williams, "Electrical records of afferent nerve impulses from muscular receptors," *Am. J. Physiol.*, 1924, 69:283–303).

EXCERPT PP. 147–149

In general, it may be said that as compared with the direct [artificially induced] response, the [naturally induced] reflex action current appears after a latency of about 9σ, then rises to a maximum which is reached from four to ten times as long after its onset as is the case in the impulsed [*sic*; should be "impulses"] directly evoked from the nerve by a single shock; and the maximum when reached is much smaller even in a maximal reflex than is evoked by maximal stimulation of the nerve.

In connection with the magnitude of disturbance the observation of Camis [1909] is important. He reported that maximal stimulation of either the peroneal or popliteal nerve alone failed to evoke as much reflex contraction of the flexor muscles as maximal stimulation of both together. In other words, neither of these nerve trunks was able alone to evoke the maximum response of which the reflex centre was capable. In view of this, we should not expect to find the response in the motor nerve in the reflex as great as when all its fibres are excited electrically. Furthermore, it must be remembered that nearly half of the fibres in the peroneal nerve are afferent and play no part in the motor discharge from the centre, and yet these fibres undoubtedly contribute a full share in the response to direct stimulation. There is some doubt whether even these two considerations taken together can explain alone the great difference in magnitude between the reflex and the direct response, considering the vigor of the reflex contraction which can be evoked by a single shock. Perhaps we shall have to seek further yet to account fully for the difference. The discrepancy in the time relations may furnish some clew.

For the strikingly more gradual development of the reflex response than of the direct, two conceivable explanations present themselves.

(1) It might be inferred that impulses arising in a reflex centre are different in kind from those evoked by an artificial stimulus directly applied to the nerve trunk. In one case the nerve fibres receive the impulses from a natural source, in the other case from a wholly unnatural source and in a manner different from any occurrence in the course of their normal functioning. Conceivably, the individual impulses arising in the neurones from reflex excitation are qualitatively different from those artificially induced and rise to their full intensity more gradually. Such a view is quite at variance with the conception of the nerve impulse which has developed from the researches of Lucas, Hill, and Adrian. Their results make the propagated disturbance in nerve appear to be a sort of explosive event whose character is always the same by whatever agent evoked, so long as the condition of the nerve remains unchanged. It further appears, so far as individual fibres are concerned, to obey the "all-or-none" law; that is, its magnitude is always the same in normal fibres regardless of the strength of the stimulus. On the other hand, it is to be remembered that all these researches on the properties of the nerve impulse have been carried out with artificial stimuli, and it is still conceivable that the reflex centre can induce in nerve fibres a different kind of activity which we have found no means of duplicating.

(2) The more gradual rise of the electrical disturbance in the case of the reflex may be quite as easily explained in a way which harmonizes perfectly with the view that the impulse is essentially the same however evoked. It has already been suggested that we have no grounds for the conclusion that in the flexion reflex the impulses in the many neurones making up the motor nerve are discharged "in a volley" rather than in "platoon fire," to use Brucke's [1877] phrase. They might conceivably start down the nerve trunk simultaneously in all the fibres. Yet it is quite as likely, if not even

probable, that the reflex times in the hundreds of separate arcs will not be exactly the same, and that the arrival of the various outgoing impulses at a given point in the nerve will be spread out over a considerable period of time. Just such a scattering in time would perfectly explain the more gradual development of the observed electrical disturbance at the point where it is recorded. It would also contribute another factor to account for the greatly reduced intensity of disturbance as compared with the direct response; for if at any given instant only a small percentage of all the fibres taking part in the reflex are at the height of their activity, at no time will there be so great a disturbance as if all were active at once. This consideration taken in connection with those already mentioned, namely, the fact that nearly half the fibres involved in the direct response are afferent and the fact that by no means all of the motor fibres are called into action by stimulation of a single afferent nerve, may well account for the smallness of the action current obtainable from the maximal reflex.

EDGAR DOUGLAS, LORD ADRIAN
(30 November 1889—   )

When Lucas's work on the nerve impulse ended in 1914, the state of knowledge had developed to the point that the impulse had been shown to be a momentary wave of activity governed probably by factors such as the all-or-nothing principle and the nerve's refractory period; that the nerve fibre worked by a succession of jerks separated by periods of enforced rest, and, although it seemed highly probable that the impulses were the messages carried in the nerves, this had not been proved. One of the young men associated with Lucas, who continued his work after his death, was E. D. Adrian. It was he who solved this vital question.

Adrian was born in London and studied medicine at Cambridge and St. Bartholomew's Hospital, London. He was graduated in 1915, and then worked in clinical neurology and physiology; from 1929 to 1937 he was Foulerton Research Professor of the Royal Society. He was appointed professor of physiology in the University of Cambridge in 1937 and on retirement in 1951 became Master of Trinity College, Cambridge, an appointment he relinquished in 1965. His work has been confined to neurophysiology and the function of sense organs and the many honors he has received indicate its worth. He was created first Baron Adrian of Cambridge in 1955.

First of all Adrian extended the work of Lucas on the all-or-nothing principle to its final proof in the nerve and was the first to provide conclusive evidence of its presence there ("The all-or-none principle in nerve," *J. Physiol., London,* 1913–1914, 47:460–474). Gotch had suggested that the disturbance in a nerve was always of the same intensity in each fibre and that a strong stimulus produced a larger potential wave merely because it activated more fibres. In other words, and with present-day hindsight, the nerve fibre unit could react in only one of two ways, either maximally, like heart muscle as Bowditch had shown, or not at all; there were no intermediate grades of response. Each pulse of activity in the nerve fibre had to be of constant intensity and had to involve all the resources of the fibre irrespective of the strength of the stimulus.

EXCERPT PP. 471–472

SUMMARY

When a nerve is narcotised locally and stimulated at a point central to the narcotised area, the strength of stimulus necessary to affect the muscle does not rise gradually, but remains approximately constant until conduction fails. This indicates, as Symes and Veley, Verworn and others have pointed out, that the ability of the propagated disturbance to pass a region of decrement does not depend upon the strength of the stimulus which sets it up. In other words there would seem to be an all-or-none relation between the strength of the stimulus and the size of the disturbance in each nerve fibre. However the experiment is not always satisfactory. Sometimes there may be a small rise in the strength of the threshold stimulus occurring suddenly just before the failure of conduction, and sometimes there may be a small gradual rise throughout the narcosis. Lodholtz has shown that the latter is due to a local fall of excitability in the nerve under the electrodes, and he has suggested that the sudden rise may be due to the premature failure of the most excitable fibres of the nerve. Experiments prove that this is the true explanation, for the strength of stimulus required to give a maximal contraction never rises, although the strength for minimal contractions may do so. It follows that the effective strength of stimulus for any one nerve fibre remains absolutely unchanged until the moment when conduction in that fibre is completely suspended. This result is independent of the total duration of the narcosis and it can be shown that the nerve is conducting imperfectly long before the moment of complete failure.

We must conclude that in any nerve fibre under normal conditions there is an all-or-none relation between the strength of the stimulus and the size of the propagated disturbance which follows it. This agrees with the fact that the size of the disturbance at any point in a normal fibre depends only upon the local condition of that point and not upon the previous history of the disturbance.

By 1914 Adrian was considering a form of signaling in the nerves. The difficulty was again the technical one of providing a means of detecting and recording the potentials carried in the nerve. In the early 1920's the amplifying powers of the thermionic valve had been realized, and Adrian combined this instrument with the capillary electrometer to analyze the nerve messages. At first he worked with groups of nerve fibres ("The impulses produced by sensory nerve endings. Part I," *J. Physiol.*, London, 1926, 61:49–72).

EXCERPT PP. 71–72

SUMMARY

The paper describes a combination of a capillary electrometer with a three valve amplifier which is capable of recording rapid changes of potential of the order of .01 millivolts with almost complete absence of disturbance from mechanical and electrical artefacts. With its aid it has been possible to record the action currents accompanying afferent impulses in the frog's sciatic nerve when the gastrocnemius is stretched by a weight, in the cat's internal saphenous nerve when the skin is pinched, in the cat's and rabbit's vagus when the lungs are inflated and in the cardiac depressor nerve of the rabbit. Numerous control observations have been made to exclude the possibility that the recorded oscillations of potential are due to any other cause than the passage of impulses in the nerve. It is probable that many of the oscillations represent action currents in a single nerve fibre, and these have the same general form and the same general time relations (allowing for temperature differences) in all the sensory nerves in which they can be isolated sufficiently for measurement. There is no evidence that an increase in the stimulus increases the size of the action currents in single fibres, but the frequency of the impulses in the nerve trunk increases and leads to interference and overlapping of impulses in different fibres.

In the same year (1926) Adrian, in collaboration with Yngve Zottermann of Stockholm, was able to report the next step in his investigation, a study of single nerve fibres. This established the identity of the nerve message with its electrical manifestation. ("Impulses from a single sensory end-organ," *J. Physiol.*, London, 1926, 61:viii.) The impulses of individual fibres were of constant size and an increase in stimulus strength increased their frequency. It was as though nerve cells communicated with each other by a sort of machine-gun fire.

EXCERPT P. VIII

. . . . We have now succeeded in recording the afferent impulses from preparations containing only a limited number of sensory fibres and in many of these it is possible to detect the impulses set up in a single fibre. The preparation used was the sterno-cutaneous muscle of the frog. The nerve to this muscle contains about 15–20 nerve fibres and there is at least one muscle spindle. When the muscle is stretched, the nerve shows a series of electric responses occurring rather irregularly at a frequency of 100 a second or more. Successive strips of the muscle are now cut away in order to reduce the number of end-organs in action, and with each section the frequency of the responses becomes smaller and signs of definite rhythms appear. Finally the records show one regular series of responses, or two or three regular series of slightly different period. We take each of these regular series to represent the impulses set up by a single end-organ. The frequency of the series ranges from about 10 to 50 per sec., increasing as the stimulus is increased. The magnitude of the responses remains the same whatever the stimulus. By recording the frequencies with stimuli of different strength it is possible to construct a 'recovery curve' for the end-organ. It appears to have the same form as the recovery curve of a nerve fibre, but the rate of recovery is about 5 to 10 times as long. The regular discharge of impulses with a constant stimulus we ascribe to the relatively slow rate of adaptation of the end-organ compared with the rapid rate of adaptation in a nerve fibre which prevents a constant stimulus from setting up more than one impulse.

A further account of nerve activity is given in Adrian's book, *The mechanism of nervous action. Electrical studies of the neurone* (Philadelphia, 1932), and it illustrates well his simple yet vivid and informative style of writing. Concerning the electrical record, it is ". . . a true index of the message in the nerve fibres, and so far there has been no clear instance of lack of agreement. In fact the correspondence has occurred so often that according to all the rules we are justified in assuming that it is universal" [p. 16]. Elsewhere he stated the following.

EXCERPT PP. 12–13

If these records give a true measure of the activity in the sensory nerve fibres it is clear that they transmit their messages to the central nervous system in a very simple way. The message consists merely of a series of brief impulses or waves of activity following one another more or less closely. In any one fibre the waves are all of the same form and the message can only be varied by changes in the frequency and duration of the discharge. In fact the sensory messages are scarcely more complex than a succession of dots in the Morse Code.

The same kind of electrical activity is found in the motor nerve fibres. When a message passes down a motor fibre from the central nervous system to arouse a muscular contraction we find again a rhythmic succession of potential changes alike in size but varying in frequency. Fig 5 [fig. 61] gives a record from a single motor fibre supplying the peroneus longus muscle in a spinal (decapitate) cat. The record was taken at the beginning of a flexion reflex evoked by pinching the foot; the movement developed slowly and the development goes hand in hand with the increase in frequency of the potential waves. Thus the effect produced on the motor nerve fibres by the excited nerve cell in the spinal cord is like that produced on the sensory fibre by the stretched muscle spindle (Fig. 3). It may be noted that in Fig. 5 the recording instrument was a capillary electrometer, not an oscillograph, and as the movement is very highly damped the true form of the potential waves is not shown, although it can be worked out by a fairly simple analysis.

EXCERPT P. 21

We come back then to our records of nervous messages with a reasonable assurance that they do tell us what the message is like. It is a succession of brief waves of surface breakdown, each allowing a momentary leakage of ions from the nerve fibre. The waves can be set up so that they follow one another in rapid or in slow succession, and this is the only form of gradation of which the message is capable. Essentially the same kind of activity is found in all sorts of nerve fibres from all sorts of animals and there is no evidence to suggest that any other kind of nervous transmission is possible. In fact we may conclude that the electrical method can tell us how the nerve fibre carries out its function as the conducting unit of the nervous system, and that it does so by reactions of a fairly simple type.

JOSEPH ERLANGER   HERBERT SPENCER GASSER
(5 January 1874—   )   (5 July 1888—11 May 1963)

As has already been seen on several occasions, until the minute and very brief changes in the electrical potential of the nerve could be recorded adequately, the study of their characteristics was necessarily limited. The method which has proved to be the most revolutionary and which has been responsible for much of the advance in the last four decades is the cathode ray oscilloscope. It employs an inertialess electron beam and its introduction into nerve physiology was due to the American physiologists, Erlanger and Gasser. With its aid they were able to suggest that a nerve is made up of different kinds of fibres.

Erlanger was born in San Francisco and was graduated in medicine from the Johns Hopkins University in 1899. He soon turned to physiology and from 1910 to 1946 was professor of physiology and head of the department at the Washington University Medical School in St. Louis. His work was mainly in the field of neurophysiology, and since 1946 he has held the appointment of emeritus professor (see Erlanger, 1964). Gasser was born in Platteville, Wisconsin, and also attended the Johns Hopkins Medical School where he received the M.D. degree in 1915. From 1916 to 1931 he worked in St. Louis and it was during this period that the fruitful collaboration between the two men took place. In 1931 Gasser was appointed professor of physiology at Cornell University Medical School in New York City, and from 1935 to 1953 director of the Rockefeller Institute in the same city. Like Erlanger, he studied in particular the physiology of the nervous system (see

Les Prix Nobel, 1946, Erlanger, p. 85, Gasser, pp. 86–87; Gasser, 1963*a*, 1963*b*).

The two men began their collaborative studies in 1921 and the following selections have been taken from the summary of the report of their preliminary findings ("A study of the action currents of nerve with the cathode ray oscillograph," *Am. J. Physiol.,* 1922, 62:496–524).

EXCERPT P. 523

The low voltage cathode ray oscillograph offers a means by which nerve action currents can be easily and accurately recorded. A description is given of the apparatus by which this may be accomplished. It consists essentially of a three-stage amplifier, giving 7,000- to 8,000-fold amplification, working into a Braun tube. The method is possible because nerve action currents can be repeated with great precision twenty times per second and the record appears as a standing wave on the screen of the tube, where it may be drawn or photographed.

A description is given of apparatus for synchronizing the nerve potential changes recorded on the ordinate with the movement along the abscissa. The rate of movement along the abscissa is controlled by a condenser and resistance, and can be made very fast. The action current of mammalian nerve has been recorded in the range of velocities between 50 and 20 meters per second.

. . . .

. . . .

The action current has a gradual start, a steep smooth anacrotic limb and a more gradual catacrotic limb. The latter like the former shows a period of great initial acceleration so that the crest is situated near the anacrotic side. In frog nerve and some mammalian nerves there are secondary waves on the catacrotic limb. Suggestions are made as to the cause of these waves.

Further studies led Erlanger and Gasser to the discovery that certain nerves transmit with more than one velocity of action current, owing presumably to the presence in them of fibres of different sizes ("The compound nature of the action current of nerve as disclosed by the cathode ray oscillograph," *Am. J. Physiol.,* 1924, 70:624–666: portions of this article have been reproduced by Fulton, 1966, pp. 243–246).

EXCERPT P. 659

. . . . the evidence we have thus far presented is so clearly in favor of their being discrete action currents originating simultaneously under the stimulating electrode and traveling along the nerve at different rates, that no other plausible way of accounting for them seems possible . . . .

EXCERPT P. 662

The waves then represent discrete action currents in different nerve fibers. In the present state of our knowledge it is, however, impossible to assign to the waves definite functions . . . .

EXCERPT PP. 665–666

These few examples will suffice to indicate the possible applications of our findings that the fibers composing a mixed nerve are not all alike in a physiological sense. To repeat, these differences may mean that the stimuli the fibers deliver are different and perhaps adequate to the structures they innervate. It should be made clear, however, that we have not yet succeeded in obtaining any direct experimental evidence that can be regarded as proving the existence of differences in the stimulating values of the impulses delivered by the different types of fibers. The results of our investigations do, however, prove that in certain of the mixed nerves the action current is compound. Furthermore they indicate the possibility, which is being investigated further, that each of the potential waves of any action current is a composite of potential changes slightly out of phase in individual nerve fibers. However this may be, we suggest for the sake of convenience that action currents from which discrete waves separate out be called *compound* and that the potential waves which lengthen on propagation be designated *simple* action currents.

SUMMARY

The action current differs in form in different nerves and with the distance it is propagated from the stimulating induction shock.

In the phrenic nerve of warm-blooded animals its form is simple; as it progresses along the nerve there occurs a gradual though slight lengthening of all of its phases and a diminution in its amplitude.

In the sciatic nerve of the bull frog and of the green frog, and in the tibial nerve of the dog the action current under or close to the stimulus also is simple in form; but as it moves along the nerve it dissociates usually into three, sometimes into four waves. In the saphenous nerve of the dog the action current usually breaks up into two waves.

The waves are regarded as discrete action currents traveling in fibers possessing different physiological characteristics. They have approximately the same duration, but different propagation rates and therefore different wave lengths. The fiber groups have distinctive thresholds of stimulation and duration of refractory phase.

Each of the waves of these compound action currents as it progresses along the nerve changes its form just as does the simple action current in the phrenic nerve. It is suggested that these changes are due in part, at least, to slight differences in the propagation rate in individual, or in many small groups of fibers, whose action currents therefore get slightly out of phase as they progress.

In 1944 Gasser and Erlanger shared a Nobel Prize in Medicine and Physiology, and on 12 December 1945 Gasser gave his Prize Lecture. In the twenty-one years since the paper of 1924, above, they had assembled much more evidence concerning the compound action current. Although it is possible that some of their conclusions may be disproved, their fundamental observation that the nerve is made up of fibre groups and differing physiological functions is unlikely to be entirely refuted. The following selections are from Gasser's Nobel Lecture, "Mammalian nerve fibers" (*Nobel lectures physiology or medicine 1942–1962* [Amsterdam, 1964], pp. 34–47).

EXCERPT PP. 34–37

. . . . During the early period [of our work] it became evident that the action potential (i.e., the variation during activity of the potential difference between two electrodes in contact with the nerve) was characterized not only by the initial rapid negative deviation which was called the "spike," but also by a subsequent sequence of low potential changes which were called the "after-potentials." The latter in their standard form consist in a negative after-potential followed by a positive after-potential. And, as we shall see later, their existence has shown itself to be useful in fiber classification.

. . . .

. . . .

. . . .

Distinctly different sets of constants clearly point to the existence of three main groups of fibers. These have been named A, B, and C. Differences have been found as between both the spikes and the after-potentials. The durations of the spikes measured in presumably single axons may be given, omitting random variations, as 0.45 msec for A, about 1.2 msec for B, and about 2.0 msec for C (Fig. 1 [fig. 65]). For technical reasons the accuracy cannot be as great for the very small fibers as for the larger ones.

The after-potentials are smallest in the A-fibers; and in low-gain records taken so that the spike may be seen at the same time, as in Fig. 1, they are scarcely visible. There is a negative after-potential ending (in the saphenous nerve of the cat) at about 12–15 msec, followed by a positive after-potential ending at about 70 msec. At its maximum the latter has a value equivalent to 0.1–0.4 per cent of the spike height. B-fibers normally have no visible negative after-potential; though one may be developed by special procedures. The potential curve as seen in the records drops promptly to a level of positivity equivalent to 1.5–4 per cent of the spike height, and then returns to the base line over a period of 100–300 msec. In the C-fibers of visceral nerves there is again a well-developed negative after-potential. It lasts 50–80 msec, and is followed by a positive after-potential larger than in A-fibers but not so large as in B-fibers. Its maximum is equivalent to about 1.5 per cent of the spike height and it is traceable for 1 to 2 seconds. About the after-potentials in C-fibers of dorsal root origin little is known.

As would be expected from the configurations of the action potentials the excitability cycles are equally distinctive. After an absolutely refractory period commensurate with the spike duration the subsequent course of the excitability follows the curves set forth in Fig. 2 [fig. 66]. A return to normal through supernormality followed by subnormality holds for the A- and C-fibers, though on quite different time scales. In B-fibers without a negative after-potential refractoriness merges into subnormality without an intervening rise of excitability to or above the resting level.

Thus far no mention has been made of the difference between nerve fibers that is the most obvious of them all: the velocity of conduction. Over the range of the three groups all velocities are known between 115 and 0.6 m.p.s. (meter per second). Within each of the three groups the variations are 115 m.p.s. to about 10 m.p.s. for A, 15 m.p.s. to about 3 m.p.s. for B, and 2 + m.p.s. to about 0.6 m.p.s. for C.

. . . . The conclusion from our first experiments, which as far as it goes is still deemed to be correct, namely that velocity is in approximately linear relationship with the fiber diameter, was derived from an analysis of what was later learned to be an incomplete listing of the fibers in the A-group. After the catalogue of the three groups was completed it became apparent that the system of analysis that had been used was not adequate to establish the conclusion as valid even for the A-group alone. To find what the source of the difficulty might be was the object of the more recent experiments.

EXCERPT PP. 45–47

There is little danger of overestimating the importance of the C-fibers in sensory nerves. As compared with A-fibers, they are far more numerous, and there is a similar variation in the relative velocities . . . .

. . . .

One finding stands out in bold outline, and the conclusion from it is amply supported otherwise: pain messages are carried both by A- and C-fibers . . . .

Due weight is not generally given to the experimental support for the representation of touch among the small fibers . . . .

. . . .

From the foregoing review it appears that attempts to identify modalities with definite segments of the velocity spectrum have not been very successful. We are left faced with evidence for conduction of single modalities at very different velocities, and inclusion of a number of modalities within a narrow band of fibers.

What then is the significance of the wide velocity range? Is it timing? Reflection on this, the most obvious interpretation of all, causes it to loom progressively larger. One need but consider the speed with which posture is controlled in preparation for the reception of oncoming detailed information and the adjustment of fine movement; or again the mode of transmission of excitation through any central ganglion. The more one sees of the exquisite precision with which events take place in the central nervous system the more one is impressed by it. The more the idea of timing grows in meaning content the more it becomes a directive for future exploration. Differential axonal velocities must play their part in the mechanism. Be this their only contribution to integration, it is still a large one.

EDGAR DOUGLAS, LORD ADRIAN
(*See p. 224*)

It is extremely hazardous to select from the large mass of modern investigators an individual to represent the group, in this instance physiologists studying the electrical phenomena of nerves. The work of Adrian, however, has been of such eminence that a relatively recent statement by him on the messages of the nerves seems appropriate for inclusion. The following selections have been taken from his Waynflete Lectures of 1946 (*The physical background of perception* [Oxford, 1947]) in which it will be noted that his opinions on the sensory impulses carried by the nerve fibre remained fundamentally unchanged from those of our earlier extract (p. 225). Like his teacher, Keith Lucas (p. 218), however, he was also concerned with the application of knowledge of peripheral nerve function to the activity of the brain.

EXCERPT PP. 13–15

The conclusion of all this is that nervous communication must be of a relatively simple character. The signalling between one group of nerve-cells and another, the signalling which must play an essential part in our thought and our intelligent activity, is based on the transmission of repeated waves of activity or impulses in the nerve-fibres. These are brief disturbances always made up of the same sequence of physical and chemical changes, and from the fortunate circumstance that the impulses are accompanied by small electric currents we can make records to show us what signals are passing from moment to moment along the fibres. We can tap the messages from one nerve-cell to another.

. . . . We can think of them [the messages] then as the units of nervous activity whatever the chemical transformations they involve . . . .

. . . . But everything goes to show that although there may be some variations there are no radical differences in the messages from different kinds of sense organ or different parts of the brain. Impulses travelling to the brain in the fibres of the auditory nerve make us hear sounds and impulses of the same kind [as those] arranged in much the same way in the optic nerve make us see sights. The mental result must differ because a different part of the brain receives the message and not because the message has a different form.

We cannot, of course, be quite certain that all the communication between one nerve-cell and another inside the brain has the same simple character, for large collections of cells might interact in other ways. We can be certain that much of it has, for it is possible to detect the impulses travelling to and fro inside the brain as well as in the peripheral nerves. And the method of communication depending on the passage of a rapid sequence of impulses down a nerve-fibre will give a reasonably flexible message, for the frequence and number of the impulses may vary and so may the number of nerve-fibres employed . . . .

The chief conclusion, however, is that the nerve-fibres carry out their work on a simple and uniform plan, and this suggests that the activity of the brain from moment to moment should be capable of definition as a spatial arrangement and no more. It must be a pattern of excitations highly complex and rapidly fluctuating but built up of the same elements in all its parts, the elements being nerve-cell activity induced by the flow of impulses along the nerve-fibres.

ALAN LLOYD HODGKIN
(5 February 1914—   )

The actual process underlying the transmission of a nervous impulse has also been investigated and research in this vital area continues today, linked historically with the earlier work of Bernstein (pp. 213–216) and Overton (pp. 216–218).

One of the ways of learning more about the phenomenon of nervous transmission would be to gain access to the nerve fibre itself, and this became possible when in 1936 J. Z. Young rediscovered the large axons of the squid, *Loligo forbesi* ("The structure of nerve fibres in cephalopods and crustacea," *Proc. R. Soc.*, 1937, 121B:319–337); these can be as large as 1 mm. in diameter compared to the maximum diameter of .020 mm. in mammals. A new field for exploration was thus revealed, and suitable intracellular microtechniques were developed almost simultaneously by Curtis and Cole (1940) in the United States, and by Hodgkin and Huxley (1939) in Cambridge, England. The scientist whose investigations of this new area of research have been and continue to be the most fruitful is the British physiologist Hodgkin.

Hodgkin was born in Danbury, near Oxford, and studied science at the University of Cambridge. Throughout the Second World War he was engaged in research on radar and thereafter returned to Cambridge in 1945 as lecturer in physiology. In 1952 he was appointed Foulerton Research Professor of the Royal Society in the University of Cambridge. His investigations have been entirely in the field of nerve impulse transmission, and there has been frequent recognition of his contributions. He shared a Nobel Prize with his co-worker A. F. Huxley and with Sir John Eccles of Canberra, Australia, in 1963.

By the use of intrafibre microelectrodes it has been shown that the basic mechanism of nerve impulse transmission is an ionic exchange that takes place between the inside and the outside of the nerve fibre. Hodgkin and his collaborators have shown that the passage of sodium ions into the axoplasm of the fibre and of potassium ions out of it creates a change in direction and enhancement of the potential difference, and that this stimulates the next section of the fibre. Thus the impulse proceeds along the nerve.

In March 1961 Hodgkin gave the Sherrington Lectures in the University of Liverpool and the following selections have been taken from them as published (*The conduction of the nervous impulse*, Liverpool, 1964). This is the only book that gives an account of the very important discoveries made by the British group of investigators of nervous transmission.

EXCERPT PP. 17–18

. . . . Many years before the introduction of the microelectrode technique physiologists believed that the electrical changes associated with the activity of nerve and muscle arose at the surface membrane. This idea was verified by experiments in which the electrical potential difference across the surface of the fibre was measured directly with an internal electrode. The earliest experiments with nerve were made with the giant axon of the squid, *Loligo*. Here, the usual method is to introduce a long capillary electrode into one end of the fibre and push it in for a distance of 10–30 mm. (Fig. 4 [fig. 63]). The presence of an internal electrode does not have any obvious effect on the activity of the nerve, since impaled axons survive for many hours and the external action potential is not altered by the insertion of an internal electrode. Another method which has a wide application depends on the fact that a very small capillary can be inserted transversely into many types of fibre without causing appreciable damage . . . . As a rule such electrodes have tip diameters of less than 0.5μ and are filled with 3 molar KCl in order to reduce their electrical resistance. Both methods have been applied to the giant axons of *Loligo* and give similar results. In such experiments it is found that the inside of a resting nerve fibre is 50 to 70 mV negative to the external solution; this standing difference in electrical potential is known as the resting potential. When an impulse travels along the fibre, the inside swings momentarily positive giving a transient action potential with an amplitude of 100–120 mV. At the crest of the action potential the inside of the fibre is 40–50 mV positive to the external solution.

Figure 5 [fig. 64] illustrates the form of the action potential in the giant axon of *Loligo*. The record on the left is from an intact axon in its natural position in the animal. When the microelectrode which had a tip diameter of about 0.5μ, was pushed through the surface, the potential jumped suddenly to a new value about 70 mV negative to the zero—this is the resting potential. The record shows the action potential which travels along the fibre, its amplitude is 110 mV and duration (at 9° C) about 1.5 millisecond. In this experiment the squid had been subjected to only slight operative procedure and the nerve was still connected to the muscles. A few milliseconds after the impulse had passed the micro-electrode it reached the muscles. The body wall then gave a powerful flap which smashed the microelectrode and terminated the experiment. For this and many other reasons it is simpler to work with an isolated axon as has been done in obtaining the record in Figure 5B. The action potential differs slightly from that in the intact animal but the essential features of the conduction mechanism are the same in both cases.

EXCERPT PP. 27–29

. . . . One of the many useful properties of giant nerve fibres is that samples of protoplasm or axoplasm as it is usually called can be obtained by squeezing out the contents from a cut end . . . . As in many other cells there is a high concentration of potassium ions and a relatively low concentration of sodium and chloride ions. This is the reverse of the situation in the animals' blood or in sea water, where sodium and chloride are the dominant ions and potassium is relatively dilute. Potassium ions are probably free inside the fibre and do not seem to be bound to proteins or other large molecules. This statement is based on evidence from a variety of experiments. In the first place it would be difficult to account for the high electrical conductivity of axoplasm (0.5–0.8 times sea water) or for osmotic balance unless the main ionic constituents of the protoplasm were free. Electrical measurements which show that the membrane behaves like a potassium electrode at high external concentrations of potassium also require that the internal activity coefficient of potassium be similar to that in the external solution. More direct evidence is provided by studies with radioactive potassium, ^{42}K, which show that the mobility and diffusion coefficient of this ion is nearly the same as in free solution and by experiments with internal potassium electrodes which give an activity coefficient similar to that in sea water.

Although there is little doubt that the potassium inside nerve fibres is mainly in the ionized form, caution should be exercised in applying this result to other ions which have a greater tendency to form complexes. Measurements of the mobility of calcium inside squid axons show that this ion moves in an electric field at a rate less than $\frac{1}{30}$ of that in free solution and Hinke's observations with Na- and K-electrodes suggest that the activity coefficient of sodium in axoplasm is about 30 per cent less than that of potassium.

The excess of potassium inside the fibre is balanced by organic anions of which, in squid fibres, isethionic acid was shown by Koechlin (1955) to be the most important . . . .

At the surface of the nerve fibre the membrane acts as a barrier and prevents the ions in the external solution from mixing rapidly with the internal solution. This membrane has a high electrical resistance, about 1000 ohm cm² in a resting axon of *Loligo*, and an electrical capacity of about 1 microfarad/cm². These are values which might be expected from a bimolecular layer of lipid with a thickness of 50Å, dielectric constant of 5 and an electrical resistivity of 2×10^9 ohm cm. The high resistivity of the membrane is in striking contrast to that of the axoplasm and external fluid, these being about 30 and 20 ohm cm respectively. During a nerve impulse the conductivity of the membrane increases about 100 fold and sodium and potassium ions move down their concentration gradients. These movements are thought to provide the immediate source of energy for conducting the impulse.

Neurochemical Transmission in Nerves

The history of ideas regarding nervous transmission along fibres having been considered, the nervous system's second kind of nervous conduction, that which takes place at the termination of the fibre, must now be discussed.

In Chapter II consideration was given to the growth of the neuron doctrine, which maintains that nerve cells and fibres are in contiguity, but not in continuity, with their neighbors. The points where they meet are the synapses, a word introduced by Michael Foster and Sherrington (Fulton, 1949, p. 55*n*.; Foster, 1897, III, 929), and electron microscopy has confirmed the belief of the neuronists that direct contact across the narrow gap of separation, the synaptic cleft, does not take place. How then does the message that has travelled along a fibre pass across this cleft to another neuron? In other words, how does synaptic conduction take place? Likewise, how does the conducted impulse find its way into the muscle fibre to bring about contraction of the muscle?

A solution to the problem of impulse transmission in the nerve fibre has been, and will continue to be, dependent partly upon advances in the physical sciences, and especially upon the development of increasingly penetrating physical techniques, and partly upon the correct interpretation of chemical phenomena; likewise the enigma of transference of messages across the synaptic cleft and the neuromuscular junction has been tackled partly by physical methods but mainly by the application of modern biochemical and pharmacological knowledge. So far little is known of the complexities of this phenomenon, and although it was recognized in the nineteenth century that its basis was perhaps in part a chemical process, substantial advances have been possible only in the last few decades.

There is no adequate account of the growth of this idea, but the following publications may be consulted: Cannon (1934), Dale (1938a, 1954), Loewi (1954), Holmstedt and Liljestrand (1936, pp. 168–201).

There is, however, another group of investigators who are studying the electrical rather than the chemical transmission across the synapse, led by Sir John Eccles (1903–   ) of Canberra, Australia, but their work is much too recent to be represented here. Eccles has reported many of his findings in a book (1964) in which there is an excellent account of "The development of ideas on the synapse," pages 1 to 10, and in a paper (1965). It seems that both types of synaptic transmission take place and that the two groups of workers concerned have declared "a truce based on a clearly defined territorial agreement" (Eccles, 1964, p. 261).

CHARLES SCOTT SHERRINGTON
(27 November 1857—4 March 1952)

Before the history of neurochemical transmission is traced the concept of the synapse must be considered, for it is at this site that nerve impulses are passed on, either by chemical or physical means or by both. The first person to discuss the matter in detail was Charles Sherrington, the renowned British physiologist, and his account will be taken as representative of a great deal of investigation both past and present.

Sherrington was born in London and studied medicine at Cambridge and St. Thomas's Hospital, London. At the former he came into contact with Sir Michael Foster and after having been graduated in medicine in 1885, he turned to physiology, and in 1895 was called to the chair of physiology at Liverpool. In 1913 he became Waynflete Professor of Physiology in the University of Oxford, whence he retired in 1936. His studies were devoted to the physiology of the nervous system and his contribution to this subject was probably greater than that of any other person. He was also a poet of some distinction (see *The assaying of Brabantius and other verse,* London, 1925) and a philosopher (see Fulton, 1947; Brown, 1947;

Ritchie, 1947; Sherrington, 1952*a*, 1952*b*; Fulton, 1952; Cohen, 1958; Granit, 1966).

Sherrington's most remarkable publication was his book, *The integrative action of the nervous system* (New Haven, 1906), in which he introduced a new and far-reaching concept of integrative nervous function. In the first chapter he dealt with the simple reflex and in so doing for the first time discussed the synapse in detail, a structure that is a meeting place for several neurophysiological ideas: the neuron theory, synaptic transmission, reflex-arc function, etc. A selection from Sherrington's fine book is presented below, and reference will be made to some of its other chapters later. At this point the work of Held (pp. 118–122) is of special relevance, since in 1897, the year in which the term *synapse* was introduced (p. 370), he described it (1897*a*, p. 288) as follows: "For the time being the nerve cell's zones of transfer appear histologically as mainly variable and variously constituted pathways between concrescing surfaces that I shall designate physiologically simply as zones for the transmission of stimuli."

EXCERPT PP. 16–18

. . . . If there exists any surface or [*sic*; should be "of"] separation at the nexus between neurone and neurone, much of what is characteristic of the conduction exhibited by the reflex-arc might be more easily explicable. At the nexus between cells if there be not actual confluence, there must be a surface of separation. At the nexus between efferent neurone and the muscle-cell, electrical organ, etc., which it innervates, it is generally admitted that there is not actual confluence of the two cells together, but that a surface separates them; and a surface of separation is physically a membrane. As regards a number of the features enumerated above as distinguishing reflex-arc conduction from nerve-trunk conduction, there is evidence that *similar features, though not usually in such marked extent, characterize conduction from efferent nerve-fibre to efferent organ*, e.g., in nerve-muscle preparation, in nerve-electric-organ preparation, etc. Here change in character of conduction is not due to perikarya (nerve-cell bodies), for such are not present. The change may well be referable to the surface of separation admittedly existent between efferent neurone and effector cell.

If the conductive element of the neurone be fluid, and if at the nexus between neurone and neurone there does not exist actual confluence of the conductive part of one cell with the conductive part of the other, e.g., if there is not actual continuity of physical phase between them, there must be a surface of separation. Even should a membrane visible to the microscope not appear, the mere fact of non-confluence of the one with the other implies the existence of a surface of separation. Such a surface might restrain diffusion, bank up osmotic pressure, restrict the movement of ions, accumulate electric charges, support a double electric layer, alter in shape and surface-tension with changes in difference of potential, alter in difference of potential with changes in surface-tension or in shape, or intervene as a membrane between dilute solutions of electrolytes of different concentration or colloidal suspensions with different sign of charge. It would be a mechanism where nervous conduction, especially if predominantly physical in nature, might have grafted upon it characters just such as those differentiating reflex-arc conduction from nerve-trunk conduction . . . . Against the likelihood of nervous conduction being pre-eminently a chemical rather than a physical process must be reckoned, as Macdonald well urges, its speed of propagation, its brevity of time-relations, its freedom from perceptible temperature change, its facile excitation by mechanical means, its facilitation by cold, etc. If it is a physical process the intercalation of a transverse surface of separation or membrane into the conductor must modify the conduction, and it would do so with results just such as we find differentiating reflex-arc conduction from nerve-trunk conduction.

As to the existence or the non-existence of a surface of separation or membrane between neurone and neurone, that is a structural question on which histology might be competent to give valuable information . . . . But in the neurone-chains of the gray-centred system of vertebrates histology on the whole furnishes evidence that a surface of separation does exist between neurone and neurone. And the evidence of Wallerian secondary degeneration is clear in showing that that process observes strictly a boundary between neurone and neurone and does not transgress it. It seems therefore likely that the nexus between neurone and neurone in the reflex-arc, at least in the spinal arc of the vertebrate, involves a surface of separation between neurone and neurone; and this as a transverse membrane across the conductor must be an important element in intercellular conduction. The characters distinguishing reflex-arc conduction from nerve-trunk conduction may therefore be largely due to intercellular barriers, delicate transverse membranes, in the former.

In view, therefore, of the probable importance physiologically of this mode of nexus between neurone and neurone it is convenient to have a term for it. The term introduced has been *synapse*.

CLAUDE BERNARD
(12 July 1813—10 February 1878)

Although the early history of the chemical mediation of nervous effects has not been investigated thoroughly, nevertheless it has been claimed that in 1877 du

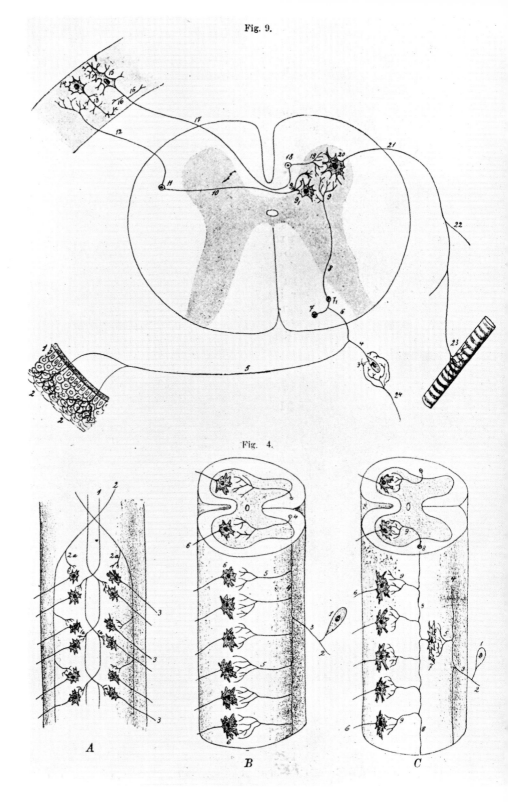

Fig. 9.

Fig. 4.

Fig. 32. Waldeyer (1891, p. 1353, figs. 9, 4). For explanation see text (p. 116).

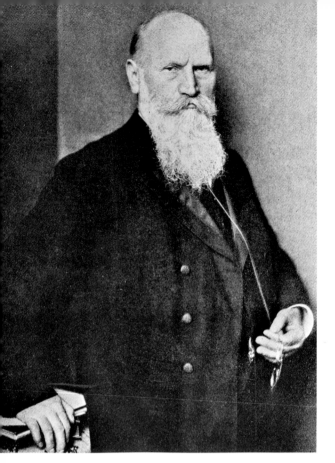

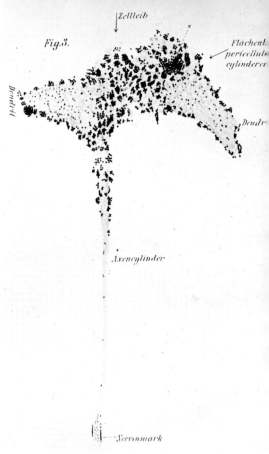

FIG. 33. Wilhelm Waldeyer. From B. J. Gottlieb and A. Berg, *Das Antlitz des germanischen Ärztes in vier Jahrhunderten*, Berlin, Rembrandt-Verlag, 1942, p. 184. By permission.

FIG. 34. Held (1897*b*, Plate XII, fig. 3). Lumbar anterior horn cell, adult dog, showing Endfüsse on cell body (X, a group of them), dendrite and axon.

FIG. 35. Held (1897, Plate IX, fig. 11). Trapezoid nucleus cell, adult rabbit. Terminal fibres (compact granules visible) break up into end basket.

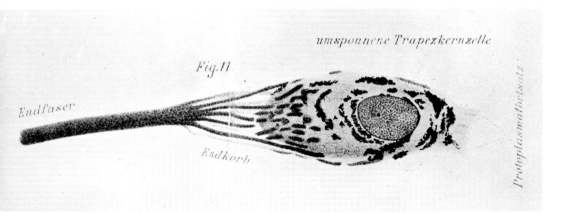

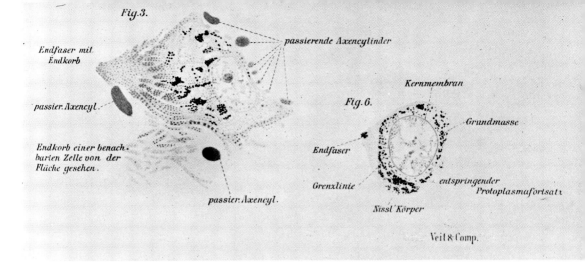

FIG. 36. Held (1897, Plate X, figs. 3, 6). Fig. 3: trapezoid nucleus cell, adult rabbit, partly enveloped by terminating fibres; intimate association between axon protoplasm and cell's ground substance clearly seen since they have a common plasma layer; terminal basket of neighboring cell. Fig. 6: same cell, nine-day-old dog; homogeneous boundary line between axon terminal and cell protoplasm.

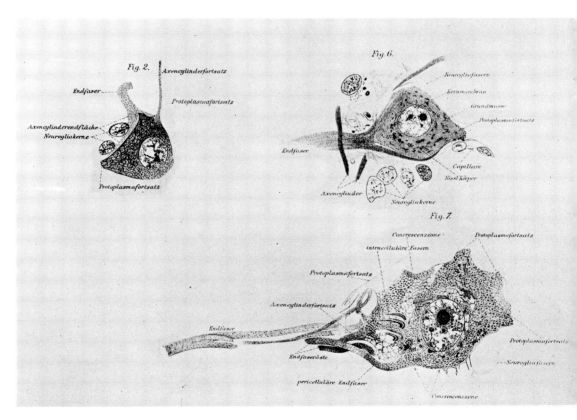

FIG. 37. Held (1897, Plate XII, figs, 2, 6–7). Fig. 2: trapezoid nucleus cell, mature cat fetus; terminating axon with concrescence and originating axon. Fig. 6: same, four-week-old dog. Fig. 7: same, adult rabbit; terminating and originating axons shown; axon terminals fuse with protoplasm on cell surface or enter cell substance.

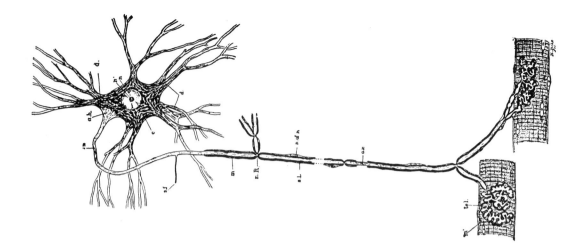

FIG. 38. Barker (1899, p. 41, fig. 17). Lower motor neuron: *a, h*, axon hillock devoid of Nissl bodies and showing fibrillation; *ax*, axis cylinder, which near cell body is surrounded by myelin, *m*, and neurilemma; *c*, cytoplasm, with Nissl bodies and lighter ground substance; *d*, protoplasmic processes (dendrites) containing Nissl bodies; *n*, nucleus; *n'*, nucleolus; *nR*, node of Ranvier; *sf*, side fibril; *n* of *n*, nucleus of neurilemmal sheath; *tel.*, motor end plate; *m'*, striped muscle fibre; *sL*, segmentation of Lantermann.

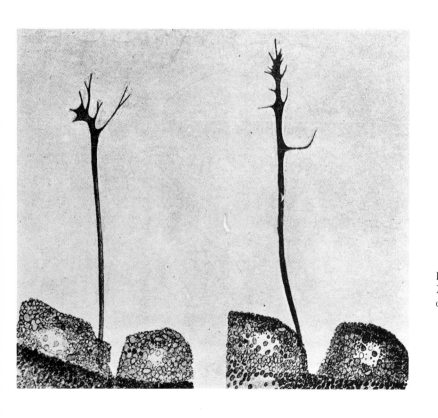

FIG. 39. Harrison (1908, p. 407, 22). Fibre growing into lymph f embryonal spinal cord cells.

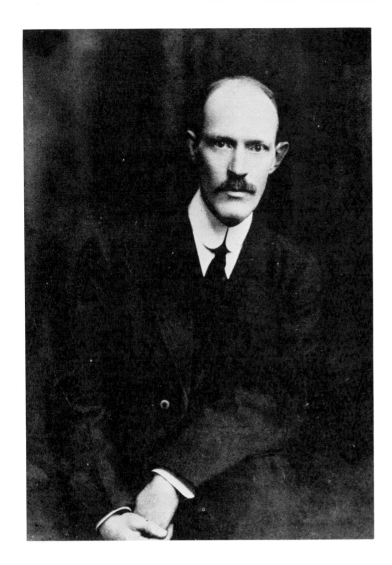

FIG. 40. Ross Granville Harrison, March 1911. By courtesy of Miss Madeline Stanton.

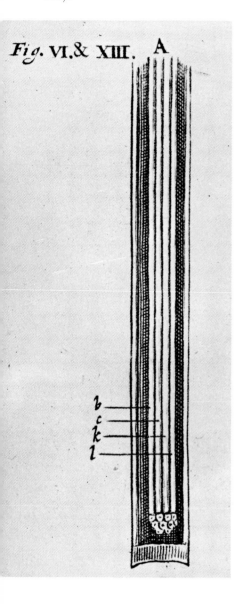

FIG. 41. Descartes (1662, p. 19, figs. 6, 13). See text for explanation p. 158).

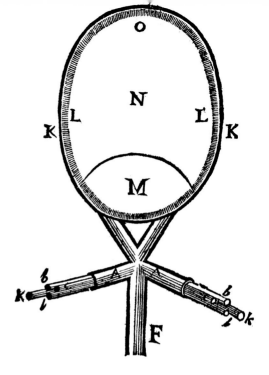

FIG. 42. Descartes (1664, p. 15). See text for explanation (p. 158).

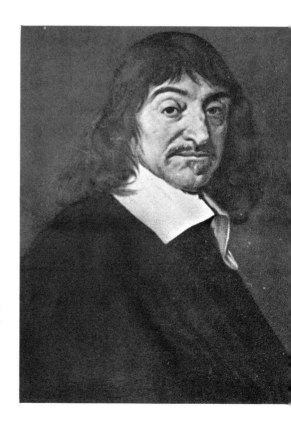

FIG. 43. René Descartes. By Franz Hals in the Musée de Louvre. By permission.

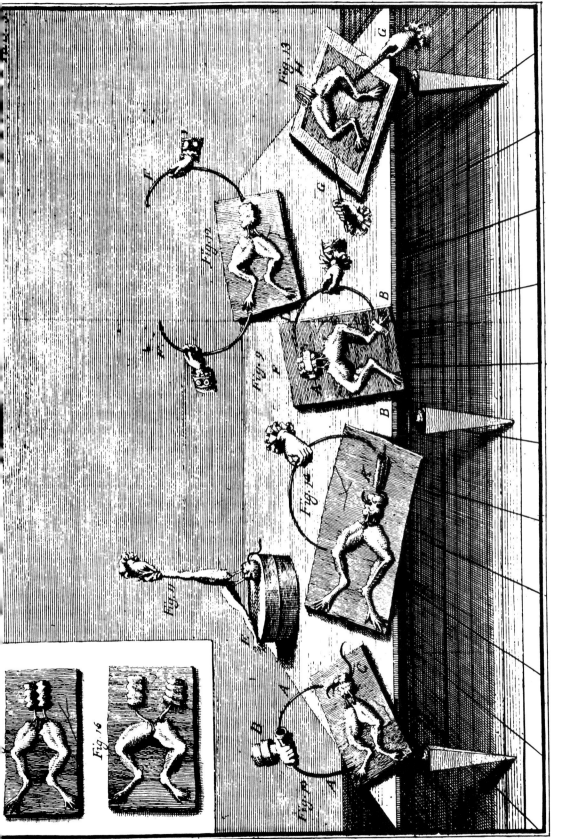

Fɪɢ. 44. Galvani (1791, Plate III). Courtesy of the Bundy Library. For explanation see text (p. 181).

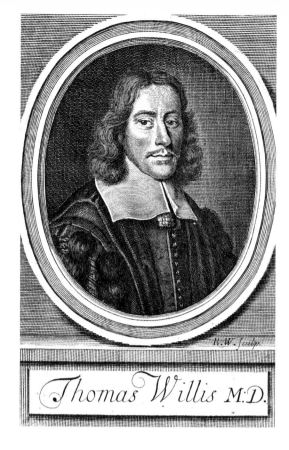

Fig. 45. Thomas Willis. From Willis (1685). Line engraving by R. White after the print by Loggan.

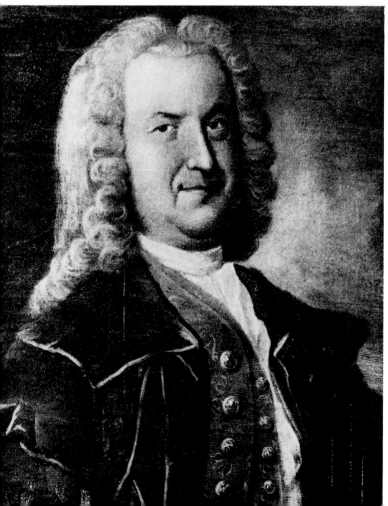

Fig. 46. Albrecht von Haller in 1746. From A, Weese, *Die Bildnisse Albrecht von Hallers*, Berne, 1909.

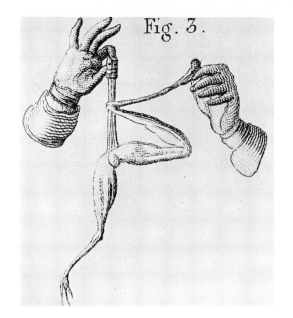

FIG. 47. Aldini (1803, Plate I, fig. 3).
For explanation see text (p. 185).

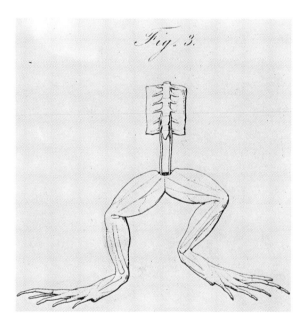

FIG. 48. Matteucci (1844, Plate I, fig.
3). Frog prepared according to Galvani's method.

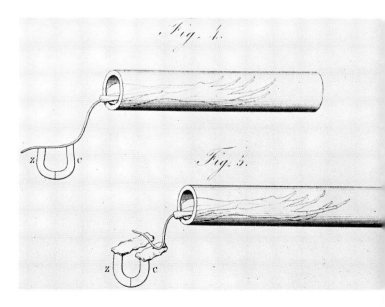

FIG. 49. Matteucci (1844, Plate I,
figs. 4–5). Galvanoscopic frog and
electromotor element.

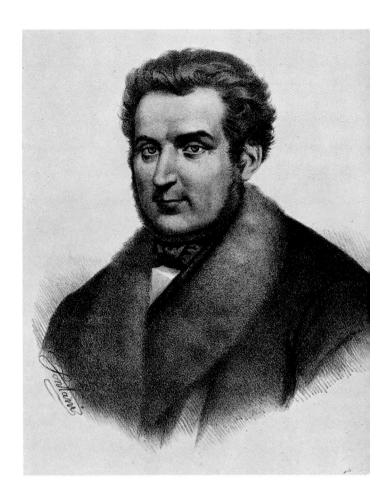

FIG. 50. Carlo Matteucci in 1853. By permission of the Wellcome Trustees.

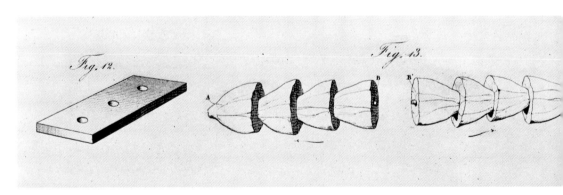

FIG. 51. Matteucci (1844, Plate I, figs. 12–13). Baseboard and electrophysiological pile.

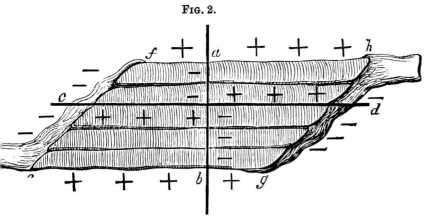

FIG. 2.

FIG. 52. Du Bois-Reymond (1853, p. 17, fig. 2). For explanation see text (p. 194).

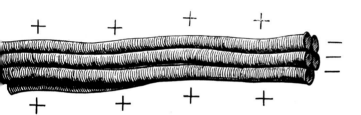

FIG. 53. Du Bois-Reymond (1853, p. 19, fig. 3). "Simplest case of the muscular Current observed . . . up to January, 1843." Primary fibres X 75. For explanation see text (p. 195).

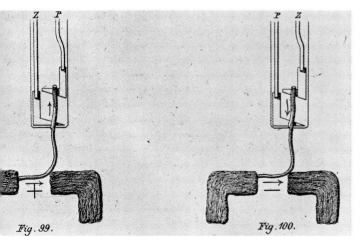

Fig. 99.   *Fig. 100.*

FIG. 54. Du Bois-Reymond (1849, Plate II, figs. 99–100). For explanation see text (p. 200).

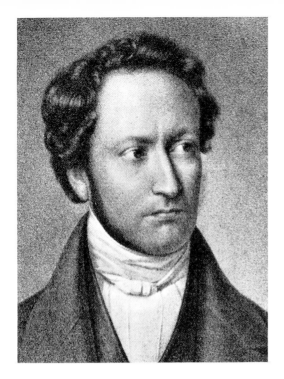

FIG. 55. Johannes Müller in 1837. Lithograph by Werner after a drawing by Rinck. From U. Ebbecke, *Johannes Müller*, Hannover, Schmorl and Seefeld, 1951. By permission Theodor Oppermann Verlag.

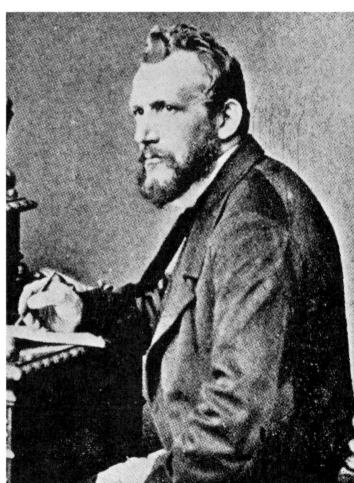

FIG. 56. Emil du Bois-Reymond. From M. A. B. Brazier, *The electrical activity of the nervous system*, London, 1960, Plate I. By permission.

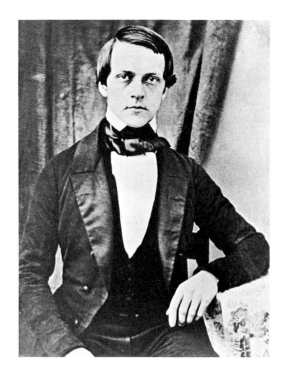

Fig. 57. Hermann von Helmholtz in 1848. From L. Koenigsberger, *Hermann von Helmholtz*, Oxford, Clarendon Press, 1906, facing p. 58. By permission.

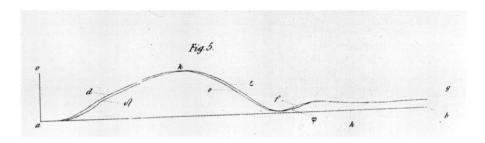

Fig. 58. Helmholtz (1852, Plate VII, fig. 5). Two curves *adefg* and αδεφγ, represent first and second periods of stimulation. For explanation see text (p. 209).

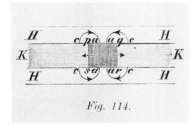

Fig. 59. Hermann (1905, p. 243, fig. 114). For explanation see text (p. 213).

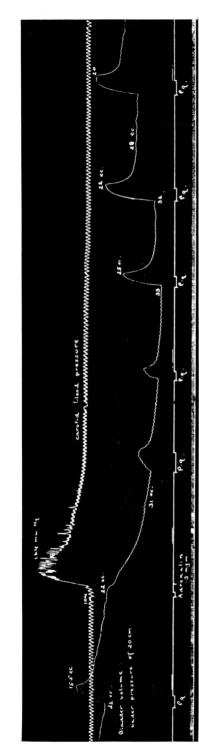

Fig. 11. Prolonged, though slight, inhibition of cat's bladder by adrenalin after 6 days' degenerative section of the hypogastric nerves. Ether. Vagi cut. Catheter up urethra. Pelvics cut above rectum and Ludwig electrodes placed on both, bladder never being exposed. Volume record under constant pressure of 20 cm. Bladder was in high tone but without rhythm.

12.36. Stimulation of both pelvics caused contraction from volume of 22 to 15·5 c.c., showing their contractile power to be greatly lessened by the degenerative section of the hypogastrics.

12.38. Adrenalin, ·3 mgm. into ext. jug. Bladder slowly relaxed from 22 to 31 c.c.

12.40'.30''. Stimulated pelvics, coil 9—bladder contracted 2·2 c.c.

12.42'.45''.	,,	,,	2·4 c.c.
12.44'.15''.	,,	,,	8 c.c. from 33 to 25 c.c.
12.46'.15''.	,,	,,	10 c.c. from 32 to 22 c.c. with persisting contracture to 28 c.c.
12.48.	,,	,,	8 c.c. from 28 to 20 c.c.

The drum was not run continuously throughout this period.

Fig. 60. Elliot (1905, p. 442, fig. 11). For explanation see text (p. 245).

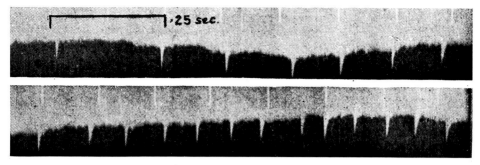

FIG. 5. Impulses in a single motor nerve fibre supplying the peroneus longus in the cat (spinal). The nerve has been cut down until only one active fibre remains (Adrian and Bronk, 1929). A flexion reflex is produced by pinching the foot and the frequency of the discharge increases as the contraction develops. Record made with capillary electrometer and amplifier. The potential changes are actually diphasic though the damping of the electrometer movement is too great to show their true form.

FIG. 61. Adrian (1932, p. 13). See text (p. 227).

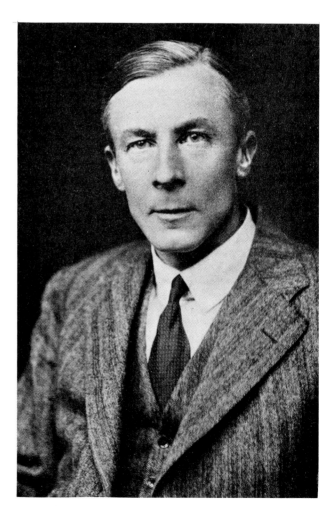

FIG. 62. Edward Douglas Adrian in 1932. From *Les Prix Nobel en 1932*, Stockholm, Norstedt & Söner, 1934, facing p. 63. By permission of the Nobel Foundation.

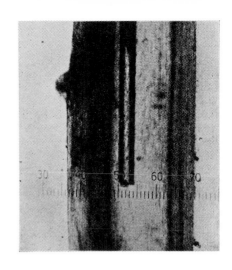

Fig. 63. Hodgkin and Huxley (1939, p. 710, fig. 1; also Hodgkin, 1964, fig. 4). For explanation see text (p. 235).

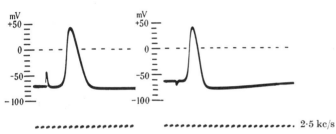

A. Axon in whole animal (8·5° C)

B. Isolated axon (12·5° C)

2·5 kc/s

Fig. 64. Hodgkin (1964, fig. 5. From an unpublished series of experiments of Hodgkin and R. O. Keynes: Hodgkin, "The Croonian Lecture. Ionic movements and electrical activity in giant nerve fibres," *Proc. R. Soc.*, 1958, 148B:5, fig. 3). For explanation see text (p. 236).

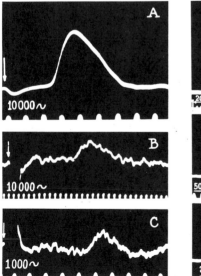

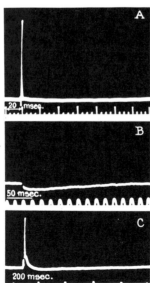

Fig. 65. Gasser (1946, p. 130, fig. 1). "Left. Spikes of all unit axons of the A, B, and C groups. Right. Spikes and after potentials of the A, B, and C groups in multiple fiber preparations."

Bois-Reymond first suggested a chemical explanation for transmission from motor nerve to voluntary muscle fibre (Dale, 1937–1938):

> There must be either a stimulating secretion in the form perhaps of a thin layer of ammonia or lactic acid or of some other substance on the outside of the contractile tissue so that violent excitation of the muscle takes place, or the influence must be electric.

However, Matteucci, thirty-five years earlier (1842, p. 339), had suggested that "the cause of these [electrical] currents may well be a chemical action."

These statements refer more specifically to fibre than to synaptic conduction and are in any case vague and unsupported by conclusive experimental data. The approach to transmission across the neuromuscular junction was to be pharmacological rather than purely chemical, and the first observations were made by the great French physiologist Claude Bernard.

Bernard was born near Saint-Julien, north of Lyons, and studied medicine in Paris. In 1841 he became assistant to the famous physiologist Magendie (see p. 299) at the Collège de France and in 1854 was appointed professor of general physiology. In the following year he succeeded his teacher as professor of experimental physiology. He became the most prominent French physiologist of his day, and his work included the investigation of gastrointestinal function, the nervous system, blood temperature, the autonomic nervous system, and the actions of toxic substances. His book, *Introduction à l'étude de la médecine expérimentale* (Paris, 1865), is a classic discussion of the experimental method and should be read by all who are involved with biological research (see Bernard, 1881; Foster, 1899; Olmsted, 1939; Olmsted and Olmsted, 1952).

While du Bois-Reymond was studying the electrophysiology of muscle Bernard was observing the effects of the South American arrow poison, curare. He demonstrated in animals that the paralysis of the striated muscles produced by it was apparently owing to a lesion in the motor nerve rather than in the muscle which retained its inherent irritability. Somehow, messages had been prevented from reaching the muscles, and, moreover, the process was reversible; on the other hand, sensory nerves were not affected. It was shown later that the nerve itself was uninfluenced by the drug because its electric excitability, its conduction velocity, amplitude of nerve impulses, and other properties were not modified. Thus the site of action of curare was not in the nerve, as Bernard thought, but at the neuromuscular junction. Nevertheless, he had demonstrated the susceptibility of the nerve-muscle preparation to a chemical or, more correctly, a pharmacological effect, and thus Bernard's work marked the origin of the notion that the junction between nerve and muscle has peculiar properties. The link with developments in the study of the neuron's morphology was obviously important here, but the junctions of nerves with muscles or nerves had not been elucidated at this time (see Chapter II).

These investigations had grown from Bernard's interest in experimental pharmacology and from his belief in the general principle that toxic agents could be used as "instruments physiologiques" in physiological analyses, as in this instance where he had been able to distinguish the motor from the sensory nerve and the muscle from the nerve on the basis of their reaction to curare. It was in part Bernard's ability to derive basic precepts and create research methods in experimental medicine which made him one of the most outstanding physiologists of the nineteenth century. Moreover, his contention that physiology was the basis of scientific medicine had a very important influence on the development of both.

The following passages are from a book published in 1857 (*Leçons sur les effets des substances toxiques et médicamenteuses* [Paris, 1857]) although his experiments on curare had been carried out earlier and some of them reported in 1850. He was stimulated to publish the details in an appendix because of similar work reported by Koelliker (1856, dated May 1856) which Bernard stated was "in harmony with my own" (p. 470). For the history of curare, see McIntyre, 1947; Thomas, 1964.

The first excerpts presented below have been taken from a lecture given on 4 June 1856 and the second group are from a similar lecture on 27 June of the same year.

EXCERPT PP. 351–353

Haller thought, and with reason, that the muscles had a contractility of their own which by itself sets in play a particular stimulus carried by the nerves. In order to prove the accuracy of this opinion it was necessary to isolate the action of the muscle from the nerve stimulus. Now I believe that curare, which produces this separation, resolves this question in the most complete and satisfying manner. It is impossible, in fact, to admit the identity of two properties, so that the same agent destroys the one whereas it leaves intact or even increases the other. From a pathological viewpoint, this separation demonstrates the possibility of the two types of paralysis—the one nervous, the other muscular.

   . . . .

   . . . .

Whatever the reflections to which this fact gives rise, it is nonetheless well established *that curare affects the nervous motor system and it alone.*
From this one must necessarily conclude:

1° *That the contractility of the muscular system is independent of the nervous system.*

2° *That the motor nerves may be injured without the sensory nerves being involved.*

EXCERPT PP. 464–469

In 1844, M. Pelouze gave me some curare which he had obtained from M. Goudot. This poison came from New Granada and had the characteristics and properties of the curare examined by MM. Boussinggault and Roulin.

When conducting experiments on live animals, I was struck by a new fact: I noted that in those animals that were poisoned with curare, the nervous system, immediately after death, loses its property of acting on the muscular system to cause convulsions. If, for example, one poisons a frog by placing a small amount of dry or dissolved curare under the skin of its back, one observes that as the poison takes effect the reflex movements are extinguished completely. If, soon after, one prepares the frog according to the procedure of Galvani by laying bare the hind limbs and by isolating the lumbar nerves [pp. 178–183], one does not obtain any contraction in the limbs from an electric stimulus applied directly to the nerves, whereas the same stimulus if applied to the muscles causes violent convulsions. Not only have the nerve trunks lost their excitability, but even the nerve branches, no matter how close to the muscles one may stimulate them.

The physiological conclusions that I have drawn from this experiment are that muscle contractility is completely distinct and independent from the nervous function which releases it, since in effect, curare permits the former to continue, while completely abolishing the latter. From this I have concluded that the question of the independence of muscle irritability, debated since Haller, has been definitively settled by means of this specific physiological analysis brought about by curare. This experiment was referred to in a work that M. Pelouze and I reported to the Académie in 1850, regarding the chemical and physiological properties of curare. [T. J. Pelouze and Claude Bernard, "Recherches sur le curare," *C. r. Acad. Sci., Paris*, 1850, 31:533–537.]

. . . .

. . . .

. . . .

It became evident that these last reflex movements in the healthy limb, produced by stimulation of the poisoned parts, must have been transmitted by the sensory nerves that remained intact. This gave me the idea that curare had destroyed only the properties of the motor nerves, but not those of the sensory nerves, and that if one does not obtain a reflex movement by pinching the skin when the animal has been completely poisoned, it does not prove that the animal is insensible, but only that the motor nerves have become universally incapable of reacting on the muscles by sensory reflex stimulus as well as by voluntary influence. The inability to move may, in fact, be owing to two causes: 1, an animal will not perform movements because it has not been forced to do so, and because neither its will power nor any sensation transmitted by the nerves brings it about. This is therefore an immobility by paralysis of the sensory nerves; 2, an animal might still remain motionless, although it has the will to move or is impelled to do so by an external stimulus. This is when the nerves are incapable of transmitting the motor influence to the muscles. In such a case, there is immobility through paralysis of the motor nerves.

It is in this latter fashion that curare acts . . . .

. . . .

From this second series of experiments, I have concluded that curare affects a physiological analysis that is not limited to the isolation of the properties of the muscular system. It also separates in a distinct manner the properties of the motor and the sensory nerves, since it is seen that it preserves the properties of the sensory nerves and destroys that of the motor nerves . . . . Finally, I have verified that this action of curare is exerted upon the motor nerves so as to destroy them by proceeding from the periphery to the center, which is the reverse of an ordinary paralysis of these nerves.

THOMAS RENTON ELLIOTT
(11 October 1877—4 March 1961)

No advance was made on Bernard's work for several decades, and there were at least two reasons for this delay. In the first place, further investigations had to await the growth of biochemistry and of techniques to handle biological materials in the field which we today call pharmacology. Moreover in the 1850's little was known about the terminations of the neuron either in contact with another neuron or with a muscle fibre, and the synapse had not yet been envisaged (see Chapter II).

Bernard's experiments were on the whole a distinct but distant predecessor of the concept of chemical mediation, but the modern work of identifying the nature and action of the transmitter substance did not commence until the beginning of the present century. In 1904 Elliott made a very significant suggestion.

Elliott was born at Willington in the county of Durham and studied medicine at Cambridge and at University College Hospital in London. It was while he held a research fellowship at Cambridge that he carried out the work to be described below. In 1910 he was appointed assistant physician to University College Hospital and in 1922, professor of clinical medicine, retiring from this position in 1939. His work was mainly on the adrenal glands, the innervation of the viscera, and on clinical topics (see Dale, 1961; Elliott, 1961a, 1961b; Holmstedt and Liljestrand, 1963, pp. 175–177).

The early work on chemical mediation was carried out on the autonomic nervous system, and Elliott was the first to suggest that a chemical transmitter which brought about the transmission of excitatory or inhibitory stimuli, might be liberated at the nerve endings. In 1904 he pointed to the similarity between the effects of adrenaline and stimulation of the sympathetic nerves, and argued that perhaps adrenaline was released at the periphery of a nerve fibre owing to the arrival there of a nerve impulse. His preliminary report ("On the action of adrenalin (Prelimi-nary communication)," *J. Physiol., London,* 1904, 31:xx–xxi) contained the follow-ing statements:

EXCERPT P. XXI

. . . . And the facts suggest that the sympathetic axons cannot excite the peripheral tissue except in the presence, and perhaps through the agency, of the adrenalin or its immediate precursor secreted by the sympa-thetic paraganglia.

. . . .

Therefore it cannot be that adrenalin excites any structure derived from, and dependent for its persistence on, the peripheral neurone. But since adrenalin does not evoke any reaction from muscle that has at no time of its life been innervated by the sympathetic, the point at which the stimulus of the chemical excitant is received, and transformed into what may cause the change of tension of the muscle fibre, is perhaps a mechanism devel-oped out of the muscle cell in response to its union with the synapsing sympathetic fibre, the function of which is to receive and transform the nervous impulse. Adrenalin might then be the chemical stimulant liberated on each occasion when the impulse arrives at the periphery.

In the following year, the details of his experiments were published ("The action of adrenalin," *J. Physiol., London,* 1905, 32:401–467) and the passages below have been taken from this paper.

EXCERPT P. 404

The Cat. As in all mammals, the nervous plexus at the base of the cat's bladder is supplied by sympathetic fibres from the lumbar spinal roots which run in the hypogastric nerves, and by sacral fibres in the pelvic visceral nerves (*nervi erigentes*). If either a pressure or volume record of the fluid contents of the bladder be taken, it is seen that excitation of the hypogastric nerves causes a brief contraction which is followed in the majority of instances by extensive relaxation. As noticed by Langley and Anderson [1895], the contraction is almost confined to the muscle at the base where the urethra debouches upon the bladder: the relaxation con-cerns the rest of the bladder, and apparently leaves the basal part unaf-fected.

Injection of adrenalin into the external jugular vein causes complete relaxation. The latent period of this inhibition by adrenalin is much less than that by electrical excitation of the nerves: consequently relaxation occurs simultaneously with the contraction at the base of the bladder, and prevents the latter from leaving its mark on a tracing of the bladder's volume (cp. Fig. 11 [fig. 60]). Otherwise the curves agree.

Often the tone of the cat's bladder is completely abolished by section of the pelvic visceral nerves, and then neither adrenalin nor excitation of the hypogastrics can alter the physiological tension of the sheet of muscle. Inhibition by adrenalin is, however, so potent that during the dominance of the drug strong excitation of the pelvic visceral nerves (cp. Fig. 11) fails to cause contraction. By this test the action of adrenalin may be revealed even when it is masked by a previous atonic state of the bladder.

. . . .

On the other hand in the urethra stimulation of the hypogastrics causes such firm contraction as will steadily uphold a pressure of more than half a metre of water.

An identical contraction is obtained by the injection of 1 mgm. adrenalin.

EXCERPT P. 426

. . . . Adrenalin excites the plain muscle concordantly with its sympathetic innervation, and the dominant form of innervation determines the main reaction of the mass, to contraction in the bird, relaxation in the mammal.

It seems then that certainly for all Mammalia, and probably for all Vertebrata, the following law is true: *The reaction to adrenalin of any plain muscle in the body is of a similar character to that following excitation of the sympathetic (thoracico-lumbar visceral, or autonomic) nerves supplying that muscle, and the extent of the reaction varies directly with the frequency of normal physiological impulses received by the muscle in life through the sympathetic nerves.*

The various experiments that have been described above establish this identity in certain organs whose innervation was previously open to discussion.

In the portion of the paper where he discussed the localization of the action of adrenaline, Elliott stated that this must be at the junction between muscle and nerve—the myoneural junction which by 1905 was a well-recognized structure.

EXCERPT P. 436

But when plain muscle develops connection with sympathetic nerves it must at the *myoneural junction* acquire a mechanism that can receive the nervous impulse, and thereupon initiate the appropriate muscular response. That part of the junction which is irritable by adrenalin is on the muscular side, in so far as its tropic centre lies in the muscular nucleoplasm. But though its parent is the muscle, it would not have been called into existence had it not been for the developing union with a sympathetic nerve cell.

Furthermore, if it were shown that the nervous excitatory impulse is of the same nature, whether travelling down a motor or inhibitor peripheral axon, then it would be the function of the myoneural junction to determine whether the change of muscular tension shall be positive or negative. And this assumption would find support in the analogy of the response to adrenalin. The one stimulus, adrenalin, applied from without in the place of a nervous impulse arriving down the axon, may provoke either inhibition or contraction; and the decision as to either change rests upon the reacting mechanism at the periphery.

The conclusion—that adrenalin excites not the muscle fibre directly, but a substance developed out of it, and in consequence of the union of the sympathetic axon with it—would seem to be clearly founded on the instances, as those of the bladder and the bronchioles where the muscle in default of sympathetic innervation is totally irresponsive to the presence of adrenalin, were it not for the class of reactions discussed on page 415 [skin muscles and apparent exceptions].

The following has been taken from Elliott's summary of this long paper.

EXCERPT PP. 466–467

. . . . Its [adrenalin's] single characteristic is the aptness to stimulate plain muscle and gland cells that are or have been in functional union with sympathetic nerve fibres.

1. In all vertebrates the reaction of any plain muscle to adrenalin is of a similar character to that following excitation of the sympathetic (thoracico-lumbar) visceral nerves supplying that muscle. The change may be either to contraction or relaxation. In default of sympathetic innervation plain muscle is indifferent to adrenalin.

2. Extent of reaction varies directly with the frequency of normal physiological impulses to rapid change of tension received by the muscle in life through the sympathetic nerves.

3. A positive reaction to adrenalin is a trustworthy proof of the existence and nature of sympathetic nerves in any organ.

4. Plain muscle, when denervated, shows increase of the capacity for irritation by adrenalin than it had previously possessed.

5. Sympathetic nerve cells with their fibres, and the contractile muscle fibres are not irritated by adrenalin. The stimulation takes place at the junction of muscle and nerve.

6. The irritable substance at the myoneural junction depends for continuance of life on the nucleoplasm of the muscle cell, not of the nerve cell.

7. Such peculiar irritability marks the profound biochemical distinction between all postganglionic nerves of the thoracico-lumbar visceral class,

whether motor or inhibitor, on the one side, and all other efferent nerves with their respective junctions on the other.

Sir Henry Hallett Dale
(9 June 1875—)

Despite Elliott's statements concerning the liberation of adrenaline at the sympathetic neuromuscular junctions, he did not pursue the matter further; either his interests turned elsewhere or the techniques then available to him could take him no further; or the comparison of adrenaline with sympathetic action was not found to be absolute.

One of the few workers who followed up his suggestion was W. E. Dixon (1871–1931) of London (see Holmstedt and Liljestrand, 1963, pp. 181–184) who suspected that a chemical substance might also be responsible for the inhibiting action of the parasympathetic vagus on the heart. In a paper published in 1907, "On the mode of action of drugs," he concluded as follows.

EXCERPT P. 457

. . . . some inhibitory substance is stored up in that portion of the heart to which we refer as a "nerve ending," that when the vagus is excited this inhibitory substance ["inhibiting hormone," as he called it] is set free, and by combining with a body in the cardiac muscle brings about inhibition.

This substance he thought was muscarine, or muscarine-like in its actions, and the next step in the elucidation of this problem was taken by H. H. Dale, now Sir Henry H. Dale, in 1914.

Dale was born in London and studied medicine at Cambridge from 1894 to 1900, where, like Elliott, he spent some time as a research student. His clinical studies were at St. Bartholomew's Hospital, London, and on their conclusion he entered the field of physiology. He spent some time with E. H. Starling and with Paul Ehrlich at Frankfurt, and then became pharmacologist and later director of the Wellcome Physiological Research Laboratory in London. In 1914 he went as head of the department of biochemistry and pharmacology to the new National Institute for Medical Research and was made director in 1928. He retired in 1942 and for the next four years was associated with the Royal Institution of Great Britain. He is now Senior Scientific Consultant to the Wellcome Trust in London. His work has been mainly in three areas: the investigation of ergot, histamine, and the choline esters (see Adrian, 1955; Loewi, 1955; Burn, 1955; Gasser, 1955; Dale, 1958, 1963; Holmstedt and Liljestrand, 1963, pp. 184–190).

While working on ergot he discovered a substance which turned out to be acetylcholine and reported his findings in a preliminary communication in 1914 ("The occurrence in ergot and action of acetyl-choline (Preliminary communication)," *J. Physiol., London*, 1914, 48:iii–iv).

The intense depressor activity of acetyl-choline was described by Hunt and Taveau [1906], who examined a series of choline-esters, and found that acetyl-choline lowered the blood-pressure in doses far smaller than the minimal pressor dose of adrenine [adrenaline]. I have been familiar for some time with a pronounced inhibitor effect on the heart, shown by some specimens of ergot, and always associated with an intense stimulant action on intestinal muscle. Both actions were abolished by atropine. Since none of the known principles accounted for this action, the chemical nature of the substance responsible for it was investigated by A. J. Ewins, who was able to isolate it and identify it as acetyl-choline.

I find that acetyl-choline in minute intravenous doses (0.0001 mgm. to 0.001 mgm.) produces a vasodilator fall of blood-pressure without significant effect on the heart. It dilates the vessels of the perfused rabbit's ear. In somewhat larger doses (0.01 to 1 mgm.) it causes also pronounced vagus-like inhibition of the heart, and various other effects of stimulating nerves of the cranial and sacral divisions of the autonomic system—secretion of saliva, contraction of the oesophagus, stomach and intestine, and of the urinary bladder. The effects, though intense while they last, are remarkably evanescent, and are repeated with striking uniformity if a series of similar injections is given. Presumably the ester is rapidly hydrolysed in the circulation into its relatively inert components. The action on plain muscle which is innervated only by nerves of the true sympathetic system, such as that of the uterus, is relatively slight. The pupil forms an exception among structures innervated by cranial autonomic nerves, constriction being absent or insignificant.

This was followed by a classic paper ("The action of certain esters and ethers of choline, and their relation to muscarine," *J. Pharmac. exp. Ther.*, 1914, 6:147–190) in which he reported his investigations on acetylcholine in detail. He also made reference to the possibility of this substance playing some role in the action of the autonomic or involuntary nervous system and even went so far as to call it "parasympathomimetic" in action, a term comparable to "sympathomimetic" (p. 184).

EXCERPT PP. 188–189

The question of a possible physiological significance, in the resemblance between the action of choline esters and the effects of certain divisions of the involuntary nervous system, is one of great interest, but one for the discussion of which little evidence is available. Acetyl-choline is, of all the substances examined, the one whose action is most suggestive in this direction. The fact that its action surpasses even that of adrenine, both in intensity and evanescence, when considered in conjunction with the fact that each of these two bases reproduces those effects of involuntary nerves which are absent from the action of the other, so that the two actions are in many directions at once complementary and antagonistic, gives plenty of scope for speculation. On the other hand, there is no known depôt of choline derivatives, corresponding to the adrenine depôt in the adrenal medulla, nor, indeed, any evidence that a substance resembling acetyl-choline exists in the body at all. Reid Hunt found evidence of the existence of a substance in the supra-renal gland, which was not choline itself, but easily yielded that base in the process of extraction. If acetyl-choline, however, or any substance of comparable activity, existed in the supra-renal gland in quantities sufficient for chemical detection, its action would inevitably overpower that of the adrenine in a gland extract. The possibility may, indeed, be admitted, of acetyl-choline, or some similarly active and unstable ester, arising in the body and being so rapidly hydrolysed by the tissues that its detection is impossible by known methods. Such a suggestion would acquire interest if methods for its experimental verification could be devised.

Otto Loewi
(3 June 1873—25 December 1961)

So far there had been suggestive evidence and discerning suggestions regarding two chemical mediators of nerve impulses in the autonomic nervous system. But until 1921 there was no conclusive experimental proof available. Meantime, the idea was held that transmission between nerve fibres was owing to a spreading of the electrical process accompanying the nerve impulse from the end of the fibre to the effector organ. However, in 1921 Loewi began his studies on neurochemical transmission.

Loewi was born in Frankfurt am Main and attended medical school at Strassburg, Munich, and then again at Strassburg where he came into contact with the great pharmacologist Schmiedeberg and the clinician Naunyn. After a brief period in 1898 in clinical medicine he turned to pharmacology and spent the next twelve years as associate professor with H. H. Meyer: seven at Marburg and five at Vienna. In 1909 he became professor of pharmacology and head of the department in the University of Graz. Following the Nazi occupation of Austria in 1938 Loewi fled to Britain and then to the United States where he held a post in the department of pharmacology at New York University College of Medicine until his death. His work included the biochemistry of metabolism and diabetes, the neurohumoral transmission, and endocrine function (see Loewi, 1961; Dale, 1962; Fredericq, 1962; Holmstedt and Liljestrand, 1963, pp. 190–196; Loewi, 1963).

By means of simple yet vital experiments Loewi gave for the first time direct experimental evidence of chemical transmission at the neuromuscular junction of the vagal and sympathetic nerve fibres to the heart. He could collect from a stimulated heart a substance which in another heart produced the same effects as the nerve action, whether vagal inhibition or acceleration by sympathetic stimulation; the substance producing the former he called *Vagusstoff*. Thus Loewi had unequivocally proved that nerves do not influence the heart directly but that a chemical mediator is responsible for the observed effects of nerve stimulation.

The way in which he arrived at the details of his experiments is an example of a "hunch" appearing to a scientist in a dream. W. B. Cannon of Boston, who was himself prominent in this field of autonomic nervous system action, gave the following account of it (1934, p. 149; there is another version in Ingle, 1963, p. 123).

In conversation Loewi has given an interesting account of the origin of his experiments. One night, having fallen asleep while reading a light novel, he awoke suddenly and completely, with the idea fully formed that if the vagus nerves inhibit the heart by liberating a muscarin-like substance, the substance might diffuse out into a salt solution left in contact with a heart while it was subjected to vagal inhibition, and that then the presence of this substance might be demonstrated by inhibiting another heart through the influence of the altered solution. He scribbled the plan of the experiment on a scrap of paper and went to sleep again. Next morning, however, he could not decipher what he had written! Yet he felt that it was important. All day he went about in a distracted manner, looking occasionally at the paper, but wholly mystified as to its meaning. That night he again awoke, with vivid revival of the incidents of the previous illumination, and after this experience he remembered in his waking state both occasions. He set up a frog heart filled with Ringer's fluid, and after inhibiting the heart by stimulating the vagus nerve, found that the fluid had acquired a new property—that of being able to induce in another frog heart typical inhibitory vagal effects. Furthermore, he found also that when the sympathetic nerves were stimulated, to make the heart beat more rapidly, the Ringer solution in contact with it became endowed with cardio-accelerator power, i.e., an agent was added to it, which, like adrenin, had sympathomimetic influence. Although, at first, these observations were not confirmed by some investigators, they have been wholly substantiated by others, and at present [1934] the support for Loewi's work may be regarded as conclusive.

Loewi's first paper appeared in 1921 ("Über humorale Übertragbarkeit der Herznervenwirkung, I. Mitteilung," *Pflügers Arch.*, 1921, 189:239–242) and the following passage is the discussion of his results.

EXCERPT P. 242

The experiments show that by stimulation of the cardio-inhibitory and cardio-accelerating nerves, which is equivalent to nerve stimulation, substances can be demonstrated in the fluid filling the heart. Therefore, these substances are formed, broken down or prepared by nerve stimulation, and at first cells do it without exception. Concerning the significance of these substances, there are two possibilities: on the one hand, they may originate directly from the effect of nerve stimulation independent of the type of cardiac activity, and thus liberate the specific reaction of the heart from the nerve stimulus which, accordingly, would be only indirectly effective. If, in the sequence of experiments, their action trails quantitatively behind that of nerve stimulation, this should not come as a surprise since it may be assumed that only an insignificant portion of the substances which are formed and separated in or at the cell passes over into the humors, and that, on the other hand, the latter causes intense dilution. From a different viewpoint, there is also the possibility that these substances are only products of the specific type of cardiac activity which is released by the nerve stimulus; under such circumstances, therefore, the identification of their action with the nerve stimulus would be only accidental, so to speak.

As regards the question of the character of the substances, we can so far merely exclude the possibility that we are dealing with potassium in the material produced by vagal irritation, since increased potassium activity would not be removed by atropine as was the case in our experiments.

In Loewi's second paper, of what was to be a series of publications on neurochemical transmission ("Über humorale Übertragbarkeit der Herznervenwirkung. II. Mitteilung," *Pflügers Arch.*, 1922, 193:201–213), he discussed the nature of the *Vagusstoff*, the substance which acted in the same way as parasympathetic, vagal stimulation.

EXCERPT PP. 208–209

The fact that the action of the *Vagusstoff* is promptly removed by atropine narrows down greatly the number of substances which must be considered and directs the investigation along very definitive lines. Of the substances so far known to occur in the body, choline and related substances are actually the only ones that need concern us.

I first explored the possibility that it was choline itself. Admittedly, its action on the heart, even in high concentration, is relatively weak and rarely leads to diastolic arrest. However, if vagal activity comes into play, it could act in areas which are not reached in the same manner by influences introduced from the outside.

Therefore, I first looked into the question if, and in what amount, choline may occur in the vagus content [of the heart] of the toad and the frog. [The heart was perfused with Ringer's solution, and the perfusate is meant when "vagus content" is used here and below.] For this purpose the vagus contents were completely dried with a weak acid in the vacuum and acetylated. The effect of the acetyl product was tested on a heart, as described in more detail by Geiger and Loewi. In eleven experiments we found choline in the control as well as in the vagus content. Since it was also observed in the diffusate from the intestine and from the uterus, it may be assumed that it diffuses out of all organs. The vagus content always contained more than that of the control: that is, from two to five times more. Titration of the volume by comparison with measured acetylcholine yielded a volume of choline corresponding to 1:1–5 million during the period of vagal action, a concentration which, under all circumstances, is ineffective in the heart. Fig. 6 [fig. 72] shows such a titration experiment which illustrates the increased volume of the vagus period as well as a comparison with acetylcholine. Because of the importance of the question I tested the results in other ways . . . .

Therefore, choline proper is not the negative inotropic, effective substance of the [*Vagusstoff*] content of the heart, although during vagal action the volume contains more of it. It is possible that we are dealing here . . . . with cholinesterase, the occurrence of which was presumed in the past (Hunt, Guggenheim) and recently became a strong probability (le Heux). However, its isolation in pure form is undoubtedly very difficult and still remains to be accomplished.

EXCERPT PP. 211–212

IV. DISCUSSION OF THE RESULTS

The question whether nerve stimulation is directly responsible for the apparent result, or whether it is brought about by the formation of chemical substances which, for their part, cause the effect, has been discussed repeatedly . . . . Finally, Bayliss also considers it possible that the nerve acts by way of the formation of a chemical substance. The present exploration established for the first time proof for the justification of such hypothesis.

Above all, two questions now come to the fore: how is the nerve able to form this substance, and where does this take place? In my opinion, the first question is still unanswerable. Concerning the second question, I premise that the inhibitory effect of the vagus can still be observed in the nicotinized heart which no longer responds to the irritation of the vagal trunk, and thus acts postganglionically. In the past it was thought that postganglionically acting agents, the effect of which was removed by atropine, react upon nerve endings, since the result of the nerve irritation by atropine, too, has been eliminated. If this were so and we applied it to our case, the vagus stimulation would lead to the formation of a substance which would stimulate the same vagus terminally. Under such circumstances, we should have to interpret the results of the nerve irritation as its direct effect. As substances which resemble the stimulation of the parasympathetic and sympathetic nerves, such as pilocarpin and adrenalin respectively, are not diminished effectively by degeneration of the postganglionic nerve fibres, the idea of the nerve ending being the site of action has been dropped. Today it is postulated, and justifiably so, that they act on some parts of the effector organ which possess chemical or physical characteristics (i.e., receptive substances). In my opinion, this hypothesis is strengthened by the fact that embryonic organs which still lack nerves respond to the parasympathetic and sympathetic poisons mentioned above in the same manner as those which have nerves. These particularly characteristic sites of action by no means need to be present in all organs, and they may even indicate a much higher degree of functional differentiation, as, for example, that represented by the well-known differentiation of muscles into red and white. By taking this point of view, I believe that the vagus and sympathetic substances do not react upon the nerve but directly upon the effector organ.

The mode of action is unknown.

Loewi's fundamental discovery with the frog's vagus was applied to parasympathetic function in other animals. By 1926 he had accepted the identity of *Vagusstoff* with acetylcholine ("Über humorale Übertragbarkeit der Herznervenwirkung. X. Mitteilung. Über das Schicksal des Vagusstoffs," *Pflügers Arch.*, 1926, 214:678–688; in collaboration with E. Navratil).

EXCERPT P. 688

. . . that the *Vagusstoff* is a cholin ester. [Footnote: Because of the extremely marked activity of the Vagusstoff, it might be thought to be acetylcholine.]

In 1935 Loewi gave a Ferrier Lecture to the Royal Society on 20 June ("The Ferrier Lecture on problems connected with the principle of humoral transmission of nervous impulses," *Proc. R. Soc.*, 1935, 118B:299–316), and in it he reviewed succinctly the growth of the idea of the chemical transmission of the nerve impulse. He had now accepted completely the fact that *Vagusstoff* was identical with acetylcholine, but the sympathetic transmitter could not be identified with the same certainty.

EXCERPT P. 300

. . . . But first, in view of what is to follow, we must characterize the transmitters released by nerve stimulation. If I may start with the transmitter of vagus-stimulation, the "Vagusstoff," its effect, on account of its chemical instability, fades very quickly and can be annulled by atropine. Both properties are shared by the "Vagusstoff" with certain esters of choline, especially with acetylcholine. The quick destruction is caused by a specific esterase present in the heart. Furthermore, I was able to show that the action of this esterase is inhibited in a specific manner by minute amounts of eserine. This must be mentioned because it was this discovery which alone made possible the later extension of the proof of the occurrence of neuro-humoral transmission to a very wide range of effects. The "Vagusstoff" behaves exactly like acetylcholine, not only with regard to the properties already mentioned, but also with regard to each of its other peculiarities. Further, Dale and Dudley succeeded in isolating acetylcholine in substance from animal organs. To my mind these facts leave no doubt that the "Vagusstoff" is acetylcholine; I propose, therefore, to refer to it as such.

With regard to the characters of the substance released by stimulation of the cardio-accelerator nerves as well as by other sympathetic nerves, it could be shown that it shares many properties with adrenaline: both, for example, are destroyed by treatment with alkali and by ultra-violet and fluorescent radiation. The effect of both is inhibited by ergotoxine. Finally, as Cannon and Rosenblueth have pointed out, the action of the sympathetic substance is potentiated by small amounts of cocaine, in themselves ineffective, in exactly the same manner as Fröhlich and I demonstrated for adrenaline thirty years ago. In spite of all analogies, however, and although personally I am convinced of the identity, I do not feel justified as yet in assuming that the sympathetic transmitter is adrenaline, and I will therefore call it "the adrenaline-like substance."

Sir Henry Hallett Dale
(*See p. 248*)

In the same Ferrier Lecture of 1935 (p. 254) Loewi reduced the history of contributions to the understanding of the chemical mediation of nerve impulses to the following sentence (p. 299), although he modestly omitted his own work: "Elliott suggested the conception; Dixon made the first experiment upon it; to Dale is due the greatest extension of its scope."

Sir Henry Dale's early work on acetylcholine, which together with that of Elliott, Dixon, and others led to Loewi's experiments, has been considered (pp. 248–250). As Loewi suggested, Dale's contribution was probably greater than that of any of the others, and in 1936 they shared the Nobel Prize in Medicine and Physiology. In his Prize lecture on 12 December 1936, Dale discussed some of the more important developments of his earlier work ("Some recent extensions of the chemical transmission of the effects of nerve impulses," *Nobel lectures physiology or medicine 1922–1941* [Amsterdam, 1965], pp. 402–413). One of these concerned the role of acetylcholine in voluntary muscle and another, the immensely difficult problem of chemical transmission in the brain.

EXCERPT PP. 411–413

. . . . I must be content today to have presented the main headings of the evidence, which, as it seems to me, is forcing upon us the conclusion, in spite of the preconceptions which made the idea initially so difficult to entertain, that acetylcholine does actually intervene as a chemical transmitter of excitation, in the rapid and individualized transmission at ganglionic synapses and at the motor endings in voluntary muscle; that, in the terminology which I have proposed, the preganglionic fibres of the autonomic system, and the motor nerve fibres to voluntary muscle, are also "cholinergic."

You will see that we are thus led to the conclusion that nearly all the efferent neurones of the whole peripheral nervous system are cholinergic; only the postganglionic fibres of the true sympathetic system are adrenergic, and not even all of these. As I have earlier pointed out, on more than one occasion, before the evidence for the cholinergic function of voluntary motor nerves was nearly as strong as it has now become, this new classification of nerve fibres, by chemical function, renders at once intelligible the formerly puzzling evidence as to the functional compatibility of different types of nerve fibre, in replacing one another in experimental regeneration. The whole of the evidence of such replacement, obtained by Langley and Anderson early in the present century, can now be summarized by the simple statement that any cholinergic fibres can replace any other cholinergic fibres, and that adrenergic fibres can replace adrenergic fibres, but that no fibre can be functionally replaced by one which employs a different chemical transmitter. The chemical function, as I have expressed it, seems to be characteristic of the neurone, and unchangeable. In that connexion, particular interest appears to me to attach to the recent observations of Wybauw, which seem to provide clear evidence that the antidromic vasodilatation, generally believed to be produced through peripheral axon branches from sensory fibres, also employs a cholinergic mechanism. If this is substantiated, and if my suggestion holds good that the chemical mechanism is characteristic of the neurone, the question at once presents itself, whether at the other ending of the same sensory neurone, in a central synapse, the same cholinergic transmission of excitation will be found.

Hitherto the evidence concerning a chemical transmission in the central nervous system, of the type which we have found prevailing at all peripheral synapses, is scattered and insufficiently uniform in its indications. The basal ganglia of the brain are peculiarly rich in acetylcholine, the presence of which must presumably have some significance; and suggestive effects of eserine and of acetylcholine, injected into the ventricles of the brain, have been described. I take the view, however, that we need a much larger array of well-authenticated facts, before we begin to theorize. It is here, especially, that we need to proceed with caution; if the principle of chemical transmission is ultimately to find a further extension to the interneuronal transmission in the brain itself, it is by patient testing of the groundwork of experimental fact, at each new step, that a safe and steady advance will be achieved. The possible importance of such an extension, even for practical medicine and therapeutics, could hardly be over-estimated. Hitherto the conception of chemical transmission at nerve endings and neuronal synapses, originating in Loewi's discovery, and with the extension that the work of my colleagues has been able to give to it, can claim one practical result, in the specific, though alas only short, alleviation of the condition of myasthenia gravis, by eserine and its synthetic analogues.

We have not attempted to bring the history of neurochemical transmission nearer to the present day. At close range it is impossible to evaluate, and even some of the passages we have included above may in the future be shown to have pointed in the wrong direction. On the other hand, statements and conclusions unappreciated today may tomorrow appear relevant if not prophetic. Such was the case with one of Dale's intuitive comments made in 1937 ("Acetylcholine as a chemical transmitter of the effects of nerve impulses. II. Chemical transmission at ganglionic synapses and voluntary motor nerve endings. Some general considerations," *J. Mt. Sinai Hosp.*, 1938, 4:416–429, The William Henry Welch Lecture, II, 10 May 1937) which indicated that acetylcholine might turn out to have a much wider role to play. Recent books such as that of Nachmansohn (1959) amply justify this shrewd statement.

EXCERPT PP. 427–428

There remains one other question, on which I ought to touch briefly in conclusion. We have seen that Feldberg and Vartiainen (1934) failed to obtain evidence of the liberation of acetylcholine when they stimulated the vagus nerve, the fibres of which pass through the vagus ganglion without synaptic interruption, or when they stimulated antidromically the postganglionic fibres from the superior cervical ganglion. They concluded that acetylcholine was liberated at the synaptic endings of preganglionic fibres, and not from nerve fibres at other points of their course. The evidence from work on striated muscle, though the point could not there be made the subject of such direct experiment, pointed in the same direction. In both cases it seemed to correspond to the liberation of acetylcholine only at those points where it would immediately make contact with structures demonstrably sensitive to its action, and would thus serve as a physiological transmitter of excitation. The survey made by Chang and Gaddum (1933) led to the conclusion that the distribution of acetylcholine in the body tissues, with certain conspicuous and unexplained exceptions, is on the whole related to this physiological function of transmitting the effects of cholinergic nerve impulses from the nerve endings. The question, however, remained open, whether this difference, between the endings of cholinergic nerve fibres in relation to effector cells or at interneuronal synapses, and the rest of such fibres, was absolute and qualitative, or merely quantitative. Barsoum (1935) found that nerves, and certain autonomic nerves especially, yield relatively large proportions of acetylcholine to extraction. There is certainly no evidence that acetylcholine applied artificially to any nerve trunk has a perceptible stimulating, or other physiological action upon it. On the other hand, there is evidence, chiefly from Italian physiologists (Calabro, 1933; Bergami, 1936), that small proportions of a substance behaving like acetylcholine are liberated from a mammalian nerve (vagus, phrenic, etc.), into a Ringer solution into which it is allowed to dip, either when the nerve is stimulated artificially, or even when normal, physiological impulses pass along it from the nerve centres. The conditions, as regards the composition of the Ringer solution requisite for success, seem to be rather artificial; and it is difficult to picture a function for the release of acetylcholine, as the impulse passes along an intact nerve, which could find a place in any yet extant theory of the nature of the nerve impulse and its propagation. It can only be said at present that the phenomena described have such interest and importance, that it may be hoped and expected that attempts to confirm them and further to explore their significance will be undertaken in other laboratories. If the liberation of a chemical mediator at a nerve ending should prove to be, not a process peculiar and limited to that ending, but merely a local intensification, to ensure transmission to a contiguous cell, of a process which actually figures in the propagation of the impulse along the nerve fibre, we should have to make yet a further revision of our existing conceptions. Some minds have undoubtedly felt difficulty in postulating a complete breach in the nature of the processes concerned in transmission, where the excitation passes from nerve ending to effector cell. This particular difficulty would then disappear, but only at the cost of a more fundamental change of conception concerning the nature of the propagated wave of excitation than any which has yet been seriously considered.

Conclusion

It is today accepted that the nerve fibre is a polarized cable-like structure that transmits potential changes resulting from the movements of sodium and potassium across its boundary membrane. The ions move along electrochemical gradients and in so doing provide the electric currents that determine the further spread of the impulse. Thus a process of depolarization is passed along self-regeneratively. Synaptic transmission can be either a chemical or an electrical phenomenon and synapses which transmit electrically, chemically, or in both ways, have been identified; Eccles (1964, pp. 261–265) has conveniently listed the properties of each variety.

This point has been reached by a large group of investigators of whom only a few have been represented here. The comparative approach has in particular been exploited and the greater part of the work has been on non-human preparations. In particular the invertebrates have proved to be of value, as shown by the contribution of Young and of Hodgkin (pp. 234–237). But plant life has provided vital data, and studies of the ionic relationships of the giant plant cells of *Nitella*, a freshwater plant, and *Valonia*, a marine algae, by Osterhout (Shedlovsky, 1964) and his colleagues (e.g., Osterhout, 1931) have provided the basis of much of our knowledge of bioelectric potentials and active transport. Moreover, Osterhout and Hill (1929–1930) using *Nitella* have given the most convincing evidence in favor of biological transmission processes being electrical in nature.

The most important technical advance in this field has been the increasing perfection of microtechniques, and this together with the various electrical recording and stimulating apparatus and the electron microscope, have opened up a wide field for future endeavor. And as Eccles has commented (1964, p. 265) regarding the synapse, ". . . the pace quickens."

CHAPTER IV

ANATOMY OF THE SPINAL CORD

Introduction

The history of the detailed anatomy of the spinal cord is relatively short compared with that of other parts of the nervous system. This is because little advance in the knowledge of its finer structure could be made before appropriate technical facilities for its more intimate examination became available in the middle of the nineteenth century. Up till then, accounts only of the macroscopic features could be given, for, since the cord is made up of nerve cells and fibres, no significant progress could be expected until the morphology of the neuron (Chapter II) had been elucidated, at least in part. However, during the period to be surveyed below, from the fifth century B.C. to the twentieth, the concept of the spinal cord changed from that of a pultaceous, avascular mass analogous to bone marrow with no neurological function, to that of a highly organized, intricate structure of great complexity with vital and specific functions.

The following material deals first with the general macroscopic, and second with the general microscopic anatomy of the spinal cord. As space does not allow consideration of more than one special constituent, the history of the pyramidal tract has been selected as a representative of all the others and it forms the third section of the present chapter.

There is no single publication that deals with the history of the cord's anatomy, although a considerable amount of historical material is to be found in Stilling (1859, *passim*).

General Macroscopic Anatomy

GALEN
(See p. 14)

Although the clinical manifestations of spinal cord injury had been observed by the ancient Egyptians, as is clear from the Edwin Smith Papyrus, and also by the

Hippocratic Writers (e.g., *On joints*, 48, Littré [1839–1861], IV, 213–217), as far as can be determined little was known about the anatomy of this structure. The Hippocratic Writers mentioned it, and they recognized that it originated from the brain and that it could be differentiated from bone marrow: ". . . the marrow called dorsal arises from the brain" (*On flesh*, 5, Littré [1839–1861], VIII, 588–591). They had ideas similar to that of Aristotle, already cited (p. 9), respecting the hot cord countering the cold brain (*On diseases*, II, 5, Littré [1839–1851], VII, 12–15). Additionally, Aristotle mentioned the subject in *The parts of animals* (II, 6, Ogle [1911], 651*b*:33–37) with evident confusion since he asserted that the spinal cord was the marrow of the vertebral bodies, an idea preserved in our term "spinal marrow":

> What has been said hardly applies to the spinal marrow. For it is necessary that this shall be continuous and extend without break through the whole backbone, inasmuch as this bone consists of separate vertebrae. But were the spinal marrow either of unctuous fat or of suet, it could not hold together in such a continuous mass as it does, but would either be too fluid or too frangible.

Herophilus's statement concerning the cord (p. 146) is important because he seems to have been the first to recognize that nerves take their origin from the cord as well as from the brain. As already indicated (p. 147), Galen considered the cord to be an integral part of the nervous system, a fact suggested by others before him, but with less assurance. A summary of Galen's writings on the cord was provided by one of the compilers of late antiquity, Oribasius (A.D. *c.* 325–*c.* 400) of Constantinople, and has been presented in translation by Cohen and Drabkin (1948, pp. 483–485).

In the following passage from Galen's *Use of parts*, XII, 11 (Daremberg [1854–1856], II), as well as elsewhere, he discussed it at length, beginning with a justification of its existence. He thought of the cord as a bundle of nerves grouped together for convenience and safety, each nerve running without interruption from the brain to periphery, or in the reverse direction, just as nerve fibres are gathered together in a nerve trunk.

EXCERPT PP. 31–32

> One should not assume that the spinal cord need not exist, nor that it would be preferable to have it located elsewhere than in the spine, nor, having been located in the spine that it was more protected from injuries than it actually is. For if the marrow did not wholly exist, one of two things would result: either all the parts of the animal located below the head would be completely deprived of movement, or it would be absolutely necessary that a nerve descend directly from the brain to each part. But, if the parts had been denied movement—the meaning of what we say will be

immediately understood—the animal would no longer be an animal; it would, so to speak, be a work of stone or clay. On the other hand, to lead a very slender nerve from the brain to each part would be the work of a creator little mindful of security. There would be danger in causing nerves to travel such a distance. I do not say merely a thin nerve capable of being broken and shattered, but even a completely different, thick ligament, artery or vein. As of these organs so of the cord, from the origin suited to each; it arises like a large trunk that escapes from the earth, and as it advances and approaches various parts this trunk gives off branches derived from the same origin and serving all the parts; also it was preferable that the cord, like a river rising from its source, extend from the brain, continuously sending forth a nerve channel to each of the parts that it meets, through which both sensation and motion are conveyed . . . .

Now let us examine a consequence of this fact, since the spinal marrow is like a second brain for the parts below the head and, like the brain, must be protected by a hard and resistant covering.

In the same treatise (XIII, 8, Daremberg [1854–1856], II) Galen described the protective coverings of the cord: bone, posterior longitudinal ligament, dura mater, and pia mater.

EXCERPT PP. 71–72

A solid ligament attaches so precisely to the anterior parts of all the vertebrae [posterior longitudinal ligament] that to the eyes of many physicians they appear fused one to another rather than attached. This ligament abuts on the anterior surface of the tunic that envelops the membranes of the spinal cord; in advancing a little anteriorly it inserts itself on each side in the cartilage that lubricates the vertebrae [intervertebral disc]. . . . Both membranes of the cord resemble exactly the appearance of those that entirely envelop the brain, except that in the spine there is no space between them such as in the head; the differences are therefore that the dura mater touches and envelops all the pia mater and a very strong and very fibrous third tunic [posterior longitudinal ligament] envelops them exteriorly.

What then are the grounds for these arrangements, for nature does nothing in vain? As the spinal cord presents conditions that are common to it and to the brain, and conditions that are special to it, so it presents a structure similar in the similar parts and a structure special and different for the special parts. The common conditions are a substance similar to that of the brain, and that is the origin of the nerves. The special conditions are that the brain, enveloped by an immobile bone, has pulsations and in consequence movements, but the cord, surrounded by mobile vertebrae, does not have movements. It was therefore right that both the cord and the brain be equipped with two membranes, one to bind together their substance, which is very soft, the other to protect and shield them against the bones that surround them; it was also right that these bones envelop them like a rampart or wall capable of receiving bodily shocks that might otherwise disunite, bruise, and injure them in some way, without being damaged.

Here now are the particular things that differentiate them. Because the brain pulsates, the dura mater is far enough away from it to permit it to dilate; the cord does not pulsate and the dural membrane is united with the thin membrane without any intervening space. On the other hand, as there is a powerful one in those of the spine, the brain does not have an external envelope other than the dura mater, but the marrow has that third fibrous tunic, thick and strong, that we have just mentioned [posterior longitudinal ligament]. Indeed, as the cord follows the successive flexions, incurvings, and extensions of the spine, it would soon be shattered if it were not enveloped by such a covering. A viscous humor lubricates this covering as well as the ligament that attaches the vertebrae, and it lubricates all the articulations.

The following brief excerpts are from Galen's further work on anatomy, *On anatomical procedures* (IX, 13, Duckworth [1962], pp. 20–22) in which he gave a detailed account of the dissection of the spinal cord.

EXCERPTS PP. 20–22

. . . . Yet the dura mater enwrapping the spinal marrow is intimately combined and connected with the dura mater which surrounds the brain, just as the thin meninx [pia mater] lying upon the spinal marrow is intimately combined with the thin meninx upon the brain. For the spinal marrow has two meninges which take their origin from the meninges of the brain . . . .

. . . . And here [at the intervertebral spaces], in accordance with the sequence of the vertebrae, the nerves spring out on both sides of them, and the nerve roots pass out through perfectly rounded foramina, the width of each single foramen corresponding to the thickness of the nerve which passes out through it . . . .

. . . . Now this sheath [pia mater] is laid upon it [the spinal marrow] absolutely tensely and intimately, and in it are numerous veins just as in the pia mater enveloping the brain. You see these veins in the large animals very clearly, plunging down into the substance of the spinal marrow, and sinking into the depth of it.

VESALIUS

(See p. 153)

During the medieval period nothing of note was added to Galen's account of the spinal cord's structure, and even the early Renaissance anatomists made few original observations. Thus in his *De humani corporis fabrica* (1543, Bk. IV, Ch. XI) Vesalius mainly reproduced the opinions of Galen, often using identical words and phrases. The following passages, however, seem to have been based upon his own dissection experience. As noted before (p. 155), Vesalius frequently relied upon Galen for ideas regarding function of the body but recorded his own knowledge of its structure.

EXCERPT P. 339 [439]

WHERE THE DORSAL MARROW IS FORMED FROM MANY THREADS

When it creeps through the middle of the thorax, that it may be rendered especially suitable for the hard nerves serving and providing motion, it descends no longer simple but divided into innumerable shoots [cauda equina] not otherwise than if you were to tie together many very slender threads stretched in a straight line to some membrane, and then by degrees you were to distribute one and then another thread from that cluster through separate foramina through which the nerves issue, until only a single thread [conus medullaris] remained, corresponding to the termination of the dorsal marrow. In that way the dorsal marrow is consumed into the nerves which slip forth through foramina carved in the vertebrae . . . .

THE NUMBER OF PAIRS OF NERVES GIVEN OFF BY THE DORSAL MARROW

The dorsal marrow, led through the vertebrae, by degrees distributes the nerves, becoming more slender in its progression. Professors of dissection count the nerves as sixty, sometimes fifty-eight, now thirty and now twenty-nine pairs [thirty-one pairs is the accepted figure today]. From the part of the dorsal marrow contained in the cervical vertebrae seven pairs are given off; from the part carried through the thoracic vertebrae, twelve pairs; from the five lumbar vertebrae, five; from the os sacrum, six, although there may be five pairs of nerves of the os sacrum if it is formed of six bones; these nerves can in some degree be called twin since they are led forwards and backwards and hardly originate from one root. The termination of the dorsal marrow slipping from the os sacrum is not considered a nerve, nor does it end in ramules which deserve the name of nerves, although I have sometimes seen that slipping from the os sacrum distributed into three very short twigs; in that case the os sacrum was formed of only five bones.

François Pourfour du Petit
(24 June 1664—10 June 1741)

Little more attention was paid to the anatomy of the spinal cord until the eighteenth century, although a few exceptions may be noted, such as Malpighi's account of "fibres" in brain and cord (p. 580). This neglect may have been owing in part to its inaccessability, or more likely, to the persistent Galenic concept that the cord was merely a convenient pathway for nerves running directly from the periphery to the brain or in the reverse direction, like nerve fibres in a large nerve. During the eighteenth century evidence was accumulating that the spinal cord had functions of its own, and this promoted interest in its internal structure.

There are only a few detailed eighteenth century accounts of the spinal cord, and we have chosen three of the more important: those of Pourfour du Petit, 1710, Huber, 1741, and, finally, the excellent account of Vicq d'Azyr, 1781.

Pourfour du Petit was born in Paris and studied medicine at Montpellier where he was graduated in 1690. He continued his studies in anatomy, surgery, botany, and chemistry in Paris and in 1693 was appointed for four years as a physician to Louis XIV's army in Flanders. During a further term of military service ending in 1713 he carried out at Namur observations on the nervous system, some of which are mentioned below. Later he practised mainly ophthalmology with an interest in the anatomy and physiology of the eye and in optics. He noted the pupillary constriction following sympathetic section and contributed further to the elucidation of the sympathetic nervous system (see Jourdan, 1820–1825, V, 399–400; Dezeimeris, 1828–1839, III, 703–704; Kruger, 1963).

Pourfour du Petit's contributions to neuroanatomy and neurophysiology are little known owing to the fact that the book containing them was published anonymously and had a limited circulation; only four or five copies are known to exist today (*Lettres d'un medecin des hôpitaux du roy a un autre medecin de ses amis,* Namur, 1710). In "La premiere lettre contient un nouveau systeme du cerveau" (pp. 1–16) he described the decussation of the pyramids (pp. 283–284) and later gave a brief account of the internal structure of the cord, one of the first of any merit.

EXCERPT P. 15

The whole spinal cord is divided along its length into two equal parts. These two parts are composed of longitudinal medullary fibres which are bound together by transverse medullary fibres. These transverse fibres are not exactly in the center of the cord, for the anterior partition [anterior median sulcus] is not as deep as the posterior. The pia mater extends into the anterior partition as far as the transverse fibres; but only some very fine blood vessels pass along the posterior partition [posterior median sulcus] for which reason it is less apparent. Consequently it is more difficult to divide the cord through its posterior part than its anterior. The vessels which enter the cord by the two partitions insinuate themselves between the transverse fibres and are distributed there; they produce the gray color. This has given rise to the belief that there is a glandular substance in the spinal cord, although there is no evidence at all of it. The vessels are distributed, moreover, in the lateral parts of the cord, and form a web among the longitudinal fibres where brown lines, which are represented in the second figure, are seen [Fig. II in fig. 73].

JOHANN JACOB HUBER
(11 September 1707—6 July 1778)

The first detailed and accurate description of the spinal cord appears to have been that of the Swiss anatomist Huber. He was born at Basel and in 1730 went to Berne to study medicine under Haller; after further study at Strassburg, he received his doctorate at Basel in 1733. In 1736 Huber joined the faculty of the University of Göttingen where six years later he became professor *extraordinarius*. Thereafter, on Haller's recommendation, he was appointed professor of anatomy and practical surgery at the Collegium Carolinum in Cassel where he remained until his death. His anatomical work was mainly on the spinal cord and nerves (Husemann, 1931).

Huber's book on the spinal cord, *De medulla spinali speciatim de nervis ab ea provenientibus commentatio cum adjunctis iconibus* (Göttingen, 1741), served as a basis for the descriptions of many later writers. A large part of it, however, dealt with the accessory nerve of Willis. The following excerpts are a portion of Huber's description of the external appearances of the cord and include the first detailed account of the spinal roots and the denticulate ligaments. His drawings of the cord are of high merit. In respect to the internal structure of the cord, however, he did not advance beyond Pourfour du Petit for the reasons to be given below.

EXCERPT PP. 2–5

II

If we remove all the coverings from the spinal marrow except that which immediately invests it very closely and is an extension of the pia mater, then almost the whole surface is observed to bristle with [spinal] nerve filaments. Those filaments gathered into definite bundles, constituting the connections of the [spinal] nerves, are different in different regions. Some are collected into short bundles and enter the dura mater directly; these are very numerous. Others which extend further before they perforate the dura mater, are fewer and even thicker and have another direction . . . . Understand first of all that consideration is not being given to the deeper structure of the nerve filaments, but only to as much of the offshoots of the pia mater as appears to the naked eye. The extreme softness of the marrow and its singular nature refusing a more intimate analysis persuade us to pass over in silence those things existing within and what can be detected by the use of the microscope.

III

To avoid all obscurity, otherwise easily arising from the differing origin and gathering of the nerve filaments, we shall consider the spinal cord divided into four different regions [like a quartered circle]. This can be done very suitably and aptly since the cord itself especially rejoices in four distinct origins [anterior and posterior on the left and right] of those [spinal root] filaments and constitutes a like number of sections. [The site of origin of the roots] extends in a straight line almost continuously through the whole downward course of the cord, with a part of each section, always double, interposed; that is, a smooth column invested solely with pia mater and lacking filaments. If now the spinal cord is incised transversely through the middle into four equal sectors, one of which accurately bisects the anterior and posterior, the other the right and left, and if they are cut exactly perpendicularly, then each will display a series of filaments going forth from the middle of its outer surface [anterior or posterior spinal roots, left and right] separated by two smooth, half surfaces [if, as on a clock, the left posterior root is at 1:30 and the anterior at 4:30, the cord surface between is made up of 1:30 to 3, and 3 to 4:30]. And so, according to the general division, there will be right and left filaments; also the nerves, produced thence and approaching for the sake of their mates, serve this distinction. Then there is a more special division of these filaments (by which they are distinguished from the cranial nerves); the anterior filaments face the bodies of the vertebrae and the posterior ones, the nearer parts of the spine [posterior wall of the spinal canal].

IV

Hence, we must also give consideration to the four sectors of the spinal cord, or the smooth columns interposed in twin series between the individual [spinal root] filaments [cf. the above comparison with a clock face]. The right surface or column does not differ from the left; but they differ from the anterior and posterior [surfaces] by their denticulate ligament, which is a little larger than they on each of its own sides as well as in width. How the anterior and posterior surfaces differ from one another has been partly said. It must be known that the anterior [spinal root] filaments arise very close to one another, and there leave a narrow, smooth space as on the posterior face, and that the anterior filaments run quickly, that is higher, towards the middle of the cord, and in the posterior more slowly or downwards . . . .

Of the rest of its insertions, it [denticulate ligament] makes its first and highest attachment with the dura mater in denticulate fashion, but not very robust nor very short, at the swelling border of the occipital bone a little above the foramen of the vertebral artery, yet lower and a little more exterior than the exit from the skull of the ninth pair of cranial nerves [hypoglossal]. The first, somewhat slender dens of the ligament goes forth from the dura mater and, free for a brief space, descends obliquely outwards before it is affixed to the innermost covering of the spinal cord, which occurs between the filaments of the first and second cervical nerves. It puts forth the rest of the dentes in that way mentioned elsewhere; they, however, not observing a special distance, that is, always in the middle of the space between the two [spinal] nerves, although inserted now higher now more deeply but not passing over the intervening space until the body of the marrow, which, however, itself, also varies, comes to an end.

FÉLIX VICQ D'AZYR
(*28 April 1748—20 June 1794*)

Despite what had been written about the spinal cord by Pourfour du Petit, Huber, and others, knowledge of its internal structure was as yet limited. Towards the end of the eighteenth century, however, anatomists turned their attention more and more to this problem, and one of the most outstanding accounts produced was that of Vicq d'Azyr whose name is still associated with a fibre pathway in the brain (p. 592).

Vicq d'Azyr, the son of a physician, was born near Cherbourg. He studied philosophy at Caen and medicine at Paris, and on completion of the latter study in 1773, established a very popular course in anatomy. Although he never held a university appointment, in addition to being a renowned anatomist, he was also a successful physician, eventually becoming the premier physician to Marie Antoinette. After having made several contributions to human and comparative anatomy, he died, probably of an acute pulmonary infection, at the age of forty-six. In consequence only the first volume of a large, projected work appeared, *Traité d'anatomie et de physiologie* ([Paris, 1786]. See Moreau, 1805; Dubois, 1806; Dufresne, 1906; Spillman, 1941).

In 1781 Vicq d'Azyr published a brief but noteworthy description of the nervous system, accompanied by excellent illustrations ("Recherches sur la structure du cerveau, du cervelet, de la moelle elongée, de la moelle épinière; et sur l'origine des nerfs de l'homme et des animaux," *Hist. Acad. roy. Sci., Paris, 1781,* 1784, pp. 495–622), and the following passages have been taken from the portion (pp. 597–603) dealing with the cord. Huber had suggested the division of the cord into columns, and Vicq d'Azyr extended the idea. The partition into a right and a left half was important from the clinical viewpoint, for it was thought to explain some forms of hemiplegia.

EXCERPT PP. 600–601

One cannot help seeing a certain amount of ashen-colored [gray] or cortical substance in the depths of the spinal cord. Petit de Namur [Pourfour du Petit] was of a different opinion; he only admitted to dark lines and to a complex of vessels furnished by the pia mater, the interlacing of which appeared to him necessarily to produce a gray color.

The ashen-colored or cortical substance of the spinal cord [central gray matter] must be divided into three parts, a middle and two lateral parts.

The middle part is transverse; it extends from right to left; thicker and larger in the cervical region, smaller and narrower in the thoracic region, it again acquires greater volume without increase in width towards the lumbar region. This configuration can perhaps be compared with that found in the middle of the letter **H**.

The two lateral parts of the ashen-colored substance [anterior and posterior horns on each side] are curved in such a way that the convex borders face one another, while their concavities are turned laterally. Two extremities can be distinguished here as well as a body that is the central part; the anterior extremity [horn] is the larger and is shaped like a little head; the posterior extremity is very narrow and it is prolonged by an almost imperceptible streak to the posterior surface of the spinal cord; it terminates precisely at the point where the filaments that make up the posterior root of the spinal nerves arise. The body of this semilunar, lateral portion of the cortical [gray] substance, which may be compared to a Job's tear [*Coix Lacryma*, a species of grass with round, shining grains resembling tears], always decreases from the head, which is anterior [in an animal], as far as the very fine termination where its journey is seen to end caudally.

The lateral, semilunar parts of the cortical substance in the upper cervical region are thicker than lower down in the same region; they are still less so in the dorsal region. Towards the lower dorsal region and in the lumbar region, the posterior extremity [horn] of this semilunar part is enlarged, and in the terminal cross sections, towards the cauda equina, it is almost equal to the head or anterior extremity. It is important to notice above all,

1° that the volume of this substance in the lower sections of the spinal cord is much greater than in the dorsal region, and likewise larger in the cervical region; 2° that the anterior [median] sulcus, which in all the rest of the spinal cord is shorter than the posterior, becomes of almost equal depth near the cauda equina.

EXCERPT PP. 602–603

It follows from this description:

1° That the spinal cord is formed of two cords, one on the right and the other on the left, side by side with the [median] sulci already mentioned separating them anteriorly and posteriorly; 2° that the white matter is, as it were, excavated in its depths to accommodate the gray or cortical substance; 3° that on opening the posterior [median] sulcus, the gray or cortical substance is reached without difficulty; and that on opening the anterior sulcus a very thin white layer, which is situated like a commissure in front of the gray substance, forms the bottom of the sulcus; 4° that on breaking the adhesions which hold the walls of the sulci together, and on cutting the white layer, or anterior commissure, the cords of the spinal cord can be separated into quite distinct bodies; and having been separated entirely the one from the other and from the cortical substance, these cords are somewhat flattened and resemble ribbons which run side by side, as seen from in front and from behind, forming the medullary columns as they are seen in the vertebral canal; 5° finally, that in another report [probably never published] it will be possible to admit that instead of two cords in the spinal cord, there are four quite distinct divisions, two of which are located posteriorly between the semilunar and convex portions of the cortical substance and divided by the posterior sulcus [posterior columns]; and two others situated laterally in the concavity of these same semilunar portions of the cortical substance, and divided anteriorly by the anterior sulcus [lateral columns].

General Microscopic Anatomy

BENEDIKT STILLING
(22 *February 1810*—28 *February 1879*)

Little advance could be made on Vicq d'Azyr's studies of the macroscopic features of the spinal cord, and the next step was to examine it by means of techniques other than simple inspection. Already in the seventeenth century the microscopic appearances of the cord had been observed by Leeuwenhoek (p. 34 and *fig.* 3 in Fig. 2). He had identified nerve fibres, and much later Ehrenberg (see p. 40) examined them with his achromatic microscope. Much of the earlier microscopy of the nervous system was devoted to the peripheral nerve, to the spinal root ganglion, and to brain tissue (Chapters II and VIII), and the first person to use new methods of examining the spinal cord in detail was the German surgeon and anatomist Stilling.

Stilling was born in Kirchhain in the Electorate of Hesse and was graduated in medicine at Marburg in 1832. He became an assistant in the surgical clinic and at the end of 1833, provincial surgeon in Cassel. Although he had no university appointment he had contact with many of the leading scientists of Germany, France, and Britain, and he was able to carry out important anatomical, physiological, and surgical studies, the most significant of which were on the structure of the nervous system (see Kussmaul, 1879; Strauss, 1910; Stilling, 1910).

In January 1842 he developed a technique for examining the spinal cord (pp. 834–837), which eventually revealed a remarkable amount of detail of its internal structure. This involved slicing the frozen, or alcohol-hardened, cord like a cucumber into a series of very thin sections (*Schickt für Schickt*) and examining them unstained with the naked eye or with the microscope, usually under a low power; he was thus the first to use serial sections. Some of Stilling's findings are recorded in the excerpts below, taken from a monograph prepared in collaboration with J. Wallach (*Untersuchungen über die Textur des Rückenmarks*, Leipzig, 1842). Stilling was also interested in spinal cord function (p. 306), and his investigations revealed to him the importance of the gray matter. He described it as "not only the anatomical but the actual physiological nucleus of the spinal cord" (p. 14) and devoted a long description to its structure.

EXCERPT PP. 14–16

If I then made a longitudinal cut through half the spinal cord, and, for example, with a sharp knife cut a thin layer from the posterior gray and white column, then prepared it on a glass slide in such a manner that I had before me a small square piece, approximately 1½ lines wide and long [see p. 41], consisting of half gray and half white matter of the posterior tracts of the spinal cord, the following was observed:

The difference between the gray and the white matter was extraordinary, as could be seen by inspection with the naked eye as well as with a low magnification. The white matter was darker and opaque; the gray, less dark, transparent, and yellowish-red. With compression [of the preparation] the fibres of the white matter were seen lying parallel to each other and parallel to the [long] axis of the spinal cord, that is, running lengthwise; the individual fibres, as already described in the first chapter, were thick, large, and clearly distinguishable. By contrast, the gray substance did not as yet permit recognition of any part of its texture, with the exception of a disproportionately large number of vessels when compared to those of the white substance.

If compression was now slightly increased, it was noticed that the structure of the fibres of the white matter became more and more distinct, very clearly distinguishable from that of the gray. But the gray substance, too, demonstrated clearly—first at a magnification of 15 or 35 (ocular No. 0, lens 1 + 2)—that it consisted of fibres, as reported in the first chapter, and, indeed, of a double layer of fibres *that proceeded in opposite directions. A large proportion ran parallel to the fibres of the white matter. The other part advanced in the opposite direction, crossing at right angles the longitudinal fibres of the gray matter and forming right angles with it as far as the fibres of the white matter.*

These transverse fibres proceeded in bundles of large or small dimension, at a diameter of $\frac{1}{8}$ to $\frac{1}{16}$ line in width, as shown in Figs. 1 and 2 [fig. 75], with a magnification of 18–35 times. *They appeared much darker than the longitudinal fibres of the gray matter,* so that they looked like the fibres of the white matter, and one might believe these transverse bundles to consist of fibres from the white matter. From later investigation it became apparent that such assumption cannot be allowed. The course of the fibres mentioned is illustrated in Figs. 1, 2, and 3–*a.* longitudinal fibres of the white matter; *b.* longitudinal fibres of the gray matter; *c.* transverse bundle of the gray matter.

In this way I now continued to slice from various parts of the spinal cord thin layers which consisted half of gray, half of white matter, and the same result was obtained from all these investigations; the gray matter consisted of fibres that proceeded in two opposite directions. *A large portion of the fibres (of the gray matter) took a course parallel to the axis of the spinal cord, as well as parallel to the fibres of the white matter; another portion proceeded in a transverse direction, parallel with the transverse diameter of the spinal cord, which crossed at right or obtuse angles to the longitudinal fibres of the first portion.*

EXCERPT PP. 17–19

We begin our consideration of the cord sections prepared in this way [this paragraph follows that on p. 834, in which part of the technique is described], and we then find a round opening, the canalis spinalis [central canal]. This is surrounded by extremely delicate fibres of the gray matter that I shall describe later in more detail in reference to their course and their relations. If we now take Fig. 7 [fig. 78] to assist us and follow it when inspecting the posterior bundles [horns], we notice that both gray posterior columns [horns] consist of a dark mass which appears separated from the white matter by clear, boundary strips. However, on closer observation we do not find any margin of separation, but:

We realize in astonishment that in the center the entire mass of the gray posterior horns appears to consist of nothing but bundles of fibres that lie parallel to each other. Their apex at the boundary with the white matter radiates in all directions, like the spokes of a wheel, and enters the white matter of the posterior and the lateral columns. The illustration demonstrates this clearly so that I need not give it a more detailed description. Since the apex of the two posterior columns [horn] varies considerably, often heart-shaped, often semicircular, and often appears drawn out into a long point that extends almost to the [external] surface of the white matter, the shape of the bundles that radiate into the white substance is of course very variable, and we have tried to illustrate this variation in Figs. 4 and 5 [figs. 76 and 77].

. . . .

. . . . we also notice in the gray matter of the anterior columns [anterior horns], that the fibres, in opposite direction to those of the posterior, spread into the anterior white matter columns. However, the kind of dispersion here is not as regular and as beautiful as in the posterior columns. Rather here in this area three, four, six, and more processes of the anterior gray matter [horn] in thick bundles, almost clublike [Fig. 7], pass through the entire [thickness of the] anterior white matter, up to its surface. Between these thick bundles one notices innumerable smaller ones (but much smaller than in the gray posterior columns) which radiate into the white matter of the anterior columns where they produce the most variable connections, as in a plexus of the finest mesh . . . .

If we can therefore compare the gray matter of the spinal cord and its fibre extensions into the white matter with the sun which emits its rays in all directions (centrifugally), I must still add that the gray tracts of the two sides *are connected and associated with each other by a peculiar radiation of fibres.* These are the bundles of transverse fibres of the gray commissure for the anterior and posterior columns [horns] that lie above and below the central canal [Fig. 7, fig. 78]. That is, we notice unmistakably, directly around the canal, extremely delicate fibres that surround the margin and closest neighborhood of the canal in a circular fashion. However, these fine, circular fibres are joined by two thick layers of bundles of horizontal fibres of the gray matter, which, the one superior, the other inferior (in man, anterior and posterior [*sic*]) to the canal, have a precisely horizontal direction, but their individual fibres radiate fanlike in both directions, into both horns of the gray substance, upwards, downwards, straight across, etc. In this way they effect the most manifold connections.

In a later publication (*Untersuchungen über den Bau und die Verrichtungen des Gehirns. I. Über den Bau des Hirnknotens der den Varoli'schen Brücke*, Jena, 1846) Stilling recorded further detailed accounts of the white and gray matter of the cord, first in prepared and then in fresh material.

EXCERPT P. 6

B. CROSS SECTION

If one prepares a fine, transparent, transverse section from a hardened spinal cord, in which all the longitudinal fibres are thus cut through at right angles or almost at right angles, such section then exhibits the following characteristics:

With the naked eye one can see its white matter in the posterior, anterior, and lateral columns to be of the same color, dull white, shading somewhat into yellow or grayish. No orderly arrangement can be distinguished. The section looks like fine, dull, ground glass whereas on longitudinal section the section has a smoother, frequently polished appearance.

Under the microscope, with fifteen magnifications and with transmitted light, the section appears as a dark-gray or blue-black mass of uniform color or grain, which is interrupted only here and there by yellow areas, but generally and rather regularly, by clear-white, thinner areas. The whole thing looks like the dark base of a coarse-grained lithograph plate.

If we suppose, as is in fact the case, that all the fibres of the white anterolateral and posterior columns proceed parallel to the [long] axis of the spinal cord, we then see under the microscope throughout the cord, only the thinnest transverse sections of the individual primary fibres with their double contours [see Fig. 2 in fig. 75]. Between the opaque cross sections of the sheaths of the primary fibres are the interstices that separate the individual primary fibres from each other. The interstices are completely transparent, since they are filled with alcohol or with transparent crystal shapes.

EXCERPT P. 8

B. GRAY MATTER OF THE CENTRAL NERVOUS SYSTEM

. . . .

. . . . [The gray matter's] constituents are partly known; they are nerve cells and fibres. One must assume that it consists of several types of nerve cells.

1. *Nerve cells of the largest kind* that I have called large spinal bodies [anterior horn cells]. They occur in groups in the anterior gray matter [horn] of the spinal cord . . . .

2. . . . .

3. *Nerve cells of the smallest size.* These seem to make up the largest

bulk of the gray matter and to be, so to speak, its primary or ground substance. They have the most general distribution in the central nervous system. I shall call them later a *fine granular mass.*

The constituents of the *substantia gelatinosa* of the spinal cord (and of the pons Varolii) also seem to be of this variety. However, the nerve cells first mentioned are spherical without processes, whereas in most of the remaining places the elements of the fine, granular gray matter have an irregular shape and processes, similar to those of the largest nerve cells.

EXCERPT P. 11

B. [FRESH] GRAY MATTER

In general it appears still lighter or more transparent than the white matter in sections of equal thickness. One recognizes that it contains fibres and nerve cells. The *fibres* are not all visible as they are in the white matter. That is, among them are many which are markedly finer and have smaller dimensions [non-myelinated fibres], about a third smaller than the fibres of the white matter (the dimensions of the latter vary, too, however; yet they do not present such wide variation).

Because of the considerable mixture of elements and the confusion caused by the preparation, one recognizes in the gray matter only fibres in continuity, and not transverse sections or very short segments of individual fibres. Those that lie together in bundles can be easily distinguished with fifteen magnifications, indeed, with the naked eye; for example, the fibres that proceed transversely through the substantia gelatinosa. The individual ones, especially those of the finer kind, can only be distinguished with certainty and explored with greater magnification (fifty to four hundred).

The *nerve cells* seem to have different sizes in fresh as well as in hardened material.

A. VON KOELLIKER
(See p. 61)

As might be expected, the results of Stilling's labors were not invariably correct, and one of his critics was the great Swiss histologist Koelliker, who stated that although Stilling's data concerning the brainstem were acceptable, those on the spinal cord were less so (*Mikroskopische Anatomie*, Vol. II, Pt. I [Leipzig, 1850], p. 462). But although errors were inevitable, Koelliker's opinion seems somewhat uncharitable when one takes into account the dimensions of Stilling's studies of the cord and the primitive techniques available to him. Koelliker, on the other hand, employed chromic acid or potassium dichromate as a fixative and so was able to add to Stilling's observations. He described the white and gray matter of the cord in more detail than any previous author and then examined the intramedullary origin and destination of the motor and sensory roots, respectively. An account of the former appears on page 272 and the latter, described in his famous textbook, *Handbuch der Gewebelehre des Menschen* (Leipzig, 1852), is presented in translation below.

EXCERPT PP. 280–281

 The *posterior nerve roots*, as already mentioned, also proceed, like the anterior ones, horizontally or slightly ascending from the posterolateral sulcus through the longitudinal fibres of the white matter as far as the posterior horns. Here they break up into individual, small or stout bundles (from 0.01–0.2''' (Figs. 141 *s* and 144 *b* [figs. 79 and 80] and each by itself takes a straight course, without any direct connection with nerve cells, through the *substantia gelatinosa* into the *substantia grisea*. In doing so they take two directions. One part bends upwards in a curve, or nearly at a right angle, and takes its further, longitudinal course in the most posterior part of the *substantia grisea* just anterior to the *substantia gelatinosa*, gradually joining the posterior columns in particular; part also joins the posterior portion of the lateral columns in order to extend further as its longitudinal fibres (Figs. 141 *r* and 144 *g*). A second part of the sensory root, always in the form of a bundle (Figs. 141 *t* and 144), penetrates between the above-mentioned longitudinal bundles more anteriorly, and finally loses itself in the posterior and lateral columns; it also enters the gray commissures. The former type of fibre is frequently quite distinct in transverse sections, especially those of the posterior columns (Fig. 141 *p, q*). I have seen them best in the lower end of the cord, distal to the lumbar enlargement, where they passed towards the *conus medullaris* as far as the region of the gray central nucleus, bent backwards only in the posterior columns; they are seen likewise in the lumbar enlargement between the *substantia gelatinosa* and the posterior commissure. Also the horizontal root fibres which run in the lateral columns are often exceedingly distinct, but they seem to be considerably less numerous than those which enter the posterior columns. The connection of the gray commissure with some of the sensory root fibres is, as regards the posterior ones, not difficult to see. These fibres, in part at least, running backwards along the posterior columns continue directly into the bundles of the *substantia gelatinosa*. However, in the anterior gray commissure I have also seen fibres which run in a horizontal direction towards the tips of the posterior horns, although not in direct connection with the sensory roots. The fibres of the commissure connect not merely with the sensory roots, but also, and in fact quite obviously, with the posterior columns and less distinctly with the lateral columns. From the anterior parts of those adjacent to the base of the posterior horns, curved bundles cross in the commissures and mix with the other commissural fibres (Fig. 141 *o, u, l*). Probably these fibres pass across to the opposite side in the commissures connecting with the posterior roots; in this case a crossing of fibres in the posterior commissure is also found, similar to the anterior halves of the cord. In consequence of these observations, the sensory roots receive their fibres mainly from the posterior and lateral columns (of the posterior halves) of their side and probably also from the same two columns of the other side through the gray commissures.

PAUL EMIL FLECHSIG
(29 June 1847—22 July 1929)

Further elucidation of the internal structure of the spinal cord was determined by advances in microscopic techniques and associated methods of tracing the pathways of nerve fibre. Knowledge of the fibre itself and of its connection with the nerve cell was also essential before the complexities of the cord could be understood. Thus detailed and accurate data had to await the neuron doctrine (see Chapter II). Meantime, Türck had introduced his secondary degeneration method (pp. 851–853) of following spinal cord tracts which was especially valuable in tracing the pyramidal tract (see p. 284). By its use he could identify six pathway segments (p. 285). Stimulated by this work, the German neuroanatomist Flechsig introduced his myelogenetic technique.

Flechsig was born in Zwickau, Saxony, and took up the study of medicine in Leipzig in 1865, graduating five years later. After two years of military service, he began work as assistant in the Leipzig Institute of Pathology where he began his studies on myelogenesis. After being chief of the histology department of the Institute of Physiology, he transferred to psychiatry and became professor *ordinarius* in 1878. As director of a mental asylum he attracted students from many countries; he retired in 1921. Flechsig's study of myelogenesis occupied most of his life, directed first to the spinal cord (e.g., the dorsal spinocerebellar tract or "Flechsig's tract") and later to the internal capsule (see p. 615) and the cerebral hemispheres. His work on projection and association centers (p. 550) was derived from the last. He also contributed to clinical and pathological aspects of neurology (see Flechsig, 1927; Pfeifer, 1930, with abbreviated bibliography; Haymaker, 1953, pp. 31–35).

Flechsig's myelogenetic method (Appendix, pp. 857–858) was based on the fact that the fibres in different parts of the developing nervous system receive their myelin sheath at different stages of growth (Nielsen, 1963). As in the case of the cerebral cortex (pp. 611–619), his application of his method to the spinal cord led to many discoveries, and the following excerpt has been translated from an early book on fibre pathways in brain and cord (*Die Leitungsbahnen im Gehirn und Rückenmark des Menschen auf Grund entwickelungsgeschichtlicher Untersuchungen*, Leipzig, 1876) in which he discussed generally the myelogenetic method and compared it with that used by Türck (pp. 851–853) which employed secondary degeneration. Flechsig's method proved to be the more valuable of the two although it was not without its limitations, as he mentioned. Like Türck's method, it was especially important relative to the pyramidal tract (pp. 611–618).

EXCERPT PP. 256–259

1. The time differences [in myelination] demonstrated by two points on the same fibre which are only a few mm. apart, in regard to the presence of the complete myelin sheath, are insignificantly small wherever it is possible to prove beyond doubt their continuity. From this we may conclude that if *apparently* continuous fibre masses vary by many months in development, a *direct association* cannot exist (without disruption by the ganglion cells). This viewpoint is important, for instance, in determining the relation of the tracts of the spinal cord to those of the [medulla] *oblongata*, as well as of the fibre bundle of the white [matter] tract to that of the gray matter, since the latter is also separated into systems by means of the medullary covering.

2. Wherever we are able to observe it, the majority of the fibres of similar type and belonging to the same system, contains myelin sheaths everywhere, which appear almost simultaneously. If, therefore, *bundles of fibres* which lie adjacent to each other vary [in their development] by months, it is highly *improbable* that they *belong to the same system*.

3. Finally, we could *perhaps* consider as a guiding principle that the fibre systems of the spinal cord and of the [medulla] *oblongata* which connect with the higher centers of the cerebrum and the cerebellum, represent without exception later formations, as far as we can judge at the moment. Thus with regard to this it becomes to a large degree improbable that the posterior longitudinal bundle [posterior columns] has anything to do with the intrinsic cerebral centers, and there are still other considerations of a similar kind.

If, in addition, we compare embryological investigations [myelogenesis] with those based upon secondary degeneration, it is seen that both are closely related to one another, insofar as the latter also reveals striking morphological features of certain fibres, or systems of fibres, in their entire course. The usefulness of both procedures is obviously not the same in all areas. The *entire extent* of all systems which degenerate for long stretches cannot be established by means of secondary degeneration, because some hardly ever do so in their entire extent. This applies, for example, to the ascending degeneration of bundles of the posterior and lateral columns; a lesion which interrupts all fibres is inconceivable here. In this case embryological investigation is more successful. On the other hand, where we are dealing with the development of single parts of systems, secondary degeneration contributes better results, since in the course of development, systems are distinct in those areas where they exhibit the same behavior in their entire course. Wherever we are able to employ both methods together, the conformity of the results obviously strengthens their essential reliability. If, for example, we observe that a bundle of fibres of the gray matter of the spinal cord develops a myelin sheath several months earlier than the pyramidal tracts, and that, when the latter degenerate, their fasciculus remains completely intact, it is logical to exclude a direct association between them. Similar examples can be cited frequently; in the course of the following presentation we shall have occasion to refer to these. Inasmuch as the usefulness of secondary degeneration is founded essentially upon an explanation based on embryological organization, the fundamental importance of the latter comes clearly to light again.

The merits of our object of investigation become immediately obvious if we compare with our own results those so far obtained by the approach used by other anatomists.

Indeed, one has frequently tried to establish a relation between the cross section of the spinal cord and the various cerebral centers and to divide the white matter of the cord into its systems. If, however, we disregard experiments by individual pathologists (Türck, Bouchard, Charcot) which have been mentioned already and which still have to be evaluated, this attempt has met with little success. Even if one succeeded in following the fibre mass from the cerebrum and the cerebellum to the [medulla] oblongata, nevertheless it could not be traced further. In the material thus far used by preference, the developing central nervous system of man and of different animals, the various fibre systems demonstrate throughout no characteristic differences that would assist us in establishing the part contributed by each one. Thus one could neither determine whether their position in the spinal cord at different levels is the same, nor, in the case of those that combine with each other, how much of each was still present at a given level; one has to be content with the statement that fibres pass from certain regions of the medulla oblongata into the anterior, lateral, or posterior columns without being able to establish their approximate position and size. It is noteworthy that we have searched unsuccessfully for precise information regarding the position of the pyramidal fibres in the lateral columns, etc., especially in reviewing such investigators as Deiters, Koelliker, Henle, and Gerlach, who endeavored through careful criticism to compile accurate information.

Only in the posterior columns has a differentiation into several compartments, based upon the caliber of the fibres and their development, been made: the columns of Goll on the one hand and the remaining portions [columns of Burdach] on the other. Beyond this, one has not proceeded further, other than to separate the white matter of the spinal cord into anterior, lateral, and posterior columns, although one was quite conscious of the fact that this division did not necessarily have anything to do with division into precise systems, but essentially was rather of a topographic nature. Indeed, in many cases the manner of communication of the coarser columns of the spinal cord and of the [medulla] oblongata has remained a controversial subject, even though one has been in a position to make serial sections over an area exceeding that required to give evidence of the association. The inadequacy of the latter procedure is based essentially upon the fact that fibre systems, which frequently change their direction, remain as a rule in the same plane for short distances only. Furthermore, owing to the identical contents of different systems and to the obscuring of their characteristic qualities, a combination of various cross section pictures is difficult to achieve.

Pyramidal Tract

The two biological processes, secondary degeneration and myelogenesis, provided a method of studying spinal cord fibres in death and in development, respectively. Türck's use of the former procedure stimulated Flechsig to investigate the latter, and together these two investigators were able to sort out some of the incredibly complicated communications and pathways of the cord. Others contributed, too, and several have left their names associated with the structures they defined; thus there is Clarke's column or dorsal nucleus (1851), Goll's fasciculus gracilis (1860), Gowers' ventral cerebellar tract (1879), and Monakow's rubrospinal tract (1909).

Each spinal cord fasciculus has its own story (that of the spinothalamic tract is related in detail by Keele, 1957, pp. 101–131), but we propose to include here the history of only one, the pyramidal tract. This was the first to be investigated fully and is one of the most important. The early history of the motor pathway, especially in regard to the decussation, has been compiled by H. M. Thomas (1910), and the first selection given below represents the early, vague concept of motor pathways rather than an understanding of the pyramidal tract of the spinal cord.

Only the anatomical delineation of the pyramidal tract in the spinal cord has been included here, its course in the cerebrum being considered in Chapter X. The last selection given is that of Flechsig, which appeared in 1877. Thereafter it was thought that the tract formed a well-demarcated corticospinal system, and that the upper and lower motor neurons mentioned by Waldeyer (p. 115) were a product of the application of the neuron doctrine to the investigations of the pyramidal tract. Similarly, it was at first thought that pyramidal fibres arose only from the Betz cells (p. 439) of the motor area of the cortex (Holmes and May, 1909). However, beginning with the scepticism of Brown-Séquard (1889), the older concepts gradually became untenable, and although the anatomy and physiology of the tract has not yet been fully elucidated, it is quite clear that the pyramidal system is by no means as simple as it was at first considered. We have not entered this disputed area but have preferred to conclude with the precise delineations made by Flechsig. The subsequent literature concerning the form and function of the pyramidal tract has been surveyed by Marshall (1936), and the whole problem is discussed by Lassek (1954).

Aretaeus the Cappadocian
(A.D. *c. 81–138* or A.D. *c. 131–200*)

It was known to the author of the Hippocratic work, *On injuries in the head,* 13 (Littré [1839–1861], III, 235), that damage to one side of the brain would produce spasms on the opposite side of the body, and centuries later Aretaeus attempted to give an anatomical explanation for this curious phenomenon.

Aretaeus was born in Cappadocia in Asia Minor and was educated in Alexandria; he probably practised there although his precise dates are not known. He is recognized especially for his descriptions of disease but he was also interested in the form and function of organs. Influenced perhaps by the Hippocratic writings, he thought that all nerves from the brain decussated. He referred to a structure at the base of the brain shaped like the letter X, and it is likely that he misinterpreted the function of the optic chiasm. The following passage is from his book, *On the causes and symptoms of chronic diseases,* I, 7 (*The extant works of Aretaeus the Cappadocian,* edited and translated by F. Adams, London, 1856). He was discussing single and paired organs and how half an organ might be affected by disease.

EXCERPT P. 306

. . . . And, indeed, this thing teaches us a lesson in respect to the diversity of power and discrimination between the right side and the left. For the inherent cause is equal; and means which occasion the affection are common in both cases, whether cold or indigestion, and yet both do not suffer equally. For nature is of equal power in that which is equally paired; but it is impossible that the same thing should happen where there is an inequality. If, therefore, the commencement of the affection be below the head, such as the membrane of the spinal marrow, the parts which are homonymous [ipsilateral] and connected with it are paralysed: the right on the right side, and the left on the left side. But if the head be primarily affected on the right side, the left side of the body will be paralysed; and the right, if on the left side. The cause of this is the interchange in the origins of the nerves, for they do not pass along on the same side, the right on the right side, until their terminations; but each of them passes over to the other side from that of its origin, decussating each other in the form of the letter X.

DOMENICO MISTICHELLI

(1675—28 August 1715)

From the time of Aretaeus and Galen to the beginning of the eighteenth century little of new was added to the anatomy of the motor pathways, although the mechanism of transmission within the cord and nerves themselves was under constant consideration during the latter part of this period (pp. 155–177). The first to offer another anatomical explanation for the crossed effects of a cerebral lesion was Mistichelli.

Mistichelli was born near Pisa and after studying medicine there he became professor of medicine at the University of Pisa. In 1709 he took up an appointment at the charity hospital in Rome. In the same year he published an essay on apoplexy (*Trattato dell'apoplessia*, Rome, 1709) in which he described a decussation of the fibres of the meningeal coverings of the medulla oblongata (fig. 74), but curiously enough not of the medulla oblongata itself which he considered to be structureless even when viewed with a microscope (Capparoni, 1939). It is interesting to note that Mistichelli had returned to Erasistratus's first concept of nerves originating from the meninges (p. 12). Hence it followed, in Galenic terms, that if an obstruction of the motor nerves occurred in one hemisphere the opposite side of the body was affected. Despite the crudity of Mistichelli's account, he had at least observed the decussation in the brainstem. The following passage has been taken from Chapter VIII. After referring to the Hippocratic works mentioned on page 141, he continued as follows.

EXCERPT P. 58

2. To explain these [Hippocratic] texts it is necessary to recall what I have recently observed, that is, that the medulla oblongata externally is interwoven with fibres that have the closest resemblance to a woman's [plaited] tresses [fig. 74]. Whence it occurs that many nerves that spread out on one side have their roots on the other; so, for example, those that extend to the right arm, through such plaiting, can readily have their roots in the left fibres of the meninges. The same may be understood of those on the left proceeding from the right; and so one may go on describing many,

if not all the other nerves, that have their origins immediately from the spinal cord.

3. Therefore the supposition is clear that, if on the right side of the [cerebral] meninges or hemisphere of the cerebrum, or the extension of the medulla oblongata, through oppressive humors, or through convulsions, strangulation, or some other defect, the transit of the animal liquid [spirit] through very small interstices is impeded, it will soon happen that the arm or leg or other left part, with which those nerve filaments are in agreement, will remain either convulsed or paralyzed, or deprived of sensation and motion, because the nerves of those parts do not receive the necessary supply of spirit from the opposed part that has been injured.

François Pourfour du Petit
(See p. 265)

Whereas Mistichelli's explanation for contralateral paralysis was vague and inaccurate, Pourfour du Petit, who published in the following year, not only gave an accurate account of the decussation of the motor pathway but supported his anatomical observations with experimental investigations.

These appeared in the anonymous book already cited (p. 265), *Lettres d'un medicin des hôpitaux du roy*, etc. (Namur, 1710, "La premiére lettre contient un nouveau système du cerveau"). While serving as a military surgeon Pourfour du Petit observed the contralateral motor paralysis resulting from an abscess following a cerebral wound and succeeded in producing comparable results in experiments on dogs; in each instance, the motor signs were opposite to the cerebral hemisphere lesion. His anatomical findings were as presented below.

EXCERPT PP. 10–12

Here, I believe, Sir, are quite convincing proofs that the animal spirit changes from one side to the other. The problem is to understand how this crossing comes about, and I believe that I have discovered the answer.

All the cortical substance of the cerebral hemispheres supplies the medullary part [white matter] which is itself but a mass of an infinite number of tubes, some of which constitute the corpus callosum while others collect together to form the middle fluted bodies [corona radiata]. The inferior part of the cerebral peduncles (of the medulla oblongata [i.e., in his terminology, midbrain, pons, and medulla oblongata]) which can be seen between the optic nerves [optic tracts] and the pons, is a continuation of the middle fluted bodies [corona radiata]. The medullary fibres of which it is composed pass through the pons, separated from each other by the pontine fibres with which they are intertwined. They collect together again at the inferior part of the pons in order to form exclusively the pyramidal bodies.

Each pyramidal body divides at its inferior part into two large bundles of fibres. But more often there are three and sometimes four. Those on the right side pass to the left and those on the left pass to the right, binding themselves together as can be seen at D in the first figure [fig. 73]. There is nothing easier than to demonstrate on a prepared brain that the medullary fibres which pass through the pons make up solely the pyramidal bodies . . . . On account of the direction of the fibres shown, it is very different from all similar efforts that have been made up to the present time. These fibres change places with one another so markedly that the description that I give of them cannot be of much value if it is not illustrated with drawings.

Ludwig Türck
(22 July 1810—25 February 1868)

Anatomists in the early nineteenth century became increasingly aware of the decussation of the pyramids as described by Pourfour du Petit, but the arrangement of the pyramidal fibres in the cord was not understood until the middle of the century. The detailed study of the internal anatomy of the spinal cord began with Stilling (pp. 270–275). He did not, however, attempt to map out individual fibre tracts, mainly because his research methods were much too primitive. However, he stimulated others to do so. One of these was Türck who applied to the problem the phenomenon of secondary degeneration which had been described by Waller in 1850 (pp. 70–74). Thus he was the first to identify accurately a spinal cord pathway, the crossed and uncrossed pyramidal tract; the description by Burdach in 1806 of the fasciculus cuneatus had been macroscopical only.

Türck was born in Vienna and attended the Medical School there, obtaining a degree in 1837. He spent the rest of his career in Vienna and it was from his pioneer endeavor that the famous Viennese School of Neuropsychiatry arose. In 1847 he became chief of the Department of Neurology, one of the first in Europe. His main work was with secondary degeneration in the central nervous system, studied by means of neurological diseases and experimental investigations. He followed tracts in the spinal cord and showed that their degeneration took place in the direction in which they conducted. Türck also worked on systemic disease of the spinal cord, neuro-ophthalmology, skin dermatomes (pp. 312–316), and various neurological diseases. His contributions to neurology, however, seem to have been overshadowed by his researches in laryngology which occupied his later years (see Neuburger, 1910; Türck, 1910; Haymaker, 1953, pp. 92–95; Lesky, 1964).

By observing the degeneration of the nerve fibres of the spinal cord after their interruption, mainly by compressing lesions, Türck was able to delineate six pathway segments on each side of the cord (two anterior, two lateral, and two posterior); one of these contained the direct or crossed pyramidal tract and another the indirect or uncrossed pyramidal tract (of Türck). In the following passage from "Über sekundäre Erkrankung einzelner Rückenmarkstränge und ihrer Fortsetzungen zum Gehirne" (*Z. kais. kön. Ges. Ärzte, Wien*, 1852, 8 [ii]:511–534), he summarized his findings. He first described and named the pyramidal pathways and then discussed the spinal cord tracts in general (see pp. 851–853 for description of his method).

It should be noted that at this time Türck believed the pyramidal tract to originate in the basal gray matter of the brain and not in the cerebral cortex. Therefore, the name he used, *pyramidal*, referred to the pyramids of the brainstem and not to the pyramidal cells of Betz in the cerebral cortex; they had not yet been described (p. 439).

EXCERPT PP. 531–533

1. If, in disease centers in the cerebrum or spinal cord, the conductivity of certain medullary tracts is inhibited for a long time owing to atrophy, granular cells [compound granular corpuscles] develop in considerable numbers and induce a metamorphosis which extends through the subsequent course [of the tracts].

2. If, in such cases, one now makes several transverse sections through the spinal cord, the medulla oblongata, the pons, and through the cerebral peduncle including its ganglia, and if one compares the affected areas *with each other* and notes their position in individual cross sections, one gains an insight into the anatomical course of the medullary tracts which show secondary degeneration. At the same time, however, one also learns something about the direction in which these fasciculi run. The results obtained, which so far correspond in part with statements made relative to the fibre pathway, but which could not be entirely elucidated with the use of known anatomical and physiological evidence, are as follows:

3. A medullary tract passes from the cerebral peduncle downwards by continuing into the longitudinal fibres of the ipsilateral half of the pons, then into the ipsilateral pyramid. At the decussation of the pyramids it proceeds to the medulla oblongata (in one case in two bundles) of the opposite side where, as the posterior half of the lateral column, it proceeds downwards to the vicinity of the termination of the spinal cord. For the sake of brevity we have named it the pyramidal-lateral-column-tract (*Pyramiden-Seitenstrangbahn* [crossed or lateral pyramidal tract]).

4. The pyramidal-lateral-column-tract conducts in a centrifugal direction a current which originates in the lenticular nucleus, the corpus striatum, the thalamus, and the medullary layer of the cerebrum. However, we

cannot say with certainty that this is a motor impulse to the opposite side of the body, but it is on the same side as the conducting [motor] tract of the spinal cord. The tract so designated is seen to manifest secondary degeneration with old, apoplectic, and [other] brain lesions in the above-mentioned parts of the brain.

5. A second medullary tract also enters as a longitudinal fibre bundle from the cerebral peduncle through the ipsilateral half of the pons; however, it does not cross as the pyramids do in the medulla oblongata but descends on the same side of the spinal cord as a medial segment of the anterior column where its secondary degeneration terminates slightly more cephalad than in the posterior segment of the opposite lateral column [crossed pyramidal tract]. We have named it the capsular-anterior-column-tract (*Hulsen-Vorderstrangbahn* [uncrossed pyramidal tract of Türck]).

6. The capsular-anterior-column-tract conducts an impulse which is transmitted in a centrifugal direction from the lenticular nucleus and corpus striatum on the side of the cerebral lesion, and simultaneously to the side of the body which is opposite the conducting [motor] tract of the spinal cord. Presumably this is a motor impulse. Thus far, the tract so designated has been found affected as a result of chronic lesions in the lenticular nucleus and corpus striatum.

7. Apart from these two tracts in the cited cases of brain disease, no other tract of the spinal cord, nor of the gray matter, was seen to have secondary degeneration.

8. It cannot be decided whether the motor impulse which originates in the cerebrum is conducted downwards in both of the mentioned tracts or by other pathways.

EXCERPT PP. 533–534

13. The remaining tracts of the spinal cord must be considered anatomically and physiologically distinct from those discussed so far. In the first place the separation of the medial and lateral segments of the anterior columns by the anterior intermediate sulcus, as seen in the cervical region of the cord, is a complete division which extends to the neighborhood of the termination of the spinal cord. Something similar probably happens in the case of the division of the posterior tract into two by the posterior intermediate sulcus, although these could only be demonstrated as far as the level of the fourth thoracic nerve. A similar separation, although not indicated externally by a fissure, exists between the anterior and posterior segments of the lateral columns. Thus, each half of the spinal cord contains six medullary bundles. Second, it is certain that no centripetal nerve current is transmitted from the lower extremities or from the lower segments of the

thorax through the tract just discussed. It might be possible that they could serve as pathways for a current which originated in the upper extremities or in the upper segment of the thorax; however, this is unlikely. It is undecided whether these tracts conduct centrifugal currents which perhaps originate in certain areas of the cerebrum or the cerebellum.

PAUL EMIL FLECHSIG
(*See p. 277*)

The myelogenetic method of examining the nervous system introduced by Flechsig (Appendix, pp. 857–858) played an outstanding role in detection of the detailed constitution and distribution of the pyramidal tracts. With its help he studied their variations and established that they originated in the cerebral cortex and not in the basal ganglia as Türck had believed. A link with physiologists investigating cortical function (p. 447) had already been made. Flechsig was thus dealing with the axons of the so-called upper motor neurons but he did not at this time detect the second component of the tract, the lower motor neuron. This was the work of the neuronists and of Wilhelm His, *Senior* (1887) in particular (p. 99), who identified the anterior horn cells and their efferent fibers in the anterior spinal roots. Waldeyer (1891) made reference to the two-neuron pathway (p. 115).

The following passages have been translated from a long article that was serialized between 1877 and 1878 ("Über 'Systemerkrankungen' im Rückenmark," *Arch. Heilk.*, 1877, 18:101–141, 289–343, 461–483; 1878, 19:52–90, 441–447). The portions dealing with the pyramidal tract in the brainstem and brain are presented in Chapter X (p. 611).

EXCERPT PP. 296–303

1. *As a rule, the right as well as the left pyramid divides into a direct and a lateral pyramidal tract (semidecussation of the pyramids)*, so that we find altogether four pyramidal tracts in the spinal cord (75% of the cases that I have examined). Thus, *each individual* pyramid divides in *all possible proportions* into the ipsilateral direct or the contralateral lateral tract and *each given manner of distribution of the left pyramid may combine with any given one of the right. The most frequent finding is that each pyramid contributes about 3–9% of its spinal cord fibres to the direct tract, and, corresponding to this, about 97–91% to the lateral tract.* Therefore the lateral pyramidal tracts contain as a rule considerably more fibres than the direct pyramidal tracts. However, in some of the individuals whom I have examined the proportion of the latter increased to approximately 90%, and, on the other hand, decreased to approximately 1% (considering that

for the time being we are only concerned with four tract cases). The last modification is immediately followed by a second main type.

2. *All of the pyramidal fibres* that reach the spinal cord are able to *cross* into the lateral tracts (*total decussation of the pyramids,* 11% of my "reliable" cases); the direct tracts are then completely missing, and we find only *two* pyramidal tracts in the spinal cord.

3. Lastly, one pyramid may—again with a great variety of proportions—be distributed in the ipsilateral direct and contralateral lateral tract (*semilateral semidecussation of the pyramids*). The number of the pyramidal tracts of the spinal cord is then *three* (in 14% of my reliable cases).

It follows from the aforesaid report that no generalized valid assertions can be made regarding either the *number* of the pyramidal tracts in the spinal cord or the *extent of each individual one* . . . .

. . . . The variable arrangement of the pyramidal tracts, considering its frequent occurrence, is a fertile source in particular for asymmetries of the direct pyramidal tracts, a behavior which already deserves attention because it results in frequent simulation of pathological conditions, partial atrophy of the medulla, etc., for structural relationships which are within normal ranges.

As regards the *longitudinal extent of the pyramidal tracts,* their position and other behavior at different levels of the spinal cord, the *lateral pyramidal tracts* can as a rule be followed to the origins of the third and fourth sacral nerves, and it is remarkable that this is so [in cases] when they receive only a small part of the pyramidal fibres. They are located throughout in the posterior halves of the lateral columns (*ps, ps',* Figs. 1, 4, 5, 6, 7 [fig. 82]) and here they form compact bundles, mostly infiltrated by a few nerve fibres of a different kind; only in the lower dorsal and upper portion of the spinal cord are numerous heterogeneous elements inserted between them which for the most part belong to the direct cerebellar tract of the lateral column. The lateral pyramidal tracts only touch the *gray matter* corresponding to the posterolateral margin of the substantia gelatinosa of the posterior horn (Fig. 1). More anteriorly, towards the processus reticulares (Lenhossek [reticular process or formation]) they are separated from the gray columns by longitudinal fasciculi of different systems. The behavior with regard to the *periphery* of the cord varies at different levels. The lateral pyramidal tracts are separated from the pia mater for the most part by a now thinner, now thicker layer of longitudinal fibres, the direct cerebellar tract of the lateral columns that will soon be described in more detail. In the upper half of the spinal cord they only touch the periphery in the area of the second to the fourth cervical nerves just lateral to the posterior roots. In the lower half of the spinal cord they reach the surface more and more, for the direct cerebellar tracts of the lateral columns become gradually thinner distally. Thus the whole external surface of the lateral pyramidal tracts lies directly against the pia mater in the lumbar enlargement (*ps*, Fig. 7). Its cross section from upper to lower end [of the cord] decreases in size consistently, which occurs because its fibres successively curve towards the gray substance. The decrease in the linear cross section appears in the enlargements, especially the cervical one, to be more extensive than in the dorsal spinal cord.

The *direct pyramidal tracts* demonstrate considerable individual variations in their longitudinal extension because sometimes they reach only to the cervical cord and sometimes to the lumbar enlargement. In general the rule prevails that the greater the number of their fibres in the uppermost cervical portion the more easily they can be demonstrated distally. In the *majority of cases* they extend to the *middle of the dorsal cord* so that in the lower regions of the cord one finds more than two pyramidal tracts only as an exception . . . . The cross section (the number of fibres) of the direct pyramidal tracts constantly decreases from above downwards, similar to that of the lateral tracts. Its location is as a rule in the medial part of the anterior columns . . . . The form of the cross section changes in individual and in region; most frequently it approaches an ellipse, the short axis of which is set transversely.

. . . .

. . . .

The pyramidal fibres do not possess a uniform *caliber*; some resemble the finest [non-myelinated], others the strongest fibres of the white columns, still others take a middle position . . . .

. . . . Therefore we must assume, on the basis of embryological findings [myelogenesis], that the pyramidal fibres of the spinal cord terminate (temporarily!) in the anterior horn of the gray substance in some manner.

If now we once more review the disclosures obtained with the help of embryology, the evidence of particular interest is that the pyramidal tracts present a *direct process of the white matter of the cerebral lobes* which extends to the lowest regions of the spinal cord, a fact which, among other things, may be the key to the elucidation of the involvement of our tracts in innumerable cerebral diseases. If, furthermore, upon the basis of our investigations we try to decide the question whether the pyramidal tracts present an *elementary fibre system* defined in the above sense, then much is still lacking to justify an unequivocal affirmative answer. Nevertheless, it is very noticeable that everything we were able to establish and report regarding the origin and the termination of the pyramidal fibres speaks *for and not against* the assumption that they fit into the mechanism of the central organs *in a consistent manner*. We have reached the assumption that:

1. All pyramidal fibres originate in the cerebral cortex; that they

2. all descend, without demonstrable interruption by other kinds of gray masses, into the anterior gray horns of the cord, homologous to the gray matter of the cerebrum; that finally

3. a temporary termination must somehow take place in the latter sites [anterior horns].

CHAPTER V

FUNCTION OF THE SPINAL CORD

Introduction

In the second century A.D., Galen contended that the spinal cord was basically a conducting structure, and through it the motor, sensory, and some of the autonomic functions of the body below the neck were mediated. It is therefore necessary to investigate the history of the discovery of the motor and sensory activities of the cord; the autonomic nervous system will not be included. It is now known that the cord is fundamentally a series of reflex centers with up and down traffic as a later addition.

This history is remarkable for the very long gap that separated the first significant investigator, Galen, from the next experimentalists of note in the second decade of the nineteenth century. Hence, apart from the work of Galen, the story is restricted to the nineteenth and twentieth centuries. The first problem presented here is concerned with efforts to differentiate the spinal roots according to their function, and then to discover how the fibres of these roots are distributed to the peripheral structures, chiefly the muscles and skin. F. A. Longet (1841, pp. 3–86) has considered in sequence the contributions of investigators to the problem of cord function from Galen to Valentin.

GALEN
(See p. 14)

One of the most important features of Galen's brilliant anatomical discoveries was his insistence upon their correlation with function, and, therefore, it might be suggested that we have done him an injustice by making an artificial separation between his descriptions of anatomy and function. However, the following excerpts may be read in conjunction with the passages on pages 260 to 263, thus offering a more complete, truer impression of Galen's contributions to the anatomy and physiology of the spinal cord.

Little or nothing was known of the function of the cord before Galen's famous experiments which, incidentally, provide us with an excellent example of his use of the experimental method. They were not to be repeated or extended until Robert

291

Whytt began his study of the spinal cord in the middle of the eighteenth century (pp. 336–342). The following excerpts, giving an account of Galen's experiments on transverse section of the spinal cord, have been taken from his *Anatomical procedures*, IX, 13–14 (Duckworth, 1962, pp. 22–26). Details are included only of those carried out in the cervical region, although he investigated all levels, using the living, unanesthetized ape or the monkey.

EXCERPT PP. 22–26

. . . . So when you have cut this [bone], and have brought the instrument to the site of the spinal marrow, then at this stage you must so manipulate it, that thereby you may feel about with your hand on it in the depth [of the wound] and rock it to and fro so as to leave no part of the spinal medulla undivided. After the incision, in all the nerves which lie below the place where the transection has been made, both the two potentialities are lost, I mean the capacity of sensation and the capacity of movement, and also all the bodily parts of the animal in which they are distributed become insensitive and motionless, a result that is inevitable, clear and intelligible . . . .

CHAPTER 14. SUMMARY AND CONCLUSIONS, WITH OBSERVATIONS ON THE EFFECTS OF TRANSECTION OF THE CERVICAL SPINAL CORD

To sum up briefly, then, the matter is as I described it before: the parts of the body which have become paralysed, and from which their movement has been taken away, are those of which the nerve proceeding to them has its root, its head, below the dividing incision through the spinal marrow. Hence, from the anatomy of the nerves, you can easily infer the derangement which will befall the animal as the result of the transection of the spinal marrow in all its several parts. Similarly, when you have read the book 'On the Causes of Respiration,' and the book 'On the Voice,' you understand what degree of damage falls upon the respiration, and upon the voice, at the transection of each single vertebra. . . . If now you know from their anatomy where the nerves of these muscles arise, then you also know for certain when any single one of these muscles will be paralysed.

But I should like to add more to what I have mentioned here, namely, that should the spinal marrow that lies between the skull and the first vertebra be severed, or the meninx whicn protects the end of the posterior ventricle of the brain be cut through, then at once the whole body of the animal becomes deprived of movement. It is just here that you will see, in the temples of the gods, the oxen receive the stab when the so-called sacrificers of oxen cut into them. But as for the incision which is made behind the first vertebra, it inflicts on the animal just the same manifestations, not because it lays open the first ventricle [*fourth* in modern terminology] but because it paralyses the feet of the animal, and arrests the whole of its respiration. And this is found also with regard to the incision which is made behind the second, third, and fourth vertebra, when in making the cut you go to work thoroughly, so that you divide the nerve which springs off at its [fourth vertebra's] junction with the fifth. However, the first [i.e., upper] segments of the neck still move themselves in the animal on which the cut has been made in such a manner. Transection of the spinal marrow behind the fifth vertebra paralyses all the remaining parts of the thorax, and arrests their movements, but the diaphragm remains almost unscathed, and so also does a small portion of the upwardly ascending part of the musculature of the thorax [*Mm. scaleni*]. The transection which takes place behind the sixth vertebra damages in the same way the upwardly ascending thoracic musculature, and the diaphragm meets with less damage than that which followed in consequence of the preceding cut. But after the transection which takes place behind the seventh vertebra, and more particularly after that made behind the eighth vertebra, the whole of the mobility of the diaphragm remains unscathed, and indeed in most instances still more so than is the case after the cut behind the sixth vertebra. Again the mobility of the upwardly ascending musculature, and the mobility of the whole neck will remain quite free from damage, but the intercostal muscles do not at the same time remain uninjured thereby. For the mobility of this musculature is destroyed and becomes totally lost when one imposes the cut upon any one of the vertebrae of the neck, and the whole hind-brain is cut off from the first thoracic vertebra. Amongst the proofs of that is the fact that the activity of the intercostal muscles becomes totally lost when one carries through the spinal medulla behind the first thoracic vertebra a cut which completely divides it, whereas a slight proportion of this activity stays retained when the cut takes place behind the second vertebra. In connection with that there is the fully analogous point that those intercostal muscles which lie higher up than the situation of the incision preserve their activity, whereas the activity of the muscles lying below the site of the incision will be abolished.

A passage in *The sites of diseases*, III, 14 (Daremberg [1854–1856], II) described the results of hemisection of the spinal cord.

EXCERPT P. 579

Dissection has shown us that the motor nerves for all the voluntarily moved parts of the animal below the neck take their origin from the spinal cord. You have been told frequently that this part is called spinal cord, but often simply dorsal [cord]. You have also seen that the nerves that move the thorax take their origin from the cervical cord, and, moreover, you have been told that transverse incisions that sever the cord completely deprive all parts of the body below this level of sensation and movement, since the cord receives the faculties of sensation and voluntary movement from the brain. You have also seen during dissection that transverse incisions of the cord that reach only its center [hemisection] do not paralyze all the lower parts but only the parts situated directly below the incision; the right when the right is cut, and the left when the left is cut.

It is thus clear that when the faculties of the brain are prevented from reaching the origin of the cord [upper cervical], all structures below, but excluding the face, will be deprived of movement and sensation.

Finally, in the *Anatomical procedures*, VIII, 6 (Kühn [1821–1833], II, 681), Galen dealt with a third type of experiment, a midline, longitudinal spinal cord incision:

If one cuts the spinal cord along the median line from above downwards, there is no resultant paralysis of the intercostal nerves nor of those of the right or the left side, even in the lumbar region or in the legs.

[César] Julien Jean [César] Legallois
(1 February 1770—c. 10 February 1814)

As already pointed out, investigation of spinal cord function was held up by the persistence of the Galenic concept that the cord was merely an ingeniously constructed pathway for the nerves proceeding from the brain to their peripheral destinations. As such it could have no independent activity. However, on rare occasions a few had turned their attention to it, as, for example, Leonardo da Vinci (1452–1519):

The frog retains life for some hours after being deprived of its head, heart, and intestines. And if you prick the said nerve [spinal cord], it suddenly twitches and dies . . . . It thus seems that here lies the fundamentum of motion and life.

But Leonardo had no influence on the development of anatomy or physiology (O'Malley and Saunders, 1952, p. 352; see also Plate 154 for illustration of the cord; Hopstock, 1921, especially p. 166).

As with the anatomy of the cord, so, too, its physiology was neglected until the eighteenth century. The work of Whytt at this time was of great importance and its relevance to the idea of reflex activity will be dealt with in Chapter VI (pp. 336–342). One of his discoveries was the fact that in the frog only a part of the cord, its upper or lower half, was necessary for reflex movements. These investigations were extended by the work of the French physiologist Legallois which stemmed from the animal experiments of Fontana, who by means of artificial respiration had been able to maintain life after decapitation.

Legallois was born at Cherneix on the coast of Brittany and studied medicine at Caen and Paris, although his studies were disturbed by the Revolution. He was graduated in 1801, and in 1813 was appointed to the staff of the Bicêtre; he died of pneumonia at the relatively early age of forty-four. Legallois was one of the first experimental physiologists of the nineteenth century, and the long line of renowned French physiologists, Magendie, Flourens, Bernard, Brown-Séquard, etc., began with him. He is remembered in particular for his observations on the site of the respiratory center in the medulla oblongata, which was the first contribution to the modern concept of brain localization (pp. 469 ff.), and for his support of the neurogenic theory of heart action. Like Whytt, he was an avowed vitalist (see C. J. Legallois, 1814–1815; E. Legallois, 1830).

On 9 September 1811, at a meeting of the Imperial Institute in Paris, Legallois presented a report of his experiments in rabbits (*Expériences sur le principe de la vie, notamment sur celui des mouvemens du coeur, et sur la siège de ce principe* [Paris, 1812]). The following selections, presenting Legallois' conclusions, have been translated from the edition of 1812.

EXCERPT PP. 282–283

From these facts, Dr. Le Gallois concluded that decapitation does nothing more than arrest inspiratory motions, and that consequently the source of all these motions is in the brain; but the source of the life of the trunk is in the trunk itself. In seeking afterwards for the immediate seat of each of these two principles, he discovered that the seat of the inspiratory movements is in that part of the medulla oblongata which gives rise to the nerves of the eighth pair [glossopharyngeal, vagus, and accessory cranial nerves] and that of the life of the trunk is in the spinal cord. Each part of the body is not animated by all of the cord, but only by the portion from which it receives its nerves, so that by destroying only one portion of the cord, only the parts of the body which correspond to that portion die. Moreover, if the circulation of the blood in a portion of the cord is intercepted, life is enfeebled and soon completely extinguished in all the parts which receive their nerves from it. There are then two methods of causing life to cease in any particular part of the body of an animal: the one by destroying the cord from which this part receives its nerves, the other by intercepting in it the circulation of blood.

It follows therefore that the support of life in one part of the body depends essentially upon two conditions; namely, the integrity of the corresponding portion of the cord, and the circulation of the blood.

EXCERPT PP. 138–141

. . . . section of the spinal cord near the occiput and decapitation destroy the inspiratory movements without causing cessation of life in the trunk; this only dies through asphyxia, and at the end of the same period of time when respiration has been prevented by any other means, presuming hemorrhage to have been arrested.

If asphyxia is circumvented by insufflation of the lungs, the life of the animal may be prolonged for a period of time, the *maximum* in this case being the same as after section of the eighth pair of nerves.

If, instead of decapitation [decerebration] being performed near the occiput, it is performed in the cranium so as to spare that part in which the prime mover of respiration resides, and to leave it in continuity with the spinal cord, the animal may live and breathe by means of its own power and without any assistance, until it dies of inanition. This is the *maximum* of its life in this instance; but, for well-known causes, cold-blooded animals are the only ones in which this happens.

Not only does the life of the trunk in general depend upon the spinal cord, but the life of each part of it in particular depends upon the portion of the cord from which it receives its nerves, so that by destroying a certain amount of the spinal cord we induce death only in those parts which receive their nerves from the destroyed part of the cord. All those which receive their nerves from undestroyed cord continue to live for a longer or shorter time.

If, instead of destroying the cord, transverse sections of it are made, the parts [of the body] corresponding to each segment of the cord enjoy sensation and voluntary movement, but without any harmony and in a manner as independent of one another as if the whole body of the animal had been cut transversely in the same places; to put it briefly, there are, in this case, as many quite distinct centers of sensation as there are segments made of the cord.

CHARLES BELL
(*November 1774—28 April 1842*)

Since at least the time of Herophilus (*fl. c.* 300 B.C.) there had been recognition of a distinction between motor and sensory nerves (p. 144), and Galen had argued (p. 147) that each kind came from different parts of the brain. However, no detailed study of this division of function was made until the nineteenth century. In 1809 Alexander Walker (1839, pp. 19–29) discussed the problem anonymously and, respecting the roots of the spinal cord, considered the anterior to be sensory and the posterior motor. About two years earlier Bell had begun to investigate the anatomy of the nervous system.

Charles Bell was born in Edinburgh, the younger brother of John Bell, the famous anatomist of that city. He studied medicine in Edinburgh but, for a variety of reasons, moved to London in 1804. After years of hard work he bought the famous Great Windmill Street School of Anatomy, initiated by William Hunter, and in 1813 he was appointed surgeon to the Middlesex Hospital. Although Bell became one of London's most outstanding anatomists and surgeons, in 1836 he accepted the chair of surgery in Edinburgh which he held until his death six years later. In addition to being a distinguished anatomist and surgeon, Bell was an excellent physiologist, pathologist, and artist, but his greatest contribution to medical knowledge was his work on the form and function of the nervous system. His scientific work was recognized with a knighthood (see Gordon-Taylor and Walls, 1958).

Like many before him (Chapter IX), Bell was of the opinion that different parts of the brain had different functions. Like the ancients, he was impressed in this regard by contrasting the cerebrum to the cerebellum, and sought evidence for their divergent functional behavior in their extensions into the spinal cord and roots. Thus he considered the cerebrum to be the center for motion and sensation and these faculties to travel in the anterior part of the spinal cord and the anterior spinal roots. He believed that "secret" or vital actions, that is, involuntary or reflex activities, were centered in the cerebellum (see Willis, p. 639), the posterior columns, and the posterior roots of the cord. He made no reference to the posterior roots as having a sensory function, and, in fact, Bell could not have observed sensory phenomena in his experiments since, as it later transpired, he had used stunned rabbits. Thus he did not make a clear distinction between the spinal roots, as is sometimes claimed. He did nevertheless provide the first experimental evidence that the anterior roots convey motor impulses, and this is as far as one can go in the matter. It should also be noted that his contribution to the idea of localization within the brain was neither outstanding nor influential.

Throughout his life Charles Bell corresponded with his elder brother George Joseph, professor of Scots Law at Edinburgh University (*Letters of Sir Charles Bell, K.H., F.R.S.L. & E. Selected from his correspondence with his brother George Joseph Bell* [London, 1870]). The following letter was dated 12 March 1810.

EXCERPT PP. 170-171

I write to tell you that I really think I am going to establish my Anatomy of the Brain on facts the most important that have been discovered in the history of the science.

You recollect that I have entertained the idea that the parts of the brain were distinct in function, and that the cerebrum was in a particular manner the organ of mind, and this from other circumstances than what I am now to detail to you.

It occurred to me that as there were four grand divisions of the brain, so there were four grand divisions of the spinal marrow; first, a lateral division, then a division into the back and forepart. Next it occurred to me that all the spinal nerves had within the sheath of the spinal marrow two roots—one from the back part, another from before. Whenever this occurred to me I thought that I had obtained a method of inquiry into the function of the parts of the brain.

Experiment 1. I opened the spine and pricked and injured the *posterior* filaments of the nerves—no motion of the muscles followed. I then touched the *anterior* division—immediately the parts were convulsed.

Experiment 2. I now destroyed the posterior part of *the spinal marrow* by the point of a needle—no convulsive movement followed. I injured the anterior part, and the animal was convulsed.

It is almost superfluous to say that the part of the spinal marrow having sensibility comes from the cerebrum; the posterior and insensible part of the spinal marrow belongs to the cerebellum.

Taking these facts as they stand, is it not most curious that there should be thus established a distinction in the parts of a *nerve*, and that a nerve should be insensible? But then, as the foundation of a great system, if I can but sustain them by repeated experiments, I am made, and a real gratification ensured for a large portion of my existence.

In August 1811 Bell published privately a small pamphlet entitled *Idea of a new anatomy of the brain submitted for the observations of his friends* ([London, 1811]) which included the passage given below supporting his contention of a functional localization in the brain. Despite Bell's request, it seems that none of his friends responded with observations on the publication, and none of them felt inspired to repeat his work.

EXCERPT PP. 20–23

In thinking of this subject, it is natural to expect that we should be able to put the matter to proof by experiment. But how is this to be accomplished, since any experiment direct upon the brain itself must be difficult, if not impossible?—I took this view of the subject. The *medulla spinalis* has a central division, and also a distinction into anterior and posterior fasciculi, corresponding with the anterior and posterior portions of the brain. Further we can trace down the crura of the *cerebrum* into the anterior fasciculus of the spinal marrow, and the crura of the *cerebellum* into the posterior fasciculus. I thought that here I might have an opportunity of touching the *cerebellum*, as it were, through the posterior portion of the spinal marrow, and the cerebrum by the anterior portion. To this end I made experiments which, though they were not conclusive, encouraged me in the view I had taken.

I found that injury done to the anterior portion of the spinal marrow, convulsed the animal more certainly than injury done to the posterior portion; but I found it difficult to make the experiment without injuring both portions.

Next considering that the spinal nerves have a double root, and being of opinion that the properties of the nerves are derived from their connections with the parts of the brain, I thought that I had an opportunity of putting my opinion to the test of experiment, and of proving at the same time that nerves of different endowments were in the same cord, and held together by the same sheath.

On laying bare the roots of the spinal nerves, I found that I could cut across the posterior fasciculus of nerves, which took its origin from the posterior portion of the spinal marrow without convulsing the muscles of the back; but that on touching the anterior fasciculus with the point of the knife, the muscles of the back were immediately convulsed.

Such were my reasons for concluding that the cerebrum and the cerebellum were parts distinct in function, and that every nerve possessing a double function obtained that by having a double root. I now saw the meaning of the double connection of the nerves with the spinal marrow; and also the cause of that seeming intricacy in the connections of nerves throughout their course, which were not double at their origins.

The spinal nerves being doubled, and having their roots in the spinal marrow, of which a portion comes from the cerebrum and a portion from the cerebellum, they convey the attributes of both grand divisions of the brain to every part; and therefore the distribution of such nerves is simple, one nerve supplying its destined part.

FRANÇOIS MAGENDIE
(6 October 1783—7 October 1855)

Bell had hoped that he would be able to formulate, as he put it, "a system captivating as the circulation," and he also wrote that "on this I shall swell myself into importance, and make myself very happy" (*Letters of Sir Charles Bell*, London, 1870, 25 May 1810 and July 1811 respectively). However, knowledge of the *Idea* was necessarily limited and Bell made no further efforts to extend his experimental evidence; nor did he refer to his ideas in an edition of his textbook on anatomy and physiology published in 1816. His subsequent interest in nerves was directed to the functions of the facial and trigeminal cranial nerves, and through this interest he made amiable contact with the great French physiologist Magendie, who was to carry out decisive experiments to demonstrate the difference between the anterior and posterior spinal roots.

Magendie was born in Bordeaux and received his medical training in Paris where he was graduated in 1808. He then became prosector in the Anatomical Institute of Paris and physician to the Central Bureau of Hospitals and at the Salpêtrière. In 1836 he was appointed professor of physiology and general pathology at the Collège de France. Here he built up his school and continued his teaching, research studies, and practice until his death, when he was succeeded by Claude Bernard (p. 241). His experimental work was extensive, but, under the influence of the *idéologue* philosophers, he was concerned more with the collection of data than with interpretation of them. He was well known for his disregard of his laboratory animals as well as the feelings of his contemporaries. Nevertheless, one of his greatest contributions was the experimental techniques he created. Magendie may also be considered to have been the founder of modern pharmacodynamics (see Olmsted, 1944; Temkin, 1946).

It is clear that Magendie had no detailed knowledge of Bell's experiments on the spinal roots, although it is possible that contact with Bell and his assistant and son-in-law John Shaw, in 1821, may have influenced him. In any event he embarked upon a series of investigations, the results of which he published in his own journal in 1822 ("Expériences sur les fonctions des racines des nerfs rachidiens," *J. Physiol. exp. path., Paris*, 1822, 2:276–279). In his report, which is commendably brief and precise, Magendie stated that he had for a long time contemplated the study of the spinal cord roots but that his attempts had failed owing to technical difficulties. At last, however, he had been able to expose the spinal cord in a six-weeks-old puppy.

EXCERPT PP. 277–279

. . . . Then I had a view of the posterior roots of the lumbar and sacral pairs, and by lifting them successively with the blades of some small scissors, I was able to cut them on one side, leaving the cord intact. I did not know what the result of this attempt would be; I reunited the wound with a skin suture and observed the animal. At first I thought that the limb corresponding to the cut nerves was entirely paralyzed; it seemed insensible to the strongest pricks and pressures and also appeared to be immobile; but soon, to my great astonishment, I saw it move in a very apparent manner, although there was a complete absence of sensation. A second and third experiment gave me exactly the same result, and I began to consider it as probable that the posterior roots of the spinal nerves had different functions from the anterior, and that they were more particularly related to sensation.

Naturally, it occurred to me to cut the anterior roots and to leave the posterior intact, but such an undertaking was easier to conceive than to perform, for how could I reveal the anterior part of the cord without interfering with the posterior roots? . . . . [He eventually overcame this difficulty.] Nothing more was needed and in a few moments I had cut all the pairs that I wished to sever. As in the preceding experiment, I cut only one side in order to have a means of comparison. One may imagine how inquisitively I followed the effects of this section; no doubts remained, for the limb was completely immobile and flaccid, although sensation was definitely preserved. Finally, so that nothing might be neglected, I cut the anterior and posterior roots at the same time; there was absolute loss of sensation and movement.

I repeated and varied these experiments on several species of animals; the results that I have just announced were confirmed in the most complete manner, both for the anterior and for the posterior limbs. I have continued these researches, and I shall give a more detailed account of them in the next issue; it is enough for me to announce today as positive, that the anterior and posterior roots of the nerves that arise from the spinal cord have different functions; that the posterior appear more particularly related to sensation, and the anterior to movement.

Magendie investigated other approaches to the spinal roots but concluded that his original method was the most reliable. In further experiments he studied the effects of strychnine (*nux vomica*), of pinching, pulling, and pricking, and of galvanic stimulation to the roots. His conclusion was that although the anterior and posterior roots were predominantly motor and sensory respectively, there seemed to be some overlapping of function; this was owing to the appearance of reflex phenomena, not understood at that time, and to the course taken by certain posterior root fibres. Magendie's report appeared in the same publication and year as his previous paper ("Expériences sur les fonctions des racines des nerfs qui naissent de la moelle épinière," pp. 366–371).

EXCERPT PP. 367–369

I then wished to submit the results of which I spoke earlier to a special test. Everyone knows that nux vomica produces general tetanic convulsions of great violence in man and animals. I wanted to learn if these convulsions would still take place in a limb in which the motor nerves had been cut, and if they would also be as strong as usual with the sensory nerves cut. The result was entirely in accordance with the preceding results; that is to say, in an animal in which the posterior roots were cut, the tetany was complete and also as intense as if the spinal nerves had been left intact; on the other hand, in an animal in which I had cut the motor nerves to one of the posterior limbs, this limb remained flaccid and immobile during the time when, under the influence of the poison, all the other muscles of the body manifested pronounced tetanic contractions.

Were contractions produced by direct irritation of the sensory nerves or the posterior spinal roots? Did a direct irritation of the motor nerves produce pain? Such are the questions that I asked myself and that experiment alone could answer.

In this regard I began by examining the posterior roots or sensory nerves. Here is what I observed: when these roots were pinched, pulled, and pricked, the animal demonstrated pain, but it did not compare in intensity with that produced when the spinal cord was only lightly touched at the place where the roots arise. Almost every time that the posterior roots were thus excited, contractions were produced in the muscles to which the nerves are distributed; these contractions were not very marked, however, and infinitely weaker than if the cord itself had been touched. If at the same time a bundle of a posterior root was cut, a mass movement was produced in the limb to which the bundle was directed.

I repeated these same experiments on the anterior bundles and obtained analogous results, but inversely; for the contractions produced by the pinching, pricking, etc., were very strong and even convulsive, but the indications of sensation were hardly apparent. These facts confirm those that I have announced; only they seem to establish that sensation is not exclusively in the posterior roots any more than movement in the anterior. One difficulty might arise, however. When in the preceding experiments the roots were cut, they were continuous with the spinal cord; was the disturbance communicated to them the true origin either of the contractions or of the pain that the animals felt? To remove this doubt, I repeated the experiments after the roots had been separated from the cord. I must report that with the exception of two animals, in which I saw contractions when I pinched or pulled the anterior and posterior bundles, in all the others I did not observe any sensory effect of the irritation of the anterior or posterior roots thus separated from the cord.

I had still another kind of experiment to make on the spinal roots, that of galvanism. Consequently, I excited them by this means, first leaving them in their natural state and then cutting them at their spinal extremity in order to place them on an insulating body. In these various instances I obtained contractions from the two types of roots; but the contractions that followed the excitation of the anterior roots were in general much stronger and more complete than those that occurred when the electric current was applied to the posterior. The same phenomenon took place whether the zinc or copper pole was applied to the nerve.

Between them Bell and Magendie established a basic neurological concept, known as the Bell-Magendie law, but the controversy that followed Magendie's paper was one of the most acrimonious and unsavory disputes of nineteenth century physiology. In the second paper cited above, Magendie recorded the following.

EXCERPT PP. 369–371

When I wrote the note contained in the preceding issue [pp. 300–301], I believed that I was the first who had thought of cutting the spinal nerve roots, but I was soon undeceived by a letter from M. Schaw [John Shaw, brother-in-law of Bell] that this young and industrious physician had the kindness to send me as soon as he had received the issue of my journal. In that letter he wrote that Charles Bell had performed this section thirteen years ago and that he had recognized that section of the posterior roots does not impede the continuance of movement. M. Schaw added that Charles Bell had published this result in a little booklet printed only for his friends and not for publication. I immediately requested M. Schaw to send me, if possible, Charles Bell's booklet so that I might render him all the justice that was his due. A few days later I received it from Schaw.

This booklet is entitled: *Idea of a NEW ANATOMY OF THE BRAIN, submitted for the observations of his friends,* by Ch. Bell, F.A.S.E. [*sic*]. It is interesting to note in it the germ of the author's recent discoveries in the nervous system. On page 22 is the passage mentioned by Schaw. I transcribe it in its entirety:

"Next considering that the spinal nerves have a double root . . . . the muscles of the back were immediately convulsed" [see p. 299].

It may be seen from this citation from a work with which, since it was not published, I could not be acquainted, that Bell, influenced by his ingenious ideas on the nervous system, had been very close to discovering the functions of the spinal roots; nevertheless, the fact that the anterior are provided for movement but the posterior belong more particularly to sensation seems to have escaped him. I must then restrict my claims to having established this fact in a positive manner.

The literature on this topic is extensive but the best surveys are by two impartial Americans, Flint (1868) and Olmsted (1944, pp. 93–122). The sum of all the evidence is, without doubt, in favor of Magendie. Bell's role was a minor one, although admittedly he carried out the first experiments on spinal roots and his work may have stimulated Magendie. His subsequent writings, however, do not enhance his position in this controversy, and the fact that he made certain alterations in earlier works republished to support his claim after Magendie's experiments, is damning evidence. Moreover, Magendie's acknowledgment of Cotugno in the priority problems concerning the cerebrospinal fluid should be taken into account.

Johannes Müller

(See p. 203)

Following Magendie's experiments and the controversy with Bell that they aroused, others attempted to verify the suggested functions of the spinal roots. In France, P. A. Béclard (1823, p. 668, par. 785) and in Germany, C. G. Schoeps (1827), for example, believed that they had done so successfully, but, as was so with other investigators, their results were inadequate and inconsistent.

Müller first became interested in the problem in 1824, but his results were not recorded until 17 March 1831 ("Bestätigung des Bell'schen Lehrsatzes, dass die doppelten Wurzeln der Rückenmarksnerven verschiedene Functionen haben, durch neue und entscheidende Experimente," *Notiz. Gebiete Nat.-Heilk., Erfurt,* 1831, 30:113–117). Despite the apparently conclusive evidence brought forward by Magendie, it was argued that the preliminary trauma to which his animals had been subjected invalidated any conclusions concerning the sensory phenomena under investigation. Furthermore, Müller found that the rabbit was an unsuitable experimental animal, since, because of fright, it often did not respond to painful stimuli, even in the intact state. Therefore he used the frog rather than any of the higher animals and stimulated both anterior and posterior spinal roots with mechanical and galvanic stimuli. He confirmed the motor functions of the anterior roots, but apart from establishing beyond doubt their absence in the posterior roots, he did not investigate the latter further although he inferred their sensory nature. Müller, like many of his German contemporaries, accorded priority to Bell. The following excerpts have been translated from Müller's original text.

EXCERPT COLS. 115–117

. . . . A good physiological experiment like a good physical one requires that it should present anywhere, at any time, under identical conditions, the same certain and unequivocal phenomena that can always be confirmed. This cannot be said of the experiments conducted to date as evidence of Bell's theory. The exhaustion owing to the injury is so great, *that the probability of error is larger than the probability of the result,* an error unfortunately inborn in so many physiological experiments.

Could one not find experiments for or against Bell's theory which are as reliable as the physiological experiments of Haller, Fontana, Galvani, A. v. Humboldt? The following will lead to the conviction that there are such proofs for Bell's theory.

By chance I finally had the idea of using frogs for the experiments in question, following the method mentioned before. They are animals which are very tenacious of life and they survive the opening of the vertebral column for a considerable time; their nerves remain sensitive for the longest time, and the thick nerve roots to the posterior extremities extend for a considerable distance in the spinal canal before they unite. These experiments were rewarded with brilliant success; they are so easy, so sure, and so conclusive that everybody can now convince himself quickly of one of the most important phenomena in physiology, and I call upon all physiologists to repeat the simple experiments that I am about to describe. The phenomena are so constant and astonishing that for simplicity and certainty of success they may well parallel the best physical *experimentum crucis.*

To open the vertebral column of the frog I use forceps with a sharp cutting edge and point. This operation can be carried out in a few minutes without any injury to the cord. Following this the frogs are very lively and hop around as before. Immediately upon opening the spine and the membranes, the thick posterior nerve roots for the lower extremities can be seen. Carefully lift these roots with a cataract needle, without seizing any part of the anterior roots, and cut them off at the point of entry into the cord. Now seize the cut end with forceps and pull the root itself repeatedly with the tip of a hairpin. Were one to repeat this experiment innumerable times in a large number of frogs, with each repetition one would remain convinced that *the mechanical irritation of the posterior roots is never followed by the slightest indication of a spasm in the posterior extremities.* The same experiment can be repeated with the same success in the very thick posterior nerve roots for the anterior extremities.

Now, with the needle lift from the spinal canal one of the anterior, equally thick nerve roots for the hind legs. The slightest touch immediately produces very marked spasms in the entire posterior extremity. These roots, too, are then cut off close to the cord, the cut end seized with the forceps and the stretched root pulled with the tip of the needle. With each irritation very lively spasms occur.

By repeating these experiments in a large number of frogs one becomes convinced that it is absolutely impossible to produce spasms in frogs by way of the posterior spinal root nerves, but that the slightest stimulation of the anterior roots immediately manifests very active spasms.

Equally conclusive are the tests using galvanism by means of a simple zinc or copper plate.

Galvanic stimulation of the anterior roots immediately causes very violent spasms but of the posterior roots it never does so . . . .

These are the experiments which leave no doubt of the veracity of Bell's theory.

I should also like to add that cutting the posterior roots off the spinal cord is often distinctly associated with manifestations of pain in the anterior portion of the trunk.

BENEDIKT STILLING
(*See p. 270*)

Although Stilling's main contribution was to knowledge of the internal structure of the spinal cord (pp. 271–275), he was also interested in the function of these structures. His concept of "spinal irritation" is no longer valid, but in a book, *Untersuchungen über die Functionen Rückenmarks und der Nerven* (Leipzig, 1842), which was primarily an attack on the unimportant ideas of Deen, he succinctly summarized his findings, revealed mainly in experiments by vivisection on frogs. Although they are not all valid—as, for example, the restriction of sensory functions to the posterior columns—they are mostly fundamental to our concepts of the sensory and motor properties of the spinal cord.

EXCERPT PP. 305–307

1. The posterior spinal roots are sensory and not motor.

2. The anterior spinal roots are motor and not sensory.

3. The posterior white matter of the spinal cord is sensory, but only when it is in connection with the posterior gray matter. It is insensitive when it is separated from the posterior gray matter.

4. The posterior gray matter is sensory whether or not it is in connection with the posterior white matter.

5. The anterior white matter is not sensory whether or not it is in connection with the anterior gray matter.

6. The anterior gray matter is likewise not sensory whether or not it is in connection with the white matter.

7. Motion arises always and only with the aid of the anterior gray matter, whether the movement is voluntary or reflex; without the anterior gray matter no such movement occurs and a transverse section through the anterior gray matter abolishes all voluntary movement below the cut.

8. The anterior white matter receives its impressions from the anterior gray, communicates them to the anterior nerve roots, and in this way causes movements, voluntary or reflex.

9. The posterior white matter receives the impressions from the posterior nerve roots, communicates them to the posterior gray matter, and in this way conducts sensation.

10. The sensation is conducted through the posterior gray substance and never without it.

CHARLES ÉDOUARD BROWN-SÉQUARD
(8 April 1817—1 April 1894)

As a result of Magendie's réport, Charles Bell claimed that the posterior columns of the spinal cord were entirely sensory in function, and although he himself vacillated on the point, a dogma arose, associated with his name; posterior columns carried sensation, anterior columns, motion, and lateral columns had to do with respiratory function. Magendie's successful operations also inspired others to repeat them, and many attempts were made to study the functional organization of the cord by sectioning techniques (see Olmsted, 1943). One of the most important of such investigations, and certainly the best known, was that of the physiologist Brown-Séquard whose name is still associated with the clinical manifestations of hemisection of the cord. Although he is remembered for this clinical entity, which he defined in 1860, his early experiments were not intended to establish it but rather to refute Bell's contention concerning the posterior columns and sensation.

Brown-Séquard was born on the island of Mauritius of an American father and a French mother. He studied medicine in Paris where he was graduated in 1846 after writing a thesis entitled *Recherches et expériences sur la physiologie de la moelle épinière*. Until he succeeded Claude Bernard in the chair of experimental physiology at the Collège de France in 1878, Brown-Séquard held appointments in Paris, Richmond (Virginia), Boston, and London. He spent much time travelling between these centers and to Mauritius, but his activity in the field of neurology and endocrinology was remarkable. He did not have his predecessor's remarkable intellect but, nevertheless, he made several outstanding contributions to medicine (see Olmsted, 1946; Haymaker, 1953, pp. 263–265).

The first spinal cord hemisections had been carried out by Galen (p. 292) but he had observed only the resultant motor signs. Others in the nineteenth century such as Deen and Stilling observed the effects of similar lesions, but it was Brown-Séquard who made the correct interpretation that sensory fibres decussate in the cord. Without being aware of it, he was, however, dealing only with the spinothalamic tract, as it is known today, because he did not appreciate the existence of the posterior column modalities; nor did he study the motor manifestations since they were already well recognized. Thus he was able to deny the popular concept that the sensory fibres of the cord lay only in the ipsilateral posterior column.

His first experiments were described in his previously mentioned graduation thesis, but in December 1849 a more detailed account was reported to the Société de Biologie in Paris ("De la transmission des impressions sensitives par la moelle épinière," *C. r. Séanc. Soc. Biol.*, 1849, 1:192–194).

EXCERPT PP. 192–193

1° As soon as a lateral half of the cord of a mammal [guinea pig] has been cut in the dorsal region, the sensibility seems very diminished in the posterior limb on the side of the section. The sensibility is totally lacking in the other posterior limb. Sometimes I have found sensibility intact or approximately so in the posterior limb corresponding to the sectioned side, while the other posterior limb was either insensitive or only slightly sensitive.

2° At the end of a five to ten minutes rest following surgery, it is always found that the posterior limb corresponding to the sectioned side is very sensitive and, in many cases, we might say in the majority of cases, this limb seems more sensitive than under normal conditions. This fact is surely very interesting, but there is yet another fact still more unexpected: the posterior limb of the side opposite the section is insensitive or only slightly sensitive.

From these observations it follows that the section of a lateral half of the spinal cord, far from causing loss of sensibility in the parts located below the section on the same side, makes them hyperesthetic, while it produces more or less complete anesthesia on the other side of the body below the section. . . .

At the meeting of 1 December 1849 we demonstrated a guinea pig in which the *right* lateral half of the cord had been cut in the presence of some members of the Society. The section was at the level of the tenth dorsal vertebra; the animal lost considerable blood. The operation, carried out in semidarkness, had been long and very painful. Under such circumstances it ordinarily happens that the two posterior limbs are found to be deprived of voluntary movement and sensibility for some time after surgery; this is what happened in this case. But at the end of five or six minutes, voluntary motion returned to the *left* posterior limb and sensibility to the *right* posterior. Approximately twelve minutes after surgery sensitivity was extreme in the *right* posterior limb and there was none in the *left* posterior. An autopsy was then undertaken at the meeting by M. Cl. Bernard, and the Society recognized that the *right* lateral half of the cord had been cut transversely at the indicated level.

EXCERPT P. 194

Therefore the spinal cord seems to have, at least in part, a crossed function in respect to the transmission of sensory impressions. This is so true that after having cut a lateral half of the cord in a mammal, then cutting the other half a few centimeters distant from the first cut, one finds the two posterior limbs insensitive or almost so. We cannot here examine the questions which are raised by these experiments; we shall make these the subject of another, expanded report. Nevertheless we believe it necessary to state that if the transmission of sensory impressions takes place in part through the posterior spinal cord, it does so chiefly through other parts of this nerve center. Indeed, not only is sensitivity [to pain] lost nowhere following section of the posterior cord, but it is rather notably increased in the parts of the body which ought to be insensitive according to the erroneous theory that the systematic physiologists persistently maintain despite the evidence with which they have been confronted, and despite M. Ch. Bell's recantation [Bell had traced the posterior columns to the pyramids and cerebrum (1844), and so had again changed his mind; he seemed still to have thought the posterior columns to be sensory.]

Another paper in the following year, 1850, gave further support to Brown-Séquard's opinions concerning the localization of pain pathways in the spinal cord. He worked with rabbits, sheep, dogs, and guinea pigs, employing pinching, pricking, galvanization, fire, and acid as painful stimuli. ("Mémoire sur la transmission des impressions sensitives dans la moelle épinière," *C. r. hebd. Séanc. Acad. Sci., Paris*, 1850, 31:700–701.)

EXCERPT PP. 700–701

Today everybody admits that the transmission of impressions received by one half of the body takes place as a whole through the corresponding half of the spinal cord [via posterior columns]. We have found, on the contrary, that the transmission takes place principally in a crossed manner, that is to say, the right half of the cord transmits, in a very large part, the impressions received by the left half of the body and vice versa.

Because of the opinion according to which the spinal cord transmits impressions in a direct line, it has been necessary to look elsewhere than to this organ for the cause of the crossed hemiplegia in diseases of the brain. An effort has been made to find it in one of the intercrossings which are observed in the medulla oblongata, in the pons and in front of it. In demonstrating that the majority of sensory fibres from the trunk and the limbs must decussate along the whole length of the spinal cord itself, our experiments offer a new and very simple solution of the problem of crossed sensory hemiplegia [hemianaesthesia].

. . . .

. . . .

If several complete sections of the same half of the cord are made, it is found that sensibility persists unchanged on the side of the section and that there is almost none on the other side.

At this moment we have three guinea pigs which for more than four months have survived a hemisection of the cord at the level of the tenth or eleventh thoracic vertebra, and an appreciable difference in the sensibility of the two posterior limbs is still noted in them, that on the sectioned side remaining always more sensitive than the other.

To explain the crossed sensory hemiplegia in cerebral diseases, it was supposed that the sensory fibres of the different parts of the body decussated in the nerve centers [brain]. It is known what disagreement exists in science with regard to the site in which this intercrossing takes place. Some authors are content to designate, en bloc, the medulla oblongata, the pons and parts adjacent to it where one finds decussations. Others, with more boldness, have indicated circumscribed parts as the special site for the intercrossing of the sensory fibres . . . .

It follows from my experiments that it is above all in the spinal cord that the sensory fibres cross, and, if there are any which come from the limbs and ascend to the brain in order to cross there, they must be very few in number.

CONRAD ECKHARD
(1 March 1822—28 April 1905)

Once it had been established that the anterior spinal roots were motor in function and the posterior were sensory, investigators began to consider their distribution respectively to the muscles and skin and the relationship between these peripheral structures and the segments of the cord. Legallois (pp. 294–296) had already suggested that segmentation of the cord occurred, but the details of this arrangement had to be worked out. Such questions as the following had to be answered: Do individual motor roots supply individual muscles exclusively? Is the skin covering a muscle supplied by the sensory root that is the fellow of the motor root supplying the muscle? At first, experiments seemed to suggest positive answers but the work of Eckhard revealed the true state of affairs.

Eckhard was born in Homberg and studied medicine at Marburg and Berlin. He was assistant to Carl Ludwig and then prosector under Ludwig Fick in Marburg. In Giessen he worked with Bischoff before being appointed professor of anatomy and physiology there. His studies were mainly on nerves and muscles and on the physiology of salivation, and he published voluminous textbooks on anatomy and physiology (Kehrer, 1905).

While working in Carl Ludwig's laboratory in Leipzig, Eckhard studied the anatomy and physiology of the joints, muscles, and nerves of the legs of the frog including the distribution of the spinal roots to the lower extremities. He reported his results in an important paper published in 1849 ("Über Reflexbewegungen der vier letzten Nervenpaare des Frosches. I. Abhandlung," Z. rationelle Med., Heidelberg, 1849, 7:281–310; the promised conclusion does not appear in this journal). In Section II of the paper, entitled "The distribution of motor fibres in the hind legs," Eckhard dealt with the problem of motor roots and gave some of the first information concerning the *myotomes*, as they were later called. In the instance of the sensory roots (Section III) he likewise drew attention to a specific distribution, the *dermatomes*.

EXCERPT PP. 303–310

1. *The fibres of one and the same spinal nerve* do not supply the same muscles in all cases; however, it is always particular muscles that can invariably be made to contract in the majority of instances of excitation of a specific nerve. The following plate [fig. 83] is a review of the muscles that could be made to contract in several experiments on individual nerve trunks.

. . . .

2. In some nerves to the limbs there are fibres for the abdominal and back muscles; thus in the seventh, there are fibres for the external oblique muscle of the abdomen, and at times in the eighth and ninth for the iliococcygeus.

3. A large number of muscles receive fibres from *several* nerve roots at the same time; almost invariably in most of the thigh muscles and sometimes from three [nerves] in some of the leg muscles; but frequently from two in several of the leg muscles. Here the question arises *whether those* [nerve] *fibres that lie in various sections of one and the same muscle originate from one or from different sites in the spinal cord?* Although this question cannot be answered definitively so long as a reliable method for the detection of the sites of origin of the spinal nerves is lacking, we can, however, in some degree narrow the problem down if (as will be adequate for our specific purpose of examining reflex movements more precisely) we express it as follows: *is it possible that the* [nerve] *fibres to one and the same muscle that lie in different nerve tracts within the spinal cord can be stimulated reflexly from different sites in the cord?* The question can be decided as follows: with the sensory and motor roots avoided the vertebral canal is opened by the method to be mentioned under III; then the spinal cord is separated into different parts by cutting transversely between the site of emergence of two consecutive nerve pairs; the parts of the spinal cord are then isolated and the posterior [sic] roots stimulated. Following this procedure I obtained twitchings in the triceps, abductor magnus and sartorius by stimulating the sensory [sic] roots in two parts of the spinal cord, one of which was connected with the eighth, the other with the ninth root; and twitchings in the triceps in two places connected with the seventh and eighth roots. It follows from this that the fibres that lie in different nerve trunks of one and the same muscle can be stimulated reflexly from different parts of the spinal cord.

4. . . . .

5. In general, the distribution of the fibres of different nerves does not

occur in such way that those of the one go to a certain group of muscles of like function while those of another proceed to a different group; indeed, there are fibres in one and the same nerve tract that go to muscles of *opposite* function in relationship to one and the same bone . . . .

III. DISTRIBUTION OF THE SENSORY FIBRES OF THE LAST FOUR SPINAL NERVES [IN THE FROG]

The main [skin] areas to which the sensory fibres of the last four spinal nerves proceed, can be easily determined. It is only necessary to open the vertebral canal, cut the sensory roots of all nerves except the one to be examined and then note those points on the skin which produce movement when stimulated . . . . The accompanying figures [fig. 83] represent the areas of distribution of the sensory fibres of the last four spinal nerves, which are as follows. The fibres of the seventh supply the side of the thigh that is turned downwards, and they are distributed more or less extensively to the skin that stretches over the anterior head of the triceps and covers the knee. In a few cases I found that it went beyond the knee to the skin that covers the dorsal side of the leg. Those of the eighth supply the anterior part of the dorsal side and the anterior surface of the leg; in addition, the dorsal surface of the two first tarsal bones, the metatarsus, the toes, and finally the web. Those of the ninth serve the posterior part of the dorsal surface of the thigh, the same part of the leg, particularly the skin which covers the first tarsal articulation; in addition, the plantar surface of the two first tarsal bones and of the middle of the foot, the plantar surface of the toes, and the web. Those of the tenth enter into the skin around the anus, neighboring parts of the back, the upper part of the dorsal surface of the thigh, and up to the midline on the trunk between the legs. The general result of this investigation is therefore: *the sensory* [nerve] *fibres do not go precisely to the parts of the skin below which lie the muscles supplied by the corresponding motor fibres.*

LUDWIG TÜRCK

(See p. 284)

It was clear from Eckhard's experiments that in their distribution to the skin of the trunk and limbs the sensory fibres of the posterior spinal cord roots formed zones arranged in specific patterns, dermatomes; the next step, therefore, was to examine these patterns more closely. The most important studies at this time were those of Türck. On 24 July 1856 he presented a preliminary account of his results in the dog to the Imperial Academy of Sciences in Vienna ("Vorläufige Ergebnisse von Experimental-Untersuchungen zur Ermittelung der Haut-Sensibilitätsbezirke der einzelnen Rückenmarksnervenpaare," *Sber. kaisl. Akad. Wiss., Wien,* Math.-Naturw. Klasse, 1856, 21:586–589).

EXCERPT PP. 586–588

I attempted to elucidate these zones by means of a physiological experiment, by dividing in the anesthetized dog, the individual nerve pairs [roots] in the vicinity of the spinal ganglia. Following this I defined the areas of skin thus anesthetized. In these experiments the individual areas could not only be clearly recognized, but a very remarkable regularity in their arrangement could also be demonstrated.

. . . .

The individual spinal nerve transmits sensibility to a considerable portion of its skin region, either exclusively or overlapping with the neighboring roots, and to such a degree that following its section the strongest mechanical stimuli have no effect, whereas sensibility is high all around it; this is a phenomenon that I have already noted in most of the roots. My investigations of those areas of the skin which one can demonstrate to be supplied mutually by two neighboring roots are not yet completed.

The areas of distribution of the individual roots in the neck and trunk present ribbon-like strips which extend round from the spinous processes to the midline anteriorly in a vertical or almost vertical direction on the longitudinal axis of the body [see fig. 85].

The areas of distribution of the spinal roots which supply the skin of the extremities, with some variations, follow exactly the pattern just reported for that of the other roots; however, this comparison only becomes evident when the extremities have been placed in a certain position to the trunk. For the anterior extremities, the lateral position is at right angles to the trunk, with full extension of all the joints and with a somewhat supinated hand. For the posterior extremities it is also that of complete extension of the individual parts, whereby the extended extremities are placed obliquely in such a way that they form an angle of approximately 45 degrees with the tail of the animal, and with a moderate rotation outwards. In the report given below these positions of the extremities have been presupposed, and, in order to facilitate a comparison with the human body, the animal was assumed to be in the erect position. The agreement of both areas can be observed in an illustration [none with this article, but see fig. 85], because the zones of the extremities behave approximately as if they had originally extended from the sides of the neck and trunk exactly like all the others and had only later become turned laterally inside out as a cover because of the formation of the extremities. Thus some individual areas were pulled so far laterally that they became completely separated from the anterior and posterior median lines of the trunk; others remained adherent to the median lines but became separated between the two (second thoracic nerve); others, situated at the borders, although able to complete the arc around the trunk, nevertheless were drawn along at their margins by the extremity which touched it when protruding. In all this, however, they preserved their original relative position to each other as well as to the trunk, so that they always kept a more or less vertical, or in the lower extremities, successively oblique direction relative to the longitudinal axis of the trunk, and so that the original curved course, too, in some still remained clearly visible [see fig. 85].

The zone of the fifth cervical nerve forms a band which proceeds right round the lowest region of the neck and contains the spine of the scapula and the point of the shoulder. Inferiorly at the anterior and posterior median line of the trunk, it borders directly upon the area of the second thoracic nerve. Between the two are inserted the areas of the sixth, seventh, and eighth cervical and first thoracic nerves. The area of the sixth cervical nerve is located in the above-mentioned position, superiorly on the extensor side of the shoulder joint and it extends in a narrow point to the elbow joint. The area of the seventh cervical nerve grasps this point like a fork at the medial and lateral side of the upper arm and extends on the radial side of the arm towards the first finger. The area of the eighth cervical nerve is distributed below it, on the posterior surface of the forearm, over the back of the hand and some fingers [see fig. 85].

In the remainder of the article Türck described briefly the sensory areas supplied by thoracic, lumbar, and sacral roots, section of which, he noted, occasionally induced a rise of skin temperature. Unfortunately his many professional activities prevented him from completing this remarkable study which he intended to apply to the human being and at his death in 1858 the material was gathered together and edited by Carl Wedl. It was summarized by Sherrington (1894, pp. 643–646). The following passages are from the Denkschrift published by Wedl ("Über die Haut-Sensibilitätsbezirke der einzelnen Rückenmarksnervenpaare," *Denschr. kaisl. Akad. Wiss., Wien*, Math.-Naturw. Klasse, 1869, 29:299–326).

EXCERPT PP. 321–322

SPECIAL REMARKS REGARDING THE AREAS OF SENSATION OF THE NERVES OF THE UPPER EXTREMITIES WITH REFERENCE TO EMBRYOLOGICAL DEVELOPMENT [FIG. 85]

The first cervical nerve does not supply any cutaneous nerves. The second, third, fourth, fifth cervical nerves have exclusive areas only. The sixth cervical nerve has an exclusive and a combined area. The seventh and eighth cervical nerves have combined areas only. The first thoracic nerve, like the sixth cervical nerve, has an exclusive and a combined area.

The line of demarcation between anterior and posterior branches corresponds approximately to the transverse processes of the vertebrae. The line of demarcation between posterior and anterior branches of the second cervical nerve reaches the external auditory canal at the side of the neck, which corresponds very well to the demarcation between anterior and posterior branches at the side of insertion of the outer ear.

However, between the fifth cervical and second thoracic nerve zones are inserted those of the sixth cervical and first thoracic nerves so that their exclusive areas merely directly touch the exclusive areas of the fifth cervical and second thoracic nerves . . . .

During that period of embryonic development when the extremities are still missing, the fissure between the zone of the fifth cervical and second thoracic nerves cannot exist; it must be formed somewhat later at a time when the extremity grows out of the trunk like a branch from the trunk. The cutaneous areas which are supplied by the fifth cervical and second thoracic nerves can only move away from each other in their median sections because new skin grows between them simultaneously with the growth of the extremity, into which the nerves of the limb which it is to cover also grow.

However, during the development of the upper extremity a cleavage of the second thoracic nerve zone also takes place so that the area is divided into a much larger section which proceeds diagonally on the back and on the external periphery of the upper arm down to the elbow, and into a much shorter one that adheres to the sternum.

The unequivocal result of the foregoing is that during foetal life the upper arm lies diagonally across the chest and coalesces with it in such manner that the elbow borders upon the area of the second thoracic nerve, and consequently the total area of this nerve, like those of other thoracic nerves, presents an uninterrupted arc proceeding around the trunk. When the upper arm detaches itself from the trunk it pulls along with it a part of the skin of the third and fourth thoracic nerve zones as a cover for its posterior surface. That portion of the third thoracic nerve zone situated towards the head grows into the transverse fissure of the second thoracic nerve and fills it. In another case this was accompanied by a similar splitting of the area of the third thoracic nerve. [See fig. 85.]

EXCERPT P. 322

In general the cutaneous nerve areas of the upper and lower extremities form girdles; they have the shape of the iron bands of armor and they overflow into the cleft of an upper and a lower area at acute angles. The angle gives a measure of its actual width which can be recognized when the extremities are placed in a certain normal position relative to the trunk. These zonal areas which surround the extremities are mostly broadened at their centers since they follow the extremity which is growing out.

CHARLES SCOTT SHERRINGTON
(*See p. 238*)

Türck had planned an extensive survey of sensory zones or *dermatomes* in the experimental animal and in man. Although he did not carry this out, others who followed him were able to verify and clarify his pioneer observations. The person who probably added most data was Sherrington who had set himself the task of learning as much as possible about the fundamental components of the spinal reflex. These are the afferent sensory and the efferent motor fibres, and in respect to the former he was especially interested in their peripheral distribution.

The following passages (from "Experiments in examination of the peripheral distribution of the fibres of the posterior roots of some spinal nerves," *Phil. Trans. R. Soc.*, 1894, 184B:641–763) include some of the basic statements made by Sherrington concerning the dermatomes. In many instances he was confirming and extending the work of Türck begun thirty-eight years previously. Sherrington studied an individual root's function by sectioning its two or three neighbors.

EXCERPT P. 758

The field of skin belonging to each sensory spinal root may be called the *sensory spinal skin-field*. These fields are segmentally arranged and do not present the same variety of configuration presented by the fields of peripheral nerves . . . .

Each sensory spinal skin-field extends to a certain extent across the neighbour skin-fields. Each has an *anterior overlap* extending into segmental fields anterior to it, each a *posterior overlap* into fields posterior; each has also *crossed overlaps* trespassing into the fellow field of the opposite lateral half of the body, both at the mid-dorsal (the *dorsal crossed overlap*), and at the mid-ventral line (the *ventral crossed overlap*). The fore and aft overlaps are throughout the body very great, and it appears that each point of skin throughout the body is supplied by at least two sensory spinal roots, in certain regions by three. The overlap of the skin-fields of the separate filaments of a posterior root is very great indeed, at least in some cases.

EXCERPT P. 759

The absolute segmental level of a point of surface is subject to Individual Variation, just as that of muscular points in the body-wall and viscera. This

Individual Variation affecting the skin is correlated with variation in the constitution of the afferent spinal roots, so that the limb plexus may be *postfixed* or *prefixed* by its sensory roots just as it may be by its motor roots. A mixed nerve may be postfixed by its motor roots and by its sensory roots in the same individual, or may be prefixed by both. There is some evidence (Frog) that a plexus may be prefixed by its motor roots when it is not so by its sensory roots, and *vice versa*.

EXCERPT P. 760

The distribution of the fibres of the sensory spinal root in the limb, as elsewhere, indicates a segmental significance in their constitution rather than a functional based on co-ordination. Without denying the existence of functional factors in the progressive development of the limb, it must be admitted that there is little evidence that the collection of fibres in each sensory root has resulted from an assortment of the fibres with a view to assisting toward functional co-ordination.

The motor roots, too, had to be examined carefully, and the anterior horn cell plus its axon represented the second part of the pyramidal tract, the lower motor neuron. In the next excerpt (taken from "Notes on the arrangement of some motor fibres in the lumbo-sacral plexus," *J. Physiol.*, London, 1892, 13:621–772) Sherrington described the distribution of the cells in the anterior horn; the term "spinal border cells of Sherrington" is still used. He was especially concerned in this instance with the cells which looked after specific muscles of the foot.

EXCERPT PP. 687–688

. . . . If the point of emergence of the anterior rootlets from the grey matter can be taken as a guide, one may say with little hesitation that the increase in size of the horn in the limb regions is due to the addition of a large lateral mass. Within this lateral mass of the horn in the case of each of the enlargements of the cord, the nerve-cells appear distinctly as two large and well-defined groups. These are the *antero-lateral* and the *postero-lateral cell-groups* of the anterior horn. There is at certain levels also a middle group lying nearer the centre of the horn, but this is far from being so large or clearly defined a group as are the other two . . . . In the cat, dog, and in Macacus as in man *antero-lateral* and *postero-lateral* groups appear really to be of distinct existence. There are three main groups of cells obvious in the anterior horn of the enlargement, a *medial* continuous with the group that in fairly unbroken fashion extends throughout the entire length of the cord; an *antero-lateral* and *postero-lateral* that are not obvious elsewhere than in the enlargements.

What is the longitudinal arrangement and relationship of these groups?

When transverse sections of the cord arranged serially are examined successively in an ascending direction, the cord at the level of the 10th sub-
thoracic nerve-root is found to present a small and simple anterior horn,
containing but one collection of large cells that could be in bold terms
described as a group. Passing upwards to the level of the rootlets of the next
segment (it must be remembered that here the rootlets form a close
unbroken row) a second group with some abruptness makes its appearance
in the horn: this is a *lateral* group. It rapidly acquires such proportions as to
dwarf the original *medial* group, but it lies quite away from that group and
is so large as to cause a prominence which even in the cat is well seen
without help from the microscope. Scarcely has this group become well
established when another group almost as suddenly appears in the horn,
again a lateral group, but lying ventral to the preceding one.

At a higher level still the original *medial* group itself becomes enlarged,
but at that level the lateral group which was the earlier met in following the
serial sections upwards is much reduced in size, and somewhat higher
disappears.

Thus as one passes from below the enlargement into it the first modification undergone by the anterior horn is that the *postero-lateral group* of cells
appear. Somewhat higher the *antero-lateral* group is added, higher still the
medial group of the horn attains its maximal development.

Examined therefore in the ascending direction the cord displays at the
same point at which the outflow of efferent fibres to the lower limb begins
(and we know that outflow begins with fibres to the intrinsic muscles of the
foot) a striking change in the constitution of the ventral horn, owing to the
sudden addition to the horn of the great *postero-lateral group* of ganglion
cells. This group therefore suggests itself as related to the intrinsic muscles
of the foot.

Myotomes, the muscle equivalents of dermatomes, were also investigated with
the precision, experimental ingenuity, and clarity characteristic of Sherrington's
method of work ("On the spinal animal," *Med.-chir. Trans.*, 1899, 82:449–477).

EXCERPT PP. 457–458

Analysis of the spinal nerve-supply of the muscles of either limb demonstrates that the muscular tissue of the limb is arranged in a number of rays,
there being one ray for each one metamer contributing to the limb. Of
these rays the tailmost in the fore-and-aft series are the longest; they extend
to the extreme free apex of the limb, whereas the foremost, the most
rostral, pass only as far as the thigh, the next hindward as far as the knee,
the next hindward as far as the ankle. In the fore limb of *Macacus rhesus*
the common *rhesus* monkey, the four hindmost, most aboral rays all con-

tribute to the musculature of the hand. When we inquire how these units of the segmental architecture of the limbs, these muscular rays, are related to the physiological or functional units of the limb musculature, it is at once obvious that the extent and boundaries of the two do not coincide. The definitely-bounded, individual, and circumscribed masses of muscular tissue which are known as "the muscles" of the limb are functional elements of its structure as a physiological machine. But each of these functional elements is compounded and pieced together out of several rays or myotomes. Moreover, the boundaries between the myotomes do not correspond with the intervals, between muscles nor even with those between muscle-groups. Degeneration experiments which enable one to follow the distribution of the individual nerve-fibres of a root show that in some muscles the number of motor nerve-fibres given by a spinal root to a muscle is too small to evoke from the muscle any contraction obvious to inspection, for cases occur where a limb-muscle receives three, four, or five motor nerve-fibres from a particular nerve-root. This I regard as strong testimony to the morphological character of the overlap.

Another feature of the distribution of the motor fibres of the spinal root to a muscle is the remarkable frequency with which it is subject to slight individual variation. In examining a series of individuals (cats, monkeys) it is almost rare to meet two consecutive members of the series in which the root distribution is not by the degeneration or experimental method demonstrably somewhat different. Thus as instance I found in some individuals *supinator brevis* innervated from the sixth and fifth cervical nerves, in others, from the sixth and seventh. In the former case the innervation of the muscle may be termed *"prefixed"* type, in the latter *"post-fixed."* In my observations I considered it sufficient to group the individuals into two classes, a *post-fixed* and a *prefixed*. The *absolute* segmental level of a muscle is variable over the range of nearly a whole segment's length; the *relative* segmental position is, however, preserved inviolably constant.

In the same article Sherrington drew important conclusions from the factual information he had collected during the preceding decade. He also gave an excellent account of the spinal ganglion cells, which, together with their motor equivalents, the motor cells of the anterior horn (see p. 274), form an arc that is the foundation of the spinal reflex (Chapter VI). Also included here is a further important detail concerning dermatomes.

EXCERPT PP. 451–453

To judge how far the reactions of the spinal organ can be really considered as segmentally arranged, it is important to have a conception as clear as possible of the spatial relations of the spinal nerve-cells. The delineation of the spinal segment usually given presents its true extension very imperfectly.

The edifice of the whole nervous system is based, as upon two pillars, upon two nerve-cells, the afferent root-cell, and the efferent root-cell. These form a fundamental spinal arch upon which all other neural arcs are superposed and functionally rest, immediately or mediately—even those of the hemispheral cortex. The afferent root-cells of the spinal axis may be arranged in three great groups: (1) cutaneous, from the sense organs of the skin; (2) "muscular," from the sense organs of the musculo-articular apparatus; (3) "sympathetic," from the viscera. Each spinal afferent root consists typically of three constituent roots—a cutaneous, a muscular, and a visceral. The efferent root-cells are conveniently grouped in two sets, one supplying skeletal muscles (1), the other entering the sympathetic chain (2) to innervate the musculature of the blood-vessels, of the skin, and of the viscera, including some secretory apparatus in the two latter.

To deal with the afferent root-cells first. The cutaneous afferent root-cells have their perikarya or cell bodies in the spinal ganglion. Probably in each one of the spinal ganglia the majority of the cells belong to nerve-fibres afferent from skin. The peripheral distribution of the collection of cutaneous nerve-cells of each spinal ganglion occupies a semi-zonal field of body surface. The zone is relatively wide and invests a little more than the entire width of one lateral half of the body, trespassing slightly across the middle line both ventrally and dorsally. In the regions of the trunk and neck and perinaeum this zonal arrangement is quite obvious, but in the regions of the limbs it is less so, and at first sight appears departed from. The skin fields of the last three cervical and the first two thoracic, of the last two lumbar and of the first two sacral ganglia are entirely confined to the limb and do not meet the middle line of the body either ventrally or dorsally. But when the skin fields of the ganglia of the limb region had been carefully ascertained the results collated showed clearly that both in the brachial and in the pelvic limbs the zonal form of the fields still obtains, each semi-zone being wrapped half round the limb instead of half around the body. Hence exist what I have termed the *ventral* and *dorsal axial lines of the limbs;* these, forming, as it were, lines of watershed between the systems of semi-zones (Pl. XIII [fig. 88]), meet at their one end the mid-ventral and mid-dorsal lines of the *body,* and may be looked upon as lateral extensions thereof. They are not hypothetical, for they are exhibited in the striping of animals. . . . These axial lines of the limbs are of much clinical importance, for they are the boundaries observed by the upper limits of the anaesthesia accompanying injuries to the spinal cord or spinal roots in the regions of the lower and upper limbs respectively.

The skin fields belonging to the spinal ganglia are wide, and that for each ganglion largely overlaps its neighbours . . . . In certain regions (e.g., the hand, the foot, the pinna of the ear) the skin receives sensory fibres from each of *three* adjacent ganglia. This explains how it is that the limb plexuses exist. The peripheral nerves of the limbs have to obtain components from more than one spinal nerve root. The innervation of the limb musculature is similarly plurisegmental. If, therefore, the spinal ganglion be considered a segmental collection of nerve-cells, those nerve-cells at their peripheral endings impinge on the body-surface over a zonal area which overlaps slightly with the contra-lateral zonal areas across the ventral and dorsal lines, and overlaps greatly with the collateral zonal areas next in front and next behind (headward and tailward) of itself. This zonal skin area may be considered a "segmental field" of skin.

All of Sherrington's work was carried out on laboratory animals, and its application to the elucidation of the motor and sensory functions of the human spinal cord followed naturally. The passages below are from another classic paper ("Experiments in examination of the peripheral distribution of the fibres of the posterior roots of some spinal nerves.—Part II," *Phil. Trans. R. Soc.*, 1898, 190B:45–186).

EXCERPT PP. 89–92

In concluding this section a few words are desirable regarding the comparison between the segmental anatomy of Man and of *Macacus* in this region. Beyond question the similarity between the two is almost minutely exact. The most salient point of difference appears in the motor distribution of the IInd thoracic root, which is not generally considered to contribute to the brachial plexus in Man. Its contribution is of almost universal occurrence in the animals used in the Laboratory . . . . As judged by the root-constitution of the phrenic nerve, therefore, the muscles innervated by the brachial region of the cord are more prefixed in Man than in the other Mammalian types coming under observation, including Monkey. It may be, therefore, that in a certain number of human brachial plexuses the IInd thoracic does not contribute to the innervation of the hand muscles; and certainly in *Macacus* the amount of contribution by it varies, for I have in some individuals failed to evoke contraction of the deep flexor of the forearm through it, though this is often readily done. On the other hand again, it is possible that the segmental position of diaphragm (or rather of phrenic nerve) may vary independently of that of the musculature (or nerve-trunks) of the limb; but this supposition is not in harmony with the rule I found deducible from the lumbo-sacral plexus, viz., "the shifting up or down of the region of outflow along the cord applies to all the efferent fibres of that length"; in other words, although each muscle (nerve-trunk) is displaced absolutely, it is not displaced relatively to its neighbours . . . .

As to the spinal skin-fields of *Macacus* and of *Man*, clinical opportunities arise for observing some of the latter sufficiently to give ground for brief examination of the correspondence between the two. The opportunities of the bedside have afforded the basis for the admirable papers of THORBURN, HEAD, JAMES MACKENZIE, STARR and KOCHER . . . . These cases go far to show that the agreement in this region between *Macacus* and Man is very close, extending even to details of individual variation . . . .

As just mentioned, the topography of certain skin-areas of painfulness and hyperalgesia, explicable by reference from visceral disease, has been investigated by HEAD, and shown by him to exhibit a segmental arrangement. This segmental scheme is, broadly taken, notably similar to that of the spinal root-fields as exhibited in *Macacus* . . . . The difficulty of minute comparison between the two is much enhanced by the frequent individual variation which I find to obtain.

One noteworthy point issues clearly from their comparison, however. In the root-fields I met certain peculiarities of contour which recurred with such constancy that I soon came to recognise them as diagnostic for certain fields . . . . The similarity is too significant for chance coincidence. Again, HEAD's weighty discovery that two fields of skin—an upper between IVth cervical and Ist thoracic, and a lower between Ist lumbar and Vth lumbar—are, as regards reference of visceral pains, virgin and blank, suffices of itself to establish the intimate connection of the two schemes. The situation of these gaps is, according to both sets of observations, the very region of most pure, of least complicated, limb character. *Exact* and *absolute* correspondence between skin-fields of *Macacus* and Man is not to be expected, if, as I have, I think, proved above, the skin and muscles of Man are more prefixed than are those of *Macacus*.

Conclusion

Further investigation of the segmental character of the spinal cord has confirmed and extended the original work of Eckhard, Türck, and Sherrington; other experimental techniques have produced much the same results. In the case of man the most important study was that of Head (Head and Campbell, 1900). Head used herpes zoster to indicate the dermatomes, for in this condition individual posterior spinal roots may be involved and the sensory pathway thus interrupted. Foerster (1933), in cases of root trauma or surgery, discovered the same overlapping described by Sherrington in the monkey (p. 316). This may seem to be a relatively simple problem, but it has not yet been entirely resolved as evidenced by the fact that overlapping has recently been denied (Keegan and Garrett, 1948). The role of sensory modalities other than pain has also attracted attention, and the segmental innervation of the skeletal muscles (myotomes) has been worked out on the basis of Eckhard's and Sherrington's early experiments. Nevertheless, some of the more intricate functional relationships of the spinal cord and its roots are still under investigation.

THE REFLEX

Introduction

The spinal reflex, although by no means the only reflex, is the commonest, and historically it is the most important. The growth of knowledge concerning it resulted from the application of the discoveries reviewed in Chapters IV and V, respectively those related to the structure of the spinal cord and those related to its motor and sensory functions, and also from data concerning the form and function of the nerve (Chapters II and III).

Until the eighteenth century the concept of a spinal reflex did not exist, and its origins are to be found in attempts to account for the differences between various kinds of muscle movements. Thus from the fourth century B.C., it was recognized that some movements were controlled by the will, the so-called voluntary movements. There were also others, however, such as those of the heart, which could not be influenced in this way; these were called involuntary movements. The significant difference seemed to be the role of the will, or soul, or consciousness, and this factor proved to be an inseparable feature of all investigations into reflex functions until the end of the nineteenth century. Another early forerunner of the reflex concept was the idea that different parts of the body, unconnected anatomically, could have between them a sympathy or consent.

These two problems, involuntary movement and sympathy, were tackled by the ancients and again by seventeenth century investigators who differed from the former only in having slightly more anatomical and physiological knowledge. This first period in the history of the reflex was one of speculation only.

The second period covers the eighteenth century and the first half of the nineteenth and is characterized by experimentation that hitherto had not been called upon in examination of the problem. At the end of the period the main components of the spinal reflex were assumed, though not yet anatomically verified. In the second half of the nineteenth century data concerning the reflex, in common with other physiological topics, accumulated at an ever-increasing rate, and at the end of the century, as if to answer the need for a coordinator and interpreter, Sherrington appeared; or so it has seemed to historians. He was without doubt the most prolific and outstanding contributor to the mechanisms of reflex activity, and his work established the modern period which is still in existence.

The detailed anatomy and physiology of the reflex pathways, especially synaptic action, are now under investigation, and their role in the incredibly complicated activities such as inhibition, respiratory reflexes, and posture is providing many avenues of research. The opinion that reflex activity was a feature of all parts of the nervous system arose from Sherrington's work. But also of importance, at least historically, is the *conditioned reflex* of Pavlov and his school that developed contemporaneously with the Sherringtonian concepts that have been found to be more acceptable in the West.

The history of the reflex has received more attention than any other aspect of neurophysiology or neuroanatomy, due in past to the interest shown in it by psychologists. The excellent paper (1881) of Conrad Eckhard (p. 310) has provided material for most of those who have since written on this subject. Fearing's book (1930) is the largest contribution to it, and Canguilhem (1955) has provided a detailed and accurate survey of the reflex concept during the seventeenth and eighteenth centuries. In the last chapter (pp. 132–159) Canguilhem reviews the many contributions to the history of the reflex during the nineteenth and twentieth centuries. E. G. T. Liddell (1960) deals only with the nineteenth century but traces the history of the anatomy and physiology of the nerve cell and fibre as a background to work on the reflex. One-third of the book deals with Sherrington, and as Liddell was his student, colleague, and successor at Oxford, he writes with authority. There have also been numerous articles dealing with the history of the reflex that will be cited below. Two in particular deserve to be mentioned here, however, that of Hoff and Kellaway (1952), which includes selected passages from the writings of early contributors to the subject, and that of Hodge (1893).

Speculation

The early history of reflex activity deals with the distinction made between voluntary and involuntary motion and with the concept of sympathy. Both were discussed in antiquity, and Aristotle and Galen as represented here provide this background to later advances.

The concept of the reflex first appeared in the seventeenth century, although it was but a very faint glimmering of present-day beliefs. As more was learned of the anatomy of the nervous system, so inquiries into its function became more extensive. But as far as the reflex was concerned this was almost entirely speculative, as might be expected in the complete absence of any knowledge of the ultimate structure of nervous tissue. Despite their ignorance of these matters, however, certain individuals in the seventeenth century, such as Descartes and Willis, were able to conceive extremely crude forms of the reflex, which were very distant from modern concepts, or even from those of the nineteenth century. They were of course inevitably dependent upon the earlier notions of involuntary motion and sympathy which they had inherited from antiquity. Nevertheless the primitive ideas of Descartes, Willis, and others were the germs of what was to become the physiology of reflex activity, one of the basic phenomena of biology.

ARISTOTLE

(See p. 7)

The earliest reference to the concept of reflex action as it is understood today, did not appear until the seventeenth century. Nevertheless, even in antiquity two preceding, associated ideas were recognized: involuntary movement and the phenomenon of sympathy.

An involuntary movement was one over which the individual had no control and was thus the reverse of a voluntary movement. Such were the movements of the vital organs or those of the body during sleep. The distinction between voluntary and involuntary movement, which is basic to the idea of the reflex, was clearly made by the ancient Greek writers. The Hippocratic Writers were aware of it, and Aristotle, in *The movement of animals*, 11 (*De motu animalium*, [translated] by A. S. L. Farquharson, Oxford, 1912), discussed the matter as follows.

EXCERPT 703b:2–21

So much then for the voluntary movements of animal bodies, and the reasons for them. These bodies, however, display in certain members involuntary movements too, but most often non-voluntary movements. By involuntary I mean motions of the heart and of the privy member; for often upon an image arising and without express mandate of the reason these parts are moved. By non-voluntary I mean sleep and waking and respiration, and other similar organic movements. For neither imagination nor desire is properly mistress of any of these; but since the animal body must undergo natural changes of quality, and when the parts are so altered some must increase and others decrease, the body must straightway be moved and change with the changes that nature makes dependent upon one another. Now the causes of the movements are natural changes of temperature, both those coming from outside the body, and those taking place within it. So the involuntary movements which occur in spite of reason in the aforesaid parts occur when a change of quality supervenes. For conception and imagination, as we said above, produce the conditions necessary to affections, since they bring to bear the images or forms which tend to create these states.

GALEN
(*See p. 14*)

The differentiation between voluntary and involuntary movements also engaged the attention of Galen. In *The movement of muscles*, I, 1 (Daremberg [1854–1856], II, 324) he stated, "In fact, the movements of the artery and of the vein are physical movements without spontaneity. [They are natural], while those of muscles are voluntary and under the influence of the soul." And whereas Aristotle had regarded movements during sleep as "non-voluntary," Galen thought they were controlled by the soul and therefore volitional (*ibid.*, pp. 362–367). He concluded that memory had an important role to play, for some voluntary actions were immediately forgotten and were therefore equivalent to involuntary ones. As Hoff and Kellaway (1952, p. 215) point out, Galen referred in this passage to a type of vitalism whereby each portion of the body was controlled by an indwelling soul (see Whytt, p. 336). The following excerpts are from *The movement of muscles*, II, 5–6 (Daremberg [1854–1856], II, 362–365).

EXCERPT PP. 362–365

. . . . Perhaps someone will say that these acts [during sleep] are accomplished unconsciously! But neither in the continual movement of the eyelids, nor in speech, nor in declamation or conversation does one give consideration to all movements of the parts, nor when one walks from Piraeus to Athens, to all the special movements of the legs. One sees persons deep in reflection who arrive without having any notion of the length of the trip or they pass by the place where they intended to stop. Therefore, is not walking an act of the soul, and is it not accomplished voluntarily? Concerning the movements of the parts moved and the tonic activity of those not moved it seems, indeed, that we act unconsciously in the walking during discussion and in sleep. Thus the reason by which you explain that persons who are awake often pay no attention to their special movements; if you will only attribute it to persons asleep or unconscious (*carus*), then you will no longer be astonished at how many voluntary acts take place even among these persons. But would it not be rash for one in ignorance of the reason to declare categorically that none of these acts occurs voluntarily?

. . . . If we have a very striking criterion for voluntary acts, as we do, let us declare that not only each of the acts mentioned but also respiration itself takes place voluntarily, so much so that it appears to satisfy this criterion. What then is this criterion by which we judge voluntary acts? I wish to give you not one indication but many indications, all of them in agreement. If you can at your desire stop the performance of acts begun and perform those that have not begun, this is by the effect of volition. If, furthermore, you are capable of performing them faster or slower, more or less frequently, is it not completely evident that the act is subordinate to the will? The will cannot stop the movement of the pulse or of the heart, or render it more or less frequent, nor accelerate it. Also one does not say that such acts are acts of the soul, but natural. Under these conditions reason directs the movement of the legs. In fact, it can stop the movement begun, then take it up once more after it has been interrupted, and render it faster or slower, more frequent or infrequent. These same things occur in the movement of respiration, which is an activity of the diaphragm and of the muscles of the thorax as we demonstrated in our book *On the causes of respiration*; it comes from the soul and not nature since the movement of the muscles is an act of the soul. In those instances in which the cause is not known it is not correct to disregard facts clearly known. Thus the proofs of voluntary acts are clearly known, but we are embarrassed to explain the means by which we unconsciously accomplish particular movements.

. . . . Hence it is evident that volition governs respiration; but it is difficult to explain why we are not aware of many voluntary acts.

CHAPTER 6

To discover these truths, we shall begin with this principle, that persons often do many things that they forget an instant later, as those who, through fear, drunkenness, or some such cause, have not the least recollection of what they did under those conditions. The reason for the forgetfulness is, in my opinion, that they did not give all the attention of their mind to these acts. Indeed, the imaginative part of the soul, whatever it may be, is that which appears endowed with memory. If this part of the soul in its perceptions collects clear impressions of objects, it preserves them forever, and that constitutes memory. If, on the contrary, it collects in an abstruse and superficial manner, it does not preserve them, and that constitutes forgetfulness. Also, in anger, deep meditation, drunkenness, madness, fear, and generally with strong emotions of the soul one does not recall later anything of what one did when in those states. Is it therefore astonishing that if during sleep, the soul acts abstrusely, the perceptions are also abstruse and consequently do not persist? Is it astonishing if in the state of wakefulness, even when the spirit is occupied with meditation and wholly absorbed in its reflections, that a very small part of this spirit, which occupies itself with walking, receives an obscure impression of the act and consequently forgets it at once and no longer recalls if the act has been performed voluntarily? In fact, if we did not retain any memory at all, we should be incapable of reflecting on any past acts; so in the case of the acts of which we have no recollections, we are unaware what their nature was; for it is first necessary to preserve them in the memory before finally reflecting on their nature. Therefore it does not appear to me at all astonishing that volition acts on respiration during sleep, and that, I do not say once awake, we respire voluntarily. This resembles what takes place in those who move the feet and the legs and talk in their sleep, and who, having then forgotten it entirely, pretend that movement of the limbs and the voice are produced without volition. Those who are delirious also speak, walk, and perform all voluntary movements, but when their fit has passed, they no longer remember what they did.

The phenomenon of sympathy, whereby certain parts of the body are in relationship or in sympathy with others, although not visibly connected, is also to be encountered in the medical writings of Greco-Roman antiquity. The Hippocratic physicians, and probably their predecessors, too, were aware of it. Thus one Hippocratic Writer stated that on account of sympathy, swelling of the breasts and of other parts might accompany a uterine lesion (*Diseases of women*, II, 174, Littré [1839–1861], VIII, 354–355). The fact that Galen thought a common blood supply would account for this sympathy indicates that we should be cautious when trying to interpret the phenomenon as an early step towards the modern reflex concept.

Nevertheless, Galen considered the idea of sympathy more closely elsewhere (*The sites of diseases*, I, 6, Daremberg [1854–1856], II, 494–504). After defining the term, he gave an example: a cervical spinal cord lesion produced aphonia because of intercostal muscle paralysis although the larynx itself was unaffected. We would not interpret this as a "sympathetic" effect but rather as a consequence of respiratory embarrassment. In the last sentence Galen referred to the phenomenon that we term "reflex" or "referred" pain, but he did not think that this was owing to sympathy.

EXCERPT PP. 494–496

. . . . When the intelligence is troubled as the result of an ailment of the stomach, be it from the vapors, or be it from malignant humors that rise to the brain, one is unable to say either that the brain was affected first or that it is completely free from the affection; but the word sympathy expresses very exactly what physicians recognize in this state. In fact, the term "sympathy" does not indicate complete absence of affection, but a disorder which is in common with another part. It would always be better and clearer to say that the part affected sympathetically suffers in consequence of the affection of another part.

. . . . Certain functions produced by a suitable material receive this material that has been prepared by other parts. It happens sometimes, and naturally, without there being a particular affection in the particular organs of the function, that this function is abolished as a result of the substance that produced it, as is seen in the case of the voice. It has been demonstrated in our treatise *On the voice* that expiration is the material of the voice and that the intercostal muscles produce it by contracting the chest. When, therefore, these muscles no longer act, the animal becomes aphonic without there being any affection in the parts pertaining to the voice itself . . . .

. . . .

Such form of injury [aphonia owing to cervical cord trauma] ought to be designated as "sympathetic," a more proper name than when [referred] pain produced in the head results from certain humors contained in the stomach.

RENÉ DESCARTES
(See p. 155)

It is clear that the ancients were far removed from even a very elementary concept of reflex action. Even their analysis of voluntary and involuntary movement did not always correspond with ours—assuming ours to be correct—and the term "sympathy" included a variety of phenomena not even distantly related to the reflex. Nevertheless, these early stirrings are worthy of notice.

The history of the modern concept of reflex activity did not begin until the seventeenth century, and the first person to discuss it, albeit in a very primitive fashion, was Descartes (Fearing, 1929). It was fundamental to his belief in automatism since he considered the body to be a machine and in certain situations to be dependent, in modern terminology, upon the transformation of an afferent sensory impression into an efferent motor stimulus.

Like his predecessors, Descartes distinguished between voluntary and involuntary movements and cited vital functions and guarding reactions to illustrate the latter. The following passage has been translated from his "Réponses de l'auteur aux quatrièmes objections," of the French theologian Arnauld, a section (pp. 289–339) of Descartes' book, *Les meditations metaphysiques . . . et les objections* [etc.], traduites par C. L. R. (Paris, 1647). Descartes' account of nerve function referred to in the following excerpt will be found on pages 157 to 158. His reference to reflected light is not, however, related to reflex action but will be mentioned later (p. 470) as an analogy.

EXCERPT PP. 304–305

. . . . I shall nevertheless say here again that it seems to me that it is a very remarkable matter, that no single movement can take place, either in the bodies of animals or in ours if these bodies do not have in them all the organs and instruments by means of which these same movements could also be accomplished by a machine; so that, even in us it is not the mind (or soul) that immediately moves the external parts, but it can only determine the course of that very subtle fluid which is called animal spirit which, constantly flowing from the heart through the brain into the muscles, is the cause of all movements of our parts, and can often cause several different ones, the one as easily as the others. Indeed, it does not always determine it; for among the movements that take place in our bodies there are some that do not at all depend upon the mind, such as the beating of the heart, the digestion of food, nutrition, respiration of those who are asleep and even of those who are awake, walking, singing, and other similar actions when they take place without the mind thinking of them. When those who fall from a height thrust out their hands to protect their heads, it is not on the advice of their reason that they perform this action, and it does not depend upon their mind, but only upon their senses which, being aware of the present danger produce some change in the brain that causes the animal spirit to pass from there into the nerves, in the fashion that is required, to produce this movement immediately, as in a machine, and without the mind impeding it.

Now since we experience this in ourselves, why then are we so astonished if the light reflected from the body of the wolf into the eyes of the sheep has the same power to arouse in it the movement of flight?

According to Descartes the human body was a machine controlled by the rational soul situated in the pineal body, and one of that body's mechanical activities was its response to potentially hurtful situations. His interpretation of nerve function has been described above (pp. 157–158), and an application of it is to be found in his well-known account of a simple reflex movement, written in 1634 but published in 1662 and 1664. The following is from the latter edition (*L'homme* [Paris, 1664], Pt. II, Art. 26) and explains "How it [the human machine] is stimulated by external objects to move in many ways"). It is an example of Descartes' simple reflex which did not involve the pineal body and therefore the soul.

EXCERPT PP. 26–28

To understand, after that, how, by exterior objects striking the sensory organs, [the body] can be stimulated to move all its parts in a thousand other ways, consider that the little threads that, as I have already said so many times, come from the most interior part of its brain and compose the marrow of its nerves, are so disposed in all those parts that serve some sensory organ, that they can very easily be moved by the objects of these senses; and that when they are moved there, even slightly, in the same instant they pull upon the parts of the brain whence they come, and in the same way open the entrances of certain pores that are in the interior surface of the brain, by which the animal spirits in its cavities immediately begin to flow and travel by the pores into the nerves, thence into the muscles which, in this machine, serve to produce movements very similar to those to which we are naturally aroused when our senses have been touched in the same way.

As, for example, if the fire A is near the foot B [see fig. 89], the particles of this fire, which as you know move with great rapidity, have the power to move the area of the skin of this foot that they touch; and in this way drawing the little thread, c, c [at base of toes and on the nerve] that you see to be attached there, at the same instant they open the entrance of the pore, d, e, at which this little thread terminates, just as by pulling one end of a cord, at the same time one causes the bell to sound that hangs at the other end.

Now the entrance of the pore or little conduit, d, e, being thus opened, the animal spirits of the cavity F, enter within and are carried by it, partly into the muscles that serve to withdraw this foot from the fire, partly into those that serve to turn the eyes and the head to look at it, and partly into those that serve to advance the hands and to bend the whole body to protect it.

The same idea was put forward in Descartes' book *Les passions de l'ame* ([Amsterdam], 1649, Pt. I, Art. 13, "That this action of external objects can lead the spirits diversely into the muscles"), and the following excerpt has been translated from it.

EXCERPT PP. 21–23

. . . . As an example of this [that sensations give rise to movement], it is easy to conceive that sounds, odors, tastes, heat, pain, hunger, thirst, and generally all objects, those of our other external senses as well as of our internal "appetites" arouse also some movement in our nerves and by means of them pass to the brain. In addition to the fact that these different movements of the brain cause our soul to have various sensations, they can also, without it, cause the spirits to take their course towards certain muscles rather than towards others, and thus move our parts. I shall prove this here only by an example. If some one suddenly places his hand before our eyes, as if to strike us, even though we know him to be our friend, that he does it only in jest, and that he will take care to do us no harm, we always have difficulty in not closing them. This demonstrates that it is not by the intervention of our friend that they are closed, since it is against our will, which is its only or at least its principal action; but that it is because the machine, or our body, is so composed that the movement of that hand towards our eyes arouses another movement in our brain which leads the animal spirits into the muscles that cause the eyelids to lower.

Elsewhere in the same book (Pt. I, Art. 36, "Example of the way in which the passions are aroused in the soul") Descartes dealt with the reaction of an individual to a frightening situation and, for the first and only time, used the word "reflect" in a biological context; no doubt he was applying an optical concept to the problem (see p. 330). The following is an example of Descartes' complex reflex action in which the pineal body takes part.

EXCERPT PP. 53–55

. . . . For that renders the brain so disposed in some men that the spirits, reflected (*refleschis*) from the image so formed on the [pineal] gland, thence go partly into the nerves that serve to turn the back and move the legs to flee, and partly into those that greatly expand or constrict the orifices of the heart, or greatly agitate the other parts whence the blood is sent to it, so that this blood, being abnormally rarefied there, sends spirits to the brain that are suitable to maintain and strengthen the passion of fear, that is, that are proper to hold open or to open a second time the pores of the brain that lead into the nerves themselves. From that fact alone, that these spirits enter into these pores, they arouse a particular movement in that gland which is established by nature to cause the soul to feel that passion. And because these pores are in relationship principally to the little nerves that serve to reduce or to enlarge the orifices of the heart, that causes the soul to feel it principally as in the heart.

A further passage from *Les passions de l'ame* (Pt. I, Art. 44, "That each desire is naturally connected with some movement of the gland, but that by practice or by habit it can be connected with others") deals with the pupillary reaction and speech, both of which are characteristic examples of "reflection" taking place without volition.

EXCERPT PP. 62–63

Nevertheless it is not always the desire to arouse some movement in us or some other effect which itself enables us to arouse it; but that depends, according to how nature or habit, have separately joined each movement of the [pineal] gland to each thought. Thus, for example, if one desires to adjust the eyes to look at a far-distant object, this desire causes the pupil to enlarge; and if one wishes to adjust them to look at a very near object, this desire causes it to contract. But if one thinks only of enlarging the pupil, one has the desire in vain; it does not expand for the reason that nature did not join the movement of the gland that serves to drive the spirits towards the optic nerve in the way required to expand or contract the pupil, with the desire to expand or contract, but instead with that of looking at distant or near objects. And when in speaking we think only of the sense of what we wish to say, that causes us to move the tongue and the lips much more rapidly and much better than if we think of moving them in all the ways required to utter the same words. The habit that we have acquired in learning to speak has caused us to connect the action of the soul which, by the intervention of the gland can move the tongue and the lips, with the meaning of the words that follow these movements rather than with the movements themselves.

Thomas Willis
(See p. 158)

The manner in which the body reacted to an external stimulus, which had been explained in purely mechanical terms by Descartes, also interested Thomas Willis. He located voluntary movements in the cerebral hemispheres and involuntary movements in the cerebellum (p. 638), and also suggested sites in the former where mental processes were located. Thus the seat of the *sensus communis* was in the corpus striatum, that of imagination in the corpus callosum, and memory in the cerebral cortex (p. 473). Willis next considered the sequence of events which took place when sensory stimuli entered the brain and then were reflected out again. This was clear allusion to the sensory and motor components of reflex action as we understand it today although it was still in very vague form. He was using the word "reflect" in much the same mechanical sense as Descartes and was describing an event which, as it involved the soul, was not the unconscious, involuntary act that we consider a reflex to be. He also employed the term to describe the function of memory which is foreign to our present-day usage. The following passage has been translated from Willis's *Cerebri anatome* (London, 1664, Ch. XI), and as Meyer and Hierons (1965, p. 143) have pointed out, reference was made to an event resembling the scratch reflex of Sherrington (p. 375).

EXCERPT PP. 72–73

. . . . *Passions* of this sort, *common sense* (*sensus communis*) and *imagination*, exist within the structure of the brain, but the *actions* are *memory, phantasy*, and *appetite* [will]. Both common sense and imagination for the most part depend on the external senses for their origin and instincts.

Regarding the former [common sense] we notice that as often as the external part of the soul has been affected, *a sensory impression*, like *an optical appearance* or like *the undulation of water*, is carried more inwardly, turning towards *the corpora striata*, and *perception* of the external *impression* occurs, *the internal impression*; if this *impression* is carried further and crosses through the *corpus callosum*, it is succeeded by *imagination*; then, if that same *flowing of the spirits* strikes against *the cortex of the brain*, as its farthest shore, it impresses on it *the image* or *character* of the sensible object; when thereafter the same image is reflected, it arouses *the memory* of the same thing.

The active powers of the soul, that is, *local motion, memory, phantasy*, and *appetite* now immediately succeed to *the passions*, or, because of other reasons, are led *apart* from them. Indeed, *the sensory impression* often striking *the corpora striata* but with the brain unaffected, *the local motions* are caused to turn back, with reciprocal tendency of the animal spirits. So it is that in sleep—with the appetite unknowing—upon the urging of pain we rub the place, moving the hand to it; but more often, after *the sensory impression* has crossed through from *the common sensorium* to *the corpus callosum*, it arouses *imagination*, the spirits are reflected thence, and having flowed back towards the appendix of the brain [brainstem and cord] arouse *the appetite* and *local motions*, executors of the imagination; sometimes some *sensory impression*, having been carried beyond *the corpus callosum* and having struck against *the cortex of the brain* itself, arouses other impressions lying hidden there, so that it induces *memory* with *phantasy*, often, indeed, *appetite* and *local motion* as accompaniments. Furthermore, because of other reasons, these *active powers* are sometimes accustomed to be irritated and excited apart from *the passion*. In man *the rational soul* affects the sensitive soul in various ways and at its pleasure draws out and brings into action now these, now those of its powers. In addition, the blood bubbling abnormally and hence striking the border of the brain more forcefully, arouses the appearance of things lying concealed there and, driving them towards *the middle of the brain*, causes the various acts of *memory* and *phantasy* to be represented.

Another of Willis's contributions to the history of the reflex was the suggestion that nerves could communicate with each other in peripheral plexuses without the necessity of first going to the brain as Galen had taught (pp. 326–329). This gave anatomical support to the concept of sympathy but later led to the erroneous belief that reflex activity need not utilize the central nervous system (p. 328).

In his book, *De anima brutorum* (Oxford, 1672, Ch. VI), Willis gave a further account of his crude concept of ingoing and outcoming messages which involved the brain and awareness. Although his suggestions regarding cerebral localization were speculative, they gave a much firmer anatomical basis for the reflex concept than did those of Descartes.

EXCERPT PP. 64–65

Therefore as soon as the brain of *the more* [embryologically] *perfected animals* becomes clear and the composition of the animal spirits is sufficiently lucid and purified, exterior objects carried to the organs of sensation make impressions; by the sequential arrangement or disposition of the animal spirits, these are then transmitted inwards towards *the corpora striata* and affect the sensorium commune; when a sensory impulse of the same spirits is carried like a surge of water farther into *the corpus callosum* and from there into *the cortex of the brain, the appearance* of the object received sensorily is carried inwards. This is immediately succeeded by *imagination*, and the remaining vestiges of its type constitute *the memory*. Meanwhile, when the sensory impression has been carried to the sensorium commune, it causes there the perception of the object that produced the sensation, just as the *direct* appearance of it going further creates *imagination* and *memory*; and *another reflected appearance* of the same object, as it appears congruous or incongruous, produces *appetite and local motions*, the executors of appetite. Thus the animal spirits look inwards for *the act of sensation*, and having been driven back, spring towards *the corpora striata*; when these spirits, now located around the origins of the nerves, arouse other spirits, they produce *desire for or flight from the object sensed*, and at the same time put it into effect by stirring up *movement* of this or that member or part. Then when this or that kind of *motion* has several times followed this or that kind of *sensation*, thereafter *this motion* usually follows *that sensation* as *the effect* follows the cause. Hence in this way through the ideas of sensations that are admitted and *the knowledge* of individual things to be done, and of local motions, by degrees *patterns* are produced. Indeed, from the beginning almost all *the motions* of the animate body are aroused by the contact of an external object, that is, when the animal spirits residing within the organ are struck by an object they are driven inwards, and so, as was said, produce *sensation*; then like a flood surging along the shore, are finally driven back. To the degree that that surge or *inward turning* of the animal spirits, partly reflected from *the sensorium commune*, is at last directed *outwards*, and partly extended into the central part of the brain, so then *local motion* succeeds to *sensation*, and at the same time a mark affixed to the brain from the sense of the thing perceived impresses there vestiges for *the phantasy* and *memory* of the same object then held and to be held thereafter.

Early Experimentation

Seventeenth century speculation on reflex activity gave way in the eighteenth century to experimentation on the same subject. Whereas Descartes and Willis had been inseparably devoted to the Greek concept of animal spirit, or its equivalent, as the mechanism responsible for nervous transmission, a century later certain individuals such as Robert Whytt were willing to discard the old terms and the equally old ideas clustering about them. Nevertheless the archaic notion of sympathy was still of service, and it proved possible to formulate basic concepts without any knowledge of nerve function.

Whytt's work was of great merit since he, more than anyone else in the eighteenth century, was responsible for clarifying the concept of the spinal reflex, despite the fact that little or no advance in knowledge of the anatomy of the spinal cord itself had taken place since the time of Willis. Whytt employed a combination of clinical and animal experimentation to substantiate his ideas and to support his brilliant analysis of involuntary movements and the reflex. Those who followed him, such as Unzer and Procháska, continued along the pathway he had opened, and his work was confirmed and extended by an experimenter of the early nineteenth century, Marshall Hall.

ROBERT WHYTT
(6 September 1714—15 April 1766)

Whereas Descartes declared the pineal body to be the reflecting mechanism, Willis favored certain areas of the cerebrum, as well as the peripheral nerve plexuses. Thus by the eighteenth century there were two opinions originating mainly from these two authors: one declared a central connection to be essential and the other, the peripheral anastomoses of nerves; but until the middle of the century, precise and conclusive experimental evidence in favor of one or the other was not available. It was Robert Whytt of Edinburgh who provided it.

Whytt was born of a well-to-do family in Edinburgh and began the study of medicine there in 1730. He also studied in London, Paris, and Leyden and received the M.D. degree at Rheims in 1736. In 1747 he became professor of the theory of medicine at Edinburgh and remained in that post until his death. Whytt's research was both physiological and clinical—an example of the latter being his first description of tuberculous meningitis—and his excellence was acknowledged by the important offices he held (see Seller, 1864; Carmichael, 1927).

Haller's conclusions regarding irritability and sensitivity (pp. 171–174) were vigorously attacked by Whytt who, as a vitalist, could not believe that a part of the body, such as a muscle, could act without the intervention of the soul, or, as he put it, "the sentient principle" or life force. He therefore devised many experiments in a futile attempt to refute Haller's statements, and in so doing he made a major contribution to the problem of the reflex.

Whytt's experimentation and writings on the reflex were extensive and indicate that he had a clear, agile, and perceptive mind, and that he brought his extensive clinical knowledge to bear upon the problem; however, he rarely used the term *reflex* and his interpretation of the phenomenon was necessarily primitive. Furthermore, the vitalism that influenced all his findings gave his conclusions an archaic flavor. Nevertheless, Whytt was the most outstanding eighteenth century investigator of the reflex, and his scientific approach was commendable since, when faced with the innumerable enigmas of neurophysiology and anatomy, he stated:

. . . these are questions we have wholly avoided, being persuaded that whatever has been hitherto said on these subjects, is mere speculation; and that to offer any new conjectures on matters so greatly involved in darkness, and where we have neither *data* nor *phaenomena* to support us, is to load a science already labouring under *hypothesis* with a new burden. [*An essay on the vital and other involuntary motions of animals*, Edinburgh, 1751, pp. 325–326.]

In his book, *Observations on the nature, causes, and cure of those disorders which have been commonly called nervous hypochondriac, or hysteric, to which are prefixed some remarks on the sympathy of the nerves* (Edinburgh, 1765), Whytt concluded (p. 5): ". . . that involuntary, as well as voluntary motion, depends upon some power or influence of the nerves," and (pp. 9–10) that "OUR bodies are, by means of the nerves, not only endowed with feeling, and a power of motion, but with a remarkable sympathy, which is either general and extended through the whole system, or confined, in a great measure, to certain parts." These statements appear in a chapter entitled "Of the structure, use, and sympathy of the nerves" (pp. 1–84), most of which has been reproduced by Hoff and Kellaway (1952, pp. 228–235) who justifiably applaud the remarkable sequence of observations on sympathetic, or reflex, activity.

The following passages have also been taken from this chapter and refer to Whytt's important conclusion that sympathy (i.e., the reflex) is dependent not upon peripheral nerve anastomoses, but upon the central nervous system, and in particular upon the spinal cord; he cited the auditory meatus cough reflex as an example.

EXCERPT PP. 50–55

15. IF, therefore, the various instances of sympathy cannot be accounted for, from any union or *anastomosis* of the nerves in their way from the brain to the several organs; and if there are many remarkable instances of *consent* between parts whose nerves have no connexion at all; it follows,

that all sympathy must be referred to the brain itself and spinal marrow, the source of all the nerves.

BUT for a more direct proof of this, we may observe, that the consent of the several parts instantly ceases, when their communication with the origin of the nerves is interrupted . . . . In like manner, when any of the muscles of the legs of a frog are pricked, most of the muscles of the legs and thighs contract, even after cutting off its head, if the spinal marrow be left entire; but when that is destroyed, altho' the fibres of the stimulated muscle are affected with a weak tremulous motion, yet the neighbouring muscles remain wholly at rest.

FURTHER, the effects of pain, and of fear and other passions, in preventing several sympathetic motions, seem to shew, that the cause of that *consent* which obtains between the parts of animals, is to be referred to the [central] origin of the nerves: And, since certain affections of the mind excited by the action of external objects on the organs of sense, produce extraordinary motions and other effects in the body, merely by affecting the brain; why may not impressions made on the nerves in other parts, produce likewise, through the intervention of the brain, various motions and other effects in distant parts of the body? The analogy is obvious.

LASTLY, notwithstanding the many sympathetic motions, which are daily observed, by Physicians, to arise from an irritation of the nerves in different parts of the body; yet, when the nerve going to any muscle is irritated, there is no motion excited in any part, except in the muscle to which it is distributed. Does it not hence appear highly probable, that the various sympathetic motions of animals produced by irritation, whether in a sound or morbid state, are owing, not to any union or connexion of their nerves, but to particular sensations excited in certain organs, and thence communicated to the brain or spinal marrow? . . . .

. . . .

FURTHER, when the *meatus auditorius* is irritated, by introducing into it a feather, or any such substance; an inclination to cough is often excited, especially if the membrance of the *trachea* has been rendered more sensible than usual by catching cold; but, when the *meatus auditorius* is violently pained, in consequence of an inflammation in it, no coughing is occasioned; From which it follows, that the sympathy between that *meatus* and the organs of respiration in the former case, cannot be owing to any connexion between their nerves, or indeed to any mechanical cause, but proceeds from a *particular* feeling, and must be referred to the *sensorium commune* [in the brain].

As a vitalist Whytt was naturally unwilling to accept Descartes' purely mechanical explanation for nervous phenomena; nor could he accept Haller's isolated irritability. Hence when he came to consider how muscles contract or, using modern terms, how the afferent impulse of the reflex response becomes efferent, he attributed the process to "the sentient principle." This he defined as ". . . the mind or soul in man, and that principle in brutes which resembles it" (*Observations*, 1765, p. 61n), which operated throughout the body by means of the nerves and the brain and made possible the muscles' response to a stimulus. "One sentient and intelligent PRINCIPLE" was the source of life, sense, motion, and reason and it affected the body "by the intervention of something in the brain and nerves" (*An essay*, 1751, p. 290). In the following passage, from the same source, Whytt explained the role of the sentient principle in a variety of happenings, including the pupillary light reflex, that until recently was known as "Whytt's reflex."

EXCERPT PP. 248–255

2. IF it were constantly observed, that such muscles only as had their fibres immediately acted upon by a *stimulus*, were excited into contraction, then indeed it might be suspected with greater shew of reason, that such motions were no more than a necessary consequence of the mechanical action of the *stimulus* upon the muscular fibres: but as we find the muscles of animals brought into action without any irritation of their fibres, whenever a *stimulus* is applied to the coats or membrances covering them, or to some neighbouring or even distant part, it seems absurd to imagine such motion owing to the mechanical action of the *stimulus* upon the fibres of the muscle, and not to the impression it makes on the sentient principle. Thus the contraction of the *sphincter pupillae* arising from the action of light on the *retina*, with which it has no communication of nerves, cannot possibly be explained mechanically, but must be owing to some sentient principle in the brain, which, excited by the uneasy sensation, determines the influence of the nerves more copiously into that muscle . . . . If a spark from a fire, or a drop of boiling water falls upon one's foot, the leg is instantly drawn in towards the body; but as the muscles employed in this action are those which run along the thigh, and are inserted about the head of the *tibia*, it is manifest that this *stimulus* cannot excite the muscles into contraction in consequence of any mechanical action upon them: and if sympathy of nerves, or continuation of membranes, shall be alleged as the cause of this motion, it may be justly demanded, why the muscles which run along the leg, and are inserted into the foot, are not more remarkably moved than those of the thigh, since they have a nearer connexion with the part to which the *stimulus* is applied; or why the extensors of the leg are not brought equally into action with its flexors. It remains therefore that the motion of the leg, in this case, be attributed to the pain or uneasy sensation excited by the fire or boiling water, for avoiding of which the sentient principle is instantly determined to put the flexors of the leg in motion, and so to remove the member from the offending cause . . . .

. . . .

3. WE consider that not only an irritation of the muscles of animals, or parts nearly connected with them, is followed by convulsive motions; but that the remembrance or *idea* of things, formerly applied to different parts of the body, produces almost the same effect, as if they themselves were really present. Thus the sight, or even the recalled *idea* of grateful food, causes an uncommon flow of spittle into the mouth of a hungry person; and the seeing of a lemon cut, produces the same effect in many people . . . .

FURTHER, that many very remarkable changes and involuntary motions are suddenly produced in the body by the various affections of the mind, is undeniably evinced from a number of facts. Thus fear often causes a sudden and uncommon flow of pale urine. Looking much at one troubled with sore eyes, has sometimes affected the spectator with the same disease.—Certain sounds cause a shivering over the whole body.—The noise of a bagpipe has raised in some persons an inclination to make urine.—The sudden appearance of any frightful object, will, in delicate people, cause an uncommon palpitation of the heart.—The sight of an epileptic person agitated with convulsions, has brought on an epilepsy; and yawning is so very catching, as frequently to be propagated through whole companies. In these cases, the motions produced in the vessels of the eyes or eye-lids, in the heart, stomach and bladder, in the secretory tubes of the salivary glands and kidneys, in the muscles employed in yawning, etc., cannot be owing to the mechanical action of the causes above mentioned upon the fibres of the parts moved: for what particular connexion is there between the optic and auditory nerves, and those which serve the heart, stomach, bladder of urine, mouth, salivary glands, and the muscles which depress the lower jaw and move the trunk of the body? All the nerves don't at last terminate in a point, but in a large space of the brain; wherefore the consent between them cannot be deduced from their contiguity, but must be owing to a sentient PRINCIPLE, which is present AT LEAST wherever the nerves have their origin, and which, accordingly as it is variously affected, produces motions and changes in different parts of the body.

In the *Essay* (1751) Whytt also considered the purposes of the reflex and concluded that one of them was to provide a defence mechanism.

EXCERPT PP. 289–290

The mind, therefore, in producing the vital and other involuntary motions, does not act as a rational but as a sentient principle . . . .

The general and wise intention of all the involuntary motions, is the removal of everything that irritates, disturbs, or hurts the body . . . . Nevertheless, as, in many instances, the very best things may, by excess, become hurtful; so this endeavour to free the body, or any of its parts, from what is noxious, is unhappily, sometimes, so strong and vehement, as to threaten the entire destruction of the animal fabric. But in the main, this FACULTY must be confessed highly useful and beneficial; since, without it, we should constantly have cherished in our bodies the lurking principles of diseases, slowly indeed and by imperceptible degrees, but not less surely, ruining our health and constitutions.

The location of the sentient principle, which in Whytt's view was the central link of the mechanism underlying sympathy, or the reflex, was also examined; reference to the problem has already been cited (p. 323). It was common knowledge that vital functions, and in some cases the whole animal, could survive decapitation for some time and thus involuntary movements were not dependent solely upon the brain. Stephen Hales (1677–1761) had told Whytt that whereas decapitation did not abolish reactions to stimulation, destruction of the spinal cord did (cf. Leonardo da Vinci, p. 294), and Whytt reported his observations on this important topic in 1755. The following passage is from this work (*Physiological essays*, Pt. II, Sec. II, "Observations on the sensibility and irritability of the parts of man and other animals," in *The works of Robert Whytt, M.D. published by his son* [Edinburgh, 1768]).

EXCERPT PP. 284–285

FURTHER, it ought to be observed, that when, after decollation, the spinal marrow of a frog is destroyed with a red hot wire, no visible motion is produced in its limbs or body, by pricking, cutting, or otherwise hurting them: only, when the skin of the thighs was dissected off, and the muscles were irritated, the fibres of those muscles were agitated with a weak alternate tremulous motion. Now, as the strong convulsive motions excited by irritation in the legs and trunk of the body of a frog after decollation, are to be ascribed to the sound state of the spinal marrow, since they cease as soon as it is destroyed; Is it not highly probable, that the weak tremulous motion in the irritated muscles of the thighs of a frog, after the destruction of the spinal marrow, were owing to the influence or power of their nerves, which still remained intire? It seems also to deserve notice, that, after the destruction of the spinal marrow, altho' the fibres of such muscles as were irritated exhibited a weak tremulous motion; yet there was no sympathy between the different muscles, or other parts of the body, as was observed while the spinal marrow was entire: from whence it seems to follow, that the nerves distributed to the several parts of the body have no communication but at their termination in the brain or spinal marrow; and that to this, perhaps alone, is owing the *consent* or sympathy observed between them.

This fundamental experiment establishing the spinal cord as an essential structure for the mediation of reflex activity was called by Eckhard (1881, p. 43) the

Fundamentalversuch of reflex physiology. It was partly owing to evidence of this sort that interest in the cord's function increased (p. 347). However, Whytt had already shown that even half a frog could survive (*Essay*, 1751).

EXCERPT P. 384

29. A frog lives, and moves its members, for half an hour after its head is cut off; nay, when the body of a frog is divided in two, both the anterior and posterior extremities preserve life and power of motion for a considerable time.

It could now follow that only a portion of the spinal cord was necessary for reflex activity. This was another of Whytt's important contributions to the development of the idea of the reflex. It is also clear from his writings that he had recognized the phenomenon we today call "spinal shock."

JOHANN AUGUST UNZER
(29 April 1727—22 April 1799)

As an idea develops it is at times advanced by men who make no original contribution to it but who are able to evaluate and present the evidence that supports it in a systematic manner. This was Waldeyer's contribution to the development of the neuron doctrine (pp. 113–117), and such was the role of Unzer and Procháska in regard to that of the reflex.

Unzer was born at Halle and studied medicine there in the University. In 1750 he moved to Hamburg where he engaged in a variety of literary activities as well as medical practice. From an early age he had been attracted to philosophical problems of human activity and wrote extensively on neurometaphysical topics. After the publication of his book on physiology at the age of forty-four (see Unzer, 1851, pp. i–viii; Kirchoff, 1921, pp. 13–15) he turned his attention to the pathology of contagious disease.

His book *Erste Grunde einer Physiologie der eigentlichen thierischen Natur thierischer Körper* (Leipzig, 1771) took him twenty-five years to prepare and can be described as a system of physiological metaphysics. In it Unzer helped to popularize the concept of the reflex, especially by the introduction of terms that are still in use. Thus he freely used the verb "to reflect," and his translator (1851) used it even more frequently; he also introduced "afferent" (*aufleitend*) and "efferent" (*ableitend*). He studied the reflex pathway more thoroughly than did Whytt and to do so accepted the teachings of Descartes and Haller's theory of irritability; the external sensory impression was the afferent and the internal sensory impression the efferent limb. His account of this, however, was still cumbersome and lacking in clarity although a little more precise than that of Whytt. Furthermore, he thought incorrectly that the central part of the reflex was either in the sensory root ganglia of the spinal cord, which acted like small brains for unconscious reflex activity, or in the cord itself, or even in the muscle.

The following passages have been newly translated; the word *reflect* occurs five times whereas in Laycock's translation of the same parts of the German text it is found on nine occasions.

EXCERPT P. 396

SECTION 399

An external sensory impression is transformed into an internal impression or it produces one if its progress, which is naturally from the nerve endings towards the brain, is turned back or reflected (*reflektiret*) so that it returns downwards from the brain to the branches and endings of the nerves. This happens in animals, which possess animal soul [sentient] forces, and it is usually observed in the brain through the agency of the external sensation of the external sensory impression.

EXCERPT PP. 410–412

SECTION 415

1. If at the place where a nerve receives an external sensory impression it is completely incorporated into a mechanical machine which is capable of certain animal movements at that same place, for example in a muscle, then the nerve immediately sets the machine into this animal motion. In such a case the nerve action needs nothing more than the external sensory impression, whether it goes further in the nerve or not. In this way a muscle fibre in an excised muscle contracts immediately at the place where a pinch of salt dissolves upon it or when it is stimulated by a needle point.

2. A nerve may cause nervous effects either by means of an external sensory impression on areas remote from the place of touching or on the touched parts themselves, but through other branches than the ones that have received the impression originally or else through its own efferent (*ableitenden*) fibrils. Then the external sensory impression in the nerve projects itself towards the brain. But it must make a detour from its original direction before it reaches the brain and is turned in such a way that by an internal sensory [impression] it excites the nerve of the other part or the branches of the nerves or the efferent nerve fibrils of the excited parts in the direction of the observer and away from the brain. This internal sensory impression, which is nothing else but the external one turned round, starts from the turning point and goes downwards from the brain through the nerves, branches, or fibrils into the mechanical machine which has to

perform the nerve action. This is irrefutably proved by experiments. If the toe of a healthy frog which is lying quietly is squeezed, this external sensory impression passes up into the brain. There it is turned back into the nerves of the extremities which act, and the animal moves all its limbs, sits up, and jumps away; for this effect is determined by the laws of external sensations. If the head is cut off with scissors and the toe is squeezed again, the same result is observed. In this case the external sensory impression from the toe must go through the nerve towards the brain, although it cannot reach it. For if the nerve to this foot in the upper limb is cut through, the external sensory impression cannot ascend so that squeezing the toe does not produce this effect. Therefore the external sensory impression in the nerves of the toe had of necessity to turn round on its way to the brain somewhere in the nerves of the extremities. It must have given the nerves an internal sensory impression which returned from the turning point through their stems, into their branches and directly into the muscles of the extremities. Except for the one toe, in this experiment, there is no stimulation of any other part of the body which might have set the muscles into immediate motion, as described in No. 1 [above], and likewise for that purpose the spinal cord needs to use no internal sensory impression. But now the nerve of the upper limb with the toe that was not squeezed and which has been set in motion solely by the internal sensory impression of the reflected (*reflektirten*) external one produced by the pressing of the other foot, should be cut and the [original] toe squeezed again. This limb will no longer move, although the other extremities, the nerves of which are still intact, will repeat the earlier movements. In this case, the events are the same as when an internal sensory impression is made on the spinal cord under the same circumstances. "For if the spinal cord is stimulated and spasmlike distortions of the whole body result, and if before this a separate nerve is cut through at the same time, the part of which the nerves have been cut will be the only part not to suffer spasms" (p. 508). The sensory impression which has been turned outwards, and which has given an internal impression to the nerves of the extremities, sets in motion only those muscles with which it is in continuity, from the turning point backwards into the nerve endings.

EXCERPT P. 493

SECTION 495

If an internal sensory impression without an act of mind is not primary but is an external one reflected in its course, it causes only the indirect nervous effects of an external impression. Its field of activity in a bound nerve is the same as that of a primary internal impression and it needs just as little brain [influence] and just as little imagination under comparable conditions. Such nervous effects of an internal sensory impression, without involvement of the mind from a reflected external one, is seen if a decapitated frog jumps up when its toe is pinched. The external sensory impression can in this case ascend unimpeded from the point of contact in the toe up to the point of injury in the [cervical] spinal cord and can be reflected in its course and returned without hindrance. In this way the same nervous effect is produced as that owing to the stimulation of the spinal cord by a primary internal sensory impression lacking involvement of the mind.

JIRI PROCHÁSKA
(10 April 1749—17 July 1820)

When Harvey described the circulation of the blood he was unable to complete the vascular circle because he had not discovered the capillaries, although he postulated a connection. The situation regarding the reflex was in a similar state of development, for whereas the afferent and efferent limbs were recognized, the central link was still unknown. Procháska who, like Unzer, contributed to the concept by clarifying it and by avoiding philosophical considerations which had veiled previous explanations, gave a clearer account of the central mechanism.

Procháska was born in Blizkovice in Southern Moravia, the son of a blacksmith, and studied medicine in Vienna. From 1778 to 1791 he was professor of anatomy, physiology, and ophthalmology in Prague and then held the same post in Vienna. He retired in 1819. Although he developed an extensive practice in ophthalmology, his research was carried out in the fields of anatomy, histology, and physiology, especially of the nervous system, and is to be found in the fourteen books and seventeen papers he published (see Unzer, 1851, pp. ix–xii; Kruta, 1949, 1962).

Procháska termed the central mechanism of the reflex the "sensorium commune" which was not related to the soul. In the absence of knowledge concerning its anatomical basis, this was necessarily vague, but there is nevertheless a degree of clarity in Procháska's writings not found in those of his predecessors. However, he also thought that the spinal root ganglia and peripheral plexuses could act as parts of the reflex pathway. He was careful to differentiate between theory and fact, and he evaluated critically all contemporary data on the problem of nerve function in general and reflex function in particular. The result was the formulation of the reflex as an example of nervous activity.

The following passage deals only with the "sensorium commune" and has been translated from *Adnotationum academicarum. Fasciculus tertius* ([Prague, 1784], Ch. IV, "Functions of the sensorium commune").

EXCERPT PP. 114–117

I. WHAT IS THE SENSORIUM COMMUNE, ITS FUNCTIONS, AND ITS SITE?

The external impressions which are made on the sensory nerves are very swiftly transmitted through their whole length to their origin; when they reach there, they are reflected according to a certain law and cross over into certain complementary motor nerves through which they are again transmitted very swiftly to the muscles and arouse certain determined movements. That place in which like a center the sensory and motor nerves run together, and in which the impressions of the sensory nerves are reflected to the motor nerves, is called, in the term now accepted by many physiologists, *Sensorium commune*.

. . . . It certainly does not seem that the whole of the cerebrum and cerebellum is concerned in the establishment of the Sensorium commune, but parts of the nervous system are rather the instruments that the soul uses directly for carrying out its so-called animal actions; the Sensorium commune, properly so-called, appears not improbably to extend through the medulla oblongata, the peduncles of the cerebrum and cerebellum, also parts of the thalamus, and the whole of the spinal cord; in short, as widely as the origin of the nerves extends. The surviving movements of decapitated animals, which could not be performed without the concordance and assistance of the nerves arising from the spinal cord, teaches that the Sensorium commune extends as far as the spinal cord, because if a decapitated frog is pricked, not only does it withdraw the pricked part, but also creeps and jumps, which could not be done without the agreement of the sensory and motor nerves; the site of this agreement must be in the spinal cord, the remaining part of the Sensorium commune.

The reflection of sensory impressions into motor, which occurs in the Sensorium commune, is not performed solely according to physical laws according to which the angle of reflection is equal to the angle of incidence, and the amount of the action followed by an equal reaction; but that reflection follows special laws inscribed, as it were, by nature on the medulary pulp of the Sensorium; we are able to understand these laws only from the effects, but we cannot at all discover them through our mental abilities. However, the general law by which the Sensorium commune reflects sensory impression into motor is that of our preservation: so that certain motor impressions may follow external impressions about to harm our body and produce movements aimed at warding off and removing the harm; on the other hand, internal or motor impressions may follow external or sensory impressions about to be favorable to us, and produce movement tending to preserve that pleasant condition longer.

MARSHALL HALL
(*18 February 1790—11 August 1857*)

Unfortunately, the work of Unzer and Procháska had little influence at the time; nevertheless, interest was growing in the form and function of the spinal cord owing in part to Whytt's investigations (p. 336). For example, in 1812 Legallois (pp. 294–296) had demonstrated its segmentation and its role as a center for sensory and motor activity. This was as important a contribution to the reflex theory as it was to the physiology of the cord itself. Furthermore, it attracted the attention of an English physiologist, Marshall Hall, who was to carry the concept a stage further.

Hall was born in Basford, near Nottingham, and received the M.D. degree from the University of Edinburgh in 1812. Thereafter he practised in Nottingham until 1826 when he moved to London. His research was mainly in the field of physiology and he was especially interested in the vascular and nervous systems. The results of his studies were widely accepted abroad, but Hall received little recognition in Britain and never held even a hospital appointment in London. His interests outside medicine were widespread. In regard to his work on the reflex he was accused of plagiarizing Procháska's work but this charge was never proved; Hall, it may be stated, was remarkably unaware of the research of others (see George, 1837–1838, for evidence against Hall; and for his support, Lewes, 1860, II, 166–167; see also Jeitteles, 1858; C. Hall, 1861; Hale-White, 1935, pp. 85–105).

Of greater importance than Legallois' work was the Bell–Magendie controversy (pp. 299–303) that focused attention upon the two pathways of the spinal cord reflex, the motor and sensory spinal roots. Hall, however, made no use of this new knowledge but became convinced that the neuraxis contained a special reflex system independent of the motor and sensory systems then receiving increasing attention (Chapter V).

Despite the controversies that centered about Hall's work, it is clear that he established the reflex as an essential and fundamental feature of nervous function. In a paper entitled "On the reflex function of the medulla oblongata and medulla spinalis" (*Phil. Trans. R. Soc.*, 1833, 123:635–665) he introduced the noun "reflex"; Whytt had used it but not in the sense we now understand, and both Unzer and Procháska, like Descartes and Willis before them, had used only the verb. Hall showed that reflex activity could be distinguished from other types of movement, that it produced what today we call "muscle tone," that it included sneezing, coughing, and vomiting, and that it could be influenced by disease. The discovery of these characteristics, and the general formulation of the reflex concept, remain Hall's outstanding contributions. However, the central link of the reflex continued to be a mystery to Hall, as it was to Johannes Müller, whose work was overshadowed by that of his English contemporary but was nonetheless outstanding and frequently in accord (Hall, 1837). These investigators were able to rely entirely upon their experimental findings and, unlike their predecessors, could discount the intervention of the soul and so exclude the metaphysical miasma that had clouded much of the previous work on the subject of reflex activity. The following passages have been selected from Hall's paper of 1833.

EXCERPT PP. 637–639

This property is characterised by being *excited* in its action, and *reflex* in its course: in every instance in which it is exerted, an impression made upon the extremities of certain nerves is conveyed to the medulla oblongata or the medulla spinalis, and is reflected along other nerves to parts adjacent to, or remote from, that which has received the impression.

It is by this reflex character that the function to which I have alluded is to be distinguished from every other . . . . There is, however, [in addition to voluntary respiratory and involuntary muscle action] a *fourth* [type of muscle action] which subsists, in part, after the voluntary and respiratory motions have ceased, by the removal of the cerebrum and medulla oblongata, and which is attached to the medulla spinalis, ceasing itself when this is removed, and leaving the irritability undiminished. In this kind of muscular motion, the motive influence does not originate in any central part of the nervous system, but at a distance from that centre: it is neither spontaneous in its action, nor direct in its course; it is, on the contrary, *excited* by the application of appropriate stimuli, which are not, however, applied immediately to the muscular or nervo-muscular fibre, but to certain membranous parts, whence the impression is carried to the medulla, *reflected*, and reconducted to the part impressed, or conducted to a part remote from it, in which muscular contraction is effected.

The first three modes of muscular action are known only by actual movements or muscular contractions. But the reflex function, exists as a continuous muscular action, as a power presiding over organs not actually in a state of motion, preserving in some, as the glottis, an open, in others, as the sphincters, a closed form, and in the limbs, a due degree of equilibrium, or balanced muscular action—a function, not, I think, hitherto recognised by physiologists.

. . . .

All the kinds of muscular motion may be unduly excited. But the reflex function is peculiar in being excitable into modes of action not previously subsisting in the animal economy, as in the cases of sneezing, coughing, vomiting, etc. The reflex function also admits of being permanently diminished or augmented, and of taking on some other morbid forms, of which I shall treat hereafter.

In the same paper (1833) Hall reported various reflex movements he could demonstrate by appropriate stimulation of the severed head of a turtle and of its torso. The following passages contain a description of his famous experiment on the reflex tone of the anal sphincter. Thus he included as well the autonomic nervous system in his contributions to reflex activity. He also introduced the term "reflex arc" for the first time. Bell had already made use of a "nervous circle" but this referred to muscle sense: "Between the brain and the muscles there is a circle of nerves; one nerve conveys the influence from the brain to the muscle, another gives the sense of the condition of the muscle to the brain" (p. 170, "On the nervous circle which connects the voluntary muscles with the brain," *Phil. Trans. R. Soc.*, 1826, 116 [ii]:163–173).

EXCERPT P. 645

This experiment affords evidence of many important facts in physiology. It proves that the presence of the medulla oblongata and spinalis is necessary to the contractile function of the eyelids, the sub-maxillary textures, the larynx, the sphincters, the limbs, the tail, on the application of stimuli to the cutaneous surfaces or mucous membranes. It proves the reflex character of this property of the medulla oblongata and spinalis, and the dependence of these motions upon the reflex function. It proves that the tone of the limbs, and the contractile property of the sphincter, depend upon the same reflex function of the medulla spinalis—effects not hitherto suspected by physiologists. [But see Whytt, p. 339.]

. . . .

An interesting experiment demonstrates the powerful influence of the reflex function over the sphincter ani in the turtle. If, after the removal of the tail and the posterior extremities, with the rectum, and of course with a portion of the spinal marrow, water be forced into the intestine, by means of Read's syringe, both the cloaca and the bladder are fully distended before any part of the fluid escapes through the sphincter, which it then does on the use of much force only, and by jerks. The event is very different on withdrawing the spinal marrow: the sphincter being now relaxed, the water flows through it at once in an easy continuous stream, with the application of little force, and without inducing any distension, even of the cloaca.

EXCERPT PP. 662–663

It appears probable that the facts of this paper may lead to some important additions to our knowledge of anatomy, by inducing an accurate inquiry into the origin, course, connexion, and distribution of the subcutaneous, or submucous, and muscular nerves, which constitute the arcs of the reflex function. There can be no doubt that a system of nerves takes its origin from the lower portion of the spinal marrow, to supply the sphincters and the organs of generation, which may be compared to those which concentre in the medulla oblongata. The medulla is also, in its whole course, the source of nerves which supply the limbs, the tail, and the panniculus carnosus, in those animals [the amphibia and the hedgehog] which possess these structures respectively.

Hall judged his contribution to the physiology of the nervous system to be of the greatest importance and even compared it to Harvey's discovery of the circulation of the blood. He claimed that he had spent twenty-five thousand hours on the problem! To emphasize the uniqueness of the special "reflex" nervous system which he postulated, he introduced several terms which fortunately have not survived. Thus "diastaltic" meant "reflex arc" and is contained in the title of his book, *Synopsis of the diastaltic nervous system* (London, 1850). In it he gave a succinct summary of his findings. The separate reflex or diastaltic system was mediated by special fibres, the excitosensory (afferent) and the excitomotor (efferent) which mingled with ordinary motor and sensory fibres in mixed nerves. It was limited to the spinal cord in which the nervous influence could spread in all directions, and psychical functions had no part to play in it.

The following passages are from this monograph.

EXCERPT P. 4

II. NEW TERMS PROPOSED

15. On analysing the facts which have been detailed, I observed that the following anatomical relations are essential:

1. A nerve leading *from* the point or part irritated, *to* and *into* the spinal marrow;
2. The spinal marrow *itself*; and
3. A nerve, or nerves, passing *out of* or *from* the spinal marrow—*all in essential relation or connection with each other.*

EXCERPT PP. 32–33

150. Such was the condition of our knowledge of the anatomy of the nervous system when I entered on its investigation, in 1830—an investigation which led to an entire distinction of the spinal system from the cerebral and the ganglionic, distinct at least in its application to physiology and pathology.

151. It was during this investigation that I discovered a *special nervous Arc*, consisting of an esodic and anastaltic [afferent] nerve, *essentially linked* with a special portion of the spinal marrow, and *through* this with an exodic catastaltic [efferent] nerve and *special muscles.*

152. It was during the continued investigation of this subject that I observed that this nervous arc is not simple, but very multiplex, and that it is not one exodic [efferent] nerve merely which is associated, through the spinal marrow, with the esodic [afferent] nerves, but that nerves exodic [efferent] in *all* directions are so associated.

153. The course of excited action may be traced along each and all of these *nerves*. But in what part of their tissue, and along what particles of the spinal marrow, their influence extends, we are utterly ignorant.

154. As each esodic [afferent] spinal nerve serves for sensation and for conveying diastaltic [reflex] action, it has been supposed that it contains distinct *fibres* for each of these two offices. And as the same exodic [efferent] nerve conveys the impulse from volition and from diastaltic action, it also has been supposed to contain *two* appropriate sets of fibres. The same opinion has been extended to the columns of the spinal marrow.

155. . . . .

156. . . . .

157. . . . .

158. It is during the *progress* of diseases of the nervous system that our knowledge of its physiology is useful, by enabling us to *interpret* the symptoms, and to determine the *Diagnosis*.

159. The conclusion at which I have arrived may now be stated in a few words:

1. Within the spinal marrow there is a *special Nervous Centre*;
2. To this centre are essentially attached certain *special Esodic and Exodic Nerves*;
3. These together constitute a system of *Diastaltic Nervous Arcs*;
4. The whole of these, taken together, constitute the *Spinal or Diastaltic Nervous System*, viewed Anatomically.

ERNST HEINRICH WEBER   EDUARD FRIEDRICH WILHELM WEBER
(*24 June 1795—26 January 1878*)   (*6 March 1806—18 May 1871*)

The paradoxical situation whereby the stimulation of a nerve produced not muscular movement, but its reverse, was difficult to conceive. Yet the concept of inhibition was to play an important role in the history of the reflex in the second half of the nineteenth century when the influences which modify the reflex began to be appreciated.

Galen had described the relaxation of antagonist muscles (p. 326), as had Descartes (1649, Art. 11), and these were the first examples of inhibition to be described, although it was not recognized as a basic biological phenomenon. Its experimental demonstration, however, was not possible until 1846 when the Weber brothers studied the functions of the vagus nerve (Hoff, 1936, 1940).

Eduard and Ernst Weber were both born in Wittenberg. The former studied medicine at Halle, the latter at Leipzig. Eduard was made prosector at the Leipzig anatomical institute in 1836 and professor in 1847, a post he held for the rest of his life. Ernst, who was the more renowned of the two brothers, became professor of anatomy and physiology at Leipzig in 1821. His research dealt mainly with the physiology of the nervous system and the special senses. There is no doubt, however, that Eduard was chiefly responsible for the work on the vagus to be cited below (Ludwig, 1878; Dawson, 1928).

In 1838 A. W. Volkmann of Halle first observed cardiac vagal inhibition ("Von dem Baue und den Verrichtungen der Kopfnerven des Frosches," *Arch. Anat. Physiol.*, 1842, pp. 367–377), but he judged it an experimental error (Hoff, 1940, pp. 467–469). The Webers, however, were greatly assisted by the rotation apparatus they used to stimulate the nerve; it produced electrical waves of similar polarity but varying frequency and became a very popular therapeutic device. Their classic experiments were described by the Webers in Rudolph Wagner's *Handwörterbuch der Physiologie mit Rücksicht auf physiologische Pathologie* ([Braunschweig, 1846], Vol. III, pt. 2, pp. 1–122, "Muskelbewegung"). Later Eduard Weber showed that unilateral as well as bilateral vagal stimulation produced cardiac arrest.

EXCERPT PP. 42–45

A series of experiments in which we approached the problem from many different angles and which I conducted in collaboration with my brother Ernst Heinrich led us to the discovery that, *when the vagus nerves, or the parts of the brain from which they originate, are stimulated, the speed of the rhythmic impulses of the heart slows down and the heart can be completely arrested.* I shall refer to these observations in more detail since they provide us with the first certain evidence that the heart beat can be influenced by the brain; second, that this influence is affected by a nerve not thought to be involved in heart function; and finally, since this kind of effect of a nerve upon muscular organs, whereby movements which occur independently are inhibited rather than stimulated or even prevented completely, is new and startling.

1). When both hot wires of a rotation apparatus, which had been set in motion and from which the armature had been removed, were brought into contact with the upper and lower end of the spinal cord of a decapitated frog, or with the surface of the upper cut end only, the heart rate did not change appreciably when the galvanic circuit was closed. However, if one of the wires was inserted into a nasal cavity of a frog not decapitated, and the other wire was brought into contact with the spinal cord cut transversely at the level of the fourth or sixth vertebra, and now, after the armature was removed from the rotation apparatus, the brain and spinal cord were galvanized, the heart, after a few beats, became completely arrested and remained motionless for a few seconds, even after the current had been interrupted. Subsequently it started to beat again slowly within a circumscribed area of heart muscle, feebly at first, and at long intervals. With every new beat the movement spread to a larger area of the heart, became stronger and the beats followed each other in ever shorter intervals, until the heart finally had reached again its previous rate and its full function. During the period of arrest the heart was not contracted, but relaxed, because it was collapsed, flat, and enlarged, similar to its appearance during diastole, and it then gradually filled with blood.

2). In order to find the part of the nervous system which caused this inhibitory effect upon the heart, we separated the head of a frog from the spine, between the occiput and the first cervical vertebra, in such manner that the heart, lungs, and intestines remained connected with the head. We then brought both hot wires of the rotation apparatus next to each other to the cut surface of the oblongata. The activity of the heart was likewise inhibited. At times, this inhibition was more complete, at times less so, depending on how fresh and strong the frog was, and also upon whether the portions of the nerve were more or less exhausted and whether the current was influenced by more or less favorable conditions. *Either the heartbeat slowed down from the moment of galvanization or, after a few slow beats, the heart stood still. But not infrequently, it stopped almost immediately and remained motionless until the vagus nerve was exhausted, owing to the continued galvanization and, therefore, to its inability to transmit impulses to the heart by means of its normal conductivity* . . . .

3). . . . . Therefore, the portion of the brain which exercises an influence upon the heart impulses in the frog extends from the corpora quadrigemina to the lower end of the calamus scriptorii in the medulla oblongata.

4). The question now arose as to what are the nerves by which this portion of the brain exercises the inhibitory influence upon the heart beat. In order to see whether these were the vagus nerves, we again exposed the medulla oblongata and by galvanization caused the heart to stop beating. As soon as it had returned to its active function we cut the vagus nerve on one side outside the skull and detached a piece as long as possible, lifted it, and touched it at its distal end to both conducting wires. No effect was observed upon the heart, for it beat thirty-three times per minute as previously. However, the heart stopped beating after a few beats as soon as one of the conducting wires remained in touch with the vagus nerve, while the other one touched the medulla oblongata, so that both vagi, one directly and the other through the medulla oblongata, were affected. Consequently, the cooperation of both vagus nerves was required when a process of slowing down and stopping of the heart, starting from the medulla oblongata, was to be produced. When, therefore, we cut both vagi and, while they were either placed on a glass plate or suspended in the air, both were touched simultaneously with the ends of the conduction wires without any influence upon the medulla oblongata, the heart stood still after a few slow pulsations.

Expanding Knowledge

By 1850 the concept of the reflex had been considerably clarified, especially through the work of Marshall Hall in England and that of Müller in Germany. The basic idea had been accepted, and, as physiology rapidly developed in the second half of the nineteenth century, the phenomenon received increasing attention (Gault, 1904; Canguilhem, 1964).

It is worthy of note that after 1850 the problem of the soul and its relationship to reflex activity was still under discussion. In fact, the whole problem of decapitated or decorticated animals and the relationship of this condition to the soul remained so unresolved as to permit the famous argument between Eduard Pflüger (1829–1910) and Rudolf Heinrich Lotze (1817–1881) in which the former maintained the existence of a spinal cord soul or consciousness. Nevertheless, important considerations of brain–cord relationships arose from investigations aimed at evaluating the perceptive qualities of the spinal cord. Interest was also centered on the influences that modified the reflex, and the most important contribution in this regard related to the effect of inhibition, first described by the Webers (pp. 351–354) and in more detail by Sechenov (pp. 361–365). The announcement of brain reflexes and conditioned reflexes was the outcome of these studies. The problems of summation, muscle tone, and coordination of reflexes were also considered, and the application of the reflex to the diseased state resulted in the discovery of a host of diagnostic reflexes, illustrated here by the abnormal knee jerk and the extensor-plantar response.

It was also during the second half of the nineteenth century that the neuron doctrine was established (Chapter II), and as soon as this knowledge was available the anatomical basis of the spinal reflex arc could be supplied (see Liddell, 1960). As the discovery of the capillaries permitted recognition of the complete circulation of the blood, so it was with the reflex. The central connection in the spinal cord, which had evaded investigators for two hundred years, was at last known. In his survey of the neuron Waldeyer, in 1891, described and figured the component parts of the spinal reflex. Moreover, the function of the neuron was gradually being elucidated (Chapter III) and this, too, meant that a clearer explanation of the reflex was possible.

WILHELM HEINRICH ERB
(30 November 1840—29 October 1921)

Marshall Hall had recognized that alteration of the spinal reflex might accompany disease of the nervous system, but he had not recognized any specific examples of diagnostic importance. One of the notable developments in the history of the reflex in the second half of the nineteenth century was the discovery that the reflex could be used as an accurate and reliable method for examining the function of certain parts of the nervous system. At first, however, the significance of these reflexes and the variations they manifested were not understood. Thus in the case of the first spinal reflex to receive detailed attention, the knee jerk, initially two different opinions concerning its basic mechanism were introduced by the German clinicians who first described it simultaneously but independently. One was Wilhelm Erb of Heidelberg.

Erb was born at Winnweiler in Bavaria and studied medicine at Heidelberg, Erlangen, and finally at Munich where he received his medical degree in 1864. At Heidelberg he became interested particularly in diseases of the nervous system and was appointed professor *extraordinarius* in 1869. After a brief interval at Leipzig, he returned to Heidelberg as *ordinarius*. It was there that he carried out most of his neurological work which covered many aspects of the subject, as may be readily recognized from the eponyms bearing his name. It was owing to his influence as much as to that of anyone else that neurology developed into a specialty (see Schultze, 1922; McGill, 1936, pp. 115–119; Haymaker, 1953, pp. 279–282).

Not only has the knee jerk been a useful addition to clinical neurology, but as well it has proved to be an important experimental phenomenon and has been used widely in studies of the higher as well as the lower centers of the nervous system (Fearing, 1928). Its etiology at first provoked much discussion, and Erb considered that it was a true reflex analagous to those derived from cutaneous stimulation and dependent upon the reflex arc. In this he was correct. His discussion of the reflex was dated 22 January 1875 ("Über Sehnenreflexe bei Gesunden und bei Rückenmarkskranken," *Arch. Psychiat. NervKrankh.*, 1875, 5:792–802), and in order to indicate its mechanism he called it the *Patellarsehnenreflex*, a term still occasionally used today.

EXCERPT PP. 792–794

In healthy subjects as well as in those with diseases of the spinal cord I have for some time observed striking reflexes in the quadriceps femoris that could be promptly and easily elicited, and which seemed worthy of some attention and practical evaluation. They can be elicited by light tapping of the tendon of the quadriceps above or below the patella and are best produced from the ligamentum patellae; they certainly indicate an especially intimate and close reflex relation between this tendon and the muscles that are part of it.

I believe that I am not saying anything to my colleagues that is startlingly new; most of them are familiar with this phenomenon. Despite that, the literature is almost completely silent on this and similar facts which are certainly not without interest. Recently I had occasion to review a very extensive section of the literature on the physiology and pathology of the spinal cord, but I did not discover any unequivocal and useful reports unless the pertinent communications have unfortunately escaped my notice.

Therefore I feel I may be justified in publishing a brief note regarding these tendon reflexes, since they have proved to be a very frequent and readily established sign of which the diagnostic importance is certainly not to be underestimated; moreover, as a rule they occur with greater exactitude and precision than do the cutaneous reflexes which they do not always parallel, and, finally, I can confirm their presence in many other tendons apart from those of the quadriceps.

The quadriceps reflex which prompted these observations can be produced as follows: if one firmly holds and supports the leg to be examined, slightly bent at the hip and knee joint with all the muscles relaxed, and then lightly and elastically taps the region of the ligamentum patellae with the finger or with the percussion hammer (exactly as for very light and elastic percussion or the fluctuation test of the abdomen), each tap is immediately followed by a slight but significant and evidently reflex contraction of the quadriceps; one can see it and feel it. This causes the lower leg to display a marked and often very strong movement, and it is extremely difficult to suppress this reflex voluntarily. The reflex is particularly striking when one examines a leg which is crossed over the other, with the lower leg swinging loosely; with each tap the lower leg is jerked upwards and this is more marked the more forceful the causative blow. If the phenomenon is produced with the subject in a sitting position and the foot placed firmly on the ground, the upper thigh and torso become agitated. In cases with increased excitability, these reflexes can be readily produced with the leg in a fully extended position. Each tap causes a peculiar, itching or tickling sensation in the tendon.

If closer attention be paid to the phenomenon, it will then be noted that it can be produced very easily through the extent of the ligamentum patellae, that it occurs hardly at all or very imperfectly on the patella itself, and only at its margins and upper corners no matter how strong the tapping; above the patella there is a triangular space, of which the apex is directed upwards, and which evidently corresponds to the quadriceps tendon that lies unconfined between the vastis, from which the reflex can also be elicited although less easily.

In this way I have often observed the phenomenon in healthy subjects or in patients with mild illnesses; *however, this phenomenon can be seen much more exquisitely and strikingly in individuals with diseases of the spinal cord,* and for a long time I have used the "patellar tendon reflex" (*Patellarsehnenreflex*) for examination of reflex excitability in spinal paralyses.

Karl Friedrich Otto Westphal
(*25 March 1833—28 January 1890*)

It appears that the knee jerk had been discovered at about the same time by another German neurologist, Westphal, who was stimulated to publish his account of it when, as an editor of the *Archiv für Psychiatrie und Nervenkrankheiten,* he read Erb's paper. He stated ". . . I myself have recognized the symptom which I called the lower leg phenomenon (Unterschenkelphänomen [called by Erb the patellar tendon reflex]) and which I have followed since 1871." Erb had noticed it between 1870 and 1871 which seems to have given him priority. Moreover, would Westphal have published when he did had he not had the advantage of reading Erb's communication while in manuscript form?

Westphal was born in Berlin and attended medical school there and in Heidelberg and Zürich. He specialized in psychiatric and neurological disorders at the Charité hospital in Berlin, and in 1874 was appointed professor *ordinarius* of psychiatry in the University and director of the psychiatric and neurological section. He is remembered especially for his handling of psychiatric patients and for his studies of the pathology of the spinal cord and nerve and of neurosyphilis (see Moeli, 1890; Siemerling, 1890*a*, 1890*b*).

Westphal's interpretation of the phenomenon of the knee jerk was at variance with that of Erb for he considered it to be a local muscle contraction induced by the sudden tension owing to the blow on the tendon. Thus the name he chose for it indicated that he thought, incorrectly, that it was not a reflex. His paper, "Über einige Bewegungs-Erscheinungen an gelähmten Gliedern" (*Arch. Psychiat. Nerv-Krankh.,* 1875, 5:803–834), contains the following account.

EXCERPT PP. 803–806

In 1871, a patient who consulted me because of moderate motor weakness in a leg and certain cerebral symptoms, informed me that when he sat on a chair and lightly tapped the area below the knee cap of the affected leg, it moved forwards with a sudden jerk (extension of the knee joint).

Because the complaints of the patient were sometimes difficult to interpret, one might have been inclined to regard this peculiar symptom as the outcome of hypochondriacal imagination. However, I easily convinced myself that I was dealing here with a phenomenon that had nothing to do with imagination and which could not be duplicated in the other leg . . . .

At first it was seen that the symptom to which the above patient had drawn my attention was not at all rare in cases of motor weakness in the lower extremities. If in such a case the lower extremities are flexed (as for example when seated, with the foot placed lightly on the ground) and one then taps the ligamentum patellae lightly, but with rapid, brief taps—best done by placing the index finger over the middle finger and then letting it fly back with a jerk, or still more effectively with a percussion hammer—the lower leg is propelled upwards with a sudden jerk, and one can distinctly observe the contraction of the quadriceps femoris which often causes the patient to feel a peculiar sensation in this muscle, which is difficult to describe. One may also produce the same sign in certain cases with the subject in a horizontal position in bed, that is, with the knee-joint almost fully extended. One can repeat this experiment several times, one after the other, with the same result; sometimes it seemed possible to do it as often as desired. If one produces a number of such light taps upon the ligamentum patellae, which follow each other rapidly, the leg is not infrequently held in a sustained position of extension. If, in certain cases in which the sign is especially obvious, one brings about a sudden strong flexion of the knee joint and, in doing this, holds the lower leg tightly in this position, the lower leg begins rhythmic reflex, extension movements which follow each other rapidly, but cease spontaneously sooner or later.

. . . . Tapping other places on the lower leg does not cause contraction of the quadriceps. If one places a finger upon the ligamentum patellae and presses it deliberately and slowly, neither a movement of the lower leg nor a visible contraction of the quadriceps occurs, no matter how strong the pressure. Such is the state of affairs in certain motor disturbances [lower motor neuron] of the lower extremities.

However, one may also bring about the phenomenon in healthy subjects and, as I noted later, laymen are aware of it as a curiosity; but one has to use much more force in these cases which, incidentally, vary in different individuals. If, for instance, one strikes the patellar ligament forcefully with the ulnar side of the hand, or with short and quick blows of the percussion hammer, there occurs in almost all cases a sudden extension of the lower leg in healthy subjects, too, and this of course is easier the less resistance (friction) it has to overcome in stretching; especially therefore when the leg that is to be examined hangs down relaxed, or is crossed over the other one and so can swing freely. In such instances I myself am unable to suppress voluntarily the motion which is caused by the contraction of the quadriceps. If one taps less hard, or if the extension of the lower leg meets with greater resistance, as when the foot is placed on the ground, one can often notice and feel in healthy subjects a contraction of the quadriceps which does not produce movement.

Joseph François Félix Babinski
(17 November 1857—30 October 1932)

As well known as the knee jerk is the reflex response to stimulation of the plantar surface of the foot. Together they are of vital importance to the clinical neurologist who employs them to detect disease of the nervous system. The abnormal form of the plantar reflex is known as the extensor or Babinski response, named after its discoverer and popularizer.

Babinski was born in Paris of Polish parents and spent all his life there. He studied medicine at the University and thereafter worked with the great French neurologist Charcot at the Salpêtrière. He was in charge of the neurology clinic of the Hôtel de la Pitié from 1890 to 1927, and there he carried on the teaching and research methods of his master who died in 1893. He was one of the most outstanding clinical neurologists of the present century and a prolific writer. His research covered many aspects of diseases of the nervous system, although he is best remembered for the abnormal plantar response (see Fulton, 1933; Charpentier, 1934; Haymaker, 1953, pp. 234–236; Kolle, 1956–1963, II, 162–171).

Although the abnormal, extensor reflex had been observed by the German neurologist Remak in 1893 (Wartenberg, 1951), it was Babinski who discerned its significance and importance. His first report of the normal and abnormal reactions to plantar stimulation was given to the Société de Biologie in Paris on 22 February 1896 ("Sur le réflexe cutané plantaire dans certaines affections organiques du système nerveux central," *C. r. Séanc. Soc. Biol.*, 1896, 3:207–208), but a fuller account appeared later ("Du phénomène des orteils et de sa valeur sémiologique," *Sem. méd.*, 1898, 18:321–322). Many years later Babinski admitted that his discovery of the extensor responses was the result of an extensive survey of diagnostic tests that might help differentiation between organic and hysterical hemiplegia (Wartenberg, 1947).

Babinski wrote many papers on the extensor response and one of them included, in addition, fanning of the toes or the "signe d'éventail" ("De l'abduction des orteils," *Rev. Neurol.*, 1903, 11:728–729). He was a keen photographer and used this medium to illustrate the toe movements (fig. 93). Since then many variations of this reflex have been reported but the sign of Babinski remains the only reliable and universally accepted one (Wartenberg, 1945). The significance of the reflex is still debated (Nathan and Smith, 1955; Walshe, 1956). The following passage has been translated from Babinski's article of 1898.

EXCERPT P. 321

Before I begin my description [of a disturbance of the cutaneous plantar reflex] I must say a few words about the cutaneous plantar reflex in the normal adult to whom I shall refer here exclusively. It is necessary for you to know that . . . in addition to other reflex movements such as flexion of the foot on the leg, of the leg on the thigh, and of the thigh on the pelvis, irritation of the sole of the foot ordinarily provokes a flexion of the toes on the metatarsus, to which I particularly call your attention. It is to be found in normal individuals in whom irritation of the sole of the foot leaves the toes immobile, at least in appearance, but—and this is an essential point—they never perform a movement of extension; this applies mainly to the big toe with which we are especially concerned.

Now, in certain pathological states the stimulation of the sole of the foot provokes extension of the toes, particularly of the big toe; I designate this modification of the reflex movement by the name of the *phenomenon of the toes.*

In general, it is not only by the direction of the movement [of the big toe] that the normal reflex differs from the pathological one. Most often extension is performed more slowly than flexion and, besides, flexion is usually stronger when one irritates the inner part of the sole of the foot than when the stimulation occurs on the outer part; this is reversed with the extension. Finally, while flexion generally predominates in the last two or three toes, it is in the first, or the first two toes, that the extension is most pronounced.

The phenomenon of the toes may present "formes frustes" . . . .

This having been said, I shall now make known to you the technique that must be used for proper observation of the reflex movement of the toes. It is important that the muscles of the foot and leg be not in a state of contraction, and to achieve this it is well not to inform the subject of the experiment about to be performed, and to have him close his eyes. The leg must be slightly flexed on the thigh with the foot resting with its outer side on a bed; or without any support, the leg lifted and held by the experimenter. When the lower leg has been placed in this position, one must wait until the muscles seem completely relaxed before proceeding with the stimulation.

It does not matter whether one stimulates lightly or energetically, simply tickles or pricks the sole of the foot. This last method is necessary in certain patients in order to provoke a reflex movement of the toes. However, by contrast, in other individuals it causes such violent movements of the various parts of the lower leg that they are difficult to analyse. In such a case it is impossible to determine the direction of movement of the toes, and, if it is noticed, one may be uncertain whether it was a reflex or a voluntary movement. This is an important question to be solved, for it is hardly necessary to remark that if, under normal conditions, the cutaneous plantar reflex never manifests itself by an extension of the toes, this motion may have been carried out by a voluntary action following the pricking of the sole of the foot; in such cases it becomes necessary to repeat the stimulation by performing it superficially.

There is still another cause for error of observation that I must bring to your attention. The toes necessarily follow the flexion of the foot on the leg after stimulation of the sole. If then the movement of flexion on the metatarsus is lacking, as sometimes happens, the toes, passively drawn towards the anterior part of the leg, may give a careless observer the illusion of movement of extension on the metatarsus. To avoid this cause of error, one must take great care to examine the metatarsal-phalangeal articulation of the big toe, in order to establish how the phalanx and the metatarsus behave in relation to one another.

Ivan Mikhailovich Sechenov
(1 August 1829—2 November 1905)

So far the reflex had been considered as a function of the spinal cord and, as Hall and Müller had shown, obeyed specific laws. Although the mind was not entirely excluded, it did not direct this phenomenon. One of the many developments in the reflex concept during the second half of the nineteenth century was the demonstration that the rest of the central nervous system also had reflex functions. Thomas Laycock of Edinburgh (1812–1876), who was well acquainted with the similar but vague ideas of Procháska (p. 345), had argued in 1845 that in view of the continuity of nervous structures "the brain, although the organ of consciousness, was subject to the laws of reflex action and in this respect it did not differ from the other ganglia of the nervous system" [1845, p. 298], and he concluded that the entire nervous system was the seat of reflex function in which the mind played no part. This revolutionary opinion was taken up by the Russian physiologist Sechenov, who provided experimental evidence in its support.

Sechenov was born in Teply Stan in the province of Simbirsk and completed his medical studies at the University of Moscow in 1856. He then visited Berlin where he studied under Müller and du Bois-Reymond, and he worked in Carl Ludwig's laboratory in Vienna in 1858, and in Heidelberg with Helmholtz and Bunsen. In 1860 he was appointed assistant professor of physiology at St. Petersburg. His famous work on brain reflexes led to an accusation of moral corruption, and for a time Sechenov removed to Paris where he worked with Claude Bernard. From 1870 to 1876 he was in Odessa and thereafter held the chair of physiology at St.

Petersburg until 1888 when he moved to Moscow where he died. He contributed to general physiology and biochemistry but mainly to neurophysiology; he was described by Pavlov as "the pride of Russian thought and the father of Russian physiology" (see Shaternikov, 1935; Haymaker, 1953, pp. 155–158; Ischlondsky, 1958; Koshtoyants, 1962; Sechenov, 1965).

Like Laycock before him, Sechenov accepted the doctrines of association psychology which were based on the identity of mental processes with sense perception (Amacher, 1964). He also made use of the Webers' demonstration of inhibition (pp. 352–354), and by means of elegant experiments he discovered a cerebral mechanism that could inhibit peripheral reflexes. By this new application of materialistic philosophy, he proceeded to point out that higher brain function, including so-called voluntary acts, was basically reflex in nature for it was a response to sensory stimulation which led to a motor act (1935, pp. 31–139, "Reflexes of the brain"). Thus the nervous system as a whole functioned exclusively by means of reflex activity: lower or spinal reflexes, and cerebral or "psychic" reflexes which included emotions and thoughts.

The work that formed the basis of this radical belief was carried out in Claude Bernard's laboratory and published in German (*Physiologische Studien über die Hemmungsmechanismen für die Reflexthätigkeit des Rückenmarkes im Gehirne des Frosches*, Berlin, 1863; reprinted in *Selected works*, 1935, pp. 153–176). One method of brain stimulation was chemical (common salt crystals), as was the peripheral stimulus that induced a time-measurable reflex withdrawal of a frog's leg from dilute acid. Sechenov was thus able to assess quantitatively the effect of brain stimulation on a spinal reflex as well as, for the first time, to demonstrate reversible, central neural inhibition.

EXCERPT PP. 162–163

1). The application of salt on the cut surface of the hemisphere produced no constant result.

2). *The application of salt on a section of the thalamus always produces a marked depression of reflex activity if the section of the brain is constant.* This effect usually develops during the first minute after the application of the salt and often without any movement of the animal (direct or reflex). In cases where salt is applied in the form of crystals this influence lasts longer. The depression of reflex activity gradually disappears when the irritating substance is removed (the most expedient way is with a few drops of water and blotting paper) and it can be produced again if the next stimulus is stronger than the earlier one. I have one experiment (it is cited immediately below) in which I managed to repeat the depression of reflex activity three times in one and the same animal . . . .

3). *The application of salt to a section of the brain behind the corpora quadrigemina, i.e., at the upper border of the medulla oblongata, likewise produces a depression of reflex activity, although much weaker than in the previous case* . . . .

4). *The application of common salt on a section of the spinal cord just below the fourth ventricle certainly has no influence on the reflex activity of this organ.*

EXCERPT PP. 166–169

. . . . The problem therefore is to define the effect of stimulation of the sensory nerve fibres on the reflex activity of the spinal cord. Now to decide this question in its entirety, one would of course have to exert influence upon all the sensory nerves of the body. Unfortunately this is absolutely impossible in such a small animal as the frog. Therefore I was compelled to limit the stimulation to a small number of nerves and in so doing to stimulate the peripheral nerve distributions in the skin and the oral mucous membrane rather than the nerve trunk itself.

It is obvious, furthermore, that the changes in reflex activity resulting from sensory stimulation cannot be observed at the time when the latter takes place, because it is followed immediately by more or less strong reflex movements. One is therefore obliged to await the cessation of these reflex movements and only then to make these observations on reflex activity.

It is obvious from what has been said above that under such limitations the experiment is incomplete.

1). Indeed, it can demonstrate only the after-effect of the sensory excitation but not its direct influence upon the reflex activity of the spinal cord;

2). it is reasonable to fear that the violent reflex movements which precede the observation must influence the final results of the test;

3). lastly, because of the violent reflex movements resulting from the sensory stimulation, new factors are introduced into the experiment which enable us to explain the depression of reflex activity, in case such occurs, entirely independent from the excitation of the inhibitory mechanisms. For it is conceivable that in the case of a strong sensory stimulus which reflexly excites all the muscles of the body the effect of this excitation, although slowly decreasing, is still in progress when the definitive observation is made. Then, with the second definition of reflex activity, the weak effect of the [sulfuric] acid would not attack nerve fibres that are still in a state of excitation. The effect of this stimulation would of course differ from that of the acid in the first test of reflex activity, since at this point the acid affects normal nerve fibres. In this case the phenomenon of reflex depression would be explained quite independently from the effect of the inhibitory mechanisms.

Fortunately, it is very easy to brush aside all these objections against the method. Firstly, it is clear that it is immaterial whether the depression of reflex activity is obtained simultaneously with the sensory stimulation or as an after-effect of it; the presence of reflex depression anyway indicates that the inhibitory mechanisms can be activated by stimulation of the sensory nerve fibres. Now, concerning the two other objections, they can be nullified by two experiments which were conducted as follows. Cut the spinal cord of a frog below the fourth ventricle and test the reflex activity of the animal in the usual manner (by means of the acid solution). Next, strongly stimulate the skin of the frog (usually the entire surface of the abdomen) with a heated metal plate or a concentrated solution of sulfuric acid in water, and when the violent reflex movements have calmed down, the reflex ability of the animal is again defined. In such cases a change in the reflex activity is never seen, no matter how strong the stimulus and the resultant reflexes. Therefore, the second objection is definitely unfounded. Now, as for the third one, the following experiment speaks against it. Cut the brain of the frog below the quadrigeminal bodies, thus leaving the animal with the medulla oblongata—that part of the nerve centre from which it is easiest, as is well known, to produce general bodily movements. If now the experiment just described is carried out in such an animal, the reflex movements occurring as a result of the stimulation of the skin are, if possible, even more violent and generalised than in the preceding case, and depression of the reflex activity results; however, it is neither constant nor marked. By contrast, this depression becomes marked if, in an animal prepared as before, the oral mucous membrane rather than the skin is stimulated with a concentrated solution of sulfuric acid in water (equal parts of each). The reflex movements which follow immediately are here less violent and much less widespread (sometimes they are hardly noticeable) than when the skin has been burned. From this the unbiased reader will clearly realize that the phenomenon of reflex depression can in no case be dependent on the fact that, with the first test of reflex ability (prior to the strong sensory excitation) the stimulus affects nerves under normal conditions; however, following their main stimulation it encounters these only in a changed state.

Therefore, the method can actually be used in the interpretation on which it is based, and the results of the two experiments cited can be interpreted as follows: *The spinal cord of the frog contains no inhibitory mechanisms for the reflex movements of the extremities; these however are definitely present in the medulla oblongata of the animal. These mechanisms, as far as they can be put into action by reflex means must besides be considered as nerve centres, in the widest sense of the word, that is, as nerve organizations which serve the transformation of one type of movement into another.*

These are the most important results which I derived from the method described in this paragraph.

It now remains for me to mention two experiments with strong sensory stimulation which were carried out in intact animals and in frogs with the thalamus sectioned. The latter case is completely identical with that in which the uninjured medulla oblongata was left in the animal; it is simply less easy in this case to obtain the depression of the reflex movement than in the other. However, in the case of the intact animal there is no depression at all, so that one could believe that the hemispheres were organizations which inhibit the introduction of reflex depression. The last experiment, with all the others described in this paragraph, demonstrates that the sensation of pain cannot play any part at all in the phenomenon of reflex depression resulting from sensory skin excitation. If this were actually the case, one would have to obtain a stronger depression with uninjured nerve centres, than in the case of cerebral injury behind the quadrigeminal bodies, since it is much more natural to assume the presence of conscience in the anterior cerebral parts than in the medulla oblongata.

In this way the last possible objection to the method has been removed.

I shall now summarize all the facts that have so far been obtained from the frog:

1). *In the frog, the inhibitory mechanisms for reflex activity of the spinal cord have their seat in the thalamus, the quadrigeminal bodies, and in the medulla oblongata;*

2). *These mechanisms must be considered as nerve centres in the widest sense of the word;*

3). *The sensory nerve fibres form one, and probably the only one of the physiological routes for the excitation of these inhibitory mechanisms.*

Ivan Petrovich Pavlov
(*14 September 1849—27 February 1936*)

The immediate reaction to Sechenov's theory of brain reflexes was one of opposition, but support for it soon came. His thesis that psychic phenomena were akin to the essentially somatic acts that constituted nervous activity found an important supporter in his fellow countryman Pavlov, who described Sechenov's monograph on *Reflexes of the brain* as "an attempt, brilliant and truly extraordinary for the time (though of course a theoretical one in the form of a physiological outline) to picture our subjective world in a purely physiological aspect" (Sechenov, 1962, p. 20).

Pavlov was born in Ryazan, Central Russia, the son of a parish priest. He studied medicine at St. Petersburg, and after having received the M.D. degree in 1883, he spent two years in Germany; he studied the circulatory system under Carl Ludwig at Leipzig, and gastrointestinal secretion with Heidenhain at Breslau. These topics occupied the first period of his professional life, and the Nobel Prize, awarded in 1904, recognized his important contributions to them. In 1891 he became director of the physiology department in the St. Petersburg Institute of Experimental Medicine and later, professor of physiology in the Military Medical Academy. His remarkable digital dexterity, his ability to plan an experiment, and his powers of observation together with enormous industry and a brilliant mind made him a physiologist of great renown. His present fame in Russia is based upon the investigation of higher nervous activity which he pursued after the age of fifty-five (see Pavlov, 1928–1941, I, 11–31; Babkin, 1950; Haymaker, 1953, pp. 152–155; Asratyan, 1953; Kolle, 1956–1963, I, 200–215).

At the turn of the nineteenth century there were two outstanding investigators of the nervous system. One was the British physiologist Sherrington who was studying its lower nervous activity, and whose teachings have been accepted and widely disseminated. The other was Pavlov who in 1902 turned his attention from gastric function to develop the idea of the conditioned reflex or response; the Russian word *ooslovny* means *conditional*, and although its equivalents appear in French and German, the English usage has substituted *conditioned*. His work, however, has not spread beyond the school that he founded. Although it is true that the conditioned reflex may be a useful tool with which to examine the nervous system and behavior, and that it has stimulated an immense amount of work, few Western physiologists have accepted Pavlov's purely objective reasoning. Sherrington, for example, admired the experimental data accumulated by Pavlov but was not impressed by his deductions from it. Some have even ridiculed him, like G. B. Shaw who remarked, "Pavlov is the biggest fool I know; any policeman could tell you that much about a dog" (Pavlov, 1928–1941, II, 24).

Attempts have been made recently, notably by Konorski (1948), to make the Pavlovian studies "a logical complement of the system of physiology of lower nervous activity" (p. 6). However, only selections from some of Pavlov's earlier publications have been presented below and no attempt has been made to follow the development of his thesis and that of the Pavlovian school, nor the cogent arguments of his opponents.

When Pavlov received a Nobel prize in 1904, contrary to custom before and since, in his oration he reviewed his work on the conditioned reflex rather than the contributions that had won him a prize. The following passages have been translated from that oration, as published in *Les prix Nobel en 1904* (Stockholm, 1907).

EXCERPT PP. 13–17

. . . . For the salivary glands the rule is that all variations of their activity observed in physiological experiments are exactly duplicated in experiments with psychic stimulation, that is, those in which a certain object does not come into direct contact with the oral mucous membrane, but attracts the attention of the animal from some distance. For example, the sight of dry bread produces stronger salivary secretion than that of meat, although the latter, judged by the movements of the animal, stimulates a much more active interest. When the animal is teased with meat or any other edible substance, the salivary glands produce a very concentrated mucous; however, the sight of substances that the animal rejects causes a secretion of very liquid mucous from the same glands. In brief, the experiments with psychic stimulation represent an exact, however diminutive, copy of the experiments with physiological stimulation of the glands by means of the same substances.

. . . .

. . . . The results agreed with our expectations; the relations that could be observed between external phenomena and variations in the glandular activity could be organized in series; they appeared to correspond to a law since they could be duplicated at will . . . .

. . . .

. . . .

. . . .

. . . . The reported facts fit well into a framework of physiological thinking. The effects of our stimuli at a distance may justifiably be designated and classed as reflexes. It is proved under close scrutiny that this action of the salivary glands is always stimulated by an external phenomenon; that is, it, like the ordinary physiological salivary reflex, is released by external stimuli; the only difference is that the latter is triggered off by the surface of the oral cavity, and the former by the eye, the nose, etc. A further difference between the two reflexes lies in the fact that our old physiological reflex is a constant and unconditioned one, whereas the new reflex continually fluctuates and is therefore *conditioned*. However, if one observes the phenomenon more closely, one may perceive the following essential difference between the two reflexes: in the unconditioned reflex those properties of the object to which the saliva is physiologically related, hardness, dryness, certain chemical properties, are effective as a stimulus; but in the conditioned reflex those properties of the object that in themselves have no relation to the physiological role of the saliva, such as their color, etc., act as a stimulus. These latter properties appear here almost as *signals* for the former. One must consider their stimulating effect as a further, more subtle adaptation of the salivary glands to the phenomena of the external world . . . . Any given phenomenon of the external world can become a temporary signal of the object that stimulates the salivary glands, if the stimulation of the oral mucous membrane by this object is several times related to the effect of the respective external phenomenon upon another receptor surface of the body . . . . On the other hand, one may deprive signals that [normally] act promptly of their effect if they are often repeated without simultaneously bringing the respective object into contact with the oral mucous membrane. If one shows the most ordinary type of food to the dog for days or weeks without allowing him to eat it, the sight of it finally ceases to produce salivary secretion. One may readily imagine the mechanism of the stimulation of the salivary glands by means of the signal phenomenon on the object, that is, the mechanism of the "conditioned stimulus," physiologically as a function of the nervous system. As we have just seen, every conditioned reflex, that is, the stimulation by the signal phenomenon of the object, is based upon an unconditioned reflex, that is, a stimulation by the essential properties of the object. One must therefore assume that that point of the central nervous system that is markedly stimulated during an unconditioned reflex draws to itself those weaker reflexes that are emitted by the external world upon other points of the central nervous system, i.e., that, thanks to the unconditioned reflex, a temporary fortuitous path is opened to the central point of this reflex for all the remaining external stimuli. The conditions that influence the opening and closing of this path, its usefulness or neglect, represent the inner mechanism of the efficacy or inefficacy of the signal phenomenon of external objects, the physiological basis of the finest reaction of the living substance, and the finest ability to adapt by the animal organism.

It is now often considered that the cerebral cortex is essential for the existence of conditioned responses, although physiologists are by no means agreed upon its precise function. The following passages have been taken from the "Summary" of an address given by Pavlov to the International Congress of Physiologists at Groningen, Holland, on 5 September 1913 ("The investigation of the higher nervous functions," *Br. med. J.*, 1913, ii:973–978). In it he discussed the relationship of conditioned reflexes to brain function, clearly an extension of Sechenov's work on brain reflexes. Furthermore, the value of the conditioned reflex as a tool to investigate the central nervous system as a whole, was indicated here by Pavlov.

EXCERPT P. 977

. . . . The advantage of using the salivary glands and not the skeletal muscles as indicators of the higher functions of the brain is clear enough. If we judged by the muscles, the important fact that these complicated nervous relations still remain after the extirpation of the anterior half of the brain would be concealed. These experiments deal a severe blow to the psychological classification of subjective states; a psychological explanation here would encounter insuperable obstacles and a quite incomprehensible series of phenomena.

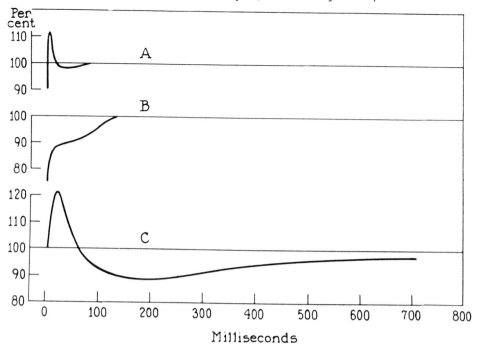

Recovery of excitability after a single response

FIG. 66. Gasser (1946, p. 131, fig. 2).
For explanation see text (p. 232).

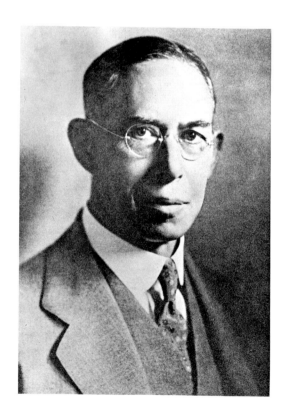

FIG. 67. Joseph Erlanger. From *Les Prix Nobel en 1940–1944*, Stockholm, Norstedt & Söner, 1946, facing p. 85. By permission, Nobel Foundation.

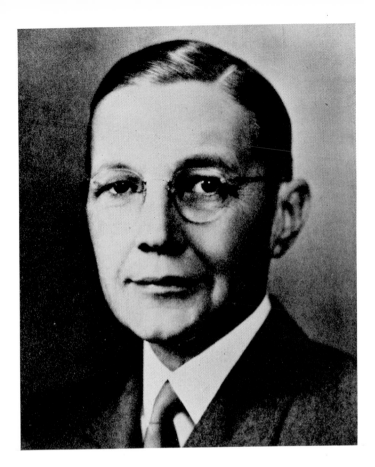

Fig. 68. Herbert Spencer Gasser. From *Les Prix Nobel en 1940–1944*, Stockholm, Norstedt & Söner, 1946, facing p. 86. By permission, Nobel Foundation.

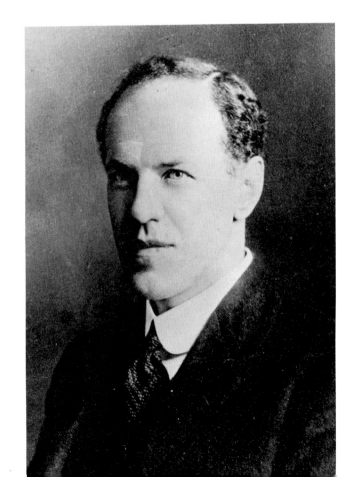

Fig. 69. Thomas Renton Elliott *c.* 1910. Courtesy of Sir Henry Dale.

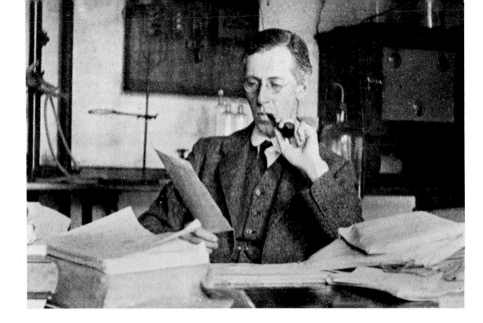

Fig. 70. Henry Hallett Dale c. 1918. By permission of the Wellcome Trustees.

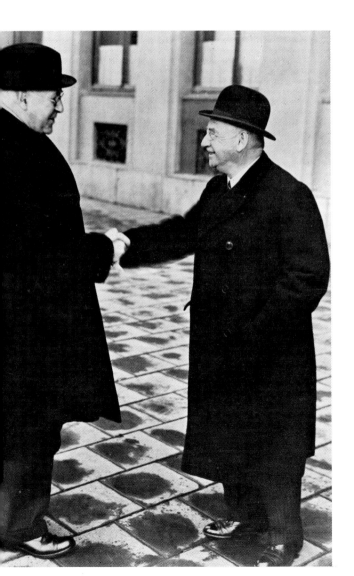

Fig. 71. Otto Loewi, right, and Sir Henry Dale, December 1936. By permission of the Wellcome Trustees.

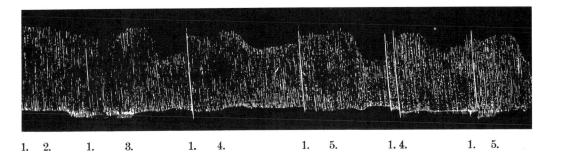

1.   2.   1.   3.   1. 4.   1. 5.   1. 4.   1. 5.

FIG. 72. Loewi (1922, p. 209, fig. 6). Frog: 1, Ringer, 2, acetylcholine, 1/100,000,000; 3, acetylcholine, 1/10,-000,000; 4, "Vagus content" (see text) of 20 min. control period, 1/40; 5, vagus content of 20 min. vagus period, 1/40; 5 corresponds approximately to 1/10,000,000; accordingly choline concentration in undiluted heart [vagus] content $1/10,000,000 \times 40 = 1/250,-000$ (see p. 253).

FIG. 73. Pourfour du Petit (1710, p. 15, Figs. I–III). Fig I depicts crossing medullary fibres. A, pons, B, pyramids, C, olivary bodies, D, lower pyramids; each divides into three fibre bundles which change sides; E–L, cranial nerves. Fig. II, spinal cord cut transversely. A, anterior partition, B, posterior partition, C, posterior nerves, E, transverse fibres, F, brown lines from posterior transverse fibres. Fig. III, cord with transverse fibres. A, junction of anterior and posterior nerves, B, longitudinal separation of posterior partition and transverse fibres seen in depths.

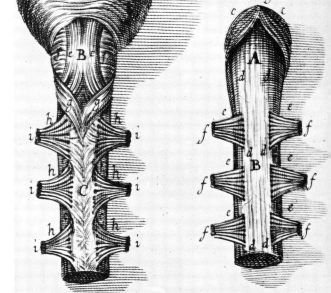

FIG. 74. Mistichelli (1709, figs. 1–2). Decussating fibres at *g* and *c*.

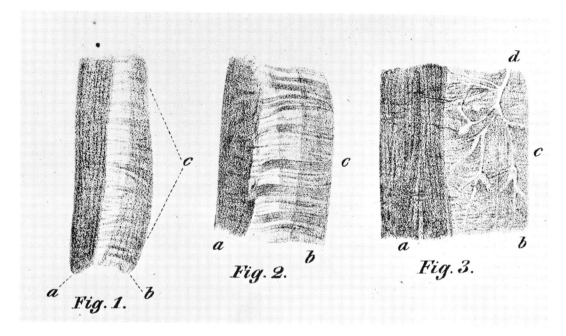

FIG. 75. Stilling (1842*b*, figs. 1–3).
For explanation see text (p. 272).

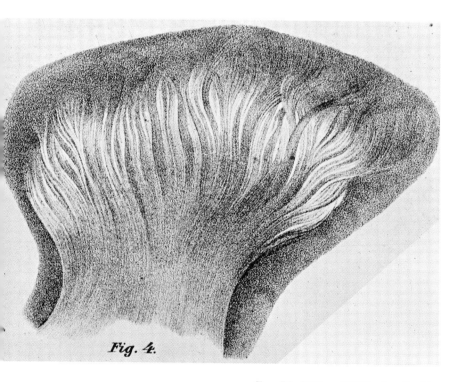

FIG. 76. Stilling (1842*b*, fig. 4). For
explanation see text (p. 273).

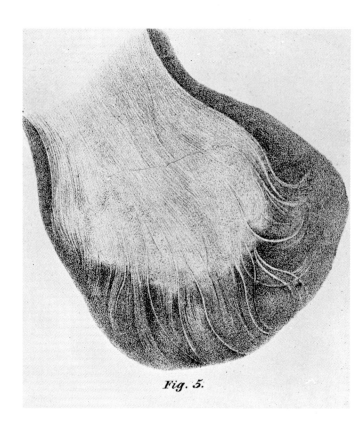

FIG. 77. Stilling (1842*b*, Fig. 5). For explanation see text (p. 273).

Fig. 5.

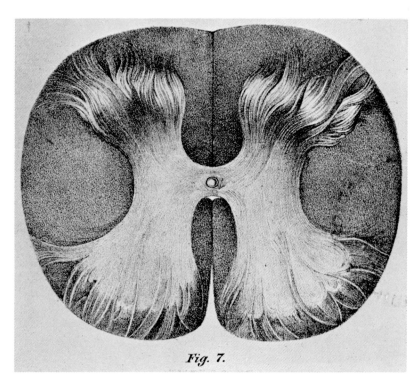

Fig. 7.

FIG. 78. Stilling (1842*b*, Fig. 7). For explanation see text (p. 272).

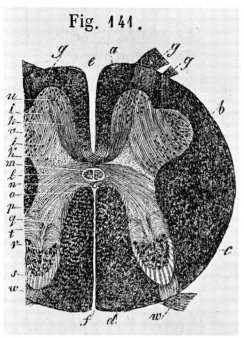

Fig. 141.

Fig. 79. Koelliker (1852, p. 275, fig. 141). Transverse section of upper lumbar cord, X *c.* 30, semidiagrammatic. *a*, anterior column, *b*, lateral columns, motor part, *c*, lateral, sensory, *d*, posterior columns, *h*, internal, *i*, external bundle of motor roots, *k*, decussation of anterior columns, *l*, gray fibres of lateral columns, *m*, central gray nucleus (? central canal), *n*, posterior gray commissure, *o*, posterior column fibres entering gray commissure, *p*, sensory fibres running to lateral columns, and *q*, entering posterior columns, *r*, longitudinal fibre bundles entering sensory roots, *s*, *substantia gelatinosa* with *w*, sensory root bundles, *t*, sensory fibres running horizontally anteriorly to gray commissure, *u* medial anterior horn cells, and *v*, lateral.

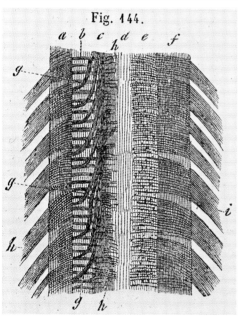

Fig. 144.

Fig. 80. Koelliker (1852, p. 280, fig. 144). Vertical section through cord midway between gray horn and point of entrance of nerve roots, X *c.* 25. *a*, posterior columns with sensory roots, *h*, crossing, *b*, *substantia gelatinosa*, *c*, posterior root prolongations that bend anteriorly to the *substantia* and run longitudinally to join posterior columns, *d*, base of posterior horn with ends of horizontal part of sensory root visible (cut across), *e*, anterior horn cells (spots) and horizontal and divided continuation of motor roots, *f*, anterior column crossed by motor roots, *i*.

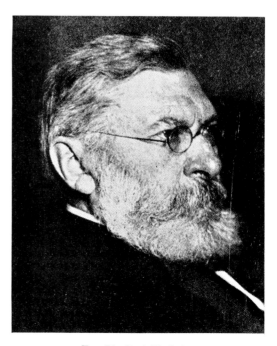

Fig. 81. Paul Flechsig. By permission, National Library of Medicine.

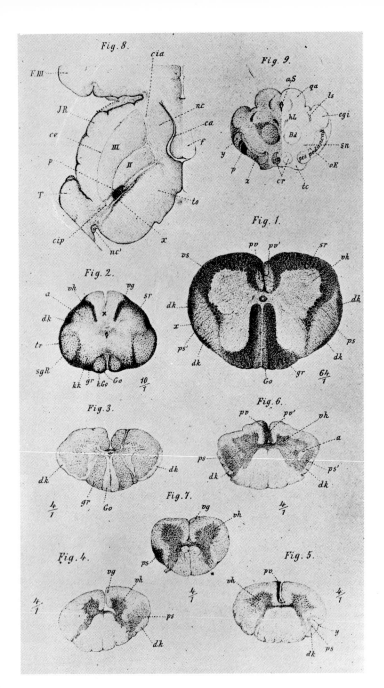

FIG. 82. Flechsig (1877, Plate VII, figs. 1–9). *ps, ps'*, lateral pyramidal tract; *pv, pv'*, anterior pyramidal tract; *dk*, direct lateral cerebellar tract; *vg*, tract of anterior column; *gr*, tract of posterior column (Burdach). Fig. 1, cervical enlargement of 35 mm. fetus; fig. 2, decussation of pyramids in 40 cm. fetus; *sgR, substantia gelatinosa*; *x*, pyramids, unmyelinated; fig. 3, cervical enlargement from case with compression of upper dorsal and lower cervical cord; fig. 4, ditto with degeneration (*ps*) of right lateral column; fig. 5, ditto with descending degeneration of left anterior and right lateral columns (*pv, ps*); fig. 6, ditto with symmetrical lateral sclerosis (Charcot); fig. 7, mid-lumbar; secondary degeneration of left lateral columns.

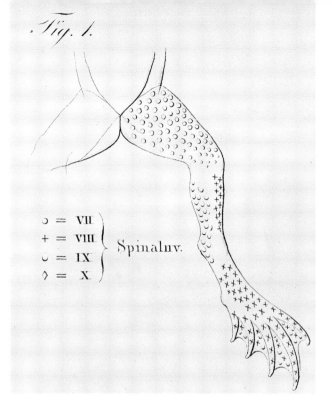

FIG. 83. Eckhard (1849, Plate V, fig. 1). Cutaneous distribution of seventh to tenth spinal roots on ventral surface of limb.

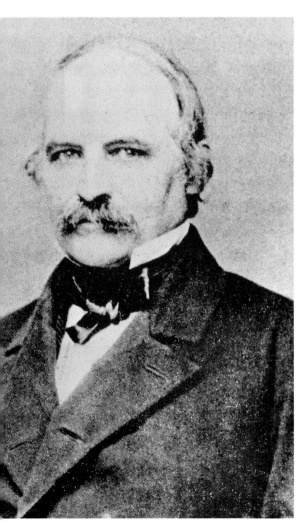

FIG. 84. Ludwig Türck. By permission, College of Physicians, Philadelphia.

FIG. 85. Türck (1869, Plate II, figs. 3–4). Fig. 3, lateral view of sensory areas of cervical (2–8 *Ha*, anterior, 3–5 *Hp*, posterior) and second to fourth thoracic (II. *B*, III. *B*, IV. *B*) roots. Fig. 4, sensory areas on medial forefoot and paw, cervical root areas, 6 to 8. *H*; 1st thoracic root area, I. *B*.

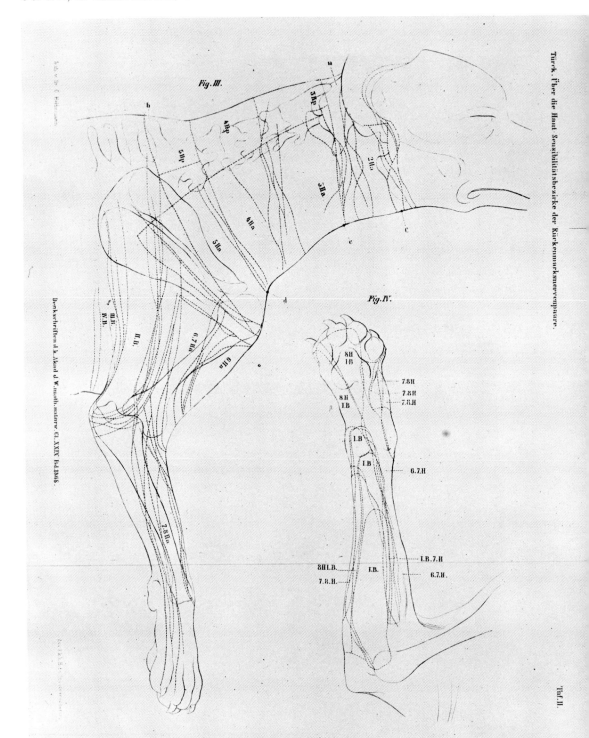

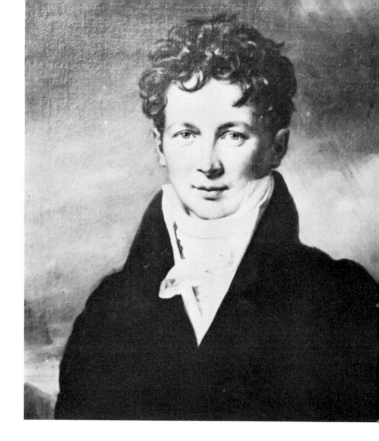

Fig. 86. François Magendie. Attributed to Guerin. By permission, Collège de France.

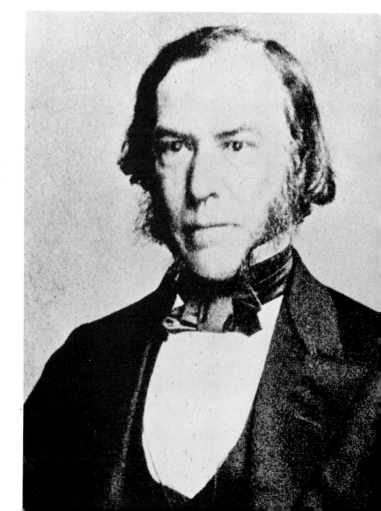

Fig. 87. Charles Edouard Brown-Séquard. By permission, National Library of Medicine.

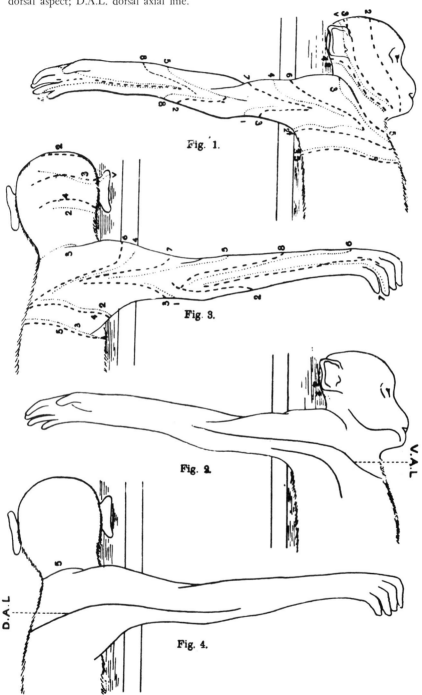

FIG. 88. Sherrington (1899, Plate XIII, figs. 1–4). Fig. 1, cervical and thoracic skin fields, anterior and posterior borders shown on ventral aspect. Numbers refer to roots; *v*, posterior border of trigeminal area; ventral axial line (V.A.L.) not shown. Figs. 3 to 4, dorsal aspect; D.A.L. dorsal axial line.

Fig. 1.

Fig. 3.

Fig. 2.

Fig. 4.

V.A.L

D.A.L

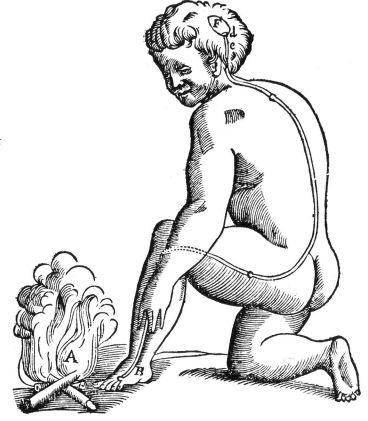

FIG. 89. Descartes (1664, p. 27). For explanation see text (p. 331).

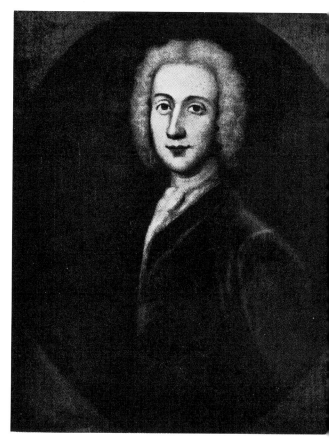

FIG. 90. Robert Whytt. By permission, Royal College of Physicians, Edinburgh.

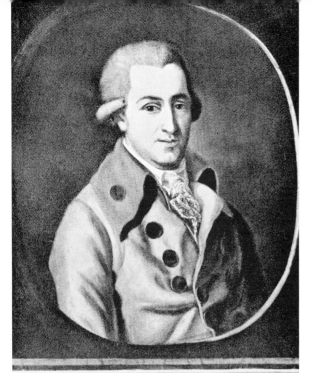

GEORGIUS PROCHAZKA.
*Med. Doct. C.R. Prof. anatomiæ publ. et physiologiæ
ac morb. oculor. publ. ac ord.*

FIG. 91. Jiri Procháska, *c.* 1788. From Kruta (1949), frontispiece. From a painting by G. Kneipa in the gallery of the Dean and Professors of the Medical Faculty of Prague. Courtesy of Professor Kruta.

FIG. 92. Marshall Hall. By permission of the Wellcome Trustees.

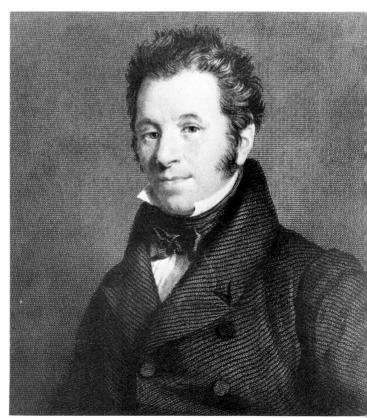

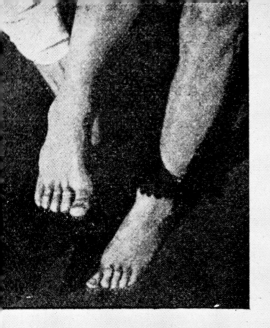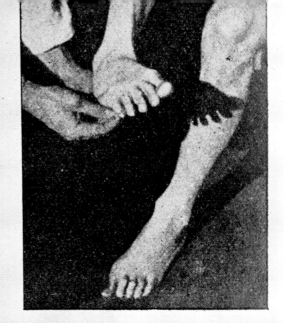

PARAPLÉGIE SPASMODIQUE.

Fɪɢ. 1. — Pied au repos.   Fɪɢ. 2. — Pied au moment de l'excitation.
Abduction des orteils, d'une intensité moyenne.

Fɪɢ. 93. Babinski (1903, p. 728).

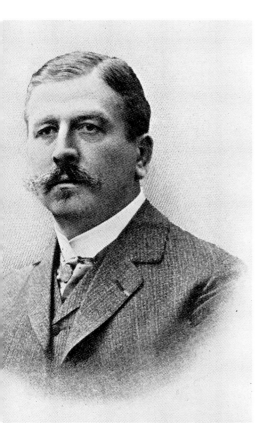

Fɪɢ. 94. Joseph François Félix Babinski. By permission of the Wellcome Trustees.

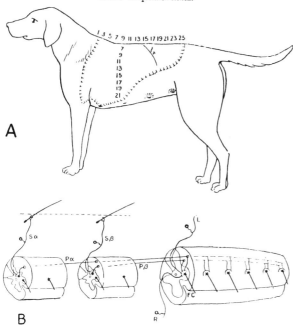

FIG. 1. The Scratch Reflex.

FIG. 95. Sherrington (1904, fig. 1). The scratch reflex.

A

B

A.—The 'receptive field,' as revealed after low cervical transection, a saddle-shaped area of dorsal skin, whence the scratch reflex of the left hind limb can be evoked. *lr* marks the position of the last rib.
B.—Diagram of the spinal arcs involved. L, receptive or afferent nerve-path from the left foot; R, receptive nerve-path from the opposite foot; Sα, Sβ, receptive nerve-paths from hairs in the dorsal skin of the left side; FC, the final common path, in this case the motor neurone to a flexor muscle of the hip; Pα, Pβ, proprio-spinal neurones.

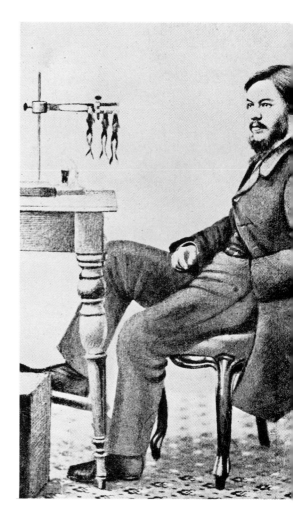

FIG. 96. Ivan Mikhailovich Sechenov in his laboratory at the medicosurgical academy of St. Petersburg. From Sechenov (1935), facing p. xviii. By permission, State Publishing House, Moscow.

In an animal from which the cerebral hemispheres have been completely removed it is impossible to form any conditional reflexes at all. It appears, therefore, that the cerebrum is the organ for the analysis of sensations, and for the construction of new reflexes and new connexions. It represents that part of the animal organism which is specialized for the purpose of retaining the animal always in a state of equilibrium with the outer world; in other words, it is an organ for direct and appropriate adjustment to the most varied combinations and changes in the phenomena of the surroundings; it is the organ which is above all others necessary for the unimpeded evolution of the organism.

. . . .

. . . .

. . . . The methods for the investigation of the higher nervous functions of animals which arise from psychological conceptions, the extrication from labyrinths, the disproving of certain hypotheses, and so forth, naturally yield a scientific material; but this is merely fragmentary, and teaches us absolutely nothing of the fundamental principles of the higher neural processes, since it needs itself to be first of all analyzed and explained. For an exact and continuous scientific investigation of the functions of the higher nerve centres, it is necessary that the fundamental and guiding principles be purely physiological ones. On the groundwork which I have just outlined it will be possible to work. The results in the hands of other investigators will show whether my premises are correct and whether they are sufficient.

Modern Period

As the nineteenth century drew to a close it became increasingly apparent that the reflex was by no means the relatively uncomplex phenomenon envisaged by earlier workers. Although the simple pathway had been delineated by the anatomists, it seemed that each successive investigation of its function opened up a new and unexpected facet. Laycock and Sechenov had extended the field to involve the whole nervous system; the problems of spinal cord "intelligence" and "consciousness" still bristled with difficulties; attempts to locate specific reflex spinal cord centers, as with the work of the phrenologists on brain function earlier in the century, led to confusion (Eckhard, 1881, pp. 163–192); and the question of the role of reflex activity in the maintenance of muscle tone seemed to have no answer. Nevertheless, partially with the aid of new techniques such as electrical recordings, a mass of useful observations was being assembled, although in piecemeal fashion. There was need for someone to extend, integrate, and interpret.

CHARLES SCOTT SHERRINGTON
(*See p. 238*)

Sherrington's fame as a renowned neurophysiologist rests more upon his work with the reflex than with any other neurological activity he investigated. He realized that the reflexes were the fundamental functional units of the nervous system, just as the nerve cell was the basic anatomical entity. Moreover, he suggested that behavior was made up of reflexes, but not exclusively, for elaborate mechanisms in the cerebral cortex were also involved. His approach to decerebrate rigidity was a masterly analysis of a phenomenon which has proved to be of primary importance to modern neurophysiology. A later topic, not represented below, was the stretch reflex which led him to consider the nature of central inhibition, both rudimentary topics of vital import to nervous system function. Nor did the problem of the ultimate unit of reflex action evade him since his genius lay in an ability to convert anatomical data into physiological fact.

In order to learn as much as possible about the overall functioning of the nervous system, Sherrington set about a detailed examination and reevaluation of its basic mechanisms. His labors during the last decade of the nineteenth century and the beginning of the present one laid the foundation for our present-day view of reflex activity. Some of his fundamental contributions are represented below but other than including a comment made in 1932 by himself and his students on an extension of this work, it is not proposed to enter the last and modern period of the history of the reflex.

Only a few of Sherrington's additions to our knowledge of the reflex can be dealt with here, but there is an excellent anthology of them, compiled and edited by one of his students, Denny-Brown (1939). As representatives, early papers on reciprocal muscle innervation, decerebrate rigidity, the final common path, and the scratch reflex, have been selected. However, Sherrington's writings are so full of new, factual information, of new interpretations, and of new ideas, all competing for presentation, that it is never easy to select relatively brief, representative passages.

The following is his conclusion concerning the spinal reflex pathway. It summarized a vast amount of experimental data gathered in the last decade of the nineteenth century and reported in 1898 ("Experiments in examinations of the peripheral distribution of the fibres of the posterior roots of some spinal nerves.—Part II," *Phil. Trans. R. Soc.*, 1898, 190B:45–186). A vital component was the synapse, a concept introduced by Sherrington which has increased greatly in importance since then; an account of it is to be found on pages 375 to 377. See also page 375 for the scratch reflex pathway.

EXCERPT P. 98

. . . . . the *afferent* nerve-fibres distributed in a given muscle arise in the *root-ganglia of exactly those spinal segments, whence emerge the motor-*

fibres for the same muscle. In other words, the sensory nerve-cells, directly connected with a given skeletal muscle, are in any one individual always of the same segmental level as the motor nerve-cells connected with the same given muscle. The simplest reflex path connected with a muscle may, therefore, be expected to lie exactly in the particular segments whence issue the motor-fibres to the muscle. In the "knee-jerk" we have evidence of a muscular reflex arc, traceable usually principally *from* and *into vastus medialis* and adjacent part of *crureus*, and this affords, as it were, a test case for the above conclusions; it confirms them perfectly; it exemplifies them by its narrow local extent, and by the segmentally horizontal, correlative position of its motor and sensory components.

In experimental *extensor rigidity* Sherrington studied and named the *reciprocal innervation* of antagonist muscles, a phenomenon recognized to some degree since the second century A.D. (Galen, p. 326). One of Sherrington's reports read before the Royal Society on 21 January 1897 ("On reciprocal innervation of antagonistic muscles. Third note," *Proc. R. Soc.*, 1897, 60:414–417) referred to part of his systematic study of mammalian reflexes. It extended the work of Sechenov (pp. 362–365), for it showed that the spinal cord possessed an inhibitory action on muscles.

EXCERPT PP. 415–416

If transection of the neural axis be carried out at the level of the crura cerebri in, e.g., the cat, there usually ensues after a somewhat variable interval of time a tonic rigidity in certain groups of skeletal muscles, especially in those of the dorsal aspect of the neck and tail and of the extensor surfaces of the limbs . . . . The extensors of the elbow and the knee are generally in strong contraction, but altogether without tremor and with no marked relaxations or exacerbations. On taking hold of the limbs and attempting to forcibly flex the elbow or knee a very considerable degree indeed of resistance is experienced, the triceps brachii and quadriceps extensor cruris become, under the stretch which the more or less effectual flexion puts upon them, still tenser than before, and on releasing the limb the joints spring back forthwith to their previous attitude of full extension. Despite, however, this powerful extensor rigidity, flexion of the elbow may be at once obtained with perfect facility by simply stimulating the toes or pad of the fore foot. When this is done the triceps enters into relaxation and the biceps passes into contraction. If, when the reflex is evolved, the condition of the triceps muscle is carefully examined, its contraction is found to undergo inhibition, and its tenseness to be broken down synchronously with and indeed very often accurately at the very moment of onset of reflex contraction in the opponent prebrachial muscles. The guidance of the flexion movement of the forearm may therefore be likened to that used in driving a pair of horses under harness . . . .

Similarly in the case of the hind limb . . . .

The same relaxation of existing contraction in the extensors can be obtained by electrical excitation of the tract in the crura cerebri, when, as sometimes happens, that excitation evokes flexion at elbow or at knee. This and the previous fact which evidences that the result is obtainable after complete removal of the whole cerebrum bear out the view arrived at in my former paper that for this reciprocal and, as I believe, elementary co-ordination, it is not essential that "high level" centres (Hughlings Jackson) be employed. I incline to think, however, that this kind of co-ordination at elbow and knee is probably largely made use of in movements initiated *via* the cerebral hemispheres as well as in the lower reflexes, on the observation of which the present Note is based. This conclusion is indicated by its occurring in response to excitation of the pyramidal fibres in the crura. In the case of the reciprocal innervation of antagonistic ocular muscles I was able to prove that it took place even in "willed movements."

Further observations on reciprocal innervation, including its more precise analysis, appeared a year later. It was now apparent that it revealed an important inhibitory function of spinal reflex activity, and Sherrington was led to consider it as the principle of muscle control in the spinal cord ("Experiments in examination of the peripheral distribution of the fibres of the posterior roots of some spinal nerves.—Part II," *Phil. Trans. R. Soc.*, 1898, 190B:45–186).

EXCERPT PP. 178–180

My own observations lead me to believe that *inhibito-motor* spinal reflexes occur *quite habitually and concurrently* with many of the excito-motor described in this paper. In graphic records of the reflex limb movements of the Frog the sudden and absolute relaxation of the muscles of one group at the very moment (to a 0.05″) of the onset of contraction in the antergetic group suggests this. Again, after spinal transection in Dog or Cat the flexion reflex being obtained in the idio-lateral limb by pressing the foot, if while that limb is drawn up by the reflex the other foot is squeezed, not only is the squeezed leg drawn up, but the limb previously flexed is, very usually, let down, relaxation of the flexors occurring concurrently with contraction of the extensors. This co-ordination I term *"reciprocal innervation."*

. . . .
. . . .

. . . . In short, my observations prove the existence of "reciprocal innervation" of antagonistic muscles as part of the machinery of spinal reflexes, and point to it as possibly a widely extensive part of that machinery. It not only affects contrasted muscle-groups, but also contrasted parts of one and the same muscle as in *quadriceps ext. fem.* and in *triceps brachii.*

Closely allied to reciprocal innervation was the phenomenon of *decerebrate rigidity,* produced in rabbits much earlier by Magendie (1823). Sherrington studied it first in 1897 and elaborated upon it later ("Decerebrate rigidity, and reflex coordination of movements," *J. Physiol., London,* 1898, 22:319–332). In this article he described the procedure of decerebration and then analyzed the resulting condition.

EXCERPT PP. 319–321

. . . . Then ensues, often almost at once, i.e., in a few minutes, sometimes however only after an interval of an hour or more, a status characterised by a peculiar rigidity of certain joints. The elbow joints do not allow then of the usually easily made passive flexion, the knee joints similarly are stiffly extended. The tail is stiff and straight instead of flexible and drooping. The neck is rigidly extended, the head retracted, and the chin thrown upward.

. . . .

. . . . The hand of the monkey is turned with its palmar face somewhat inward. The hind-limbs are similarly kept straightened and thrust backward; the hip is extended, the knee very stiffly extended, and the ankle somewhat extended. The tail in spite of its own weight, and it is quite heavy in some species of monkey, is kept either straight and horizontal or often stiffly curved upward. There is a little opisthotonus of the lumbosacral vertebral region. The head is kept lifted against gravity and the chin is tilted upward under the retraction and backward rotation of the skull . . . . When the limbs or tail are pushed from the pose they have assumed considerable resistance to the movement is felt, and unlike the condition after bulbar section on being released they spring back at once to their former position and remain there for a time more stiffly than even before.

The phenomenon of this decerebrate rigidity occurs with little variation in the monkey, dog, cat, rabbit and guinea-pig. In all these species the effect upon the fore-limb seems more intense than on the hind-limb. In the hind-limb the knee is the principal joint affected. In the rabbit the phenomenon in the hind-limb has so far as my observations go been particularly well seen. It is noteworthy that the wrist and ankle are comparatively slightly implicated in the rigidity, the ankle more than wrist. I have never in any instance been able to satisfy myself that the digits are implicated at all.

The rigidity is immediately due to prolonged spasm of certain groups of voluntary muscles. The chief of these are the retractor muscles of the head and neck, the elevators and dorsal flexors of the tail, and the extensor muscles of the elbow and knee, and shoulder and hip. This prolonged spasm I have seen maintained in young cats, with some intermissions, for a period of four days. It is increased, and even when absent or very slight may be soon developed, by passive movements of the part . . . .

Administration of chloroform and ether, if carried far, quite abolishes the rigidity. On interrupting the administration the rigidity again rapidly returns.

Section of the dorsal columns of the spinal cord does not abolish the rigidity. Section of one lateral column of the cord in the upper lumbar region abolishes the rigidity in the hind-limb of the same side as the section. Section of one ventro-lateral column of the cord in the cervical region destroys the rigidity in the fore and hind-limbs of the same side.

EXCERPT P. 332

"Decerebrate rigidity" is but a type of extensor spasm of which allied examples follow various other lesions of the cerebello-cerebral region.

The development of "decerebrate rigidity" in a limb is largely determined by centripetal impulses coming from the limb in question.

The contraction of the muscles active in "decerebrate rigidity" can be readily inhibited by stimulation of various regions of the central nervous system, and, among others, of the sensori-motor region of the cerebral cortex.

The activity of the rigid muscles can be readily inhibited by stimulation of various peripheral nerves, and, among others, of the afferent nerve-fibres proceeding from skeletal muscles.

Reflexes obtained from the cerebrate animal exhibit contraction in one muscle-group accompanied by relaxation, inhibition, in the antagonistic muscle group ("reciprocal innervation"), and this in such distribution and sequence as to couple diagonal limbs in harmonious movements of similar direction.

In the original publication of 1897 ("Cataleptoid reflexes in the monkey," *Lancet*, 1897, i:373–374) Sherrington had stated that "not the least interesting part of the reflexes under consideration is a remarkable glimpse which they allow into the scope of reflex inhibition as regards the coördinate of movements of the limbs," and he later called it a state of reflex standing. Thus the whole field of reflexes and their role in the maintenance of body posture during rest and movement was opened up. Moreover, decerebrate rigidity proved to be an excellent research tool. It was one of the most momentous disclosures in the history of neurophysiology.

Sherrington's analysis of the reflex response led to many of the concepts and terms which have long since been absorbed into neurophysiology and which formed a basis for subsequent work and underlie modern research. Thus he described the *final common path* in his address to the Physiological Section of the British Association for the Advancement of Science, at Cambridge in 1904 ("Correlation of reflexes and the principle of the common path," *Rep. Br. Ass. Advmt. Sci.*, 74th meeting, trans. Sec. I.—Physiology, pp. 728–741) and he used his famous experiments on the *scratch reflex* in the spinal dog to illustrate its mechanism. In the last paragraph he discussed the wider significance of reflex arcs in the nervous system as a whole. Reference has already been made (p. 334) to a possible example of the scratch reflex in the writings of Willis.

EXCERPT P. 730

But at the termination of every reflex arc we find a final neurone, the ultimate conductive link to an effector organ, gland or muscle. This last link in the chain, e.g., the motor neurone, differs obviously in one important respect from the first link of the chain. It does not subserve exclusively impulses generated at one single receptive source alone, but receives impulses from many receptive sources situate in many and various regions of the body. It is the sole path which all impulses, no matter whence they come, must travel if they would reach the muscle-fibres which it joins. Therefore, while the receptive neurone forms a private path exclusive for impulses of one source only, the final or efferent neurone is, so to say, a public path, *common* to impulses arising at any of many sources in a variety of receptive regions of the body. The same effector organ stands in reflex connection not only with many individual receptive points, but even with many various receptive *fields*. Reflex arcs arising in mainfold sense-organs can pour their influence into one and the same muscle. A limb-muscle is the *terminus ad quem* of nervous arcs arising not only in the right eye but in the left, not only in the eyes but in the organs of smell and hearing; not only in these, but in the geotropic labyrinth, in the skin, and in the muscles and joints of the limb itself and of the other limbs as well. Its motor nerve is a path common to all these.

. . . . The terminal path may, to distinguish it from internuncial common paths, be called *the final common path*. The motor nerve to a muscle is a collection of such final common paths.

EXCERPT PP. 731–733

Good opportunity for study of this correlation between reflexes is given in the 'scratch reflex.' When the spinal cord has been transected in the neck, this reflex in a few months becomes prominent. Stimuli applied within a large saddle-shaped field of skin (fig. 1A [fig. 95]) excite a scratching movement of the leg. The movement is rhythmic flexion at hip, knee, and ankle. It has a frequency of about four per second. The stimuli provocative of it are mechanical, such as rubbing the skin, or pulling lightly on a hair. The nerve-endings which generate the reflex lie in the surface layer of the skin, about the roots of the hairs. A convenient way of exciting these is by feeble faradisation . . . .

Prominent among the muscles active in this reflex are the flexors of the hip . . . . A series of brief contractions succeed one another at a certain rate, whose frequency is independent of that of the stimulation. The contractions are presumably brief tetani. The stimulus to the hair-bulbs of the shoulder throws into action a lumbar spinal centre, innervating the hip-flexor much as the bulbar respiratory centre drives the spinal *phrenicus* centre. In the case of the respiratory muscle the frequency of the rhythm is, however, much less.

This reflex is unilateral: stimulation of the left shoulder evokes scratching by the left leg, not by the right. Search in the spinal cord for the path of the reflex demonstrates that a lesion breaking through one lateral half of the cord anywhere between shoulder and leg abolishes the ability of the skin of that shoulder to excite the scratch reflex, but leaves intact the reflex of the opposite shoulder.

. . . . We thus arrive at the following reflex chain for the scratch reflex: (i) The receptive neurone (fig. 1 B, sα [fig. 95]), from the skin to the spinal grey matter of the corresponding spinal segment in the shoulder. This is the exclusive or private path of the arc. (ii) The long descending proprio-spinal neurone (fig. 1 B, pα), from the shoulder segment to the grey matter of leg segments. (iii) The motor neurone (fig. 1 B, fc), from the spinal segment of the leg to the flexor muscles. This last is the *final common path*. The chain thus consists of three neurones. It enters the grey matter twice, that is, it has two neuronic junctions, two synapses. It is a *disynaptic* arc.

. . . .

. . . .

. . . .

It is obvious from this that the final common path, fc, to the flexor muscle can be controlled by, in addition to the before-mentioned arcs, others that actuate the extensor muscles, for it can be thrown out of action by them. The final path, fc, is therefore common to the reflex arcs, not only from the same-side foot (fig. 1 B, l) and shoulder skin (fig. 1 B, sα; sβ), but also to arcs from the opposite foot (fig. 1 B, r), in the sense that it is in the grasp of all of them. In this last case we have a conflict for the mastery of a common path, not, as in the previous instance, between two arcs both of which use the path in a pressor manner although differently, but between two arcs that, though both of them control the path, control it differently, one in a pressor manner heightening its activity, the other in a depressor manner lowering or suppressing its activity.

EXCERPT PP. 740–741

. . . . The reflex arcs (of the synaptic system) converge in their course so as to impinge upon links possessed by whole varied groups in common—*common paths*. This arrangement culminates in the convergence of many separately arising arcs upon the efferent-root neurone. This neurone thus forms a final common path for many different reflex arcs and acts. It is responsive in various rhythm and intensity, and is relatively unfatigable. Of the different arcs which use it in common, each can do so exclusively in due succession, but *different* arcs cannot use it simultaneously. There is, therefore, interference between the actions of the arcs possessing the common path, some reflexes excluding others and producing inhibitory phenomena, some reflexes reinforcing others and producing phenomena of 'bahnung' [facilitation, introduced by Exner in 1882]. Intensity of stimulation, species of reflex, fatigue, and freshness, all these are physiological factors influencing this interaction of the arcs—and under pathological conditions there are many others, e.g., 'shock,' toxins, &c. Hence follows successive interchange of the arcs that dominate one and the same final common path. We commonly hear a muscle—or other effector organ— spoken of as innervated by a certain nerve; it would be more correct as well as more luminous to speak of it as innervated by certain receptors . . . . This temporal variability, wanting to the nerve-net system of medusoid and lower visceral life, in the *synaptic* system provides the organism with a mechanism for higher integration. It fits that system to synthesize from a mere collection of tissues and organs an individual animal. The animal mechanism is thus given solidarity by this principle which for each effector organ allows and regulates interchange of the arcs playing upon it, a principle which I would briefly term that of 'the interaction of reflexes about their common path.'

Laycock and Sechenov had suggested that nervous system activity was compounded of reflex responses, and from this concept Pavlov developed a system of conditioned reflexes fundamental to present-day Russian physiology. But it was to Sherrington that we owe the idea of an integrative nervous system in which there are independences, yet, at the same time, interactions of reflexes; thus two reflexes when weak may be neutral to each other but when strong may be in opposition. Like the neurons, which are the basis of reflex activity, reflexes are both independent yet dependent. Furthermore, the relationship of the reflex to psychological as well as to physiological events is a vital theme.

It is upon this foundation that much of modern neurophysiology has been built, and the inestimable value of the book which embodied this new approach to the reflex arc and to the nervous system as a whole is clearly understandable. *The integrative action of the nervous system* (New Haven, 1906) represents the Silliman Lectures which Sherrington gave at Yale University in 1904. In the last lecture he dealt with the broader application of the reflex to neural activity.

EXCERPT PP. 390–391

Volitional control of reflexes is a question of co-ordination not explicitly before us previously in these lectures. Its analysis has not indeed proceeded far. We may premise that some extension of the same processes outlined in Lectures V and VI, as operative in simultaneous combination and in successive combination of reflexes, must be operative in this control. There we saw reflexes modifying each other, and the more complex reactions being built up from simpler and more restricted ones. Some extension of the same process should, in view of our inferences regarding the nature of the dominance of the brain (Lecture IX), apply here also.

It is significant that, although the reflexes controlled are so often unconscious, consciousness is adjunct to the centres which exert the control. A biologist, Professor Lloyd Morgan, has urged that "the primary aim, object, and purpose of consciousness is control. Consciousness in a mere automaton is a useless and unnecessary epiphenomenon." A somewhat similar thought rose incidentally to our lips in a previous lecture (Lecture IX). The pleasure–pain accompaniment of reflexes has often been interpreted as carrying that meaning. Certain it is that if we study the process by which in ourselves this control over reflex action is acquired by an individual, psychical factors loom large, and more is known of them than of the purely physiological *modus operandi* involved in the attainment of the control. Hence, psychological studies have been more numerous than physiological in this field. It is found that kinaesthetic sensations of the movement to be acquired or controlled, though helpful, are less important than the resident sensations from the part in its "resting" state. These latter, with the power to focus attention upon them, appear, in a number of instances, to be a most necessary condition for the acquirement of the control. And in the monkey, voluntary control of a limb is largely lost when the limb has been rendered apaesthetic.

A biological inference arises at this point. We have admitted that the organs to which psychosis is adjunct, namely, the brain, and especially in higher vertebrates the cerebral hemispheres, supply the surest touchstone to rank in the scale of animal creation. That is to admit, in other words, that development of these organs constitutes, on the whole, the best criterion to the success of an animal form in the competition which lies at the root of animal evolution. These organs, we have just seen, are the organs of nervous control; and that control is exercised mainly in the perfecting and readjusting of manoeuvres of ancient heritage. The way in which we ourselves acquire a new skilled movement, the means by which we get more precision and speed in the use of a tool, the handling of an instrument, or marksmanship with a weapon, is by a process of learning in which nervous organs of control modify the activities of reflex centres, themselves already perfected for other though kindred actions. Our process of learning is accompanied by conscious effort. These nervous organs of control form, therefore, a special instrument of adaptation and of readjustment of reaction to better suit requirements which may be new. New adaptations whence the individual may reap benefit are thus attained. The more complex an organism, the more points of contact it has with the environment, and the more frequently will it need readjustment amid an environment of shifting relationships. These nervous organs of control being organs of adjustment will be more prominent the further the animal scale is followed upward to its crowning species, man. And these organs which give adjustability to the running of the reflex machinery, as such, seem themselves— perhaps, by reason of their constant relative newness—to be among the most plastic in the body. In man and the species near him, these organs are most developed, and their mechanisms are cerebral. These cerebral mechanisms constitute the clearest criterion of evolutionary success.

In 1932 Sherrington and four of his most distinguished students, Creed, Denny-Brown, Eccles, and Liddell published a book on *Reflex activity of the spinal cord* (London, Oxford University Press, 1932) which presented "a concise account of elementary features of reflex mechanism, as illustrated particularly by the mammalian spinal cord" (p. v.). They were concerned only with physiological mechanisms and purposely avoided questions evoking the biological significance of reflexes.

Richard Stephen Creed (20 December 1898—7 July, 1964; see *Br. Med. J.*, 1964, ii:193) was a demonstrator and lecturer in physiology in the University of Oxford. Derek Ernest Denny-Brown (1 June 1901—   ) is professor of neurology at Harvard University and director of the Neurological Research Unit, Boston City Hospital, Massachusetts. Sir John Carew Eccles (27 June 1903—   ) was appointed professor of physiology in the Australian National University at Canberra in 1951. Edward George Tandy Liddell (25 March 1895—   ) succeeded Sherrington in the Waynflete Chair of Physiology in the University of Oxford in 1940, from which he retired in 1960.

Their book represents an extension of Sherrington's original work on the reflex and epitomizes for us the best of the Sherringtonian school of physiology. The authors were concerned mainly with the vitally important interplay of excitation and inhibition on the motor neuron. Here Sherrington had investigated a basic anatomical unit of the nervous system, the simpler reflex arc, in terms of function and hoped to derive general integrative principles from it. The following selection comprises the authors' concluding remarks.

EXCERPT PP. 157–159

We may ask in conclusion whether from the attempted analysis of the simpler reflexes anything like a general principle emerges fundamental to co-ordination. In some degree there does. That important and practically omnipresent factor in co-ordination, namely adjustment of quantity of contraction, presents itself (and the more so as the scale of reflex complexity is ascended) as the resultant commonly of two interacting antagonistic central processes, excitation and inhibition. The degree of activity of a motoneurone corresponds with the algebraical sum of the opposed influences of excitation and inhibition convergent upon it.

It is true that for physiological experiment the nervous system, purposely curtailed in extent, even to retention of perhaps but one afferent channel, and that one active only while artificially stimulated, exhibits reflex excitation freed in many cases from concurrent inhibition. It is true also that that central excitation can be graded, by grading the stimulus, and that so also can inhibition. But under intact natural conditions we have to think of each motoneurone as a convergence-point about which summate not only excitatory processes fed by converging impulses of varied provenance arriving by various routes, but also inhibitory influences of varied provenance and path; and that there at that convergence-place these two opposed influences finally interact.

The two convergent systems themselves, one excitatory, one inhibitory, make of the entrance to the final common path, which we may accept the motoneurone as constituting, a collision-field for joint algebraically summed effect. In the higher vertebrate rarely is either member of this paired system, excitatory-inhibitory, wholly quiet when its fellow is active, for their relation to stimuli is reciprocal. The opposition between the effects of the two on the motoneurone is quantitative, and the grade of functional activity or inactivity of the motoneurone reflects this quantitative interaction. Whether the excitatory has the upper hand, or whether the inhibitory, commonly both are at work, and the functional state of the motoneurone indexes the net result from the two.

This statement can find justification and illustration in such a simple instance as that of the extensor muscles. With them we know that the mechanical action of the muscle itself affects reflexly the activity of its own motoneurones. The muscle's contraction by pulling on its own tendon can and does produce reflex excitation of itself (*autogenous excitation*), indeed this appears as one of its reflex tone. Active contraction of the muscle can also stimulate certain receptors in it which develop reflex inhibitory restraint (*autogenous inhibition*) of its own motoneurones. The ataxy of *tabes dorsalis* with its impairment of tone and its unchecked muscular momentum illustrates well how constantly each natural act rests for its normal execution on a collaboration between concurrent excitation and inhibition.

The picture of an excitatory system convergent upon the motoneurone and gathering impulses from manifold sources and paths, varying in extent and power with the set or sets of receptors in action and with the series of centres involved, offers no difficulty and the text-books furnish for it abundant diagrams. In respect, however, to the inhibitory system which the principle of action now before us requires us to envisage as more or less a counterpart and counterpoise to the excitatory against which it acts, a certain ambiguity enters the picture. Central inhibition is by experiment clearly shown to have a locus closely circumjacent to the motoneurone itself, i.e., in terms of reflex direction immediately upstream from that. There the convergent inhibitory system will certainly act. But as to whether on its way thither the inhibitory system also at other links in its neurone chain, for instance further upstream and headward (for some of its chains are long), develops inhibition which can influence the motoneurone remains still obscure. Except at the locus of the motoneurone central inhibition is little known to actual experiment, apart from somewhat indirect evidence for the bulbar vasomotor and respiratory centres.

Fundamental in the co-ordinative regulation of the motoneurone is the combined action on it of the summed excitations of the moment pitted against the concurrent summed inhibitions. Each individual motoneurone is individually dealt with thus. Hence these two opposed and separately gradable influences which by antagonistic interaction also mutually grade together, make the motoneurone and therefore the motor unit their unit of operation. The foundation of the quantitative grading is based on the individual motor unit. The musculature as a whole being composed additively of motor units the co-ordinative taxis takes expression in the musculature as a whole as an additive effect.

The range of excitation and inhibition experimentally observable in the individual motoneurone is more extensive than the mechanical response of the muscle-fibres can follow. The rate of firing of the motoneurone under summed excitation can exceed the rate which produces full tetanic tension of the motor unit. Heights of excitation therefore occur in the nervous centres greater than the skeletal muscle-fibre can commensurately express. If this seems wasteful of central activity we may remember that additional excitation exerted on a motoneurone whose muscle-fibres are already driven maximally for tetanic contraction is not necessarily wasted. That surplus remains still a contribution to co-ordination because further excitation offers a further resistance to inhibition. Conversely, an added inhibition in the case of an already quiescent neurone although in one sense wasted, is a further protection which coordination may need against excitation. In times of crisis the dilemma lies between strong actions and the very strength of the action taken may serve to safeguard it against interruption.

CHAPTER VII

THE CEREBRAL CONVOLUTIONS

Introduction

The most striking feature of the cerebral hemispheres is the arrangement of convolutions or gyri on their surfaces. Yet, paradoxically enough, it was one of the last macroscopic structures of the brain to be examined carefully. The reason for this neglect lay in the ancients' acceptance of the ventricular system as the site of cerebral activity. Thus the cortical covering of the deeper structures was held to have no important function, and, moreover, the convolutions, like loops of small intestine, appeared to lie in no particular order. The "chaos of the convolutions" was accepted almost universally until the beginning of the nineteenth century when attention was drawn by the phrenologists to the possibility of localization of function in the gyri. Morphological, embryological, and comparative studies rapidly followed this stimulus, and in fifty years the task of describing the convolutional patterns in man and in animals was largely accomplished. However, during this period, after the defeat of the phrenologists, correlation with function was almost completely neglected and remained unstudied until the 1860's by which time interest in the microscopic structure of the cortex had also developed. Thus study of the convolutions waned as cortical localization and histology became increasingly popular. In consequence many vital problems related to gyral patterns cannot yet be answered.

The history of this part of neuroanatomy can be considered in two stages: first, early observations of the gyri and sulci and their possible functions; second, the period of great activity during the first three quarters of the nineteenth century. We have made no attempt to select passages for reproduction beyond this point since no accurate evaluation of such later contributions can yet be made. The only adequate accounts of the history of the gyri are to be found in Rasmussen (1947, pp. 66ff.) and Schiller (1965).

Early Recognition

THE EDWIN SMITH SURGICAL PAPYRUS

Very little is known of the Ancient Egyptians' knowledge of human anatomy (see Grapow, 1954). On the whole it seems unlikely that they learned any detailed anatomy *per se* from the embalming techniques, and as they favored the heart rather than the brain as the primary organ of the body, they emptied the cranial cavity unceremoniously through the nose, orbit, or foramen magnum. They could therefore have learned no brain anatomy from this source. But there were observations to be made on patients with head injuries, and it is a report of such a case that gives the first written record of brain structures.

The Edwin Smith Surgical Papyrus (1930, Vol. I, *Hieroglyphic transliteration with translation and commentary*) was written probably in the seventeenth century B.C., but its contents date from the Pyramid Age (*c.* 3000–2500 B.C.); explanatory notes or glosses were added by the later editor. In it are described cases of trauma, several of which involved the head, and of these Case 6 (pp. 164–174) is of particular interest. The author reported a patient with "a gaping wound in the head with compound-comminuted fracture of the skull and rupture of the meningeal membranes," and in doing so (p. 164) he referred to the cerebral convolutions, brain pulsation, and the anterior fontanelle to which the later editor added the meninges and possibly the cerebrospinal fluid. The word "brain" appeared here for the first time in any language and, as in Greek, it implied "marrow of the skull." The comparison of cerebral gyri with the wrinkles of the surface scum on a molten metal is a useful one and indicates that a technical medical vocabulary was not yet available. There have been differences of opinion, however, concerning certain translations (Grapow, 1954, pp. 27–29).

EXCERPT PP. 165–166

If thou examinest a man having a gaping wound in his head, penetrating to the bone, smashing his skull, (and) rending open the brain of his skull, thou shouldst palpate his wound. Shouldst thou find that smash which is in his skull [like] those corrugations which form in molten copper, (and) something therein throbbing (and) fluttering under thy fingers, like the weak place of an infant's crown before it becomes whole—when it has happened there is no throbbing (and) fluttering under thy fingers until the brain of his (the patient's) skull is rent open—(and) he discharges blood from both his nostrils, (and) he suffers with stiffness in his neck, (conclusion in diagnosis).

EXCERPT P. 171

GLOSS A

Explaining: Smashing his skull (and) rending open the brain of his skull.

As for: "Smashing his skull, (and) rending open the brain of his skull," (it means) the smash is large, opening to the interior of his skull, (to) the membrane enveloping his brain, so that it breaks open his fluid in the interior of his head.

GRECO-ROMAN ANTIQUITY

In the writings of Greco-Roman antiquity now available to us, the first mention of the convolutions of the brain was made by Praxagoras of Cos (*fl.* 300 B.C.; see p. 142) and by his pupil Philotimus (see Steckerl, 1958, pp. 1–6). Galen (*Use of Parts*, VIII, 12, Daremberg [1854–1856], I, 561–562; see also Steckerl, 1958, pp. 54–55) referred with scorn to their opinion:

"Indeed they consider the brain as a kind of excrescence put forth by the spinal cord and they consequently claim that it is formed of long convolutions. However, the parencephalon [cerebellum] being the body which touches the spinal cord shares little of the same structure whereas the anterior part of the brain shows it to a well-marked and very evident degree."

But the most important reference to the cerebral convolutions occurred in the writings of Erasistratus (*fl. c.* 260 B.C.; see p. 10) and was preserved in a book written by Galen (pp. 630–631). Erasistratus made an apt analogy between the appearances of the gyri and the coils of small intestine seen when the abdomen is opened, a description used again and again by subsequent writers. He also stated that man's brain was more convoluted than that of animals because of his superior intellect. Unfortunately this opinion was rejected by Galen (see Vesalius, p. 386) and thus throughout the rest of antiquity and the medieval period.

Rufus of Ephesus (*fl.* A.D. 98–117; see p. 13) termed the brain surface *varicose* (see p. 13), and Galen himself made brief reference to the cerebral convolutions when describing those of the cerebellum (pp. 629–631). On the whole Galen took little notice of the external features of the brain because his theory of brain function involved only the ventricular system and the deeper structures. This attitude was followed for many centuries and Erasistratus's correct reasoning was entirely submerged.

ANDREAS VESALIUS
(See p. 153)

Galen's brief observations on the cerebral convolutions were not supplemented by the pre-Vesalian anatomists, and even Vesalius himself added little to the description; he did, however, give the first account of a specific sulcus, the *callosal sulcus* which, however, he did not name (see p. 579). Regarding possible function, he first cited Galen's opinions and then suggested that the sulci existed between the gyri so that the pia mater with its blood vessels could extend deeply into the cerebral mass. Thus nourishment could be provided to a much larger area of brain tissue than if the same vessels lay on the surface of a smooth, non-convoluted cerebrum. This teleological argument was echoed for several centuries. Vesalius also referred to a difference in color between the gray and white matter (p. 578) but did not identify the cortex further. The following excerpts have been translated from *De humani corporis fabrica* ([Basel, 1543], Bk. VII, Ch. IV).

EXCERPT P. 630

. . . . Furthermore, the gyri and convolutions of the brain, which Erasistratus very nicely compared to the twistings of the thin intestines, are found with the same frequency over the whole surface of the brain. There are many sinuses penetrating deeply into the substance of the brain, in appearance much like the twistings of the thin intestines, and I believe that they cannot be compared to anything more happily than to clouds as they are usually delineated by either untrained art students or by schoolboys. Nevertheless, one must not spend too much effort in seeking a resemblance since in this respect there is nothing unusual about man's brain, and these convolutions appearing in its substance are also to be found in the brain of the ass, horse, ox, and other animals which I have examined. It may be concluded, however, that nature insinuated these gyri much deeper into the substance of man's brain because of its greater abundance.

THE USE OF THE BRAIN'S CONVOLUTIONS

You may learn the shape of these twistings by observing the brain of some animal at breakfast or dinner. Both physicians and philosophers are in great dispute over their use, debating whether or not they provide man with intelligence. Thus Galen, opposing the conclusion of Erasistratus, declared the following: "Even asses have a very complex brain, although it would seem that, relative to their lack of intelligence, it ought to have been wholly simple and uniform. It would be better to consider intelligence (whatever that may be) as dependent upon a proper proportion of the substance, not upon complexity of composition. Nor do I believe it necessary to relate the perfection of received intelligence to either the amount or the quality of animal spirit." At this point, considering it sufficient to have indicated that the convolutions do not control intelligence, Galen applied the reins to his discourse, just when we most needed his opinion. We do not at all deny what Galen says, but he ought to have added that the convolutions reveal the great ingenuity of the Creator who formed them not otherwise than for the nourishment of the substance of the brain. If the substance of the brain had been continuous without all that folding of membranous fibres, it would not have been sufficiently firm for the distribution through it of veins and arteries as in the other parts of the body. There is so much of it and it is so thick that although the veins and arteries extended only on its surface would suffice for replenishing the innate heat, the deeper parts of the brain would be deprived of nourishment. Foreseeing this, nature impressed those sinuous foldings throughout the substance of the brain, so that the thin membrane, filled with numerous vessels, could insert itself into the substance of the brain and so very dexterously administer nourishment.

Archangelo Piccolomini
(*c. 1526—19 October 1586*)

Although the differences between the gray and white matter of the cerebrum were observed by earlier anatomists, for example Vesalius, the distinction was first clearly made in 1586 by Piccolomini. He was born in Ferrara and worked in Rome where he practised medicine and was professor of anatomy. Compared with Vesalius and some other Renaissance anatomists he is a slight figure; nevertheless, he made some original observations, and was widely quoted in the seventeenth century (see Pierro, 1965).

In the following passage which is from *Anatomicae praelectiones explicantes mirificam corporis humani fabricam* (Rome, 1586), Piccolomini used the term *cerebrum* when referring to the cerebral gray matter and *medulla* for the white matter. His reference to "certain lines" in the cortex is of considerable interest and may possibly refer to lamination; the *striae Piccolhomini* are the *stria medullaris* of the floor of the fourth ventricle.

EXCERPT P. 252

I call the cerebrum [gray matter] that whole ashen-colored body, darkening from white, which very closely encompasses the medulla. The medulla is the whole of the white and more solid body which is concealed within the ashen-colored one. Thus the cerebrum differs and is distinguished from the medulla by color, because the cerebrum is ashen-colored but the medulla white; in consistency, because the cerebrum is softer and the medulla a little harder and more compact; in location, because the medulla is in the middle of the cerebrum which wholly covers it over; also the ashen-colored body is distinguished from the white by certain lines. The cerebrum commences everywhere by convolutions and extends as far as the corpus callosum and that middle white part. The medulla commences at the corpus callosum and is, I say, that whole, internal, middle, and white body which is lengthened out and slips forth into the spine of the back [spinal cord].

Not only are the cerebrum and its medulla distinguished and separated from one another by the above indications, but also by the efficiency of one's dissection. For occasionally, working with slow deliberation and dexterity [with a fresh brain], I have separated the cerebrum from the corpus callosum and the whole middle, white part called the medulla.

THOMAS WILLIS
(See p. 158)

Although Willis's account of the cerebral gyri and sulci did not advance much beyond that of his predecessors, and although he repeated Vesalius's explanations of function, his overall contribution to this topic was significant and threefold.

First of all, he suggested a direct correlation between convolutional complexity and intelligence, for according to his theory of localization of function in the brain (pp. 472–473) the cortex of the gyri housed memory. Willis had thus gone back to the original opinion of Erasistratus (p. 631). Second, he reinforced this idea by examining the convolutional patterns in animals; he was therefore the first to make comparative studies of the gyri. And third, he gave the cortex a specific function; as well as storing memories it produced the animal spirits which, up till that time and according to the teachings of Galen, had been the duty of the "white matter." As Willis was an iatrochemist, he preferred to interpret the production of the animal spirits as a chemical process. We know now that he was wrong in all this, but he did, at least, direct some attention to the cerebral cortex which previously had not been considered to have any particular use.

The following passage is from the *Cerebri anatome* (London, 1664, Ch. X).

EXCERPT PP. 65–68

3. Furthermore, the whole *structure of the brain,* within its aforesaid individual compartments, *appears* yet *more divided* and *variegated;* for the whole of its exterior surface is rendered uneven and twisted *by gyri* and *convolutions,* almost like those of the intestines. These gyri, passing from the anterior part of the brain towards the posterior in a twisted and almost spiral course, go about both hemispheres so that they may mutually receive all the convolutions in a continuous course. In a more moist brain or one preserved for a longer time, the pia mater, investing and gathering everything together, is easily avulsed; then when the gyri or folds have been laid open and separated from one another, the substance of the brain is seen to be, as it were, ploughed into furrows from which arise cliffs or ridges of uneven height, not in straight rows but crossing one another; thus in the bottom of each furrow a convolution arisen from the right side may be

carried to the left, then the next following, issued from the left side may rise up on the right, and so the whole brain is variegated by a successive order of such inequalities.

If it be asked what *the gyri* and *convolutions* contribute to the brain or for what end its whole twisted structure exists, we say that the brain is so constructed for *a more abundant reception* of the spiritous *nourishment* and for *a more suitable diffusion* of the animal *spirits* for their uses. In regard to the brain's *nourishment*, which must be subtle and highly elaborated, it ought not be admitted by too wide an approach but rather by minute pores and passages. Therefore in order that a sufficient amount of such spiritous liquid be supplied, not only is it imbibed everywhere on the flat surface of the brain and its cortical substance, but that surface or cortical substance is made rough and uneven by the folds and gyri so that the spaces for receiving the liquid might be extended as widely as possible. Indeed, the twistings of the brain, like land everywhere dotted with heights and ant-hills, acquires a much wider extension than if its surface were formed flat and even. In addition, these *twistings of the brain more suitably hide* and preserve all *the blood vessels* that are very slender and smooth and twisted together in various plexuses; if they were distributed externally and uncovered, they would be exposed to very frequent injury.

But a no less important reason and necessity for the twistings in *the brain* arises from *the distribution* of the animal *spirits*. Since for the various acts of *imagination* and *memory* the animal spirits must be moved back and forth repeatedly within certain distinct limits and through the same tracts or pathways, therefore numerous folds and convolutions of the brain are required for these various arrangements of the animal spirits; that is, the appearances of perceptible things are stored in them, just as in various storerooms and warehouses, and at given times can be called forth from them. Hence these folds or convolutions are far more numerous and larger in man than in any other animal because of the variety and number of acts of the higher faculties, but they are varied by a disordered and almost haphazard arrangement so that the operations of the animal function might be free, changeable, and not limited to one. Those gyri are fewer in quadrupeds, and in some such as the cat, they are found to have a particular shape and arrangement so that this beast considers or recalls scarcely anything except what the instincts and demands of nature suggest. In the smaller quadrupeds, and also in birds and fishes, the surface of the brain is flat and even, entirely lacking in gyri and twistings. Hence it is that animals of this sort understand or learn few things by imitation and those almost only of one kind, so that they lack distinct cells separated one from another in which the different appearances of things and ideas are kept apart.

4. The reason that in the more perfect animals the individual twistings are made of *two substances*, that is, *cortical* and *medullary*, seems to be that one part serves for *the production* of animal spirits, the other for their *distribution*. It seems most likely that *the animal spirits are created* wholly or in large part *in the brain's cortical substance*, for this more immediately strains out and receives the subtle liquid from the blood; then imbuing it with a volatile salt, exalts it into pure and perfected spirits . . . . Meanwhile the medullary substance of the brain seems throughout like that of *the medulla oblongata* and *the spinal marrow*, and it is well known that the medullary parts serve for *the operation* and *distribution* of the animal spirits but not at all for their *generation* . . . . It is clear that this part is *the emporium* rather than *the factory* of the spirits, since the animals that excel in *memory, imagination,* and *appetite* are furnished a more abundant medulla of the brain, as is observed in man and the higher quadrupeds; but those that seem to have little need for these faculties, as the smaller quadrupeds, as well as birds and fishes, have a larger cortex to the brain and the medullary part is very small . . . .

After the animal spirits have been created by the constant flow of blood within the cortical substance of the brain they, having originated in that same place and having obtained a watery vehicle, at once flow more inwardly and soon enter *the medulla* of all the twistings, *filling the furrows* and their *ridges*; carried farther thence, through the special tracts of medulla of each into the medullary substance, which is placed under all the twistings as a common base for them, finally the spirits are carried into *the corpus callosum* as into a very wide field where those newly produced spirits go forth under a free and open sky.

Detailed Study

Despite the fact that Willis had drawn attention to the surface of the cerebrum, there were no further extensive studies of the cerebral convolutions until the end of the eighteenth century. Anatomists gave them scant mention, and artists continued to depict them as an irregular mass of folds with no pattern, resembling, as Erasistratus first suggested (p. 385), the haphazard arrangement of coils of the small intestine. The fissure of Sylvius (de le Boë, 1614–1672; see Baker, 1909) was mentioned for the first time by Caspar Bartholin (1641, p. 262) who gave the credit of discovery to Sylvius who did not, however, publish the following description until 1663.

All the surface of the cerebrum is very deeply marked by gyri similar to convolutions of small intestine and especially be a distinct fissure or hiatus that begins at the roots of the eyes *oculorum radices* [i.e., near the orbits]. It runs posteriorly above the temples as far as the origins of the brain stem (*medullae radices* [i.e., on a level with]). It divides the cerebrum into an upper, larger part and a lower, smaller part. Gyri occur along the whole length and depth of the fissure and even with the origins of smaller convolutions at the most superior part of it [*Opera medica* (Geneva, 1681), "Disputationum medicarum," IV, ix, 7; 1st ed. (Leyden, 1663), pp. 43–44].

In 1781 Vicq d'Azyr (1784, pp. 505–506) gave a detailed description of the fissure of Sylvius and referred occasionally to the convolutions; for example: "The posterior and inferior cerebral convolutions of the posterior lobes appear to me to be less voluminous than those of other regions [*ibid.*, p. 512, footnote *m*]." In his famous *Traité d'anatomie et de physiologie* (I, 1786) he referred to the convolutions in many of the legends to his excellent illustrations; thus in Plate III he showed anterior, middle, posterior, and inferior groups of convolutions, but he thought the two hemispheres were not symmetrical and concerned himself mostly with comparing the sizes of convolutions, not with their arrangement.

J. C. Reil (p. 593) also dealt with the gyri in his accounts of the brain's anatomy. In 1809 he described the area now known as the *Island of Reil:* "I shall call the *island* the longitudinal, oval base of the Sylvian fissure on which rest small, short, hidden convolutions that are encircled by a sulcus [1809*a*, p. 144]." And a little later he wrote: "The *island* has a longitudinal, rounded shape, and consists of a few small, hidden, and subordinate convolutions that have their own grouping and turn towards a central point. It is slightly elevated and sits on the cerebral ganglion [basal gray masses] and its curious outer wall. Around it passes a sulcus that continues posteriorly and superiorly between its two walls as the Sylvian fissure [1809*b*. pp. 196–197]." Reil also stated that the convolutions were the seat of mental processes: "Around these centers [basal gray masses] are all the convolutions of the hemispheres like the rays of this sun or like rivulets that absorb their life spirits from the ocean; around these [centers] lie the main instruments of the soul; around them originate the organs of artistic perception, of the ability for induction and representation [1809*b*, p. 207]."

There is no doubt that the controversial teachings of Gall and Spurzheim which maintained that psychological functions were represented on the cerebral surface, directed considerable attention to the convolution of the cerebral hemispheres. Thus the detailed studies of the convolutional pattern began in the early decades of the nineteenth century, and by the use of comparative and embryological data an extensive body of knowledge was accumulated. But today, very nearly one hundred years after the last selection of the present chapter, much work still remains to be done, notably on the gyral patterns and the mechanism of gyrus formation.

Franz Joseph Gall   Johann Caspar Spurzheim
(*9 March 1758—22 August 1828*)   (*31 December 1776—10 November 1832*)

The first person to draw widespread attention to the convolutions and to instigate the early nineteenth century studies of them, was Gall and, to a lesser extent, his pupil, Spurzheim. Gall is usually remembered for his doctrine of phrenology but he was, in fact, an expert anatomist; although he made few original observations, the attention he drew to the structure of the central nervous system was of the greatest importance, a fact usually obscured by his notoriety as a phrenologist.

Gall was born in the village of Tiefenbrunn in Baden and studied medicine at Strassburg and later at Vienna where he was graduated in 1795. Between 1790 and 1795 he began to work on a new concept that the brain was made up of as many *organs* as there were faculties and feelings, and as these were to be found on the surface of the brain they effected the bony covering. Thus palpation of the cranium (*cranioscopy* or, later, *phrenology*) could reveal the moral and intellectual qualities of the individual. Spurzheim who first studied theology and then attended medical school in Vienna joined Gall in 1804 as secretary and assistant. Together they left Vienna in 1805 because of opposition to their teaching, and settled eventually in Paris where they carried out further anatomical research and taught their doctrine. They parted company in 1814 and Gall remained in Paris until his death, whereas Spurzheim spent the rest of his life attempting to popularize phrenology in Europe and in the United States. He died in Boston (see Fossati, 1858; Temkin, 1947; Ackerknecht and Vallois, 1956).

Their contribution to the study of the cerebral convolutions was to describe them briefly, to discuss their comparative anatomy, and to suggest a mechanism for their formation. Concerning the last of these three, they thought that the gyri were produced by a process of folding and that in hydrocephalus the reverse took place. Although this proved to be incorrect, their long discussions and the opposition that arose (see, e.g., J. Gordon, *Observations on the structure of the brain*, Edinburgh, 1817, and Spurzheim's reply, *Examination of the objections*, [etc.], Edinburgh, 1817) helped to direct attention to structures which, until this time, had been largely neglected by anatomists. Furthermore, their concept of localization of psychological qualities on the brain surface, although erroneous in detail, was correct in principle, and it led eventually to cortical localization (pp. 488 ff.). Essentially it was another form of physiognomy, varieties of which had existed for centuries. Moreover, it focused attention on the convolutions. Gall did not, however, attempt to correlate the *organs* he recognized on the cranial surface with the underlying convolutional patterns, despite the fact that he thought they were on the brain surface.

Spurzheim collaborated in only the first two volumes of the important work, *Anatomie et physiologie du système nerveux en général, et du cerveau en particulier*

(Paris, 1810–1819), the first volume of which dealt only with anatomy and incorporated a memoir submitted to a commission of the Institut de France in 1808, published with its report and the authors' comments as *Recherches sur le système nerveux en général, et sur celui du cerveau en particulier* .... (Paris, 1809). The following passage occurs in Volume II of *Anatomie et physiologie* (1812).

EXCERPT P. 259

.... The convolutions are the expansion of the cerebral fibrils and fibre bundles. The convolutions, as far as they constitute an organ, receive their fibrils from different regions and from different accessory systems of supply as, for example, from the so-called thalami, from the so-called corpus striatum, or from different parts of these structures.

Gall gave more details when he was discussing the influence of the brain on the skull (Vol. III). He correlated his research into brain anatomy with the system of phrenology, a term introduced by Spurzheim but never used by Gall, and emphasized for the first time gyral symmetry.

EXCERPT P. 3

The gyri or convolutions do not all adopt the same direction. Some have a straight course from before backwards, others run transversely from above to the side, and others again have an oblique course. Almost all meander a little, some form pyramids, others twist themselves in spirals, etc. The basic forms of these convolutions are the same in all human brains, and they are congruent in the two hemispheres of the same brain; in a word, they are symmetrical. In small brains like those of the dog, horse, ox, sheep, etc., this symmetry is perfect; in man some small divisions vary in their forms.

All the forms of the main divisions, when these latter have developed considerably, declare their presence on the skull under the same type. Beyond that, there are the different forms and the different directions of the organs that I have drawn on the surface of the skull.

This explains the relation or the correspondence which exists between craniology [i.e., palpation of the head] and organology [the localized organs on the cerebral surfaces], or the doctrine of the functions of the brain (cerebral physiology); [this is] the sole aim of my researches.

Gall and Spurzheim were also interested in the comparative anatomy of the brain, for they considered that the obvious differences between various animals, and between animals and man, could have significance for their theory of localization of moral and intellectual functions in the brain. The following is from Volume II, and indicates that the authors were considering an evolutionary scale related to convolutional patterns and that this evidence was being used to support a theory of brain localization.

EXCERPT PP. 253–254

It can be shown that the same gradation exists in the structure of the brain of different species. As a matter of fact, I have shown in the preceding chapter that the existence of this moral quality or that intellectual faculty depends only on the presence of certain specific parts of the brain and not at all on the total mass of the brain. But it is none the less certain that the number of these faculties is directly related to the integral parts of the brain . . . .

In birds, the two hemispheres are already much more extensive, although one cannot yet discern distinct convolutions. The cerebellum still exists alone in the middle or fundamental area, but it seems already to be composed of several rings placed side by side.

In the small species of mammals, the shrews, the mice, the rats, the squirrel, the weasel, etc., one can distinguish no convolutions at all. But as they are already clearly formed in other less small species of rodent, the beaver, the kangaroo, etc., one may assume that they are found in the smaller species which I have just named.

In the bigger mammals, the cat, the pine marten, the stone marten, the fox, the dog, and the monkey, these convolutions become more and more distinct, and numerous, but their form varies according to species.

In the dolphin, the elephant, and in man, the convolutions are more numerous and deeper than they are in the beaver, the kangaroo, the cat, etc., and their shape and direction varies from species to species . . . .

The number of integral parts or convolutions of the brain varies in the same way in the different species of mammals. In certain types, the anterior lobes of the hemispheres are flattened or contracted; in others these same lobes are larger or more elevated; in still others, the inferior parts of the anterior lobes are almost entirely absent. The middle lobes and the other convolutions present the same variations.

In this way, the integral parts of the brain grow in number and in development as one passes from a less perfect animal to a more perfect one, until one reaches the brain of man which, in the anterior-superior, and superior-anterior frontal region is endowed with parts of the brain which are denied to the other animals; by which man enjoys higher qualities and faculties of judgment and moral sense.

When we see that nature follows such a course, how can it still be doubted that each part of the brain has different functions to fulfill, and that as a consequence, the brain of man and animals must be composed of as many special organs as the man or animal has distinct moral or intellectual faculties, inclinations, and aptitudes for work?

Like Reil, Gall and Spurzheim thought that the convolutions were the seat of intellectual processes as is evident from the following passage (1810, Vol. I, 309–310): ". . . the convolutions must be considered as complementary to the organs of the faculties of intelligence [and] one must at least admit that the convolutions are of an essential nature and necessary for intellectual functions." It is therefore astonishing that they made no effort to study the gyri in detail.

Friedrich Tiedemann
(23 August 1781—22 January 1861)

At last anatomists began to realize that the cerebral convolutions were not distributed in a haphazard manner and that they ought to be studied carefully like any other anatomical structure. It soon became clear that there were two methods of investigating them, in addition to observing their patterns in the adult human brain. The first was to extend the work of Willis and of Gall and Spurzheim who had drawn attention to the need for examining the convolutions in animals, and the second was to trace the pattern in the developing human fetus. Each of these approaches, it was learned, would help to decide whether the arrangement in man was variable or constant and would help to ravel its complexities. The German anatomist Tiedemann made important early contributions to both methods.

Tiedemann was born at Cassel and studied at Marburg, Bamberg, Würzburg, and Paris and eventually was appointed professor of zoology and human and comparative anatomy in the University of Landshut. In 1816 he moved to Heidelberg as professor of physiology, in 1849 to Frankfurt am Main, and finally to Munich in 1856. His work in anatomy was distinguished and the research he carried out on the chemistry of digestion, in collaboration with Leopold Gmelin (1788–1853), confirmed the finding of gastric hydrochloric acid by William Prout (1785–1850) (see Flourens, 1862).

Tiedemann's book, *Icones cerebri simiarum* (Heidelberg, 1821), contained five plates illustrating the brain of various animals, and the accompanying legends and brief text substantiated the opinion of Gall and Spurzheim that convolutional patterns varied in different orders and within the genera of certain orders.

But his investigations of the fetal brain were of greater importance to the history of the cerebral convolutions. They appeared in 1816 (*Anatomie und Bildungsgeschichte des Gehirns im Foetus des Menschen* [Nuremberg, 1816]), and the following passages, which describe the external features of the developing brain, have been translated from this edition. Tiedemann's accounts of comparative and embryological methods of investigation are to be found in the Appendix.

EXCERPT PP. 141–143

In the fourth month, the hemispheres are 10 lines [see p. 41] long and 5 in breadth anteriorly and 8 posteriorly. They are very noticeably prolonged posteriorly and cover not only the corpora striata and the thalami, but also the anterior part of the quadrigeminal bodies. Their superior surfaces are smooth and exhibit here and there a few slight depressions into which the pia mater sinks. Each hemisphere is divided on the lateral surface and inferiorly into a large anterior lobe and a conjoined middle and posterior lobe by a slight depression, the Sylvian fissure. From this fissure, in which the lateral artery of the brain [middle cerebral artery] lies, the large and hollow olfactory nerve arises and runs gradually medially and anteriorly . . . .

In the sixth month, the hemispheres of the brain are 1 inch and 6½ lines long, 1 inch in breadth anteriorly, and 1 inch and 3 lines posteriorly. They cover not only all of the quadrigeminal bodies, but even the greater part of the cerebellum. On the medial and facing surfaces of the two hemispheres more furrows, depressions, and rudimentary gyri are already visible, whereas the superior and lateral surfaces are still smooth. The hemispheres show the anterior, middle, and posterior lobes when seen from below. The two great anterior lobes of the brain are demarcated from the middle lobes by the Sylvian fissures which run laterally. In this fissure lies the large middle cerebral artery which is a continuation of the internal carotid trunk. From the fissures arise the great olfactory nerves which run medially and anteriorly and end in enlargements. The middle lobes are rounded and prominent and are separated from the posterior lobes by an indentation.

In the seventh month, the cerebrum is 1 inch 10 lines long, 1 inch 2 lines wide anteriorly, and 1 inch 5 lines wide posteriorly. It has increased so much in size that it not only covers over the quadrigeminal bodies and the cerebellum, but it also overhangs the latter a little. Indentations and depressions which are the rudiments of the convolutions and sulci, are seen here and there. The folds of the pia mater sink into them. The fissures of Sylvius are deep and ascend far up the brain, while bending a little posteriorly . . . .

In the eighth month, the hemispheres are 2 inches 11 lines long, 2 inches 1 line wide, and 1 inch 10 lines high; they cover over the cerebellum and project beyond it. On the inferior surface, the anterior, middle, and posterior lobes are clearly defined. They show everywhere many furrows and depressions into which the pia mater sinks. The depressions are most numerous, and the convolutions are thereby most prominent, in the anterior and middle lobes, but they are less numerous in the posterior lobe.

In the ninth month the hemispheres are 3 inches 4 lines long and 2 inches 7 lines wide. Their shape is now exactly that of the adult human and they are provided with many fissures and convolutions.

Now from this it follows that the cerebral hemispheres originate from the side and from in front; that originally they are a thin, medullary membrane reflected from within and posteriorly; that they gradually increase in size and thickness; and that in this way they extend from before backwards over the corpora striata, the thalami, the quadrigeminal bodies, and the cerebellum and cover over these parts. The same formation takes place in the cerebral hemispheres of animals, except that it is arrested permanently in different animals at the different stages of formation which the brain of the human fetus passes through in its successive development. The proof of this is furnished by the examination of the cerebra of animals.

Tiedemann next described briefly the external surface of the brain of various animals (pp. 143–148). The ape had the largest cerebral hemispheres and more convolutions than other animals. He concluded (p. 148), "So the brain of the human adult is distinguished from that of all animals by the size and height of its hemispheres, and by the greater number of sulci and convolutions."

RICHARD OWEN
(20 July 1804—18 December 1892)

The comparative approach now received considerable attention, and an active worker in this field was Owen, the English zoologist. Owen was born at Lancaster and received his medical education at Edinburgh. He began a private practice in London but in 1827 was appointed assistant conservator to the Hunterian Museum of the Royal College of Surgeons. In 1835 he was made Hunterian Professor of comparative anatomy and physiology, a post he kept till 1856 when he became superintendent of the Natural History Department of the British Museum from which he retired in 1884. Owen was one of the foremost anatomists and zoologists of his day and his writings are voluminous (see *Proc. R. Soc.*, 1894, 55: i–xiv; Owen, 1894).

Owen's interest in the comparative study of gyral patterns was aroused in 1833 when he wished to find out if there were consistencies characterizing species or families of mammalia, and two years later he published his findings, "On the anatomy of the cheetah, Felis Jubata, Schreb" (*Trans. Zool. Soc. London*, 1835, 1:129–136), in which he noted primary or constant sulci and secondary or less symmetrical ones.

EXCERPT PP. 135–136

That the disposition of the superimposed mass of the *cerebrum* varies in the different orders of *Mammalia,* and in some of the orders is found to vary also in the different genera, is now well known to comparative anatomists . . . .

. . . .

In the description of the outward configuration of the cerebral hemispheres in the *Cheetah* and other feline species, I have limited myself to noting those convolutions only which, after a careful comparison of the materials at my disposal, appeared to be subject to least variety. But even with this limitation a very small portion of the cerebral surface remains undescribed; and the constancy manifested in the disposition of the remainder, as to the form, extent, and symmetrical arrangement of the convolutions, argues strongly in favour of the conclusion that the folding of the hemispheric substance in the progress of its development, follows a determinate law; and that the tracing of the additional convolutions, as they successively present themselves in succeeding complexities of the *cerebrum*, may not only tend to advance zoology by bringing to light additional instances of affinities between the different groups of *Mammalia*, but ultimately lead to the determination both of the amount and locality of the convolutions in the human brain which are analogous to those of the inferior animals.

In his famous textbook, *On the anatomy of vertebrates* (Vol. III, London, 1868), he considered the problem again, and in so doing summarized his observations made in 1835.

EXCERPT PP. 115–116

. . . . In 1833 I communicated the results in regard to the convolutions of the cerebrum in the *Felidae*, distinguishing the 'folds' by letters, and the 'fissures' by figures; and finding that their homologues could be traced from species to species in that family, I distinguished most of them by names. I further entered upon their classification, and defined the 'primary' and 'secondary' fissures and folds, showing that the 'secondary fissures were in general less symmetrical than the primary ones' and that the differences observable in the brains of the *Felidae* were due chiefly to the absence of more or less of the secondary convolutions in the smaller species; 'in the common Cat the principal fissures, or anfractuosities, are less obscured by fissures of the second degree than in the larger Felines' . . . . Prior to the appearance of both these works [Leuret and Gratiolet, and Foville], I had continued my observations as opportunities presented themselves; and gave the result of such extended comparisons in the Course of Lectures delivered at the Royal College of Surgeons of England in 1842: my diagrams there, in which homologous convolutions are indicated by colours, may still testify in part to the extent to which the comparisons had been carried; the main aim which I had in view being the determination of the homologous and superadded convolutions in the more complex prosencephalon of Man.

The following excerpt is from the Hunterian Lectures given in 1842 ("Lectures on the anatomy and physiology of the nervous system," *Med. Times*, 1842, 7:1, 35, 75–76, 101). It summarized Owen's opinions on the gyri.

EXCERPT P. 101

The cerebral hemispheres progressively increase as we pass from the orders rodentia, chiroptera, and edentata, to the carnivora, the ruminants, the pacaderms, the quadrumena, and the cetacea, to man. The extent of the superficial vascular cineritious matter of the hemispheres is increased in the same gradation, chiefly by the progressive number, depth, and complications of the folds and convolutions.

A symmetrical arrangement, more or less regular or complex, can always be traced between the foldings of the two hemispheres, and the more regular in proportion to the simplicity of the convolutions; the foldings of the cerebral substance follow likewise, both in the embryonic development of a complex brain, and in the progressive permanent stages presented by the mammalian series—a regular determinate law; some convolutions [primary] being more constant than others, and these being traceable through the greatest number of brains, and recognizable even in the human brain, where at first sight they are obscured by so many accessory convolutions.

François Leuret
(29 December 1797—5 January 1851)

Of the many individuals who were now attempting to understand the convolutional patterns, the French anatomist and psychiatrist Leuret was one of the most outstanding. He was also interested in the approach to the problem through comparative anatomy, and he extended Owen's observations to mammals other than the cats.

Leuret was born at Nancy and attended medical school in Paris. After having been graduated, he studied mental disorders under Esquirol and specialized in psychiatry at the Bicêtre, as well as directing a private mental asylum. He held these appointments until his death, and he made a number of contributions to psychiatric therapy. His most important work was *Anatomie comparée du système nerveux considéré dans ses rapports avec l'intelligence,* but he survived to complete only the first volume (Paris, 1839), and the second, compiled by Gratiolet, appeared fifteen years later (see Trélat, 1857; Semelaigne, 1930, I, 214–226).

Leuret proposed that the known variations in convolutional patterns from species to species could be used as a criterion of differentiation. He therefore examined one hundred and four mammals and arranged them in ascending order of convolutional complexity; the first group contained the mouse, mole, hedgehog, and other rodents; the fourteenth and last group contained the monkeys. It is clear, too, that he had also by this method grouped them in an order of ascending intelligence.

Leuret furthermore discovered that the larger gyri were connected by means of supplementary convolutions.

The Italian anatomist Luigi Rolando (p. 480) also studied the cerebral convolutions and described the fissure which is still known by his name ("Della struttura degli emisferi cerebrali," *Mem. r. Accad. Sci. Torino*, 1831, 35:103–146). In the following passages from Volume I of *Anatomie comparée* Leuret proposed the term "fissure of Rolando."

EXCERPT PP. 397–400

Fourteenth Group: Monkeys, and above all macacs, do not have the undulate and voluminous convolutions of the elephant and the whale; in addition, at first sight they seem to be farther away from the human than these latter; but even superficial observation will soon dispel this illusion. The common form of the monkey's brain, its posterior development, and the expanse and angle of slope of the Sylvian fissure, make it similar to the cerebrum of a full-grown human embryo while the brain of the elephant, and, more so, that of the whale, when considered from these different points of view incline towards the shape of the brain of other animals.

The monkey has three anterior, three posterior, two upper, one medial, and some supraorbital convolutions.

The medial convolution I, I, I, I, I (fig. 5, pl. xv [fig. 98]) in front closely resembles that of the fox; it proceeds to the anterior part of the brain where it unites with the third anterior convolution, following which it runs posteriorly on the corpus callosum, provides a large communication + which ascends to the upper convolutions (+ fig. 4 and S +, and fig. 2 S +). Then it descends in front of the cerebellum, passes around the cerebral peduncle, and continues to reappear below, very close to the optic nerve (I, fig. 3, and I, fig. 5) in the form of the hippocampal lobe. Not only does this lobe advance to the medial convolution, but it provides two extensions which proceed above the cerebellum, as in the otter, the porpoise, and some other animals in which the cerebellum is to a large extent covered by the cerebrum.

The Sylvian fissure (S.S., fig. 2 and fig. 4) deviates posteriorly owing to the presence of two superior convolutions, S,S,S,S, and S′, S′, S′, fig. 4, of which the posterior S′, S′, S,S,S, + [postcentral], proceeds above and posteriorly in order to unite with the medial convolution, while the anterior one provides three convolutions that are directed towards the anterior part of the brain (I A, II A, III A, fig. 2 and fig. 4). Between these two convolutions exists a furrow (S, R, fig. 2 and fig. 4) that separates them along their entire length; it is as constant as the Sylvian fissure. I have called this furrow the fissure of Rolando, because this anatomist described it in man in whom it is still more developed than in the monkey.

Behind and below the Sylvian fissure there are three other convolutions, I P, II P, III P [temporal gyri], of which the latter two are clearly separated only in the monkeys that are more intelligent than the baboon.

The orbital convolutions O, O [pl. xv, fig. 1] are constant; they are larger and better divided than in lower animals, but they do not have the same regularity as the others.

If the monkey brain may, to a certain extent, be considered a rough model of that of man, that of the macac is a rough model of that of the monkey. However, one finds there, although in rudimentary form, all the convolutions of the genuine monkeys.

The number, form, organization, and relations of the cerebral convolutions were not left to chance; in each family of animals the brain was shaped in a determined way, and the divergence in opinions that have been expressed on this subject arises from failure to examine the brain carefully in a sufficiently large number of animals. Observation demonstrates that this is so; inference ought to have led to it. How, indeed, can one believe that the most important organ in the economy, that by which the manifestations of the intellect function, to which one attributes instincts and passions, would not have a fixed organization as unchangeable as that of the other parts?

Each group of brains has a type proper to it, and that type is above all indicated by the shape of its convolutions. In foxes, there are sharp and well-differentiated divisions; in cats, fewer divisions, but still definite and very simple forms; in the family of bears and martens, a tendency towards another form and preservation of some convolutions that I shall call primitive by reason of their simplicity, and a disposition of others to join each other and to present undulations. Then, a new type, less numerous fundamental separations and greater variety in details for different groups, to which belong the wombat, the kangaroo, the goat, the pig, the seal, the whale; then, suddenly an addition to the common forms, new convolutions for the elephant with a development infinite in detail. In the monkey, a type still more detailed, closer to that of man, but incomplete and rudimentary.

Usually, in one and the same family, the more the brain grows and the more it is divided up, the more it also acquires undulations. The fox, the domestic cat, the stone or beech marten, the ferret, the goat, and the chinese pig each represents the first step on a ladder, the top of which is occupied by the dog, the lion, the otter, the deer, and the wild boar. In its species, the elephant is at the top; I do not know the animal that could be placed at the opposite extreme. Among its species, the macac is right at the bottom, the monkey higher, and man much above the monkey. However, there are larger brains without an improvement over small brains that belong to the same class. Thus, the ox is not more perfect than the sheep, the whale not superior to the porpoise.

Leuret's conclusions concerning the convolutions were as follows.

EXCERPT PP. 451–453

1. . . . .

2. In the majority of mammals the brain is provided with convolutions.

3. Mammals in which cerebral convolutions are lacking all belong to orders in which structure is least perfected.

4. The cerebral convolutions of mammals are always the same in the same animal.

5. Mammals can be classified according to the similarity of their cerebral convolutions.

6. The classification established according to convolutions differs in several essential ways from that based upon the formation of the organs used for grasping food. It brings together animals with similar ability, whereas it separates animals with different abilities.

7. The cerebral convolutions are of several well-defined types, although the transitions from one type to another can be followed with the aid of intermediate types.

8. Three animals, the elephant, the lemur, and the monkey, have convolutions, the analogues of which are found only in man.

9. There is no direct relationship between the presence and development of the convolutions with brain volume. However, it is generally true to say that larger brains have convolutions which are more numerous and, above all, are more undulate.

10. The fox, the wolf, the dog, and the jackal are the animals in which the cerebral convolutions are very simple.

11. . . . .

12. . . . .

13. The herbivorous whole-hooved ruminants have less simple and more undulate cerebral convolutions than the carnivores, that rather resemble, from a general aspect, the cerebral convolutions of man.

14. . . . .

15. . . . .

16. . . . .

17. Of all mammals, the elephant and the whale have the most voluminous and undulate convolutions, but the elephant is superior to the whale as far as its convolutions are concerned, and these are common to the monkey and also to man.

LOUIS PIERRE GRATIOLET
(6 July 1815—16 February 1865)

The investigations carried out by Leuret were continued by Gratiolet, also of Paris, whose contribution to the anatomy of the cerebral convolutions was even greater than that of his predecessor.

Gratiolet was born at Sainte-Foy-la-Grande in the department of the Gironde. He began his studies in Paris in 1829 and was graduated in medicine in 1845. Meantime he had become interested in comparative anatomy and eventually, in 1862, was appointed professor of zoology in the University of Paris. His researches were especially into neuroanatomical problems, but he also contributed to the fields of physiology and anthropology (see Grandeau, 1865; Broca, 1865; Alix, 1868).

Like those before him, Gratiolet also applied the comparative approach to the problem of convolutional patterns. By tracing the gradual appearance of gyri in various types of primates ranging upwards from the smooth-brained marmoset monkey to the chimpanzee and to man, he was able to detect the gyri which appeared first, that is the primary gyri, and those which were secondary in order of appearance. He also introduced a system of nomenclature which replaced the previous cumbersome terms and which rapidly became popular and was widely adopted in Europe. To Gratiolet is also owed the limits of each cerebral lobe and their names, taken from the overlying bone; they remain today as convenient topographical areas. His most important observations were published in 1854 and summarized three years later in the second volume of Leuret's book (p. 399), *Anatomie comparée du système nerveux* (Vol. II [Paris, 1857], 101–124). The 1854 publication was entitled *Mémoires sur les plis cérébraux de l'homme et des primates* (Paris, 1854) and the following passages have been translated from it. The first has been taken from the summary and is an account of the lobes and main convolutions in the primate brain.

EXCERPT PP. 88–89

We can distinguish five lobes on the external surface of the cerebral hemisphere of the primates. One of these lobes is *the central lobe* [insula]; it forms the end point of the axis around which the lateral ventricles are coiled. The other lobes are situated around this central lobe and are superficial to it; they spread out and encircle this intermediate group, so that it is hidden at the bottom of a deep valley. This valley is called the fissure of Sylvius.

It is easy to distinguish, 1, the frontal lobe which forms the anterior extremity of the cerebral hemisphere. 2, the parietal lobe. These two lobes are situated above the fissure of Sylvius. 3, the temporosphenoidal lobe, situated below it. 4, the occipital lobe, which forms the posterior extremity of the hemisphere and which is separated from the parietal lobe by an almost straight fissure, the *external perpendicular sulcus* [parieto-occipital sulcus, Huxley].

The convolutions of the brain are marked out on the different lobes in a very simple way. We divide the frontal lobe into two lobules: the orbital lobule, of which the sulci, with the exception of the sulcus which accommodates the olfactory lobe [bulb], are very irregular, and the frontal lobule which can be easily subdivided into three horizontal, parallel tiers, thus:

1, the inferior frontal tier, or surciliary convolution (*pli surcilier*) [fig. 99, 1; hereafter numbers and Roman and Greek letters refer to fig. 99]; 2, the middle frontal tier [2]; finally, 3, the superior frontal tier [3]. It is apparent that the third is the most important of the three. It is simple in the apes, but subdivided in the highest orders of each group of primates; in the white man it breaks up into three large, winding convolutions. This partition, traces of which can be seen in the orang and the chimpanzee, is manifestly a sign of relative perfection.

The parietal convolutions have an upward slant which approximates more or less to the perpendicular; they are three in number. 1, the *first ascending convolution* [precentral, 4]. This convolution meets, at the top, the end of the superior frontal convolution. 2, the *second ascending convolution* [postcentral, 5]. The upper part of this convolution forms a bend, then expands slightly and extends to the external, perpendicular sulcus. This upper portion of the second ascending convolution [B] has certain characteristics, with the help of which we can easily distinguish the true macacs, where it is long, from the rhesus and cheropithics where it is much reduced in size. We give to it the name of the lobule of the second ascending convolution. 3, the *curved convolution* [angular gyrus, 6 and 6']. This convolution originates sometimes in front of the summit of the fissure of Sylvius, as in the long-tailed apes, the macacs, the dog-faced baboons, the saïs, sajous, and the squirrel monkeys; sometimes at the summit of the cleft itself as in the semnopithics, the gibbons, the orangs, and the ateles, and sometimes behind this summit, where it is found in man. This convolution has an ascending portion which belongs to the parietal lobe, and an ascending branch which belongs in part to the temporal lobe [A].

The temporal convolutions are also three in number. They are parallel to each other and to the fissure of Sylvius. One distinguishes easily *the superior temporal convolution* [7] which borders the fissure of Sylvius inferiorly and which we name, also for that reason, the *inferior marginal convolution*. (2), the *middle temporal convolution* [8]. This convolution is separated from the superior temporal convolution by a very deep sulcus, the parallel sulcus; the middle temporal convolution continues to the descending branch of the angular gyrus [6 and 6']. (3) the *inferior temporal convolution* [9]. This convolution runs parallel to the preceding ones and is not always very distinct; its posterior extremity traverses the occipital lobe.

The occipital lobe, in its turn, is subdivided into several individual parts, in three principal tiers, that is to say, the inferior [12], middle [11], and superior tier [10], all three of which are horizontal and parallel. But its layout is very irregular, and only the lower tier is at all clear.

Thus, by a singular coincidence, the frontal, parietal, temporal, and occipital lobes each includes three, ordinarily well-defined convolutions. These, besides the irregular gyri of the orbital lobule, give to the external surface of the brain *twelve principal convolutions* surrounding the fissure of Sylvius.

As well as these convolutions, we should also note four others which pass from the occipital lobe to the temporal and parietal lobes.

I name them *transitional convolutions (plis de passage)*.

The first transitional convolution [α], the superior one, joins the second ascending convolution to the summit of the posterior lobe.

The second [β] joins the summit of the angular convolution to the superior tier of the occipital lobe.

The third [γ] is intermediate between the middle temporal convolution and the middle tier of the occipital lobe.

Finally, the fourth [δ] joins the lower tier of the occipital lobe to the middle convolution of the temporal lobe.

Of these four convolutions, the last two are constantly superficial, but the two superior convolutions merit careful consideration. Thus in one instance, they are found together, as in the long-tailed ape, the semnopithics, the gibbons, the orangs, man, and the ateles. [Discussion of variation in these gyri follows.]

EXCERPT P. 90

Thus, consideration of these convolutions is of extreme importance; it is a simple and certain way of revealing their nature, and it resolves one of the greatest difficulties which arises in the general comparison of the brain of man with the brain of the primates.

The next passage has been taken from Gratiolet's account of the cerebral convolutions in man.

EXCERPT PP. 57–59

The shape of the human brain is known. The singular height, the width of the frontal lobe of which the anterior extremity instead of tapering off in a sharp point ends in a surface, the length of which corresponds to that of the frontal one; the size of the angle which the planes of the orbital cavities form with each other; the lowering of the Sylvian fissure. The abundance and general complication of the secondary folds distinguish this brain at a glance from that of all the primates.

But if one compares the proportions of the parts, these differences, extensive and characteristic as they are, nevertheless allow such analogies to continue to exist between the *human* brain and that of all the *monkeys* and the same general description does for both.

Here we have the same principle divisions, the same lobes, the same folds. Not all the parts are similar, but they are all homologous.

A colored illustration of a human brain seen in profile will make these similarities very close [Pl. XII, fig. 1. Lateral views of sixteen varieties of primates, including man. Coloring shows the relative sizes of the groups of gyri]; as typical for this comparison, I have selected a brain in which the secondary gyri were intentionally concealed; in this way one can compare it more easily with the brain of higher monkeys.

A basic fact must be noted; it is the receding position of the root of the first ascending gyrus [precentral] (Pl. I, fig. 1, 2, 4.4.4. [fig. 99]). This gyrus which, in all the pithecans originates above the angle of the Sylvian fissure, starts in man approximately two centimeters posterior to this point.

From this it follows that the posterior border of the anterior [frontal] lobe recedes and that this lobe thus becomes larger while pushing back the parietal lobe, the posterior limit of which is, by the way, much less well defined than in monkeys, for reasons that we shall soon explain.

For the same reason, the anterior borders of the occipital lobe are poorly defined. Nevertheless it is evident, even in the adult, that it is markedly reduced; this reduction is still more apparent in the brain of the human fetus which we have illustrated. (Pl. XI, fig. 1, 2, 3.)

The temporosphenoidal lobe is of medium bulk and the parts which are located above the Sylvian fissure considerably exceed those that are below. Finally, the central lobe [insula] is large and occupies the greatly enlarged base of the Sylvian fissure.

Lobes of the medial surface.—The lobes of the medial surface are also very remarkable. The hippocampal sulcus is almost horizontal; the internal perpendicular sulcus [parieto-occipital] fissure changes course, and, pushed back by the development of the frontoparietal region slopes slightly posteriorly; the medial occipital lobe enclosed between these two sulci is triangular and is covered by shallow gyri. The quadrilateral lobe [cuneus] is very large.

The occipitosphenoidal lobe relatively is rather reduced; besides, it recalls, in general and in particular, the arrangement which the monkey's brain demonstrates, but it is much less hollowed out in the part which corresponds to that of the cerebellum.

Cerebral convolutions.—Such is in general the relationship of the lobes to one another; the gyri by which they are covered in turn deserve to be carefully inspected.

Convolutions of the lateral surface.—The gyri of the lateral surface, covered with sulci capriciously tucked in, have a very complicated appearance; but with a little care a way can be seen through this labyrinth and a considerable complication disappears.

One can then distinguish with the greatest of ease, 1, the orbital lobe which is remarkable for the size of the olfactory sulcus; 2, the inferior frontal convolution or the "surcilier" gyrus [1.1.1.]; 3, the middle frontal convolution which surrounds the "surcilier" convolution 2.2.2.; 4, lastly, the upper frontal gyrus which is subdivided into two or three large and sinuous folds which go through the summit of the first ascending convolution 3'.3'.3'.

It would be impossible to give an adequate description of these folds in the human species if one did not compare a large number of individuals one with another. Indeed, they vary in the most capricious manner, they are distinguished or mingle in a thousand different ways, and nothing indicates more the importance of these gyri than the almost infinite irregularity of their variations.

In individuals who belong to the white race the "surcilier" convolution (inferior frontal) is well defined in most cases, as one may see in the brain illustrated in Plate I, fig. 1 [1.1.1.]. As to the middle gyrus 2.2 it is generally speaking twisted in a very complicated way and blends in such manner with the superior frontal gyrus that it is frequently very difficult to define its exact borders.

This is, let us say, the most common arrangement; however, we must not consider that it is absolutely characteristic.

EMIL HUSCHKE
(14 December 1797—19 June 1858)

Although much of the early work on the arrangement of cerebral gyri and sulci was carried out in France, certain individuals in Germany also interested themselves in this neuroanatomical problem. One of these was Huschke of Jena. Huschke was born at Weimar and attended medical achool in Jena where in 1824 he was appointed professor of anatomy and embryology. He remained there for the rest of his life and made several contributions to the study of anatomy (see Rüdinger, 1881).

Huschke's most famous book was on the anatomy of the brain, *Schaedel, Hirn und Seele des Menschen und der Thiere nach Alter, Geschlecht und Raçe* (Jena, 1854). It reflects his adherence to the cult of *Naturphilosophie*, and it is also declared to have been the first published medical work to contain photographs.

The following selection describes "the system of convolutions in apes and man." Huschke thought that the brain was an electrical machine and that each part, including the convolutions, had a specific role to play. It was an example of the overenthusiastic application of early electrophysiological knowledge to problems of brain function. He made certain important general statements regarding the gyri and the sulci.

EXCERPT PP. 134–135

If I summarize all these investigations for the elucidation of a natural system of the human cerebral convolutions, the following general postulates and laws of development may be established:

1) In the beginning, the convolutions of the cerebrum run longitudinally; the transverse convolutions are secondary and they arise in the divisions or sinuosities of the longitudinal convolutions, except here and there where they represent connections of two primary convolutions that are still joined together and which have not yet separated completely. In this case they would have a lesser, in the other case a greater importance; there the indication of incomplete polarization, here the terminal points of the separated primary convolutions.

Therefore, as much as the cerebellum corresponds to the cerebrum in its overall structure as well as in the direction of its principal convolutions, it is, however, contrary to it; the cerebrum is developed longitudinally, the cerebellum transversely.

2) The first longitudinal convolutions (*primary convolutions*) are circular, rising obliquely posteriorly, and they are open inferiorly and anteriorly. This gaping area corresponds to the Sylvian fissure. The anterior half of the circle of each primary convolution, therefore, lies for the most part in the frontal brain, and the posterior half belongs to the parietal. Of the two parts, the posterior hemispheres in most mammals (? all) are larger and also give off more subdivisions than the anterior.

3) Every hemisphere has three to four primary convolutions inserted concentrically into each other, which, for the time being until their final anatomical and physiological elucidation [is possible], are best designated as first (the inferior one), second, third, and fourth convolution. From the first to the fourth, they increase in width and in the extent of their arc.

4) . . . .

5) Their *horseshoe form* is related to the same shape of the *base* or *root of the corona radiata* in that this also represents a circle which is open inferiorly and externally; and the Sylvian fissure therefore is likewise in

exact communication with that behavior of the corona radiata, just as the optic nerve runs downwards and so causes the cleft in the retina. Perhaps it is simultaneously associated with the circular form or contortion which the corpus striatum, the thalamus, and also the infundibulum and pituitary body display.

6) The *position of the Sylvian fissure* is not uniformly oblique in all mammals. It is almost vertical in the herbivorous (sheep, ox, horse) and it is at the same time very small and shallow. It is longer and more oblique in the *feris* (cat, panther, lion, dog, fox, otter, polecat, bear, coati, raccoon, etc.); that of the pig and the elephant is midway between these two. It reaches its greatest length in the monkey and its greatest width and most *horizontal* position in the human. Here it proceeds backwards along the entire upper portion of the squamous suture of the parietal bone, whereas in the marten it merely adopts the situation of the pterygoid squamous suture.

In general, a vertical position seems to indicate a smaller frontal and a greater parietal brain, and *vice versa*.

7) The length and oblique position of the Sylvian fissure parallel the ever-increasing substance of the *first* primary convolution, whereas the rest are forced back and displaced in proportion.

8) The more tortuous the primary convolutions, the deeper the sulci between them, the more impressions and branches, the more asymmetrical their structure, the more perfect is an animal species. For the most part this is the case in the larger species of one genus or family (perhaps with the exception of the ox in which the convolutions are not more perfect than those of the sheep, and of the whale which, according to Leuret, does not seem to be superior to the dolphin).

The statement that the number and complexity of the convolutions is in proportion to the intellectual functions of an animal, is limited to the animals of one and the same class, insofar as each class has its own peculiar type and a scale of this type corresponding to the different species (Leuret).

William Turner

(7 January 1832—15 February 1916)

In the decade 1856 to 1866 a great deal of information concerning the cerebral convolutions was accumulated, as can be seen, for example, in a standard textbook of anatomy such as that of Quain; the editions of 1856 and 1866 illustrate this change. By 1866 the Edinburgh anatomist Turner could state that "we can now localise the different gyri, and give to each its appropriate name" (*The convolutions of the human cerebrum topographically considered*, Edinburgh, 1866, p. 7). Broca (p. 494), however, was not quite so optimistic.

Turner was born in Lancaster and studied medicine at St. Bartholomew's Hospital and Medical School in London. He joined the Anatomy Department of Edinburgh University in 1854 and thirteen years later was appointed professor of anatomy. He retired in 1903 after a distinguished career in teaching and research, as well as making further contributions in the fields of anthropology and university administration (see Turner, 1919).

In the monograph cited above, Turner differed from Gratiolet on a number of important points; for example, he established the fissure of Rolando as the posterior limit of the frontal lobe. Detailed study of individual gyri was still required and Turner helped to supply some of these data. The following selection is his account of the intraparietal fissure that he described for the first time.

EXCERPT PP. 12–13

The intra-parietal fissure (*IP* [figs. 100 and 101]).—This fissure is figured in all the more accurate drawings of the human and quadrumanous brain, though no special description has been given of it. It lies within the parietal lobe, from which circumstance I have termed it intra-parietal. It may be recognised at the sixth month of intra-uterine life. It is situated immediately behind and ascends parallel to the ascending parietal gyrus, and then bends almost horizontally backwards, and extends for a varying distance in different brains; in some cases it may be traced between the first and second bridging convolutions, as in the right hemisphere of figs. 1 and 2. Its ascending part separates the supra-marginal gyrus (A) from the ascending parietal (5); its horizontal part separates the supra-marginal gyrus from the ascending parietal lobule (5'). Not unfrequently one or more secondary gyri bridge it across superficially; a frequent seat for such a connecting convolution is at the angle of junction of its ascending and horizontal portions, excellent representations of which may be seen in the brains of the Bushwomen figured by Professors Gratiolet and Marshall. The intra-parietal fissure is usually separated from the horizontal part of the fissure of Sylvius by that portion of the supra-marginal gyrus which joins the lower end of the ascending parietal convolution. In Gratiolet's Bushwoman it may be seen, however, that they are continuous with each other; and I have observed the same arrangement in more than one European brain (see fig. 1).

When the hemisphere is viewed in profile, three fissures may be traced passing for a greater or less distance upwards and backwards on its outer face. These are from before backwards, the ascending limb of the Sylvian fissure, the fissure of Rolando, and the intra-parietal fissure—of which the fissure of Rolando always mounts the highest. They may, more especially the first-named, be continuous with the horizontal limb of the Sylvian fissure, and then seem as it were to radiate from it, but not unfrequently they commence at some little distance above it, and it is owing to their position and direction that the ascending frontal and parietal convolutions are so accurately defined.

It now seemed that the asymmetry of the gyri of the two hemispheres occurred particularly in the secondary ones; the primary, such as the fissures of Sylvius and Rolando, were relatively constant. Moreover, the intelligent, the male, and the European appeared to have a more complex pattern than the mentally impaired, the female, and the savage. But even today evidence is insufficient to substantiate these early impressions. The influence of Darwin's theory of evolution, published in 1859, was also an important stimulus to work on the gyri. It was considered by some that man's dominance in the scale of animals was reflected in his convolutional pattern.

The realization that gyri were, on the whole, constant in design led naturally to consideration of their possible function. Perhaps they did after all take part in cerebral activity. It is significant that at this time (the early 1860's) evidence was accumulating to establish the theory of cortical localization of function (see Chapter IX). In the following excerpt Turner discussed this problem.

EXCERPT P. 27

The precise morphological investigations of the last few years into the cerebral convolutions have led to the revival in Paris of discussions, in which the doctrine of Gall and his disciples—that the brain is not one but consists of many organs—has been supported by new arguments, and the opinion has been expressed that the primary convolutions, at least, are both morphologically and physiologically distinct organs. Hence both the physiologist and pathologist have been induced to take an interest in a subject which, at the first glance, might seem as if it lay almost exclusively within the province of the morphological or descriptive anatomist. For, instead of the vague and too often loose descriptions of the seats of morbid products to which, through the imperfection of anatomical modes of expression, they were not unfrequently compelled to resort, they have at last been provided with a method of description and a system of nomenclature of that precise character that a lesion affecting the surface of the hemisphere can now be localized with great exactness, the particular convolution or convolutions it affects can be distinctly expressed, and the means can thus be afforded of making an exact comparison of the morbid appearances seen after death in one brain with those which may be observed in others. By combining the results obtained from the examination of a large number of diseased brains, and studying them in connexion with carefully recorded clinical histories of the cases taken during life, it will in time be seen if a lesion in a given convolution is always associated with a particular train of symptoms. If this should be found to be the case, then some authority may be claimed for the view that the convolutions are physiologically distinct organs. Already some steps have been taken which seem to lead in this direction. The observations of M. Paul Broca [see p. 494], that, in some cases under his charge, loss of the cerebral faculty of speech (aphasia) co-existed with a lesion of the posterior third of the inferior left frontal gyrus, seem to point to that convolution as the seat of the faculty of spoken language. Dr. Sanders has also communicated to the Medico-Chirurgical Society of our city a case in which a similar defect in the power of speech occurred along with a lesion in the same locality. Such observations have put this aspect of the subject into that stage that, to use the words of Dr. Sanders, "it requires and invites fresh investigation."

ALEXANDER ECKER

(10 July 1816—20 May 1887)

A further important contributor to the morphology of the convolutions was Ecker of Freiburg, the last to be considered here. Ecker was born in Freiburg, Baden, and he studied medicine both there and at Heidelberg where one of his teachers was Tiedemann (p. 395). In 1844 he was appointed professor of anatomy and physiology in the University of Basel, and six years later became professor of anatomy, physiology, and anthropology (see Ranke, 1887). His influence regarding gyral anatomy was widespread on account of his small book on the subject (*Die Hirnwindung des Menschen nach eigenen Untersuchungen insbesondere über die Entwicklung derselben beim Fötus*, Braunschweig, 1869 and 2nd ed. 1883). Ecker's descriptions are more detailed than those of Turner but the factual information led him to make no inferences concerning possible function. The following excerpt has been newly translated from the introduction; it gave more precise definitions of the general types of gyri and sulci.

EXCERPT PP. 3–4

If we make an introductory survey of the convolutions in general, we can divide them into, first of all, chief or primary, then into secondary, and finally into tertiary convolutions.

The chief or primary convolutions are similar to huge mountain ridges the features of which give a characteristic appearance to the scenery, as has been so truly stated. The secondary gyri are produced by a primary convolution forming sulci and splitting longitudinally into narrower secondary convolutions so that secondary mountain ridges come into being by the formation of valleys perpendicular to them.

We can call the deeper sulci separating the primary convolutions from each other the primary sulci and we may call those which separate the secondary convolutions from each other, secondary sulci. Finally, we can give the name tertiary convolution to the small protruding mountain ridges which come out of the valley walls of the primary convolutions into a primary sulcus and give the bottom of the valley or sulcus a zig-zag course as they insert themselves chiefly between those of the opposite side. On the whole, they can be clearly seen only when the edges of the primary sulci are pulled apart; they come to light immediately in brains in which the primary convolutions have disappeared owing to senile or other atrophy through the great infiltration of the pia mater. Whereas the groups of primary convolutions are always fairly regularly arranged, many variations occur in the region of the secondary and tertiary convolutions. This may be because of the fact that sometimes only a few, sometimes many, secondary sulci are present, which is especially responsible for the variety in the number of convolutions, or because in the one case hidden tertiary convolutions reach the surface and in the other convolutions on the surface usually sink into the depths. In the first case the sulci are bridged over and in the second, sulci come into being where usually there are none.

Ecker described each gyrus and sulcus in turn, and the following account of the central sulcus (fissure of Rolando) appeared in the section of his book which dealt with primary fissures.

EXCERPT PP. 8–10

This sulcus which, as mentioned already, was first described in detail by Rolando [see p. 480], is always and without exception present in the human brain and it is characteristic for the human brain as well as for most apes. At the same time it is one of the first, but not the first, to appear in the fetal brain, for normally it is recognizable at the end of the fifth month. Because of its constant occurrence and because it is never, or very rarely ever, bridged over by a secondary convolution during its course, it forms the surest point of departure for finding the convolutions. It begins near the medial [sagittal] edge of the hemisphere and runs from there obliquely forwards and downwards to end near the upper edge of the posterior limb of the Sylvian fissure; thus the sulci of the two sides together form an acute angle open to the front. As the frontal lobe increases in size and the brain in general reaches a state of higher development, this angle seems more acute and the course of the sulcus posteriorly seems to be become steeper. Even the very position of the sulcus seems, under the conditions men-

tioned, to be sometimes pushed more posteriorly. Along its whole length
the sulcus is limited by two convolutions, the *anterior* and *posterior central*
[pre- and postcentral] convolutions (A.B.) Fig. 2 [fig. 102], which at both
ends of the sulcus run into one another in the form of a bow; that is, at the
medial edge of the hemisphere and on the upper edge of the fissure of
Sylvius. This forms a natural boundary between the frontal and parietal
lobes on the upper surface of the hemisphere, and I therefore count the
anterior central [precentral] convolution as belonging to the frontal lobe
and the posterior [postcentral] as part of the parietal.

Conclusion

Despite an increased interest in the cerebral surfaces, resulting from the rapidly
growing knowledge of cortical localization from 1870 onwards (Chapter X), and
the demand from surgeon and diagnostician for precise data, investigation of the
convolutions lagged behind the study of cortical histology. However, further extensive comparative studies have been carried out, techniques of measuring the total
cerebral surface area have been developed, and a number of theories explaining the
process of gyral formation have been put forward. Ariëns Kappers (Kappers, Huber,
and Crosby, 1936) whose work on the phylogeny of the gyri has been the most
outstanding, pointed out that deeper cerebral structures as well as the cortex must
be considered when investigating the gyri. "It must not be forgotten that higher
development is associated many times with an increase in the deeper parts of the
brain mass, and a more highly developed brain may have relatively fewer fissures or
sulci than the smaller brain of a lower mammal" (p. 1519). The complexity of the
problem, therefore, increases.

But no fundamental advance of importance has taken place since the intensive
period of study illustrated by our second group of selections. Too few measurements of cortical area and correlation with intelligence, for example, are available
to allow any precise conclusions. It seems possible, however, that individual convolutional irregularities may be as specific as fingerprints and that some relation
between morphology and function exists. On the other hand, the latter possibility
has been viewed cynically by some. Thus it has been suggested that sulci may be
related to functional areas in three ways: they may form the boundaries of an area,
they may cut through the middle of an area, or they may bear no special relation to
an area. It certainly seems clear that true functional regions rarely correspond to
anatomical boundaries.

In 1890 D. J. Cunningham, professor of anatomy and surgery at Trinity College,
Dublin, stated in an important paper on the formation of cerebral convolutions
that "the descriptive anatomy of the human cerebrum is now very nearly complete;
what still remains to be done is the establishment of our knowledge upon a proper
morphological basis." In the instances of the sulci and gyri this task is far from
completion.

CHAPTER VIII

THE MICROSCOPIC STRUCTURE
OF THE CEREBRAL CORTEX

Introduction

Although Piccolomini in 1586 had differentiated the cerebral cortex from the underlying white matter (pp. 387–388), little attention was paid to this distinction until the middle of the next century. At that time the early microscopists attempted to investigate the structure of the cortex but they were uniformly unsuccessful, except that they verified its intensely vascular nature that had already been advanced as an explanation for its gray color.

The history of the microscopic structure of the cerebral cortex, like that of the neuron, did not begin properly until the 1830's when the achromatic microscope was applied to the problem. Since then data has accumulated at an ever increasing rate, but so far only a small part of the problem has been solved, and decades, if not centuries, of work lie in the future. It is now known that the cortex is an incredibly complicated structure but that it has some useful landmarks. For example, there are six definable layers, from without inwards: molecular (10%), outer granular (9%), pyramidal (30%), inner granular (10%), ganglionic (20%), and fusiform (21%). Moreover, some cells, such as the motor cell of Betz, are characteristic. Likewise, it seems that a few cortical areas, probably about eight in number, are morphologically as well as functionally distinct.

The history of the microscopical investigation of the cerebral cortex can be conveniently considered in four chronological periods of advancement. The first includes the early crude attempts by the pioneer microscopists to probe its structure, and the much more accurate observations made with the achromatic microscope soon after its invention. The second contains the discovery of cortical layers, and the third the discovery of individual constituents of the cortex such as the Betz motor cell. The fourth and final period deals with attempts to reveal the functional arrangement of cells and fibres (cyto- and myeloarchitectonics, respectively); these efforts are still being made and no doubt there will be further periods of development.

Just as the following account will overlap that of the neuron, so there is also an overlapping of the next chapter that deals with cortical function. Secondary literature on the history of knowledge of the morphology of the cerebral cortex is limited, but there is an excellent collection of primary sources by Bonin (1960);

they deal, however, more with cortical localization than with structure. See also other books by Bonin (e.g., 1950) for historical information on the cerebral cortex.

Early Microscopy of the Cerebral Cortex

As soon as the microscope was widely accepted and relatively reliable models became available in the middle of the seventeenth century, the cortex of the cerebral hemispheres was examined. It seems certain, however, that none of the pioneers saw the nerve cell in the cortex despite the claims made in favor of, for example, Malpighi and Leeuwenhoek. As was the case with respect to early studies of nervous tissue elsewhere in the nervous system, no real advance was possible before the achromatic microscope was invented. Thereafter the cell was identified with certainty.

Nevertheless, representatives of the early workers in the field must be included in any survey of the history of knowledge of cortical histology because of the widespread influence they had on contemporary views of the form and function of the nervous system.

MARCELLO MALPIGHI
(10 March 1628—29 November 1694)

Malpighi may not have been the first to examine the cerebral cortex with a microscope but he was the first to record an account of what he saw. He was born at Cruvalcuore near Bologna and attended the Medical School of the latter city where he was graduated in 1653. Three years later he was appointed public lecturer in medicine in Bologna but in the same year was called to Pisa to lecture. In 1660 he returned to Bologna but from 1662 to 1666 taught at Messina in Sicily. Apart from his last years in Rome, as physician to the pope, he spent the rest of his life in Bologna where much of his famous work on the microscopy of animals and plants was carried out. He was one of the most outstanding biologists of the seventeenth century and his name is still applied to several histological structures. His discovery of the capillaries in 1661 was probably his greatest achievement (see Atti, 1847; Pizzoli, 1897; Foster, 1901, pp. 84–120; MacCallum, 1905; Cardini, 1927; Adelmann, 1966).

After having examined glandlike organs such as the liver, spleen, and kidneys, Malpighi turned his attention to the brain which he, like the Hippocratic Writer (*On glands*, 10, Littré [1839–1861], VIII, 564–565), considered to be a gland. It has been repeatedly stated that Malpighi described the cells of the cerebral cortex and the fibres of the white matter. It is possible that he saw the latter, but the structures that he called "minute glands" were not cells; Malpighi had misinterpreted the avascular areas outlined by the cortical network of blood vessels (Clarke and Bearn, 1968). He had only a crude microscope and used no staining or fixing techniques, and the fact that the "glands" were seen better in a boiled than in a fresh brain suggests that they were not histological structures. Moreover, in Malpighi's description it is never clear when he was using a microscope and when he was not.

The report of his examination of the cerebral cortex and white matter appeared in *De viscerum structura exercitatio anatomica* ([Bologna, 1666], "De cerebri cortice," pp. 50–70) and the following passage from Chapter I has been translated from it.

EXCERPT PP. 51–54

. . . . It should be recognized that [the cortex of the cerebrum] does not arise from concreted blood, but, as it appears to me, is like a special kind of parenchyma containing minute passages through which the collected watery part of the blood is strained out as through a sieve. I have been able to acquire further knowledge of this substance by repeated dissections and long investigation, but that very minute and indivisible structure, through the nature of which the greatest power is set in motion, yet evades me; nevertheless these things which are being revealed may extend a pathway towards the final problems, but they will not cause me to doubt what I have thus far said.

In the cerebrum of perfected [higher] sanguineous animals I have discovered that the spread-out cortex is formed from a mass of minute glands; these originate in the gyri of the brain and, extended like tiny intestines, end at the white roots of the nerves, or, if you prefer, they originate there. They are so exactly fitted to one another that their mass forms the surface of the brain. They have an oval shape which, however, is everywhere compressed by the adjacent glands so that certain obtuse angles are formed producing countless spaces of almost equal size. On the external surface they are covered by the pia mater and its blood vessels, which penetrate deeply into their substance. From the inner side extends a white "nervous" fibre with resemblance to a vessel, and which can be observed owing to the brilliant whiteness of these bodies; hence the white medullary substance of the cerebrum arises from connected bunches of many fibrils. If the nature of the cortex may be explained by a homely example, let it be the structure of the pomegranate, for in the symmetrical compaction of its seeds we have the appearance of the innumerable cerebral glands composing the cortex, and the fibres bursting forth from each seed and carried through the membrane have a rough resemblance to the cerebrum's medulla. I recall that I saw some unripe dates which, attached [to their stem] on one side and the other, resembled the cerebral glands, and the vessels or fibrous bodies to which they were individually attached, if bundled together, compared to the other [structure], the partly hard, medullary body.

These cerebral glands are observed only with difficulty in the raw brain, even in the large brain of perfected animals, because they are lacerated when the pia mater is pulled off; their shining whiteness makes it difficult to distinguish the coterminous borders, and their softness, the spaces among them. They appear more readily in the boiled brain, because their substance is thickened by boiling, and the spaces among them become more open, especially of the furrows on the sides; they become even more apparent when the pia mater has been pulled off, especially if they are examined while still warm. You will be able to distinguish these glands [from the spaces] if you pour ink over them and then wipe it away gently with a piece of cotton, because in this way the spaces are blackened so that the outlines of the glands are more easily discerned. Since these glands are to be found in all animals, you can easily see them in the cerebrum of fishes and fowl, although only when boiled. . . . These cortical glands in their complicated arrangement form the exterior gyri of the brain and are attached to the medullary fibres or little vessels originating from there, so that wherever the gyri are cut transversely a well-defined mass of glands is always observed spread over the medulla; it is to be seen even more clearly in the cerebellum.

ANTONY VAN LEEUWENHOEK
(*See p. 30*)

Another person who made a study of the cerebral cortex with a microscope was the famous Leeuwenhoek, who, like Malpighi, is said to have seen cortical cells, or "globules" as he called them. It seems certain that he did not identify the cell, however, and as already mentioned (p. 29), he was probably looking at fat cells or globules, or optical artifacts. Nevertheless, his observations, in common with those of Malpighi, influenced his contemporaries and his account of them has therefore been included here. It is contained in a letter written to the Royal Society of London from Delft on 25 July 1684 (*Opera omnia, seu arcana naturae* [Leiden, 1722], "De structura cerebri diversorum animalium: etc.," I, 29–41; it appeared in English as "An abstract of a letter of Mr. Anthony Leewenhoek, Fellow of the Society; concerning the parts of the brain of several animals . . ." *Phil. Trans. R. Soc.*, 1685, 15:883–895. The following is a translation of part of the complete letter as it appears in the *Opera omnia*.

EXCERPT PP. 30–32

In my examination of the turkey's brain I began with those parts that are usually called cortical. Except for various minute blood vessels and little globules, they are formed of very pellucid, crystalline and, as it appears to the observers, oily material that, because of its limpid and pellucid substance, deserves more correctly to be called the vitreous rather than the cortical substance of the brain. When I had separated this substance into very small particles I soon observed a slight, thin liquid or ichor issuing from it. It was composed of far smaller globules of which, in my judgment, not even thirty-six equalled the size of one globule of those making our blood red; although this trickle of liquid did not extend farther from the brain than perhaps $\frac{1}{10}$ part of the diameter of a hair, it was nevertheless mixed with the aforesaid globules. I observed this fluid material to be especially in the brain of turkeys that had been dead for some time. This experience taught me that part of this liquid issued from certain small vessels and, furthermore, that many of the small vessels had perhaps degenerated into watery material. In addition to those small globules there were some larger ones of which I judged six to equal one globule of our blood. Therefore I believed that these two kinds of small globules had flowed forth from minute vessels that I had injured, perhaps rupturing them, and that certain of them had been a thin, fluid material in the living animal, but rendered cold and immobile in the vessels, and in this way produced those globules as slightly thickened, coagulated parts of it. In addition, some clear and irregular globules were scattered through this, of which some equalled the size of one of our globules of blood, others were larger; through this clear material and globules very slender blood vessels were sprinkled in large number, and only in that quantity of the brain that would constitute not even one large-sized grain of sand. Many of these blood vessels were so minute that, insofar as it was possible to see with the eyes, if a single, oval, red blood cell of chickens and birds had been divided five hundred times, clearly not even so could one of those parts be contained in the hollow of these blood vessels. . . . I decided in this way that the dark color of the cortical part of the brain, by which it differs from the white part that is called the medullary part and is designated by a special name, takes its origin as follows: that first the larger part of it is formed of a substance of pellucid particles that are so closely attached together that they produce a vitreous or watery clearness, and then that this darkish color is produced by the transit of a great many minute blood vessels through it. I also observed throughout many very small particles that I judged to be globules and equal in size $\frac{1}{6}$ part of one of the globules coloring our blood.

These particles were not translucent and gave the brain a darkish color, and I suspected that they might have run forth from some blood vessels I had cut in the course of my dissection.

FREDERICK RUYSCH
(23 March 1638—22 February 1731)

The third seventeenth century account of the ultimate constituents of the cerebral cortex was that of Ruysch who used the technique of blood vessel injection.

Ruysch was born at The Hague and studied medicine at Leyden where he became interested in anatomy and botany and was not graduated until some years later, at Franeker in 1661. Four years later he took the chair of anatomy at Amsterdam where he carried out his renowned injection experiments and assembled a remarkable collection of specimens that are now in Leningrad. The details of his techniques, however, were never disclosed (see Portal, 1770–1773, III, 259–293; Hazen, 1939).

Ruysch concluded from his experiments that the cerebral cortex was made up of blood vessels only and he reported his results on 21 August 1699 when replying to a letter from M. E. Ettmüller of Leipzig (1673–1732), *Frederici Ruyschii responsio ad expertissimum virum Mich. Ernestum Ettmullerum . . . in epistolam ejus anatomicam problematicam de corticali cerebri substantia,* [etc.] (*Opera omnia anatomico-medico-chirurgica,* Vol. I [Amsterdam, 1737]). He was very proud of his discovery and commented upon it as follows: "Among all the discoveries that I have made within the last forty years, the following is the greatest, namely, the discovery that the cortical substance of the cerebrum is not glandular, as many anatomists have described and depicted it, nay, have positively asserted, but wholly vascular" (*Thesaurus anatomicus sextus* [Amsterdam, 1744], p. 8, in *Opera omnia,* Vol. III [1744]).

EXCERPT P. 18

Now that I have presented the opinions of the most famous anatomists regarding the cerebral cortex, it only remains to add my own opinion to theirs.

After I have injected the blood vessels with such skilled dexterity that the most minute branches have been filled and appear to us like bolsters [a mass of hair?], we clearly observe the cortical substance of the cerebrum to be formed from nothing but blood vessels combined in various ways . . . . while the very minute arteries extending from the internal surface of the pia mater take on the appearance of moss. So, too, I now declare, indeed, demonstrate, that the cortical substance of the cerebrum presents the appearance of moss and of a mass of hair [?], and that this appearance is, so to speak, nothing other than the protuberant extremities of little blood vessels. As it was also noted by me in regard to the spleen, so in their extremities these little blood vessels seem to take on another nature and disposition, for they become so delicate and moist that unless injected with a liquid, scarcely, and not even scarcely, can they be investigated without danger of their destruction. These moist, protuberant extremities of the blood vessels seem to compare to the fibres or medullary tracts of the cerebrum, and I believe they have the same function that authors ascribe to the glands.

Sometimes, for the sake of the curious, I have removed the whole cortical substance from the medulla without notable harm to the medullary substance.

Ruysch's opinion agreed in part with Leeuwenhoek's but throughout the rest of the seventeenth century and during most of the eighteenth, it rivaled that of Malpighi, and they were both repeated over and over again. There were no further observations of note during this period; Fontana (p. 37) described "globules" of the retina in 1781 (II, 213–221), but whether they were retinal nerve cells or optical artifacts cannot be determined.

CHRISTIAN GOTTFRIED EHRENBERG
(See p. 39)

One of the immediate results of the new approach to the cerebral cortex made possible by the achromatic microscope, was the report of Ehrenberg who, as well as describing the peripheral nerve fibre and the cell of the posterior root ganglion (pp. 41–42), gave the first accurate account of cells of the cerebral cortex. It appeared in the article published in 1833 and previously cited (p. 39). The following brief passages have been taken from it. His material was unfixed and unstained.

EXCERPT P. 451

. . . . The cortical substance of the cerebrum consists of a dense, very fine, vascular network which in many parts contains blood granules; its surface is covered by a layer of sinewy, tenuous fibres (called pia mater) interwoven with blood vessels. Apart from the very dense and delicate vascular network of the cortical substance I distinguish in it a very finely, granular, smooth mass in which here and there large granules (*Körner*) are deposited in the form of nests or layers. The larger granules are free but the very fine, smaller ones (*Körnchen*) appear connected in rows by delicate filaments wherever their smallness, softness, and transparency permits us to convince ourselves of these conditions.

EXCERPT PP. 456–457

Regarding the nerve endings, I am taking the liberty of drawing attention to what seems to me to be a not unimportant observation. I have already mentioned that, to begin with, I noted in the cortical substance of the brain, in addition to the vascular network and the delicate cerebral substance of the surface, an irregular layer of free, colorless, large globules (*Kügelchen*) which Leeuwenhoek perhaps differentiated [p. 32], but which have been ignored by more recent investigators. Completely identical, large granules (*Körner*) have long been known as constituents of the retina, and here, too, they are in connection with a very dense vascular network formed by the division of the [retinal] artery and the central [retinal] vein, while the retina itself is the free end of the optic nerve.

Ehrenberg then went on to suggest that the globules were a product of the blood, perhaps "excreted" red blood cell nuclei, which is reminiscent of Ruysch's conclusion (pp. 420–421).

GABRIEL GUSTAV VALENTIN
(*See p. 43*)

Another young microscopist of the 1830's was Valentin who, like Ehrenberg, was referred to in Chapter II. Working under much the same circumstances, without staining or fixing techniques, he made more detailed observations of the cortical cell. The following passage is from the publication of 1836 previously cited (p. 43), and fig. 5 should be referred to.

EXCERPT PP. 164–165

4. The globules [*Kugeln* = nerve cells] of the *covering mass* [*Belegungsmasse* = cortex] exhibit different shapes in different areas in each individual animal, as well as in various species of animals. Sometimes they are round or rounded, sometimes oblong, at times rounded at one side, terminating at the other side in a tail-like appendix [fig. 5]. They always consist of a granular parenchyma, the grayish-red, very small corpuscles of which are interwoven in a semisoft, viscous, transparent, connective substance akin to areolar tissue. In the center, or near to it, is a round or oblong

nucleus which consists of a boundary and a very clear interior. Corresponding to the center of this *nucleus*, yet close to its surface, is a single, round or oblong, solid corpuscle [nucleolus].

In the continuous covering formation [cortex], the external contour of the globule is always round in areas where it can be seen distinctly. Generally in the interstitial covering formations [junction with white matter?] it seems round only so long as the globule is not separated from the neighboring primary fibres. However, when isolated, it presents the shape just described. The more its shape approaches the oblong, or terminates in a tail-like end, the more and more obviously oblate the globule becomes. The parenchyma itself has long been described by investigators as the tissue of the grayish-red substance [cortex] *per se*. The large nucleus is more imbedded in the interior of the parenchyma. The corpuscle [nucleolus], which in its position corresponds to the center of the *nucleus*, is situated completely on the surface of the globule, and indeed, forms, as can be noted when it is examined, a kind of very small projection or hillock.

The Discovery of the Cortical Layers

The early microscopists had been able eventually to show that whereas the white matter of the cerebral hemispheres consisted of fibres only, the gray matter was made up of cells and fibres. They had not, however, become aware of any special arrangement of the latter. But, in fact, the presence of distinct cortical layers could be identified with the naked eye, and the first suggestion of them was made in the eighteenth century by Gennari, Vicq d'Azyr, and Soemmerring, who each detected a white line in the occipital cortex. Moreover, the first detailed observations on the lamination of the cortex were also made without the aid of the microscope by Baillarger in 1840. Thereafter the rapidly developing science of microscopy allowed increasingly precise investigations of the complex morphology of the cerebral cortex. In this respect the contributions of Gerlach (pp. 88–90), Golgi (pp. 90–96), and other neurohistologists who added to our knowledge of the neuron must be recognized here.

FRANCESCO GENNARI
(4 October 1752—4 December 1797)

The first indication that the cortex might not be uniform in structure and that it might manifest regional differences came from the work of Gennari, an Italian medical student. Not much is known of Gennari. He was born at Mataleto de Langhirano, near Parma, where he attended medical school and received a medical degree in 1776. He had already distinguished himself as an anatomist at this time, and he died at the early age of forty-five (see Fulton, 1937; Paoletti, 1963).

On 2 February 1776 Gennari sectioned a frozen human brain and with the naked eye noticed a white line in the cortex (*Lineola albidior*) which was more readily visible in the occipital region. This is known today as the line of Gennari, and it forms a reliable landmark for the area striata of the occipital cortex. He described it in a book, *De peculiari structura cerebri nonnullisque ejus morbis* (Parma, 1782), which seems to have been unknown to Vicq d'Azyr who mentioned the line in 1781 (1784, 1786, Planche IV, *ccc* legend on p. 5). The German anatomist S. T. Soemmerring also described it (1788, p. 70) but referred to Gennari.

The following passage is a new translation from Gennari's book of 1782.

EXCERPT PP. 72–75

A THIRD SUBSTANCE OF THE BRAIN. PAR. XLVI

I have found no anatomist who has taught that there is in the brain, in addition to the cortical and medullary substances, that other which I am accustomed to call the *third* substance of that organ. Especially when the brain has been dissected horizontally in layers, if one inspects the cortex where it is attached to the medullary substance [white matter], a whitish substance [*n*. Pl. III, fig. I, *hhhh*, and fig. II, *ddd* (fig. 105)], like a line, appears which is wholly unlike both the cortex and the medullary substance. However, it is not always to be found in exactly the same place since it appears sometimes very close to and sometimes more distant from the medullary substance; nor does it always have the same dimension and color, for sometimes it is wider and darker, sometimes it is narrower and a little brighter; in one instance it can be discerned with difficulty, in another not at all (because it is often formed of very fine parts), so that I have found [*n*. sometimes I have found this substance to be double, that is, two little lines (Pl. III, fig. I, **hhhhhh**). It is also found in the sheep, cat, hare, etc.] it to vary [*n*. it disappears with inept dissection, especially if oblique] not only in different brains but also in different parts of the same brain. I can recall finding it scarcely ever or only faintly in the anterior part of the brain, but it becomes more and more observable as it is carried to the posterior part. In the medial part of the posterior lobes of the brain, not far from that part which rests on the tentorium, is the place (and this should be especially noted) in which I have observed [*n*. very often on tracing this little line, it seemed to be carried to the innermost substance of the hippocampus] this substance of which I speak, collected into a small, very white *line*, extended very neatly but nowhere within the cortex [*n*. . . . I saw this little line for the first time on the 2 February 1776] itself. Just as the use of so many other things is as yet concealed from us, so I do not know the purpose for which this substance was created.

JULES GABRIEL FRANÇOIS BAILLARGER
(*26 March 1809—31 December 1890*)

In the 1830's interest in the structure of the cerebral cortex increased, partially owing to the stimulus from phrenology that had drawn attention to the cerebral surface as a possible functional area, and partially owing to the revelations of the new microscopists such as Ehrenberg and Valentin (Chapter II). This attention given to the cortex paralleled contemporary studies on the convolutions of the cerebrum (Chapter VII). Among medical scientists one of the few stalwart supporters of Gall's phrenology was the French psychiatrist Baillarger. He was the first to show that the cortex was made up of layers and that fibres connected it with the internal white matter.

Baillarger was born in Montbazan, Indre-et-Loire, France, and studied medicine in Paris where he received his degree in 1837. Having been influenced by the great psychiatrist Esquirol, he turned immediately to psychiatry, and in 1840 was appointed physician to the Salpêtrière where he worked for twenty years. He was especially interested in clinical psychiatry and made important contributions to the problems of hallucination and aphasia (p. 496), and to the classification of mental disorders (see Ritti, 1892; Semelaigne, 1930, I, 332–342; Fulton, 1951; Haymaker, 1953, pp. 10–13).

Occasional suggestions that the cortex was laminated had already been made, but Baillarger, in an unsuccessful attempt to correlate morphological variation with mental disease and intelligence, made the first important contribution. He examined thin sections of cerebral cortex by transmitted light and was able to identify the six alternately transparent and opaque layers recognized today (p. 423); he enumerated them from within outwards, the reverse of the present-day convention. Moreover, he traced the line of Gennari in the fourth or inner granular layer to all parts of the cortex; this extension is known today as "the external line of Baillarger" and Gennari's line is the part of this layer in the visual cortex. Deep to it was "the internal line of Baillarger" at the inner margin of the fifth layer.

Baillarger reported his results in 1840 ("Recherches sur la structure de la couche corticale des circonvolutions du cerveau," *Mém. Acad. roy. Méd. Paris*, 1840, 8:149–183) from which the following excerpts have been translated.

EXCERPT P. 150

The structure of this cortical layer which has received little attention, seems to me to be also worthy of some notice.

The first question which I shall examine is this:

Is the gray substance of the convolutions formed by only one or by several layers?

EXCERPT PP. 151–154

The researches which I have undertaken have made me recognize that the gray cortical substance of the convolutions of the brain is formed of *six layers*, arranged thus:

The first, from within outwards, is gray, the second white, the third gray, the fourth white, the fifth gray, and the sixth whitish (pl. 1, fig. 6, left half [fig. 106]).

These six layers, alternately gray and white, which remind one of the structure of a galvanic pile, can be seen with the naked eye in most places; but they can be demonstrated very clearly by the following method which is based upon the fact that the gray substance allows light to pass through it, whereas the white substance is opaque.

By a vertical cut I remove a very thin layer of gray cortical substance; I place it between two glass plates which I unite with wax to prevent all movement; I then expose it to the light of a lamp and examine it by that transmitted light.

If the layer of gray substance studied in this way is homogeneous and simple, it will allow light to pass through completely; if there are one or several white layers in its thickness, they will be recognized by their opacity.

Here is what I observed:

From within outwards six layers are counted.

The first is transparent, the second opaque, the third transparent, the fourth opaque, the fifth tranparent, and the sixth opaque or half-opaque (pl. 1, fig. 6, right half).

If one stops examining by transmitted light, one sees that the opaque layers (second, fourth, and sixth) are white, and that the other three (first, third, and fifth) are gray (pl. 1, fig. 6).

The cortical substance of the convolutions of the brain is thus formed of six layers, gray and white alternately, from within out; this, to recall the comparison of Vicq-d'Azyr, makes it resemble a gray ribbon with three white bands in it.

The procedure I have indicated not only serves to confirm in another way what can be demonstrated by simple inspection. There are cases where it is the only way of recognizing the structure of this part.

Thus, in the brains of young children, the gray substance of the convolutions appears completely homogeneous, even when examined with the magnifying glass. But if it is studied as I have indicated, one finds the six layers, the existence of which could not have been suspected, alternately transparent and opaque.

Without insisting on all the varieties which this organization of the cortical layer can present, I shall indicate, however, some which account for several past errors.

1° It frequently happens that the two intermediate white layers (second and fourth layers, pl. 1, fig. 6, left half) are very close to each other, so that the gray substance that separates them (third layer) is very thin or can be recognized only here and there; then the two white layers appear to form only one, which explains why M. Cazauvieilh has, as a matter of fact, seen only one (pl. 1, fig. 8).

2° Sometimes the two white layers are very close to the white cortical substance. The gray substance that separates them (first layer) has almost disappeared. This arrangement, which occurs only rarely, is frequently seen in conjunction with the preceding one. The first four layers thus seem to form only one thicker layer that constitutes the inner plane of the gray substance. When examined by transmitted light, vestiges of the first and third atrophied layers can be recognized frequently (pl. 1, fig. 9).

Consequently, it can be understood why Gennari and other authors have located the yellow substance [the line of Gennari: see pp. 424–425] between the central white matter and the cortex and not within the substance of the latter. I shall return to this point later.

3° The white line described by Vicq-d'Azyr [line of Gennari], which divides the gray substance of the posterior lobes, is very obvious and seems to be unique. With closer attention, one can be convinced that above or below [i.e., deep to] this very important white line, there is a second, very small and scarcely visible line; but if the area is examined by the transmitted light, it is easily recognized (pl. 1, fig. 10).

I shall remark that the gray matter of Ammon's horn is stratified as in the convolutions. This is additional evidence that this structure, as has been correctly stated, is nothing more than an internal convolution.

I have seen the six layers of the cortical gray matter in more than thirty brains taken at random and belonging to subjects of different ages who had died from a great variety of diseases. I have found them in the brains of the mammals I have been able to examine. I must therefore consider that their presence in the normal state is constant.

Another vital contribution to the history of the cerebral cortex was Baillarger's statement regarding the connections between gray and white matter. It had been postulated since the time of Malpighi that "ducts" of the white matter were connected with "glands" of the cortex, but Baillarger pointed out that white matter nerve fibres extended to the gray matter, thus suggesting that the latter had an important role to play in the nervous system.

EXCERPT PP. 154–155

On examining a very thin section of gray matter by the method already mentioned, one can readily recognize the existence of a great number of fibres penetrating from the central white matter into the cortical substance.

. . . .

. . . .

. . . .

In summary, the white matter, at the summit of the convolutions, is entirely united to the gray matter by a large number of fibres.

A simple juxtaposition of these two substances is thus inadmissible.

In the depths of the sulci, the fibres sent by the white matter into the cortex are so short and infrequent that in certain brains it is apparently possible to separate them without rupture; this is never possible at the summit of the convolutions.

ROBERT REMAK

(See p. 46)

Although Baillarger carried out his observations on cortical stratification with the naked eye, he was aware from reported microscopic studies that whereas the white matter of the cerebrum was made up of fibres, the cortex consisted also of cells. It was Remak (pp. 46–52), however, one of the most outstanding microscopists of the nervous system, who confirmed microscopically the cortical stratification of Baillarger. The following excerpt has been translated from his paper, "Anatomische Beobachtungen über das Gehirn, das Rückenmark und die Nervenwurzeln" (*Arch. Anat. Physiol.*, 1841, pp. 506–522). As elsewhere (p. 52), he referred to a possible connection between nerve cell and fibre, a conjecture as yet unproved.

EXCERPT PP. 509–511

As I have already described in the paper cited above [1839], the gray cortical substance of the cerebrum in adult mammals and adult man shows a stratified structure. First, a relatively thick layer of a gray or grayish-red substance follows the white cortical matter; then a whitish intermediate layer is succeeded by a thin layer of gray matter which, on account of its similarity to the gelatinous substance of the spinal cord, I have called *gelatinous substance* . . . . The gelatinous substance is followed by the central white matter. Thus the gray cortex consists of four *layers,* if one includes the white stratum, and is composed of *two white* and *two gray* ones that alternate with each other. In some of the gyri, and principally in those that are adjacent to the corpus callosum, one can readily recognize with the naked eye or with a magnifying glass an intermediate white layer internal to the first gray layer that lies below the white cortical layer; and following that one may distinguish between the gray cortex and the central white matter a total of *six* layers of different thickness alternating with one another.

With reference to the surface of the gyrus, the primary fibres which originate in the central white matter penetrate the gray cortex and proceed perpendicularly in a straight line through its different layers. The closer they approach the surface of the gyri, the smaller does their diameter become and the more they separate from one another, so that the elements of the gray matter lie between them. As already stated above, it seemed to me at times as if some of these fibres had become finer, that they were infiltrating all layers of the cortex in a straight line, and that they were passing into the primary fibres of the white cortical stratum at a curved angle. Most of the primary fibres disappear successively from view in all the cortical layers, and finally the remaining ones disappear in the most external cortical layer close to the surface of the gyri and very close to the white cortical layer, although I could not say with certainty whether they pass into the elements of the gray matter (ganglion cells and their processes). Hannover [p. 60] has already spoken in support of such a probability. However, because of my experience, I have become suspicious of the *direct* transition of the dark-edged primary fibres into the brain cells (ganglion corpuscles); it seems rather more probable to me that the dark primary fibres (*Primitivröhren*) extend into the long or short pale processes of the brain cells. This much is certain, that the primary fibres form neither ramifications nor loops in the gray cortex. The earlier reports in this connection by Valentin and myself were obviously owing to an insufficient number of preparations, and to investigations that lacked sufficient scope.

The primary fibres which radiate from the central white matter towards the surface of the gyri are *crossed* by primary fibres in their course through the layers of the gray cortex, and pass through it in a direction parallel to the surface of the gyri, and, with respect to their course, are evidently analogous to the primary fibres surrounding the gyri at their surface. These latter which, in contrast to those *radiating* from the central white matter, might be called *crossing fibres*, proceed so sparsely through the gray layers of the cortex that they escape observation almost entirely. They appear densely crowded together, however, in the white intermediate layers, and the whitish color of these areas in the gray cortex is based precisely on the fact that the bulk of the primary nerves which, as is well known, produces their white appearance in all portions of the nervous system, is fortified by the crossing fibres. By the way, with regard to the latter I have no proved observations to show whether they deviate in some parts from their course and mix with the radiating fibres in the direction of the surface of the center, or whether they, too, pass into the elements of the gray matter.

Remak's illustrations, published in 1844, were the first to depict the microscopic structure of the cerebral cortex, albeit very crudely. They appeared in "Neurologische Erläuterungen," *Arch. Anat. Physiol.*, 1844, pp. 463–472, and the following explanations have been translated from the text of this article.

EXCERPT P. 468

The sixth figure of the accompanying plate [fig. 107] illustrates a slightly enlarged cross section of the posterior lobe of the cerebrum of a sheep. It shows that the gray matter is composed of six layers, as I have indicated [pp. 428–429], and that a white layer is on the outermost surface (white cortical layer), followed by gray and white ones alternately.

The seventh figure is a schematic cross section of the same gray matter to exhibit its fibre contents, as far as I was able to establish it convincingly with my studies at that time. Thus it shows the gray matter permeated by fibres (crossing fibres) which take a course parallel to the surface of the convolution and which, owing to the fact that they lie closely together, produce the white color of the white cortical layer (*a*) as well as in both white intermediate layers (*c, e*). More spherical elements are found in the three gray layers (*b, d, f*). Those fibres that radiate from inside the brain (*g*) disappear slowly on their way to the outer gray layer (*b*), and I was unable to prove with certainty that the primitive tubes [nerve fibres] extend into the ganglion cell.

RUDOLPH ALBERT VON KOELLIKER
(*See p. 61*)

As in the instance of examination of the nerve cell and fibre elsewhere in the nervous system (see Chapter II), new experimental methods embodying the use of staining and fixation procedures were to lead to a more detailed and more precise knowledge of the cerebral cortex. Thus the renowned histologist Koelliker, using material fixed in chromic acid, was able to describe its constituent cells and fibres in much greater detail, and he made important contributions to the disposition in layers.

The following passage has been translated from his famous *Handbuch der Gewebelehre des Menschen* (Leipzig, 1852). In it Koelliker, like Remak, referred to the possible connection between nerve cell and fibre, which was a vital step in the establishment of the neuron theory (p. 62).

EXCERPT PP. 298–300

The finer structure of the *gray substance* of the convolutions is fairly clear (see my *Mikroskopische Anatomia* [Pt. I, Leipzig, 1850], Pl. IV, fig. 2). It is most conveniently divided into three layers, an external *white,* a *middle pure gray,* and an internal *yellowish-red.* The last, which is almost equal to the other two in thickness, usually has a clear, often white band in its outermost portion, and in it sometimes has a second, thinner and less white layer more internally so that there are four or even six consecutive layers: 1) yellowish-red layer, internal part, 2) first white band, 3) yellowish-red layer, external part, 4) second white band, 5) gray layer, 6) superficial white layer. The gray substance contains in its entire thickness both nerve cells and nerve fibres, and besides these a great deal of granular stroma, exactly like that of the cerebellum. The *nerve cells* are not easy to investigate, except in chromic acid preparations, and in all three layers they are alike in that by far the majority possess one to six processes which branch repeatedly and finally end in exceedingly fine pale fibrils of about 0.004′′′ [see p. 41] in diameter, which differ, however, as to size, number, etc. In the *superficial white* layer the cells are sparse and small (from 0.004–0.008′′′) with 1–2 processes, and they lie singly in abundant, finely granular ground substance. The *middle* or *pure gray* layer is the richest in cells which are gathered one against the other, also in a granular ground substance. Their size varies very considerably, some of them being very small, from 0.003–0.005′′′, and often appearing to be nearly all nucleus; but, on the other hand, many are found to be much larger, up to 0.016 and 0.02′′′ (Fig. 149 [fig. 108]). Their shape is pyriform or fusiform, with three or many angles, also perhaps more rounded, there being usually 1–6 processes in the vast majority of cells, but usually 3, 4, or 5. Where this is not the case, they may have been torn off during the preparation, for the mutilation of cells which are on the whole very fragile happens extremely easily. Finally, in the innermost *yellowish-red* layer the cells are again rather sparse, though still very abundant, otherwise being the same as those in the gray substance, and sometimes having pale and sometimes pigmented contents; the latter occur especially in the inner layers and in old persons.

It can be easily demonstrated that the *nerve tubes* [fibres] of the gray substance of the convolutions arise from the medullary [white] substance of the hemispheres and penetrate the yellowish-red layer, bundle after bundle, directly and all parallel with one another. Here a great many of the fibres detach themselves from each other and pass through the yellowish-red layer in all directions, but especially parallel to the surface and consequently cross the main bundles. When these fibres proceeding horizontally are more closely gathered together, they form the above-described whiter or clearer bands in this layer. The more external band lies exactly where the bundles which enter the gray substance are lost. As these proceed further towards the external surface they decrease in size all the time because they give off lateral fibres and because they become thinner and lose their elements, until when they reach the gray layer they are lost from sight; however, if they are followed more carefully, they can still be seen as intricately entwined fibrils which have hardly any signs of dark contours. There is a certain, though small, number of fibres, which do not lose their width and dark contours but continue through it in a straight or oblique course so that they can proceed horizontally further into the external white layer. In this layer is found a considerable number of finer, the finest and the finest of all fibres (Fig. 150 [fig. 109]) crossing one another in various directions, and they are in several layers one upon the other. Their origin is obviously traced to those arising from the grayish-red layer and are probably derived, as Remak assumes, at the base of the brain from the knee [anterior extremity] of the corpus callosum. How these fibres are related to the cells in the white layer is uncertain, although this much is certain, that many return into the grayish-red substance from which they originated, or in other words they form *loops* which Valentin described first and which I have noticed very frequently and distinctly in chromic acid preparations treated with sodium hydroxide. I have also seen in the gray-reddish substance isolated loops with limbs close together and with their convexities facing the surface of the brain. . . . Despite all my searches, I have not found a connection between the nerve cells and fibres in the cerebral cortex, but the presence of such a connection seems to be nowhere more likely than here where the nerve fibres, especially in the pure gray layer, look so much like processes of the cells in which, in fact, they end. There is here an immense number of nerve fibres which are so thin and pale that they could hardly be considered as such if they were not straighter than the processes and if they did not show delicate varicosities, especially when treated with sodium hydroxide. If anywhere in the central nervous system a source of nerve fibres exists, it is here, although when the fragility of the structures is realized, it would be quite understandable if this had not yet been observed.

THEODORE MEYNERT
(14 June 1833—31 May 1892)

After 1850 the field of neurohistology developed rapidly and many studies of the cerebral cortex were made. It then became clear that the types of cells and their arrangements varied in the many different cerebral regions. Rudolf Berlin of

Stuttgart, 1833–1897 (*Beitrag zur Structurlehre der Grosshirnwindungen,* Erlangen, 1858), was the first to suggest a classification into a few common varieties: pyramidal, small and irregular or granular, and spindle-shaped cells. This was the beginning of cytoarchitectonics, which attempts to subdivide the brain into regions of specific structure, although the subject did not receive close attention until the beginning of the twentieth century. But the work of one of Berlin's contemporaries, Meynert of Vienna, was of much greater importance. His contributions, made possible by better techniques and the advancing knowledge of the neuron, proved to be fundamental to all histological studies of the cerebral cortex that followed them. He provided the first detailed survey of the cerebral cortex.

Meynert was born in Dresden and studied medicine at Vienna where he was graduated in 1861. He spent all his professional life in Vienna and in 1873 was appointed professor *ordinarius* of nervous diseases. His career was typical of that of several nineteenth century alienists whose activities were divided between neuroanatomy and clinical psychiatry. In particular he studied the cerebral cortex and its connections and from his work on brain morphology which was an attempt to establish a scientific basis for psychiatry comparable to that of neurology, he was led to an anatomical classification of mental diseases which, however, has not survived. Meynert's influence was widespread and Flechsig, Wernicke, Forel, and Freud were indebted to him for inspiration. Like certain other investigators of the nervous system such as Sherrington and Henry Head, he was a tolerably good poet and he also possessed artistic propensities (see Anton, 1930; Haymaker, 1953, pp. 64–67; Kolle, 1956–1963, II, 96–105; Bonin, 1960, pp. xi–xii).

Meynert's first task was to study the cortical cells systematically. He concluded that there were five not six layers, for he combined Baillarger's second and third (p. 436); thus his fourth layer is the fifth of Baillarger and of most modern workers. But in the calcarine cortex of the occipital lobe he found eight. His results on many aspects of the cortex were published in a long, rambling article ("Der Bau der Gross-Hirnrinde und seine örtlichen Verschiedenheiten, nebst einem pathologisch-anatomischen Corollarium," *Vjschr. Psychiat.,* Vienna, 1867, 1:77–93, 198–217 and 1868, 2:88–113) in which the cortical layers were discussed on pp. 198–213; a more succinct account of the layers will be given later (p. 436). The following passage summarized the whole article. It referred to his observations on the variation of cell types in the cerebral cortex and to the possible association of cell morphology with function. His work thus elaborated that of Berlin and it was the first outstanding advance in cytoarchitectonics. With reference to Meynert's allusions to cortical function, it should be recalled that he wrote this paper (1867–1868) before cortical localization of function was established experimentally by Fritsch and Hitzig in 1870 (pp. 507–511). The description of the association fibres (*fibriae propriae*) or "radiations of Meynert" is likewise of great significance, and paragraph 9 alluded to the relations between the cortex and the basal ganglia.

EXCERPT PP. 111–113

1) Over the major portion of its surface the cortex includes three types of elements: 1. pyramids of graduated caliber, 2. small, irregular, and 3. spindle-shaped cells.

2) One cortical area (the uncinate convolution) consists of pyramids only. An extensive motor disturbance (epilepsy and epileptic-like convulsions) is followed by a constant disorder of it.

3) A cortical area, which is a direct site of origin of central elements (olfactory lobe), is distinguished by the accumulation of smaller, irregular cortical cells which are also found in the retina. There is yet another area of many-layered development of these components, the connections of which are unknown. (Eight-layer type.)

4) The spindle-shaped elements prove to be dependent, in regard to their form and stratification, upon the course of the fibrae propriae [arcuate fibres] of the individual convolutions.

5) A cortical area in the center of the cortical convexity is accompanied for the most part, by a flat, independent accumulation of spindle-shaped elements; the related white matter has an excessive abundance of fibrae propriae. This area is distinguished by a connection with the organs of higher senses, a function which presupposes the most elaborate combination of perceptions of different colors; speech joins this region, as is revealed by pathological processes.

6) A cortical area which demonstrates in the human the least developed function, is atrophied as far as its substance is concerned. (Olfactory lobe.)

7) The central organ of speech is a cortical area in which the function in the human reaches an incomparable level and in man attains the greatest dimension. (The insula.)

8) The special construction of the olfactory lobe is an example of the fact that peripheral variations are related to corresponding differences in the structure of the cortex.

9) Although on account of their continuity, elementary form and their union with the fibrae propriae of the cortex, the claustrum and amygdaloid nucleus prove to be a morphological entity, and, since the walls of the Sylvian fissure are similarly constructed, the comparative anatomic method demonstrated nevertheless that the claustrum pursues, in contrast to the amygdaloid nucleus, a completely independent degree of development. Since this variation in degree is related to variations in function, there must exist functional variations between similarly constructed cortical areas which can depend only on the variety of the peripheral connections.

10) Regarding the agreed lamination, presumably of motor and of sensory elements which fill such an extensive and major area of the cerebral cortex, one can hardly presume, with the foregoing in mind, that this area deserves everywhere the perfection of similar function; today it has become almost a postulate, owing to physiological psychology. Since the revelation that simple sensory perceptions include final impressions as long

as they possess, like tactile, visual, and acoustic ones, the character of spatial perception, we cannot but attribute their occurrence to the cerebral cortex.

However, as far as these conclusions are based upon perpetual relations of perceptive motions and sensory impressions, a continuous simultaneous occurrence of sensory and motor elements in the cerebral cortex is most probable. There is, therefore, a sameness in the stratification of all territories which serve spatial perception, regardless of what local variation in sensory modality to which it is connected might be. The time has come to extend the investigation of this train of thought, as soon as continued studies have further elucidated and outlined the diffusion of this agreed stratification.

On the basis of these studies, Meynert divided the brain into two parts, depending upon their cortical structure: the *neo-pallium*, also known as the *isocortex* of the Vogts (see pp. 453–456), the non-olfactory cortex or the *pallium* of *Koelliker*, where the outer layer was mainly gray matter: the *archipallium* also known as the *allo-cortex* of the Vogts, the olfactory cortex, or the *rhinencephalon* of Koelliker, where the outer cell layer was made up mainly of white fibres. In the article of 1867–1868 the following summary of this fundamental division appeared on page 111.

STRUCTURAL DIFFERENCES OF THE CEREBRAL CORTEX

Cortex with gray outer surface			Cortex with white outer surface		
5-layer type		8-layer type	Cortex with granule cells (Olfactory lobe)	Defective cortex, consisting of pyramidal and spindle-shaped cells (Septum pellucidum)	Defective cortex consisting of pyramidal cells (uncinate convolution and Ammon's horn)
Simple form (general type)	Combined form (owing to heaping up of the claustrum)	Lower cortical layer of the cuneus, upper cortical layer of the lingual gyrus, occipital pole			
The walls of the Sylvian fissure, the posterior orbital convolution in its lateral portion, the tip of the temporal lobe					

For Meynert the cerebral cortex was a complex center for all cerebral processes, because it was connected with other structures and parts of itself by means of projection, commissural, and association fibres (see Chapter X, p. 602). Sixteen years after the article of 1867–1868, he published *Psychiatrie: Klinik der Erkrankungen des Vordeshirns, [etc.]* (Pt. I, Vienna, 1884) which contains an excellent account of cortical lamination, of which a selection is presented below (also see

Meynert's chapter "Vom Gehirne der Säugethiere" in Stricker, 1869–1872, II, 703–710).

EXCERPT PP. 55–56

As I reported in 1867, the ganglion nerve cells of the gray matter form regular, concentric layers which vary according to their locality.

The most widely distributed type of cortical layer is, first of all, found in all convexity convolutions. In general, in a transverse section of the cortex they demonstrate to the naked eye a uniformly gray appearance that contains a washed-out, less pigmented area in the center of some of the widest parts of the cortex. With approximately one hundred magnifications transparent sections of these convolutions show five layers enumerated from the pia mater.

The 1st layer consists essentially of the ground substance and its connective tissue-like elements. The latter are collected mostly at the cortical surface. Small, irregularly angular cells are scattered in this layer. This is the neuroglia layer.

2nd. There follows a layer which is well demarcated externally by densely stratified small, apparently pyramidal-shaped bodies with their apices turned towards the cortical surface, and which measure approximately 10 μ in height. Internally, too, this layer has a rather sharply defined border which is not owing to a change in the size of the cortical elements but to the lesser density of their distribution. This is the layer of small pyramids.

3rd. In the next layer there begins a column-like arrangement of nerve cells which lie less close transversely owing to the accumulation of nerve bundles starting at the basal aspect of the small pyramids. In the course of increasing internally these insert themselves between groups of pyramids. The pyramids attain a height of 40 μ or even 60 μ, with increasing caliber, depending upon the width of the convolutions. In addition to the ramified process from the apex, the length of which may extend to the outer small pyramidal layers, and four to seven ramified lateral basal processes, one can recognize a middle basal process (Fig. 24, lowest row of layer 3 [fig. 110]) which proceeds in the opposite direction, parallel to the apex processes, towards the medullary substance. The nuclei of the pyramids appear for the most part as a smaller model of the pyramid in shape, extending frequently into the processes of the pyramid. This is the layer of the large pyramids, that is, the layer which contains them.

4th. There is an abrupt change of caliber between the third and fourth layer which is made up of small, multiform elements with predominantly spherical-angular shapes. This is the granular formation.

5th. Between this layer and the white matter of the convolution and not distinctly separated, is the large pyramidal layer, consisting near its outer margin of rather large although shorter pyramids. However, the more internally (towards the medulla) one goes, the more exclusively do transverse, spindle-shaped nerve cells of approximately 30 mm. length occur; because of exterior processes which proceed towards the granular layer, they may attain the appearance of vertically compressed pyramids. However, one never notes here anything like a middle basal process.

The white matter forms the sixth layer of these convolutions. It is much permeated by spindle-shaped cells which are equivalent to those of the fifth layer. The axis cylinder as well as the medullary sheath varies very much in caliber, from considerable fineness to the thickness of spinal cord fibres. The central fibres lack Schwann's sheath and Ranvier's nodes (Boll) characteristic of the medulla of peripheral nerves.

The white matter is infiltrated by granules (cubic cells, Boll) which, in their arrangement (in the adult brain, physiologically never continuously) imitate the course of the nerve fibres.

In the entire cortex we find only three kinds of corpuscles: 1, the pyramidal form; 2, the granular (mixed) form of small nerve cells; and 3, the spindle-shaped type. In the illustration (Fig. 24) the first formation is found in the second and third layers, the granules in the fourth, and the spindles in the fifth layer. In Fig. 25 [fig. 111], however, the pyramids are seen in the second layer, the granular elements in the second, fifth, and seventh layers, the spindle-shaped in the eighth layer. The pyramids and the spindles differ essentially from each other owing to their position. The elements of the pyramidal layer, which have their longitudinal axis parallel to each other, are vertical (actually radial) to the cortical surface. The longitudinal axis of the spindles, however, lies parallel to the cortical surface. In the entire central organ a morphological law is evident, enabling the formative activity to affect the direction of the nerve cells in such manner that this direction of their longitudinal axes is parallel to the course of the fibre system which originates from them.

The Discovery of Certain Individual Cortical Constituents

A variety of cellular elements had now been identified in the cerebral cortex and two important influences stimulated anatomists to examine them with even greater care. One was the widespread interest in the cell and the fibre, engendered by the controversy between those who on the one hand, like His, Forel, and Ramón y Cajal and their followers, believed in their independence, and those on the other, like Gerlach and Golgi and his school, who maintained that they were connected by means of a network of fibres; this was the famous neuron versus net dispute (pp. 87–183). The other influence was the attention then being given to the cerebral cortex as a functional structure (pp. 447–457). The discovery of the cortical motor cell and some of the findings of Ramón y Cajal typify for us this period of intense activity.

Vladimir Alexewitsch Betz
(1834—30 September 1894)

Despite Meynert's careful studies of the cerebral cortex, which involved a search for variation in cells and their arrangement, he appears to have overlooked one of the most characteristic cortical cells, the pyramidal or motor cell. This was the first nerve cell of the brain to receive individual attention, and it was the Russian anatomist Betz who, in 1874, gave the first adequate account of it.

Betz was born in Kiev where he attended medical school. He was appointed first as prosector in the University of Kiev and received the chair of anatomy in 1868 which he was to occupy for twenty-one years. He resigned this position to become principal physician to the southwestern Russian railway and appears not to have carried out any further anatomical research (see Benedikt, 1895, 1906, pp. 204–205, 255–256).

Betz discovered the cells that are now known by his name in Meynert's fourth cortical layer (i.e., next to the deepest) of the precentral gyrus of man, chimpanzee, and other primates and of the dog, and he reported his findings in a paper entitled "Anatomischer Nachweis zweier Gehirncentra" (*Zbl. med. Wiss.*, 1874, 12:578–580, 595–599. Unfortunately the inaccurate German text and numerous printing errors render parts of it obscure).

As the title indicates, Betz recognized two areas, motor and sensory: "Based upon the present findings, it may be asserted that there are 2 cerebral areas which may be designated as 2 centers, one motor and the other sensory [p. 598]." In a later paper ("Über die feinere Structur der Grosshirnrinde des Menschen," *Zbl. med. Wiss.*, 1881, 19:193–195, 209–213, 231–234), basing his conclusions upon observation of five thousand human brains, Betz discussed the cerebral cortex which he thought had five layers. Although the histological atlas he planned did not appear, it is said that his collection of preparations is still preserved in the University of Kiev (Petrov, 1954, p. 27). Betz must therefore be considered an important early pioneer of cortical cytoarchitectonics for, as he said (1874, p. 578), he "arranged [the material] in topographical order."

However, he is remembered mainly for the *Betz cells* and in the article of 1874 (p. 578) he first of all stated his intentions:

> . . . I set myself the problem of establishing criteria which might permit
> us to demonstrate the presence or absence of certain parts of the brain in

man and in animals, by assessing the quality and quantity of the histological elements of each gyrus.

Betz not only studied the morphology of the pyramidal cells but he also postulated their function by relating his findings to those of Fritsch and Hitzig who in 1870 had identified the motor area of the dog's brain (pp. 507–511). The following selection has been newly translated from the German.

EXCERPT PP. 578–580

The sulcus of Rolando divides the cerebral surface into two parts; an *anterior* in which the large pyramidal nerve cells predominate, and a *posterior*—including the temporal lobes—in which the cell layers are the same. This state of affairs applies to the orbital convolutions as well as to the medial surface of the hemisphere; in the latter the border of the above-mentioned partition is the anterior margin of the lobus quadratus [cuneus].

. . . .

Now, the area which we have designated as the *anterior* one, contains cell formations which, until now, have never been described. They appear in the above-mentioned sites and are the largest pyramidal nerve cells of the entire nervous system; I should like to call them "giant pyramids." They are predominately in the fourth cortical layer and are from 0.05–0.06 mm. wide, and from 0.04–0.12 mm. long. Each of them has two main processes, and 7 to 15 secondary protoplasmic processes [dendrites] which in turn branch out into smaller ones. At its origin, one of the main processes is thick, as is the case in the pyramidal cells of the cortex [?]. It then tapers as it proceeds to the periphery of the cortex and, in its course, gives off branches. The other process, however, is thin; it starts in the nucleus of the cell, and proceeds directly into the axis cylinder which becomes thicker after a short distance and acquires a nerve sheath; it thus undoubtedly continues as a nerve. The cells of this *anterior* cortical region do not form a continuous layer but rather are imbedded as nests of one, two, three, or more cells. These nests are from 0.3–0.7 mm. distant from each other. In such a nest one may find at times as many as five cells of different sizes and of the dimensions stated above. Furthermore, these cells are sparser in the lower half of the anterior central [precentral] convolution but more plentiful and closer together in its upper end and in the part on the medial surface of the hemisphere.

In young individuals and in an eleven-year-old brain I found fewer nests; the cells were smaller and also had fewer protoplasmic processes. In very old brains (seventy years old and slightly younger) these cells acquire a seemingly special nucleus which consists of yellow granules that are resistant to carmine dye. In children and young individuals these cells have a uniform protoplasm which can be evenly stained with carmine and in which no derangement can be shown. These cells are more numerous and apparently larger in the *right* hemisphere than in the left. In the above-designated places there exist in the white matter a countless number of thick axis cylinders which stain readily with carmine and are therefore distinct from the other thin, small nerve filaments which cannot be stained in this way. In their manner of stratification and thickness, these filaments resemble the axis cylinders of the anterior horn of the spinal cord.

These giant pyramids occur in the stated areas in every human brain, in the idiot, in the chimpanzee, in the gray, brown, small Persian Pavian, and in the green monkey.

Such consistency in the region where these cells can be found, manifested as a very definitive cortical layer, as well as in a specific cerebral convolution, prompted me to devote my attention to that particular part of the animal brain, mainly the *dog's*, in which Fritsch and Hitzig achieved such brilliant physiological results, i.e., the lobe which borders the cruciate sulcus [see pp. 507–511]. *I now found such cells of the same shape and in exactly the same position in nests in the dog, precisely in the lobe just mentioned.* So in the dog, as well as in man, they are imbedded in the fourth cortical layer and *occur only in this lobe and in the anterior half of the posterior* [postcentral] *convolution bordering it.* In the dog, they are somewhat smaller, but nevertheless are the largest in its entire nervous system. They also possess two large and many small processes, and the inner process runs into a genuine nerve filament. In the area where they are found there are also many axis cylinders visible in the white substance which run in the same direction as in the human. Undoubtedly these cells have all the attributes of the *so-called "motor cells"* and very definitely continue as cerebral nerve fibres.

WILLIAM BEVAN LEWIS
(21 May 1847—14 October 1929)

The existence of the giant pyramidal cells of the cerebral cortex was not widely accepted until the British psychiatrist Lewis verified the findings of Betz and added further morphological details.

Lewis, or Bevan Lewis and Bevan-Lewis, as he later called himself, was born at Cardigan in Wales and received his medical training at Guy's Hospital Medical School, London, where he was graduated in 1868. Thereafter he worked at the West Riding Lunatic Asylum as pathologist and assistant medical officer and carried out his researches on the cortex. He later became professor of psychiatry in the University of Leeds and director of the asylum there (see Lewis, 1929*a*, 1929*b*).

His first paper, written with Henry Clarke, medical officer to the West Riding Prison, appeared in 1878 ("The cortical lamination of the motor area of the brain," *Proc. R. Soc.*, 1878, 27:38–49). Like Betz, the authors recognized the five-layered cortex of Meynert and gave a detailed description of "the ganglionic cells of the fourth layer." These were the Betz cells first illustrated in this paper (fig. 113). They were thus the first to define a functional area on histological grounds and thereby opened the way for the study of precise cortical areas.

A few months later Lewis published another paper ("On the comparative structure of the cortex cerebri," *Brain*, 1878, 1:79–96) which extended the earlier observations in man and compared them to the motor area in the cat and to certain cortical regions in the sheep. The following passages have been taken from this latter article in which the account of the Betz cell is briefer than in the earlier publication.

EXCERPT P. 80

. . . . There is a five- and a six-laminated cortex, each typical of a certain definite area: but, whilst the six-layered formation is found extensively spread over the convolutions of the parietal and other regions, the *five-laminated* type is pre-eminently characteristic of the motor area of the brain. Another highly important feature of this region is the presence of large ganglionic cells which under the title of "giant cells" were made the subject of special attention by Professor Betz over three years ago. Our examinations tend to convince us that these cells have a motor significance, and that in their configuration, size, and distribution, they present us with a thoroughly unique formation. These great elements are constituents of the fourth cortical layer; and as the question with regard to lamination centres around the mid-regions of the cortex, this fourth layer will necessarily share the larger amount of our attention.

EXCERPT PP. 81–82

GANGLIONIC CELLS OF THE FOURTH LAYER

I. Form.—The pyramidal form is frequently seen, whilst a plump body elongated towards either pole, so as to approach somewhat the fusiform, is a very typical variety. On the other hand, the truly fusiform or bi-polar cell is rarely met with. The great irregularity in marginal conformation is attributable, in a great degree, to the extension of the protoplasm of the cell to some distance up the numerous branches. Each cell contains a large round or oval nucleus within which a nucleolus can always be demonstrated. These cells are peculiarly prone to pigmentation.

II. Size.—The measurement of a large number of these cells from a limited area on the ascending frontal gyrus gave an average length of 60 μ, an average diameter of 25 μ; the extremes being 30 μ and 96 μ for length, 12 μ and 45 μ for breadth. Taking a very large selection of cells from *various points* of this convolution, we found the average measurement to be 71 $\mu \times$ 35 μ. The largest cell met with measured 126 $\mu \times$ 55 μ. The dimensions of the nucleus were 13 $\mu \times$ 9 μ. (The *micromillimeter* [μ] = .001 of a millimeter.)

III. Processes.—The average number of secondary processes was seven, the largest number fifteen. Sections taken across the long axis of the cell exhibited the cell as the centre of an extensive area over which its branches spread, radiating outwards and downwards from all points of its margin. In these sections as many as eighteen branches might be detected occasionally. This being the mode of branching, it will be readily apparent that the absolute number of processes cannot be determined with any degree of certainty.

IV. Distribution.—The result of our examination on this point has been to demonstrate the very important fact that these ganglionic cells occupy certain *definite areas* remarkably constant in position; and it appears to us that these large *cell-groupings* are especially and exclusively a characteristic feature of the motor area, as defined by Ferrier [pp. 512–518]. The authors do not question the fact that ganglionic cells of smaller size are found distributed over the cortex at a distance from this region of the motor centres; but we have never found in these latter realms the *large groups* or *distinct areas* to which we now draw attention.

EXCERPT PP. 83–84

To recapitulate, we have presented to us a series of distinct groupings of these great cells, arranged chiefly along the *parietal aspect* of the ascending frontal convolution, interrupted by two groups which occupy the *frontal aspect* at the origin of the superior and middle frontals, and which at these points run into an extensive area, disposed over the posterior third of the two latter convolutions. The cells are largest in those groups found at the upper end of the ascending frontal, and diminish in size towards the lower extremity of this convolution, as shown by the following table:

	Average Size of Ganglion Cells	Largest Cell
Left Ascending Frontal (upper extremity) ...	60 $\mu \times$ 25 μ	90 $\mu \times$ 45 μ
Upper Frontal (area at posterior end)	45 $\mu \times$ 20 μ	69 $\mu \times$ 27 μ
Left Ascending Frontal (lower extremity) ...	35 $\mu \times$ 17 μ	41 $\mu \times$ 18 μ

Thus, throughout the region examined, these cells form an *interrupted series*, differing essentially from the continuous layers above them; and the groups thus formed are distributed over certain areas, closely corresponding to several of the motor centres of Ferrier. Each group is subdivided into numerous secondary clusters of from two to five cells—the "nests" of Betz. The all-important fact to bear in mind with regard to these elements is their *interrupted distribution*, a feature which is still maintained in districts where their diminution in size no longer warrants our calling them "Giant cells."

S. RAMÓN Y CAJAL
(*See p.* 109)

In the last quarter of the nineteenth century there were notable advances in neurohistology, occasioned chiefly by the introduction of more versatile and more reliable staining techniques. Thus, contributions to our knowledge of the constituents of the cerebral cortex were especially noteworthy, and the work of Meynert, Betz, Lewis, and many others in identifying the various cells and fibres was continued apace. But the most prominent investigator at this time was Ramón y Cajal (Conel, 1953).

Golgi's work on the cortex was also outstanding, for much of the evidence supporting his nerve net theory came from it (pp. 91–96), and his staining technique (pp. 842–845) was of vital importance as it was essential to apply to the cerebral cortex a stain that would delineate as much as possible of the cell and its processes. Ramón y Cajal employed it to outline the neuron with outstanding success, together with the methods of Nissl (p. 850) for cell bodies, of Weigert (p. 845) for myelinated fibres, and of others. Of his many discoveries, two were of special significance: the longitudinal cell and the afferent fibre.

His first important paper on the histology of the cerebral cortex appeared in 1891 ("Sur la structure de l'écorce cérébrale de quelques mammifères," *Cellule*, 1891, 7:123–176) and was a detailed study of the rat, mouse, rabbit, and guinea pig. In it he described for the first time the spindle-shaped longitudinal cell of the first, or molecular, cortical layer. This was later termed *Cajal's cell* by the Swedish anatomist Retzius, and it is a measure of Ramón y Cajal's sardonic humor that he referred to it in later years as "Cajal's cell of Retzius."

EXCERPT PP. 135–137

SPINDLE-SHAPED CELLS (FIG. 1, PL. I [FIG. 115])

These elements are slender, have a smooth contour and are enormously elongated. In the eight-day old rabbit in which they stain very well, they have a perfect spindle shape, they are horizontal, and they spread out in an anterior–posterior direction, a circumstance which means that we must study them in sections cut in the same plane.

The protoplasmic expansions [dendrites], two in number, leave the poles of the cells, and proceed in opposite directions; they are prolonged horizontally for a considerable distance, and it is because of this extreme length that one is rarely able to find them in sections of all the [cortical] elements. Finally, after a variable and almost rectilinear course, they turn at right angles and ascend almost to the surface of the cerebrum, where they seem to end freely (Fig. 1, *d*). During their horizontal course, these expansions give off small collateral, protoplasmic branches, which also appear to terminate in the most superficial part of the molecular layer. However, this ending has not always been seen quite distinctly because of irregular deposits of silver chromate which very frequently contaminate the external boundary of the molecular layer.

The axis cylinder issues neither from the body of the cell nor from the thickest part of the protoplasmic expansions; it is because of this that we were not able to distinguish it in our first preparations, which besides were incomplete. But continuing our observations with the help of more successful impregnations, we were astonished to see that the axis cylinder was double, sometimes triple, and that it issued from the protoplasmic branches, at a great distance from the cell body.

When the axis cylinder is double, which happens frequently, each neural expansion gives birth to its protoplasmic prolongations at the obtuse angle which these make so that they can ascend. (Fig. 1, *a*.) Then the expansions run in opposite and anterior–posterior directions traversing a considerable extent of the molecular layer; these are ordinarily prevented from pursuing their full course. A large number of ascending collaterals issue at right angles, or nearly so, from these axis cylinders which appear to end in varicose terminals, after having branched several times. These branches, which to us seem to end freely, always remain within the territory of the first zone, and they complicate considerably the structure of this cerebral layer.

Sometimes, in addition to these two axis cylinders which are anterior–posterior in direction and which we have just described, another can be seen to arise along the rectilinear course of the polar protoplasmic branches, like any secondary protoplasmic branch. These supernumerary axis cylinders most often ascend and behave like the main axis cylinders (Fig. 1, *b*).

The spindle-shaped cortical cells are not very numerous. We found six or seven in a half-centimeter long, anterior–posterior section of the cortex from an eight-day-old rabbit. We think, however, that they are more abundant, for the infrequency and difficulty of staining them must be taken into account. Very often the molecular layer gives no reaction because of an excess of hardening in the mixture; or it is contaminated with irregular precipitates; at other times only the neural fibrils are stained and it is impossible to determine their origin.

As far as one can rely upon it, preparations simply colored with carmine, with nigrosin, etc., reveal these elements with some clarity. They are, in fact, few in number, although in certain parts of the cortex they seem to be very numerous. Their spindle-shaped body is very pale and attracts neither carmine nor osmic acid; they are thrown into relief by a dark and granular background. The nucleus is elongated and lies in the axis of the cell (Fig. 4, *c*).

In the same paper of 1891, Ramón y Cajal described the afferent or exogenous fibre of the cerebral cortex and was thus able to account for the last important cortical element which remained unidentified; Koelliker called it *Ramón's fibre*.

EXCERPT PP. 148–150

6. FIBRES FROM THE WHITE MATTER WHICH ARBORIZE IN THE GRAY MATTER

All authors since Gerlach admit the ramification in the gray matter of sensory nerve fibres originating from other regions of the nervous system, perhaps from the sensory nerves. Golgi also supported this opinion; he supposes that the ramifications of these fibres, probably sensory, contribute to form the diffuse net of the gray matter. Other authors, such as Monakow for example, admit not only that some fibres ramify, coming from other divisions of the nervous system, and penetrate to the gray matter, but that all cerebral regions give rise to association fibres, and the brushlike ending of fibres of the same kind comes from other parts of the centers.

But the information from these authors is very vague; it seems that they have been led to admit the existence of these fibres more by theoretical induction than by direct anatomical observations. Golgi, who indubitably has seen them in the cerebellum as appears from his drawings, neither represents them nor describes them specially in the cerebral cortex; the general description that he gives of them, when considering the origin of nerves, makes it doubtful whether he has actually seen them in the cortex, or whether he has not mistaken them for the axis cylinders of incompletely stained pyramidal cells.

These doubts have been caused by the very great difficulty experienced in staining these fibres. We have never found it possible to impregnate adult brains when Gogi's three methods of impregnation are used. We had already despaired of ever being able to demonstrate their existence, when, recently, in the brain of an eight-day-old mouse, and in that of a newborn rabbit, they were revealed to our gaze with perfect clarity.

Let us say first of all that we possess a sufficiently safe criterion which allows us to recognize them. They are ordinarily the biggest fibres among those that cross the gray matter of the cerebral cortex; their thickness considerably surpasses that of the axis cylinders of the giant pyramidal cells; further, they are differentiated from the latter because their course is sometimes oblique, sometimes horizontal or zig-zag (Fig. 16, *a, b* [fig. 114]).

These fibres come from the white matter across which we have followed them for some distance. They bend to a right or obtuse angle in order to enter the cortex, and after a variable course, but which is almost always oblique, they divide into two or three large, divergent branches. These branches go off obliquely and proceed over a large area; then they branch many times and finally their finest rootlets end in diffuse, free, varicose arborizations, usually close to small or medium-sized pyramidal cells. All these fibres, and their main branches, possess a very thick myelin sheath. Because of the great thickness of the myelin, and above all because of their irregular course, now horizontal, now oblique, they can be distinguished from the axis cylinders of the pyramids, whose course, as may be said, is nearly straight and descending (radiating bundle of medullary fibres).

After having seen them in small mammals, it is not difficult to recognize them in sections of human convolutions, after staining with the Weigert-Pal method. In our opinion, all the extraordinarily large fibres with oblique or horizontal courses, which cross the gray matter in the middle and lower zones of the cortex are of this kind. It is easy to discover the complete encircling with myelin as well as the very long interannular segments.

The main elements of the cerebral cortex had now been identified, but Ramón y Cajal carried out many subsequent studies on them. His descriptions of the cortex are still the most authoritative accounts and are used by modern investigators. The fullest is to be found in *Histologie du système nerveux de l'homme et des vertébrés* (translated by L. Azoulay, Vol. II [Paris, 1911], 519–861). In his last publication he provided his final opinion, "Neuronismo o reticularismo?" *Archos. Neurobiol.,* 1933, 13:608. See also *Studies on the cerebral cortex* [limbic structures], translated by L. M. Kraft, London, 1955.

. . . . In all respects the problem of the connections between nerve elements of this layer [cerebral cortex] remains highly obscure. The large number of axons that arrive as frequently from the white matter as from the various cortical zones also contributes to it. Perhaps association and callosal fibres intermingle with them.

In summary, at this very moment the little we know about the kinds of neuro-neuronal connections in the cerebral cortex agrees in principle with the arrangement of the connections made in other parts of the brain.

The elucidation of the manner of connection between the innumerable endogenous, exogenous, collateral, and terminal branches originating in thalamic, callosal, and association fibres in every way constitutes at present an overwhelming problem. It will put to the test the sagacity and patience of many generations of future neurologists.

Cortical Architecture Related to Function

The labors of Ramón y Cajal and his followers in particular, and those of many other groups of neurohistologists made possible the next development in the study of the structure of the cerebral cortex. Towards the end of the nineteenth century two related lines of investigation, cortical histology and cortical localization (Chapter IX), converged, for it was only to be expected that a correlation between form and function should be attempted. The result was a new approach, a study of the architecture of cells, cytoarchitectonics, and of fibres, myeloarchitectonics, so that maps of the cerebral surfaces could be constructed to delineate areas of distinct morphology and function. However, the origins of cytoarchitectonics can be traced to the work of Berlin (p. 433) and Meynert (pp. 432–437), and to that of Betz (pp. 438–440) and Lewis (pp. 440–446) each of whom had deduced that the giant pyramidal cells, and therefore the specific cortical region containing them, were motor in function. Moreover, Flechsig's work (pp. 548–554) on the delineation of cortical areas from the study of the relative times of myelination of the developing white matter fibres, also supported this approach, and the Swede, Carl Hammarberg (1865–1893), for the first time indicated the precise histological differences between the motor and sensory areas of the cortex (*Studier öfver idiotiens klinik och patologi jämte undersökningar af hjärnbarkens normala anatomi*, Uppsala, 1893).

The investigation of cyto- and myeloarchitectonics began properly in 1903 when the three most important contributors, Campbell in England, and Brodmann and the Vogts in Germany, published preliminary accounts of their work. Unfortunately, many of the workers in this field considered the cortex to be a mosaic of discrete organs, reminiscent of the phrenologists' charts but based on histological and functional differentiation which, however, could not always be verified by others. Although this excessive parcellation is no longer acceptable, there is no doubt that the many inquiries carried out have provided extremely useful data concerning the human and animal cortex; it has been accumulated for the wrong reasons but is nonetheless valuable *per se*. The study of cortical architectonics proceeds today, and it is still a rewarding pursuit with the same objective of identifying areas specific both in form and function (see historical material in Campbell, 1905; Fulton, 1937; Lorente de Nó, 1949; Hassler, 1962).

ALFRED WALTER CAMPBELL

(18 January 1868—4 November 1937)

One of the earliest to take up the study of cytoarchitectonics was the Australian, Campbell. He made one of the first and most adequate comparative studies of the cytoarchitecture of the anthropoid cerebral cortex. His work was characterized by a strict adherence to facts and lacks the speculation that dilutes the data of the German cytoarchitectonists. The drawings that accompany his work are among the best ever produced, and they have been reproduced repeatedly.

Campbell was born near Harden in New South Wales, Australia, and studied medicine in Edinburgh. After having been graduated in 1889, he began to specialize in mental diseases and travelled widely in Europe. While occupying posts in clinical psychiatry and neuropathology in Liverpool, he came in contact with Sherrington who stimulated his interest in the cerebral cortex. After detailed study of that subject (1900–1903), Campbell returned to Australia in 1905 and spent the rest of his career in the clinical practice of psychiatry and neurology in Sydney (see Campbell, 1938; Fulton, 1938a, 1938b; Haymaker, 1953, pp. 16–18).

Campbell's classic book, *Histological studies on the localisation of cerebral function* (Cambridge, 1905), is based upon a detailed examination of human and anthropoid brains; the latter had been used by Grünbaum and Sherrington in their localization experiments (pp. 518–523). However, Campbell's first paper on the subject was in the form of an abstract of a communication read to the Royal Society on 3 December 1903 ("Histological studies on cerebral localisation," *Proc. R. Soc.*, 1903, 72:488–492). His essential aim was "to further the establishment of a correlation between physiological function and histological structure" [p. 488], and he dealt with the central gyri, the occipital, temporal, and limbic lobes from human and anthropoid ape material. He recognized twenty regions in the human brain and described the cellular (cytoarchitectonic) and the fibre (myeloarchitectonic) structure of each.

EXCERPT PP. 488–490

III.—THE PRE-CENTRAL OR MOTOR AREA

The pre-central or motor type of cortex is confined—roughly speaking— to the pre-central or ascending frontal convolution and a small coterminous portion of the paracentral lobule, its distinctive histological characters are a wealth of nerve fibres far superior to that of any other part of the cerebral cortex, and the presence of the "giant cells" of Betz or "ganglionic cells" of

Bevan Lewis. It is important to notice that its structure differs absolutely from that of the post-central or ascending parietal gyrus.

On examining the brains of two chimpanzees and one orang it was found that a similar area could be mapped out, not only agreeing closely in point of structure and distribution with that in the human brain, but coinciding absolutely with the field which Sherrington and Grünbaum [pp. 518–523] have recently found responsive to unipolar faradization in the same animals.

. . . .

. . . .

. . . .

IV.—POST-CENTRAL AND INTERMEDIATE POST-CENTRAL AREAS

This area is readily defined in both man and the man-like ape, and is limited in its distribution to the post-central or ascending parietal gyrus and its paracentral annexe, the floor of the fissure of Rolando forming a definite anterior boundary.

Since its cortical structure differs markedly from that of the motor area, and at the same time exhibits features common to known sensory areas (the visual and auditory), its supposed motor function is denied, and it is maintained on the following additional grounds that it constitutes the terminus where fibres conveying common sensory impressions primarily impinge. Physiologically it is "silent" under the influence of electrical excitation, and also partial ablations give rise to no interference with movement (Sherrington and Grünbaum [pp. 520–521]). Its fibres, like those of sensory spinal tracts, myelinate early (Flechsig and Vogt). It is the terminus for the "cortical lemniscus" (Tschermak). Personal observations in three cases of Tabes Dorsalis, a disease affecting the sensory system of neurones essentially, have disclosed profound cortical alterations concentrated in this area. Similar observations in cases of amputation of an extremity have revealed changes situated on a corresponding surface level with those noted in the pre-central or motor area.

It is suggested that confusion concerning the function of the central gyri has arisen in the past, from the fact that the tracts of fibres pertaining to these gyri run in such close association below the Rolandic floor, that a lesion affecting the conduction chain of one gyrus is rarely free from the damaging influence of involvement of the other.

Intermediate Post-central Area.—This is a skirting zone in which the structural type is intermediate between that of the post-central area and the remaining parietal gyri.

It may serve for the transmutation and further elaboration of impressions primarily received in the post-central area.

KORBINIAN BRODMANN

(17 November 1868—22 August 1918)

The name of Brodmann is remembered today in association with a map he published in 1907 of the fifty-two cerebral cortical areas that he differentiated ("Beiträge zur histologischen Lokalisation der Grosshirnrinde. VI. Mitteilung: Die Cortexgliederung des Menschen," *J. Psychol. Neurol., Lpz.*, 1908, 10:231–246, see p. 236 [fig. 116]). He was a pupil of the Vogts and was specially charged with the investigation of cortical cell architecture.

Brodmann was born in Liggersdorf, Hohenzollern, and studied medicine in Munich, Würzburg, Berlin, and Freiburg im Breisgau. He received a medical licence in 1895 at Freiburg and in the following year met Oskar Vogt (p. 453). Thereafter he devoted his life to the study of the nervous system and eventually joined Vogt in Berlin in 1901 at the Neurobiological Institute. During the next nine years he studied the architectonics of the brain but in 1910 moved to Tübingen. He died soon after joining Kraeplin, Nissl, and Spielmeyer in Munich (see Haymaker, 1953, pp. 13–16; Kolle, 1956–1963, II, 38–44; Bogaert, 1961).

Brodmann's contribution to the comparative histology of the cerebral cortex was immense because the field, when he first entered it, was very confused. He selected the comparative approach for the task of subdividing the cortex, and from his work stems the comparative mammalian cytoarchitectonics of today. His concept of an increasing differentiation during evolution seems to have been amply confirmed. He also investigated the myeloarchitecture of the cortex and eventually was able to divide the entire cortical surface into fifty-two areas which he grouped into eleven regions, or principal fields. The numbers he gave to the areas are still used, but it is impossible to discover how Brodmann established the subdivisions in man as he gave no detailed account of them in the human brain.

Nevertheless, his work on the monkey brain stood practically unchallenged until recently when considerable confirmation derived by modern techniques was reported (Bonin and Bailey, 1947). Admittedly Brodmann's results "have been accepted by physiologists as of divine authority and a vast superstructure has been built on this shaky foundation" (Bailey and Bonin, 1951, p. 192), but this does not necessarily detract from the acceptability of many of them. Furthermore, Brodmann's pioneer work proved to be an important stimulus to others.

As was so with Campbell and the Vogts, Brodmann's first important paper appeared in 1903 ("Beiträge zur histologischen Lokalisation der Grosshirnrinde. I. Mitteilung: Die Regio rolandica," *J. Psychol. Neurol., Lpz.*, 1903, 2:79–107; see also "II. Mitteilung: Der Calcarinatypus," *ibid.*, pp. 133–159); however, the following passages have been translated from his famous book, *Vergleichende Lokalisationslehre der Grosshirnrinde in ihren Prinzipien dargestellt auf Grund des Zellenbaues* (Leipzig, 1909).

His aims he stated thus: "Although my localizing studies stemmed from a purely anatomical point of view and I wished only to attempt the solution of anatomical questions; the objective from the beginning was the advancement of knowledge of function and of pathological manifestations [p. 285]." Reference should therefore be made to selections from this book that deal with cortical function (pp. 447–457). Brodmann tackled his anatomical investigations in systematic fashion.

EXCERPT P. 10

Accordingly, our subject is divided into two main parts:

(1) the investigation of the cell layers of cortical sections and their modifications in the mammalian series—*comparative corticoarchitectonics* (*Cortextektonik*).

(2) The arrangement of the surfaces of the hemispheres in various mammals in fields on the basis of cytoarchitectonic differences—*comparative and topographical localization of the cerebral cortex*.

In Chapter IV of the same book, Brodmann dealt with brain maps, first dividing the cerebral cortex into eleven main histological regions.

EXCERPT PP. 127–129

In contrast to a description of the cortical fields according to lobes and gyri as reported in earlier communications, we shall, in the following, divide the surface of the hemispheres of various animals into large, structurally uniform main zones; these coincide only partially with the morphological formations of earlier nomenclature, the lobes, lobules, and gyri, each of which comprises a number of tectonically related areas. The reasons for this are related to comparative anatomy and are based upon the following reflection. One may very well classify the hemispheres in man and in those animals with gyri which are closely related to him, by morphology and roughly according to homologous lobes. However, what corresponds in lower orders, for instance in small rodents and insect eaters, to the frontal or the temporal lobe of primates is utterly impossible to identify by external inspection. It is, however, possible to identify histological structures, and a whole series of zones with identical or homologous structure can be demonstrated in all mammals.

Therefore, we designate large areas of similar structure as uniform, structural zones, so-called "principal regions" (*regiones*) and contrast these with the individual areas (*areae*). Consequently, in the future we no longer differentiate only among the regions of the frontal lobe, the temporal lobe, the occipital lobe, etc., but as a starting point take principal regions in which the individual areas are distributed according to their histological individuality.

One can distinguish such homologous regions in large numbers everywhere in the human and in other mammals. They are: 1. Postcentral, 2.

Precentral, 3. Frontal, 4. Insular, 5. Parietal, 6. Temporal, 7. Occipital, 8. Cingulate, 9. Retrosplenial, 10. Hippocampal, 11. Olfactory regions. Some of these principal regions are markedly developed in higher animals and exhibit a clear segmentation into individual areas, but in the lower orders they are simple in structure; other regions present the reverse situation for they are specifically more abundantly divided up in lower and more primitive species than in the more highly organized animals. Certain zones, such as the olfactory region, are very much reduced in size and developed only rudimentarily in individual groups so that they could not be included at all in the cerebral map, whereas in other classes, particularly in the large ones, they occupy a considerable part of the whole cerebral surface.

. . . . As can be seen, they [the main regions] coincide only partially with the regions in the customary arrangement; we should like to emphasize above all that the morphologically uniform *"Rolandic region"* is broken down into two separate main zones, the precentral and postcentral region, each of which in turn comprises several areas. In addition, and in order to forestall erroneous interpretation, we must stress again that not all of these principal zones are distinguished from each other by sharp lines of demarcation, but in part flow into one another, as for example the parietal and temporal region.

Having delineated the main regions, Brodmann next outlined the fifty-two areas of which they were composed. The following is an account of area 4, known today as this, and also as the motor or precentral area. Apart from the pre- and postcentral areas and possibly the calcarine cortex, recent workers have not confirmed the sharp limits which Brodmann thought existed between regions (see, for example, Penfield and Boldrey, 1937).

EXCERPT P. 134

*Field Four—Area gigantopyramidalis—*is one of the most distinctly differentiated and also cytoarchitectonically the most significantly outlined structural areas of the entire human cerebral cortex.

It comprises a circumscribed cortical region which narrows inferiorly like a wedge along the central sulcus and lies exclusively upon the central gyrus anteriorly and the adjacent part of the paracentral lobule (approximately its median third). Medially, it covers approximately the middle third of the paracentral lobule. Laterally it occupies the entire width of the anterior [pre-] central convolution next to the edge where any two surfaces of the cerebral hemispheres are in contact. It sometimes transgresses upon the base of the first frontal convolution and ventrally it soon confines itself to the posterior half of this gyrus. From approximately the middle of the central sulcus it narrows increasingly (individual variations) and withdraws completely into the deep cortex, that is the caudal lip of the central gyrus, at which point the sharp demarcation rather far above the lower end of the central fissure ends in and fuses with Field 6.

EXCERPT PP. 135–136

As has been known since Lewis and Clarke [p. 440], no insignificant localized differences, apart from individual variations, occur within the zone thus circumscribed in respect to number, size, and distribution of the giant pyramids. Lewis and Clarke wished to attribute corresponding col-umn-like collections of these cells to the physiological centers for leg, trunk, arm, and face, but later their reports did not meet with universal confirma-tion and also required a review by physiological experiment. It can be considered completely settled *that in general the size and number of the Betz giant cells decrease from the top to the bottom, that is, laterally from the paracentral lobule, and that the dense cell nests also gradually disappear towards the ventral end of the central sulcus to allow a more isolated arrangement of these cells. In addition, it must be noted that the distribu-tion of the giant pyramids in the upper third of the zone is also predomi-nantly cumulative on the convexity of the convolution, whereas ventrally they become almost exclusively solitary, with respect to the layer. On the whole, the cortical thickness likewise becomes less ventrally. However, despite the regional differences just mentioned, the cytoarchitecture pre-sents no adequate criteria.*

OSKAR VOGT   CÉCILE VOGT
(6 April 1870—31 July 1959)   (27 March 1875—3 May 1962)

Brodmann's work on the cytoarchitectonics of the cerebral cortex had been inspired by Oskar and Cécile Vogt whose investigations of the correlation between cortical patterns, expressed in terms of cell and fibre morphology and of function, were more extensive than those of any other workers in the field.

Oskar Vogt was born in Husum, Schleswig, and studied at Kiel and Jena. His interest immediately turned to the anatomy of the nervous system and to psychia-try, which he studied under Binswanger, Forel (p. 104), and Flechsig (p. 277). In Paris he worked with Dejerine from 1896 to 1898, and there met Cécile Mugnier who was born in Annécy, in the province of Savoy, and studied medicine in Paris. They were married in 1899 and worked together for the remainder of their active lives; as their relative contributions are inseparable, the term "the Vogts" refers either to his or to her work. They established a laboratory, the Neurobiological Institute, in Berlin, eventually taken over by the University, and they practised neurology and psychiatry to finance it, carrying out their anatomical researches as well. In 1931 the Kaiser Wilhelm Institute for Investigation of the Brain was built for them in Buch, a suburb of Berlin, but six years later they moved to a privately endowed brain research institute near Neustadt in southern Germany where they worked together until Oskar Vogt's death (see Haymaker, 1951; Kolle, 1956–1963, II, 45–64; Bruetsch, 1960; Hopf, 1962; Freund and Berg, 1963–1964, II, 435–443).

Oskar and Cécile Vogt first of all studied the cerebral myelinated fibres (myeloarchitecture) and then their relationships to the cortical nerve cells, the study of which they had delegated to their pupil Brodmann. At the same time they mapped physiological areas in the monkey's cortex and, like Brodmann, correlated these with structure and used his subdivisions (pp. 450–453). They believed that physiological differences would be reflected in structure and that the interplay between the two hundred or so functional areas which they eventually isolated represented human intellect and behavior.

Despite their extensive contributions to knowledge of the cerebral cortex, the teaching of the Vogts on this subject has had little influence on neurological thought. Their contention that every recognizable difference in cortical structure represented a functional differentiation has been accepted by few and their method of delineating areas structurally could rarely be repeated by others.

As with Campbell (pp. 448–449) and Brodmann (pp. 451–453), their first important observation on the cortical organization was in 1903 ("Zur anatomischen Gliederung des Cortex cerebri," *J. Psychol. Neurol.*, 1903, 2:160–180), and in this paper Oskar Vogt outlined some of their basic aims. The importance they attached to thalamocortical connections has been justified by recent research. Although their minute parcellation of the cortex is no longer accepted, their contribution to our knowledge of cortical histology and function must at least be acknowledged.

EXCERPT PP. 179–180

The trend of ideas which has been discussed in the foregoing, and the preliminary results, especially of our cytoarchitectonic investigations, are those upon the basis of which a refinement of the anatomical organization of the cerebral cortex must appear desirable. At the same time it becomes sufficiently evident from our exposition which path will lead us to this goal. *Structural peculiarities, that is systems of fibres and architectonic features, must be criteria for the separation of cortical territories.* Might such peculiarities be soon determined so systematically that in the foreseeable future a corresponding cortical organization could become possible?

What can we do in this direction, first with the help of investigations of fibre systems? An (elementary) fibre system, according to our definition, is the sum of all those nerve fibres that one nerve center sends to another. From this it follows that, from the standpoint of a fibre system, we shall be able to differentiate more cortical centers, the more special subcortical centers connected with the cerebrum can be distinguished. Therefore the exploration of the subcortical centers will have an effect upon the cortical organization. This is particularly true for the thalamencephalon. The more areas we can distinguish here, the more cortical fields will be separated. Now, C. Vogt and I shall soon show in our neurobiological studies that the simple investigation of the medullary fibres of the young thalamencephalon leads to the differentiation of numerous centers. Their number will certainly increase when the findings in the young brain are supplemented by the study of secondary degenerations and by architectonics. Then, the fibre system principle of division of the cortex will also yield excellent results.

In this respect it is certain that the systematic anatomy of fibres must still make considerable progress before it can contribute to a more precise delineation of cortical fields. However, if others continue to work diligently and we ourselves succeed in carrying through the program that we have outlined in our introductory neurobiological reports, such results will not be wanting.

The preceding expositions have shown several instructive examples for the functional capacity of the *cytoarchitectonic* principle of division. After we have succeeded in overcoming certain initial technical difficulties, we shall then apply this principle extensively. For our part, we shall do so. At the same time, other investigators, too, are working assiduously in this direction.

No greater difficulties confront *myeloarchitectonic* studies than confront cytoarchitectonic ones. In this area, too, other workers apart from us hope to report soon facts that lead to the promotion of a structural organization of the cortex [e.g., Brodmann, pp. 451–453].

Of course, along with this, all these three principles of division should go hand in hand, furthering and complementing one another.

If this happens, the anatomical exploration of the brain will, in our opinion, soon pave the way for organization of the cortex, which promises to permit urgently needed elucidations for the establishment of analogies, for the anatomical recognition of special physiological fields, and lastly for conclusions relating to localization from individual peculiarities or perhaps also from genetic stages of development.

In all complex problems in the solution of which various subdisciplines participate, there are alternate periods during which cultivation by one or the other subdiscipline is particularly suited to explain this problem. Such a period appears to us to exist at the present time for the anatomy of the brain regarding the important question of localization in the cerebral cortex. This is our guiding thought.

Sixteen years after their first publication of 1903 the Vogts reported on the results of their work on the myelo- and cytoarchitectonics of the cerebral cortex ("Allgemeinere Ergebnisse unserer Hirnforschung," *J. Psychol. Neurol.*, 1919, 25:273–462). The following is from their concluding remarks.

EXCERPT PP. 455–456

All that remains to be discussed is what general scientific importance for the architectonic division of cortical fields must be derived from all our investigations to date.

1. According to our earlier reports, the cerebral cortex demonstrates a *laminar* and an *areal* disintegration. Under these circumstances the question might arise, whether we had based the presentation of cortical architectonics upon stratification or upon division into fields. One might consider taking up the individual main layers one by one and describing correlatively the topical variation of each layer. With reference to this, we must first note that the homology of the principal layers of the isocortex with those of the allocortex [terms introduced by the Vogts to differentiate the non-olfactory from the olfactory cortex, respectively] encounters difficulties which for the time being are insurmountable. Therefore, the architectonics of the allocortex would have to be omitted from such a presentation. In addition, we would lack any means for the exact localization of that cortical area where a layer manifests a definite variation, since the topographical orientation according to the sulci—as we have seen above—is completely unreliable. *The only sure topography is provided by architectonic differentiation* . . . . Thus it seems a matter of urgency *to bring the organization of the cortex into line with architectonic description.*

2. Originally we proceeded from fibre-system studies. These required a definition of the elementary fibre system, and we found this in the "entity of all those nerve fibres that transmitted from one nerve center to another." This definition presupposed the knowledge of nerve centers. However, these were unknown to us at the time. We looked for them and today we believe—as far as the cerebrum and the subcortical cerebral parts are concerned—that we have discovered them in the architectonic cortical fields and the architectonic nuclei of the subcortical gray masses.

Our architectonic cortical fields show partly qualitative, partly only somatotopic differences. Our entire knowledge of the gray of the central nervous system points everywhere to a division into somatotopic areas. This is not only true for the cerebrum and the spinal cord, but also for the cerebellum, the thalamus, and the striatum. As far as somatotopical differences occur in the architecture of the cerebral cortex, they may be considered without hesitation as the fibre-system centers for which we were looking. But also where architectonic areas are qualitatively different—differences in their connection with conductors outside the gray matter must be assumed *a priori*—perhaps only quantitatively—so that we must also recognize special, fibre-system centers in such areas, even if perhaps at first field complexes must be made the starting point for fibre-system studies.

Now, these conclusions have been completely confirmed by our experiments to date.

Conclusion

Extensive studies of cyto- and myeloarchitectonics continued under the influence of Brodmann, the Vogts, and others. Thus C. von Economo and G. N. Koskinas produced a monumental work on cortical areas (*Die Cytoarchitektonik der Hirnrinde des erwachsenen Menschen*, Vienna, 1925), based on the work of Brodmann but identifying more than twice his number of areas; it helped to dispel some of the confusion produced by the Vogts' multiplicity of areas. O. Foerster ("Motorische Felder und Bahnen," in Bumke and Foerster, *Handbuch der Neurologie* [Berlin, 1936], VI, 1–357) attempted to correlate the Vogts' areas in the human brain with motor response to strong electrical stimulation.

Unfortunately, too much emphasis has been laid upon anatomical data, and that concerning function lags behind owing in part to a lack of techniques for its investigation. Furthermore, although cytoarchitectonic studies have provided the physiologist with important information, they have also deceived him into believing that precisely limited areas could be defined and that a mosaic of cortical "organs" comparable to those of the phrenologists might be identified. The most outstanding attack on cytoarchitectonics was that of K. S. Lashley and G. Clark ("The cytoarchitecture of the cerebral cortex of Ateles: a critical examination of architectonic studies," *J. comp. Neurol.*, 1946, 85:223–305) which proved its unreliability but at the same time concluded that "many localized structural differences are a product of developmental variations unrelated to the ultimate functions of the areas. Marked local variations in cell size and density among individuals of the same species may constitute a basis for individual differences in behavior" (p. 300).

It seems certain, however, that a knowledge of morphology must be supplemented with further data, such as electrical and chemical, before an adequate interpretation of cortical form and function can be made.

CHAPTER IX

BRAIN LOCALIZATION

Introduction

The most important development in the history of brain physiology came about when attempts were made to show that the brain, rather than being an amorphous, functionless mass as was demanded by Aristotle's cold-sponge concept (pp. 9–10), was comprised of many parts, each of which had a specific function. The gradual realization that the cerebral cortex, for example, had detectable morphological differences, both macroscopical and microscopical, as illustrated in Chapters VII and VIII, naturally suggested that perhaps its function likewise lacked uniformity.

Although cerebral localization is now usually considered to be synonymous with the localization of cortical function, in the first part of the present chapter the term is used in its more general sense. Thus the first two sections are concerned with those investigators who sought to locate function in the cerebral hemispheres and in most cases were primarily concerned with the problem of mental functions and the seat of the soul. Such crude theories, based either entirely on speculation or on speculation derived from clinical or anatomical observations, have subsequently been proved erroneous. Nevertheless, the ideas they propagated were of the greatest importance because of their influence, which in some instances was universal. The period of conjecture ended early in the nineteenth century with the phrenology of Gall and Spurzheim, the downfall of which resulted mainly from the application of the experimental method to the problem.

However, from Gall's idea that function was located on the surface of the brain grew the modern concept of cortical localization, and the rest of the chapter deals with this concept; no attempt has been made to follow the development of functional localization elsewhere in the cerebral hemispheres; for example, the hippocampus, basal ganglia, the visual pathways, and nuclei, etc., are not considered.

The third period of development represents the clinical studies that kept Gall's beliefs alive during the middle of the nineteenth century, and which finally proved that he had been right, although for the wrong reasons. Significant clinical studies have continued to the present day, but the real origin of cerebral cortical localization as we know it was in 1870, when the experimental investigation of the cortex was again carried out, but with a much greater knowledge of brain anatomy and techniques than had been available earlier in the century. We are still in this period of development, although most investigators have moved away from the earlier concepts of precise localization and of cortical maps and mosaics. It is represented here by some of the major contributions to knowledge of various parts of the cortex, both physiological and anatomical. Finally, the more recent opinions on the holistic functioning of the cortex are illustrated, and these help to indicate that the enigma of cortical localization is still, after many centuries of endeavor, very far from a satisfactory solution.

For the early literature, see Hunt (1868–1869), Dodds (1878); Riese and Hoff (1950–1951) and Riese (1959, pp. 73–151) relate the story from the point of view of the modern cortical equipotentiality theory rather than from an objective, unbiased standpoint. Bonin (1960) has also presented excerpts from the work of some of those who contributed to the idea of cortical localization.

Ancient Speculation

Apart from some of Galen's opinions on the motor and sensory functions of the brain (pp. 149–150), those ancients who opposed Aristotle's concept of cardiac supremacy (pp. 8–10) were concerned principally with a search for the seat of the soul within the brain and with the related problem of the cerebral localization of mental functions. Pythagoras (6th century B.C.) placed the rational part of the soul in the brain and one of the Hippocratic Writers (pp. 4–5) deemed the brain the site of all mental phenomena; although another writer knew that a lesion of one side of the brain produced contralateral spasms (*On wounds in the head*, 19, Littré [1839–1861], III, 254–255), no inferences were made from this astute observation, nor was it discussed further in antiquity except by Aretaeus (pp. 281–282). These opinions were followed by Plato (pp. 5–7), the Alexandrian anatomists (pp. 10–12), and later by Galen although there was no agreement as to the precise location of the soul within the brain. Galen or one of his followers may have enumerated the possibilities (*On the history of philosophy*, XXVIII; Kühn [1821–1833], XIX, 315).

From such ideas of antiquity arose the concept of three mental functions: first, that of the *sensus communis*, or the gathering together of all forms of sensory perception to produce imagination; second, of reasoning; and third, of memory. Although these arose from interpretations of Galen's writings, he believed, on the whole, that mental faculties were in the substance of the brain, whereas the medieval tradition which was eventually to become universally accepted, favored the cerebral ventricles. Thus developed the doctrine of the ventricular localization of psychological functions which was transmitted through both Arabic and Western traditions well into the seventeenth century. However, in the middle of the sixteenth century opposition to it appeared, and this is represented here by Vesalius who also gave an account of ventricular localization (see Sudhoff, 1913; Pagel, 1958).

GALEN
(*See p. 14*)

As well as locating mental activity in the brain at large, Galen also referred to the functions of specific parts of the brain. His division of nerves into sensory and motor, following Herophilus (p. 146), and his statement that they originated respectively from the anterior and posterior parts of the brain (p. 148), was in itself a simple form of brain localization. Moreover, his application of anatomical and physiological knowledge of the localization of disease processes is in keeping with our present-day method of arriving at a neurological diagnosis.

"Those then who know by dissection the origin of the nerves going to each part will better heal each part that is deprived of sensations and movement" (*The sites of diseases*, III, 14, Daremberg [1854–1856], II, 581).

In the following passage (*The sites of diseases*, IV, 3, Daremberg [1854–1856], II, 590) this topic is discussed in greater detail. The last sentence makes reference to the ventricular localization of mental processes which was to become a universal concept a few centuries after Galen's death.

EXCERPT P. 590

. . . . The motion of the tongue is derived from the seventh pair of nerves [twelfth cranial nerve] which arises from the brain near the origin of the spinal cord. Now, if the two parts of the brain, the right and the left, find themselves affected in this area, there is danger of apoplexy [i.e., bilateral hemiplegia]. If it is one portion only, it terminates in paraplegia [hemiplegia] which at times destroys motion in one half of the tongue only, and sometimes attacks the internal parts of the head, now these, now others, and sometimes an entire portion of the body as far as the feet. One may then observe that the tongue has been the only part of the face involved in the aforesaid lesion, without its sense of touch or taste being injured. The reason for this is evident to you who have seen that the nerves which leave the anterior part of the brain proceed towards the face, and those from the posterior part [as well as from the spinal cord] are distributed over all the parts below the face in the intact animal; the pair which converges on the muscles of the tongue, muscles which accompany voluntarily the motions of this organ, are also part of these latter nerves. It is therefore natural that when the anterior portion of the brain alone is affected, the movement of the tongue remains intact while all other parts of the face lose their sensory and voluntary motions in one part, either on the right or on the left. If the entire anterior part of the brain is injured, its upper ventricle [lateral ventricles] is necessarily also affected by sympathy, and the intellectual functions are damaged.

Galen also employed experiments to test local brain function. Compression of the brain and heart have been cited already (p. 16), but he gave further details of the former, together with the effect of cutting into the ventricles of the brain (*Anatomical procedures*, IX, 12, Duckworth [1962], pp. 18–19). The more serious effects produced by compression or incision of the fourth ventricle were no doubt owing to involvement of vital centers. This technique of brain compression was to be used much later by Auburtin, in the nineteenth century, to study the local cerebral control of speech (p. 492).

EXCERPT PP. 18–19

. . . . Should the dissection be thus performed, then after you have laid open the brain, and divested it of the dura mater, you can first of all press down upon the brain on each one of its four ventricles, and observe what derangements have afflicted the animal. I will describe to you what is always to be seen when you make this dissection, and also before it, where the skull has been perforated, as soon as one presses upon the brain with the instrument which the ancients call 'the protector of the dura mater.' Should the brain be compressed on both the two anterior ventricles, then the degree of stupor which overcomes the animal is slight. Should it be compressed on the middle ventricle, then the stupor of the animal is heavier. And when one presses down upon that ventricle which is found in the part of the brain lying at the nape of the neck, then the animal falls into a very heavy and pronounced stupor. This is what happens also when you cut into the cerebral ventricles, except that if you cut into these ventricles, the animal does not revert to its natural condition as it does when you press upon them. Nevertheless, it does sometimes do this if the incision should become united. This return to the normal condition follows more easily and more quickly, should the incision be made upon the two anterior ventricles. But if the incision encounters the middle ventricle, then the return to the normal comes to pass less easily and speedily. And if the incision should have been imposed upon the fourth, that is, the posterior ventricle, then the animal seldom returns to its natural condition.

Whereas Herophilus had favored the ventricles for the seat of the soul, and thus of psychological activity, Galen preferred the brain substance itself, although the last sentence of the selection on page 14 shows that, as is so often the case, he could have more than one opinion on a subject. Thus he stated (*The sites of diseases*, III, 9, Daremberg [1854–1856], II, 561–562):

As for me, arguing in accordance with the evidence revealed by dissection, it seems to be acceptable that the soul itself resides in the body of the brain where it produces reasoning, and the memory of sensible images is preserved there.

He also discussed the relative merits of the ventricles and the substance of the brain as the seat of the soul in *The opinions of Hippocrates and Plato*, VII, 3 (Kühn [1821–1833], V, 600–611) and decided in favor of the latter. The ventricles, however, prepared the animal spirits which were the instruments of the soul.

Galen dealt with the subdivision of mental functions in greater detail elsewhere (*The differentiation of symptoms*, 3, Kühn [1821–1833], VII, 55–62), and this was to form the basis of a system of cerebral localization that persisted for centuries. These functions consisted of imagination, reason, and memory.

EXCERPT PP. 55–56

. . . . Thus the sensitive soul has five distinct functions; seeing, smelling, tasting, hearing, and touching. The motor soul has one closely related instrument and one kind of movement, as has been demonstrated in the book, *On movement of muscles*, but it has various special instruments so that it may seem to have various forms. The remaining function of the soul, which arises from the principal faculty, is divided into imagination, reason, and memory.

In the same chapter Galen discussed mental disturbances and argued that each of the faculties of the mind, imagination, reasoning, and memory, could be affected separately. From this it could be maintained that each must be represented in a separate part of the brain. However, Galen decided against such localization, although later writers who established the cell or ventricular doctrine may have used this to support their claims.

EXCERPT PP. 60–62

. . . . Therefore let us examine the injuries of the principal [mental] functions, and first of the imagination. Injury of this is also like another paralysis which is called torpor and catalepsy, just as another injury, distorted and wandering movement, which is called delirium; another deficient and weakened movement, as in coma and lethargy. Nay more, a kind of paralysis of function, madness; that which is like deficient movement of it, stupidity and folly; and that which is like aberration is called delirium. For very often delirium is found in both at the same time, in distorted imagination and inept reason; however, sometimes it is only in one of them, just as occurred in the case of the sick physician Theophilus who, although he otherwise conversed sagaciously and recognized those present, believed that there were pipers in the corner of the house where he was lying, and that they continually played their pipes, producing music; he believed that he observed some of them standing, others sitting, continually piping day and night, so that he cried out, constantly ordering them to be ejected from his home. Later, after he had convalesced and recovered from this kind of delirium, he told everything which each visitor had said and done, and he remembered the appearance of the pipers. To some there is no appearance of a vision [hallucinations], but when the reasoning faculty of the soul has been affected, they are afflicted with frenzy, as occurred to one who, when the doors had been bolted, threw vessels through the windows; afterwards he asked passersby to order him to throw things, and clearly gave the names of the different vessels; in this manner he obviously demonstrated that he was injured neither in the imagination nor in the memory of names. Why then did he wish to throw down and smash everything? He was unable to understand this, but through his activity he indicated his delirium. As regards the memorative faculty of the soul, the symptoms appear not only in those who are ill, but also in those who escape illness; this may be learned from Thucydides who declares that some preserved from a pestilence so far forgot all that had preceded as not only to forget their own households but even themselves.

Nemesius of Emesa
(*fl. c.* A.D. 390)

Those who followed Galen were, on the whole, content to accept his opinions without question, and it is therefore of considerable interest that in the problem of the localization of mental phenomena his teachings were not followed implicitly. Whereas he had preferred the brain substance, a deviation in favor of the ventricular system now took place and the three faculties of *sensus communis* and imagination, reasoning, and memory were located in the lateral, third, and fourth ventricles respectively. Rudiments of the idea seem to have originated with Poseidonius (4th century A.D.), a surgeon of Byzantium, but they were elaborated by Nemesius.

Nemesius, Bishop of Emesa, in Syria, was a Christian philosopher but there is no available information on his life. He is known only for his book, *On human nature*, which was an interesting attempt to interpret Greek scientific knowledge of the human body from the standpoint of Christian philosophy, and it was held in high regard by Albertus Magnus and Thomas Aquinas. In this work he discussed the form and function of the brain, based on Greek, and mainly Galenic, sources, but he placed the mental functions in the ventricles or cells and so produced the ventricular or cell doctrine which dominated psychological considerations until the seventeenth century (fig. 117). See Haller (1774, pp. 113–114); Domanski (1900); Jaeger (1914). The following selections are from a new translation of *The nature of man* (*Cyril of Jerusalem and Nemesius of Emesa*, translated and edited by William Telfer [Philadelphia, 1955]).

EXCERPT P. 319

Now the faculties of the soul can be distinguished as imagination, intellect, and memory, respectively.

EXCERPT P. 321

. . . . Now, as organs, the faculty of imagination has, first, the front lobes of the brain and the psychic spirit contained in them, then the nerves impregnated with psychic spirit that proceed from them, and, finally, the whole construction of the sense-organs. These organs of sense are five in number, but perception is one, and is an attribute of the soul. By means of the sense-organs, and their power of feeling, the soul takes knowledge of what goes on in them.

EXCERPT PP. 331–332

The Creator devised each of the other sense-organs to be dual, and located each of them in a certain place and portion of the body; for he gave us a pair of eyes, a pair of ears, and two nostrils for smelling. Also, in every living creature he implanted two tongues. In some creatures, for example, snakes, the two tongues are separate, and in others, as in the case of men, the two are joined up and made one. For this reason he made there to be two ventricles in the front, only, of the brain, so that the sensory nerves running from each ventricle should constitute the sense-organs in pairs. It was of his abundant care that he made them in pairs, so that if either were affected, the other would be there to preserve that particular sense.

EXCERPT P. 338

As regards the faculty of imagination, its possibilities and organs, its subdivisions and what they have in common and wherein they differ, has been sufficiently, if summarily, treated, to the best of my power. As regards the faculty of intellect, on the other hand, its subdivisions are judging, approving, refuting, and essaying, while it expresses itself in recognition of objects, in virtues, in various kinds of knowledge and the principles of the several arts, as well as in deliberation and choice. It is this faculty, also, which divines the future for us through dreams, a form of prognostication which the Pythagoreans say is the only true form, following the Jews in this. The organ of the faculty of intellect is the middle part of the brain and the vital spirit there contained.

EXCERPT PP. 341–342

So, then, the faculty of imagination hands on to the faculty of intellect things that the senses have perceived, while the faculty of intellect (or discursive reason) receives them, passes judgement on them, and hands them on to the faculty of memory.

The organ of this faculty is the hinder part of the brain (called also cerebellum and hinder-brain) and the vital spirit there contained. Now, if we make this assertion, that the senses have their sources and roots in the front ventricles of the brain, that those of the faculty of intellect are in the middle part of the brain, and that those of the faculty of memory are in the hinder brain, we are bound to offer demonstration that this is how these things work, lest we should appear to credit such an assertion without rational grounds. The most convincing proof is that derived from studying the activities of the various parts of the brain. If the front ventricles have suffered any kind of lesion, the senses are impaired but the faculty of intellect continues as before. It is when the middle of the brain is affected that the mind is deranged, but then the senses are left in possession of their natural functions. If the front ventricles and the middle of the brain are affected together, both thought and sensation break down. If it is the cerebellum that is damaged, only loss of memory follows, while sensation and thought take no harm. But if the middle of the brain and the cerebellum share in the damage, in addition to the front ventricles, sensation, thought, and memory all founder together, with the result that the living subject is in danger of death.

Avicenna

(See p. 20)

Although the basic form of the idea introduced by Nemesius remained the same, there were several variations of it and many authors presented the concept pictorially. It not only dominated thought in the Christian West but it also proved acceptable to the Moslems, for it was essentially a simple solution of the complicated problem concerning the mind and its functions. The ventricular doctrine therefore appeared in the writings of Avicenna, although considerably elaborated. It is found in his book, *On the soul* (F. Rahman, *Avicenna's psychology. An English translation of Kitāb al-Najāb, Book III, Chapter VI, with historical-philosophical notes and textual improvements on the Cairo edition* [London, 1952]).

EXCERPT P. 31

One of the animal internal faculties of perception is the faculty of fantasy, i.e., *sensus communis*, located in the forepart of the front ventricle of the brain. It receives all the forms which are imprinted on the five senses and transmitted to it from them. Next is the faculty of representation located in the rear part of the front ventricle of the brain, which preserves what the *sensus communis* has received from the individual five senses even in the absence of the sensed objects.

It should be remembered that receptivity and preservation are functions of different faculties. For instance, water has the power of receiving an imprint, but lacks that of retaining it. Next is the faculty which is called 'sensitive imagination' in relation to the animal soul, and 'rational imagination' in relation to the human soul. This faculty is located in the middle ventricle of the brain near the vermiform process, and its function is to combine certain things with others in the faculty of representation, and to separate some things from others as it chooses. Then there is the estimative faculty located in the far end of the middle ventricle of the brain, which perceives the non-sensible intentions that exist in the individual sensible objects, like the faculty which judges that the wolf is to be avoided and the child is to be loved. Next there is the retentive and recollective faculty located in the rear ventricle of the brain, which retains what the estimative faculty perceives of non-sensible intentions existing in individual sensible objects. The relation of the retentive to the estimative faculty is the same as that of the faculty called representation to the *sensus communis*. And its relation to the intentions is the same as that of representation to sensed forms.

However, Avicenna's most important work was his *Canon*, the influence of which rivaled the writings of Aristotle and Galen in the medieval period and beyond. The ventricular or cell doctrine was discussed in detail in Book I (O. C. Gruner, A *treatise on the Canon of Medicine of Avicenna incorporating a translation of the first book* [London, 1930]).

EXCERPT PP. 134–138

176. *The Interior Senses.*—There are five groups of interior faculties: the composite, the imagination, the apprehensive or instinct, the retentive or memory, and the ratiocinative. The first two are taken together by the physician [Galen], but not by the philosopher [Aristotle].

177. *The Composite sense* (= *Common sense:* Hiss-i-mushtarik) is that which receives all forms and images perceived by the external senses, and combines them (into one common mental picture).

178. *Imagination.*—(*Phantasy*). This preserves the percepts of the composite sense after they have been so conjoined, and holds them after the sense-impressions have subsided. The common sense is the recipient and the imagination is the preserver. The proof of this belongs to the philosopher.

The chief seat of the activities of these two faculties is the anterior part of the brain.

179. *The Cogitative Faculty.*—The faculty which medicine calls cogitative is taken in two senses in philosophy. It is regarded sometimes as "imaginative faculty" [*mutakhayyal:* animal] and sometimes as "cogitative faculty" [*mutafakkira:* human]. In the view of the philosopher, the former is where the apprehensive faculty comes into play, and the latter is where reason controls or decides that a given action is advantageous. There is also the difference that the imagination deals with sense-form percepts, whereas the cogitation uses the percepts which have been stored in the imagination and then proceeds to combine and analyse them, and construct quite different images: e.g., a flying man, an emerald mountain. The imagination does not present to you anything but what it has already received through the sense-organs.

The seat of this faculty is in the mid-portion of the brain.

180. *The apprehensive faculty.*—This faculty is the instrument of the power called *instinct* in animals. ("*Animal prudence.*") By it, for instance an animal knows that a wolf is an enemy, and the kid distinguishes its dam as a friend from whom he need not flee. Such a decision is not formed by the reasoning powers, but is another mode of apprehension. Friendship and enmity are not perceived by the senses, nor do the senses comprehend them; and they are not perceived by the reason either. Man employs the same faculty on very many occasions exactly as does an irrational animal.

. . . .

. . . .

. . . .

181. . . . .

182. *The Retentive Faculty. Memory* (Ḥafiẓa, Dhakira). The power of memory is as it were a treasury or repository for those supra-sensuous ideas discovered by the apprehensive faculty, just as the imagination is the treasury or repository for the sense-impressions of forms and sensible images (formed by the common sense). The seat of this faculty is in the posterior region of the brain.

VESALIUS

(See p. 153)

In the middle of the sixteenth century the ventricular localization of psychological functions was still being taught, for Vesalius in *De humani corporis fabrica*

(Basel, 1543, Bk. VII, Ch. I) told how he had been made to learn it. His reference to "Some Philosophic Pearl" was to the book, *Margarita philosophica* (Freiburg im Breisgau, 1503), an encyclopaedia of learning written by Gregor Reisch. Figure 117 from this work is one of the best known attempts to depict the idea and consists of medieval speculation superimposed upon a crude representation of Greek anatomy.

Vesalius opposed this relic of ancient teaching and his own interpretation of the functions of the ventricles will be cited with his account of the ventricular system (pp. 714–718).

EXCERPT P. 623

. . . . I have not yet forgotten how when I was following the philosophical course in the Castle School, easily the leading and most distinguished school of the University of Louvain, in such commentaries on Aristotle's treatise, *On the soul*, as were read to us by our teacher, a theologian by profession and therefore, like the other instructors at that school, ready to introduce his own pious views into those of the philosophers, the brain was said to have three ventricles [this is not found in Aristotle's treatise]. The first of these was anterior, the second, middle, and the third, posterior, thus taking their names from their sites; they also had names according to function. Indeed, those men believed that the first or anterior, which was said to look towards the forehead, was called the ventricle of the sensus communis because the nerves of five senses are carried from it to their instruments, and odors, colors, tastes, sounds, and tactile qualities are brought into this ventricle by the aid of those nerves. Therefore, the chief use of this ventricle was considered to be that of receiving the objects of the five senses, which we usually call the common senses, and transmitting them to the second ventricle, joined by a passage to the first so that the second might be able to imagine, reason, and cogitate about those objects; hence cogitation or reasoning was assigned to the latter ventricle. The third ventricle [our fourth] was consecrated to memory, into which the second desired that all things sufficiently reasoned about those objects be sent and suitably deposited. The third ventricle, as it was more moist or dry, either more swiftly or more slowly engraved them as into wax or a harder stone. Then, as those commentaries taught, according to the ease or difficulty of engraving, this ventricle preserves these things entrusted to it for a shorter or longer period of time. Yet that third ventricle neither retains nor engraves these things for itself but for the second ventricle, so that as often as this latter decides to reason about something entrusted to the bosom of memory, the third ventricle swiftly transmits whatever this is into the second ventricle, returning it as something that ought to be in the workshop of reason. Furthermore, that we might more aptly consider each thing that was thus taught, an illustration was shown us taken from some Philosophic Pearl [fig. 117] presenting to our eyes the aforesaid ventricles which each of us studied very carefully as an exercise and added a drawing of it to our notes. We were persuaded that this figure included not only the three ventricles but also, as we were led to believe, it displayed all parts of the head including the brain.

Modern Speculation

While the ventricular localization of mental processes was still widely accepted, new ideas appeared that were in fact often a modification of old beliefs. Thus Willis placed the three traditional psychological functions in the brain substance, but, unlike Galen, he gave them precise locations. Meantime the whereabouts of the seat of the soul was still a major and perplexing problem that remained throughout the seventeenth and most of the eighteenth century; the literature on it is vast (see Schubert, 1877; Arnett, 1904; Révész, 1917). Only one representative has been chosen, Descartes, whose suggested solution although entirely incorrect nevertheless had extensive repercussions. In opposition to the ancients, he upheld the existence of a single soul, a development of thought that received increasing support in the eighteenth century. Like Galen, Descartes drew attention away from the cerebral cortex.

At the end of the eighteenth century evidence was accumulating, some, for example, in the works of Procháska, that the brain was made up of many functional units and from this resulted the phrenology of Gall and Spurzheim. Again, most of these considerations were speculative, or as in the case of Gall, were theories based on erroneous clinical observations. Nevertheless, Gall's work was of vast importance since his idea of cerebral surface localization was a direct predecessor of the modern idea of cortical physiology. In order to consider the work of those who opposed Gall and almost completely extinguished his idea of cerebral localization, selections from the writing of Flourens are included here, although more properly they belong to the period of experimental studies. Furthermore, as Flourens' ideas cannot properly be considered without mentioning those of Rolando, this latter investigator will also be included in the present section.

RENÉ DESCARTES
(See p. 155)

The first important departure from the medieval tradition of brain localization was made by Descartes who, as is widely known, selected the pineal body as the seat of the soul.

This suggestion was of the greatest importance because it deviated from the universally accepted Platonic concept of the tripartite soul. Plato had divided the soul into three parts, the vegetative in the abdomen, the sensitive in the heart, and, like Pythagoras, the reasoning or rational soul in the brain, but Descartes' solution was to consider the body as a machine and thus dispense with the first two. The third portion of the soul or mind, which in man controlled the bodily machine, was in the pineal body, a location Descartes arrived at more by speculation than by accurate anatomical observation. As such, the pineal received sensory impressions and instigated movements, as already illustrated by his crude concept of the reflex (pp. 329–333). Descartes was therefore the first to locate function in the brain precisely (Jefferson, 1949).

The first selection (*L'homme*, Paris, 1664, Pt. V, Arts. 105–106) deals with the body as a machine.

EXCERPT PP. 105–107

Now, before I pass to the description of the rational soul, I desire that you reflect again a little on all that I have said of this machine; and that you consider, first of all, that I have not supposed in it any organs or springs that are not such that one can very easily persuade himself that there are wholly similar ones in us as well as in many irrational animals . . . . In view of the fact that all the membranes and all the fleshes also appear to be composed of many fibres or threads, and also the same may be remarked in all plants, so that it is a property seemingly common to all bodies that grow and are nourished by the union and junction of the small parts of other bodies, they could imagine no greater likeness in respect to the brain . . . .

I desire that after you have considered all the functions that I have attributed to this machine, such as the digestion of meats, the beating of the heart and arteries, nourishment and growth of the parts, respiration, wakefulness and sleep, the reception of lights, sounds, odors, tastes, heat, and such other qualities in the organs of the external senses, the impression of their ideas on the organs of "common sense" and "imagination," the retention of imprint of these ideas in the memory, the internal movements of the "appetites" and "passions," and, finally, the external movements of all the parts which follow so appositely the actions of the objects that are presented to the senses, as well as those of the passions and of the impressions that are met with in the memory, and that imitate as perfectly as possible those of a true man; I desire you, I say, to consider that these functions follow completely naturally in this machine solely from the disposition of its organs, no more no less than the counterweights and wheels of a clock produce its movements and those of another automaton, so that for this reason it is not necessary to conceive in it any other vegetative or sensitive soul, or any other principle of movement and life than its blood and its spirits, agitated by the heat of the fire that burns continually in its heart, and that there is no other nature than all the fires that are in inanimate bodies.

The next selection is from *Les passions de l'ame* (1649, Pt. I) and contains Descartes' reasons for selecting the pineal body as the control center of the body and mind. It followed closely the contents of a letter which he had sent to Father Mersenne on 26 January 1640.

EXCERPT PP. 45–51

ARTICLE 31

THAT THERE IS A SMALL GLAND IN THE BRAIN IN WHICH THE SOUL EXERCISES ITS FUNCTIONS MORE PARTICULARLY THAN IN ITS PARTS

It is also necessary to know that although the soul is joined to the whole body, there is, however, a certain part in which it exercises its functions more particularly than in all the others. It is commonly believed that this part is the brain, or it can be the heart: the brain, because the organs of sensation are in relationship with it; and the heart because the passions are felt in it. But on examining the matter with care, it seems to me to have been clearly recognized that the part of the body in which the soul exercises its functions immediately is not at all the heart, nor, as well, the brain as a whole, but only the most internal of its parts: this is a certain very small gland situated in the middle of its substance and so suspended above the channel by which the spirits in its anterior cavities have communication with those of the posterior, that the slightest movements which take place in it can greatly alter the course of these spirits; and reciprocally that the least changes which occur to the course of the spirits can greatly alter the movements of this gland.

ARTICLE 32

HOW ONE KNOWS THAT THIS GLAND IS THE PRINCIPAL SEAT OF THE SOUL

The reason that persuades me that the soul cannot have any other place in the whole body than this gland, where it immediately exercises its functions, is that I consider that the other parts of our brain are all double so that we have two eyes, two hands, two ears, and, finally, all the organs of our external senses are double; and that inasmuch as we have only one solitary and simple thought of one single thing during the same moment, it must necessarily be that there is some place where the two images which come from the two eyes, or the two other impressions which come from a single object by way of the double organs of the other senses, may unite before they reach the soul, so that they do not present to it two objects instead of one. It can easily be conceived how these images or other impressions could unite in this gland through the mediation of the spirits that fill the cavities of the brain. There is no other place in the body where they could be thus united unless it be in this gland.

. . . .

ARTICLE 34

HOW THE SOUL AND BODY ACT UPON ONE ANOTHER

Now let us concede that the soul has its principal seat in the little gland that is in the middle of the brain, whence it radiates throughout all the rest of the body through the intervention of the [animal] spirits, the nerves, and even the blood which, participating in the impressions of the spirits, is able to carry them through the arteries into all the parts. And recalling what was said earlier of our body's machine, that is, that the little threads of our nerves are so distributed into all its parts that on the occasion of the various movements that are aroused in it by perceptible objects, they open the pores of the brain in various ways so that the animal spirits contained in its cavities may enter diversely into the muscles by means of which they are capable of being moved; also that all the other causes that can move the spirits in various ways suffice to direct them into different muscles. Let us add here that the little gland that is the principal seat of the soul is so suspended between the cavities which contain the spirits that it can be moved by them in as many different ways as there are different sensory aspects of object; but that it can also be moved in different ways by the soul which is of such nature that it receives as many different impressions, that is to say, that it has as many different perceptions as reach it from the different movements in this gland. Also as the body's machine is so reciprocally composed that from that alone this gland is variously moved by the soul, or, by such other cause as may be, it drives forth the spirits that are about it towards the pores of the brain which lead them by the nerves into the muscles by means of which it causes them to move the parts.

THOMAS WILLIS

(See p. 158)

The scheme of localization projected by Descartes was not, however, accepted by Willis who evolved a plan of his own. He believed that whereas the cerebellum controlled involuntary movements such as those of the heart and the lungs (p. 638), the cerebrum was the domain of voluntary movements and also of sensation. The cerebral hemispheres were provided with three centers, the corpus striatum which received all sensations and was thus the seat of the *sensus communis,* the corpus callosum where imagination took place, and finally the cerebral cortex where memories were stored. Thus the three classical psychological functions were no longer represented in the cerebral ventricles but in precise portions of the brain substance. It should be understood, however, that Willis, in common with seventeenth century anatomists, was applying the term "corpus callosum" to all parts of the white matter, in addition to the structure known by this name today.

Reference has already been made to the functioning of the system in the selections from Willis's writings dealing with the reflex (pp. 333–335), and memory is discussed in the passage on the cerebellum.

The following selections have been taken from his book, *De anima brutorum* (London, 1672, Cap. IV). It is clear that Descartes was applying his knowledge of optics to the system he evolved and it is interesting that Willis also suggested optical analogies. His selection of the corpus striatum as an important cerebral center is significant, for as late as the 1860's Hughlings Jackson considered it to be the brain's motor center.

EXCERPT PP. 43–44

As to the different functions and operations of *the spirits* so established in separate provinces, first, we attribute to them a twofold aspect, that is, *inwards* for *sensation* and *outwards* for *movement.* But more particularly it is possible to conceive of *a middle part of the brain,* a kind of interior chamber of the soul equipped with dioptric mirrors; in the innermost part of which images or representations of all sensible things, sent in through the passages of *the nerves,* like tubes or narrow openings, first pass through *the corpora striata* as through a lens; then they are revealed upon *the corpus callosum* as if on a white wall, and so induce perception and at the same time a certain imagination of the things sensed. As often as the representations or images expressed there bring in nothing except mere knowledge of the object, soon after, as by another surge progressing from *the corpus callosum* towards *the cortex of the brain* they are hidden in its folds; with the disappearance of *phantasy* they constitute *memory* of the thing. But if the sensible appearance impressed upon the imagination promises anything of good or evil, thereupon the spirits are aroused and look back to the object by the stroke of which they were agitated. They swiftly command the other spirits within the passages of the nerves and those residing in the moving parts to grasp and move it away. Thus *the sense* brings in *imagination,* this, *memory* or *appetite,* or both at once; and finally, *appetite* brings in *local motions* which set in flight the appearing good or evil. For each of these kinds of animal functions, indeed, for the different acts of each kind to be performed, *the animal spirits,* which are the immediate instruments of them all, have special or distinct tracts or pathways. If there is any obstruction within them, at once some function is hindered or some member of *the sensitive soul* cut off, and, as it were, becomes powerless.

EXCERPT PP. 47–48

As concerns *the functions* and *uses* of *the corpora striata*, even though we are unable to see with the naked eye or manipulate with our hands any of those things which are carried on within the secret conclave of the brain, nevertheless, by the effects and by comparative analogy, that is, of *the faculties* and *acts* with *the techniques of the machine*, we can at least conjecture how the operations of the animal functions are performed within these or other parts of *the brain*; especially because it appears plainly that the functions of *the internal movements* and senses as well as of *the external* are performed by the aid of the animal spirits within certain distinct, arranged pathways or kind of slender tubes.

And so, since it appears from the aforesaid that *the corpora striata* are so placed between *the cerebrum* and *cerebellum* and the whole *nervous appendix* [brain stem with spinal cord] that nothing is carried from the former into the last or, on the contrary, can be carried back thither from it, unless it pass through those bodies, and since special passages lead from the separate *organs of movements, sensations, and other functions* into the very wide center; and since, in addition, passages lie open from these into *the corpus callosum* and into all the medullary tracts of *the brain*, nothing seems more probable than that these parts [corpora striata] are that *common* sensorium that receives and distinguishes all the appearances and impressions and transfers them in suitably ordered arrangement into *the corpus callosum*, represents them to the imagination presiding there, and transmits the force and instinct of those spontaneous *movements* begun in *the brain* into *the nervous appendix* for performance by the motor organs. Because of these multiple and various functions so many *medullary striations* or *internal nerves* are produced within the corpora striata for the various extensions and *radiations* of the animal spirits that it may be concluded that *the sensitive soul,* just as all its powers and equally its exercise of them within *the brain,* as well as in *the nervous system,* is merely *organic* and therefore extended and in some way corporeal.

JIRI PROCHÁSKA
(See p. 345)

For the next one hundred years after the contribution of Willis, there was no noteworthy advance in the problem of brain localization. Even at the end of the eighteenth century attempts were still being made to locate the sites of the *sensus communis* and mental processes in the brain. One of the most important at that time was to be found in the writings of Procháska who divided the nervous system into the *sensorium commune*, made up of the brainstem, spinal cord, and nerves, and the rest of the brain, the seat of the intellect; an account of this division is in a selection which deals with his work on the reflex (pp. 345–346). But on the whole Procháska did not proceed far beyond Willis and he was not able to localize precisely the various areas for mental function which he postulated, although he suspected that adequate dissection would give the answers. Nevertheless he is an important link in the development of the idea of brain localization.

The following passages have been translated from his famous book, *Adnotationum academicarum, Fasciculus tertius* ([Prague, 1784], Cap. V, "Functiones animales," Par. III, "Whether or not there is a special site in the brain for each part of the intellect."

EXCERPT PP. 141–143

His own consciousness and a certain capacity for feeling convinces each one that thought occurs in his brain. But since each brain is composed of many variously shaped parts, it appears likely that nature, which attempts nothing in vain, decided upon differing uses for those parts, so that the different parts of the mind seem to require different parts of the cerebrum and cerebellum for their functions. Since, however, the *Sensorium commune*, by certain laws peculiar to itself and without the consciousness of the mind, reflects sensory impressions into motor, and because we have declared the *Sensorium commune* to be comprised of the spinal marrow, medulla oblongata, and the whole origin of the nerves, it follows that, with the exception of the *Sensorium commune*, the cerebrum and cerebellum and their parts are the organs of the faculty of thought. However, because these organs are wholly lacking in some animals, it may be conjectured that in such the faculty of thought is also lacking and that they live solely because they have been endowed with that nervous force of the *Sensorium commune* and of the nerves. Hitherto it has been impossible to determine what parts of the cerebrum and cerebellum provide primarily for these or those parts of the intellect . . . .

And so it is by no means improbable that each part of the intellect has its organ in the brain, with one for perceptions, another for judgment, and perhaps still others for will, imagination, and memory, all of them working together admirably and arousing one another to action. However, I believe that of them the organ for imagination is especially remote from the organ for perceptions, because with the organ for perceptions lulled to sleep and at rest, the organ for imaginations may remain in action and produce dreams. But dreams have this quality, that although the total of discerned ideas represented is often very ridiculous and wholly erroneous, we are not at first convinced of their absurdity and falsity, until upon awakening we recognize correctly through the organ for perceptions that all these phantasies are false.

Franz Josef Gall   Johann Caspar Spurzheim
(*See p.* 392)

The next step in the localization of psychological functions was to provide specific areas for each of them, and it was taken at the end of the eighteenth century by Gall, the inventor of cranioscopy or, as others called it, phrenology. Together with Spurzheim he established the idea, already current in some quarters, that the brain was the organ of the mind and was itself made up of multiple organs. Each organ or area represented a mental or moral activity and, as they were on the surface of the brain, their hypertrophy or atrophy could be detected through the skull by palpation. Gall believed that there were twenty-six or twenty-seven such organs, and he based his classification of mental traits on an analysis of behavior. However, his followers increased the number and Spurzheim, for example, divided the various capacities of the human mind into (1) feelings, which included the sentiments and propensities, and (2) the intellectual faculties, including the reflective and perceptive activities. It was assumed that each had a separate localization and that each could be charted precisely on the cranium (fig. 118).

Phrenology did not survive as a scientific approach to brain physiology, but Gall's primary concept of functional localization, even though it was based upon false premises, has been proved correct. He had evolved a systematic theory of the relationship between brain structure and psychological faculties and this led later in the century to the division of the cortex into functional regions. Unfortunately, his contribution to this vital concept and to neuroanatomy was obscured by the uncritical and overenthusiastic activities of his many followers. He had, nevertheless, vaguely discerned the concept of cortical localization, although he employed incorrect reasoning.

Gall began his teaching in 1796 and expressed his ideas at length in *Anatomie et physiologie du système nerveux en général, et du cerveau en particulier* (4 vols. [Paris, 1810–1819]; Spurzheim collaborated in only the first two volumes). The following passages are from Volume II (1812), Section VI, "On the plurality of the organs."

EXCERPT PP. 258–259

SECOND ANATOMICAL PROOF

THE ANALOGY WHICH EXISTS BETWEEN THE ORGANIZATION OF THE BRAIN AND THAT OF THE OTHER NERVOUS SYSTEMS PROVES THAT THE BRAIN IS COMPOSED OF MANY ORGANS

The nervous system of vegetative or automatic life, the spinal cord or the instruments of the nervous system of voluntary movements, the nervous system of the sense organs, are each composed of particular organs that preside over a particular viscus, a particular voluntary movement, or over a particular sense. Each of these subdivisions has its origin, its accessory system, and its final expansion in a viscus, in one or many muscles, or in an external sense organ. By means of this arrangement, each particular nervous system has its own function, and the function of none of these systems can be replaced by that of another.

The same law presides over the arrangement of the brain. The convolutions are the expansion of the cerebral fibrils and of the fibre bundles. The convolutions, as far as they constitute an organ, receive their fibrils from different regions and from different accessory systems of supply as, for example, from the so-called thalami, from the so-called corpora striata, or from different parts of these structures.

In the first volume [p. 242] we have indicated several of the neural bundles, the enlargements and expansions of which form the convolutions of the hemisphere and we have had them engraved. Moreover, all brain lesions do not manifest their effect on the opposite side as is the case with lesions of the parts which are the continuation of the pyramidal bodies [pyramidal tract]; one must conclude from this that the cerebral parts do not all have the same origin, or in other words that parts of the cerebrum exist in which the fibrils cross each other at their origin and that others exist in which the fibrils do not cross.

This coincidence of the structure of the brain with that of other nervous systems clearly proves that nature when forming the brain had the intention of creating several organs just as she had this end in view when forming the subdivisions of the other nervous systems.

Having concluded that there were many functional areas or *organs* in the brain, Gall, in the same volume, discussed their relationship with one another.

EXCERPT PP. 262–263

Expressions [such as]: "all the parts are bound together and uniformly connected, and rely one upon the other," are equally far from representing what exists in nature. They are fragments of the opinion which states that the brain is but a pultaceous mass. Without doubt, this hypothesis does not recognize the existence of parts independent one from the other of which each has its own functions; but it would be also quite inconceivable that a single organ absolutely homogeneous throughout could present phenomena so different and give rise to manifestation of moral qualities and intellectual faculties so various and so dissimilar.

But the white matter of the brain is not entirely and uniformly blended; nowhere does a fusion of cerebral parts exist. On the contrary, fibres and fibre bundles are seen very distinctly everywhere. These fibres or fibre bundles have a constant and uniform direction, different however in each region; they form their own expansions and their own convolutions; they develop at different stages of life; their number varies greatly in different kinds of animals, etc. It is true that all these parts are connected to each other, but do these connections prove that each is not an independent organ? "All the organs of the animal body," says Reil, "have a kind of union between them and none can exist without the other; the preservation of one depends upon the existence of the other, but this fact must not lead us to the false conclusion that the proximate cause of an organ's action can be found elsewhere than in itself. This is by no means the case; each organ is independent and acts by itself by virtue of its own powers and it contains directly within itself the proximate cause of the phenomena which it offers." For the rest, in consequence of these objections, neither any sense organ, nor any viscus could be a special and appropriate organ; for all are connected with each other and in general with the organism.

The part of Gall's work that was of most significance for the theory of cortical localization was that on the faculty of language and speech. Moreover, it was the starting point for his ideas. He separated verbal memory from the faculty of language, but he connected their cerebral organs and placed them both in the frontal convolutions. As a boy, he had observed that individuals with a retentive memory had protruding eyes, and in his system he argued that the areas representing the memory of words were on the orbital surfaces of the frontal lobes which rested upon the posterior half of the supraorbital plate; hypertrophy of them, therefore, pushed out the eyes. It was upon this false assumption and upon others like it that Gall based his system.

The following passages have been taken from Volume IV of his *Anatomie et physiologie* (1819).

EXCERPT P. 48

XIV. UNDERSTANDING OF WORDS, UNDERSTANDING OF NAMES, MEMORY OF WORDS, VERBAL MEMORY

HISTORICAL

. . . .

Although I had no kind of preliminary knowledge, I was forced to the idea that eyes so formed are the mark of an excellent memory. It was only later that I said to myself, as I have already reported in the preface to the first volume [Vol. I, p. II], if memory manifests itself by an external characteristic, why should not the other faculties also have their visible external characteristics? That is what provided the first impetus for all my researches and was the occasion for all my discoveries.

EXCERPT PP. 50–51

SITE AND EXTERNAL APPEARANCE OF THE ORGAN OF MEMORY OF WORDS AND NAMES

When discussing the sense organ of anyone, I said that the anterior convolutions of the middle lobe are in contact with the posterolateral parts of the orbit. When these convolutions are very well developed, that part of the sphenoid bone which forms the posterior third of the external wall of the orbit, is pushed forwards; this diminishes the depth of the orbit and renders the eyeball prominent.

It is however by no means probable that the middle lobe is assigned to these faculties. The fruit-eating animals have only internal convolutions, and they learn words and names as well as the carnivorous animals. Besides, memory has too little analogy with the carnivorous instinct to permit us to suppose that the convolutions of the middle lobe, which are located above the ear, constitute the organ of the carnivorous instinct, and the anterior convolutions of the same lobe the organ of the memory of words.

Now if it happens in fact that the eyeball is pushed out of the orbit by a considerable development and by a great prolongation of this lobe, the resultant appearance of the eyes would no longer be the sign of an excellent memory. This is perhaps the reason why certain persons with large eyes projecting from the head, and in the prime of life and health, do not always have a more than ordinary memory. It is at least generally certain that some persons learn by heart with ease but have a treacherous memory for names, while others easily fix names in their minds but have great trouble in remembering quotations, however inconsiderable, whether prose or verse. I have not yet succeeded adequately in discerning all these varieties; however, in ten judgments that I may make, I shall be mistaken only once at the most. I should be still less likely to be mistaken if the organ of this faculty were not placed in such a region that it can extend itself in all directions from above downwards, anteriorly, laterally, and from below upwards.

I regard as the organ of memory of words that part of the brain which rests on the posterior half of the orbital roof [the central portion of the posterior third of the orbital surface of the cerebral hemisphere, immediately anterior to the tip of the temporal lobe]. In the engravings we have not given special numbers to the part of the faculty of speech.

However, it is certain that frequently it is only the posterior half of the orbital roof which is depressed by the great development of the part of the brain indicated; and in this case, the posterior part of the orbit must equally lose its depth and the eyeball must be pushed forwards. This form of the eyes is often encountered without the circumstances that I shall indicate when speaking of the faculty of speech, taking place at the same time; it is for this reason that I deal with this latter organ separately.

EXCERPT PP. 55–56

XV. THE UNDERSTANDING OF THE LANGUAGE OF SPEECH; TALENT
IN PHILOLOGY, ETC.

. . . .

The largest part of the middle portion of the inferoanterior convolutions lying on the superior wall of the orbit or on the vault, is well developed; this wall is not only flattened but even depressed. There results a particular position of the eyes. In this case, the eyes are at the same time protruding and depressed towards the cheeks in such a way that there is some space between the eyeball and the upper orbital margin. The eyeball thus depressed acts on the lower orbital margin and increases its concavity. This marked excavation in the living subject with the eyes open produces the appearance of a little pocket full of water, from which comes the term "pocketed eyes" [*yeux pochetés*].

Persons who have eyes like this not only possess an excellent memory for words but they have a particular disposition for the study of languages and in general judgment of all that pertains to literature. They compile dictionaries, write history; they are very suitable for the functions of librarian or conservator; they gather the scattered riches of all centuries; they compile learned volumes; they scrutinize antiquities and, no matter how little they may have of the other faculties, they are the admiration of all the world on account of their vast erudition.

LUIGI ROLANDO
(20 June 1773—20 April 1831)

While Gall and Spurzheim were expounding their theory, further evidence was being collected to prove that the brain was not an amorphous mass. This came from the famous experiments of the Italian anatomist and physiologist Rolando. Although his work was to be an early precursor of the experimental studies on cerebral localization carried out later in the nineteenth century, it is convenient to consider it here in its chronological context and to refer to it later. Its relationship to Flourens (pp. 483–488) also demands that it should be included here.

Rolando was born in Turin and received his medical training there. In 1804 he was called to the University of Sassari in Sardinia as professor of practical medicine and physician to King Victor Emmanuel of Sardinia. He spent ten years there and returned to Turin to occupy the chair of anatomy until his death. He investigated mainly the nervous system, and together with Flourens (p. 483) was a pioneer in the application of experimental techniques to the study of its function. As well as his work to be cited below, his experiments on the cerebellum (pp. 653–656) were outstanding (see Carron du Villards, 1830; Bellingeri, 1834).

Rolando was one of the first to study the effects of an electrical current on the brain. His method, however, was crude and most of his results were no doubt owing to the spread of the strong current he used to peripheral muscles. The other techniques he employed were likewise primitive and his results were necessarily inconclusive; he himself drew few conclusions from them and little notice was taken of them at the time. He was, nevertheless, an important pioneer in the experimental approach to brain physiology and his findings, although open to valid criticisms, suggested correctly that the cerebrum, and in particular its internal fibres, was in some way associated with voluntary motor function, a fact well known but which had not at that time been experimented upon extensively. However, his results were refuted by Flourens (see p. 484) and on this account had little or no influence.

The passages below have been translated from his book, *Saggio sopra la vera struttura del cervello dell'uomo e degl'animali, e sopra le funzioni del sistema nervoso* (Sassari, 1809). Flourens, who carried out similar investigations, published an annotated French translation of Rolando's experiments (1823, and 1824, pp. 273–302) in order to refute a charge of plagiarism.

EXCERPT PP. 31–38

With the idea of remarking what effects might be induced by a current of galvanic fluid directed from the brain to the various parts of the body, I trepanned the cranium of a pig and then introduced a conductor of the Voltaic pile into the hemispheres of the brain and touched now one part now another, while the other wire was applied to different parts of the body. From these experiments, repeated on various quadrupeds and fowl, I obtained only violent contractions, and I observed that these were much stronger when the metallic conductor penetrated into the cerebellum.

The hemispheres of the pig's brain, however, had been not a little lacerated from the repeated introductions of the point of the conductor, so that the corpora striata and the ventricles were somewhat damaged; nevertheless, the animal lived for twelve hours in a condition of stupor and would have lived longer if it had not been subjected to further injury.

. . . .

A very agile kid, the cranium of which I trepanned in two places, provided me with more satisfactory results. I introduced a probe through one of the two openings made with the trepan so that I was able to cut almost all the filaments of the medullary substance which has acquired the name of *corpora striata* and traverses the gray matter. I also attacked the corpus callosum and the septum lucidum, but the animal remained upright and moved, turning away from the injured side; a half hour later I made a similar lesion on the left hemisphere, but I cut the aforesaid filaments closer to their origin, where they still preserve the name of crura of the brain. Although there was considerable loss of blood, nevertheless the animal remained erect and for perhaps two hours stood immobile and upright; it moved only when a strong shove forced it to change its position, and minor irritations, fairly loud noises, and the presence of food did not arouse any movement. After about two hours it began to take a few steps, to lean against the wall, or to place itself in a corner, and it spent two or three hours in this way in a condition of stupor or like an animal deeply asleep; towards evening it lay down and slept probably the whole night since it was found in the same place in the morning. I sacrificed it after thirty-six hours in order to examine the injured parts.

. . . . The most curious phenomena, however, were those offered by a large pig in which, with a knife, I cut most of the fibres that are seen to pass from the thalami to the corpora striata. Hardly had this been done when it was seen that it could move its front legs as formerly, but it seemed that when the animal sought to move them in one direction, almost of themselves they moved in the other. Shortly thereafter it was found to be in a very deep stupor, during which, snoring loudly, it stood on its feet continuously for twelve hours leaning against the wall; if it moved slightly away, it immediately sought some support. After this, laying itself down, when it arose it remained on its feet a very short time; it was sacrificed after twenty-six hours for examination of the injuries mentioned.

Similar experiments were repeated on a large number of animals such as goats, sheep, and guinea pigs, and varied in many ways with the principal purpose of observing what phenomena were produced by the lesions of the bigeminal prominences [quadrigeminal bodies], the thalami, the fornix and its appendices. The results were that every time a large number of fibres that cross the corpora striata were cut or lacerated, and either the corpus callosum or the fornix injured, there always occurred a state of lethargy and coma, and at other times symptoms of *catalepsy*. In the guinea pigs, however, and in other small animals the signs of coma did not seem so pronounced, but I observed some no less singular phenomena.

When the hemisphere was injured, the animal walked and ran continuously in a circle away from the [injured] side, and when a similar injury was made on the other hemisphere, it began to turn in the opposite direction; at other times through similar injuries the animal ran without any direction because it bumped into all the objects placed before it, and finally, according to the alteration produced, I observed that it was as if it had no control of its hind legs and turned on these as on a pivot by means of its front legs.

I made a number of experiments on kids, lambs, pigs, deer, dogs, cats, and guinea pigs with the idea of observing what results would occur from injury to the bigeminal prominences, but I rarely obtained a constant effect, which will not cause astonishment if one considers the special interlacing of the numerous medullary filaments met with in these parts (see fig. 2); since it is extremely difficult to recognize what bundles of fibres have been lacerated in such operations, and what have been cut or injured in such others, it is not possible to determine the consequences clearly and distinctly when such dissimilarities appear in the results. In fact, in some of the aforesaid larger animals I have observed that upon laceration now of the bigeminal prominences, now portions of the thalami, phenomena are manifested indicating that the animal's muscles do not move according to the direction that appeared in its movements, but with an irregular uncertainty not otherwise than if drunk; now they walk to the side, now they lift their feet higher than is necessary, and at another time drag them.

For many reasons I am prevented from giving in detail the observations that these and other experiments have furnished me, and I shall refer only to one of the more astonishing of them that was furnished by some guinea pigs. These, injured in their bigeminal prominences, and at the same time the neighboring part of the thalamus, at first turned about as usual, then lay down on one side moving the legs constantly, but more the front ones as if to walk, and, if they placed themselves on the side other than that on which they fell, immediately they turned over and placed themselves in the first position with, I should say, the same quickness to be observed in those dolls with leaden feet and a body formed of a very light substance, which every time they are placed upside down or extended on a level surface, immediately through the force of gravity rise up on their heavier base. If the guinea pigs were supported on that side on which they were lying, they walked a little, and when some of them began to walk by themselves after ten to fifteen days, and seemed almost recovered, the slightest shove was sufficient to cause them to fall on this side; never on the other except through a proportionate force; some experiments in which the pineal gland was injured and, in fact, separated from its peduncles, did not furnish any data through which it was possible to conjecture about its usefulness.

PIERRE FLOURENS
(13 April 1794—8 December 1867)

Although the phrenology of Gall and Spurzheim met with widespread support, it also encountered powerful opposition and the most effective was that of the French physiologist Flourens. He, more than anyone else, was responsible for the downfall of phrenology in informed circles, although it has continued to be practised as a variety of physiognomy to the present day.

Flourens was born in Maureilhan, near Montpellier where he attended the Medical School. After graduation he went to Paris where he was introduced to the great naturalist Cuvier and other prominent scientists. He began work immediately in physiology, which his distinguished countryman, Magendie (p. 299), had developed and he became one of the outstanding founders of the French school of experimental physiology. He held most of the important positions in this subject which were then available in Paris, mainly owing to Cuvier's support. Flourens' contributions were principally to the physiology of the nervous system, thus rivaling Magendie who had also chosen this field of study; however, Flourens investigated problems of embryology, the functions of the semicircular canals, bone growth, the action of ether as an anaesthetic, and comparative physiology. When he retired in 1848, he was professor of comparative anatomy (see Bernard, 1840–1849; Olmsted, 1953).

It has been said that Flourens did for the central nervous system what Magendie and Bell did for the peripheral. He concluded that the cerebral hemispheres were the seat of intelligence and sensation, the cerebellum of motor function, and the medulla oblongata of vital functions. We are concerned here only with the first of these three; that dealing with cerebellar function is discussed on pages 656 to 660. Flourens did not believe the cerebrum to be partitioned but that the special senses and intellectual faculties were represented in its whole extent. Thus he opposed the teachings of Gall (Flourens, 1843) and was responsible for a hiatus in development in the concept of cortical localization, but his work was of such great importance to brain physiology in general that it merits representation here. When assessing the results of his experiments it must be kept in mind that his techniques, like those of Rolando, were crude, that the examination of his animals was superficial, and that he worked mainly with birds, the cortical physiology of which is still imperfectly known today. Although his results are therefore open to question, he is usually credited with anticipating the holistic theory of brain function (pp. 558–574). His reputation was such that his conclusions were accepted almost universally for a generation. He refuted Rolando's findings which had indicated that the cerebral hemispheres controlled motor function (pp. 480–483), and he described them as "vague, confused, and incoherent phenomena" (Flourens, 1824, p. 281, footnote). Furthermore, "the animal, far from suffering from the lesions of the cerebral lobes, is not even conscious of them" (*ibid.*, p. 284, footnote 1). Flourens' own experiments, which were very similar to those of Rolando, led him to opposite conclusions, although similarities in results are obvious.

His first paper on cerebral function was read before the Académie des Sciences in 1822 and was published the following year ("Recherches physiques sur les propriétés et les fonctions du système nerveux dans les animaux vertébrés," *Archs. gén. Méd.*, 1823, 2:321–370). The following is Flourens' famous account of the pigeon from which both cerebral lobes had been removed.

EXCERPT P. 352

It held itself upright very well; it flew when it was thrown into the air, it walked when it was pushed; the iris of its eye was very mobile but nevertheless it did not see; it did not hear, it never moved spontaneously, it nearly always assumed the appearance of a sleeping or drowsy animal, and when it was irritated during this kind of lethargy, it took on the appearances of a waking animal.

In whatever position it was placed it recovered its equilibrium perfectly and did not come to rest until it had done so.

I placed it on its back and it got up, I put water into its beak and it swallowed it; it resisted the efforts I made to open its beak, it struggled when I disturbed it; it passed excrements; the least irritation disturbed and annoyed it.

When I left it to itself, it remained calm and absorbed; in no case did it give any sign of volition. In a word, it was an animal condemned to perpetual sleep and deprived even of the faculty of dreaming during this sleep; such, almost precisely, had become the pigeon of which I had removed the cerebral lobes.

The following are some of Flourens' conclusions from this and other experiments.

EXCERPT P. 363

2. On the other hand, if the cerebral lobes are removed, vision is lost for the animal no longer sees; volition is lost for it no longer wishes [to move]; memory, for it no longer remembers; judgment, for it no longer judges; it strikes itself twenty times against the same object without learning to avoid it; it stamps on the ground when struck blows rather than fleeing.

A movement once started continues, but it never begins spontaneously; it only flies if thrown into the air; it only walks if it is pushed; it only swallows if food is forced into its beak: but, remarkable to relate, flight, walking, or swallowing once begun, continue and take place with perfect regularity and accuracy.

EXCERPT P. 368

3. The nervous system is not a homogeneous system; the cerebral lobes do not act in the same way as the cerebellum, nor the cerebellum like the spinal cord, nor the cord absolutely like the nerves.

4. But it is a single system, all of its parts concur, consent, and are in accord; what distinguishes them is the appropriate and determined manner of acting: what unites them is a reciprocal action through their common energy.

These observations were extended and reported in Flourens' book published in 1824 (*Recherches expérimentales sur les propriétés et les fonctions du système nerveux dans les animaux vertébrés*, Paris, 1824). The following passages describe Flourens' needle-pricking experiments.

EXCERPT PP. 17–20

EXPERIMENTS TO DETERMINE THE PROPERTIES OF THE DIFFERENT PARTS OF THE CEREBRAL MASS

1. In a small rabbit, I removed both frontal bones; the animal lost little blood and it was as well after the operation as before it.

I cut through the dura mater on both sides, carefully avoiding injury to the blood vessels which I saw running on it; I likewise cut the pia arachnoid and removed both membranes; I pricked the cerebral hemispheres throughout their length without producing anywhere the least sign of muscular contraction.

2. In a pigeon, I removed the cerebral hemispheres in successive layers; the animal remained stationary.

3. . . . .

4. . . . .

5. I removed the whole left cranial vault in a young dog; I pricked and cut the cerebral lobe and the cerebellum of this [left] side; the animal was neither disturbed nor agitated.

6. In a much older dog, I pricked the quadrigeminal bodies; weak convulsions resulted. I pricked the medulla oblongata and they became violent.

7. In a rabbit I first pricked the corpora striata and the thalami in all directions and then removed them completely in successive slices; no agitation accompanied this double procedure.

8. . . . .

9. . . . .

10. . . . .

11. Thus, 1° the cerebral hemispheres are not at all likely to excite immediate muscular contractions.

Flourens produced a great deal of experimental evidence and the following are some of the more important conclusions he derived from it.

EXCERPT P. 35

8. Likewise if one [cerebral] lobe is removed, the animal retains its memory; if two are removed, it is lost.

With one lobe removed, it can hear; with two removed, it no longer hears.

It can see when one lobe is still intact; it can no longer see when this is lost.

Memory, vision, hearing, volition, in a word all sensations disappear along with the cerebral lobes. The cerebral lobes are therefore the sole organ of the sensations.

EXCERPT PP. 97–98

17. Animals deprived of their cerebral lobes no longer have sensation, judgment, memory, or volition; for there is volition only if there is also judgment; judgment if there is memory; memory if there has been sensation. The cerebral lobes are, therefore, the exclusive site of all sensations and of all the intellectual faculties.

18. But do all these sensations and all these faculties occupy the same site in all these organs concurrently or is there a different site for each one of them?

The following conclusions answered the question.

EXCERPT PP. 99–100

4. Thus, 1° one may remove, be it from the front, from the back, from the top, or from the side, a certain amount of the cerebral lobes without loss of their functions. A very limited portion of these lobes suffices therefore for the exercise of their functions.

2° Relative to this removal, all functions decline and are gradually extinguished; and, beyond certain limits, they are completely lost. Therefore, the cerebral lobes contribute in their entirety to the full exercise of their functions.

3° Finally, as soon as one sensation is lost, so all of them are; as soon as one faculty disappears, all of them vanish. There are therefore no different sites for the different faculties nor for the different sensations. The faculties of feeling, judging, or desiring one thing reside in the same place as that of feeling, judging, or desiring something else, and consequently, this faculty which is essentially single is located essentially in one organ alone.

5. Nonetheless each of the various [special] sense organs has a distinct origin in the cerebral mass.

EXCERPT PP. 121–122

GENERAL AND DEFINITIVE CONCLUSION OF THIS REPORT

1° The cerebral lobes are the exclusive site of sensations, perceptions, and volitions.

2° All these sensations, perceptions, and volitions concurrently occupy the same area in these organs. Therefore the ability to feel, to perceive, and to desire constitute only one essentially single faculty.

3° The cerebral lobes, the cerebellum, and the quadrigeminal bodies may lose a portion of their substance without losing the exercise of their functions. They are able to recover it after having lost it completely.

4° The spinal cord and the medulla oblongata have everywhere an *ipsilateral action* only. The quadrigeminal bodies, the cerebral lobes and the cerebellum alone have a *crossed action*.

In the last analysis, the cerebral lobes, the cerebellum, the quadrigeminal bodies, the medulla oblongata, the spinal cord, the nerves, all these essentially different parts of the nervous system have specific properties, appropriate functions, and distinct actions; and despite this marvellous diversity of qualities, functions, and actions, they nevertheless constitute but a single system.

One stimulated point in the nervous system stimulates all others, one weakened point weakens all; they have reaction, change, and energy in common. Unity is the outstanding principle which rules. It is everywhere, it dominates everything. The nervous system therefore forms but a single system.

Clinical Studies

Rolando's experimentally imperfect evidence of cerebral function and Gall's revolutionary concept of mental and moral processes located in the cerebral hemispheres had each been refuted by the authority of Flourens, and for decades the great physiologist's conclusions were accepted universally. At the same time the excesses of the phrenologists, based on the widespread teachings of Spurzheim, of the Combes of Edinburgh, and of other popularizers, helped to turn the scientific world against Gall's basic thesis of cerebral localization, but one or two French physicians did not abandon him. Bouillaud, for example, from his experience of patients with brain disease, thought that Gall's localization of speech functions to the frontal lobes was correct, and Bouillaud's tenacity and perseverance, together with that of his son-in-law Auburtin and the timely support of the French anthropologist and surgeon Broca, led eventually to the acceptance of the first functional localization, that of speech. Thereafter it was only a matter of time before others were also suggested.

Meantime support for cortical localization also came from the clinical observations and theoretical deductions of Hughlings Jackson who had been influenced by the reasoning of the philosopher Spencer; the latter's reference to the subject is included in this section, for although it was not based on clinical studies it nonetheless was an important contribution because of its effect upon Jackson.

These events took place between 1825 and 1870, and they set the scene for the most important development in the history of cerebral localization, the experimental studies, to be considered in the next section, which began in 1870 and continue today. Clinical studies have also continued parallel with those based on animal experiments, but apart from one or two references to them they will not be included.

JEAN-BAPTISTE BOUILLAUD
(*16 September 1796—29 October 1875*)

Flourens' work was verified by a formidable array of experimental physiologists that included Longet, Magendie, Lorry, Matteucci, Deen, Weber, Budge, Schiff, and Vulpian. On the other hand, Gall's opinion concerning the localization of the faculty of language in the frontal lobes soon found a skillful advocate in the person of the French physician Bouillaud. He represented a link between the phrenologists of the early nineteenth century and the birth in its last quarter of cortical localization as we recognize it today.

Bouillaud was born near Angoulême, Charante, and studied medicine in Paris where he received the M.D. degree in 1823. He was greatly influenced by the famous surgeon Dupuytren, and Magendie inspired in him an interest in physiology. In 1831 Bouillaud was appointed to the chair of clinical medicine in the Paris faculty, and joined the staff of the Charité Hospital in 1848 in succession to Laennec. He worked widely in the field of clinical medicine in which his publications on diseases of the heart and nervous system and on medical nosography are best known. His ability was recognized by many appointments and honors. It may be added that Bouillaud, as a child of the Revolution, always voted with the left, and that the character of Dr. Bianchon in Balzac's *La cousine Bette* was modeled from him (see Rolleston, 1930–1931; Dejeant, 1930; Herrick, 1940).

Bouillaud's important contribution was that of pointing out how frequently loss of speech was associated with a lesion of the anterior lobes of the brain. On the 21 February 1825 he read before the Royal Academy of Medicine a paper entitled "Recherches cliniques propres à démontrer que la perte de la parole correspond à la lésion des lobules antérieurs du cerveau, et à confirmer l'opinion de M. Gall, sur le siège de l'organe du langage articulé" (*Archs. gén. Méd.*, 1825, 8:25–45). The following selection has been translated from it.

EXCERPT PP. 25–28

There is no physician at all familiar with clinical research who has not had frequent occasion to observe lesions of locomotor function caused by brain disease. In this way inflammations and cerebral compressions produce respectively spasmodic movements and more or less extensive paralysis. It is therefore not without great astonishment that one reads in M. Flourens' work on *Les propriétés du système nerveux* that the brain exercises no direct and immediate influence on muscular phenomena. If there were not facts galore that counter this assertion, the slightest reasoning would suffice to refute it. Indeed, a great number of movements that we carry out are directed by intelligence and volition. Now, M. Flourens himself admits that the brain is the unique site for desire and intellect; thus, it is the brain which determines and regulates the muscular contractions in which these two functions are involved. Besides, all one has to do is to glance at the anatomical connections of the brain with the spinal cord to be convinced that it must play an important role in the various actions in which muscular contraction predominates. Besides, this truth could not be contested, I repeat, by anybody who has collected a certain number of observations on cerebral disease.

But it is not enough just to know in a general way that the brain is indispensable for the production of several muscle movements; the question remains to determine if the various parts of which the brain is composed each controls special movements; and finally to investigate if there exist several cerebral nervous centers which are affected by muscular motions. Now, the multiplicity of cerebral organs when considered from this latter point of view become an infinitely probable fact, or rather a strictly demonstrable one if it is remembered that partial lesions of the muscular functions caused by a localized effect of the brain are not infrequently encountered. Thus, for example, one often observes a paralysis only of the upper or of the lower limb owing to a deep lesion of a given part of the cerebral mass.

For a long time attempts have been made *to localize* the functions of the brain, considered as a *center* of motion . . . .

It would be wrong to believe that the limbs are the only parts for movements of which certain special *centers* exist in the brain. Indeed, it is the same with all the organs charged with the execution of muscular motions under the direction of intelligence; among others are the tongue and eye, two admirable structures which play such important roles in the mechanism of intellectual functions. In this report I shall limit myself to the influence of the brain on the movements of the tongue, considered as the instrument of speech; and to movements of other muscles which cooperate with it in the production of this important phenomenon. Later on, I shall try to elucidate this same influence upon the movements of the eye.

I do not know why it has not been taught that the movements of the organs of speech must have a very special center in the brain; this truth seems so simple and obvious to me. To prove it conclusively it is necessary to state on the basis of observation, that the tongue and its related organs in the act of speech can be separately paralyzed, that is to say, without other parts being affected simultaneously; and that they can preserve the function of their movements whereas other parts, such as the limbs, are deprived of them. This is what I shall prove first. I shall try subsequently to determine the site of the nervous center which directs the mechanism of the organs of speech.

It is not enough, however, that there exists in the brain a particular *force* destined to regulate and to *coordinate*, the marvellous movements by which man with his articulated voice communicates his thoughts, and expresses his ideas and depicts, so to speak, the movements of his soul; it is important to discover the seat of this force in the brain. Now from my personal observations and from those I have collected from other authors, I believe that the nervous principle in question, which may be termed the legislating organ of speech [*organe législateur de la parole*] resides in the anterior lobes of the brain.

General conclusions. 1.° In man the brain plays an essential role in the mechanism of a large number of movements; it directs all those which are subject to the control of intelligence and volition.

2.° There are in the brain several special organs, each of which directs specific muscular movements.

3.° The movements of the organs of speech, in particular, are controlled by a special, distinct, and independent cerebral center.

4.° This cerebral center occupies the anterior lobes.

5.° The loss of speech depends now upon the loss of the memory of words, now upon the loss of the muscular movements by which speech is composed, or, what comes perhaps to the same thing; now upon a lesion of the gray matter and now upon that of the white matter of the anterior lobes.

6.° The loss of speech does not involve loss of the movements of the tongue considered as an organ of prehension, mastication, or swallowing of food, or the loss of taste; which presupposes that the tongue has three sources of distinct action in the nerve center, a hypothesis, or rather a fact, which agrees admirably with the presence of a triple nervous organ in the tissue of the tongue.

7.° Several nerves have their origin in the brain proper, or rather communicate with it by means of anastomotic fibres; the nerves which animate the muscles which cooperate in the production of speech, for example, have their origin in the anterior lobes, or at least have essential communications with them.

Simon Alexandre Ernest Auburtin
(*15 October 1825—? 1893*)

Bouillaud's paper of 1825, and others which followed it and repeated his thesis with additional evidence and persuasion, received little recognition. The odium associated with the extravagant claims of phrenology, mainly owing to Spurzheim, was too powerful, and any attempt to justify Gall's theory of localization was, for the time being, unacceptable. Moreover, Flourens' opinions, supported by his wealth of experimental observation and that of his supporters, and by his authority, held sway. But gradually the idea of localization of function in the cerebrum began to receive increasing attention.

In the very year that Bouillaud's first paper had been published, 1825, his son-in-law, Ernest Auburtin, was born in Metz. He received his medical degree in Paris in 1852, and became *Chef de Clinique* at the Hôpital de la Charité. His interests were in topics already investigated by his father-in-law, such as cardiac and rheumatic diseases. His name disappeared from the *Annuaire Médical* in 1893 so suggesting a demise about that time (Lautour, 1948). He took up Bouillaud's discarded work and eventually the whole question of cerebral localization was reconsidered in a famous series of discussions at the meetings of the Société d'Anthropologie de Paris in 1861 (see Stookey, 1963).

On 21 February 1861 Pierre Gratiolet (see p. 403) read a paper entitled "Sur la forme de la cavité crânienne d'un Totonaque, avec réflexions sur la signification du volume de l'encéphale" (*Bull. Soc. Anthrop. Paris*, 1861, 2:66–71). This and one by Broca which followed it ("Sur le volume et la forme du cerveau suivant les individus et suivant les races," *ibid.*, pp. 139–204) explored the relationships between brain size and intelligence. In the ensuing discussion of these papers, 4 April 1861 (*ibid.*, pp. 209–220), Auburtin maintained that function, not of the whole brain but of parts of it, should be studied. Moreover, like Bouillaud, he argued in favor of the localization of speech functions to the anterior lobes. At the time there was a patient in the Hôpital St. Louis with a traumatic frontal cranial defect, but with intact speech and intelligence, of whom Auburtin reported the following observations, in some degree reminiscent of the animal experiments of Galen (p. 461). Auburtin then announced his support for Bouillaud's original contentions.

EXCERPT PP. 217–220

. . . . During the interrogation [of the patient] the blade of a large spatula was placed on the anterior lobes; by means of light pressure speech was suddenly stopped; a word that had been commenced was cut in two. The faculty of speech reappeared as soon as the compression ceased. It has been claimed that this observation proved nothing because pressure could be transmitted to the other parts of the brain; but this pressure was directed in such a way that only the anterior lobes were affected, and, besides, it produced neither paralysis nor loss of consciousness. Again it has been objected that similar results have been obtained in individuals with defects in other parts of the cranial vault, and in particular in that celebrated beggar whose skull cap had been entirely lost because of necrosis, and who revealed his skull to passersby in order to secure alms. In these individuals, in fact, compression exerted on the middle part of the brain suddenly suppressed speech, but at the same time it suppressed all other functions of the brain and produced complete loss of consciousness. In the wounded patient in the Hospital of St. Louis, on the contrary, compression applied with moderation and discretion did not affect the general functions of the brain; limited to the anterior lobes it suspended only the faculty of speech.

These facts, which I could easily multiply, have been compared with others in which a lesion of the anterior lobes left the faculty of speech intact. However, these lesions affected only one anterior lobe and only a part of it. Now, it is possible that the right lobe, remaining intact, may partially supply the functions of the more or less diseased left lobe.

Besides, the anterior lobes are of considerable size and the precise point where the faculty of speech resides has not yet been determined. A lesion of these lobes, even an extensive one, could therefore destroy several convolutions without changing the part or parts that direct speech. So that a contradictory observation might be valid, it would be necessary that both anterior lobes be totally destroyed; if the patient then continued to talk, the theory which I entertain would be proved to be false. I believe that there is not a single fact of this kind in science.

On the other hand, it has happened several times that, because speech was destroyed but intelligence preserved, a lesion of the anterior lobes was diagnosed at the patient's bedside, and later this diagnosis was confirmed at autopsy. There are facts of this kind relating to apoplexies and others relating to softenings.

For a long time during my service with M. Bouillaud I studied a patient, named Bache, who had lost his speech but understood everything said to him and replied with signs in a very intelligent manner to all questions put to him. This man, who spent several years at the Bicêtre, is now at the Hospital for Incurables. I saw him again recently and his disease has progressed; slight paralysis has appeared but his intelligence is still unimpaired, and speech is wholly abolished. Without doubt this man will soon die. Based on the symptoms that he presents, we have diagnosed softening of the anterior lobes. If, at autopsy, these lobes are found to be intact, I shall renounce the ideas that I have just expounded to you; however, I can only argue according to the facts which exist in science today. Now, to the best of my knowledge, no one has ever seen a lesion limited to the middle and posterior lobes that has destroyed the faculty of speech.

Auburtin defined his position as follows:

". . . I shall content myself with the examination of one particular function of the anterior lobes of the brain, for it is sufficient to demonstrate a single localization in order to establish the principle of localizations, and I ask for no more than this" (*ibid.*, p. 213).

PIERRE-PAUL BROCA
(28 July 1824—8 July 1880)

The proof demanded by Auburtin was very soon available. One of the participants in the discussion at the Société d'Anthropologie was Broca, the renowned French anthropologist and anatomist whose name is still associated with the left inferior frontal gyrus. He was able to support the opinions of Bouillaud and Auburtin, and he suggested precise localization of speech functions.

Broca was born at Sainte-Foy-la-Grande near Bordeaux and educated at Bordeaux and Paris; he received his M.D. in 1848. After being *professeur agrégé* of the faculty of medicine in Paris, he was appointed to the chair of "pathologie externe" at the School of Medicine in 1867 and held several hospital appointments. His main work was in the field of anthropology, and some have claimed that he was its founder; he created the Société d'Anthropologie de Paris in 1859. But, in addition, he was anatomist, pathologist, and surgeon. (See C., 1880; Dally, 1884; Genty, 1936; Haymaker, 1953, pp. 259–263; Huard, 1960, 1961).

Shortly after the discussions at the Société d'Anthropologie referred to above (p. 492), Broca encountered a patient who proved to be the test case for Bouillaud and Auburtin's theory. This was the famous "Tan," so named because this was the only word he could utter on account of chronic aphasia or, as Broca termed it, *aphemia*. He died on 17 April 1861, and the next day Broca presented briefly the clinical and pathological features of his case to the Société d'Anthropologie ("Perte de la parole, ramollissement chronique et destruction partielle du lobe antérieur gauche du cerveau" (*Bull. Soc. Anthrop. Paris*, 1861, 2:235–238). A frontal lobe lesion which Auburtin had predicted was present.

At the next session, on 2 May 1861, Broca joined in the discussion on the volume and form of the brain (*ibid.*, pp. 301–321) and made the following observations on cerebral localization.

EXCERPT PP. 319–321

It seems to me that the principle of cerebral localizations has been established by both physiology and pathology which demonstrate the independence of functions, and by anatomy which demonstrates the diversity of organs. Nothing permits us to determine yet the precise relations of these various organs and of these different functions, nor to estimate their number, nor to know whether the principle of localizations extends to the secondary functions and to the secondary organs, and if it will ever be possible, for example, to label each convolution as the phrenologists have tried to do . . . . But these precious descriptions [of gyri] that we owe above all to M. Gratiolet [see pp. 403–407], have as yet not found their place in the classical textbooks of anatomy, and, of twenty *enlightened* physicians who perform autopsies, there is perhaps not one who, upon finding a circumscribed lesion in a cerebral lobe, is capable of giving the name of the convolution or of the diseased convolutions. It will therefore be a long time before we have enough positive scientific facts to establish a system.

During the last session [18 April 1861] I showed you the brain of a man [Tan] in which a lesion of the frontal convolutions had abolished the faculty of speech. I felt obliged to present to the Society this rare and curious fact which by strange coincidence has fallen into my hands at the same time that Mm. Gratiolet and Auburtin were discussing the site of the faculty of speech. But, while I inclined towards M. Auburtin's opinion, I did not intend to take part in the debate. I am expressing myself neither for nor against specific localizations; I seek only to present a general principle by considering the cerebral convolutions, not one by one, but in groups or, if you wish, by areas. Now, the parallel which I have tried to draw between the anterior and the posterior lobes of the hemispheres has been fully confirmed by the recent remarks of my eminent opponent [Gratiolet]. He has given us important details on the relative development of the occipital, parietal, and frontal lobes, according to age, sex, and race, and upon the direction of the frontoparietal suture considered as the posterior limit of the frontal convolutions. They provide valuable support for the opinion of those who place the site of man's highest faculties, the intellectual faculties to be accurate, in the anterior lobes; and those of sensation, inclination, and passion in the parietal and occipital lobes. And our colleague does not think otherwise, for he tells us specifically: "It is in the frontal lobe that the majesty of the human brain in some measure resides." Now, the majesty of the human brain is owing to the superior faculties which do not exist or are very rudimentary in all other animals; judgment, comparison, reflection, invention, and above all the faculty of abstraction, exist in man only.

The whole of these higher faculties constitute the intellect, or, properly called, understanding, and it is this part of the cerebral functions that we, M. Gratiolet and I, place in the anterior lobes of the brain.

By August 1861 Broca had examined the brain of Tan more carefully and had arrived at several precise conclusions. He therefore presented the material to the Société Anatomique of Paris ("Remarques sur le siège de la faculté du langage articulé; suivies d'une observation d'aphémie (Perte de la parole)," *Bull. Soc. anat.*

Paris, 1861, 36:330–357), and in so doing gave the theory of cerebral localization one of its most important stimuli. It has been argued that Auburtin rather than Broca should be given the greater credit for this (Stookey, 1954, 1963), but there is no doubt that the honors should be equally divided. Broca was by far the greater figure and Auburtin was merely perpetuating the views of Bouillaud, as he did in respect to various topics in clinical medicine. It should be noted, however, that when the brain of the test case Tan and others used by Broca in his arguments were examined by Pierre Marie (1906), the lesions were not nearly so precise and localized as had been claimed. Even so, the beliefs of Auburtin and of Bouillaud, who had himself supported Gall, were given incontrovertible proof by Broca.

EXCERPT P. 353

If one seeks to be more precise, one will state that the third frontal convolution is the one which presents the most extensive loss of substance; that it is not only cut transversely at the level of the anterior extremity of the Sylvian fissure, but it is also entirely destroyed in the whole of its posterior half; that by itself it has suffered a loss of substance equal to about half the total loss; that the second, or middle [frontal] convolution, although very profoundly injured, still retains its continuity in its most internal part; and that consequently, according to all probabilities, the disease has begun in the third frontal convolution.

The other parts of the hemispheres are relatively healthy.

EXCERPT PP. 356–357

. . . . I now have only a few words to add in order to set forth the results of this observation.

1,° Aphemia, that is to say, loss of speech [renamed aphasia by Trousseau, 1861], before all other disturbance of intellect, has been the result of a lesion in one of the anterior lobes of the brain.

2,° Our observation therefore confirms the opinion of M. Bouillaud who places the seat of the faculty of articulate speech in these lobes.

3,° The observations collected so far, at least those which are accompanied by a clear and precise anatomical description, are not numerous enough to allow one to consider this localization of a specific faculty in a particular lobe to be definitely demonstrated, but it can at least be considered extremely probable.

4,° It is a much more doubtful question to know if the faculty of articulate speech is dependent upon the whole anterior lobe or particularly upon one of its convolutions; in other words, to know if the localization of cerebral faculties happens by faculty and by convolution, or only by groups of faculties or by groups of convolutions. Further observations must be collected with the object of solving this question. It is necessary for this purpose to indicate exactly the name and the place of the diseased convolutions and, if the lesion is very extensive, to seek, wherever possible by

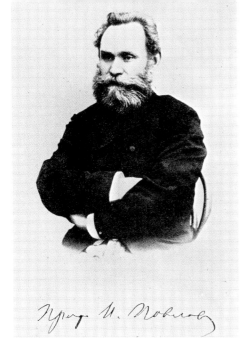

Fig. 97. Ivan Petrovich Pavlov. From *Grosse Nervenärzte*, ed. K. Kolle, Vol. I, Stuttgart, Thieme, 1956, facing p. 200. By permission.

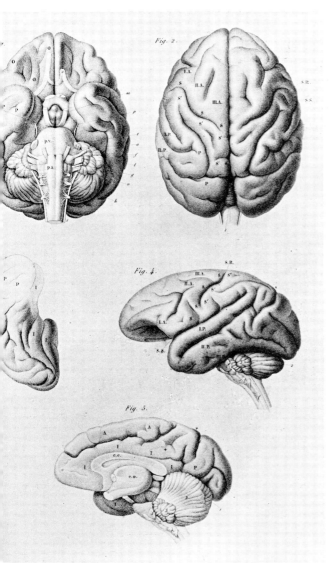

Fig. 98. Leuret (1839, Plate XV). Brain of baboon.

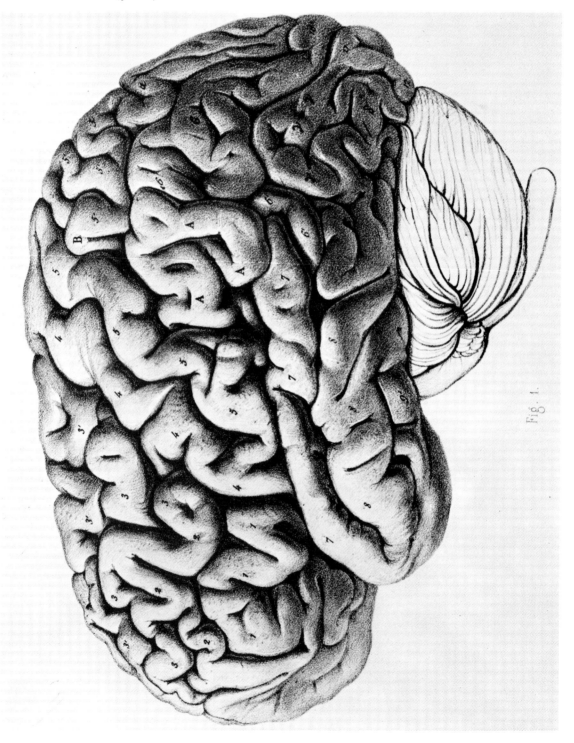

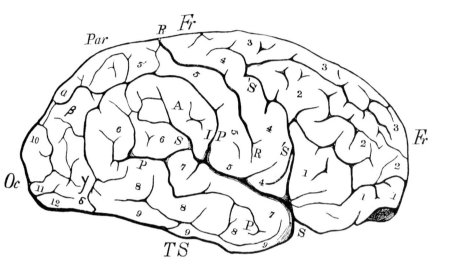
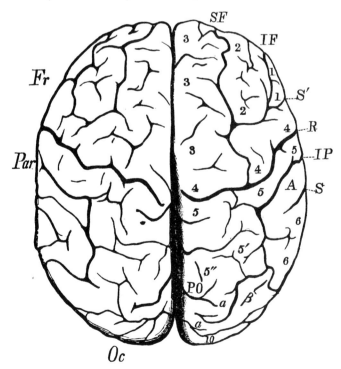

FIG. 102. Ecker (1869, p. 7, fig. 1).
Lateral view: c, central fissure, A, pre-
central, B, postcentral gyrus; F, frontal,
P, parietal, O, occipital, T, temporal
lobes.

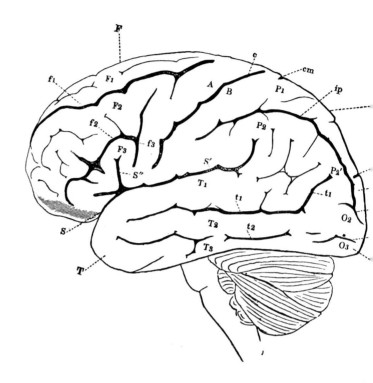

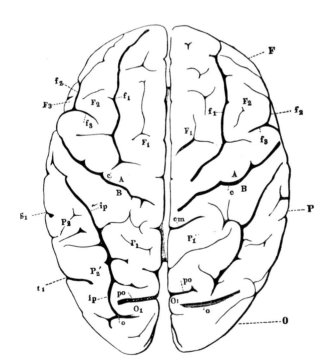

FIG. 103. Ecker (1869, p. 9, fig. 2).
Brain from above. Symbols as in fig.
102.

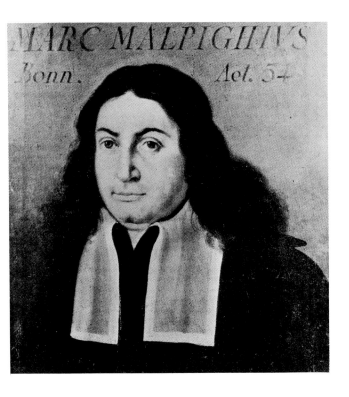

Fig. 104. Marcello Malpighi in 1682. From M. Pijoan, "A new and hitherto unpublished portrait of Marcello Malpighi," *Bull. Hist. Med.*, 1933, 1:81–84. By kind permission of the editor.

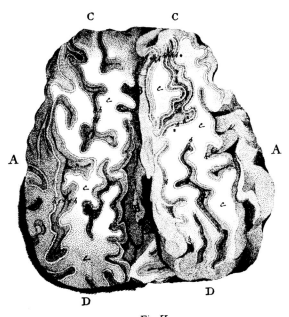

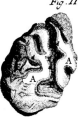

Fig. 105. Gennari (1782, Plate III, figs. 1–2). For explanation see text (p. 424).

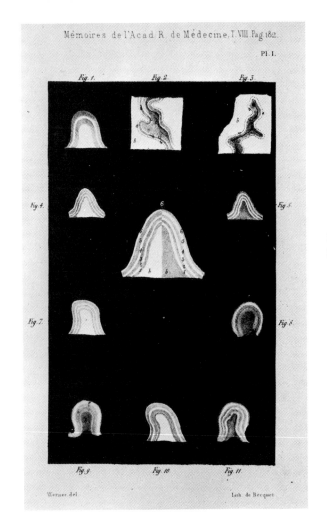

Mémoires de l'Acad. R. de Médecine. T. VIII. Pag. 182.
Pl. I.

Fig. 1.   Fig. 2.   Fig. 3.

Fig. 4.   Fig. 5.

Fig. 7.   Fig. 8.

Fig. 9.   Fig. 10.   Fig. 11.

Werner. del.   Lith. de Becquet

FIG. 106. Baillarger (1840, Plate I).
For explanation see text (p. 426).

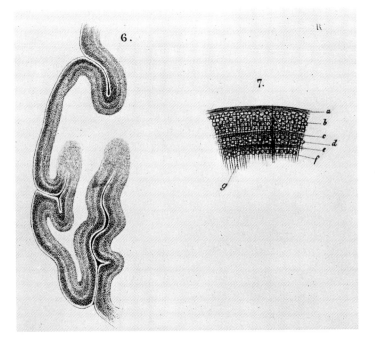

FIG. 107. Remak (1844, Plate XII,
figs. 6–7). For explanation see text (p.
430).

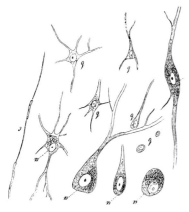

Fig. 108. Koelliker (1852, p. 299, fig. 149). From internal portion of human cortex. Nerve cells: *a*, large, *b*, small, *c*, axis cylinder.

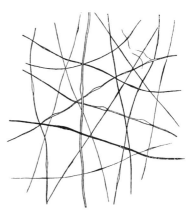

Fig. 109. Koelliker (1852, p. 300, fig. 150). Finest fibres of superficial human white matter, X 350.

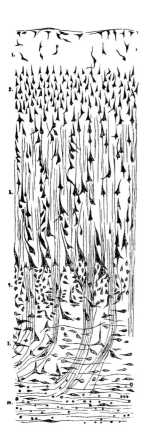

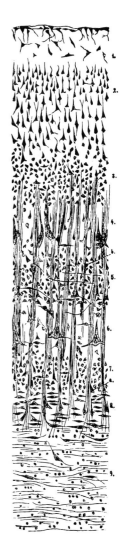

Fig. 110. Meynert (1884, p. 53, fig. 24). Section through third longitudinal frontal gyrus adjoining a fissure (five-layer type cortex): 1, superficial layer of neuroglia, 2, small pyramids, 3, large pyramids (formation of Ammon's horn), 4, granular layer, 5, spindle-shaped cells (claustrum formation); M, white matter.

Fig. 111. Meynert (1884, p. 69, fig. 25). Section of calcarine fissure cortex: 1, neuroglia; 2, pyramids; 3, external granular layer; 4, external bare layer with solitary cells; 5, middle granular layer; 6, inner bare intergranular layer with solitary cells; 7, inner granular layer; 8, spindle-shaped cells; 9, white matter.

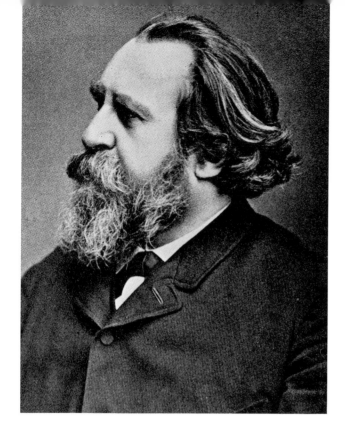

Fig. 112. Theodor Meynert. From *Grosse Nervenärzte*, ed. K. Kolle, Vol. II, Stuttgart, Thieme, 1959, facing p. 98. By permission.

Fig. 113. Lewis and Clarke (1878, Plate II). First illustration of the human Betz cell.

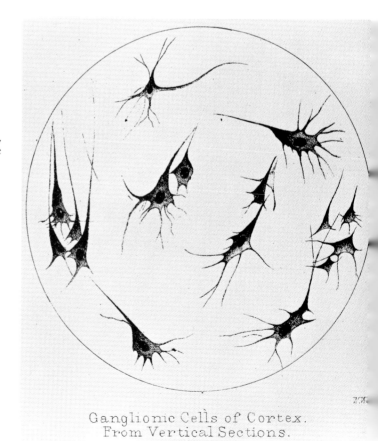

Ganglionic Cells of Cortex.
From Vertical Sections.

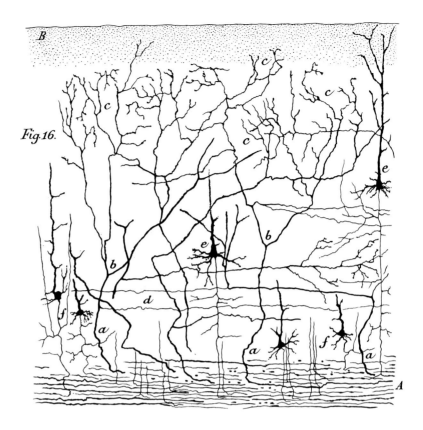

FIG. 114. Ramón y Cajal (1891, Plate III, fig. 16). Transverse section of supraventricular region of brain, fifteen-day-old mouse. Large fibres from white matter branch in the gray: *a*, ascending, bifurcating at *b*; *c*, various terminal branches; *d*, very long collaterals of ascending fibres; *e*, large pyramids; *f*, globular elements. A, white matter, B, molecular layer.

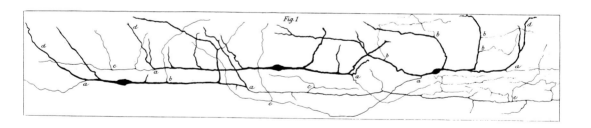

FIG. 115. Ramón y Cajal (1891, Plate I, fig. 1). Longitudinal section of molecular layer of cerebral cortex, eight-day-old rabbit; Golgi's rapid method. Three spindle-shaped cells: *a*, polar or principal axis cylinder; *b*, supernumerary axis cylinder giving off several dendrites; *c*, branches of axis cylinder.

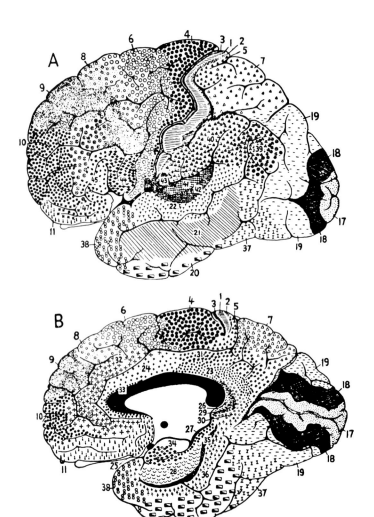

F<small>IG</small>. 116. Brodman (1908, p. 236). Cortical fields of lateral and medial surfaces of human cerebrum.

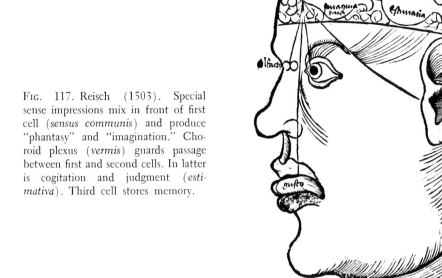

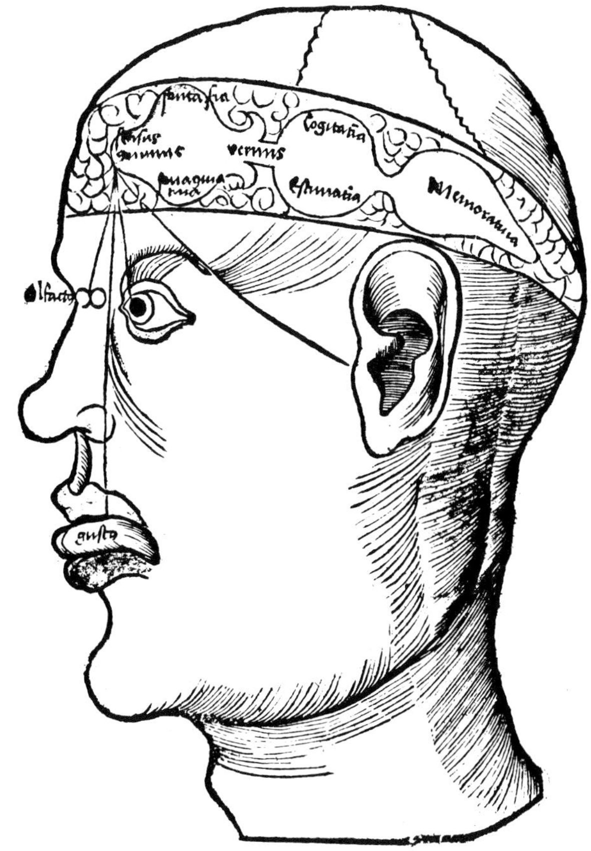

FIG. 117. Reisch (1503). Special sense impressions mix in front of first cell (*sensus communis*) and produce "phantasy" and "imagination." Choroid plexus (*vermis*) guards passage between first and second cells. In latter is cogitation and judgment (*estimativa*). Third cell stores memory.

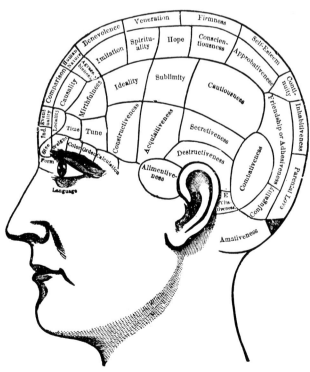

FIG. 118. *Human nature library*, New York, July 1887, p. 11, Fig. 6. The phrenological organs.

Fig. 6. THE PHRENOLOGICAL ORGANS.

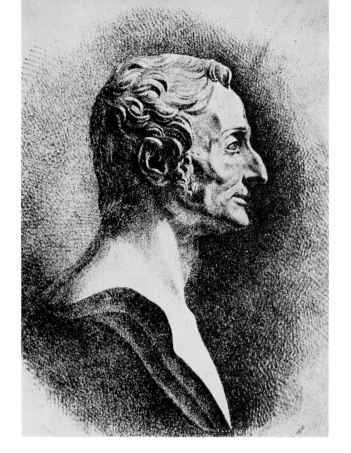

FIG. 119. Luigi Rolando. From P. Capparoni, *Profili bio-bibliografici di medici e naturalisti celebri italiani*, II, Rome, 1928, Plate XXII. By permission of the Istituto Farmacologico Serono, Rome.

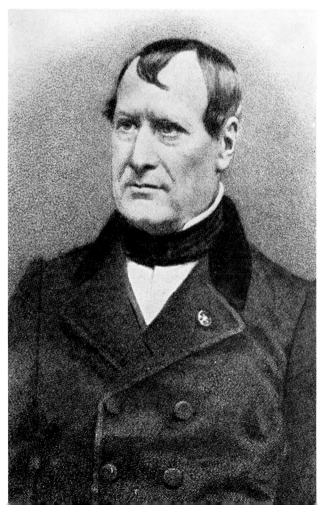

FIG. 120. Pierre Flourens. By permission of the Wellcome Trustees.

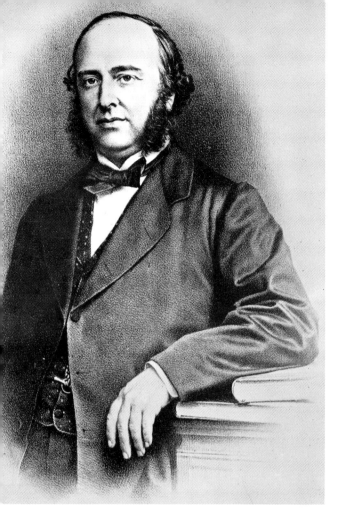

Fig. 121. Pierre-Paul Broca. From an engraving after a portrait (1867) by Lafosse. By permission of the Wellcome Trustees.

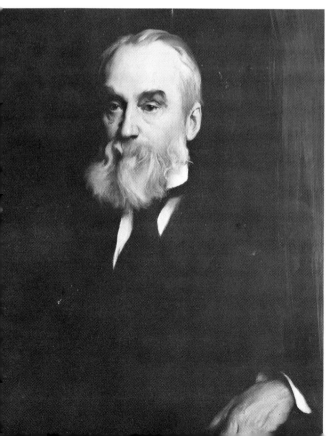

Fig. 122. John Hughlings Jackson. From a portrait in the Royal College of Physicians of London. By permission.

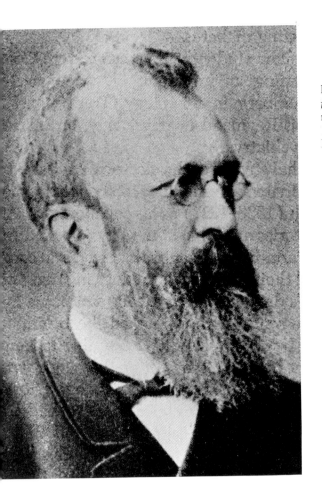

FIG. 123. Eduard Hitzig. From *The founders of neurology*, ed. W. Haymaker, Springfield, Illinois, Thomas, 1953, p. 139, and by permission of Dr. Webb Haymaker.

FIG. 124. Fritsch and Hitzig (1870, p. 313). For explanation see text (p. 510).

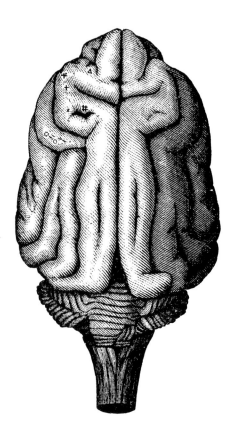

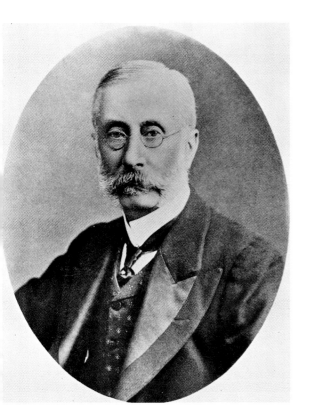

FIG. 125. David Ferrier. By permission of the Wellcome Trustees.

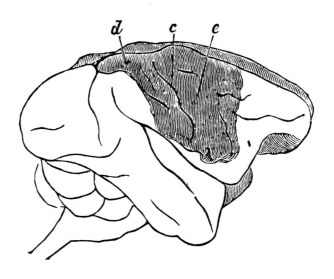

FIG. 126. Ferrier (1876, p. 201).

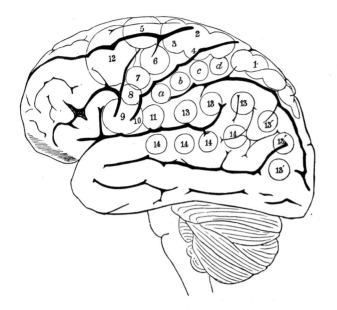

FIG. 127. Ferrier (1876, p. 304, fig. 63). Lateral view of human brain. For explanation see text (p. 517).

FIG. 128. Grünbaum and Sherrington (1902, Plate IV). Brain of chimpanzee: left hemisphere from side and above. "Motor" area stippled but much is hidden in sulci; overlapping of body areas frequent. "Eyes" areas represent conjugate eye movements.

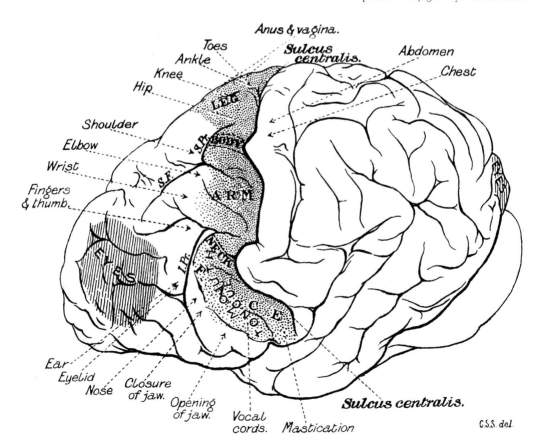

anatomical examination, the place or rather the convolution where the disease appears to have begun.

5,° In our patient, the initial site of the lesion was in the second or third frontal convolution, most likely in the latter. It is thus possible that the faculty of articulate speech is located in one or other of these two convolutions; but one cannot know this yet on account of the fact that previous observations are silent on the state of each convolution taken in turn, and one cannot even foresee it since the principle of localizations by convolutions is not yet firmly established.

6,° In any case, it suffices to compare our observation with those that have preceded it [i.e., of the phrenologists], to discard today the idea that the faculty of articulate speech resides in a fixed spot, circumscribed and situated under it-does-not-matter-which bump of the cranium; the lesions of aphemia have been found most frequently in the most anterior part of the frontal lobe not far from the eyebrow and above the orbital roof; whereas in my patient they were much further back and much nearer to the coronal suture than the supraciliary ridge. This difference of location is incompatible with the system of bumps [phrenology]; it will, on the contrary, be perfectly compatible with the system of localizations by convolutions, because each of the three great convolutions of the superior part of the frontal lobe runs successively in its antero-posterior direction through all the regions where the lesions of aphemia have so far been found.

Two years later, Broca further confirmed the principle of cortical localization ("Localisation des fonctions cérébrales.—Siège du langage articulé," *Bull. Soc. Anthrop., Paris*, 1863, 4:200–202) and stated (p. 202):

Here are eight instances in which the lesion was in the posterior third of the third frontal convolution ["the convolution of Broca" (Ferrier)]. This number seems to me to be sufficient to give strong presumptions. And the most remarkable thing is that in all the patients the lesion was on the left side. I do not dare draw conclusions from this. I await new facts.

. . . .

. . . .

. . . . Will it be possible to provide the same demonstration for other less circumscribed faculties? Perhaps this will be very difficult.

HERBERT SPENCER

(27 April 1820—8 December 1903)

It was perhaps unfortunate that the early clinical investigators chose the complex function of speech as an illustration of cortical localization. This topic is still a much disputed subject, and the precise localization of speech "centers" initiated by Broca retarded rather than facilitated its elucidation. Nevertheless, the interest that was brought to bear on the whole question of functional localization in the cortex was of the greatest significance.

So far speculators such as Gall, experimentalists such as Rolando, and clinicians such as Bouillaud, Auburtin, and Broca had contributed to the problem. But philosophers also took part, and the most important of these was the Englishman Spencer. His contribution itself was not great but it influenced the renowned neurologist John Hughlings Jackson.

Spencer was born at Derby and became first a railway engineer but abandoned this occupation about 1845. Thereafter he spent the rest of his life writing on psychology, biology, sociology, politics, and philosophy, although he had not had any formal training in these subjects (see Spencer, 1904; Elliot, 1917).

Herbert Spencer's philosophy is no longer acceptable and his huge *Principles of psychology* first published in 1855, which attempted to systematize psychological knowledge synthetically and to establish verbal formulae, was unscientific and is now obsolete. His reputation as a psychologist rests on the second edition (1870–1872), but in the first he introduced a number of original and revolutionary ideas. For example, his description of developmental levels of human intellect found expression in Hughlings Jackson's fruitful and fundamental concept of levels in the nervous system. Another of Spencer's suggestions was that the brain had localized function. The following passages illustrate this and are taken from *The principles of psychology* ([London, 1855], Ch. VII, "The feelings"). Spencer was discussing phrenology, and although he accepted its fundamental proposition, "it is in many points quite indefensible" (p. 611).

EXCERPT PP. 607–608

That, in their antagonism to the unscientific reasonings of the phrenologists, the physiologists should have gone to the extent of denying or ignoring any localization of function in the cerebrum, is, perhaps, not to be wondered at: it is in harmony with the course of controversies in general. But no physiologist who calmly considers the question in connection with the general truths of his science, can long resist the conviction that different parts of the cerebrum subserve different kinds of mental action. Localization of function is the law of all organization whatever: separateness of duty is universally accompanied with separateness of structure: and it would be marvellous were an exception to exist in the cerebral hemispheres. Let it be granted that the cerebral hemispheres are the seat of the higher psychical activities; let it be granted that among these higher psychical activities there are distinctions of kind, which, though not definite, are yet practically recognizable; and it cannot be denied, without going in direct opposition to established physiological principles, that these more or less distinct kinds of psychical activity must be carried on in more or less distinct parts of the cerebral hemispheres. To question this, is not only to ignore the truths of physiology as a whole; but especially those of the physiology of the nervous system. It is proved experimentally, that every bundle of nerve-fibres and every ganglion, has a special duty; and that each part of every such bundle and every such ganglion, has a duty still more special. Can it be, then, that in the great hemispherical ganglia alone, this specialization of duty does not hold? If it be urged that there are no marked divisions among the fibres of the cerebrum, I reply—neither are there among those contained in one of the bundles proceeding from the spinal chord to any part of the body: yet each of the fibres in such bundle has a function more or less special; though a function included in that of the bundle considered as a whole. And this is just the kind of specialization which may be presumed to exist in different parts of the cerebrum. Just as there are aggregated together in a sciatic nerve, a great number of nerve-fibres, each of which has a particular office referring to some one part of the leg, but all of which have for their joint duty the management of the leg as a whole; so, in any one region of the cerebrum, each nerve-fibre may be concluded to have some particular office, which, in common with the particular offices of thousands of neighbouring fibres, is merged in some general office which that region of the cerebrum fulfils. Indeed, any other hypothesis seems to me, on the face of it, untenable. Either there is some arrangement, some organization, in the cerebrum, or there is none. If there is no organization, the cerebrum is a chaotic mass of fibres, incapable of performing any orderly action. If there is some organization, it must consist in that same "physiological division of labour" in which all organization consists; and there is no division of labour, physiological or other, of which we have any example, or can form any conception, but what involves the concentration of special kinds of activity in special places.

John Hughlings Jackson
(4 April 1835—7 October 1911)

One of Spencer's devoted students, friends, and admirers was the British neurologist Hughlings Jackson, who helped to verify the correctness of his theoretical arguments favoring the cerebral localization just cited.

Jackson was born at Providence Green, Hammerton, Yorkshire, and he attended the York Medical School which is no longer in existence. In London he secured appointments to the London Hospital and in 1862 to the recently established National Hospital for Paralysis and Epilepsy where he became its most brilliant staff member and served for forty-five years. The majority of his clinical studies were carried out at these hospitals. Jackson was remarkable for his powers of clinical observation and for his deductive philosophic grasp. By means of these and without conducting any experiments, he was able to formulate several neurological concepts which are still fundamental to our knowledge of the nervous system, and to organize some of the chaotic mass of clinical neurological knowledge then becoming available. He often admitted his indebtedness to Spencer and also to Thomas Laycock (1812–1876); he was also importantly influenced by Brown-Séquard (see Broadbent, 1903; Hughlings Jackson, 1911*a*, 1911*b*; Hutchinson, 1911; Mercier, 1912; Taylor, 1912; Haymaker, 1953, pp. 308–311; Kolle, 1956–1963, I, 135–144).

Jackson argued that the nervous system was a sensory-motor machine divided into coordinated centers, and after careful consideration and observation of the "convulsions beginning unilaterally" ("Jacksonian epilepsy"), he suggested the probability of motor centers for various movements within the territory of the middle cerebral artery. This was pure constructive reasoning based entirely upon clinical and pathological studies. Although he postulated cortical representation of function, he did not suggest a fixed mosaic pattern, and he did not envisage the precise, circumscribed "centers" of Broca and Wernicke. It seems today that Jackson's approach was nearer the truth.

Many of his writings are scattered in obscure journals, although most of the important papers have been collected (*Selected writings of John Hughlings Jackson*, 2 vols. [London, 1931]). Often one idea must be traced through several articles to observe its development. This, together with his turgid style and the absence of summaries, makes his writings difficult to appreciate.

The first selection has been taken from an early paper ("Loss of speech," *Clin. Lect. Rep. Med. Surg. Staff London Hosp.*, 1864, 1:388–471). Jackson took Auburtin and Broca's idea a step forward by saying that if one function, speech, could be localized in the brain, why not more than one? The case he reported reminds us of Gall's comparable childhood observation which influenced him in later life (p. 478).

EXCERPT PP. 457–459

CASE XXXV.—LOSS OF SPEECH, WITH HEMIPLEGIA ON THE RIGHT SIDE

I have lately called to mind a case I knew something of when I was a boy. I was one day, about eighteen years ago, being driven to ——, one very cold morning, on my way to school. When about half-way, five miles, the driver, who had his daughter with him, about seventeen years old, asked her if she had got her keys; and as she did not reply after several inquiries, he stopped, and then found that she could not answer him. He then turned back. On reaching home, I remember being struck by a self-contradictory expression made use of by the patient. She said "I can't talk." I have since learned from the nurse who attended her, that she soon gradually lost speech altogether, and became paralysed on the right side. For three weeks she did not utter a word, but was apparently conscious, and must have swallowed well, as I have been told that her appetite was very good. The first word she ever uttered was in reply to a question—addressed to her in order to get her to talk—she said "waistcoat." It had no bearing on the question.

She regained the use of her limbs; was married about twelve years after the attack, and died a year later of convulsions in labour.

She never quite regained her power of speech, and used, even to the last, frequently to call things by the wrong names. I remember in particular, that she often made mistakes in the names of the members of her family. Her articulation was curious. She altered words, but pronounced the real or fictitious syllables of them pretty well. For instance, I once heard her call a "pigeon" a "gippin." This seems like a reversion of the syllables of the word. When a defect like this is very great—when it occurs in every word—the patient would be unintelligible. It is clearly not a defect of articulation from want of power in the lips, tongue, and palate, but rather a want of power in that part of the brain which superintends the formation (by the combination of syllables) of words, which have been selected by the general faculty of language to express (in articulate language) the particular idea to be enunciated.

Total loss of power to form words is the Aphemia of Broca; and the clumsy talking I have mentioned is, I think, but an irregular step towards recovery.

M. Broca says, that aphemia may be considered to be either the loss of a purely mental faculty, or merely a kind of locomotive ataxy. It seems to me, that a loss of guiding power in the articulatory apparatus, is at least a great part of the defect in the confused talking of which I am now speaking. It certainly exists without any obvious paralysis of the lips, tongue, or palate . . . .

. . . .

I mention the resemblance of the relation of the talk of chorea to that of incomplete aphemia, and of the bearing on it of the peculiar muscular movements in chorea in order to widen the subject for future investigation. For I think it is clear, that in chorea there is frequently disease of that part of the brain, which superintends the movements of the tongue in uttering syllables; and again, the frequent one-sided nature of the movements of the limbs, and their often dying out into definite hemiplegia points to disease of, or at least near to, the corpus striatum. Again I think from many circumstances, that embolism is a frequent cause of chorea. I do not say, plugging of the trunk of the middle cerebral, but probably of some of its ramuscles, which supply convolutions near the corpus striatum. There is no more difficulty in supposing that there are certain convolutions superintending those delicate movements of the hands, which are under the immediate control of the mind, than that there is one, as Broca suggests, for movements of the tongue in purely mental operations.

In 1870 Jackson collected a number of his observations and hypotheses and published them in an important paper ("A study of convulsions," *Trans. St. Andrews med. Grad. Assoc.*, 1870, 3:162–204; also published as a separate monograph [London, 1870]; reprinted in *Selected writings*, Vol. I [London, 1931], 8–36). In it one can follow his progress towards the idea of cortical representation of movement. His belief that the corpus striatum acted as a motor center was, however, incorrect. It should also be recalled that at this time nothing was known of the electrical properties of the cortex, despite Jackson's use of the term "discharge."

EXCERPT PP. 163–164

I chiefly wish to show in this article that the most common variety of hemispasm is a symptom of disease of the same region of the brain as is the symptom hemiplegia; viz., the "region of the corpus striatum." The loose term "region of the corpus striatum" is advisedly used. Hemiplegia shows damage (equivalent to destruction) of the motor tract, hemispasm shows damage (equivalent to changes of instability) of the convolutions which discharge through it. Palsy depends on destruction of *fibres*, and convulsion on instability of *grey matter*. As the convolutions are rich in grey matter I suppose them to be to blame, in *severe* convulsions at all events; but as the corpus striatum also contains much grey matter I cannot deny that it may be sometimes the part to blame in slighter convulsions. Indeed, if the discharge does begin in convolutions, no doubt the grey matter of lower motor centres, even if these centres be healthy, will be discharged secondarily by the violent impulse received from the primary discharge. Now both these parts—the corpus striatum and many convolutions—are supplied by one artery, the middle cerebral or Sylvian, and this artery circumscribes the region I speak of.

EXCERPT P. 186

1.—*The seat of the internal lesion.* The fact that the symptoms are local implies, I hold, that there *is* of necessity a *local* lesion. I submit that one-sided spasm, or spasm beginning in one side, implies *local* change in the central nervous system as surely as one-sided palsy does. It may be plausibly asserted that there is no local lesion in those chronic cases of convulsion where the spasm is general and also contemporaneous, or nearly contemporaneous. But in a case like Case 4, where the fits always start on one side and always in the very same fingers, it is simply incredible that there is no persistent local lesion. The fact that the patient is seemingly quite well betwixt the paroxysms does not negative this view in the least. No fact is better recognised than that a large part of one cerebral hemisphere may be *destroyed* when there are no obvious symptoms of any kind.

EXCERPT PP. 189–191

If a small number, or, let us say, a square inch, of convolutions were cut away by the knife, there would be no loss of power, no paralysis. This is admitted. How then can discharge of this square inch produce violent convulsions? If lack of the part leads to no *loss* of function, how can discharge of that part lead to *excessive* function?

As nervous processes ascend in complexity, the number of fibres of necessity increases, and at the same time the number of ganglion cells. Moreover, the ascent is not one of aggregation—different independent processes being tacked upon others. It is an evolution of the higher out of the lower, of course with additions. The facts supplied by cases of hemiplegia show that *each* part of the corpus striatum "contains" movements of the whole of the face, arm, and leg, although no doubt in each part the muscles of the face, arm, and leg are represented in different degrees, and are grouped in different order. In hemiplegia the loss is of a *certain* number of possible Simultaneous movements of the face, arm, and leg—the sum of a number of possible co-ordinations in Space. Similarly a convulsion on one side is the abrupt development of a certain number of possible Successions of movements of the face, arm, and leg—the sum of a number of possible co-ordinations in Time.

Now palsy results from destruction of *fibres*, and of course the *fewer* the fibres which go to a muscular region from a particular part of the nervous system, the *more* that region is paralysed by a destroying lesion in that part. In the ascent from the comparatively simple processes of the corpus striatum to the highly complex ones of the convolutions there will necessarily be a great increase of fibres, and hence large destroying lesions in the hemisphere will result in no palsy, whereas palsy will follow lesions equally large in the corpus striatum. But the increase of complexity necessitates many ganglion cells, results in a large supply of explosive matter, and hence excessive discharge, producing severe convulsions, occurs, when this grey matter becomes unstable.

Then it may be said that one convolution will represent only the movements of the arm, another only those of speech, another only those of the leg, and so on. The facts above stated show that this is not the plan of structure of the nervous system. Thus, to take an illustration, the external parts, x, y, and z, are each represented by units of the corpus striatum. But the plan of representation is not that some units contain x largely only, as x_3, others y largely only, as y_3, but that *each* unit contains x, y, and z—some, let us say, as x_3, y_2, z, others as x_2, y_3, z, etc. When we come to the still higher evolution of the cerebrum, we can easily understand that, if the same plan be carried out, a square inch of convolution *may be wanting,* without palsy of the face, arm, and leg, as *x*, *y*, and *z* are represented in other convolutions; and we can also easily understand that *discharge* of a square inch of convolution must put in excessive movement the *whole* region, for it contains processes representing *x*, *y*, and *z*, with grey matter in exact proportion to the degree of complexity.

In 1873 Jackson published a paper "On the anatomical and physiological localisation of movement in the brain" (*Lancet,* 1873, i:84–85, 162–164, 232–234 [no continuation as promised]) and reprinted it in 1875 together with an article by William Gowers (*Clinical and physiological researches on the nervous system,* No. 1, "On the localization of movements in the brain," London [1875]). In a lengthy preface to the reprint Jackson reviewed the development of his thoughts concerning localization.

EXCERPT PP. I–III

In former papers I have considered convulsion as a *symptom of disease* of the brain; and also, for the purposes of anatomy and physiology, *as an experiment made on the brain by disease.* This plan is complex. In the paper now republished, therefore, I considered convulsive seizures and certain cases of paralysis with regard only to the Localization of Movements in the Brain. In this Preface I shall show that I have for more than ten years, and before the experiments of Hitzig [see pp. 507–511] and Ferrier [see pp. 513–518] were made, held that convolutions contain nervous arrangements representing movements. It is in accordance with this belief that I have long considered chorea, and more lately convulsion, to be movements resulting from "discharges" of the cerebral cortex. The careful investigation of such motor symptoms, with a view to the localization of movements, is a subject in which I have for some years felt deeply interested. So far back as seven years ago I suggested that the facts of convulsive seizures should be used for purposes of Localization. In the *Medical Times and Gazette,* Aug. 15, 1868, I published a note on "Localization," various kinds of convulsive seizures being the facts brought forward. At that time, however, I believed the corpus striatum to be the part discharged in *convulsions* beginning unilaterally, although then and several years before I believed the convolutions also to contain processes representing movements. What at this time interested me most was, not so much the Localization of movements in the cerebral hemisphere, in the sense that, for example, the movements of the foot are localized here and those of the arm in another place, but the facts of the cases as they bore on a broad principle of Localization. I considered them as part of the evidence that the most special or most voluntary movements have the Leading Representation. For in disease the most voluntary or most special movements, faculties, &c., suffer first and most, that is in an order the exact opposite of Evolution. Therefore, I call this the Principle of Dissolution—Dissolution as the opposite of Evolution.

EXCERPT PP. X–XII

The reader will observe that I did not in the paper here reprinted try to *prove* that the convolutions contain processes representing movement. *I had for years assumed that convolutions contain processes representing movements and impressions.* In fact, I cannot conceive of what other materials the cerebral hemisphere can be composed than of nervous arrangements representing impressions and movements. I have long taken this for granted when considering what is commonly called the Physiology of Mind, especially with regard to speech, as well as when speaking of convulsions and chorea.

. . . . In fact, in every paper written during and since 1866, whether on chorea, convulsions, or on the physiology of language, I have *always* written on the assumption that the cerebral hemisphere is made up of processes representing impressions and movements. It seems to me to be a necessary implication of the doctrine of Nervous Evolution as this is stated by Spencer.

When speaking of convulsions (a mass of movements) as being owing to discharges of *convolutions* ("Study of Convulsions," *St. Andrew's Medical Graduates' Transactions*, vol. iii., 1870), "I say . . . . Surely the conclusion is irresistible, that 'mental' symptoms from disease of the hemisphere are fundamentally like hemiplegia, chorea, and convulsions, however specially different. They must all be due to lack, or to disorderly development, of sensori-*motor* processes."

In innumerable places I have written to the same effect explicitly or implicitly. To have long believed this is no proof of its truth; but I think that, to say the least, it adds something of plausibility to the evidence in favour of the interpretation Hitzig and Ferrier give of the results of their experiments. I had been driven to the conclusion that the convolutions *must* represent movements and impressions long before their experiments were made. So far as I can imagine, there is nothing else they can represent. I cannot conceive what even the very highest nervous centres can possibly be, except developments out of lower nervous centres, which no one doubts to represent impressions and movements. These are audacious expressions, and therefore I am very anxious to show that my opinions are not mere after-thoughts.

Experimental Studies

Experiments on the cerebral hemispheres, including stimulation of the cerebral cortex, had been undertaken sporadically from the beginning of the nineteenth century. Thus Rolando (pp. 480–482) had shown the importance of the cerebrum for motion and its response to electrical stimulation, but his conclusions were overshadowed by the more influential yet not wholly correct teachings of Flourens (pp. 483–488). Because of Flourens' important influence on Gall's concept of cerebral localization, and since Flourens' work neutralized that of Rolando, these latter two investigators could not be considered separately. Hence they have been dealt with in chronological sequence in the second section of the present chapter. Charles Bell (pp. 296–299) ought also to be mentioned at this time, since his work on the spinal roots (Bell, 1811) stemmed from a belief that different parts of the cerebrum and cerebellum had different functions (Olmsted, 1943). Furthermore, the discovery, by Legallois (pp. 294–296), in the same year, 1811, of the respiratory center in the medulla oblongata, was perhaps the earliest example of precise localization of function within the brain.

In addition, other isolated attempts at cortical excitation had been made, but the weight of authority was in favor of Flourens' negative results. At this time knowledge of the physiology of the nerve impulse was developing side by side with technical advances required for the successful investigations of cortical responses to electrical stimulation. As adequate apparatus and methods became available the field developed rapidly and the electrophysiological literature from 1870, the beginning of modern cortical physiology, expanded accordingly. The selections given below are arranged according to anatomical division. The first deal mainly with the motor area and are followed by those illustrating investigations of the occipital, temporal, and frontal lobes. This second group is predominantly physiological but anatomy also contributed in the form of myelo- and cytoarchitectonics, as did clinical neurology; this last contribution was extensive but is represented here mainly by the work of Henschen (pp. 533–535). Finally, the movement away from circumscribed and mosaic-like cortical "centers" to a more integrative concept of function has been illustrated by the work of those who opposed the localizers, that is, the antilocalizers.

As in the case of earlier experimenters such as Rolando and Flourens, the two most important factors in experimental studies, such as excitation and ablation, were the mechanical techniques employed and the powers of observation of the experimenter, coupled with his ability to devise methods of assessing the many disorders of function in his animals. Thus it is not by chance that when the selected studies of the cortex contained in the present work have been placed in chronological order, they are also found to be in a sequence of functional disorders of increasing complexity and difficulty of examination. Motor defects were relatively easy to evaluate in animals, but sensory, visual, auditory, and mental signs have presented increasingly difficult problems to the observer. In the early part of our present period the clinical examination of the patient was limited enough, and that of the experimental animal was therefore necessarily more primitive. Hence, in the earlier research reports there is no doubt that functions said to be normal may, in fact, not have been so.

The varying organization in different species of animals is an important aspect of mammalian cortical localization, and the neglect of a comprehensive comparative approach to the problem has been partly responsible for past errors and for the delay in determining the full pattern of representation. Thus in the case of the motor cortex a recent careful study of the rat has led to a reexamination of the monkey with consequent modifications of previous concepts. There is no doubt that some of the confusion experienced by early investigators stemmed from their neglect of species differences and their willingness to compare findings in animals with those that might be found in man.

Another factor that must be recalled when evaluation of early experiments on cortical stimulation and ablation is made, concerns the anatomy, both macroscopic and microscopic, of the cortex. Until the neuron theory was adopted (Chapter II), until something was known of nerve function (Chapter III), and until the various technological advances associated with them had been made, no investigations of the cerebral cortex could be adequately precise. Thus ability to locate a cortical lesion exactly and to avoid damaging adjacent tissue unwittingly, is an essential basis for any experiment. Still another factor of vital importance has been the need to avoid postoperative complications, especially inflammatory ones. Their occurrence owing to primitive surgical techniques has been another complicating factor (A. E. Walker, 1957*a*, 1957*b*).

A. Mainly Motor Functions

The pioneer stimulators of the cerebral cortex found the elicited motor responses the easiest to study, and likewise the deficiencies of motion produced by ablation. The early papers on the experimental study of cortical function therefore dealt more extensively with the motor areas. Only five contributors to this ever expanding field of knowledge have been selected for consideration.

Eduard Hitzig
(*6 February 1838—28 August 1907*)

Gustav Theodor Fritsch
(*5 March 1838—12 June 1927*)

In 1870 a new era in the concept of cortical localization began and we are still in it today. It was opened by two young Germans, Hitzig and Fritsch, who were able to confirm experimentally the conclusions that Hughlings Jackson had arrived at solely by means of clinical observation and reasoning, which many had thought

ingenious but fanciful. They demonstrated that electrical stimulation of the cerebral cortex induced motor responses and for this purpose used techniques not
available to earlier workers.

Hitzig, who was the more outstanding of the two, was born in Berlin and
received his degree there in 1862. He first of all engaged in private practice in Berlin
and was thus employed when he collaborated with Fritsch. In 1875 he was
appointed professor of psychiatry in Zürich and four years later moved to Halle,
first of all as the director of a psychiatric clinic and later as director of a new
university neuropsychiatric clinic; he retired in 1903. His main work concerned
cerebral physiology and he was a typical example of the German nineteenth
century pure experimental physiologist (see Wollenberg, 1908; Anton, 1914; Haymaker, 1953, pp. 138–142).

Fritsch came of wealthy parents and attended medical school in Berlin. With his
private income he was able to travel widely and interested himself in activities apart
from physiology. Eventually he became chief of histology and photography in du
Bois-Reymond's institute and in particular investigated the electric fish. In 1870 he
was appointed professor *extraordinarius* of physiology in the University of Berlin
but was not promoted further (Grundfest, 1963).

The experiments of Hitzig and Fritsch were carried out in the former's bedroom
and consisted of stimulation of the dog's exposed cerebral cortex with a pair of
blunted electrodes carrying a stimulus from the closing, opening, or commutation
of the current of a galvanic pile of sufficient intensity to cause a distinct sensation
when applied to the tip of the tongue. It seems likely that a continuous current of
about 1 mA. with a maximum of 11 V. was used (A. E. Walker, 1957*a*). From the
resultant muscular movements the experimenters were able to map crudely the
motor part of the cortex (fig. 124). Their famous article, dated 28 April 1870, was
entitled "Über die elektrische Erregbarkeit des Grosshirns" (*Arch. Anat. Physiol.*,
1870, pp. 300–332), and the following selections have been translated from it.

EXCERPT P. 308

These investigations were prompted by observations which one of us
[Hitzig, see *Berl. klin. Wschr.*, 1870, 7:137–138] had the opportunity of
carrying out in man, regarding movements of voluntary muscles; these were
produced, for the first time, by direct stimulation of the central organ in the
human subject. It was found that by passing constant galvanic currents
through the posterior part of the head, one could easily produce movements of the eyes, which, by their very nature could only have been
produced by the direct stimulation of cerebral centers. Inasmuch as these
movements only occur with galvanization of this particular part of the
head, they could be considered as owing to stimulation of the quadrigeminal bodies, which seemed likely, or of adjacent parts. However, when
actions were employed to increase the excitability, these ocular movements
also occurred with galvanization of the temporal region. The question

therefore arose, whether this method caused the eye movements by circuits or currents penetrating to the base, *or, whether the cerebrum, contrary to the generally accepted view, is endowed with electric excitability.*

Since a preliminary experiment which one of us conducted in the rabbit had a generally positive result, we set up the following investigation, in order to reach a definitive solution to this question.

The results of their experiments on dogs were as follows.

EXCERPT PP. 310–314

Part of the convexity of the cerebrum is motor (we are using this expression in Schiff's sense), *another part is non-motor.*

In general, the motor part is located in the anterior, the non-motor in the posterior part. By stimulating the motor part electrically one obtains combined muscular contractions of the opposite half of the body.

With the use of very weak currents, these contractions can be localized to specific, strictly limited muscle groups. By stimulating the same or closely adjacent parts with stronger currents, other muscles were immediately involved, as well as muscles of the same side of the body. *When employing extremely weak currents, the possibility of isolated excitability of a narrowly delimited muscle group is, however, restricted to very small foci,* which we shall call centers for the sake of brevity. As a rule, a very minute shifting of the electrodes still causes a movement of the same extremity; however, if, for example, extension occurred first, such extension elicited flexion or rotation. With the described method of stimulation and with the use of extremely low currents, we found that the surface of the cerebrum lying between the areas designated by us as centers, could not be stimulated. However, if we increased either the distance from each other of the two electrodes or the strength of the current, we were able to produce contractions; but these involved the entire body in such manner that it was impossible to differentiate clearly whether they were unilateral or bilateral.

The location of the centers, which we shall soon define more closely, is very constant in the dog. The precise demonstration of this fact met with some difficulties at the start. However, we disposed of these by first locating the area where the weakest current that would still excite, resulted in the most marked contraction of the group in question. We then stuck a pin between the two electrodes into the cerebrum of the living animal and, following removal of the brain, compared the individual points thus marked with those of the alcohol-preserved preparations from previous experiments. How constantly the same centers are located is best revealed by the fact that we repeatedly succeeded in locating the desired centers at the center of a single trephine hole without opening the skull further. Upon removal of the dura, the muscles which depend on the center contracted with the same certainty as if the entire hemisphere had been exposed . . . .

To facilitate repetition of our experiments we shall report the following exact data regarding the localization of the individual motor centers, and, in doing so, we adhere to Owen's nomenclature [Owen, 1868, p. 118].

The center for the neck muscles (see Δ in the fig. [fig. 124]) is situated in the middle of the prefrontal gyrus, exactly where the surface of this gyrus conceals, in the region of the lateral end of the frontal fissure, the center for the extensors and adductors of the muscles of the foreleg (see + in the fig.). A little posterior to the latter and closer to the coronal fissure (see + in the fig.) are the central areas which guide the flexion and rotation of the limb. The area for the hind leg (see # in the fig.) lies also in the postfrontal gyrus but medial to that of the foreleg and slightly more posterior. The facial nerve (see ⌀ in the fig.) is innervated by the middle portion of the suprasylvian [second basal] gyrus. The point in question often exceeds 0.5 cm. in size and extends from the main bend above the Sylvian fissure forwards and downwards.

We must add that it was not possible in every case to set the neck muscles in motion from the first mentioned point. However, we have often succeeded in exciting to contraction the back, tail, and abdominal muscles, starting at the parts between the points marked. And yet it was impossible to establish definitively a circumscribed point from which they could be individually excited. We found that the entire portion of the convexity posterior to the facial center was absolutely inexcitable, even when subjected to disproportionate intensities of current.

Having described in detail the results of cortical stimulation, Fritsch and Hitzig carried out an experiment to produce the reverse situation. In two dogs they removed an area of cortex which by prior stimulation had been shown to represent the right foreleg. They observed the following.

EXCERPT PP. 329–332

I. While running the animals set down their right anterior paw clumsily, now more medially, now more laterally than the other, and they then slid slightly laterally on this paw but never with the other, so that they fell to the ground. No movement was lost completely; however, the right leg was drawn up somewhat less.

II. Very similar phenomena while standing. Besides, it happens that the anterior paw is put down with the dorsum instead of with the sole, without the dog realizing this at all.

III. While sitting on his buttocks and with both anterior paws on the ground, the right anterior paw gradually slides laterally until the dog lies completely on his right side.

However, he can always get up immediately under all circumstances. The skin sensation and the sensation of deep pressure show no detectable changes in the right anterior paw.

. . . .

. . . .

. . . .

However this may be, it is certain that an injury of this center alters only the voluntary movement of the limb which surely depends upon it, but does not abolish it, so that the motor impulse has therefore other areas and pathways still ready to be brought into play and to hurry to the muscles of that leg . . . . Moreover, it is equally certain that such an injury, although its importance decreases when the reports by Flourens, Hertwig, and others are considered, produces demonstrable symptoms, provided the correct area is affected; indeed, the symptoms become most obvious in the limb of which the muscles contracted with previous electrical stimulation of the [cerebral] substance, which was then destroyed.

Thus it becomes evident that in the previous extensive mutilations of the cerebrum, either other parts had been selected or insufficient attention had been given to the performance of finer movements. Furthermore, it may be concluded from the sum of all our experiments that, contrary to the opinions of Flourens and most investigators who followed him, the soul in no case represents a sort of total function of the whole of the cerebrum, the expression of which might be destroyed by mechanical means *in toto*, but not in its individual parts. *Individual psychological functions, and probably all of them, depend for their entrance into matter or for their formation from it, upon circumscribed centers of the cerebral cortex.*

ROBERTS BARTHOLOW
(28 November 1831—10 May 1904)

Fritsch and Hitzig and Ferrier had studied the response of animals to cortical stimulation, and Ferrier had inferred (pp. 513–518) that the human brain had similar properties. The next step in the proof had to await the opportunity of the clinic; but just as Broca's case appeared at an appropriate moment (pp. 494–497), so did the chance of exploring the human cortex electrically. It came to the American, Bartholow, in 1874.

Roberts Bartholow was born at New Windsor, Maryland, of Alsatian and English parentage and received the M.D. degree from the University of Maryland in 1852. Eventually, in 1864, he settled in practice in Cincinnati, Ohio, where he was also appointed professor of medical chemistry and the practice of medicine at the Medical College there. He spent his later life in Philadelphia where he was professor of materia medica at the Jefferson Medical College. He wrote mainly on therapeutics and his books were widely popular (see Holland, 1904).

In 1874 Bartholow had under his care a patient, Mary Rafferty, with a large cranial defect which exposed the posterior parts of each cerebral hemisphere. Hence he was able to stimulate her brain, but the experiments were terminated by the girl's death from meningitis. He published an account of his observations without comment ("Experimental investigations into the functions of the human brain," *Am. J. med. Sci.*, 1874, 67:305–313), and the following selections have been taken from it.

EXCERPT PP. 309–311

Apparatus and Method of Experiment.—Galvanic current from a 60 Siemens and Halske cup battery. Faradic current, primary, from Galvano-Faradic company's double cell battery. Insulated needle electrodes of various lengths.

As portions of brain-substance have been lost by injury or by the surgeon's knife, and as the brain has been deeply penetrated by incisions made for the escape of pus, it was supposed that fine needles could be introduced without material injury to the cerebral matter. The needles being insulated to near their points, it was believed that diffusion of the current could be as restricted as in the experiments of Fritsch and Hitzig and Ferrier . . . .

. . . .

Observation 2. To test faradic reaction of the surface of the dura mater.—Two needles insulated were introduced into left side until their points were well engaged in the dura mater. When the circuit was closed, distinct muscular contractions occurred in the right arm and leg. The arm was thrown out, the fingers extended, and the leg was projected forward. The muscles of the neck were thrown into action, and the head was strongly deflected to the right. These effects were produced by the current from one cup, the wooden cylinder entirely inclosing the bobbin. (Current of least volume and intensity from one cup.)

The same phenomena precisely occurred when the right posterior lobe was acted upon by a current of the same strength. The head was deflected strongly to the left, and the extensors of the left arm and leg were thrown into action.

Observation 3. To test faradic reaction of the posterior lobes.—Passed an insulated needle into the left posterior lobe so that the non-insulated portion rested entirely in the substance of the brain. The other insulated needle was placed in contact with the dura mater, within one-fourth of an inch of the first. When the circuit was closed, muscular contraction of the right upper and lower extremities ensued, as in the preceding observations. Faint but visible contraction of the left orbicularis palpebrarum, and dilatation of the pupils, also ensued. Mary complained of a very strong and unpleasant feeling of tingling in both right extremities, especially in the right arm, which she seized with the opposite hand and rubbed vigorously. Notwithstanding the very evident pain from which she suffered, she smiled as if much amused.

The needle was now withdrawn from the left lobe and passed in the same way into the substance of the right. When the current passed, precisely the same phenomena ensued in the left extremities and in the right orbicularis palpebrarum and pupils. When the needle entered the brain-substance, she complained of acute pain in the neck. In order to develop more decided reactions, the strength of the current was increased by drawing out the wooden cylinder one inch. When communication was made with the needles, her countenance exhibited great distress, and she began to cry.

The above experiment terminated in a left focal convulsion which became generalized and lasted five minutes. After death the brain was fixed and examined.

EXCERPT P. 312

. . . . On the left side the needle had entered the upper parietal lobule of Ecker . . . the gyrus centralis posterior of Henle . . . the postero-parietal lobule of Turner, one inch from the longitudinal fissure, and had penetrated a depth of one inch. The track of the needle was marked by some diffluent cerebral matter two lines in diameter.

On the right side the needle had entered the same convolution, but more posteriorly, and one inch and a half from the great longitudinal fissure. The needle on the right side had also penetrated to a greater depth—one and a half inch—and its track through the lobe was marked, as on the other side, by a line of diffluent cerebral matter.

DAVID FERRIER
(13 January 1843—19 March 1928)

The revolutionary findings of Fritsch and Hitzig resultant from their stimulation and ablation experiments were not accepted immediately. They were diametrically opposed to the opinion of the majority of physiologists, including such authorities as Flourens, Magendie, Deen, Longet, Eduard Weber, and Budge; and furthermore both investigators were young and unknown. It seemed that only the early and primitive work of Rolando (pp. 481–483) gave them support, although admittedly tenuous.

However, confirmation was soon forthcoming from the British neurologist Ferrier, who repeated the experiments of Fritsch and Hitzig, but mainly in the primates, with the express purpose of reproducing experimentally the "discharging" and "destroying" lesions of Hughlings Jackson and so putting to the test his opinions regarding unilateral epileptic convulsions and cortical localization (pp. 500–507). It was owing to Ferrier's work that those opinions were placed upon a sure basis of experimental fact.

Ferrier was born at Woodside near Aberdeen and educated at the Universities of Aberdeen, Heidelberg, and Edinburgh. He received his medical degree at Edinburgh in 1868 and moved to London in 1870. In 1872 he was appointed to the staff of King's College Medical School and to that of the National Hospital, Queen Square, in 1880; in 1873 he had worked temporarily at the West Riding Lunatic Asylum in Wakefield, Yorkshire. A chair of neuropathology was created for him at King's College Hospital Medical School in 1889, and in 1911 he was knighted. Ferrier divided his interests between clinical neurology and neurophysiology, but his chief contributions were to the latter and they were mainly concerned with cortical function (see Sherrington, 1928; Stewart, 1928; Viets, 1938; Haymaker, 1953, pp. 122–125).

Whereas Fritsch and Hitzig had used the galvanic electrical current, Ferrier employed the faradic, and his method, which was itself an important experimental advance, was followed by all subsequent observers until the introduction of improved techniques in the 1920's. He first of all confirmed the findings of Fritsch and Hitzig and then made comparable investigations in the monkey in which he mapped the cerebral cortex and showed that the precentral, superior temporal, and parietal lobe gyri formed the excitable area; above all, he delineated the motor cortex, his "motor-region." His results appeared first in an article entitled "Experimental researches in cerebral physiology and pathology" (*West Riding Lun. Asyl. med. Rep.*, 1873, 3:30–96), and in 1876 he published a book, *The functions of the brain* (London, 1876), in which he repeated his earlier results and extended them. It was one of the most important publications in the field of cortical localization. A later and detailed review of his results, and of those who followed him, appeared in his Croonian Lectures of June 1890 (*The Croonian Lectures on cerebral localisation*, London, 1890). The following selections have been taken from his book of 1876.

EXCERPT PP. 199–202

SECTION II.—THE MOTOR CENTRES

72. It has been shown in the preceding chapter that electrical irritation of the brain of the monkey at certain definite points in the convolutions, which, speaking generally, bound the fissure of Rolando, gives rise to certain definite and constant movements of the hands, feet, arms, legs, facial muscles, mouth, and tongue, etc. Similar, and in many respects completely homologous movements, were shown to result from irritation of the frontal regions of the external convolutions in the brain of the cat, dog,

and jackal, and of the anatomically corresponding frontal regions of the smooth brain of the rodents; the regions characterised by similarity of movements having been indicated in the figures and description by the same letters of designation.

. . . .

. . . .

The question, however, with which we are more particularly engaged is the determination of the physiological significance of these regions. The mere fact of the excitation of movements is, as we have already seen, no proof that the regions stimulated have a motor significance, for the stimulation of a sensory centre may give rise to reflex or associated movements. Whether the centres now under consideration are directly motor, or only give rise to movements in a reflex or indirect manner when stimulated, is a question which has been answered differently by different investigators on this subject. The definite purposive character clearly perceivable in many of the movements, and their correspondence with the ordinary volitional activities and peculiarities of the animals, apart from other considerations, point rather to the conclusion that they are the result of the artificial excitation of the functional activity of centres immediately concerned in effecting volitional movements, and as such truly motor. As the question, however, is one capable of being answered by direct experiments, we may proceed to the consideration of these. If these regions are centres of voluntary motion, paralysis of voluntary motion ought to follow from their destruction, and any apparent exception to this result must be capable of satisfactory explanation, consistently with this view, if it is the correct one.

The following experiments on monkeys give no uncertain reply to the questions stated.

The first experiment I have to record is instructive, as showing the respective effects of irritation and destruction of the convolutions bounding the fissure of Rolando. The right hemisphere of a monkey had been exposed and subjected to experimentation with electrical irritation. The part exposed included the ascending parietal, ascending frontal, and posterior extremities of the frontal convolutions. The animal was allowed to recover, for the purpose of watching the effects of exposure of the brain. Next day the animal was found perfectly well. Towards the close of the day following, on which there were signs of inflammatory irritation and suppuration, it began to suffer from choreic spasms of the left angle of the mouth and left arm, which recurred repeatedly, and rapidly assumed an epileptiform character, affecting the whole of the left side of the body. Next day left hemiplegia had become established, the angle of the mouth drawn to the right, the left cheek-pouch flaccid and distended with food, which had accumulated outside the dental arch; there being almost total paralysis of the left arm, and partial paralysis of the left leg. On the day following the paralysis of motion was complete over the whole of the left side, and continued so till death, nine days subsequently. Tactile sensation, as well as sight, hearing, smell, and taste, were retained. On *post-mortem* examination it was found that the exposed convolutions were completely softened, but beyond this the rest of the hemisphere and the basal ganglia were free from organic injury (fig. 52 [fig. 126]).

In this we have a clear case, first, of vital irritation producing precisely the same effects as the electric current, and then destruction by inflammatory softening, resulting in complete paralysis of voluntary motion on the opposite side of the body, without affection of sensation.

EXCERPT P. 204

To these experiments I might add others, in which, from extension of the lesion, at first circumscribed to the sensory centres (angular gyrus, etc.) some limited paralysis exhibited itself, as of the wrist and hand. Such cases always coincided with softening of the respective motor centre, as already determined by the electrical exploration. In all cases, so long as observation could be maintained, the progress, as regards the paralysis, was always from bad to worse, there being no appearance of compensatory action, or return of the faculty of movement when the centre was effectually disorganised. No evidence could to my mind more convincingly prove that destruction of the cortical substance of what we may justly term the motor centres in the monkey causes paralysis of the movements determined by the electric stimulus, and that this paralysis is entirely dissociated from sensory paralysis in any form. It has been shown that paralysis of tactile sensation may cause paralysis of motion, by abolishing that which is the usual guide to muscular movement. In these experiments the power of movement alone was destroyed, sensation remaining acute and unimpaired.

In the same book Ferrier mapped the cortical functions in the monkey brain and then transferred them to a diagram of the human brain (fig. 127). This cortical map, reminiscent of the phrenologists' charts, was the first of its kind and it influenced investigators considerably. Today the precise and circumscribed areas that Ferrier found in the monkey and then extrapolated to man (pp. 305–308) are not accepted, but the belief in *centers* was an important and inevitable phase in the development of the concept of cortical localization. He was not alone in his unwarranted use of data from animal studies in an attempt to elucidate the human cortex (see Krause, pp. 523–526). In this regard the famous remark of Charcot should be recalled. At the International Medical Congress of 1881 in London Ferrier demonstrated one of his monkeys which had been rendered hemiplegic by cortical ablation. On seeing the affected limbs Charcot exclaimed, "It is a patient!"

EXCERPT PP. 305–308

121. In the accompanying figures [only fig. 63 (fig. 127) has been repro-
duced] I have indicated approximately the situation of the centres or areas
[in man] homologous with those experimentally determined in the brain of
the monkey. An exact correspondence can scarcely be supposed to exist,
inasmuch as the movements of the arm and hand are more complex and
differentiated than those of the monkey; while, on the other hand, there is
nothing in man to correspond with the prehensile movements of the lower
limbs and tail in the monkey.

In fig. 63 [fig. 127] a lateral view of the left hemisphere of the human
brain is given, and the same letters placed on regions approximately corresponding to those on fig. 64 [lateral view of monkey brain].

. . . .

(1), placed on the postero-parietal lobule, indicates the position of the
centres for movements of the opposite leg and foot such as are concerned in
locomotion.

(2), (3), (4), placed together on the convolutions bounding the upper
extremity of the fissure of Rolando, include centres for various complex
movements of the arms and legs, such as are concerned in climbing, swimming, etc.

(5), situated at the posterior extremity of the superior frontal convolution, at its junction with the ascending frontal, is the centre for the
extension forwards of the arm and hand, as in putting forth the hand to
touch something in front.

(6), situated on the ascending frontal, just behind the upper end of the
posterior extremity of the middle frontal convolution, is the centre for the
movements of the hand and forearm in which the biceps is particularly
engaged, viz., supination of the hand and flexion of the forearm.

(7) and (8), centres for the elevators and depressors of the angle of the
mouth respectively.

(9) and (10), included together in one, mark the centre for the movements of the lips and tongue, as in articulation. This is the region, disease
of which causes aphasia, and is generally known as Broca's convolution.

(11), the centre of the platysma, retraction of the angle of the mouth.

(12), a centre for lateral movements of the head and eyes, with elevation
of the eyelids and dilatation of pupil.

(*a*), (*b*), (*c*), (*d*), placed on the ascending parietal convolution, indicate the centres of movement of the hand and wrist.

Circles (13) and (13′) placed on the supra-marginal lobule and angular
gyrus, indicate the centre of vision.

Circles (14) placed on the superior temporo-sphenoidal convolution, indicate the situation of the centre of hearing.

The centre of smell is situated in the subiculum cornu Ammonis.

In close proximity, but not exactly defined as to limits, is the centre of taste.

The centre of touch is situated in the hippocampal region.

Being a clinician as well as an experimentalist, Ferrier was aware of the clinical implications of his findings, and, like Hughlings Jackson, he was interested in extending his knowledge of cortical function by observing the effects on it of disease processes. The following is from his Gulstonian Lectures for 1878 (*The localisation of cerebral disease*, London, 1878).

EXCERPT P. 23

The conclusion, therefore, which I would provisionally draw from the results of experimental physiology, and proceed to justify by a consideration of the facts of human pathology, is, that there are certain regions in the cortex to which definite functions can be assigned; and that the phenomena of cortical lesions will vary according to their seat, and also according to their character—viz., whether irritative or destructive, two classes into which they may all be theoretically reduced. And, as the experiments of physiology necessitate the strictest topographical accuracy in the position and limits of individual centres, it is of vital importance that the same accuracy should be observed in respect to the situation of lesions in the human brain.

ALBERT SIDNEY FRANKAU GRÜNBAUM   CHARLES SCOTT SHERRINGTON
(*Known as* A. S. F. LEYTON *from 1915*)   (*See p. 238*)
(*5 June 1869—21 September 1921*)

Although Ferrier and others had defined a motor area of the cerebral cortex, it was thought by some (e.g., Mott, 1894) that only a mixed sensory-motor region existed. By the end of the nineteenth century many investigations of the cortex had been carried out, but those that established the pre-Rolandic motor area separate from the sensory region posterior to it were the work of Grünbaum and Sherrington.

Grünbaum was born in London and studied medicine at Cambridge and at St. Thomas's Hospital, London. After study in Vienna (1896) he took up an appointment with Sherrington at Liverpool. In 1904 he moved to Leeds as professor of pathology and in 1919 was made director of the clinical laboratory at Addenbrooke's Hospital, Cambridge. In 1915 he changed his name to Leyton. His main work was in the field of cancer research (see Grünbaum, 1921*a*, 1921*b*; G. H. Brown, 1955, p. 438).

Grünbaum and Sherrington worked with lightly anesthetized, anthropoid apes, the orang, the gorilla, and the chimpanzee, and employed unipolar faradization from an inductorium that allowed finer localization than would have been the case with the usual double electrode. Apart from the motor eye fields, the excitable areas delineated were confined to the pre-Rolandic convolutions. Their first report was read to the Royal Society on 21 November 1901 ("Observations on the physiology of the cerebral cortex of some of the higher apes (Preliminary communication)," *Proc. R. Soc.*, 1902, 69:206–209). The following selection has been taken from their account of the "motor" area.

EXCERPT PP. 206–208

II. "MOTOR" (SO-CALLED) AREA

This area [see figs. 128 and 129] we find to include continuously the whole length of the precentral convolution. It also enters into the whole length of the *sulcus centralis*, with the usual exception of its extreme lower tip and its extreme upper tip.

In all the animals examined, we have found the "motor" area not to at any point extend behind *sulcus centralis*. Feeble reactions can occasionally, under certain circumstances, be provoked by strong faradisation behind the *sulcus centralis*, but these are equivocal, and appear under conditions that exclude their acceptance as equivalent to "motor-area" reactions.

On the mesial surface of the hemisphere the "motor" area has extended less far down than was expected. It has not extended to the calloso-marginal fissure. Certain areas near that fissure have yielded us movements, e.g., of shoulder, body, wrist, and fingers; but we hesitate, for reasons to be given in a fuller communication, to class these with those of the "motor" area proper.

We have found the precentral convolution excitable over its free width, and continuously round into and to the bottom of the *sulcus centralis*. The "motor" area extends also into the depth of other fissures besides the Rolandic, as can be described in a fuller communication than the present. The hidden part of the excitable area probably equals, perhaps exceeds, in extent that contributing to the free surface of the hemisphere. We have in some individuals found the deeper part of the posterior wall of the *sulcus centralis* to contribute to the "motor" area.

In the "motor" area we have found localised, besides very numerous other actions, certain movements of the ear, nostril, palate, movements of sucking, of mastication, of the vocal cords, of the chest wall, of the abdominal wall, of the pelvic floor, of the anal orifice, and of the vaginal orifice. We have met with various examples of inhibition effects produced by this cortex, such as described by one of us [C. S. S.] previously in the cortex of the lower apes.

We find the arrangement of the representation of various regions of the musculature follow the segmental sequence of the cranio-spinal nerve-series to a very remarkable extent. The accompanying figure (Plate 4 [fig. 128]) indicates better than can a verbal description the degree of adherence to this sequence.

We do not find that the exciting current for the "motor" cortex requires to be extremely strong for the anthropoid brain. "Epilepsy" is easily evoked from the cortex of the anthropoids.

Our experiments show that the *sulci* in the region of cortex dealt with can in no sense be considered to signify physiological boundaries. Further, the variation of the *sulci* in these higher brains is so great from individual to individual that, as our observations show, they prove but precarious, even fallacious, landmarks to the details of the true topography of the cortex.

. . . .

Extirpation of the hand area by itself has been followed by severe paresis of the hand, the hand being for a few days practically useless and seemingly "powerless." In a few weeks use and "power" were remarkably regained in the hand, so that it was once more used for climbing, &c. The animal ultimately not unfrequently fed itself with fruit, making use of that hand alone. Even small ablations in the pre-central gyrus have led to severe though quickly diminishing pareses. On the other hand, ablations of even large portions of post-central gyrus have not given any even transient paresis.

The second paper of Grünbaum and Sherrington was read on 11 June 1903 ("Observations on the physiology of the cerebral cortex of the anthropoid apes," *Proc. R. Soc.*, 1903, 72:152–155). In particular they noted facilitating influences (*Bahnung*) that were to be of great significance.

EXCERPT PP. 152–153

Repeated observations on excitation of the cortex of the pre-central convolution confirm an opinion we had formed at the time of our former communication, and indicated in the diagram then furnished, but not verbally expressed. This is to the effect that the anterior limit of the "motor" field is not of sharp, abrupt character, but fades off forward somewhat gradually. This edge extends further forward under *Bahnung* [facilitating influence]. Under general conditions producing lowered excitability of the cortex it retires backward in the direction of the central fissure.

In a similar manner the boundary of the area for any particular movement, may by *Bahnung* be extended beyond its average limit. The special form of movement provoked from a given spot of cortex is thus influenced by the particular forms of movement excited from neighbouring points just antecedently.

. . . . In short, neither the ablation or the excitation methods gave any evidence that the remaining part of the arm area had taken on the functions of the ablated hand area. The recovery of hand movement seems, therefore, not due to either the adjacent cortex of the same hemisphere, or to the corresponding hand area of the opposite hemisphere, taking on the functions of the ablated cortical hand area.

Faradisation of the cortex of the post-central convolution, though not like the pre-central itself eliciting movement, when employed at certain places facilitates the elicitation of movement by faradisation at certain points at about the same horizontal level in the pre-central convolution. In other words, from certain parts of the post-central convolution, a facilitating influence (*Bahnung*) can be exerted upon somewhat adjacent parts of the pre-central convolution.

Removal of the adjacent levels of the pre-central convolution does not render the post-central convolution "excitable"; that is to say, destruction of the pre-central convolution does not make it the more possible to obtain movements under faradisation from the post-central convolution.

Their final paper on the motor area of the primate cerebral cortex appeared in 1917 ("Observations on the excitable cortex of the chimpanzee, orang-utan, and gorilla," *Q. Jl. exp. Physiol.*, 1917, 11:135–222). As well as presenting a detailed account of functional areas, the authors analyzed the "functional instability" encountered with stimulation of the same cortical point. This has since been shown to correspond closely to the findings in man. Much of this work had been done earlier, but owing to a disagreement with Sir Victor Horsley, Sherrington delayed publication of it until the former's death in 1917 (Fulton, 1952a).

FUNCTIONAL INSTABILITY OF CORTICAL MOTOR POINTS

This raises the question of the functional instability of a motor cortical point. In addition to the influence of depth of narcosis, freedom of blood supply, local temperature, and such effects of experimental exposure of the cortex as "drying" or inspissation of applied Locke's solution, the motor responses of a cortical point may be easily and greatly modified by precurrent, especially closely precurrent, stimulation either of itself or of neighbouring, especially closely adjacent, cortical points. The motor response from a given point, though it may, as the maps of cortical localisation usually depict, remain approximately the same throughout a lengthy experiment, even from hour to hour, when similar stimuli are repeated at intervals not too brief, may yet vary considerably in result of precurrent stimulations not too distant in time and place. Experiments in which a large field of cortex is examined systematically point for point by electrical stimulation to determine the functional localisation are likely to display the influence of previous stimulation of one point upon another.

Three phenomena of this kind, presumably all closely akin, make themselves evident in an examination of the motor cortex, namely, *facilitation of response, reversal of response, and deviation of response.* Of these the first, noted by various observers and particularly fully studied recently by T. Graham Brown in the chimpanzee as well as in macacus and other monkeys, is characterised by a change of the cortical point's response in the direction of increase, with or without other modification. It may be induced by stimulation of the point itself or by the stimulation of other points. Reversal of response is a change supervening which may culminate in complete reversal of the sense of the movement of the response, e.g., extension of a joint may become flexion of that joint. Deviation of response is a change which alters the character of the response, so that instead of the original movement appearing, some other movement, e.g., of another joint or part, appears in place of the original. All these changes are temporary. They may be taken as expressions of what has been termed the functional instability of a cortical motor point.

1. *Facilitation of Response.* Facilitation of response has been a usual accompaniment of our observations on the anthropoid motor cortex. Comparing our experience of it there with our experience of it in macaque and callithrix, facilitation seems to be somewhat more extensive in the anthropoid than in the lower forms of monkey. Thus, as was remarked in our preliminary communication, it affects the delimitation of the whole of the anterior border of the motor field. That border is not of sharp and abrupt edge, but seems to fade off forward rather gradually. Facilitation makes it extend farther forward than it does without facilitation. Thus if the anterior border is delimited by stimulating a series of cortical points in succession from behind forward, the anterior limit of the field is found to lie farther anterior than if determined by stimulating a series of points starting well in front of the limit and followed from before backward. In a similar way the boundary of the area for any particular movement may by facilitation be extended beyond its average limit; in this latter case, deviation of response comes in as well.

2. *Reversal of Response.* The mutual influence exerted by points moving the same joint but in opposite directions was dealt with in the paper by T. Graham Brown and one of us [1912].

3. *Deviation of Response.* A cortical point can also influence the motor response of another whose response is neither diametrically opposed to nor identical with or very closely similar to its own.

EXCERPT P. 144

The main point which we here wish to emphasize in preface to the subjoined list of motor responses and maps of cortical points belonging to them as observed in experiments [details of their stimulation experiments now follow] is that in looking through such data we would wish the reader to bear in mind that the fixity of such localisation is as regards minutiae to some extent probably a temporary one, i.e., obtained at the time of observation, but in our opinion might not be precisely the same were examination possible at a number of different times and in a number of different experiments. As regards minutiae of localisation in the motor cortex, our experience agrees with that of those who find, as Shepherd Franz [1915] expresses it, that the motor cortex is a labile organ.

The conclusion of the authors concerning the motor cortex was as follows.

EXCERPT P. 219

10. The motor cortex may be regarded as a synthetic organ for compounding and re-compounding in varied ways movements of varied kinds of scope from comparatively small, though in themselves well coordinated, fractional movements. For this synthesis the motor cortex is provided with, i.e., has at call, these partial or fractional movements and postures. The cortex obtains these partial movements, perhaps by analytic powers of its own, from the bulbo-spinal mechanisms, but the higher of the synthetic results of the bulbo-spinal mechanism exhibit, as judged from cat and dog, certain only of the kinds of compound movements which the motor cortex gives. From the recomposition of these partial movements into wholes of varied pattern and sequence there result motor acts which, taken in their entirety, making use of the same fractional pieces, attain with them aims of varied scope by varying the spatial and temporal combinations of them.

FEDOR KRAUSE
(*10 March 1857—22 September 1937*)

So far the study of functional representation in the cerebral cortex had been carried out in animals, except for one or two investigators such as Bartholow (pp. 511–513) who made a few isolated observations in man. Obviously, not until the techniques of neurosurgery had developed sufficiently could the human cortex be examined carefully at operation. The first to attempt this in any detail was the famous German surgeon Krause.

Krause was born in Friedland, Silesia, and studied medicine in Berlin. After having been graduated, he worked with Koch and Langenbeck and then moved to Halle as assistant to the great surgeon Richard Volkmann, from 1883 to 1889. Gradually he turned from general to neurological surgery. He was appointed head of the surgical clinic at Altona in 1892 and eight years later became chief surgeon of the Auguste-Hospital in Berlin where he spent the rest of his active career and carried out most of his pioneer neurosurgery in cooperation with the renowned neurologist Hermann Oppenheim. In 1930 he retired to Rome. Krause has been claimed as the founder of German neurological surgery (see A. E. Walker, 1951, pp. 248–249; Kolle, 1956–1963, III, 199–206; Behrend, 1957).

Like other contemporary neurosurgeons, such as W. W. Keen of Philadelphia and V. Horsley of London, Krause attempted to map out the motor region. In lightly anesthetized patients on whom he was operating, usually for a cortical scar, he explored the motor area carefully with unipolar faradic stimulation while three assistants observed the responses. Krause's findings were recorded in an illustration (see fig. 131) which first appeared in his famous *Chirurgie des Gehirns und Rückenmarkes nach eigenen Erfahrungen* ([Berlin, 1908–1911], II, 185, fig. 66). It is interesting to note that when he reproduced it twenty years later (Krause and Schum, 1931, facing p. 454) there were only five additions. As Scarff (1940) has pointed out, however, it is quite possible that Krause, like his fellow map-makers (see Ferrier, pp. 513–518), supplemented his findings from those of the experimental physiologists upon animals, such as the results of Grünbaum and Sherrington (pp. 518–523).

Nevertheless, Krause's painstaking work was an important pioneer investigation that rivaled and perhaps excelled the more publicized reports of others. The following selection has been translated from the 1908–1911 edition of his book. It is clear from it that his primary aim was to provide a useful surgical technique rather than to conduct physiological experiments per se. In keeping with all other early investigators on animal or human material, he did not follow the motor area on to the medial surface of the hemisphere, an error that was not corrected until 1940 (Scarff, 1940).

EXCERPT PP. 183–184

According to my experience I must say that there is only one procedure which in man gives certain information concerning the central region; that is, electrical stimulation . . . .

My results obtained by the faradic stimulation of the human brain are indicated in fig. 66 [fig. 131]. All the foci belong to the anterior central [precentral] convolution. It shows that those for the lower extremity are arranged on the upper surface of the brain near the longitudinal sinus, and it can be inferred from animals that they extend on to the medial surface of the hemisphere; approximately the upper quarter of the central convolution is claimed for the lower extremity. About one half of the middle portion responds with contractions in the contralateral upper extremity from the shoulder down to the fingers. Finally, in the lower quarter the areas for the facial and masticatory muscles are added; here also should be found those for the muscles of the larynx, the platysma, and the tongue.

In animal experiments it has been established that the area for the turning of the head and eyes to the opposite side is in the posterior portion of the second and in the adjacent part of the first (upper) frontal convolution . . . just above the area for the fingers [fig. 131] . . . . Craniocerebral diagnosis [in man], together with the results of faradic stimulation, showed the area to correspond completely with the foot of the second frontal convolution.

EXCERPT P. 187

. . . . The excitable areas are separated from one another by smaller or greater portions of cerebral cortex which were not stimulated even by strong currents. This is clearly shown in the figure [fig. 131].

The focal fields (*Focusfelder*)—if I may use this expression—that is, centers for parts of the limbs, are not arranged in the same way in the anterior central convolutions of different individuals. In some they lie more laterally and nearer the Sylvian fissure, and in others nearer the midline. Individual excitable points for parts of a limb or for parts of the facial and masticatory muscles are always found next to each other in a focal field.

The following are some of Krause's observations on stimulation of the brains of epileptics.

EXCERPT PP. 188–189

Moreover, it is to be observed that the excitability of the cerebral cortex becomes exhausted by the faradic current, sooner in some individuals and later in others, so that a response is no longer obtained by the repeated stimulation of an area previously excited and only returns after a long rest.

Very frequently the stimulation of an area has been followed not only by the movements shown in fig. 66, but an immediate accompaniment of muscle contractions occurred, owing to release by faradization of the neighboring parts of the cortex. For example movement of the thumb was concluded by extension of the index finger at the proximal joint with flexion of both terminal phalanges and ulnar flexion of the wrist joint . . . .

Hence only those points are called foci of the cerebral mantle in which electrical excitation is most definitely expressed and most easily initiated.

Our scheme gives only a summary of the foci, which have been identified by numerous stimulations. Physiological excitation undoubtedly follows its own particular course and in comparison with it, electrical stimulation even in its finest graduations is an extraordinarily crude procedure . . . .

Finally one should not be misled by the assumption that all the identified foci or even the great majority of them, are present in each human.

. . . . on the basis of all my experience, *the faradic investigation of the cerebral cortex in the operating room represents an indispensable method of investigation*; it offers the only possible way to obtain accurate information regarding the central convolution.

B. Visual Functions—Occipital Lobe

As in the case of the motor area of the cerebral cortex, early in the history of investigation of cortical localization attention was drawn to the visual cortex of the occipital lobe.

Bartolomeo Panizza
(15 August 1785—17 April 1867)

In most of Flourens' pigeons from which he had removed portions of the cerebral hemispheres, some degree of visual impairment, often complete, was a common consequence (pp. 483 and 488). Little notice was taken of this, however, and in any case Flourens did not believe that local cerebral function existed. Vision was one of the general sensory activities of the cerebrum and the majority of physiologists supported this opinion. It was the Italian anatomist Panizza who first carried out animal experiments which demonstrated that the occipital lobe was essential for vision (Petella, 1901).

Panizza was born at Vicenza and studied at Padua, Bologna, Florence, and Pavia. After serving in the Napoleonic army he worked with Scarpa and then was appointed professor of anatomy at Pavia in 1817, a post he occupied for forty-nine years. He worked in the fields of anatomy and physiology and showed special interest in problems relating to the cranial nerves and to the blood and lymphatic systems of the reptile (see Verga, 1869; Berlucchi and Traschi, 1963).

Panizza also traced the optic pathways in animals and used his experimental observations to elucidate human pathology by noting the occurrence of an occipital lobe or deep hemispheral lesion in patients with visual defects not of peripheral origin. His classic paper, which thus combined experimental and clinical investigations on the optic pathways, was published in 1855 ("Osservazioni sul nervo ottico," *G. I. r. Ist. Lombardo Sci. Lett. Arti*, 1855, 7:237–252). The following passages from it describe some of his experiments. First he examined the effect of the removal of the optic lobe in the raven upon its vision; he did not attempt any precise cortical localization. Next he created the reverse situation in which the eye was removed and the changes in the optic pathway were observed; this, in the hands of Gudden (pp. 854–857), became a very important method of examining the brain anatomically.

EXCERPT PP. 239–240

I have undertaken some experiments to explain the truth and importance of the relations of the optic nerve with the above-mentioned parts [thalamus, cerebral peduncles, tuber cinereum, etc.]. I chose the raven as a bird that, in addition to being a lively and robust animal, has a thin cranium so that it may be cut easily with an ordinary knife and the brain exposed without any damage to its functions. When a cerebral hemisphere had been laid bare, with a probe I lifted up its posterior lateral part and, by means of a slender nervotome formed like a lance, I touched and injured the optic lobe, now in a transverse direction, now from front to back. Every time that I ceased some slight touch, the animal gave no sign of resentment, but when I wished to penetrate the substance with a needle, not only were there indications of sensitivity but also convulsive movements . . . . I verified what the distinguished *Flourens* and others have already observed regarding vision, that is, the loss of vision in the opposite eye not only after a deep injury, but also from a slight lesion, since the integrity of the optic lobe appears absolutely necessary for the exercise of such function. Indeed, when the raven that had sustained the aforesaid injury was set free, although it walked as swiftly as before, nevertheless with each step it bumped against the wall and against objects placed on the side corresponding to the affected eye [owing to hemianopia]; it did not see a finger or other object placed near that eye although the iris preserved its movement. Kept alive for two days, it ate and displayed its customary liveliness and readiness in movement although the cerebral hemisphere was denuded; the vision of the affected eye remained consistently obliterated. After the animal had been exsanguinated, a linear injury was found in the middle of the upper surface of the right optic lobe, two-thirds of a line [see p. 41] deep and one line long with a very slight effusion of blood on the tip of the part injured. Using the same precautions in other ravens, I have injured the posterior part of the right thalamus above the optic lobe; the result was the same, that is, loss of vision [hemianopia] in the opposite eye, persistence of the movements of the iris, and free movements of the whole body; at postmortem the injury to the thalamus, more or less near the optic lobe, could scarcely be found.

EXCERPT P. 242

In another experiment I blinded one eye of various chicks and ducklings just born or a few days old. Kept alive for many months, some over a year, the optic nerve in all of them was found to be atrophied and more or less ashen-colored and gelatinous, a condition that was present also in the square wing (*aja quadrata* [? quadrate lobe, also called cuneus]); or, broken down into two ashen-like bundles, it embraced the opposite nerve so that one might say that the right nerve passes divided to the left, and these ashen-like bundles, accompanied from there from the square wing [? cuneus], seem to me to be the total crossing. In addition, I have observed that the part that is rendered most atrophied is the optic lobe, the surface of which becomes entirely ashen-like; nonetheless I sometimes saw a slight diminution of the optic lobe while the thalamus was much diminished as well as all the rest of the nerve. As regards the healthy eye, ordinarily I saw the corresponding optic lobe much developed and the remainder of the nerve not in proportion; however, cases are not lacking in which I found the nerve [optic] tract between the thalamus and the eye much enlarged, but not the optic lobe. All these anomalies are explained by knowledge of the different connections by which the aforesaid nerve is related to the above-mentioned parts of the encephalon, relations that are found in harmony with the anatomico-physiologico-pathological observations.

In mammals the relationships of the optic nerves with the parts of the brain are almost the same. The bigeminal eminences [quadrigeminal bodies] (especially the *nates* [inferior bodies]), the thalamus and its appendices, the medullary bundles extending from the convolutions of the posterior part of the cerebral hemisphere, certain fibres from the cerebral peduncle, from the lateral walls of the infundibulum of the third ventricle and from the *tuber cinereum*, run together to give origin to this nerve. These relationships are the same in the rabbit, the ox, the lamb, the horse, the dog, and man; it is more apparent in the horse than in all the others how the thalamus runs together there and how the fibre bundles issuing from it to form the optic nerve are found to be continuous with the fibre bundles [optic radiation] issuing from the external side of the same thalamus [lateral geniculate body], that then go to compose the fibre apparatus of the superior and posteroinferior cerebral convolutions.

Hermann Munk
(3 February 1839—1 October 1912)

The astute observations of Panizza received little or no attention because at the time Flourens' opinion that there was no localized function in the cerebral hemispheres (pp. 483–488) was predominant. However, as soon as the study of cortical function was established in the 1870's, the part of the brain representing visual perception was investigated. Panizza had shown that the posterior lobes were responsible and Ferrier had concluded from his early experiments that in the monkey the angular gyrus was the visual center; presumably in his ablations he had interfered with the blood supply of the underlying optic radiation. The work of Munk, however, indicated that the occipital and occipitoparietal regions were the seat of all visual perceptions. His contribution to this subject had a profound effect upon those engaged in studies of cerebral anatomy, physiology, and pathology, and also upon psychologists.

Munk was born in Posen and studied in Berlin and Göttingen as a student of Müller, du Bois-Reymond, Virchow, and Traube. He was graduated from the University of Berlin in 1859 and spent his whole professional life in the physiological laboratories there. In 1869 he was appointed professor *extraordinarius* of physiology and in 1876, director of the Institute of Physiology at the Berlin Veterinary School. The greater part of his research dealt with neurophysiological problems, especially those concerning the cerebral cortex (see Pagel, 1901; Rothmann, 1909, 1912).

The techniques of ablation used by Munk were more precise than those of his predecessors and he was able to remove small areas of animal cortex and observe the effects. He believed in the precise and multiple division of the cerebral cortex into functional areas. He was able to confirm Panizza's belief that visual function was localized in the occipital lobe of the brain, and he also located auditory function in the temporal lobe. At first Munk thought the visual area was on the lateral convexity of the occipital lobe, but later, perhaps influenced by Henschen (see pp. 533–535), he favored the medial surface. He differentiated mental or psychic blindness (*Seelenblindheit*), now known as agnosia, from cortical blindness (*Rindenblindheit*). Contrary to most opinion, he thought that removal of the whole occipital lobe was necessary to produce cortical blindness, and this was shown to be correct only in 1936 (Klüver, 1936). Of equal importance, Munk demonstrated experimentally the projection of the retina on the visual cortex, an idea put forward by Meynert some years earlier (see p. 436).

The most important feature of Munk's experiments was the thoroughness with which he examined his animals. For example, he was able to substantiate his conclusions concerning psychic blindness when it was suggested that the visual defect he had produced was owing to scotomata rather than to agnosia (Loeb, 1884). His observations on psychic deafness owing to temporal lobe ablation were equally acute.

The following excerpts are from an early paper read to the physiological society in Berlin on 27 July 1877 ("Zur Physiologie der Grosshirnrinde," *Berl. klin. Wschr.*, 1877, 14:505–506). Figure 132 has been taken from Munk's book, *Über die Functionen der Grosshirnrinde. Gesammelte Mittheilungen aus den Jahre 1877–80* ([Berlin, 1881], fig. 1, p. 29), but it is common to all his experiments. Distribution of Area A_1 produces psychic blindness and of B_1, psychic deafness; A and B are the total visual and auditory areas respectively.

EXCERPT PP. 505–506

In dogs of medium size I removed from the convexity of the parietal, occipital, and temporal lobes approximately circular pieces of cerebral cortex of about 15 mm. diameter and 2 mm. thickness; in some they were removed first from one hemisphere and later symmetrically from the other, and in some symmetrically from both hemispheres simultaneously. The experiments showed that the portion of cerebral cortex explored contained an anterior, purely motor [fig. 132, DCE] and a posterior, purely sensory area, the outline of which is approximately indicated by a line which one might imagine being drawn vertically from the terminal end of the Sylvian fossa towards the falx [fig. 132, areas A and B]. Ablations in front of the line are always followed by motor disturbances, noted first by Fritsch and Hitzig; ablations behind this line have never produced even a trace of this. By contrast, in the region of the posterior sensory area, mind-blindness is regularly produced if the ablation involves the occipital lobe close to the upper posterior tip (area A_1 [fig. 132]); psychic deafness, if the ablation involves the temporal lobe close to its lower tip (area B_1). In the former case the animal lost the memory of visual images [memory pictures], in the latter the memory of auditory images. Following ablation in front of or below area A, or between it and area B, no changes whatsoever could be noted in the operated animals.

Furthermore, it could be demonstrated that the motor disturbances as well as mind-blindness always disappeared gradually and completely without the least trace within four to six weeks, so that the operated animals could no longer be distinguished in any way from the normal ones. In the animals affected with mind-blindness, one could follow in minute detail how these animals learned to see again exactly as in their earliest years. This has led to the concept that the visual area of the cerebral cortex extends far beyond the occipital lobe and the auditory area likewise beyond that of the temporal lobe. Moreover, in the visual or auditory area the memory images are deposited, so to speak, in a central point with ever increasing radius, perhaps in a sequence similar to perceptions arriving at consciousness. Following ablation of area A_1 or B_1, which for the time being house all or most of the memory images, the remainder of the visual or auditory areas in the neighborhood of A_1 or B_1 are occupied by new memory images.

. . . .

. . . . When after the course of 8 to 14 weeks the equally developed, intact and mutilated dogs of the same litter were sacrificed, we noted at autopsy that in the blinded dogs the occipital lobe, which had previously been identified as the visual area, and in the deaf-mute dogs the temporal lobe, previously identified as the auditory area of the cerebrum, were actually retarded in development compared to the normal. However, obviously in compensation, the temporal lobe was developed beyond the normal in the blind dogs, the occipital in the deaf dogs, so that the total volume of the hemisphere was not appreciably diminished. By comparing the blind with the deaf dogs, it was noted that the temporal lobe was markedly shifted towards the falx in the blind dogs and the occipital lobe towards the temple in the deaf dogs . . . .

Regarding the results of the repeated ablation experiments, I believe I should first emphasize that also in all further investigations, without any exception, interference with the occipital lobe (area A) was followed exclusively by mind-blindness, and with the parietal lobe exclusively by motor disturbances. Not only is the visual function, acoustic function, etc., localized in general in the cerebral cortex, but individual memory images, too, have their definite seat there. This has recently been beautifully demonstrated in two experiments in which, following ablation of area A, with the loss of all other memory images of visual perception, a single memory image was found to be preserved intact; in one case the image of a pail from which the dog was accustomed to drink, in the other that of a hand movement, to which the dog, prior to surgery, had been trained to respond by giving his paw. In the more recent experiments, too, no changes were noted for the most part in the operated animals following extirpation in front of or below area A. However, sometimes a slight visual disturbance of this kind, and exclusively of this kind, could be distinguished in that the dog was less able to follow with the eye contralateral to the lesion the throwing of pieces of meat than with the homolateral eye.

Since injury of the longitudinal sinus is not accompanied by untoward effects and complications, the cerebral cortex of the medial surface of the hemisphere could be investigated. Here ablations of the occipital lobe have yielded the same results as those in front of or below area A.

In the past it has not been possible to observe the return of auditory perceptions, and more recently I have tried repeatedly but in vain to accomplish this . . . . However, I have now finally succeeded in verifying the gradual recovery from mind-deafness also; in one dog I was able to ascertain from day to day how it learned to hear anew, and this in no way different from its earliest youth, until, in the course of approximately one month it differed in no way from a normal dog.

In order to test the concept that following ablation of area A the environment of this area is filled by the new memory images of vision, numerous experiments were carried out with secondary ablation of the areas in front of and below area A in dogs that had been rendered mind-blind and had recovered from it. However, all these experiments ended unhappily; . . . . Frequently the dogs that had been rendered mind-blind succumbed to such disease [intracranial inflammation] sooner or later, often only after months, by which time the dogs had learned to see again perfectly and had behaved normally for many weeks. In the less severe cases merely a visual disturbance was observed, but a visual disturbance with the dog not only being mind-blind again—having lost for the second time the newly gained memory images of visual perception—but completely blind. It could hardly be prompted to move, did not avoid the obstacles in its way, stumbled against everything, etc. [cortical blindness]. In the more severe cases the blindness was accompanied by chronic convulsions and ataxia, in the severest cases also by coma. Only in the most severe cases did death occur, and a pronounced meningitis, spreading through the entire cerebrum and including the anterior lobes, was noted. In the other cases the disturbances gradually regressed, and the dog regained its previous state completely in the less severe cases, whereas in the more severe cases only the motor disturbances disappeared while the blindness remained. Autopsy demonstrated in the less severe cases moderate meningitis of the occipital lobe, in the severer cases a marked meningitis of the occipital and a lesser one of the parietal lobe. Apparently the pathological process had rendered the environment of area A incapable of functioning, partly temporarily, partly permanently. Consequently this is the part of the cerebrum in which the direct effect of the sensory perception upon movements takes place; in the dog it is the cerebral cortex. According to Herr Goltz it is located behind the cerebral hemispheres in the frog. And, as had been concluded earlier, the location of visual perception is in a large expanse of the cortex of the occipital lobe, whereas only a portion of this part of the cortex is filled with the memory images of visual sensation.

Munk also studied the effects of electrical excitation of the occipital cortex and found that the results corresponded closely with those achieved by ablation. The following is from an article, "Of the visual area of the cerebral cortex, and its relation to eye movements," which appeared in *Brain* (1890, 13:45–67).

EXCERPT PP. 64–65

. . . . At any rate, it is of unmistakeable value, that the conformity of the experiments by both methods [ablation and excitation] warrants the assumption that there is some certainty in the knowledge acquired. And this conformity extends even farther than I have yet mentioned. For the results, which the stimulation of the antero-lateral extremity of the visual area offers, is only completely comprehensible, on the assumption that the antero-lateral part of the retina of the corresponding side is in connection with that extremity, and the results of excitation of the middle of area A [visual area] are only rightly to be understood on the assumption that the centre of distinct vision of the opposite retina belongs to this area; and that the part indicated has been accurately hit upon in this latter stimulation, when both eyes remain at rest, or only one eye moves; but not quite accurately, if both eyes move . . . .

. . . . The projection of the retinae upon the visual areas presents itself now in its full significance as the substratum for the localisation of the visual perceptions, since the involuntary eye-movements, which are brought about through the radiating fibres supply the necessary complement.

SALOMEN EBERHARD HENSCHEN

(*28 February 1847—4 December 1930*)

Further precision in the localization of visual function was achieved by the Swede, Henschen. He localized it to the calcarine fissure on the medial surface of the occipital lobe and, furthermore, suggested that the upper lip represented the upper retinal quadrant and the lower lip the lower quadrant. He was, however, in error when he said that macular vision was anterior rather than posterior in the fissure. He traced in detail the component parts of the visual pathway from retina to cortex, and although here, too, several of his conclusions were erroneous, his contribution to our understanding of the anatomy and physiology of visual perception was of great importance.

Henschen was born in Uppsala and studied in Stockholm. He took his postgraduate training in Germany, and in 1882 he was appointed professor of clinical medicine at Uppsala. Early in his career his interests turned to diseases of the brain and their application to anatomical and physiological problems. His work was entirely clinicopathological and not experimental and was directed to the explanation of cerebral cortical function. In 1900 he became professor of medicine in the Caroline Institute in Stockholm. He had an argumentative and militant personality and was frequently involved in controversy. He was also outspoken and publicly denounced the Nobel Committee for not awarding him a prize, which he considered he merited (see his autobiography in Grote, 1925, pp. 35–76; Lenz, 1924; Ingvar, 1931).

Henschen represented an extreme form of localizational thought. He maintained that each retinal cell was projected onto a cortical cell, and later he even speculated on the location of single ideas or memories in single cells, an idea still held by some (Nielsen, 1936). In 1892 he read a paper before the Congress of Experimental Physiology in London that was published the next year ("On the visual path and centre," *Brain*, 1893, 16:170–180); the following passages have been taken from it.

EXCERPT PP. 176–179

We now enter upon the consideration of the occipital lobe. A number of observations have been made in literature upon occipital lesions. Most of them were accompanied with hemianopsia, but only a few of them are of use in the accurate study of the localisation of the centre of vision. In 20 cases the lesion was diffuse in the medulla of the occipital lobe. None of them localise the visual centre to a circumscribed portion of the lobe, because the visual path was destroyed by the lesion, but many of them go to prove that it does not extend further than the occipital lobe. All cortical or sub-cortical circumscribed lesions, on the contrary, are of great importance in the localisation of the visual centre. The first question that arises is, Does the centre of vision lie on the lateral, mesial, or ventral surface? . . . . Firstly, a lesion on the mesial surface causes hemianopsia only if the cortex of the calcarine fissure, of the fibres derived from it, are affected. Secondly, a lesion limited to the calcarine cortex can induce a complete hemianopsia, and of this the most instructive case is, I believe, one now published in my book, which includes all guarantees for an exact conclusion. It was stationary, uncomplicated, and the clinical examination, as well as the *post-mortem,* was accurate. The lesion was limited to the cortex in the depth of the calcarine fissure, and the hemianopsia was complete and absolute. Besides, many other negative cases confirm this result, and, in particular, one of my own, with a bilateral destruction of the margo falcata [possibly an area immediately anterior to the parieto-occipital sulcus on the medial surface of the hemisphere], without defect in the field of vision, proves that the visual centre is not to be looked for there, as Nothnagel and others have affirmed. As to the still more accurate limitation of the visual centre in the cortex of the calcarine fissure, the cases, on the whole, are not sufficiently definite to decide, but there are not at present any absolute reasons for extending it further than the lips of the fissure. In some cases a complete hemianopsia resulted without a lesion in the frontal part of this cortex; in others without any affection of the most posterior part; but in all cases the middle part of the fissure was implicated.

. . . .

Organization of the Centre of Vision.—The next question is: How is the centre of vision organised? At first there exists a projection in the calcarine fissure. I have mentioned above that my researches have led me to the conclusion that the fibres of the dorsal retinal quadrant lie dorsally both in the frontal and occipital visual path. The interesting case of Hun's proves that there is the same arrangement in the calcarine cortex. Thus the upper lip represents the upper retinal quadrant, and other cases strengthen this opinion.

. . . .

. . . .

. . . .

Of as great interest is the question as to whether the same elements represent homologous points of the retina, or not, and how they are situated in relation to each other . . . . These facts seem to prove that the elements of both retinal halves are represented in the calcarine cortex by different cells, which lie beside each other. As to the perception of colours, the commonly received opinion that it is situated on the ventral surface will not admit of criticism. Some of my own cases prove positively that colour perception is also situated in the calcarine cortex.

In 1924 Henschen summarized the history of the anatomy and physiology of the central visual apparatus and detailed his own contributions to the problem ("On the value of the discovery of the visual centre. A review and a personal apology," *Scand. scient. Rev.*, 1924, 3:10–63). The following brief passages are from it.

EXCERPT P. 18

This case verified my supposition, namely, that every limited lesion of the calcarine cortex causes a corresponding limited blind spot in the visual field, or, that there exists a mathematical projection of the peripheral retina in the calcarine cortex, which I gave the name "Cortical retina."

EXCERPT P. 30

The kernel of my researches and conclusions can be formulated as fol-lows: *The visual field coincides with the area striata.* These words include, for the present, the statement, that our senses have a peculiar and sharply limited anatomical seat and organisation in the brain, *the statement also including, at the same time, a revolution of earlier views and also an important progress in our knowledge of the organisation of the brain and its functions.*

MECHYSLAV MINKOWSKI
(*14 April 1884–   *)

Although localization of visual function in the occipital lobe had become more exact during the nineteenth century, the area of cortex responsible had not been located with anatomical precision. It was the work of Minkowski which made this possible, as well as providing answers about the complex arrangement of the visual pathway.

Minkowski was born in Warsaw and studied medicine there and at Munich and Breslau; he received his diploma at Kasan in 1907. His postgraduate work was carried out with Pavlov at St. Petersburg and in Greifswald and Berlin. He spent all his active career in Zürich where he succeeded Monakow (pp. 619–623) as profes-sor of neurology, 1928–1954, and director of the University Institute of Brain Anatomy and Polyclinic for Nervous Diseases. His most important work has been in the field of cortical function, especially the visual areas. Minkowski came of a family of brilliant scientists and must be differentiated in particular from his brother Oskar who studied diabetes (*Who's Who in Switzerland, 1964–1965*, p. 399).

Working with dogs, Minkowski confirmed Henschen's localization of the visual area of the posterior and medial surfaces of the occipital lobe rather than in Munk's areas A and A_1 (fig. 132), and he was the first to prove experimentally that the striate area of the occipital cortex was the cortical visual center. Complete and bilateral removal of this area produced complete and permanent blindness. He also found that the upper halves of the retinae were related to the anterior half, and the lower halves to the posterior half of the striate area; thus, for example, a lesion of the latter produced a superior homonymous hemianopia. In opposition to Henschen he suggested that each retinal point was projected not on a single cortical point but an extensive area so that only widespread lesions produced complete destruction of the representation of any point. Thus most of each retina was represented in the contralateral striate area, and the small central region remaining had bilateral representation.

Of equal importance was his discovery of the organization of the lateral geniculate body. The crossed and uncrossed fibres from the retina terminated in different cell layers and this allowed the projection of the ipsilateral and contralateral homonymous retinal halves on each striate area.

The following conclusions have been taken from his article of 1911 ("Zur Physiologie der Sehsphäre," *Pflügers Arch.*, 1911, 141:171–327).

EXCERPT PP. 306–307

There exists a constant projection of the retina upon the cortical retina [the name given by Henschen (p. 533) to the calcarine cortex upon which the retina projects], *and in such manner that the upper parts of the retina are located in its anterior portion, the lower parts in the posterior. However, the projection is not of a geometrical but of a physiological nature: each identifiable element of the retina is not connected with one, but with an entire area of identifiable elements of the cortical retina, although with some of these more closely than with others. This area is the larger, the stronger the physiological claims to the respective element of the retina, or the closer it is to the point of central vision; the latter is represented like an island within the area of the cortical retina, but in a particularly extensive area. The corresponding parts of both retinas have a common projection field within the confines of the cortical retina.*

If a portion of the cortical retina is cut out, recovery occurs only inasmuch as such elements of the cortical retina which were earlier in loose connection with the elements of the retina predominantly involved (constituting for these only cortical excitatory side stations), now enter into an especially close relationship with these (becoming cortical excitatory main stations). The rapid rate of this recovery and its absence with extensive, partial surgery, demonstrate that it takes place essentially in anatomical paths which already exist, and not in ones newly formed.

This assumption offers an adequate explanation for the fact that on the one hand small ablations, particularly those from the central portion of the retina, do not necessarily lead to a demonstrable disturbance of vision, and, on the other hand, more extensive surgical interventions which start at the poles of the cortical retina and spread over a large area of it, will cause a permanent scotoma of constant position and shape in the contralateral eye.

Minkowski was also concerned with the occipital center for eye movements.

EXCERPT PP. 318–320

Since the oculomotor effect from electric stimulus of the occipital lobe is preserved following frontal incision which severs the occipital lobe from the motor region, the existence of a corticofugal pathway which connects the occipital lobe directly with the subcortical motor nuclei is physiologically assured. Anatomically as well, the occurrence of such a pathway cannot be doubted . . . .

From my experimental studies it follows that the opticosensory area is identical with the area striata; anatomically expressed, this means that those fibres of the optic radiation which carry primary visual sensation terminate totally in this cortical area; on the other hand, the electrical stimulation experiment demonstrates that the opticomotor field does not coincide with the area striata but is found outside it, although in its immediate vicinity; it must therefore be assumed that the corticofugal optic radiation originates, if not exclusively, nevertheless predominantly, outside the cortical retina.

GORDON MORGAN HOLMES
(22 *February* 1876—29 *December* 1965)

At a time when controversy over the visual cortex was widespread it was in one way fortunate, although at the same time regrettable, that a large number of brain injuries became available for examination. Animal experiments had provided basic data which had to be checked with human material, thus extending the clinical approach of Henschen (pp. 533–535). The First World War, like the Russo-Japanese War (1904) in which occipital lobe lesions had been investigated, provided cases of penetrating cranial wounds that helped to substantiate the work of the experimentalists. One of those who took advantage of this opportunity was the Anglo-Irish neurologist Holmes.

Holmes was born at Castlebellingham, County Louth, Ireland, and educated in Dublin, Berlin, and Frankfurt am Main. He served as neurologist to the Charing Cross Hospital in London and in 1909 was appointed to the National Hospital, Queen Square, from which he retired in 1941. He was one of the leading members of the British school of neurology during the first three or four decades of the present century, and his work, both experimental and clinical, covered a large part of neurology; that part dealing with visual and cerebellar function (pp. 677–681) is especially well known. His services to medicine were rewarded with a knighthood in 1951.

In addition to verifying the findings of Minkowski and others, Holmes solved the vexing question of the localization of central vision representation in the striate area. He reported his findings, based on a large series of cases, in the Montgomery Lectures delivered at Trinity College, Dublin, in June 1919 ("Lecture I—The cortical localization of vision," *Brit. med. J.*, 1919, ii:193–199) from which the following selection has been taken.

EXCERPT P. 194

CORTICAL LOCALIZATION OF CENTRAL VISION

If the evidence from these and similar cases shows that the upper halves of the retinae are represented in the upper or dorsal parts of the calcarine areas and the lower in the lower or ventral, we may now turn to the consideration of the cortical localization of macular or central vision . . . .

. . . .

. . . .

. . . .

. . . .

This case illustrates the type of blindness that is produced by superficial injuries of both occipital poles—that is, by wounds that injure the posterior parts of the striate areas. In all such cases we find peripheral vision intact and central vision abolished. They are consequently evidence that central or macular vision is represented in the more posterior parts of the visual areas, and that this region is not concerned with peripheral sight.

The evidence to be obtained from unilateral lesions confirms this opinion and also supports the conclusion we have already arrived at, that the upper parts of the retinae are connected with the upper parts of the visual cortex and the lower with the lower.

Homonymous paracentral scotomata are frequently produced by injuries of the polar region of one occipital lobe.

EXCERPT P. 196

This series of cases illustrates the evidence that my observations can furnish on the cortical localization of central and pericentral vision. It proves that the macular and perimacular regions of the retinae are represented at or near to the occipital poles of the hemispheres. It is probable, indeed, that the portion of the area striata which frequently spreads over the occipital pole and on to the lateral surface of the brain may be the centre of macular sight. The frequency of paracentral scotomata is consequently accounted for by the more exposed position of this part of the visual area than of that which lies on the mesial surfaces of the hemispheres. It seems very probable, too, that the maculae have anatomically larger representations in the cortex than the less highly specialized peripheral zones of the retinae, and in this we may find the explanation of the frequency of small areas of blindness in the neighbourhood of the fixation point, though the causal lesions may be relatively gross.

EXCERPT P. 197

Such observations as these, which are only selected illustrations from a large number of cases, indicate that there is a definite areal representation of the retinae in the visual cortex. There can be little doubt, too, of the general principles of this localization; the macular regions are represented posteriorly and the periphery of the retinae more anteriorly in the occipital lobes, while the upper and lower portions of the retinae are projected on to the corresponding parts of the visual cortex. Further, the mesial horizontal segments of the retinae are probably projected in the neighbourhood of the floors of the calcarine fissures.

And not only is each segment of the retinae represented in a definite portion of the visual cortex, but this representation is fixed and immutable, so that if a part of the visual cortex be totally destroyed there will be a permanent blindness of the corresponding segment of the visual fields. Only so can we explain the persistence of such a small scotoma as in Case V, which, when examined three and a half years after the infliction of the wound, was found almost identical in size and position as within the first few days of the injury. In Case III, too, the blind area remained unaltered between one and ten months after the injury. There is no place here for the theory of vicarious representation of the function of parts destroyed by other regions of the brain.

C. Auditory Functions—Temporal Lobe

The amount of attention which the early investigators of cortical function gave to the different parts of the cerebral hemispheres was inversely proportional to the difficulty of observing the effects of stimulation or ablation. Thus the temporal lobes, which Ferrier, Munk, and others had shown to be responsible for auditory function, were neglected because of the difficulty of examining hearing in animals.

Only one early contribution to this part of the physiology of the cerebral cortex has been selected.

E. A. [SIR EDWARD ALBERT SHARPEY-] SCHÄFER   SANGER MONROE BROWN
     (2 June 1850—29 March 1935)   *(10 February 1852—1 April 1928)*

The first detailed study of the temporal lobe cortex was carried out by Schäfer and Brown in 1888.

Sharpey-Schäfer was born in London as E. A. Schäfer and attended University College Hospital Medical School where he received his medical qualification in 1874. There he worked with William Sharpey, the first British physiologist of note, whose pupils founded important schools of physiology in Cambridge, Oxford, Edinburgh, and Baltimore. In 1918 Schäfer, because of his indebtedness to his teacher and in memory of his son, Sharpey-Schäfer, who had been killed in the First World War, added "Sharpey" to his own name. He was appointed Jodrell Professor of Physiology at University College in 1883, and after holding the post for sixteen years accepted the chair of physiology in the University of Edinburgh. He retired in 1933. His early work was in the field of histology, but from 1883 he turned his attention to investigation of the cerebral cortex, the endocrine glands, and a number of neurophysiological problems (see Hill, 1932–1935; Sharpey-Schäfer, 1935a, 1935b).

Brown was born in Bloomfield, Ontario, but spent his professional career in the United States. He received the M.D. degree from New York University in 1880 and practised psychiatry in several mental hospitals before being appointed professor of neurology at the Post-Graduate Medical School of Chicago in 1890. He later held appointments at Rush Medical College in the same city, in medical jurisprudence and hygiene and in clinical medicine as well as in clinical neurology in the University of Illinois. His name is associated with a type of hereditary cerebellar ataxia with spasticity ("On hereditary ataxy," *Brain*, 1892, 15:250–268), but his only experimental work was that in collaboration with Schäfer (Brown II, 1928).

Schäfer and Brown observed the effect in monkeys of the removal of portions of the temporal lobe cortex ("An investigation into the functions of the occipital and temporal lobes of the monkey's brain," *Phil. Trans. R. Soc.*, 1888, 179B:303–327). Unlike Ferrier, they noted no alteration in auditory function but in some of their animals they observed a profound mental change. Little attention was paid to the latter observation at the time, and it has been only very recently that the relationship between the temporal lobe and mental function has received close attention.

In their sixth monkey extensive bilateral ablation of temporal lobe cortex led to transient mental changes. Case 12, a female Rhesus monkey, had the superior temporal gyrus gray and white matter removed bilaterally by means of a two-state operation (fig. 133), with the following effects.

EXCERPT PP. 318–319

Result.—As soon as the animal was recovered from the effect of the anaesthetic her hearing was tested, and, although still somewhat lethargic, she was found to give attention even to slight sounds, such as kissing or sucking noises made with the lips. This was repeatedly tried, and she invariably responded by looking up.

This Monkey made a rapid recovery; indeed the double operation produced no perceptible effect upon its general health. But the creature shows the same change of disposition that was manifest in Monkey No. 6. She appears to have lost, in great measure, intelligence and memory. She investigates all objects, even the most familiar, as if they were entirely unknown, tasting, smelling, and feeling all over everything she comes across. She is tame, and exhibits no fear of mankind, but shows uncontrollable passion on the approach of other Monkeys, so that it is now necessary to shut her up in a cage by herself. Like Monkey No. 6, she now invariably devours her food by putting her head down to the platter, instead of employing the hands to convey it to her mouth. Moreover, her appetite is insatiable, and she crams until her cheek-pouches can hold no more. She evidently still sees, hears, tastes, and smells perfectly well, but her understanding of the impressions which she derives from her senses is unquestionably small. Cutaneous sensibility shows no appreciable diminution.

The peculiar idiotic condition into which this Monkey was thrown by the operation was more persistent than in the case of No. 6. Recovery proceeded but gradually; and, although in many points improvement was manifest, there was never, during the whole time that the animal was kept, that complete return of intelligence which was observed in No. 6 (which had, it will be remembered, a much more extensive bilateral lesion). Her appearance remains stupid, and her movements lethargic; she is still savage towards her fellow Monkeys; her attention is not easily attracted, either by sights or sounds, although an abrupt movement or a sudden and unusual noise will produce signs of perception. She usually takes her food up with her hands, but is still markedly greedy, taking, when she can get it, much more food than a normal Monkey of the same size.

From their experiments Schäfer and Brown concluded that the seat of auditory function was not in the temporal gyri alone, and this was in keeping with the findings of Luciani and Seppilli (1885). They also discussed the problem of the mental changes and their etiology.

EXCERPT PP. 324–325

Our experiments upon the temporo-sphenoidal or temporal lobe have been all, with one exception, performed bilaterally, for we very early came to the conclusion that no definite results were to be obtained in Monkeys regarding the senses of hearing, taste, or smell from unilateral lesions of the brain. Roughly speaking, we may class our experiments under two heads: (1) partial or local extirpations of portions of the lobe, (2) complete removal of the whole lobe. The partial extirpations comprised (*a*) the antero-inferior part of the lobe (cases 1 and 2), (*b*) the superior temporal gyrus (cases 1, 3, 7, and 11). They have produced in our hands no appreciable effect, neither loss of taste, smell, nor hearing, and, so far as could be determined in Monkeys, no diminution in the acuteness of any of these senses. Animals with the antero-inferior portion of the lobe, including the subiculum, completely cut away smell their food, immediately detect a malodorous substance, such as aloes or asafoetida, with which it (e.g., a raisin) may have been smeared, and cast it aside without tasting. A raisin into which quinine has been inserted is smelt, eagerly bitten, and immediately rejected with expressions of disgust. Animals with both superior temporal gyri completely destroyed give evidence of the possession of acute powers of hearing; they turn at the slightest rustle, look up at the smallest noise, even immediately after the operation and when still drowsy from the prolonged influence of the anaesthetic, and follow with the head and eyes the direction of footsteps along a corridor outside the room in which they are confined. Some of these animals we have had under observation for many months; they have been seen and tested by many people, and the absence of the gyrus has been attested by *post-mortem* examination.

EXCERPT P. 327

. . . . It must, however, be remarked that in the latter instance [case 12] the operation was conducted in such a manner as to produce a very profound lesion of that part of the hemisphere. The fissures bounding the gyrus (Sylvian and parallel) were drawn open, and the whole of the convolution, in its entire extent and depth, completely shelled out on both sides of the brain. A very great amount of vascular disturbance was thereby necessarily produced, and this must have affected, for a time at least, other portions of the brain.

Probably, therefore, the most reasonable explanation of the general depression of the intellectual faculties which these operations produced is to be found in this vascular disturbance. This, without actually causing the complete paralysis of function of the remainder of the cerebrum, which would have been evidenced by motor paralysis, may yet have sufficed to interfere with the active performance of its functions sufficiently to produce the results described. Thus, in both cases the movements were slow, the senses dulled, the memory very defective, and the disposition changed. It would obviously be unreasonable to assume, certainly in the second case, that these alterations are caused by the local lesion, but it appears to us that they may not unreasonably be explained on the hypothesis we have put forward. The gradual recovery of intelligence in both these animals is extremely interesting, and recalls instances which have been recorded in the human subject in which a gradual recovery has taken place after almost total abolition of the intellectual faculties.

D. Mental Functions—Frontal Lobe

If it could be accepted that the brain was the seat of intellectual functions, it was reasonable that attempts should be made to localize them to one or several precise parts of the brain, as for any other cerebral activity. In other words, it seemed that a new form of phrenology might be possible. This problem, as might be expected, has proved to be one of the most difficult of those facing the neurophysiologist and psychologist, and it will continue to face them well into the future.

When the scientific investigation of cortical function became practicable at the end of the nineteenth century, attention was turned to the question of mental activity and its possible site or sites. There seemed to be considerable old and new evidence to implicate the frontal lobes. Eventually three opinions developed, one supporting local specialization of the cortex and a second taking the contrary view that psychological processes were determined by an aggregate of cortical activity. The latter was upheld by the antilocalizationists such as Monakow (pp. 565–570) and by Munk who observed that "intelligence is located everywhere in the cerebral cortex and nowhere in particular." The third idea has become known as the holistic theory whereby certain activities such as intelligence, for example, are continuously distributed throughout the cortex; Flourens, Goltz, Ferrier, and Lashley have favored this controversial doctrine. On the whole, modern opinion supports the last two views, although it is clear that the frontal lobes are involved with thought processes more than some other parts of the cerebral hemispheres, and that they guide and integrate the personality. Their precise role and their relationships with others structures are still a matter for speculation. Deterrents to early workers in this field were, of course, the absence of a satisfactory definition of psychological functions, the inadequate methods available for their examination, and the paucity of human data.

One of those who claimed that the frontal lobes were the seat of mental activity will be represented below, and the attitude of the opponents can be seen in the sections on Goltz and Monakow. Despite the fact that we can no longer agree with all the conclusions of the early investigators, nevertheless they accumulated a mass of useful data regarding mental activity. For a survey of the development of neurological concepts of intelligence, see Halstead (1947, pp. 19–29; see also Chap. II, pp. 67–93) and Bianchi (1920, pp. 67–93).

Leonardo Bianchi
(*5 April 1848—13 April 1927*)

Hitzig was one of those who believed in the precise localization of psychic activity, but the person who contributed more than anyone else at this time to our knowledge of frontal lobe function was the Italian neurologist Bianchi. He maintained that the frontal lobes were "an organ of intellect" and a controller of the highest levels of integration.

Bianchi was born in San Bartolomeo and after having been graduated in medicine at the University of Naples in 1871, he was given an appointment there in 1882 in the new Institute of Psychiatry. Eight years later he was made professor of nervous and mental diseases and worked in the fields of neurology and psychiatry for thirty-seven years. Of his various researches, those into the function of the frontal lobes were the most important; they reveal his remarkable powers of observation (see Mieli, 1921–1923, Pt. II; Lord, 1928; Haymaker, 1953, pp. 110–114).

By 1895 there were at least three theories of frontal lobe function: (1) it was the motor center for contralateral eye movements and for attention (Ferrier); (2) it was the center for the highest intellectual processes (Wundt, Hitzig, Bianchi); and, (3) it was the motor center for the dorsal musculature (Munk, Luciani). One of Bianchi's early papers on the frontal lobes appeared in 1895 ("The functions of the frontal lobes [translated from the original MS by A. de Watteville]," *Brain*, 1895, 18:497–522), and the following is a part of his conclusions. He had found that the removal of one lobe produced little effect on the monkey, and hence rejected the contentions of Munk and Ferrier.

EXCERPT PP. 521–522

Overlooking the possible contention of some objectors, that the serious mental disturbances observed in the mutilated animals, depended on interference with the senses of taste and smell, my hypothesis is that the frontal lobes are the seat of co-ordination and fusion of the incoming and outgoing products of the several sensory and motor areas of the cortex. As the nervous waves from peripheral organs of reception (retinal rods, tactile organs, &c.) are transmitted from neurons of the first order to neurons of the second (mesocephalon, thalamus), and from these again to neurons of the third order (cortex), thus we may suppose that from the last-mentioned, nerve impulses travel to the frontal neurons of the highest order. The frontal lobes would thus sum up into series the products of the sensori-motor regions, as well as the emotive states which accompany all the perceptions, the fusion of which constitutes what has been called the *psychical tone* of the individual. Removal of the frontal lobes does not so much interfere with the perceptions taken singly, as it does disaggregate the personality, and incapacitate for serialising and synthesizing groups of representations. The actual impressions, which serve to revive these groups, thus succeed one another disconnectedly under the influence of fortuitous external stimuli, and disappear without giving rise to associational processes in varied and recurrent succession. With the organ for the physiological fusion which forms the basis of association, disappear also the physical conditions underlying reminiscence, judgment, and discrimination, as is well shown in mutilated animals. Their agitation and motor incoherence depend upon the reflection of nerve impulses set up by stimuli through small sensori-motor arcs, without the intervention of the previously accu-mulated psychical co-efficients.

Fear is an immediate result of psychical disaggregation, from defective sense of personality, and unbalanced perception and judgment . . . . Cour-age rests upon the treble basis of self-conscious force, rapid perception of the enemy's powers for offence or defence in relation to one's own, and the influence of certain feelings; our animals show an absence of all these characteristics . . . . On the one hand, their effective nature, friendliness, and sociability is impaired; on the other, their avidity becomes reckless and insatiable.

Twenty-five years later Bianchi published a detailed account of his many observa-tions on the function of the frontal lobes in animals and man (*La meccanica del cervello e la funzione dei lobi frontali*, Turin, 1920).

EXCERPT PP. 232–235

Briefly summing up the psychology of monkeys mutilated in the frontal lobes, the following results have been confirmed:

1. Defect of the perceptive power, consisting of only partial perception of objects of the external world, lacking some of the specific and differential features, whence arises failure to recognize objects already known and new objects that have a relation of similarity, analogy, etc., with those known. Thus some objects are mistaken for others similar only in color or shape . . . .

2. Memory, weak and unreliable, is extraordinarily reduced, not only for recent but also for past acquisitions. The mutilated monkey does not make use of past experience; he always repeats the same actions without profiting from the failure of the preceding act and without altering his actions to reach a determined object . . . . In consequence of not utilizing past experience, the mutilated monkeys have lost that biophylactic power that guides life in its passage through the difficulties of the physical environ-ment and those [created by] his fellows with whom he lives.

3. The associative power is strongly depressed; the power of acquaint-ance and of acquisition that the normal monkey displays in the varied circumstances of its existence, especially in captivity from which new adap-

tations arise, is withdrawn or shut off from the mutilated monkey. Judgment is poor and immediate, often erroneous through lack of the element of comparison . . . .

What is more important is that in monkeys in which the operation was successful, there is complete lack of any initiative whatsoever. The movements performed by these animals lack any evident objective. They are the effect of internal impulses that readily become automatic, or they are immediate reflexes from simple impressions that do not find a field of association or of coordination to achieve a determined goal. . . .

. . . .

. . . .

4. Mutilation of the frontal lobes produces a not less noteworthy modification in the emotional and sentimental manifestations of the life of the Cebus . . . . What is completely lacking with frontal mutilation are the higher sentiments, those which represent a complex of the primitive emotions with new and numerous factors: friendship, gratitude, jealousy, maternal and protective feelings, dominance and authority, and above all that of sociability, a sense of its own dignity, and the sense of ridicule; all these disappear with mutilation of the frontal lobes, while the primitive emotions remain, now and then even intensified, but unadapted to the struggle for existence in which these inferior beings succumb . . . .

5. In all cases conduct is demonstrated as incoherent. This incoherence takes origin from the defective imagination and memory, the inability to represent an objective and to sustain it in the focal point of the consciousness . . . .

EXCERPT P. 314

The behavior of mutilated monkeys [i.e., by removal of frontal lobes] displays suppression of all manifestation of the spirit of initiative and of inquisitiveness. This is proof that through the experiment the imaginative power, evocative power, and determination of thought have been suppressed. This syndrome includes irrational fear, errors of judgment, indifference towards things and living beings, a tendency to collect useless and filthy things (as do some idiots as well as the demented), and *tics*. Perceptive indifference, lack of all initiative, of any objective, inability to develop a thought logically, strong emotional episodes (fear, anger, and sometimes aggressiveness, whence emotional reaction) are common facts in the life of imbeciles. All this phenomenology is sufficiently demonstrative of what I believe to be the function of the frontal lobes.

EXCERPT PP. 354–355

My experiments have demonstrated that although the fundamental and intermediate emotions are preserved (some altered) after ablation of the

frontal lobes, the higher sentiments or emotions, as these have been outlined in the monkey, are absent or profoundly disturbed, in correspondence
to what is observed to follow severe lesions of the same lobes in man.
Although in the mutilated monkeys conduct is reduced to single reflexes,
dissociated and inconsequential, hence lacking biophylactic power, the
organic reflexes of the primitive emotions (fear, anger) prevail. On the
other hand, in the same unmutilated animals there prevails a more protective conduct, of an evident affective intonation, and in consequence more
logical, based upon perceptions, experiences, and judgment, and the organic reflexes of the primitive emotions are proportionately much reduced.
This is confirmed most strikingly in the sentiment of sociability, abolished
in the monkeys with ablation of the frontal lobes. Sentimentality is therefore revealed as especially a function of the frontal lobes. Its structure,
formed of emotions, of ideas variously associated, of impulses, of inhibitions, permits us to presuppose organs differing from those of the primitive
emotions. The results of phylogenetic and ontogenetic inquiries in relation
to the evolution of the brain, and especially of the frontal lobes, as well as
clinical and experimental observations, are in some measure in convincing
agreement.

In this book Bianchi also showed that his earlier findings were still valid, and he
provided the following succinct conclusion to them.

EXCERPT PP. 89–90

The first experiments that I undertook on dogs permitted me to express
myself in an initial communication in the sense that, for the time being, it
was possible to conclude that the *unilateral* mutilations of the prefrontal
lobe of the experimental animals were not followed by any noteworthy
symptoms; and that the bilateral mutilations in the dogs had produced a
distinct change in character, especially prominent in all the psychic manifestations; defective perceptive judgment, exaggerated fear through defective critical power and through inability to avail themselves of their physical powers, actually preserved; amnesia and a psychically blind behavior,
defective initiative and resourcefulness, lack of finality in complex movements, revealed by incoherent conduct and lessened vivacity (lowering of
the psychic tone), so that any ordinary person would have judged these
animals to be imbecile.

E. ANATOMICAL STUDIES

So far in this chapter only the function of the cerebral cortex has been considered. However, while the physiologists and clinicians were tackling this problem,

the histologists were investigating the structural elements of the cortex and their complex arrangement (Chapter VIII). A correlation of the two groups of data was a natural development (for Meynert's views that initiated this association, see p. 432). Two outstanding and early attempts to discover the anatomical basis for function will be presented below. Whether or not a correlation may be possible eventually, it is now realized that for the present available techniques are inadequate to provide a conclusive answer.

PAUL EMIL FLECHSIG

(*See p. 277*)

The method of myelogenesis invented by Flechsig has already been discussed but only in relation to the anatomy of the spinal cord pathways (pp. 277–280 and 857–858). In its application to the brain, which he began to investigate in 1893, it was based upon observation of the appearance of myelinization in the subcortical, white matter of the developing human fetus and infant. As this varied, in time Flechsig was able to identify groups of fibres and their dependent cortical areas in a chronological sequence of development; function was possible only when myelinization was complete. He was thus able to isolate *projection* or motor and sensory areas that were dependent upon fibres that matured early, chiefly before birth, and neighboring *association* areas controlling intellectual functions, of which the fibres matured after birth; these terms were already in use (Meynert, 1872, pp. 602–605). Each group of fibres was subdivided into subsidiary, functional systems, so that it was possible to map the cortex; the numbers that Flechsig gave to the areas were changed as his experience grew. Figure 134 is his best known diagram and comes from the long report he made to the Zentralkomitee für Hirnforschung in 1904 ("Einige Bermerkungen über die Untersuchungsmethoden der Grosshirnrinde, insbesondere des Menschen," *Ber. Verh. k. sächs. Ges. Wiss. Leipz.*, Math.-Phys. Klasse, 1904, 56:50–104, 177–248); it shows the cortical areas he identified and numbered. His results did not always coincide with those derived from other techniques of which he took little heed.

As might be expected, Flechsig's work caused a great stir and it provoked much beneficial discussion and experimentation; one of his principal opponents was Bianchi who refuted Flechsig's conclusions concerning the frontal lobes.

His contribution to the history of cortical localization has thus been an outstanding one, even though many of his conclusions have since been disproved. An account of his myelogenetic technique applied to the cerebral cortex is to be found in a paper ("Developmental (myelogenetic) localisation of the cerebral cortex in the human subject," *Lancet*, 1901, ii:1027–1029), and the following excerpts have been taken from it (see fig. 134).

EXCERPT PP. 1027–1028

In the cerebral convolutions, as in all other parts of the central nervous system, the nerve-fibres do not develop everywhere simultaneously, but step by step in a definite succession, this order of events being particularly maintained in regard to the appearance of the medullary substance . . . . Thus there come into existence sharply circumscribed areas differing in the stages of development of their elements which I call myelogenetic cortical areas. These fields are constant in arrangement; they repeat themselves in essentially the same position and extent in all individuals of approximately the same age. The contours do not change perpetually with the progress of the medullary investment, but show during a certain period the same type, a fact which obviously depends upon the general character of the myelogenetic differences . . . .

In my first memoir on the subject I estimated the number of the myelogenetic cortical areas at 40. Further researches have shown that some of these must be combined into one, so that I at present distinguish only 36. I find it useful to denote the areas simply by numbers (1 to 36) corresponding to their respective places in order of development, and therefore wholly chronological. In order to present a comprehensive view, and having regard to differences of a general nature, I have classified them in the three following chronological groups: (1) regions of early development (primordial zones), (2) regions of intermediate development (intermediary zones); and (3) regions of late development (terminal zones).

. . . .

The general significance of the myelogenetic localisation of the cortex may be put into words as follows. Every area possesses a special anatomical position and, therefore, also a special functional importance. For a great number of the areas this can now be absolutely proved. (The objection that the recognition of thirty-six different "organs" in the cortex means a falling back to the phrenology of Gall, and other objections of a like kind, may be met by a simple reference to the fact that it was the myelogenetic parcelling out of the surface of the brain which for the first time provided tangible and comprehensive anatomical data for the scientific solution of the questions involved, and which revealed points of difference that had not up to that time been even suspected.) The average size of a cortical area (about twenty square centimetres = three and a quarter square inches) is very considerable when compared to the much smaller dimensions of the medulla oblongata with its many centres.

Flechsig's conclusions concerning his cortical areas were at times speculative and, as he mentioned, he was occasionally accused of returning to phrenology. However, the basic divisions of the cortex into motor, sensory, and association areas was correct and, as all of his work has not yet been fully evaluated, other parts of it may also be acceptable. It certainly had a profound influence upon subsequent theories of cortical function and contemporary comments on it were frequent (Barker, 1897*a* and *b*; Ireland, 1898; Sabin, 1905).

A brief but excellent account of Flechsig's cortical centers is to be found in a paper delivered to the 13th International Congress of Medicine held in Paris in 1900 ("Les centres de projection et d'association du cerveau humain," *XIIIe Congrès International de Médecine, Paris, 1900, Section de Neurologie,* pp. 115–121), from which the following selection has been translated (see fig. 134). Thus far Flechsig had identified only eighteen to twenty areas.

EXCERPTS PP. 117–121

The anatomy of the normal adult brain provides only very uncertain information compared with that of the fetus and the newly born. In the latter one can in a certain way differentiate between several of the cortical areas from the start.

1° There are about eighteen to twenty myelogenetic areas for which a well-developed corona radiata can be easily distinguished. In other regions the presence of a corona radiata cannot be demonstrated either in the infant or in the adult. The latter therefore does not expand later; it never expands.

2° Those areas which have no corona radiata are rich in long association systems, whereas these systems are found only in small numbers in those areas which abound in coronae radiatae.

3° One may therefore, purely from an anatomical standpoint, divide the cortical areas into projection and association centers. The presence of isolated projection fibres in association centers does not detract from this classification, since the name implies merely the predominance of one of these elements. Only if in the two kinds of cortical areas the long association and projection systems were represented in equal proportions, would it be no longer possible to uphold this classification . . . .

PROJECTION CENTERS

Recently, I have distinguished four of these centers:

The area of bodily sensation,

The visual area,

The auditory area,

The olfactory and taste area.

According to my recent discoveries, each of these areas (with the exception of the auditory area) is formed by the grouping together of several myelogenetic cortical areas. The area of bodily sensation has eight, and each of the others three. Furthermore, the area of bodily sensation (still called the tactile area, or area of general sensation) occupies a somewhat more extensive area than that I had attributed to it; at the 1st frontal convolution it spreads a few centimeters farther anteriorly. The most anterior segment (about 2 cm. long) of the supramarginal gyrus must be part of it. The subangular gyrus constitutes a new projection that I have subsequently discovered; the structure of its cortex has the special characteristics of sensory centers.

ASSOCIATION CENTERS

At first I distinguished four association centers:
The frontal center,
The parietal center,
The temporal center,
The insular center.

Later I grouped the parietal and the temporal into a single center: the large posterior association center. The verified existence of a projection center in the subangular gyrus places the union of these two centers in the posterior portion of the second temporal convolution. They proceed one with the other for only a short distance. Therefore it seems to me that there is every reason to preserve the old division into temporal and parietal center.

In these parietal and temporal centers it is particularly easy to note a subdivision into peripheral zones that reach their complete development earlier, and into central areas that only mature much later. In the frontal association center the same subdivision is evident, but the arrangement is more complicated. The peripheral zones are in contact with the sensory centers and are joined to them by numerous arcuate fibres. The insula and the precuneus seem to consist of nothing but peripheral zones. Perhaps the peripheral areas constitute transitional forms between the areas abundant in corona radiata and those which lack them. At times, although very rarely, one finds in these peripheral zones atypical bundles of the corona radiata which represent aberrant projection fibres of the sensory centers. Such isolated discoveries do not at all prove the general and regular presence of bundles of the corona radiata in the peripheral zones.

The central territories of the association zones (especially the mid portion of the angular gyrus, the third temporal convolution and the anterior half of the second frontal convolution) are, according to all appearances, the nodal points of the long association systems, while the peripheral zones exhibit these characteristics only feebly. The central areas are all terminal ones; essentially they are characteristic of the human brain. Their isolated destruction is never accompanied by a motor or sensory defect. The motor phenomena of excitation which may accompany lesions of them must be interpreted as actions from a distance.

The central regions of the association areas are centers which are in more or less direct relation, each with several sensory areas, but some with all of them; they probably combine the activities in themselves (association).

Following their bilateral destruction, the intellect appears to be diminished; the association of ideas is especially disturbed. Therefore, the central areas, based upon their appearance, are of the utmost importance for the exercise of intellectual activities, for the formation of mental images composed of several sensory qualities, for the performance of acts such as the naming of objects, reading, etc. These functions are regularly disturbed in the case of inflammation of the posterior association centers. Clinical observation establishes and justifies the legitimacy of our division of the cerebral cortex into sensory centers (projection centers) and association centers.

With great diligence and much ability Flechsig worked incessantly on his myelogenetic method, and he was able to extend his theory of association and projection areas. As he was not at the time aware of all the cortical connections, some of the areas he designated as associational have turned out to be, in fact, projectional. But his contention that the posterior association center was a primary sensory area combining parietal, occipital, and temporal cortex and serving as a directing center for the whole brain, is now accepted; it seems to be a mechanism that integrates the external world. On the other hand, when Flechsig stated that a lesion of it produced dementia, he was probably being deceived by sensory aphasia.

In 1920 Flechsig published his last important work on the subject (*Anatomie des menschlichen Gehirns und Rückenmarks auf myelogenetischer Grundlage*, I [Leipzig, 1920]), and the following excerpts have been taken from it (see fig. 135).

EXCERPT PP. 44–47

If one now reviews the results of pathological research which we have only hinted at here, one can hardly come to any other conclusion than that these facts point to ipsilateral organization of the cerebral cortex as regards its function and to myelogenetic differentiation as regards its anatomy. Secondary degeneration and clinical findings agree that in man the cortical areas, the destruction of which causes dysfunction of sensation or atrophy, constitute only a small portion of the cerebral surface and that these areas agree satisfactorily with the primary sensory fields as I have outlined them myelogenetically, whereas the remainder of the cerebral surface is essentially of a different nature . . . .

Everything taken into account, the cerebral cortex appears as a complex of multivalent functional areas which, at least at the start of extrauterine life, exhibits a high degree of independence. Its separate existence is reflected in the fact that *all the conducting tracts* of the pallium are structurally organized into myelogenetic fields . . . . Therefore, *the fundamental principle of the development of areas is applicable* not only to the projection systems but *to all cortical conducting tracts*, so that one must attribute the importance of special centers to all *myelogenetic* areas, purely from the *embryological* standpoint.

A question of the greatest importance is raised in reference to the association systems of the primary sensory areas as to whether each individual sensory area is directly connected with all cortical areas, or with most of them, by arcuate fibres and long association systems, or if this cannot be presumed, whether each individual sensory area communicates directly with one or several other primary areas.

Both points can be answered in the negative with almost complete certainty . . . .

. . . .

That each individual sensory area uniformly embraces the marginal zones that are related to it cannot be denied immediately; indeed, one might be inclined to affirm the necessity of such an organization for the interpretation of certain psychic phenomena which are related especially to memory.

This consideration suggests again the question whether or not the primary sensory areas, that is the projection fields of the individual sensory tracts, must not be considered universally as centers of larger cortical areas, which ought to be considered, although not anatomically, yet functionally as entities, insofar as they participate in their entirety in sensations, that is, perceptions of a definitive sensory quality. In other words, whether or not in the human, too (according to Munk's reports on animals), the entire cerebral cortex must be divided functionally into as many territories ("secondary sensory areas") as primary sensory areas exist. On closer inspection, all hope must be abandoned of arriving in this way at an exact division of the human cortex. Apart from the fact that it is completely impossible to delineate by any means in man the exact extent of the cortical excitation from a given sensory stimulus, the terminal fields also can only be each classified in a definitive sensory area by force.

Therefore, it seems to me that an adequate number of actual experiments exist to justify devising a general theory of the cerebral surface in the human, based on myelogenetic and pathological observations.

It will be a paramount project for the neuroanatomists to establish the number of the myelogenetic cortical fields for as many animal species as possible! For the time being, and concerning the human brain, it is conclusive only so far as a clear, total image has been obtained . . . .

The successive occurrence of sensory spheres in the series of vertebrates which has been demonstrated by Edinger is distinctly reflected in man in the cellular development (cytoarchitectonic) of the different cortical regions—myelogenetically, the principle is less striking.

If I now discuss briefly the reactions which the disclosures of my myelogenetic method had upon macroscopic anatomy, there remains hardly any doubt that not only the understanding of external forms has often been advanced, but also that important viewpoints have been established for the cruder division of the cerebral cortex, so that it will become necessary to devote considerable attention to their nomenclature.

Korbinian Brodmann
(See p. 450)

Contemporaneously with Flechsig, Brodmann was also studying the myeloarchitecture of the subcortical white matter and, by observing cytoarchitectonics in addition, he was able to subdivide the cerebral cortex of the monkey on a purely morphological basis. However, his main purpose was to advance the knowledge of cortical function and pathology (p. 450); hence he aimed at a correlation between cortical form and function which would further substantiate the theory of localization within the cortex.

In his famous book, *Vergleichender Lokalisationslehre der Grosshirnrinde in ihren Prinzipien dargestellt auf Grund des Zellenbaues* (Leipzig, 1909), Brodmann discussed the comparisons between the two groups of experimental data, and argued that because there were histological variations, so variations in function must also exist in the cortex. The following passages have been translated from Chapter IX, "Versuch einer physiologischen Cortexorganologie"; the first of them deals with general principles. The work has been translated by Bonin [1960] also.

EXCERPT PP. 304–306

2. LOCALIZED FUNCTION

Perhaps the considerations developed here make the localization of higher psychological processes impossible, in the sense of the limitations of the parallel physiological processes on which they are based. On the other hand, our histotopographical findings, which are in many respects identical with the evidence derived from the arrangement of the fibre systems and from clinicopathological experience, emphatically show that despite this objection, the circumscribed localization of certain central nervous system activities in the cerebral cortex is to be assumed.

The specific histological differentiation of the cortical areas proves irrefutably their *specific functional differentiation*—for it is based as we have seen on a division of labor. The great number of specially prepared structural areas suggests *a special separation of individual functions*. Moreover, the outlines of the fields which in all cases are sharp, finally allow us to conclude that *a strictly circumscribed localization* of the physiological activities which correspond to the area is necessary.

(*a*) THE PRINCIPLE OF ABSOLUTE LOCALIZATION

Although psychologists have often expressed themselves against this idea, on the basis of the anatomical facts already mentioned which are in favor of several cortical structures of this kind, they are compelled to adhere to the principle of absolute localization.

The strictly delimited structural zones that stand out as special morphological organs on the surface of the cortex cannot be explained in any other way than by the assumption that *an equally strictly circumscribed specific function is localized in them; in other words, each organ of this kind carries a function exclusive to itself and different from the activities of all other organs.* It does not necessarily follow, however, that in such a "center" only a single, elementary activity has its seat; for instance, that in a sense center there are only sensory elements pertaining to peripheral stimulation (visual, auditory, sensory, etc.). On the contrary, it is probable that within the same organs, an association of these elements occurs. Thus a concatenation of the elements with higher complex functions occurs in the same place, and, moreover, simultaneously with the actual sensory elements, other activities are connected with such a cortical sensory apparatus.

We cannot therefore regard such a sensory center as merely a repetition or a reflection of the peripheral sensory surface, as for example the retina, but with Wundt we consider it "a center" in the true sense of the word; that is, an organ in which different peripheral functions taking part in the sensory activity in question are centralized and confined. To make this clear, in the case of the visual center, for example, not only the functions of light sensitivity, but also those of associated emotional activity of the eyes, as well as those of certain visual reflexes, and so on, can be localized. The essential part of this view is that such elementary cortical activities which are coordinated with a peripheral sense apparatus will always remain limited to a circumscribed structural area of the cortex; that is, circumscribed in the strict sense of the word. The physiological boundaries are just as sharp and constant as the morphological ones, and also the specific conducting pathways have their origin or their exit fixed within these absolute and constant limits.

(*β*) THE PRINCIPLE OF RELATIVE LOCALIZATION

In addition to the sharply circumscribed organs, we have also found in the cerebral cortex structural areas with variable boundaries. Their tectonic features are blended more or less with those of the neighboring areas with which they partially overlap. This fact suggests the possibility of a more or less overlapping of some functions in the cerebral cortex. Certain pathophysiological evidence also speaks in favor of this. But by such an overlapping, we do not refer to the elementary functions mentioned above which are inseparably connected and in any case are located together in one center. We mean by this, cortical activities which belong to different localities in the periphery of the body and which are partially represented within the cerebral cortex. In this sense, we can speak of a *relative* localization in the sense that a physiological activity is not strictly limited to its own area but that other functions can be partially served by it as well. (*Principle of multiple functional representation of cortical areas.*)

Brodmann later discussed specific areas of localization, and in the following passages first of all pointed out that there was complete agreement between anatomical and physiological data concerning the motor area. He subsequently considered the visual area.

EXCERPT PP. 311–313

If one finally compares my other histological brain maps with the localized areas based on the stimulation results of C. and O. Vogt, one can also recognize in other mammals, and especially in the lower ones, some agreement between the anatomical boundaries and those resulting from physiological stimulation.

Thus we come to the conclusion *that there exists in the most diverse types of animals a cortical area of great physiological importance, the electrically defined motor zone, which agrees sufficiently with an area defined by anatomical methods.* This fact is sufficient for our present consideration. It forms a valuable criterion for evaluating methods which are questioned. One will probably be able to clear up small variations, but on the one hand they may be owing to inadequate techniques and inadequate observation. Yet, on the other hand, it may also be reasonable to consider that a more extensive anatomical area represents a larger entity of which the smaller "stimulation zones," represent only part of its function. In this respect it is not yet clearly determined that areas that can be stimulated electrically must be identical with the "motor region" in the strictest sense of the word—i.e., the center of voluntary movements.

Great difficulties will be encountered when we turn to other areas of function. As I have said, there is chiefly a lack of sufficient knowledge concerning the localization of the most fundamental activities. Especially in the case of man, we are not in possession of any unrefuted localization, even approximately determined, for the main sensory areas.

(B) THE VISUAL AREA IN MAN

With regard to the localization of the visual area, views differ widely. While some localize vision exclusively to the medial surface and wish to have it limited to the "calcarine cortex" in the narrowest sense of the word (Henschen [see p. 533]), others assume a much wider extension of the cortical visual area and include nearly all of the occipital cortex, including the convexity (von Monakow, Bernheimer, Förster). In this instance it seems that histological localization is indeed most suited to decide the issue. Our area striata represents a well-characterized region that is sharply delimited topically. Besides, in the whole animal kingdom it can be demonstrated so constantly and irrefutably, that without doubt one can claim for it a principal function as specific as it is elementary, and pertaining to all mammals. On the other hand, clinicopathological experiences suggest the idea that there exists a closer relationship of the area of cortex with the main sensory function usually localized in this region which is the perception of visual sense impressions. However, the localization of the visual area carried out by Henschen on the basis of simultaneous clinical and pathological observations also agrees very well in detail with the area striata [see p. 533]. This agreement may well be able to decide the issue between the two competing hypotheses of localization in favor of Henschen's view which is more in keeping with the anatomical findings. Neuropathologists must take note of this in the future.

Brodmann concluded the chapter, and the book, as follows.

EXCERPT PP. 320–321

I have come to the end of my deliberations. As can be seen, the views on anatomical and physiological localization are quite compatible. Both lead in principle to the differentiation of surface areas, that is, to a topographical division of the surface of the hemispheres into different organs. In some respects, the agreement is also satisfactory with regard to the special localization of single "centers." However, in other respects, the physiological views will have to suffer correction from the irrefutable anatomical facts. The majority of histological organs still lacks a localization of function. Here a large field of fruitful activity has been opened to physiology through the newly won findings of anatomical localization.

Nevertheless, one thing must be stressed emphatically: in future a functional localization of the cerebral cortex is hardly possible without the guidance of anatomy in man and animal. In all its spheres, physiology has its surest guide in anatomy. He who wishes to work on physiological localization will, therefore, have to take for the basis of his researches the results of histological localization. With more reason than ever, we should remember the words spoken by that great master of brain research, Bernhard Gudden [see p. 606], who thirty years ago referred to the one-sided and dangerous specialization of ablation: "Every physiological result loses its meaning if it conflicts with a proved anatomical fact . . . Therefore first anatomy and then physiology, but if physiology first, then not without anatomy."

F. Antilocalizationists

As already mentioned, there were those who wished to localize intellectual processes in precise areas of cortex whereas others felt that in the light of the advancing knowledge of histology, physiology, and pathology of the cortex the whole cortical organ was responsible for them. Thus a link with the concept of nervous tissue containing a diffuse nerve net (Chapter II) can be made here. If neurons were in continuity with one another, generalized rather than localized functions of the brain might be expected. Thus Golgi (pp. 91–96), the greatest proponent of the net theory, subscribed to the unitarian action of the nervous system. The same dichotomy of opinion existed with regard to the localization of all functions in the cortex, so that there were on the one hand the localizationists such as Hitzig, Munk, Henschen, and Brodmann, and on the other, their opponents, the antilocalizationists.

The latter were lineal descendants of Flourens (pp. 483–488) whose teaching of what became the holistic theory of equivalence of all parts of the cerebral hemispheres was predominant before 1870; his findings had been frequently confirmed, and as little was known of the histology of the brain, morphological differences of the cortex were as yet unknown. The antilocalizationists represented the expected opposition to the localizationists, and today it seems that their beliefs may be nearer the truth. They denounced the excesses of the localizationists, which were in part a result of the ignorance at that time of the cortical connections with deeper structures, and they argued against the popular designation, cortical "centers," and the cortical maps that depicted them. However, we must recall that although the concept of strict localization may have been in part erroneous, it contributed a great deal to the diagnosis and treatment of disease processes of the brain.

At present it seems that both these interpretations of cortical activity may be acceptable. Modern techniques suggest that both "the concept of regional specialization of relatively simple function and the unitary point of view of complex behavior in man are not antagonistic, but indeed, complementary" (Chapman and Wolff, 1961, p. 470).

Friedrich Leopold Goltz
(14 August 1834—4 May 1902)

One of the earliest and certainly one of the best known opponents of cortical localization was the German physiologist Goltz.

Goltz was born in Posen and educated in Danzig and Königsberg. In 1870 he was appointed professor *extraordinarius* of physiology in the University of Halle and professor *ordinarius* in the University of Strassburg in 1872. He held the latter appointment until his retirement in 1900. His research work was devoted almost exclusively to investigating the effects of cerebral ablation and of spinal cord section. His acute powers of observation and penetrating mind led him to vital and invulnerable conclusions (Ewald, 1903; Haymaker, 1953, pp. 131–135).

It was natural to conclude from the localizationists' doctrine that if circumscribed functional areas of cortex could be isolated by electrical stimulation and their function confirmed by operative ablation, removal of large portions of the cerebral hemispheres would produce severe defects of movement, sensation, and intellect. Yet Goltz, by a series of experiments on dogs, was able to show that this was not entirely the case. He gave increased publicity to his views by exhibiting these dogs, and subsequently their brains, at various physiological meetings in Europe. Two of them survived widespread cortical extirpations for fifty-one and ninety-two days respectively, and a third was shown at the International Medical Congress in London in 1881 and sacrificed there after an eighteen-month survival; the original lesion was examined by an international group of experts (see Goltz, 1881; for examination of brain, see also Langley, 1883–1884; Langley and Sherrington, 1884–1885; Klein, 1883–1884).

In 1887 Goltz reported the findings in a dog following cerebral hemispherectomy ("Über die Verrichtungen des Grosshirns," *Pflügers Arch.*, 1888, 42:419–467), and at the Physiological Congress in Basel in September 1889 he demonstrated another which had survived a three-stage operation for nine months. Again the brain was examined by independent observers and it was shown that all the left hemisphere, including the corpus striatum, had been removed (Langley and Grünbaum, 1890). Neither dog manifested the severe defects of movement and sensation which the localizationists demanded, although some might question the reliability of Goltz's examination of his dogs' sensation. Goltz described the motor state of the second dog as follows (from Langley & Grünbaum, 1890).

EXCERPT P. 607

If I let the dog run about freely in the room, he tends to move towards the left in large circles. But, if called, he comes in a straight line towards the person calling him. It is easy even to make him move in a circular direction towards the right, if he is attracted by pieces of meat held in front of him. He gazes fixedly at food held before him with the right 'intact' eye just in the same way as a normal dog. The condition of the right eye is that of hemiamblyopia as described by Loeb. He can execute movements besides those of walking. He can run. He can stand on his hind legs. The other muscles of his body are as little paralysed as those of his limbs. In eating and licking he moves his tongue symmetrically like an uninjured dog. He is very watchful and barks loudly; consequently it is impossible that the right half of his larynx should be paralysed. When anybody he knows approaches him in a friendly way, he wags his tail and shows his pleasure by movements of the ears, head, body, and limbs in just the same way as a normal dog.

There can therefore be no doubt that those who assert that after extirpation of one cerebral hemisphere in the dog, a *lasting* paralysis of the opposite half of the body *must* remain, are completely mistaken.

In 1892 Goltz published his last important paper on the problem of the decerebrated dog ("Der Hund ohne Grosshirn. Siebente Abhandlung über die Verrichtungen des Grosshirns," *Pflügers Arch.*, 1892, 51:570–614), and he included in it a final assessment of the three famous dogs which had survived for fifty-one days, ninety-two days, and eighteen months respectively; the article is long and rambling, but in the excerpts below Goltz deals mainly with the first two dogs and then discusses the decerebrated dog in general.

Later in life he was willing to accept some of the evidence of the localizationists, and Brodmann in 1911 called him a "half-localizationist." Thus Goltz declared that "the lobes of the hemispheres certainly do not have the same function," but at the same time he did not relinquish earlier beliefs such as, "I do not at all accept a circumscribed visual area" and, "the assumption that circumscribed cortical centers have different functions is untenable" ("Über die Verrichtungen des Grosshirns," *Gesammelte Abhandlungen*, Bonn, 1881, pp. 169 and 173). He thus reached a position closer to the one held today than did any of his contemporaries and he anticipated some of the concepts of Lashley (pp. 570–575) and the holistic theory of total brain function.

In the following excerpts Goltz pointed out the direct relation that exists between the amount of cortex removed and severity of the resulting mental changes. His concept of inhibition owing to irritation from the brain wound is also mentioned, but it was displaced by Monakow's diaschisis (p. 566). Although several of his conclusions were erroneous, his work helped to temper the enthusiasm of the localizationists, and he was an important pioneer of the modern holistic theory of cortical function. The main criticism of Goltz is that he was willing to take the unwarranted step of applying the findings in his dogs to the physiology of the human brain.

EXCERPT PP. 595–601

These two dogs [survival of fifty-one and ninety-two days "following removal by excision of the entire cerebrum"] were capable, at least at first, of performing movements on the spot extremely well after removal of the cerebrum. The one that survived for ninety-two days could trot around in a normal manner only one day after surgery. However, in both animals the ability to move around normally decreased later on and, at the same time, a marked and generalized emaciation took place. Still later they could move only when assisted. At the time when they still had sufficient strength, both could rise on their hind legs and stand on three limbs. The compensating movements of the body and of the eyes which occur when such an animal is placed upon a moving turntable could be demonstrated particularly well in the dog that survived surgery for ninety-two days. Proof of unimpaired auditory acuity could be established only in this dog. Neither of them could see. One of them was totally blind because, as was seen in autopsy, both his optic tracts had been cut. As mentioned already, the other one lost both eyes from a perforating inflammation [of the eyes]. Unimpaired sense of taste was noticeable in one of them when a test was conducted with meat that had been rendered bitter. This test was not carried out on the other dog. By means of tactile stimuli both dogs could be easily made to perform a number of movements. One of them chased away a fly from his head by shaking his head. When a blanket under which the other dog was sleeping was pulled off, he awoke and raised his head. When he got up he stretched very much as a normal dog does upon awakening. Neither of them allowed his extremities to be moved. They not only soon returned a limb which was in an uncomfortable position to its proper position, but also expressed their displeasure by growling.

The vocal expressions of these two dogs were as varied as in the third one [eighteen months' survival]. They could whimper, whine, squeak, complain, bark, and howl. It was particularly easy to make them furious when they were handled somewhat roughly or lifted from the ground. In addition, they expressed their dissatisfaction by barking, kicking, and biting when they were washed. When excreting feces and urine, their bodies adopted the same position as in young dogs.

Their ability to take offered food voluntarily was not as skillful as that of the third dog which may therefore be called the pearl among them. But they too were cooperative which made day-to-day feeding easy. They both succeeded in lapping up milk in small quantities. Once one of them when doing this took up a piece of meat which it then proceeded to chew and swallow in a normal manner. The same animal repeatedly licked his nose, which was smeared with butter, until it was clean. When chewing the meat that was stuffed into their mouths they behaved with equal facility. But only the one that was observed the longest [eighteen months] regained the ability to seize and chew larger heaps of meat by opening and closing his mouth voluntarily.

If we look at the performance of these three dogs without a cerebrum, it becomes immediately clear that the legend which has been perpetuated in all textbooks regarding the behavior of mammals without this structure has merely the value of a legend, and one of many that have been proposed in the field of neurophysiology. After all, until now a higher mammal without a cerebrum has never been observed for any length of time; nevertheless a picture was fabricated, based upon experience with very young mammals and birds, that combined all the features which a dog without a cerebrum might be expected to manifest.

Primarily included in these features and apparently accepted beyond a shadow of doubt was the conjecture that a mammal without a cerebrum could neither eat nor drink . . . . The theory, valid until now, that decerebrated mammals swallow only what is pushed down their throats must be abandoned. Dogs without a cerebrum voluntarily grab food near to them and ingest it . . . .

In addition, it has been said that animals without a cerebrum are mute . . . . However, nobody surmised that an adult dog without a cerebrum could be vocal in so many ways.

. . . .

Those who nevertheless persist in their opinion that an animal without a cerebrum is nothing but a complicated, albeit insensitive, machine, have additional problems to solve. Dogs that have lost only a large portion of both cerebral hemispheres behave just as stupidly as those that have lost the entire cerebrum. Consequently, if one now denies psychological activity, one admits that large parts of the cerebrum have nothing to do with psychological processes.

. . . .

The idea that animals without a cerebrum no longer feel anything is probably based primarily upon the oft-repeated opinion that such animals do not readily move spontaneously. That this assumption is incorrect for other animals such as frogs and pigeons has been convincingly demonstrated, especially by Schrader. Our decerebrated dogs were, as has been reported, only too inclined to move spontaneously, so that the resulting use of energy was partially to blame for their emaciation.

. . . .

. . . .

I do not believe it will be necessary for me to stress that I am not interested in gaining supporters for the opinion that dogs without a cerebrum retain manifold sensations. He who considers it more scientific to call the decerebrate dog an insensitive automaton will not be influenced by me. But I do insist that he observe the functions of this automation, and furthermore that he not imagine that they could function exclusively from a minute area in the cerebrum, the so-called center; I maintain that the function still operated in our decerebrated dogs even though they no longer possessed all those much lauded centers. A dog minus the so-called foreleg center should, if the foreleg is bruised, no longer howl nor attempt to bite the hand of the attacker. This statement is incorrect. A dog which has lost the so-called sensory area for vision should show no sign of guarding when the eye is touched with a needle, etc. All these assumptions are incorrect, for a dog that has no sensory area whatsoever still functions in areas which he is supposed to have unequivocally lost. A dog without the auditory area should be mute and deaf. This is wrong again, for a dog which, apart from the auditory area, has also lost all the remaining and much praised sensory areas is anything but deaf-mute. Others insist that dogs without the so-called motor centers become paralyzed. This prejudice along with all the rest must be rejected. A dog without a cerebrum is anything but paralyzed. He is only too lively in his fits of passion.

EXCERPT PP. 603–604

. . . . In my first report I have already supported the hypothesis that the disorders that may be observed immediately after mutilation of the cerebrum are partly related to an inhibition suffered by those parts of the brain located behind the cerebrum and owing to irritation from a cerebral wound. . . . . But what becomes of the cortical centers when an entire cerebral hemisphere has been excised, including the corpus striatum? Before the threatening knife they escape with incredible speed into the other hemisphere. However, the joyous roving of these miraculous centers has still not come to an end. Following destruction of the entire substance of the pallium they are always back in place. Our dogs without a cerebrum barked and snapped when their paws were squeezed. This is not supposed to be possible without a sensory area. Therefore, the sensory perceptions must have sneaked out from the substance of the pallium and escaped into other parts of the brain . . . .

A dog without a cerebrum can in many ways present less disorders than one that has lost only a quarter of the cerebrum. No responsible scientist is going to pretend that one quarter of an organ has more functions than all of it. The inevitable conclusion is that the severe disturbances that occur immediately after removal of the anterior quarter of the cerebrum are not exclusively a decrease in function, but that part of it can be related to inhibitory functions, the origins of which must be looked for beyond the cerebral substance of the pallium.

EXCERPT PP. 607–612

In my opinion the most important decreased function which can be noted following cerebral surgery is the absence of all evidence from which we assess the animal's understanding, memory, reflection, and intelligence . . . .

. . . . The fact still remains that he [the decerebrated dog] also could not utilize the auditory, olfactory, and tactile senses enabling him to act intelligently, although his nerve tracts serving these three senses were completely intact. The dog did not understand what was said to him. He responded to threats as little as to caresses. However, he had the ability to hear, for he could be awakened from slumber by noise and seemed to mind noise when he was awake.

I would like to cite the following observation as proof that the dog no longer had a memory, or capacity for reflection, and that he learned less from experience than the most stupid, unoperated animal . . . . The stupidest, unoperated animal would soon have learned that feeding followed lifting from the cage, and it would have been pleased when it was gently led to the feeding place. However, our decerebrated dog, as soon as he was seized and lifted out of the cage, behaved on the last day of his life in the same enraged fashion as he had months before. This fit of temper, expressed by kicking, barking, and biting, only subsided when he was put upon the table. Schiff has already pointed to this behavior of decerebrated animals in other experiments. They do not learn from past experience. They do not have experiences, for only he who has memories can have experiences. The decerebrated dog is essentially nothing but a child of the moment.

If the decerebrated dog does not learn to realize that feeding follows being lifted from the cage, he will understand more complex proceedings even less. An unoperated dog is grateful when he has been liberated from a restraint, when one takes off his muzzle, loosens his leash, or removes a splinter from his skin. The decerebrated dog does not know the expression of joy. He bites the hand which tries to set him free, for he does not understand the loving service that is about to be given him.

Such a dog is incapable of expressing pleasure. However, he enjoys the advantage of not knowing jealousy and envy. If one throws a piece of meat to an intact dog in the presence of another dog, he does not take the time to chew the piece he catches. He swallows it unchewed and with great effort, because he does not want to miss the next piece which his fellow dog, at whom he squints jealously, might snatch away from him. And even if no other dog is present, he does not permit himself time to chew properly, as long as he sees a supply after which he hungers. Envy and greed deprive him of the pleasure of slowly chewing and digesting the offered food. The decerebrate dog knows neither envy nor greed. . . .

When the present report is published an attempt will undoubtedly be made to deny the obvious shipwreck of the doctrine of the small, outlined centers, by inventing auxiliary hypotheses. The sad shambles of the wreck of the old theory will be patched up so that it may become seaworthy again. "Be fertile and multiply," the centers will be told, and the host of the outlined cerebral centers which is already increasing daily will be fortified by as many reserve centers in the midbrain and hindbrain, ready to go into battle when the upper ones in the cerebrum meet with an accident.

. . . .

I am not at all fundamentally opposed to the question of the localization of cerebral functions. It must be advanced by useful ablation experiments. I myself initiated the demonstration as to how to excise cerebral lobes. I do not believe in the merit of additional experiments with electric stimulation, so long as we cannot possibly know what actually was stimulated. . . . Only the third dog described in such detail was capable of walking without help until his death, and even at the end he still had the energy to stand up on his hind legs. But during the last months of his life he did not walk as naturally and energetically as during the first weeks after the last surgery. This weakness was owing to a marked emaciation of the entire posterior part of the body which occurred in all three dogs. . . . It must be somewhat difficult for the partisans of the centers, who are always ready with the assurance that the smallest disjointed remnant of a center is endowed with the most marvellous functions, to convince us that whole centers are able to conceal their functions from us. For my part, there is no mystery in the fact that considerable residual parts of the cerebrum seemingly are without any function.

CONSTANTIN VON MONAKOW
(*4 November 1853—19 October 1930*)

Another important investigator who contested the parcellation of the cerebral cortex by the localizationists was the Swiss neuropsychiatrist Monakow.

Monakow was born in Bobrezowo in northern Russia but in 1869 became a naturalized Swiss subject. He studied medicine in Zürich and was associated with Gudden and Hitzig as well as studying under Westphal, Oppenheim, Virchow, du Bois-Reymond, and Munk. He eventually established his own brain research institute in Zürich and when it was taken over by the University in 1894, Monakow was appointed professor *extraordinarius*. He retired in 1928. Minkowski (p. 535), his successor in Zürich, has pointed out (Minkowski, 1931) that Monakow's life can be divided into three periods: in the first he studied the thalamocortical connections (see pp. 619–623) and carried out other important neuroanatomical investigations such as establishing a morphological foundation for Munk's observations (pp. 528–533); in the second he investigated cortical localization; and in the third he wrote on the philosophical, ethical, and moral implications of his earlier neurobiological work and took no further active interest in neurology (see Winkler, 1923, with short bibliography; Waser, 1933, a novel based on his life; McGill, 1936, pp. 129–140; Haymaker, 1953, pp. 336–340; Kolle, 1956–1963, III, 149–163).

The second period, during which Monakow studied cortical localization, ended in 1914 with the publication of the large work, *Die Lokalisation im Grosshirn und der Abbau der Funktion durch kortikale Herde* (Wiesbaden, 1914). He introduced a new element into the problem, for he emphasized the importance of the time factor in the analysis and interpretation of cortical localization. This was his *chronogenic localization* of functions such as movement and language which was distinct from the geometrical localization of symptoms. He believed that, as the brain developed, "chronological layers" rather than spatial ones were formed, and that the cortex functioned not by the activity of circumscribed areas but by the interplay of many parts. Evolving nervous functions could not be precisely localized and the temporal element was further exemplified by his theory of diaschisis, or transient neural shock, which replaced Goltz's irritational inhibition (p. 560). The immediate symptoms are an unreliable guide to the functions of a destroyed cortical area but diaschisis, which is still accepted today, produces transient symptoms at a distance by diminishing or abolishing function. Monakow insisted on the fundamental distinction between this effect and the residual symptoms owing to local anatomical destruction. Thus recovery of cortical function, partial or complete, could be more satisfactorily accounted for than by the formation of new centers, and the temporal sequence of function could be more readily understood, although the effect of retraining must also be considered. "He thus introduced concepts which make clinical neurology a truly biological science or organismal dynamics of human behavior [Haymaker, 1953, p. 339]." Concerning intelligence, he concurred with the aggregation theory of Munk (1890) whereby the cortical properties, instead of being distributed throughout the cortex as the holistic doctrine demanded, were discretely distributed.

Monakow summarized his idea of diaschisis as follows ("Lokalisation der Hirnfunktionen," *J. Neurol. Psychiat.*, 1911, 17:185–200); full translation by Bonin (1960, pp. 231–250).

EXCERPT P. 200

No matter how the further investigation of the problem of localization may turn out, I am convinced by our latest studies of functional dissolution, that diaschisis or some similar consideration cannot be neglected. Diaschisis represents, in association with other forms of shock, a dynamic basic principle, for it creates a bridge between a nervous phenomenon which is distinctly and precisely localized, and one which is not. Thus in reality it is nothing but a collapse of the complicated activity of brain tissue, a collapse in nerve cells which show no anatomical damage and which are distant from the focus in both space and time. This collapse leads to a struggle which may end in victory or defeat for the involved elements or connections. We find an attenuated reflection of it in the conflict between the normal nerve impulses of daily life, from the simplest reflexes up to the highest psychical activity.

Monakow's vast monograph on cortical localization, published in 1914, gathered together his investigations and opinions which had resulted from the second period of his life's activities. The following excerpts are from the final chapter.

EXCERPT PP. 900–905

Now, in conclusion, referring once more to the importance of the frontal lobes for higher psychical functions, I would like to recall first that this question has always been answered in a variety of ways depending on what position the individual investigator took in reference to the localization of cortical function. The tendency to accommodate psychological or complicated physiological factors in specific, delineated areas has recently found renewed support in certain circles, because of the investigation of cytoarchitectural differences in the structure of the different cortical areas [e.g., Brodmann, see p. 554]. Significant variations have been revealed in discussions of this subject during the past decade. At the time of Flourens, and even later until Hitzig and Munk discovered the somatic cortical areas (sensory areas), no opposition was encountered by the statement that with local, superficial defects the remaining cortex in its entirety took over the undiminished functional activity, and that there did not exist a separate cortical site for the different functions. Later on, attempts were made to distribute the sensory centers in as many cortical areas as possible, so that they filled the entire convexity and, at the same time, provided the components for the mental digestion of what was perceived (Meynert, Hitzig, Exner, Luciani). Still later, the size of the sensory areas was continually restricted (Henschen, Flechsig, Ramón y Cajal), and in lieu of this, areas which lie at the periphery of these regions were supplied with higher nervous functions and designated as actual intelligence centers (Flechsig). In this manner a purely physiological division of function, as we deduce it, was placed rather arbitrarily into areas which were more sharply separated anatomically. Unfortunately, so far neither the imagination nor the biological knowledge of the investigators, based on physiological, anatomical, and pathological data, have been sufficient for these experiments to substantiate or clarify more closely this manner of localization.

At present we find ourselves in a period of investigation when the theory of separate association and projection centers proposed by Flechsig [pp. 552–554], while not yet refuted, begins nevertheless to be essentially transformed, even taking into account the anatomical and, above all, the *embryological* processes intrinsic to it. The temporal, that is, the embryological moment in function was accepted for the first time from a biological standpoint in Flechsig's theory. Although at first only partly accepted, it met with considerable attention and was particularly influenced by the work of R. Semon. The methodological errors which had formerly been committed by the majority of physiologists and brain pathologists, and of which Flourens, Goltz, and many others had warned in the past, were again recognized. Now the so-called *chronogenic localization of function* is adopted. The latter concept of localization includes in the local representation, the various nervous functions, along with the most far-reaching attention to *the phase of their first appearance*, and with the participation *also of subcortical centers*. It was selected tentatively for this work as a basis for the physiological as well as the pathological phenomena of localization and it was enriched by the principle of diaschisis [p. 566].

At first it was rather difficult to offer an exact proof for this new theory in view of the sparsity of material, especially clinical, available for the purpose. However, it seems to me that it is steadily gaining ground despite opposition from some quarters.

In my opinion, only simple physiological processes which occur simultaneously (the most important are the reflexes) can be localized precisely. Those that take place in the present do so gradually, and they always presuppose the activity of several centers, that is, apparatus. Their whole activity, that is, their function as such (for example, locomotion), cannot like an island be localized in an area. The individual components, however, each simultaneously takes up time and can (theoretically) be localized in this [temporal] manner. What then are these components and how can they be separated so that they may be "ripe for dissecting"? That is the basic question. Well, sensory stimulations and points of innervation for specific muscle groups, that is, combinations of movements of various parts of the body, are each localized intimately in groups. However, the direct results from these simultaneous combinations of stimuli are registered *moment by moment as resulting from the use of organs and parts of the body*, and fashioned into a so-called "engram." It offers a more extensive and related sphere of stimulus to very different cortical areas (points) which can be claimed in another sense than that mentioned above. Certainly there can be no question here of localization in the form of island-like areas. The majority of the higher functions work with such complicated components (engrams) and in increasingly and continually perfect combinations, that "localization" is possible here in the widest sense only. I am certain of one thing, however, in relation to the anatomical representation of the higher, and even the highest, nervous functions in the cortex. In all physiological interrelations of the structures in question and of the successive manifestations of nervous function, the stimulating processes which start in earliest childhood (also those in a latent phase) must pass through special and distinct paths of innervation which are still anatomically identifiable, although incredibly complicated.

Of course, these pathways will include an incredible number of joint components, elements which act now as a stimulus, now as a (more reciprocal) inhibition. I am sure that the majority, and above all the smaller nerve cells in the cerebral cortex which are not closely differentiated histologically, are jointly involved in the most varied way in the higher processes of innervation. Of course, the combination in which the elements are used is changing constantly, or at least frequently. In other words, the specificity of the nerve cell elements decreases steadily towards the surface of the cerebrum, and the differentiation of combined stimuli, depending on a chronogenic moment, now takes place in such manner that temporal layers of stimuli (engrams from all periods of life) provide the basis for the variety of the higher physiological, that is, psychological, functions.

According to all evidence, the driving force for the formulation and the more subtle arrangement of the higher functions is also essentially of an "embryological" nature (memory stimulus). Even the highest mental functions continue to develop and to group themselves on the basis of simple sensory stimuli and types of movement. These simple types of stimuli, however, possess their entrance or exit, which are well defined anatomically. Those functions, too, which probably have an anatomical basis in the cortical areas (cytoarchitecturally and through their external shape) will demonstrate any *morphological* peculiarity or symptom; in other words, the more complicated tasks might eventually, after all, be best expressed by specific structural peculiarities, even if only in a general way. In my opinion, however, and for reasons which I have stated above, it is completely inadmissible to consider such crude localization as that by sulci or by cytoarchitectural areas (intellectual centers restricted as regards space) as some researchers have tried to do experimentally.

. . . .

However, if we should now like to form a physiological idea of the importance of the differing structure of the cortex, even if only hypothetically, we must, to repeat once more, proceed on those paths which have been laid out for us by *embryology (in the broadest sense of the word), that is by the evolution of function* as well as by the experimental and anatomical method. Utilizing these pathways we arrive, beyond myelogenetic and histogenetic localization, first at a method which divides almost the entire cortex into two basic layers: *a*) a ventral one, which establishes the association of the cortex with the projecting fibres and long association fibre systems (the layer of multiform and of spindle-shaped elements, as well as the large and the giant pyramidal cells); and *b*) a dorsal one, which consists of histologically little-differentiated, small elements (stratum molecularis, superficial cell layer, and the upper pyramidal layer to the beginning of the middle granular layer; with the exception of the large pyramidal cell) and that which, in schematic terms, includes the cortical association systems. This latter, incidentally, is no longer in direct relation to the white matter of the cerebrum. *Localization based on anatomy and physiology* (representation of sensory organs and parts of the body) *in the entire cortex would be limited to the ventral layer* (IV—VI of Brodmann). In these, manifold (but not chessboard-like) delineated areas would be assumed which are in direct connection with the subcortical centers by special, joined projection bundles, among these, of course, being those in which representation takes place according to body surface and sensory organs (similar to the spinal cord and brain stem). Among the ventral cortical layers should also be classified, although, of course, not by linear demarcation, all carriers of stimuli of a proprioceptive nature, as far as they are served by the numerous cerebellar, mesencephalic, and spinal components which can no longer be localized according to body areas.

The more thorough investigation of these relations which are still rather obscure anatomically will be with us for a long time before we dare approach the exploration of the more immediate physiological importance of the functional factors of the dorsal cortical layers which are most probably of the highest value.

KARL SPENCER LASHLEY
(*7 June 1890—7 August 1958*)

As a development of the ideas put forward by the antilocalizationists such as Goltz and Monakow, the theory of equipotentiality of the cerebral cortex has become of increasing importance. Those who have sought this and an integrative function of the cortex are best represented by the American psychologist Lashley. He was perhaps the most important proponent of the holistic theory, which is still controversial.

Lashley was born in Davis, West Virginia, and was educated at West Virginia University, the University of Pittsburgh, and at the Johns Hopkins University. From 1917 to 1926 he worked in the psychology department of the University of Minnesota, and after a number of appointments in the United States and in Europe, became professor of psychology at Harvard University in 1935. He retired in 1955. His major contribution was to brain mechanisms and intelligence, and in particular to the science of behavior based on comparative neurology and measurement. He combined the physiological method of cerebral ablation with the learning techniques of psychology, thus helping towards the comparative study of the brain (see Lashley, 1958; Walshe, 1958; Carmichael, 1959; Boring, 1960; Cobb, 1960).

Lashley is known especially for his theory of functional equivalence of the cerebral cortex. He supported Goltz's conclusion according to which if a cerebral lesion is of considerable size its site is not of importance, since he believed that each part of the cortex has a role to play in learning and retention. The following excerpts are from a classic review, "Integrative functions of the cerebral cortex" (*Physiol. Rev.*, 1933, 13:1–42).

EXCERPT PP. 24–27

. . . . Opposed to the mosaic theory of the functional activity of specialized fields is the concept that within the special area all parts are, in certain respects and for certain functions, equivalent. This view has been expressed by Goltz [pp. 558–565] with reference to intelligence and the entire cortex, by Lashley . . . as the equipotentiality of parts, by Bethe (1931) in the theory of "sliding coupling," by Börnstein (1932) and Matthaei (1930) and seems implicit in the systems of Bianchi (1922) and of von Monakow [pp. 565–570], at least as applied to restricted fields. Three principal lines of evidence have been presented in favor of the theory: the functional equivalence of receptor surfaces, the spontaneous reorganization of motor reactions, and the survival of functions after destruction of any part of nervous centers whose total destruction abolishes them.

. . . .

. . . .

Direct experimental evidence on the equivalence of parts of cerebral fields has been presented . . . . The significant point in these observations is that a limited lesion does not abolish any identifiable parts of the function, leaving others intact, but lessens efficiency in all aspects of the function.

The same type of result appears after extirpation of parts of the motor cortex of monkeys. Destruction of small areas in general produces only temporary focal disturbances and large amounts must be destroyed in order to produce lasting defects . . . .

These three lines of evidence indicate that certain co-ordinated activities, known to be dependent upon definite cortical areas, can be carried out by any part (within undefined limits) of the whole area. Such a condition might arise from the presence of many duplicate reflex pathways through the areas and such an explanation will perhaps account for all of the reported cases of survival of functions after partial destruction of their special areas, but it is inadequate for the facts of sensory and motor equivalence. These facts establish the principle that, once an associated reaction has been established (e.g., a positive reaction to a visual pattern), the same reaction will be elicited by the excitation of sensory cells which were never stimulated in that way during the course of training. Similarly, motor acts (e.g., opening a latch box), once acquired, may be executed immediately with motor organs which were not associated with the act during training.

EXCERPT P. 34

The evidence reviewed here can scarcely be regarded as crucial upon any question of the cerebral mechanism of integration, but the picture which it gives us of cerebral activities lacks the precision which was anticipated by earlier workers. There is evidence of mutual dependence of parts in which the specialization of structures seems less important than the mere mass of functional tissue. There are indications that within the entire cortex, for certain functions, and within specialized areas, for others, the subordinate parts are all equally capable of performing the functions of the whole. Even where the highest degree of specialization exists, as in the visual and motor areas, the facts of equivalence of stimuli or equivalence of motor responses preclude any narrowly localized specialization of intercellular connections.

Herrick [1930] has expressed the significance of such data as follows: there is "first, a known localization of stable structural elements whose functions are also known, and, second, a localization of fields within which various recurring patterns of performance or schemata are known to be fabricated and within which inhibition, modification, or conditioning of these patterns takes place." The evidence seems most consistent with the view that these schemata are dependent upon some dynamic patterns of organization such as that proposed by Bethe [1931] for spinal coordination.

The following excerpts are from a paper by Lashley on "Functional determinants of cerebral localization" (*Arch. Neurol. Psychiat.*, 1937, 38:371–387); they deal with the problem of the functional significance of all localization.

EXCERPT PP. 386–387

Knowledge of such [integrative] processes in the cortex is still too limited to permit of anything but vague speculations concerning their nature, largely inferred from the phenomena of behavior. The direction of the speculations, however, is important for the development of further research. It has been assumed that the properties of experience are represented at the level of some simple nervous activity or in single loci: sensations in the sensory areas, volitional patterns in the motor regions or particular forms of intelligent behavior in restricted coordinating centers. Such conceptions of localization are oversimplified and must be abandoned. Nothing is known of the physiologic basis of conscious states, but there is some reason to believe that these states can be correlated only with the summated activity of all centers simultaneously excited. The position of Goldstein, that the functions of every center are dependent on its relations to the rest of the intact nervous system, cannot be too strongly emphasized in considering problems of neuropsychology. Conceptions of the organization of mind or of behavior are based on a logical analysis of the activities of the total organism, and the final synthesis of nervous states which constitute these activities must transcend the excitation of any single center.

. . . .

. . . .

SUMMARY

In the foregoing discussion I have sought to illustrate a physiologic approach to the problem of cerebral localization. Various lines of evidence indicate that the spatial distribution of excitations within a nerve center may form the basis for several types of integration, such as the regulation of intensity of discharge, the establishment of fields of force to determine spatial orientation, and the control of the serial timing of activities. Each of these functions implies a different mechanism of organization and, consequently, a spatial separation of the fields in which the different processes operate. Experimental and clinical data indicate that the dissociation of functions resulting from cerebral lesions is in harmony with the assumption that cerebral localization is determined by the separation of such incompatible mechanisms.

Lashley believed that not only does the cerebral cortex act in an integrated fashion but that in addition there is integration between it and all parts of the brain. Later work has cast doubts on his conclusions, but his experimental techniques were themselves a major contribution. The best summary of his views on brain function in general and on cortical function in particular is to be found in a paper presented in July 1949 to the Society for Experimental Biology at a symposium in Cambridge, England ("In search of the engram," *Symposia of the Society for Experimental Biology, No. IV, Physiological mechanisms in animal behavior* [Cambridge, 1950]).

EXCERPT PP. 478–479

4. The trace of any activity is not an isolated connection between sensory and motor elements. It is tied in with the whole complex of spatial and temporal axes of nervous activity which forms a constant substratum of behavior. Each association is oriented with respect to space and time. Only by long practice under varying conditions does it become generalized or dissociated from these specific coordinates. The space and time coordinated in orientation can, I believe, only be maintained by some sort of polarization of activity and by rhythmic discharges which pervade the entire brain, influencing the organization of activity everywhere. The position and direction of motion in the visual field, for example, continuously modify the spinal postural adjustments, but, a fact which is more frequently overlooked, the postural adjustments also determine the orientation of the

visual field, so that upright objects continue to appear upright, in spite of changes in the inclination of the head. This substratum of postural and tonic activity is constantly present and is integrated with the memory trace.

. . . .

5. The equivalence of different regions of the cortex for retention of memories points to multiple representation. Somehow, equivalent traces are established throughout the functional area. Analysis of the sensory and motor aspects of habits shows that they are reducible only to relations among components which have no constant position with respect to structural elements. This means, I believe, that within a functional area the cells throughout the area acquire the capacity to react in certain definite patterns, which may have any distribution within the area. I have elsewhere proposed a possible mechanism to account for this multiple representation. Briefly, the characteristics of the nervous network are such that, when it is subject to any pattern of excitation, it may develop a pattern of activity, reduplicated throughout an entire functional area by spread of excitations, much as the surface of a liquid develops an interference pattern of spreading waves when it is disturbed at several points. This means that, within a functional area, the neurons must be sensitized to react in certain combinations, perhaps in complex patterns of reverberatory circuits, reduplicated throughout the area.

6. Consideration of the numerical relations of sensory and other cells in the brain makes it certain, I believe, that all of the cells of the brain must be in almost constant activity, either firing or actively inhibited. There is no great excess of cells which can be reserved as the seat of special memories. The complexity of the functions involved in reproductive memory implies that every instance of recall requires the activity of literally millions of neurons. The same neurons which retain the memory traces of one experience must also participate in countless other activities.

Conclusion

In 1937 (p. 386) Lashley declared that "nearly a century of psychologizing concerning the cerebral cortex had added practically nothing to knowledge of its fundamental activities." Clearly much factual information concerning its function has been derived from experimental investigations in animals, and more recently in man, as well as from clinical and pathological observations. Thus the operation of cerebral hemispherectomy carried out by Dandy for the removal of neoplasms (W. E. Dandy, "Removal of right cerebral hemisphere for certain tumors with hemiplegia," *J. Am. Med. Assoc.*, 1928, 90:823–825; "Physiological studies following extirpation of the right cerebral hemisphere in man," *Bull. Johns Hopkins Hosp.*, 1933, 53:31–51) and by Roland Krynauw ("Infantile hemiplegia treated by removal of one cerebral hemisphere," *J. Neurol. Neurosurg. Psychiat.*, 1950, 13:243–267) in cases of infantile hemiplegia has contributed a great deal of new data concerning human cortical function, some of which has resulted from exposure of the cortex in the course of the operation. Likewise the work of the American physiologist Philip Bard on decortication of the cat (e.g., Bard and Rioch, 1937) ought to be mentioned. It has revealed that the cortex has much to do with the elaboration of acquired modes of behavior. Some consider its physiological significance equal to that of Lashley's work. But as this data has been accumulated, the incredible complexity of the cortex becomes increasingly apparent. Furthermore, the early and naive concept of the cortex functioning in relative isolation can no longer be sustained. It is now clear that its activity must be associated with all parts of the brain, and the elucidation of this integration will provide a source of study for many decades if not centuries to come.

Early investigators had hoped to find in the cortex a structure that would prove to be the controlling mechanism of the nervous system and through it of the whole body. However, the conclusions reached by Wilder Penfield, the Canadian neurosurgeon who has been responsible for much of the recent knowledge of the human cortex, in his Ferrier Lecture of 1947 illustrated how modern researches have destroyed this expectation. His opinions were based on the examination of over three hundred living, human brains.

EXCERPT P. 346

One must conclude that there is strong evidence in favour of the existence within the central nervous system of a place where neuronal circuits converge, thus making possible both sensory summation and the initiation of discriminative action. And yet there is nothing to suggest that this place is in the cerebral cortex.

. . . .

There is represented within special areas of the cerebral cortex, special aspects of sensation and special mechanisms of motor control which are indispensable to the individual for an understanding of his environment and for the establishment by him of coordinated action. There is localization also of neurone circuits which seem to be devoted to the recollection of past experience and the interpretation of present perception. But all of these elements would seem to belong to no more than a 'middle level' of elaboration in the total function of the brain.

CHAPTER X

THE CEREBRAL WHITE MATTER

Introduction

The white matter of the spinal cord has already been considered in Chapter IV and although it forms with the white matter of the brain an inseparable unit, nevertheless their histories must be dealt with separately.

The white or medullary substance of the brain was not clearly differentiated from the gray matter until 1586 (see Piccolomini, pp. 387–388), but whereas little or nothing was known of the cerebral and cerebellar cortex at that time, and knowledge of it only increased with the development of the microscope, a certain number of cerebral and white matter structures had already been identified. The history of the white matter begins in antiquity, but, on the whole, little advancement in its knowledge was made until a reliable microscope became available in the nineteenth century. Admittedly macroscopic tracing of white matter bundles was carried out in the seventeenth and eighteenth centuries, but here, too, no real progress could be made until the ultimate unit of the nervous system, the nerve cell body with its processes, was recognized. Thus the history of the white matter pathways in the brain, like that of the spinal cord tracts (Chapter IV), is inseparably connected with the history of the neuron (Chapter II).

The acquisition of knowledge concerning cerebral white matter may be divided into two parts: a period of early investigations when anatomists were chiefly making macroscopic studies, and a modern period dating from the 1870's when new techniques of microscopy, staining, and specimen preparation were introduced into neurohistology, and when new methods such as those of Flechsig and Gudden were invented to try to pierce the maze of intracerebral nerve fibres. This period continues, and further advances in anatomical, chemical, and physiological techniques can be expected. One example of the last, the physiological neuronography of Dusser de Barenne, is included below.

As noted earlier (p. 29), although the nerve fibre was not identified with certainty until 1781 (see Fontana, pp. 36–38), the terms *nerve fibre, thread,* and *filament* had been in use for centuries (Berg, 1942) and referred either to bundles of primary fibres or to the theoretical fibre in the same way that reference was made to the postulated but unidentified atom. Moreover, Descartes, who is not represented below, suggested the presence of tubes (*tuyeaux*) in the brain, passing from the pineal body to certain of its parts; these were almost certainly speculative and satisfied a demand that most seventeenth century investigators felt for structures to conduct the still-accepted animal spirits of antiquity. It is often impossible for us to know what early authors had in mind when using the word *fibre*, but it is essential to recognize that their concept of it was certainly not equivalent to ours.

In several of the selections presented below there are also accounts of the corpus striatum and the thalamus, unavoidable in view of their intimate association with the white matter. Since the basal ganglia and thalamus are not discussed elsewhere in this book, some of the passages relating to them are fairly long.

The only secondary source of value on the history of the cerebral white matter is a book written by John Gordon (1817) of Edinburgh as a violent attack upon the anatomical claims of Gall and Spurzheim. In it he referred to most of the important prenineteenth century contributions to the subject.

Early Investigations

GALEN
(See p. 14)

A differentiation between the white and gray matter was never made in antiquity and on the whole more attention was paid to the ventricular system than to the solid brain substance surrounding it. Nevertheless, some of the more obvious intracerebral white and gray masses were described, especially by Galen: the corpus callosum, fornix, thalamus, corpora quadrigemina, etc.

Galen mentioned the corpus callosum on a number of occasions (*e.g., Anatomical procedures,* IX, 3 and 4), but it should be realized that he was referring to a more extensive structure than is implied today by the term, which was really the term's usage until the nineteenth century. It could include not only the midline connection of the white matter but also the white matter in the cerebral hemispheres that it connects. Another recognized structure was the fornix, and the following is Galen's account of it (*Anatomical procedures,* IX, 4; Kühn [1821–1833], II, 724–725).

EXCERPT PP. 724–725

Observe, therefore, how it [the fornix] ought to be laid bare, since the part covered by this body is no ordinary part of the brain, but, indeed, a kind of third ventricle in addition to those already mentioned as divided and separated from each other by the septum [lateral ventricles]. Lay it bare where the veins, breaking out as if through holes [interventricular foramina], enter the anterior ventricles, for the middle region, at the same time with the anterior ventricles, is revealed at these holes; and it is necessary, by gently placing a probe, the wide part of a *spatha*, as it is called, or even of a *spathemela* * through and underneath both holes, to elevate the body [anterior columns of fornix] resting on the veins. When you have done this for each hole, the probes will meet and reveal this body which rests on the veins that run through in concealment. It [the fornix] is like the vault of a domed building, but many call this kind of building not fornical but camerate. As those who have observed this body have called it fornix-shaped; among those who are unaware of it, some contend that this vaulted body does not exist in the brain; others with an incorrect knowledge of it believe that the reference is to what has been placed above the septum [corpus callosum], although that is not [truly] vaulted. The former body may in some way be called vaulted, and if you cut it, as in the anterior ventricles so here, too, a callus will appear. The veins that are supported at the base go through the cavity of the fornix; outwardly it appears convex, that is, when the bodies lying upon it where it rises as far as the fold of the meninx have been removed; but inwardly it is hollow like the highest part of a vault.

Andreas Vesalius
(See p. 153)

Throughout the medieval period no advances were made in knowledge of the white matter, and even the early Renaissance anatomists usually paid attention only to the ventricles because of the prevalent doctrine of mental function (pp. 463–465). Other intracerebral structures were ignored.

However, the account of the corpus callosum given by Vesalius in 1543 (*De humani corporis fabrica* [Basel, 1543], Lib. VII, Cap. V, pp. 632–633) was better than that of Galen and, as well as describing the structure, he also suggested its possible functions. These were purely mechanical for the corpus callosum not only connected the two halves of the brain but it also preserved the patency of the ventricular cavities and supported the fornix.

EXCERPT PP. 632–633

THE SITE AND NAME OF THE CORPUS CALLOSUM

A little earlier I related that all the substance of the cerebrum and cerebellum surrounded by the thin membrane [pia mater] is yellowish and almost ashen-colored in that part that faces the membrane [this was his only reference to the cortex]. However, there is a part of the external

---

* A long-shafted instrument at one end of which is an olivary point and at the other a spatula used for the preparation and application of medicaments. See J. S. Milne, *Surgical instruments in Greek and Roman times* [Oxford, Clarendon Press, 1907], pp. 58–61.

surface of the cerebrum [the corpus callosum] that is not covered by the thin membrane, but like the inner substance, that external surface is gleaming white and harder than the substance on the remaining surface of the brain [the corpus callosum is, in fact, covered with pia mater]. It was for this reason that the ancient Greeks called this part *tyloeidēs* (*callosus*), and, following their example, in my discourse I have always referred to this part as the corpus callosum. Then, too, because of its shape, since it is bent like an arch in its lower part, and because of its use, some of the Greeks call it *psalidoeidēs* (archlike), and I shall look upon it as a structure of the brain because it is correctly considered as such by many. If you look at the right and left brain, the lower part of the middle of the base of the brain, the very highest region of the brain, and also if you compare the front and rear, the corpus callosum is observed to be in the middle of the brain; for the part of the corpus callosum that is farthest to the rear is a little nearer to the front of the brain than the forward part is to the rear. It comes into view of those dissecting when they manually separate the right side of the brain slightly from the left, for with the brain so separated, that which unites its parts there, the corpus callosum, is observed gleaming white, long, and arched. That surface of its body which comes into view when the brain has been separated is observed to be humped almost in the same way as the top of the head protrudes above the highest part of the forehead, occiput, and the sides of the head, although the obliquity of the corpus callosum is not so noticeable as that of the top of the head.

THE BEGINNING OF THE CORPUS CALLOSUM, OR ITS CONTINUITY WITH THE REMAINING SUBSTANCE OF THE BRAIN

When, as I said, the brain has been separated, it reveals the smooth and even upper surface of the corpus callosum, and also demonstrates this body to be continuous with the cerebrum, not to be arisen from the surface of the substance of the cerebrum which is softer and yellowish but from the deeper substance which is seen to be harder and white.

. . . .

. . . .

THE USE OF THE CORPUS CALLOSUM AND SEPTUM [PELLUCIDUM]

This portion of the cerebrum is not so large and thick that it requires special vessels, although it is, nevertheless, of great importance to the living. Indeed, it relates the right side of the cerebrum to the left; then it produces and supports the septum of the right and left ventricles; finally, through that septum it supports and props the body formed like a tortoise [fornix] so that it may not collapse and, to the great detriment of all the functions of the cerebrum, crush the cavity common to the two [lateral] ventricles of the cerebrum. There are, furthermore, two sinuses cut as a somewhat deep line into the substance of the cerebrum at the upper surface of the corpus callosum [callosal sulci]; in addition to the fact that that part of the cerebrum is unsuitable for the production of a callus body, because it must arise from deeper substance, these sinuses are believed to serve for the defluxion of pituita from the higher parts of the cerebrum; and receiving it they cause it to flow over the humped surface of the corpus callosum to the anterior.

Marcello Malpighi
(See p. 416)

The first detailed examination of nervous tissue was made by the renowned Italian biologist Malpighi. His account of the cerebral cortex has already been presented (pp. 416–418); in that account he referred to the white matter, but he also reported elsewhere and in more detail his investigation of it "through dissection with the use of a microscope." As previously noted, his microscope was very primitive, and from his description it is very likely that he observed bundles of axons rather than individual nerve fibres. Nevertheless, Malpighi provided the first definite proof that white matter was composed of "fibres" which he could trace from the brainstem to the cortex where they were imbedded like the roots of a plant. It was characteristic of his style of writing that he made analogies between plant and animal structures. He used the term "corpus callosum" synonymously with "medulla cerebri," or white matter of the brain.

The following passage has been taken from a letter Malpighi wrote to Dr. Carlo Fracassati of Pisa in November 1664 ("De cerebro epistola," pp. 1–46 in *Tetras anatomicarum epistolarum* [Bologna, 1665]).

EXCERPT PP. 11–18

Regarding the marrow of the brain [white matter] or the corpus callosum, that rough substance appears to be more solid than the cortex and to be surrounded by veins and arteries; it seems to be for filling the intervening spaces. Nevertheless, such supposition is false, as I was able to observe clearly with a microscope in the brain of fishes and less clearly in other more perfect animals, for it became evident to me that the whole of this white part of the brain is divided into roundish fibres, not unlike those white bodies or little intestines [*intestinuli*] of which the substance of the testicles is formed. . . . All the fibres dispersed through the brain and cerebellum seem to have origin from the trunk of the spinal marrow [cord] contained within the cranium [brainstem] like a noteworthy collection of fibres; for they ramify hither and thither from four reflected crura of the marrow until they end in the cortex in branching extremities. This course is more apparent in the cerebellum because the fibres are extended in the form of a tree and on the extreme branches, almost like leaves, the cortex is delicately placed; it is not attached to anything, however, so that it resembles a free leaf. In the brain [cerebrum] the vault or "tortoise" [fornix] of the ventricles is composed of fibres constructed in the form of an arch and sloping towards the sides, as appears in the illustration of fishes in which a portion of the fibres may also be observed passing above the ventricle towards the cortex but in the opposite direction, so that there is a passing and crossing over the lower fibres described above. All these are thought probably to have some continuity with the anterior origin of the spinal marrow [brainstem] . . . .

. . . . If you desire to have a rough likeness of the fibres extended in the brain, you can gain one that is not too incongruous from the cabbage and similar plants. The fibres arising from the single trunk of the spine represent the stem; from this they are dispersed into the leaves which spread out in a circular shape to form a cavity not too unlike the ventricles. These fibres of the brain extend lengthwise not, however, parallel but often meeting and apparently gathered into a bundle; soon, however, they again divide and are carried above the other lateral fibres so that they resemble a loose net; this is particularly apparent in the dogfish. I observed a remarkable bundle of fibres which still arouses my attention: it [the pons] passed across the anterior portion of the spinal marrow [brainstem] which it tightly surrounded like a girdle and finally ended in two roots [middle cerebellar peduncles] that extended through the sides of the cerebellum.

Man's perception cannot determine whether the same number of fibres which have their roots in the brain are continued in the spinal marrow [cord] and there united more closely together to form a more solid trunk, or whether the spinal marrow is only partly the offspring of the brain. From the anatomy of certain fishes, since the spinal marrow is of greater size and more solid and compact but the brain smaller and softer and its fibres loosely united, it is probable that the fibres of the spinal marrow of the cerebrum and of the cerebellum [i.e., brainstem] are the same in number. The old statement that the brain is an appendix to the spinal cord, which was recalled to light and confirmed by the famous Bartholin, agrees with this view or at least that the trunk of the nerves contained in the spine gives off roots in the cortex after having sent them in a somewhat twisted manner through the brain and cerebellum, and that branches in the form of nerves starting from the back [spinal nerves] and the head [cranial nerves] traverse the whole body.

THOMAS WILLIS

(See p. 158)

When Malpighi was writing his letter to Fracassati in November 1664, the classic book on the anatomy of the brain composed by Willis had already appeared (*Cerebri anatome*, London, 1664). In it Willis described what was then called the *medulla oblongata*, but unlike the modern usage, this term referred to all the deep white matter, the ventricles, the basal ganglia and thalami of the cerebral hemispheres, and the three parts of the brainstem. It may be visualized as a capital "Y" with a limb in each cerebral hemisphere and the stem corresponding to the brainstem. Each limb comprised a lateral ventricle and the deep gray and white matter (basal ganglia, thalamus, and related fibre pathways of which the most important was the internal capsule) closely associated with it. Willis clearly differentiated between motor and sensory components of the white matter and even suggested that ascending and descending fibres could be detected in the corpus striatum which he also described. This, however, was conjecture and Steno (1669, pp. 11–12), who castigated those who speculated beyond available data, justifiably condemned Willis for it. The following passage is from Chapter XIII of the *Cerebri anatome*.

EXCERPT PP. 81–83

We pass from *the brain* to an explanation *of its trunk* to which *the cerebrum and cerebellum* are attached like *outgrowths*. This part is commonly called *the medulla oblongata*, under which name we include all that substance that extends from the innermost cavity of the corpus callosum [ventricles, basal ganglia, and thalami] to the junction at the base of the head with the occipital foramen [magnum] where the same structure [medulla oblongata], continued farther, ends in *the spinal cord*.

The surface of *the medulla oblongata*, although rendered uneven through certain protuberances and processes, nevertheless is not varied with gyri or convolutions like *the cerebrum* and *cerebellum*, nor is its exterior substance ashen-colored like the cortex, and the internal medulla is white. *All its structure* is a kind of *medullary one*, although it does not appear pure and gleaming but is much darkened *by fibres* and *villi* stretched out and going forth in different ways. Indeed, its *fibres* are shaped differently or *stretched out lengthwise*, and sometimes *circular*.

Its *form* is *bifurcate*, and as if in emulation of [the appearance of] the Parnassus of the poets, resembles the letter **Y**. Its *limbs* arising more anteriorly from each hemisphere of the brain and inclining one to the other, near the center of the cranium join together into one trunk which, however, has a line drawn through its middle so that it seems as if made from two stems; this can be distinguished in its whole length.

The *medulla oblongata* seems *a broad,* almost *a royal, highway* into which *the animal spirits* constantly flow from their twin sources, that is, *the cerebrum* and *cerebellum,* and are carried into *all the nervous parts of the body;* when these *spirits* are disposed in order in this common passage or, so to speak *diatasso* in regular series, they serve *two purposes,* that is, either they may be directed *outwards* towards the nerves, at which time they exert *the locomotive faculty;* or flow *inwards* towards their sources when *the acts of sensation,* or rather *perceptions of sensible things,* are performed.

Within this open way a wider and widely open passage leads directly into *the spinal marrow* through which the spirits, executors of spontaneous motion, issue forth to the nerves in the several members. Meanwhile, from the same tract of the medulla oblongata smaller pathways are here and there carried outwards through particular nerves, arising within the cranium from the same medulla [cranial nerves]. Furthermore, many different things grow on this *medullary trunk,* that is, *various processes* and *protuberances* into which the spirits, directed to certain special functions, are separated lest all the spirits moving swiftly on the same pathway collide and so interfere with one another's function.

While we suppose *the animal spirits* to be gathered within the medulla oblongata in this way for performing the acts *of motions* and *sensations,* we declare that *they are not produced* there but only *carry on* their functions there. For, created only in the cerebrum and cerebellum, as they proceed *from one* or *the other,* they perform their *functions,* either *involuntary* or *spontaneous,* as will be indicated more fully later.

That we may explain here everything that relates to *the medulla oblongata,* let us observe it from start to finish and consider its several courses, diversions, and crossroads. *The medulla oblongata* begins where *the corpus callosum* is believed to end, that is, where the medullary substance of the cerebrum is thickest near the projections of each hemisphere; *bodies of a darker* and somewhat obscure *color* and like *streaked* ivory [corpus striatum] are joined to that medulla on both sides. *These two bodies* [corpora striata] are *the extremities* or apices of the legs *of the medulla oblongata;* there is a close and immediate communication between them and the cerebrum. Each of them seems like a cylinder rolled into an orb [caudate nucleus], which, however, constitutes the top, not spherical but oval, of each leg, and bent somewhat downwards to the posterior. A large portion of its surface is joined to the medullary substance *of the cerebrum,* but a part remaining free *from the brain,* rises separately and produces that protuberance displaying itself in [the floor of] each lateral ventricle [caudate nucleus, head and tail]. If *these bodies* [including also the lenticular nucleus], are sectioned longitudinally through the middle, they appear marked *with medullary streaks* like *rays*; these *streaks* have a *double purpose* or tendency, that is, *some descend* from the top of this body as if they were tracts from *the cerebrum into the medulla oblongata,* and *others ascend* from the lower part and meet up with the former, as if they were *the passages of the spirits from the medulla oblongata into the cerebrum.* It is worthy of observation, furthermore, that in the whole *brain* no other part is to be found similarly *streaked.*

The famous Danish anatomist Steno had referred (1669, pp. 4–5) to the fibres of the white matter in his essay on the brain, read in 1665 but not published until 1669.

> . . . . To say that the white matter is but a uniform substance like wax in which there is no hidden contrivance, would be too low an opinion of nature's finest masterpiece. We are assured that wherever in the body there are fibres, they everywhere adopt a certain arrangement among themselves, created more or less according to the functions for which they are intended. If the substance is everywhere of fibres, as, in fact, it appears to be in several places, you must admit that these fibres have been arranged with great skill, since all the diversity of our sensations and our movements depends upon this. We admire the skillful construction of the fibres in each muscle; how much more then ought we to admire it in the brain, where each of these fibres, confined in a small space, functions without confusion and without disorder.

Steno had suggested, moreover, that one way of studying the white matter was "to follow the nerve filaments through the substance of the brain to find out where they go and where they end" [p. 8]. He gave no account of dissections based on this suggestion, but Willis, in his *De anima brutorum* (Oxford, 1672, Ch. IV), published three years later, mentioned his experience with this method. This is of some importance since Vieussens (pp. 585–590) is usually given priority for the technique of scraping the white matter to display its fibre bundles.

EXCERPT P. 44

> . . . . Who can be sufficiently astonished at the innumerable arrangements of *nerve fibres* distributed in wonderful order into the different parts of the entire body; *the animal spirits,* like scouting forces, continually running hither and thither through them performing the functions of *sensation* and movement? Furthermore, those that dwell within *the head* itself, the superior legion of *the sensitive soul* although more freely ranging are by no means disorganized, but their forces confined by certain bounds

and limits, so to speak within the compressed space of a single chamber, attend to infinite varieties of *actions* and *passions*.

In regard to these matters, earlier in our description of *the brain* and *nerves* we distinguished in more detail the different sites of all the faculties [see p. 473], and we indicated that *the voluntary* and *involuntary* controls of the animal function, different from one another, also related to the different controls of *the cerebrum* and *cerebellum* with their respective appendices *of nerves*. Furthermore, we demonstrated that *the spirits* themselves, authors of each function, have special pathways not only within the confined channels of *the nerves* but also in the expanded emporia of *the head*, that is, *medullary tracts*, almost *intrinsically nerves*, extended very elegantly hither and thither. But since it is objected that we have not described them all and perhaps not sufficiently precisely, therefore, in order that those *medullary passages* may be better observed, we have recently undertaken another and slightly more accurate *anatomy of the brain*. This was done by gently scraping its parts with the point of a knife, removing its *softer*, brownish *substance* bordering everywhere on the cortex of the brain, but leaving *the whiter* and harder. In this way many *medullary* cords, like separate nerves communicating remarkably with one another and with other white or *medullary* bodies in different parts of *the brain* and *medulla oblongata*, were brought into view. Since this anatomical procedure clearly revealed the more hidden passages of the spirits and the movements relating to the secrets of the animal government, it permitted us to exhibit here one or another new figure of *the revealed brain*, and in special places with *the substance removed*. In these figures the common passages as well as the special pathways for the spirits are plainly seen, carrying them *directly* through the beaten track of *the medullary trunk*, and *indirectly* through the more circuitous routes of the prominences into *the corpora striata*.

RAYMOND DE VIEUSSENS
(1641—1716)

Although Steno had first suggested (p. 823) that the intracerebral white matter might be examined by following its fibres, as practised today in the dissection of fixed brains, and although Willis had used the technique (pp. 582–585), it was the French physician and anatomist Vieussens who employed the method to the greatest advantage.

Vieussens was born in the village of Vieussens in the district of Rouergue and educated mainly at Montpellier where in 1671 he was appointed physician to the hospital of Saint Eloy. He studied the anatomy and pathology of the cardiovascular system, and in 1684, after ten years' work on five hundred cadavers, he published his famous book on the anatomy of the nervous system, *Neurographia universalis* (Lyons, 1684), by which he hoped to advance the work of Willis whom he greatly admired (see Portal, 1770–1773, IV, 5–36; Sachs, 1910; Major, 1932; Levy-Valensi, 1933, pp. 621–624; Kellett, 1942).

His investigations of the white matter in the brain were the best that had been carried out but, for reasons that are not obvious, they have not been given all the credit they deserve even though they were received at the time with great enthusiasm. The terminology he introduced, particularly of the basal ganglia, presents considerable difficulties, and in the following selections from the *Neurographia universalis* all the obscurities have not been resolved. This may have made his writings less popular than they otherwise might have been. The first passage (from Lib. I, Cap. X) contains general statements about the white matter of the brain.

EXCERPT PP. 55–56

The white substance of the brain, which herein I shall sometimes call medullary substance and sometimes medulla, is composed of innumerable, connected fibres divided up into many bundles. It appears clearly when the white substance is boiled in oil, for then it can be readily separated out into the innumerable fibres which, as I said, form it when connected together. So long as these fibres are in their natural site they are so close to one another that there is no perceptible space between them and they constitute a continuous body, just as the fibres within a wooden staff may be separable from one another, but compose a continuous body, that is, the staff.

Although the white substance which we are now discussing is connected in the cerebrum, cerebellum, and medulla oblongata to the ashen-colored body [gray matter] with which it coalesces, nevertheless they differ from one another by the width of the sky; for, in addition to the fact that they are of different colors, the white substance is harder than the ashen-colored and has minute pores . . . .

Furthermore, the varying shapes of the parts from which the aforesaid [white] substance of the cerebrum is formed seem to prove clearly that [the gray and white matter] differ from one another since the ashen-colored substance appears to be a concretion of longish, rounded particles and globules, as we said a little earlier; but the medulla is formed of long fibres of a variety of shapes that are so interfolded and interrelated that they give the appearance of a spongy body which the animal spirit may permeate in many different and rather inexplicable ways, so that within it the spirit undergoes many different and inexplicable motions; because of their different arrangements different thoughts are aroused in the mind, as will be explained in Chapters XXI and XXII.

The following passages (Lib. I, Cap. XI) include a description of the corpus callosum and the deep cerebral structures, known then as the medulla oblongata (see p. 582); the "anterior processes of the medulla oblongata" were the limbs of the letter Y and contained mainly the corpus striatum and thalamus on each side. The centrum ovale which is still occasionally associated with the name of Vieussens is also described; Vieussens admitted that the name was not entirely appropriate as the oval shape was distorted posteriorly where the occipital poles are separated by a midline indentation.

EXCERPT PP. 57–58

The structure of the aforesaid corpus callosum cannot be properly observed until first the whole convex part of the cerebrum has been cut away [horizontally] bit by bit, and when this has been done and its parts and site investigated the medulla of the cerebrum is clearly brought into view; its whole extent appears separated into many tracts and is involved irregularly with the cortex by which it is everywhere covered.

When the convex part of the cerebrum has been dissected and removed piece by piece as far as the rear of the corpus callosum, if its medullary substance lateral to the corpus callosum is cut with a small anatomical knife [horizontally] from anterior to posterior, the underlying anterior [lateral] ventricles will be uncovered and their size and shape, similar in some degree to an oval figure, will clearly appear. The corpus callosum forms almost the whole roof of the ventricles; the walls, however, are constructed of medullary fibres which emerge from the ashen-like substance [gray matter] of both cerebral hemispheres. The upper fibres, that is, those that occupy the convex part [of the hemisphere] first bend laterally on each side, and then the lower medullary fibres with which they join, bend medially. In their course they very closely embrace the anterior processes of the medulla oblongata [ventricles, basal ganglia, thalami] and its legs [crus cerebri]; indeed, they join together so that the medullary fibres, coalesce and curve on themselves in the middle region of the cerebrum and are separated from one another, as it were, by the intervention of the hollow of the septum lucidum [ventricles] and fornix. Those ventricles which are usually called the anterior [lateral], from which it is well understood that all the medullary fibres of the aforesaid organ (if you will except those that end in the transverse and somewhat oblique medullary tracts stria terminalis and/or anterior commissure) run together when they emerge from the cortex and are, so to speak, united around the anterior processes of the medulla oblongata and its legs; whence they run into the aforesaid hollow so that there they end in one spongy body which occupies the oval extent of the aforesaid ventricles; we call it the centrum ovale [of Vieussens] even though it is indented posteriorly so that it touches the rear part of the corpus callosum and is united to it; hence it does not exactly resemble an oval shape.

EXCERPT PP. 66–67

When first the surface of the anterior processes of the medulla oblongata has been scraped, the exterior and smaller medullary tracts, to which they are related, come into sight.

But when they are scraped more deeply the interior and thicker of them reveal themselves as tracts which are so disposed that, with the ashen-like substance [basal gray masses] as an intermediary, they are distinguished from one another. With their striations to some extent they resemble distinct bodies. It was without doubt as a result of this that the famous Willis called the aforesaid [anterior] processes of the medulla oblongata, corpora striata; but we, having given consideration to their location, call them the upper anterior corpora striata [caudate nucleus and lenticular nucleus] so that we may distinguish these from the rest of the corpora striata of the medulla oblongata [thalami].

The next selections (Lib. I, Cap. XIII) deal with the basal ganglia and the white matter pathways which are associated with them. As already mentioned, Vieussens' nomenclature is difficult to follow, and the attempts made below to identify in modern terms the structures he described are probably not entirely successful. His illustrations demonstrate in a striking fashion the white matter pathways (figs. 138 and 139), but they are very inaccurate and they do not greatly assist the understanding of the text; Gordon (1817, p. 96) called them "diagrams."

EXCERPT PP. 83–84

. . . . [the white matter tracts] which have been so disposed that, mixed with the ashen substance [gray matter], they somewhat resemble bodies marked by striae; therefore, insofar as regards shape and site, we call this interior substance of the base of the brain the lower external corpora striata. We divide them into anterior and posterior [corpora striata and thalami respectively after they have been shaved down to the level of the internal capsule and the lenticular and caudate nuclei. The upper anterior and posterior external corpora striata are the same structures before being shaved down], because on each side white matter resembling a thick nerve has been placed transversely and somewhat obliquely between them; we therefore call this a transverse and somewhat oblique medullary tract [stria terminalis]. This medullary tract, which is seen in Plate XIV [fig. 138], and which is double, appears to be formed of certain white fibrils emerging from the lobes of the base of the brain and at the same time coalescing; this coalescence is with the lowest part of the commissure resembling a thick nerve [anterior commissure] so that by its intervention not only the lower external corpora striata communicate with one another, but also the animal spirit occupying the upper part of the brain is able to enter into some association or have some communication with the animal spirit that exists in its base. One may readily understand this if first he observes that each semicircular center between the anterior and posterior upper corpora striata [corpora striata and thalami] and each medullary tract placed between the anterior and posterior lower exterior corpora striata is like so many receptacles for the animal spirit, communicating with one another by the aid of the the commissure resembling a thick nerve [anterior commissure].

The white or medullary tracts that form the lower external and anterior bodies [corpus striatum] end on each side in the aforesaid transverse and somewhat oblique medullary tract [stria terminalis]; but the white tracts that are observed in the lower external and posterior corpora striata [corpora striata and thalami] terminate in the white tracts produced from the middle of the centrum ovale [e.g., pyramidal tract], see Plate XIV [fig. 138].

EXCERPT PP. 86–87

When the lower external corpora striata [corpora striata] have been observed, if the base of the brain is scraped so deeply that they, with the two transverse and somewhat oblique medullary tracts are removed, the other lower corpora striata are uncovered which, considering their location, we call the lower internal corpora striata. These differ from the external ones because the external are hidden within the lobes of the base of the brain, but the internal occupy the anterior part of the base of the medulla oblongata and may be distinguished by no transverse medullary tracts.

Furthermore, the white tracts of the lower external corpora striata [corpora striata] are led out from the medullary substance to the lower part of the brain (Pl. XIV), but the white tracts to which the lower internal corpora striata relate [corona radiata and internal capsule] extend from the lower region of the centrum ovale.

The lower internal corpora striata having been observed and scraped inwardly, other corpora striata come into sight which are intermediate to the upper corpora striata and the lower internal corpora striata which are found in the medulla oblongata; therefore we call them the middle corpora striata ([internal capsule] Pl. XVI). These differ from the rest because their white tracts are formed of many medullary fibres, and therefore they are thicker than the white tracts of the other corpora striata. Furthermore the white tracts [corona radiata] to which the middle corpora striata relate are led out from the middle part of the centrum ovale; nor are they terminated within the boundaries of the brain like the medullary tracts [anterior commissure] of the upper anterior corpora striata and the layers of the lower bodies, external as well as internal. On the contrary, when they emerge from the ashen-like substance into which they have been inserted, they extend by a somewhat flexible course to the anterior region of the spinal marrow [cord], so that they disappear partly into the spinal marrow and partly into the anterior origins of the spinal nerves (see Pl. XVI).

Where the aforesaid medullary tracts [pyramidal tract, etc.], which are observed in the corpora striata, extend to the spinal marrow, before they emerge from the skull they pass over the other medullary fibres of the annular process [pons] so that the medullary tracts emerging from the middle corpora striata [internal capsule and crura] and the medullary fibres of the annular process [pons] meet and cross one another; indeed, they communicate with one another (Pls. XIV and XVI).

Here it must be noted that the white tracts that are observed in the corpora striata described above, acquire an inconstant rather than a constant site like the medullary fibres of the processes led out from the medullary center of each cerebellar hemisphere [cerebellar peduncle], described in the preceding chapter [see pp. 587–588], and not like the fibres from which the medulla of the cerebrum and cerebellum is formed; so that extending to the origins of the nerves the animal spirit, which is moved in many distinct and indescribable ways in the medulla of the brain, as well as of the cerebellum, enters the aforesaid white tracts and medullary fibres of the aforementioned processes [cerebellar peduncles], like frequented and paved ways, and travels in them according to certain determined movements, as will be explained in Chapter XIX.

Félix Vicq d'Azyr
(See p. 268)

As well as patiently scraping out the fibre bundles in the cerebral white matter, eighteenth century anatomists also used the old technique of slicing in various directions. One of the most successful studies of the brain that resulted from this method was that of Vicq d'Azyr whose name is still associated with the mammillothalamic tract—the bundle of Vicq d'Azyr. Like Varolio, he preferred to dissect the brain from the base and he introduced many new sections to reveal in particular the complexities of the deep gray masses and the white matter around them. In the first and only volume of his projected *Traité d'anatomie et de physiologie* (Paris, 1786) he gave an excellent account of his work with a detailed consideration of that of his predecessors (Pt. I, pp. 85–87). He was, however, more concerned there with illustrations of brain dissections already published; there is a briefer description of the cerebral white matter in "Recherches sur la structure du cerveau, du cervelet, de la moelle elongée, de la moelle épinière; et sur l'origine des nerfs de l'homme et des animaux" (*Histoire de l'Académie royale des Sciences, 1781* [Paris, 1784], pp. 495–622) from which the following passage has been taken. In it he referred to the line of Gennari without seeming to be aware that it had already been described (pp. 424–425). His reference to fibres elsewhere in the cortex is also of interest.

EXCERPT PP. 510–512

After a very firm brain has been dissected and a portion of one of the hemispheres has been removed, if an incision is made with a scalpel in the white substance, and if it is torn rather than incised in the same direction as far as the cortical substance, then the white substance is observed to be divided from itself in the direction of the surface of the brain as if it had been formed of fibres approaching one another. In the thickness of the gray or cortical substance very thin, radiating white striations may be observed mixed with it almost like the tubular and cortical substances of the kidneys. Steno has already remarked on the extensions of the white substance into the cortical substance; it is possible that that appearance is not owing only to the action of the vessels torn by that operation, which leave traces of their broken or pulled fibrils imprinted on the soft substance of the brain. Whatever the cause of this, I believe that I ought to speak of it, and I have delineated the mingling of the two substances in the convolutions of the brain.

If during the preparation of the centrum ovale of Vieussens, one examines the shape of the posterior cerebral convolutions that are placed against the falx above the cerebellum [tentorium], ordinarily several of them may be observed that are remarkable because the cortical substance there interrupted in its length by a white linear tract [line of Gennari, see p. 424] that follows all the contours of the convolutions, and gives to this portion of the cortex the appearance of a streaked ribbon; I have not found this arrangement at all in other regions of the brain.

The white matter, considered from a horizontal incision above the posterior prolongation of the lateral ventricles [occipital horn], where that extension is found which is incorrectly called the *spur*, presents in most subjects one or two white *tracts* that have the same contours as the spur itself; they are placed in the middle of the white substance from which they differ in their firmer consistency and deeper color. Of these two *tracts*, one is internal and very slender, the other is external and a little wider.

Having sought to discover how the different cerebral regions composed of white substance communicate, the following account seems to me a possibility.

The medullary substance of the inferior and middle cerebral convolutions is continuous: 1°, under the form of white striations, in the corpora striata that it penetrates; 2°, with a rather considerable white matter center, placed under the posterior division of the fissure of Sylvius; it rises along Ammon's horn, of which it partly forms the sheath, and thus it communicates with the posterior part of the corpus callosum. Between the posterior division of the fissure of Sylvius and the corpora striata, there is a white portion [external capsule] narrower than the preceding, with which it communicates below, and above it is joined to the centrum ovale, lateral and medullary of the middle lobe. In the middle, the corpus callosum communicates with the white substance of all the lobes; laterally this same substance sinks between the thalamus and the corpora striata as far as the base of the brain [internal capsule], and the white *tract* that we have already said is extended from front to rear between this eminence and the fissure of Sylvius, is found again at the external border of the corpora striata. It is thus that the general communication of the white substance is established in the brain from front to rear, from above downwards, and in all directions, concealed at its surface and interrupted in various places by the gray substance of which we have already spoken in detail.

When describing the anterior and posterior commissures (p. 535), Vicq d'Azyr mentioned "small white cords which extend from the mammillary tubercles towards the anterior tubercles of the thalami" (p. 535). These are the mammillothalamic tracts of Vicq d'Azyr (p. 562). He also referred to them as "the white and almost horizontal *tractus* which ends in the mammillary bodies anteriorly and the medulla oblongata posteriorly." He also discussed the various types of inter- and intracerebral, white matter fibre connections.

EXCERPT PP. 535–536

It seems to me that the commissures are intended to establish sympathetic communications between the different parts of the brain, just as the nerves do between the different organs and the brain itself, a consideration which can apply to all kinds of connections observed between the different parts of the brain. These communications can in general be divided into two classes: the first run from one hemisphere to the other, the second between different regions of the same hemisphere; in this latter class must be included the *taenia semi-circularis* [arcuate fibres], the pillars of the fornix, the peduncles of the pineal gland, and the white cords which proceed from the mammillary bodies towards the anterior tubercles of the thalami [bundles of Vicq d'Azyr]; by means of these structures impressions can be readily transmitted from the base of the brain to its center and towards its sides. I include in the first class the corpus callosum, appropriately named by some anatomists *the great commissure of the brain,* the quadrigeminal bodies, the anterior and posterior commissures, the legs of the brain [cerebral peduncles], the pons, the valve of Vieussens [anterior medullary velum], the soft commissure of the thalami [interthalamic adhesion], the gray and soft substance of the infundibulum, and that which closes the third ventricle anterior to the optic nerve [tuber cinereum]. As for these latter communications, it is worth remarking that they connect the right hemisphere with the left by means of the gray and soft substance [cortex] which also has, as one sees it, its connections, and which must play an important role in the unknown mechanism of its functions. The *corpora fimbriata* [fimbria] terminate below near the *taenia semi-circularis* and it can hardly be doubted that this junction between organs, intended the one as a communication from hemisphere to hemisphere, the other as a connection between different parts of the same half of the brain, conspicuously augments the number and the influence of sympathies; without the parts that I have enumerated when speaking of the first type of commissures, the brain would be completely divided into two absolutely independent parts, the one from the other. When dealing with the origin of each nerve I shall show that the fibres which form them are very numerous and the majority proceed to very different regions, and that whether with reference to the nerves or with reference to the structure of the brain, everything is arranged in the system to multiply the connections of different parts of the brain so that inconveniences which would result from difficulty occasioned in any part of the brain, are prevented.

Johann Christian Reil
(28 February 1759—22 November 1813)

As well as seeking new ways of exploring the brain, anatomists at the end of the eighteenth century were also discovering methods of preparing the organ for dissection. This was a simple but very significant advance in the anatomy of the brain since instead of being faced with a jelly-like specimen that rapidly decomposed, the investigator could now dissect a firm organ at his leisure. It seems probable that certain procedures assisting better dissection were used in the seventeenth century, as can be determined by the firm shape of the brain in some illustrations, such as those of Willis, and it is known that Vieussens used boiling oil as a form of hardening (p. 586) and that Malpighi employed boiling in water. But the first person to use preservatives and hardening agents consistently and to write about them was the German anatomist Reil.

Reil was born in Rhaude, a village in east Friesland, and attended the Universities of Göttingen and Halle. At the latter he occupied a number of positions before he was appointed professor *ordinarius* of medicine and director of the clinic in 1788. In the following year he was made town physician of Halle. When the University was closed by Napoleon in 1806, Reil engaged in anatomical studies and in 1810 moved to the newly founded University of Berlin. He died of typhus contracted during field work following the Battle of Leipzig. His contributions to the anatomy of the brain are of great importance and were made chiefly between 1806 and 1808. In addition he is known for his writings on brain function, and he upheld the idea that the brain possessed a special energy and, although anatomically independent, had an ability to integrate all activities of the body. His philosophy thus combined both mechanistic and vitalistic interpretations, and the influence of Kant and *Naturphilosophie* are clearly apparent in his writings. His work in the fields of psychiatry, public health, and military medicine were also important (see Neuburger, 1913; Reil, 1960; A. Lewis, 1958, 1965).

Reil criticized Vicq d'Azyr's method of hacking the brain into many pieces and claimed that his own technique (pp. 830–832) was much superior. He soaked the brain in alcohol with potash or ammonia added, and the resultant specimen permitted a more detailed examination of the deep structures than had been possible previously; his account of the internal anatomy of the brain was therefore of special importance and the most outstanding of its time. Some of his comments on cerebral white matter are given below. His account of the cerebellum is dealt with on pages 647 to 652. The first selection below has been translated from an article originally published in 1795, "Über den Bau des Hirns und der Nerven" ([Gren's] *Neues J. Phys., Lpz.,* 1795, 1:96–114); the original article has not been seen, but it was reprinted in Reil's book *Kleine Schriften* (Halle, 1817, pp. 113–132) under the same title to which was added "In einem Schreiben an Gren." In *Kleine Schriften* Reil expressed the belief that the brain in general was a distinct organ with distinct functions that could not be localized; it was not just a source for the nerves. The following is his account of the cerebrum. As with most of these early anatomists, the terminology used creates difficulties of comprehension, some of which have not been surmounted and some obscurity remains.

EXCERPT PP. 118–122

ON THE CEREBRUM

The spinal cord [brainstem], divided by a sulcus, continues under the cerebellum, forming the *crura cerebri.* Lying on its upper part are several protuberances with which it is connected, the corpora quadrigemina posteriorly, the thalamus in the center, and the corpora striata anteriorly and laterally. The sulcus divides it, and both peduncles separate at an acute angle like a fork; after the optic nerve has clasped the brainstem, each peduncle then spreads like an unfolded fan almost horizontally below the large [lateral] cerebral ventricle and towards the lower and lateral parts and the peripheries of the cerebrum. Its medullary fibres radiate anteriorly and laterally, surrounded by gray matter (in the corpora striata), into the entire anterior lobe of the cerebrum to form its convolutions as far as the Sylvian fissure. In various animals there is added to it on both sides an arched branch from the anterior commissure, which is connected in the anterior lobes of the cerebrum with the convolutions of the medullary peduncles [?] and with the olfactory nerves. Its radiations proceed laterally through the thalamus into the lateral parts of the brain, and afterwards curve markedly posteriorly around the optic nerve and form the convolutions of the tip of the posterior lobe of the brain.

The corpus callosum, the largest transverse ligament of the cerebrum, may also be considered the junction point of the medulla. It consists of layers and transverse fibres in its center; however, as soon as it spreads laterally and towards the peduncles of the cerebrum, it increases in bulk so that one can visualize it as if composed of spheres which come together at their points from both sides in the center of the corpus callosum. Its uppermost layers and fibres are the shortest, and they immediately curve upwards and markedly medially; they radiate forth by extending more and more fanlike, and form the convolutions on the medial surfaces of the cerebral hemispheres against the falx. The next layers and fibres are less curved and form the convolutions of the upper lateral surface of the cerebrum. Finally, the innermost continue more horizontally above the large cavity of the cerebrum [lateral ventricle] to form the convolutions on the lateral surface of the brain, and laterally they meet the convolutions of the anterior commissure and the medullary peduncles. As the corpus callosum radiates like a cone, so it also extends in its anterior and posterior extremities and pushes into the apices of the cerebral lobes in front and behind with the convolutions [formed by] the medullary peduncles of the cerebrum.

The anterior commissure extends horizontally almost like a cylinder from the center of the brain towards its sides, and for a considerable distance does not increase very much in thickness, but then starts to thin considerably, like an upside-down cone. It radiates and forms the convolutions of the lateral part and the lower surface of the middle lobe, and progresses below the lateral angle of the large cerebral cavity.

. . . .

Now the white matter radiates from the mentioned parts almost in straight lines towards the surface of the cerebrum. A part of the latter protrudes more and ends in the convolutions, in the midst of which it lies like a seam, or like the leaves of a rock lichen. Its sharp ends are covered with a fold of cortex. The larger part terminates deep in the foldlike sulci between the convolutions, also covered with cortex. Therefore the cerebral fibres, as well as the fibres of the cerebellum, are all covered by cortex at their ends. By a special procedure [*Kunstgriff* = knack] one can easily separate the cortex everywhere from the medulla. Then one may note, between the protruding edges of the medullary foldlike sulci, their upside-down cavities with the shape of arched convolutions.

The structure of the white matter is laminated, and the laminae are made of fibres all radiating towards the surface. By a special manipulation one can cut the white matter into laminae, but not as easily and regularly as can be done in the cerebellum, because in the latter the laminae are even and smooth, while in the cerebrum they are crooked and bent.

The cortex, too, has fibres; however, they do not everywhere adjoin the medulla in a straight line but rest perpendicularly upon the various surfaces, windings, and sulci of the white matter so that they surround the latter almost like the halo of a saint's head, at various acute and obtuse angles. The fibres of the cortex, too, lie in laminae that unite at various acute and obtuse angles.

Apart from this the cerebrum has various other connections in different directions: the posterior commissure, the peduncles of the pineal gland that radiate to the anterior commisure and the anterior peduncles of the fornix, the fornix, its anterior peduncles continuing to the *corpora corticantia* [mammillary bodies].

Therefore the cerebrum is a second protuberance of the spinal cord that radiates everywhere from the mentioned parts towards its surface. All the ends of its fibres are covered with cortex, just as the opposite ends of the nervous system, that is, the extremities of the nerves are also not naked but enveloped by different coverings. If we postulate a point anywhere in the nervous system, for instance in the medulla oblongata, we may assume that the nervous system continues to radiate from this point towards both its ends, that is, towards the [peripheral] ends of the nerves and the ends of the fibres on the cerebral and cerebellar surface. In reverse, a radiation can also occur from all these nerve endings to this point and so all proceed in circles.

The anatomical studies carried out by Reil after the closing of the University of Halle in 1806 were reported in a number of papers in the *Archiv für Physiologie, Halle*, which he edited in collaboration with J. H. F. Autenrieth. For example, almost half of the space in the ninth volume (1809) was devoted to his articles; reference to his description of the island of Reil has already been made (p. 391).

After writing the 1795 article cited above, Reil perfected his method of preparing the brain (pp. 830–832) and, armed with it, he paid special attention to the white matter such as the corpus callosum and the cerebral peduncles; he thought of these as special white matter systems. The following excerpts have been translated from "Das Hirnschenkel-System oder die Hirnschenkel-Organisation im grossen Gehirn"

(*Arch. physiol.*, *Halle*, 1809, 9:147–171. A condensed version of this appeared in Max Neuburger's *Johann Christian Reil* (Stuttgart, 1913, pp. 85–86). Reil's report dealt with the cerebral peduncles which, according to his concept, seem to have extended through most of the brainstem and above it, probably corresponding to the pyramidal tracts.

EXCERPT PP. 150–151

One may divide each cerebral peduncle into a basal area [basis pedun-culi] and its tegmentum. This [division] is particularly clear during its [the peduncle's] passage through the pons and cephalad. Each part is organized completely differently. If one cuts through the cerebral peduncles above the pons [midbrain level], one finds on cross section a laminated structure in the basal area, but the tegmentum is less organized, and in it a circular area which lies directly above [posterior to] the basal area is distinguished [red nucleus]. The basal area comprises only the cerebral peduncle, but the tegmentum has a complicated arrangement.

EXCERPT PP. 161–163

. . . . The cerebral peduncle in its entire course, beginning with the pyramids, has a laminated, ribbon-like structure . . . . Each little rod [fasciculus] consists of innumerable medullary rods as thin as poppy seeds and is covered by a delicate sheath of connective tissue (*Zellgewebe*. [See p. 576]). The corona radiata in its course diverges more and more and extends into an almost perfect circle [i.e., encircling the central gray masses and ventricles] which radiates throughout the cerebral lobes . . . . The ante-rior rods are long, delicate, numerous and they lie densely packed; the middle or lateral ones are the shortest and thickest, and they are cylindrical and form predominantly the crest [of the corona radiata]; the posterior ones are the longest that are made up of fibres, and those descending to the lateral cornu are again somewhat shorter. These and the ones that proceed to the posterior cornu are not interwoven with gray matter because they do not pass through the cerebral ganglia. The corona radiata lies in the [internal] capsule; that is, at the posterior border of the thalamus; the gray matter penetrates between the little rods.

In his next paper ("Das Balken-System oder die Balken-Organisation im grossen Gehirn," *ibid.*, pp. 172–195) Reil described the corpus callosum and then pro-ceeded to discuss the connection of this system with the peduncular one.

EXCERPT PP. 182–184

How do the corpus callosum and the crus cerebri systems join with each other? Probably one should not search too anxiously for continuity of the fibres in the anatomy of the brain, since contiguity suffices for conduction. Both extend in a radial fashion and are contiguous at the periphery. The cerebral peduncles proceed from below and spread in the shape of an upside-down cone; the corpus callosum system proceeds from above, sinks down between the peduncular system and covers, so to speak, the [cone-shaped] goblet. Very likely the type of union between the two differs: 1. In the anterior cornu, especially in the area of the genu [of the corpus callosum] both make contact and between them lies white matter which has less structure and forms a binding material; 2. More posteriorly the lateral layers of the corpus callosum anastomose with the system of the cerebral peduncles; 3. At the posterior border of the thalamus and at a distance of two lines [see p. 41] from it the fibres of the corpus callosum sometimes cross those of the system of the cerebral peduncles and there form a delicate junction; 4. Finally, the last and most posterior part of the corpus callosum descends as the tapetum over the cerebral peduncle organization. Both lie as two different strata, unprotected and one upon the other . . . .

The systems of the cerebral peduncles and corpus callosum and the radiation of the lateral limb of the capsule, which is part of the system of the cerebral peduncles, constitute the nucleus of the cerebrum in the inside of which lie the cerebral ventricles. Between this nucleus and the convolutions there lies yet a middle substance [external capsule] which passes over the nucleus and is especially visible below and above the Sylvian fossa.

FRANZ JOSEF GALL   JOHANN CASPAR SPURZHEIM

(See p. 392)

An important but often overlooked stimulus to the study of neuroanatomy during the first two decades of the nineteenth century was the work of Gall and his assistant Spurzheim. Together they carried out many investigations and in their day were renowned for their anatomical skill and knowledge. However, the stigma of phrenology hangs over them and because of this their contribution to neuroanatomy is frequently underestimated.

Gall always insisted that the study of phrenology was only a means of learning more about the structure of the brain and that his dissections represented a supplementary effort towards this end. In the course of them he revealed much data that was already known, but he also made certain discoveries of his own. His main contribution to the history of the present subject arose from the controversy he stirred up and the studies by others that were thus initiated. For example, the virulent attack by John Gordon (1817), mostly unjustified, was answered by Spurzheim (*Examination of the objections made in Britain against the doctrines of Gall and Spurzheim*, Edinburgh, 1817). The controversy was concerned largely with nerve "fibres" and it served to publicize further in English-reading countries Gall's studies on the anatomy of the brain.

Gall, who was continuing the work of Vicq d'Azyr, Reil, and others, was especially interested in the intracerebral white matter connections, perhaps because connections between his postulated surface organs (pp. 476–480) were essential for coordinated mental activity. He suggested that, according to their arrangement in the hemispheres, there were two systems of fibres, the diverging (*divergent* or *sortant*, the apparatus of formation) and the converging (*convergent* or *rentrant*, the apparatus of connection). The former were equivalent to our afferent and efferent projection fibres which run to and from the cortex in a radiating mass, out of and towards the brainstem. The latter correspond to our association fibres which are entirely intracerebral and are greatly developed in man; the short ones, the arcuate fibres and the long ones, the interconnections of the parts of different lobes of the same hemisphere. The commissural fibres which connect the two hemispheres together mainly through the corpus callosum were included by Gall with the associational type.

This differentiation of the cerebral white matter into projection and association fibres was a very important advance, although refuted viciously by Gordon (1817). The distinction was adopted in different ways by later anatomists and applied to the cerebral cortex by Flechsig (pp. 548–554). In the first volume of Gall's work, *Anatomie et physiologie du système nerveux*, etc. (Paris, 1810), prepared with the help of Spurzheim, Section IX deals with the brain (pp. 191–220). The diverging or projection fibres are first described, after which follows a section on the converging or association type presented below in translation.

EXCERPT PP. 201–204

ON THE MECHANISMS OF CONNECTION (COMMISSURES) OR OF THE NERVE MASS OF THE BRAIN, ASSOCIATIONAL OR CONVERGING

We have demonstrated that the different parts of the nervous systems of the vertebral column [spinal cord], of the nerves of the head [cranial nerves], and of the cerebellum are not only in connection with each other and with neighboring systems by communicating branches, but, moreover, that the congenerous systems of the two sides are joined together and placed in reciprocal action by transverse layers of fibres (commissures). We call this organization *apparatus of connection or of junction*, though we do not doubt that they contribute to the formation of the whole, like the *mechanisms of formation*.

All parts of the cerebrum are connected with analogous parts of the other hemisphere by a similar mechanism and are thus united for mutually influencing and the attainment of a common end. Some of these parts being much larger and more distinct than in the other systems, they have not escaped the attention of the most ancient anatomists. Galen describes the *corpus callosum*. For a long time the name commissure has been given to this part, and it has even been thought that it produced a communication and a reciprocal action. "The commissures," said Vicq d'Azyr, "seem to be destined to establish sympathetic communications between the different cerebral parts."

However, mechanical views have in general been adhered to. No one has dreamed of seeking the relationship of each of the commissures with the parts of the brain nor where their origin ought to be located; nor has it been determined whether or not all parts of the cerebrum are connected with one another in the same way; nor why the connections between like parts differ so much in different animals. Finally, apart from some vague ideas about the commissures of the spinal cord, it has not been established that these connections are subject to a general law; also nothing that we have said about them relative to the nervous system has been proposed by others. Our researches have provided us with a very precise and very satisfying solution of this matter.

Previously we followed the mechanisms of formation, either the projecting or the diverging nerve filaments, as far as the gray matter on the outer surface of the convolutions. We recognized very distinctly that all the extremities of the nerve filaments penetrated into the gray matter, which for this reason is whiter on the inside than on the outside. But we have not been able to discover what eventually happens to these fibres; we do not know if they end in this place or if they turn back and run towards the interior. However, it is very likely, according to general laws, that new nerve filaments arise in the gray layer in the same way as this takes place wherever gray matter is found; and that there results from it the production of a nervous system that augments the fibres with which it is in intimate connection.

It is certain that one can clearly demonstrate the existence of two systems in the brain and that the associational (*rentrant*) system contains more numerous fibres and larger bundles than the projectional (*sortant*) system. Indeed, finer and softer filaments are noticed in the convolutions formed by two nerve layers of the projection system; but they can only be followed as distinct and visible fibres in the posterior convolutions of the middle lobe. These fibres are seen in the depths of all convolutions as they run between the fibres of the projection system and are interwoven with them [acurate fibres]. In this way the two systems form a very firm tissue on the external

limits of the cavities [cerebral hemispheres] or in the depths of the appendages or convolutions.

The filaments of the association system unite beyond the tissue [cortex]
into larger filaments and, in proportion as they run towards the interior,
they form fasciculi and layers that are brought together in the midline
between the two hemispheres, proceeding by the medial border of the
hemisphere in white nerve layers united to the fasciculi and layers of the
congenerous system of the opposite hemisphere; thus they form various
connections, junctions, and commissures.

These fibres and nerve fasciculi everywhere cross each other in different
and even opposite directions; they form special and separate layers that
carpet the interior of the cavities [hemispheres]; they are softer and whiter
than the fibres and the fasciculi of the projection system. These particulari-
ties serve therefore to vindicate us against those who have stated that the
two systems of fibres in the brain is a chimera.

But are we justified in deriving these mechanisms of connection from the
gray matter of the external surface, and in considering them as associational
(*rentrant*)?

Up to the present we have proved that the nervous systems are everywhere produced by the gray matter. For the white color of all the connecting fasciculi teaches us that they do not contain the gray matter, or at least
they contain very little. The connections are even situated outside the
hemispheres where for a certain distance they travel, so to speak, empty.
The long anterior connection, or anterior commissure, that crosses the
thick mass of gray matter of the corpora striata, is no longer in communication with this substance as we shall soon demonstrate. Therefore the origin
of this system cannot be derived from its point of connection or junction.
From my point of view it is only possible to attribute to the connections
the purpose of producing action and reciprocal reaction and unity of action
between the same parts of the two hemispheres. Finally, this second system, which is additional to the diverging [projectional] system, serves to
explain perfectly why the two hemispheres contain a mass of nerves much
larger than that which reaches them from the corpora striata, which several
anatomists, including Cuvier, have regarded as simple appendages. That
opinion of Vicq d'Azyr, according to which the gray matter of the nerve
fibres is a covering which shelters external impressions, having collapsed,
one can no longer avoid considering the *cortical* substance or the gray
matter of the whole surface of the cerebellum and cerebrum as the origin of
the connecting mechanisms.

Up to the present there has been mention in anatomy of three commissures, namely: the great commissure, *commissura cerebri maxima; corpus*

callosum, callous body; the *anterior* and *posterior commissure*; several authors have also mentioned a fourth commissure, the *median* [interthalamic adhesion], between the anterior and posterior, but others have denied its existence.

. . . .

. . . .

. . . .

. . . . We maintain the general idea that all parts have their connections, and we seek to discover to which part each connection belongs.

Modern Period

Despite the pioneer work of Reil, Gall, and others, there was still considerable confusion and vagueness in the first half of the nineteenth century concerning the intracerebral white matter; this can be readily detected in writings of that period and it occasionally makes them difficult to follow. This, however, is only to be expected when one recalls the complex fibre pathways of the central parts of the brain; even today their complete elucidation has not been achieved. In fact, no further advance in the knowledge of white matter anywhere in the nervous system could be made until more was known of its constituent part, the nerve fibre. This data became available in the 1830's when the achromatic microscope was introduced (Chapter II) and some of the early investigators, Ehrenberg for example (pp. 39–43), examined cerebral nerve fibres. As the techniques of microscopy and of preparing and staining specimens developed, anatomists began to study the incredibly complicated intracerebral white matter with greater precision, but no real progress was made until the 1870's.

Theodor Meynert
(See p. 432)

The modern period of the study of white matter was opened by Meynert who carried out one of the century's most important investigations of its disposition. In a systematic survey of the brain of the bat (*Vespertilio pipistrella*) Meynert extended the relatively crude division of fibre systems introduced by Gall, and for the first time he used the terms "association" and "projection" in their modern sense. He published his findings in a chapter of Stricker's textbook of human and animal histology (*Handbuch der Lehre von den Geweben des Menschen und der Thiere*, Vol. II [Leipzig, 1872], "Ch. XXXI, Vom Gehirne der Säugethiere," pp.

694–808). Although the following excerpt concerned a lowly animal, it proved to be a useful adjunct to the study of the more complex human brain.

In summary Meynert thought cerebral white matter was comprised of (1) arcuate fibres, (2) corpus callosum, (3) cerebellar peduncles, afferent, (4) projection systems, and (5) anterior commissure. Meynert's reference to the projection of external sensory stimuli on the cerebral cortex should be noted, because it anticipated the idea of topical representation in the cortex of the receptor surfaces of the sense organs, as for example in the case of the retina (see p. 536). Thus the term "projection" fibre or system. A number of Meynert's terms are confusing, however. Thus, he uses the phrase "central gray cavities (*centrale Höhlengrau*)" for the basal gray masses that are grouped around the ventricles.

EXCERPT PP. 697–699

To understand the conducting tracts, it is appropriate to think of the cerebral cortex as a cap covering the outside of the brain (Figs. 230, 231, and 232 *F, O, Tp, R, H* [fig. 141. N.B. All figures on single plate.]). This results from the grouping of innumerable sensory, formed elements which inhabit the cortex, the *nerve cells*. The sensory nerves are their antennae, the motor their claws. As [the fibres from] the convolutions must for the most part pass through the foramen magnum in order to reach the organs [they supply], there is a raylike convergence of them from all sides towards the brainstem and spinal cord and towards the central gray matter (*Höhlengrau*). But after the central nerve fibres have traversed the latter, they *diverge* in the form of the peripheral nervous system to all parts of the body. By means of this arrangement, contact is made between the sensory shell of the cerebral cortex and the various sensory impressions from the outside world, that is, the image which is at the same time projected on to the cortex. It thus seems that the name *projection system* is appropriate for this extensive part of the nervous system. The cerebral cortex is thereby thought of as the projection surface on which the external world is projected (P_1, P_2, P_3).

As extensive body movements are the source of certain kinds of sensation (sensation of movement), so they are also a part of the external world projected upon the brain. But the muscles are, in still another sense, a *projection;* namely, through the central and peripheral pathways of the motor nerves along which the *cerebral cortex* reflects back, as it were, the state of excitation received from the external world.

P_1, P_2, P_3 in Fig. 1 [i.e., Figs. 230–232, see fig. 141] represent the successive links of this projection system which is again and again interrupted by gray masses. Of these links, the [first and] upper link (P_1, P'_1 and *Br*) is a myelinated system arising diffusely in and radiating from the cortex, the peripheral end of which reaches the gray matter of the second category, the gray ganglia (Figs. 230, 231, 232 *Cs, Th, Qu*). From the interrupting nodal point of these *ganglion masses* springs the second link of the projection system P_2, the *cerebral peduncle system*, the peripheral [central] end of which is found in the gray matter of the third category, the gray matter around the central cavities. The third link of the projection system is the nerves of which the origins are found in the above-mentioned central gray matter, extending from the site of origin of the third cranial nerve in the gray matter around the aqueduct of Sylvius to the nuclei of origin of the lowest coccygeal nerves in the spinal cord. These, probably without exception, end peripherally in recognized microscopic end organs which have been dealt with in several chapters of this textbook.

The region through which the *first link* of the *projection system* takes its course is the *cerebral hemisphere*, within which in an obvious manner it is accompanied by two myelinated formations, the *fibres of the corpus callosum* and the arch system (*Bogensystem* [association system]).

While the projection system establishes the contact of the cortical cells with the external world, so the cells communicate with themselves in three ways inside the cerebral hemispheres, so that the part of the protoplasm of the primordial cell (*Eizelle*) from which the innumerable cells of the cerebral cortex are formed, again combines in a morphological union which represents nothing else than a reunion. This opinion is very clearly based on the midline union of the corpus callosum fibres in fetal life, after they have pierced the inner wall of the vesicles of the hemispheres. The corpus callosum bundles (Figs. 230 and 231 *T.*) unite *identical parts of the cortex* of the two halves of the *cerebral hemispheres.*

The different parts of the cortex of one and the same hemisphere are, of course, connected in continuity by means of the gray fibre network which is made up of anastomotic processes. It is, however, the most valuable proof for the law of isolated conduction which is likewise in operation here, that the parts of the cortex are also connected together by myelinated fibres, the fasciculi of the fibrae propriae or arcuate fibres. These (Figs. 230 and 232 *aa*) are composed of fasciculi with long and short courses and form a continuous layer for the inner surface of the cortex. Since the connection of functional cortical territories must be related to a connection of their states of excitation by means of this medullary system, so its fasciculi, with regard to their significance, deserve the name of *association system.*

A fourth category of cerebral white fibre bundles serves to unite the *cerebral* and *cerebellar cortex* which come together in the superior peduncle as a distinct formation lying superficially in the region of the pons. But because of the indirectness of their course between the two cortical substances and because of the intimate and long connection with the projection system of the cerebral hemispheres, it is impossible in this general survey to give a clear account of them or to sort them out.

The *gray masses* lying below the lobes of the cerebrum are (excluding the *central gray matter* as regards the second point):

1. *Masses which interrupt* [the fibres of] the projection system, and
2. *Regions where there is reduction* in size [of the projection system]. Thus the first link, the greater part of which is in the form of the corona radiata, enters the various masses of the cerebral ganglia, where its size is reduced to the insignificant dimensions of the spinal cord columns.

This reduction [in size] of the projection system in its course below the cerebral hemispheres relates not only to the *total number of fibres* but also to the *number of special fasciculi* that can be distinguished inside the projection system.

At its point of entry into the ganglia the first link of the projection system breaks up into as many parts as there are distinct gray nuclei. Figs. 230 to 232 make obvious such special masses: the *corpus striatum* and the lenticular nucleus (*Cs*) with the fibres P_1 entering them; thalamus (*Th*) and quadrigeminal bodies (*Qu*) with the radiating fibres P'_1 and *Br* entering them close to the distinct fasciculus of the fornix, *f*, which is the projection bundle from the cortex to the anterior tubercle of the thalamus. Hence the upper link of the projection system shows a *multiplicity* of terminating tracts. However, the *second link of the projection system*, the *cerebral peduncles*, at its exit from the [basal] ganglion masses is reduced to a *double* pathway, anterior and posterior, of the brainstem, that is, the *feet* of the peduncles (Figs. 230 and 232 P_2 [basis pedunculi]) and the *tegmentum* of the peduncles (Figs. 231 and 232 *Tg*). These continue in the anterior (Fig. 231 P_2 *a*) and posterior part (Figs. 230, 231, and 232 P_2 *r*) of the pons and medulla oblongata, and finally pass into the white matter of the spinal cord which is a morphologically *homogeneous* area.

Meynert's name is occasionally associated today with the dorsal supraoptic or dorsal inferior hypothalamic decussation, the commissure of Meynert. It is composed mainly of fibres from the globus pallidus and subthalamic nucleus and passes to the zona incerta. It is usually thought to be associated with Gudden's commissure, the ventral inferior hypothalamic decussation, but there is evidence to suggest that in the cat, at least, the distinction between the two cannot be made on anatomical or morphological grounds (Weaver, 1937). Meynert mentioned this fibre pathway in his publication of 1872 cited above.

EXCERPT P. 732

2. There is a commissure which is immediately behind the inferior optic ganglion and enclosed within the tuber cinereum. Its fasciculi turn back into the central gray matter but their mode of termination is as yet unknown.

BERNHARD ALOYS VON GUDDEN
(7 June 1824—13 June 1886)

Although Meynert's work and that of others was of the greatest significance in the history of the white matter, there was a limit to the information that could be derived from unaided microscopy. New methods of tracing the nerve fibre fasciculi were needed, and the one introduced by the German psychiatrist and neuroanatomist Gudden was to be of particular importance.

Gudden was born in Kleve, near the German–Dutch border, and he studied at Bonn, Berlin, and Halle; he received the M.D. degree from Halle in 1848. He then held a number of appointments in German mental asylums and in 1869 became professor of psychiatry in Zürich. In 1870 he was given the same post at Munich and, in addition, was made director of the Kreis-Irrenanstalt there. He is best known for his contributions to the anatomy of the brain, especially the visual pathways. Some account of his less successful direction of the Kreis-Irrenanstalt has been given by August Forel (1935, 1937). Gudden was murdered by the mad King Ludwig II of Bavaria (see Grashley, 1886, 1887; Haymaker, 1953, pp. 45–48; Kolle, 1956–1963, I, 128–134; Dewhurst, 1964).

In 1849 Gudden began his work on the brains of newborn animals and perfected a method whereby he could produce secondary atrophy of nerve centers and their connections by removing a sense organ, such as the eye, or a cranial nerve. He did not, however, publish this work until 1870, and meantime Panizza had described similar but much cruder experiments in adult animals (see pp. 526–528). Gudden's new technique is particularly well illustrated by his work on the optic and olfactory pathways although he and his students also applied it to the investigation of many intracerebral pathways. Thus Monakow studied the corticothalamic connections (pp. 619–623), and his work as well as that of Gudden was surveyed by Seguin in 1883; see also Nissl (1895).

Gudden combined other techniques with his own, and one which he used extensively was that of serial sectioning introduced by Stilling in 1842 (pp. 271–275). In an article published in 1874 ("Über die Kreuzung der Fasern im Chiasma Nervorum opticorum," *Albrecht v. Graefes Arch. Ophthal.*, 1874, 20 [ii]:249–268), Gudden reported his investigations of the optic chiasma in the rabbit, using serial sectioning and secondary degeneration. He referred briefly to the commissure of Gudden, the ventral inferior hypothalamic decussation, which he had already mentioned at a meeting of Swiss psychiatrists on 25 September 1872: "the posterior commissure certainly exists but it has no physiological relationships with the optic nerve and, on the contrary, it is quite independent of it" (p. 249). Gudden, in addition, made reference to a law, also known by his name, which states that lesions of the cerebral cortex do not cause atrophy of peripheral nerves, or, in other words, that degeneration of the proximal end of a divided nerve is directed towards the cell body. Having discussed the chiasma in fish, amphibia, and in birds, he turned to mammals and man.

EXCERPT PP. 252–258

IV. MAMMALS AND MAN

The greater difficulties [encountered] in the investigation of the chiasm in mammals and in man are caused by the much finer and non-laminated interlacing of the optic nerve fibres . . . . So far studies have been carried out on:

1) [Serial] sections,
2) Teased preparations,
3) Chiasms of mammals and humans who were blind in one eye.

1) . . . .

. . . .

He who wishes to use [serial] sections for his studies must take care 1) that he has at his disposal an absolutely complete series, 2) that all the sections are very thin and that their axis cylinders (may they be ever so fine) are clear and distinct. To obtain such a series of uniformly thin sections by hand requires practice and skill. I have prepared such sections, which left nothing to be desired, with the help of a microtome which the instrument-maker Catsch, in Munich, made for me according to my instructions. I stained these with carmine, making sure that they did not come in contact with alcohol. (See my report, "Über ein neues Microtom" in *Arch. f. Psychiatrie*, 1875, 5:229–234.) Serial sections from rabbits, dogs, monkeys, and humans were studied.

The examination of transverse and longitudinal sections of the chiasms of these animals and of man does not contribute much knowledge concerning the course of the fibres. More successful, however, are horizontal sections. Despite the fine, and as Michel so characteristically put it, "basket-like reticular entanglement of fibres," it can still be demonstrated with relative ease in these that the decussation of the optic nerves is complete in the rabbit. This is easy because in this animal the direction is the same for all optic fibres that originate on one side. In the rabbit, the optic nerves lie close together and form a very acute angle at their exit from the chiasm. Since in this case the fibres also cross at an acute angle, it can be definitely demonstrated that an anterior commissure is not present. The so-called posterior commissure [fig. 142, *comm. inf.*, Gudden's commissure] is situated immediately in the posterior angle of the chiasm of the optic nerves.

So far, but not a single step further, I agree with the Biesiadecki–Michel assumptions on the completeness of the chiasm. In dogs, monkeys, and man the situation is quite different.

If, however, I had satisfied the highest possible standards in the examination of sections and had tracked down at least a few individual axis cylinders in their entire course through the chiasm, I should have been forced to agree with Meynert's above-quoted report. The fibres of the optic nerves are too thin and too densely packed; besides, most of them pass through so many sectional planes that they are lost sight of in their long course. However, in the rabbit, as well as in higher mammals and in man, it is not absolutely necessary to seek this highest objective; without solving [the problem] one can obtain a sufficiently accurate result, *provided one traces section for section, fasciculus for fasciculus* . . . . The fasciculi that cross each other lie chiefly in the lower half of the chiasm and those that do not cross, in the upper half. Fig. 13 [fig. 142] represents an illustration prepared by Dr. A. Solbrig from a section taken from the middle of the upper half of the human chiasm. I do not pretend that it necessarily convinces us of the partial decussation . . . . In the rabbit, the examination, as stated already, was facilitated by the uniform direction of all the nerve fibres which originate in the optic nerve. In the dog, monkey, and the human, these courses deviate from each other in two directions: they mix, intermingle, cross over, and cover each other in some areas, and although this arrangement indicates from the first that the decussation is not complete, it nevertheless forms an obstacle for the tracing of the individual fasciculi—a fact that does not require any further discussion—together with jeopardizing the evidence of actual incompleteness [of decussation].

The anterior angle of the chiasm in the rabbit is similar to that in the dog. What was said about the anterior commissure [of the chiasma] in the rabbit therefore applies also to the dog. In the monkey and man the angle is acute and its point rounded. For this reason it is hardly possible to decide whether there is a decussation at an angle of almost 180° or an actual commissure, so long as one cannot trace the individual axis cylinders. Yet, using an analogy, it is permissible to favor the assumption that they do not exhibit an anterior commissure. In support of this opinion we point to the observation that the same fibre course that is present in its anterior angle can be noted in the major part of the lower surface of the human chiasm. The existence of the posterior commissure [Gudden's] can be easily established. In Fig. 13 the fasciculi are cut through diagonally. In man the commissure joins the optic nerve directly in its middle portion only, and a thin strip of gray substance is inserted laterally. (At least this was the case in the chiasms which I have examined.)

2) I have never prepared teased preparations to elucidate the arrangement of the nerve fibres in the chiasm, and I shall therefore pass on directly to 3), which, incidentally, constitutes the main point of my study.

3) Complete atrophy of the optic nerve traceable to the primary centers [central nuclei] and beyond, can only be induced by destroying the retina completely in earliest infancy, and preferably immediately following birth. However, what can be accomplished at will in the purest and most convincing manner by experiment, is rarely offered by chance. Those who are interested in the details of this type of investigation for the elucidation of

the nervous system in the newborn animal and its use in man, are referred to my reports in the *Archiv f. Psychiatrie* [see Appendix, pp. 854–857]. Since then I have expanded the method with considerable success to include the cerebellum and the spinal cord.

There are ways and means other than destruction of the retina to achieve complete atrophy of the optic nerves. One can be equally successful by removing the central organs of the optic nerve. In this way Mandelstamm repeated an experiment that I had conducted earlier, with the difference that he, instead of superficially removing the anterior quadrigeminal body, removed all of them and also the lateral geniculate bodies and the thalamus. The central organs of the optic nerves lie in the anterior quadrigeminal bodies, the lateral geniculate bodies, and in parts of the thalamus yet to be outlined. However, removal of the anterior bodies in the rabbit causes incomplete, and removal of all centers, complete atrophy of the optic nerves . . . . Last year Professor Kollmann undertook upon my suggestion the examination of retinas of sacrificed rabbits of the second series. The successful sections showed complete preservation of all layers with the single exception of the fibre layer. Conducting fibres always atrophy, regardless of which of the two centers by which they are connected is destroyed. By contrast, if one of two central organs is destroyed, the other one atrophies only if it is not the stimulating one but the one stimulated. This may be a law that can be traced through the entire nervous system and that allows only apparent exceptions. As I said, the optic nerves atrophy whether the retina or the visual centers are destroyed; the centers atrophy when the retinas are destroyed; but the retinas do not atrophy when the centers are removed [Gudden's law]. However, if the problem is to elucidate the conditions in the chiasm only, it is obviously more practical to undertake the much easier and much more certain destruction of the retina than that of the center. Mandelstamm operated upon rabbits. That the optic nerves in this animal cross completely has already been proved beyond any doubt by my experiment that I published in the *Archiv. f. Psychiatrie* ["Experimentaluntersuchungen über des peripherische und centrale Nervensystem," 1870, 2:713–715 (Versuch IX)]. The axes of the eyes of the rabbit have a lateral direction, those of the dog a straight-ahead one. If I were previously tempted to assume a complete decussation in the dog, too (although I never specifically stated so), continued experimentation has shown me that this assumption is completely inaccurate.

Gudden also described the transverse peduncular tract (tractus peduncularis transversus), known to him since 1849, which is present in only a small proportion of human brains and which seems to be associated with visual function (see Monakow, 1870). This discovery was one of the first to result from his new experimental technique, and although he claimed priority for it, Gall and

Spurzheim had described and figured the tract in 1810 (I, 233–234); they called it "entrelacement transversal du gros faisceau fibreux." Gudden rectified this error by giving a bibliographical account of the tract with his later experiments ("Über den Tractus peduncularis transversus," Arch. Psychiat. NervKrankh., 1881, 11:415–423). The following excerpt has been translated from Gudden's paper entitled "Über einen bisher nicht beschriebenen Nervenfasernstrang im Gehirne der Säugethiere und des Menschen," Arch. Psychiat. NervKrankh., 1870, 2:364–366.

EXCERPT PP. 364–366

A nerve fibre bundle that to my knowledge has not been described before, can be recognized on both sides of the anterior margin of the anterior quadrigeminal body, that is to say, in the medial third. It increases in size and then advances laterally and downwards to the lower part of the cerebral peduncles where it fills out the angle between the arms of the posterior [quadrigeminal] body and the medial geniculate body like an oval cord. Its direction is therefore perpendicular to the fibre tracts of the cerebral peduncles. It has a tendency to sink into the latter, approximately at its center, but, for the most part can be followed easily in the direction of the point of origin of the oculomotor nerve to the medial ridge of the peduncles, since it can be recognized by its slight ridge, which in turn is caused by the elevation of the superficial fibre layer. I shall call it the Tract. peduncularis transversus.

As I have stated, I have not seen this fasciculus described anywhere, and I have looked for it in vain among the illustrations of the comparative anatomists at my disposal. Only in the Anatomie comparée du système nerveux by *Leuret* and *Gratiolet* can it be found, shown in the sheep brain, in Plate VII, Fig. 2. However, it is obvious that it originated with the artist and not with the anatomist.

For the moment I shall refrain from offering an opinion as to whether or not the fasciculus originates in the anterior quadrigeminal bodies, nor do I want to discuss its subsequent course and the central organ to which it advances. With regard to this investigation, to which I intend to refer in a future extensive report on the rabbit brain, it is more difficult to deal with and more delicate than might be at first assumed. But I should like to say that it depends for its existence on the retina and that its development, if the latter is suitably destroyed, can be barely detected. The importance of this finding will be obvious to the expert.

I noted the fasciculus first in my examinations of the rabbit brain . . . .
. . . .
. . . .

It is also present in the human brain, but it is fragile and one often looks for it in vain. I have preserved several brains in which it was well and significantly defined . . . . The position and course are the same, with the exception that in the human brain (and also in the cow) the fasciculus is seen more laterally and presents itself at the end of the anterior margin of the anterior quadrigeminal body.

PAUL FLECHSIG
(See p. 277)

Another revolutionary method of sorting out the intracerebral pathways was the myelogenetic technique of Flechsig (see pp. 857–858). Its value for the elucidation of the internal structure of the cerebrum has been greater than that of Gudden's atrophy method (pp. 606–609), and Flechsig's pioneer work on spinal cord tracts (pp. 278–280) resulted from his use of it, as did his outstanding contribution to the problem of cerebral cortical localization (pp. 548–555).

The details of the method have been recorded elsewhere (pp. 857–858), but essentially it consisted of observing the times of myelinization in developing nervous tissue. As this varied in different pathways, a means of differentiating them on an embryological basis was thus available. Flechsig used it extensively in several classic studies of the cerebral white matter. For example, he successfully traced the pyramidal tract from pyramid to cortex; previously it had been thought that motor fibres ended in the basal gray masses. It is usually claimed that he was the first to identify the most central portion of the pathway, between the motor cortex and the internal capsule, but Gudden deserves this distinction for he described the connection while reporting a case of general paralysis of the insane to the Gesellschaft jungeren Ärzte in Zürich on the 30 December 1871 (*KorrespBl. schweizer Ärzte*, 1872, 2:78–82).

The following excellent description of the intracranial portion of the tract has been taken from a long article ("Über 'Systemerkrankungen' im Rückenmark," *Arch. Heilk.*, 1877, 18:101–141, 289–343, 461–483) dealing with "system diseases" of the spinal cord; portions relevant to the pyramidal tract in the spinal cord have been already cited (pp. 280–282).

EXCERPT PP. 290–295

ORIGIN OF THE PYRAMIDAL TRACTS IN THE CEREBRAL HEMISPHERES
AND THEIR COURSE TO THE MEDULLA OBLONGATA

Earlier authors unanimously reported that the pyramids of the medulla oblongata continue upwards into the anterior portion of the pons, the cerebral peduncle, the internal capsule, the lenticular nucleus, the caudate nucleus, etc. However, traces of the pyramidal fibres are already lost in the pons when purely anatomical methods are used, because here much bigger fibre bundles that have anatomical relations of a different kind are seen in cross section. Thus until now there has existed (since the investigators of secondary degeneration devoted little attention to this point) no absolutely exact reports as into how large a segment of the pons seen in cross section, or of the cerebral peduncle, or of the internal capsule, etc., the pyramidal tracts extend. Consequently we have no satisfactory ideas regarding their relationships with the cerebral [basal] ganglia or with the cerebral cortex. It is precisely for a problem like this that embryology proves to be a reliable guide since, without any assistance whatsoever, it is capable of bringing us closer to the desired goal in an unexpected way. In accordance with this I shall describe the origin of the pyramidal tracts in the cerebrum, based in the first instance, *solely* upon my investigations *in the fetus and the newborn*. Since I have only recently collected the pertinent observations and I am reporting them now for the first time in detail, it seems appropriate to begin with some comments on the *process of evolution* of the pyramidal tracts. The following peculiarities make it possible to identify them above the medulla oblongata from among the many different fibres that decussate and are accompanied on their way to the cerebrum.

The pyramidal tracts in the *spinal cord* and the *medulla oblongata* follow all the other longitudinal bundles of fibres (myelin covering, etc.) in development (cf. Fig. 1, Pl. VII ps, pv, etc. [fig. 82]). They are thus the fibre bundles *in the anterior part of the pons* and in the *cerebral peduncle that are first enveloped by a myelin covering* (Fig. 9, Pl. VII*p*; the differences in clarity are very probably accurately reproduced [fig. 82, p. 82. Section through midbrain at exit from cerebrum. 51 cm. fetus. Natural size]). Therefore they run in these regions during certain stages of development which, according to my observations so far, begin [at an age] corresponding to a body length of 47–51 cm., as myelinated bundles among otherwise completely non-myelinated ones. The rates of development in the *internal capsule* are slightly less valuable for anatomical use.

In accordance with my investigations, which have not yet been concluded, of all the fibre bundles related to the capsule, running in *the white matter of the hemispheres*, certain bundles (at *circa* 42–44 cm.? body length) that radiate from the thalamus to the cortex, particularly to the parietal lobes (in Fig. 8, Pl. VII; these are shown at x in section [fig. 82. Section of left hemisphere. 51 cm. fetus. Natural size]) obtain their medullary sheaths first. They are followed very soon (perhaps simultaneously) by bundles of fibres that radiate from the medullary laminae and from the medial components of the lenticular nucleus transversely through the internal capsule into the thalamus. Shortly thereafter (with a fetus of *circa* 46 cm.? length) the fibre bundles, which I consider to be the pyramidal tracts, begin to surround themselves with myelin. That particular stage of development at which the myelin sheaths have just become distinctly visible in the tracts (*circa* 46–51 cm. body length) is the best to follow in the cerebral hemispheres. I was able to observe the following in several individuals that were at this stage. Having entered the anterior portion of the pons, each pyramid divides into a number of smaller bundles. In the cerebral peduncle these again join into a compact tract [crus cerebri] that has an approximately rhombic-shaped cross section, somewhat *larger* than that of the corresponding pyramid at the upper end of the medulla oblongata. Following its entrance into the internal capsule, it mostly remains compact because it is only obliquely interwoven by some other fibre tracts (for example, the clear strip in the dark area at *p* in Fig. 9, Pl. VII) directly after its entry into the hemisphere. *Without making any connections with the gray substance of the cerebral ganglia, this bundle*, the cross section of which is now for the most part elliptical in shape (cf. *p*, Fig. 8, Pl. VII), first of all pushes between the lenticular nucleus and the thalamus. At higher levels, between the lenticular and the caudate nucleus, it reaches the *centrum semiovale* and radiates in diverging fashion towards *the cortex of the hemispheres, chiefly* to the upper parts of the *central convolutions* and to their closest neighborhood.

If we look more closely at the position of the pyramidal tracts in the places just described, we find no extensive, foreign longitudinal bundles of fibres in the *anterior portion* of the lowest parts of *the pons*. But the more cephalad, the more numerous [foreign] bundles become, so that in the upper portions of the pons, the pyramidal tracts are surrounded, especially laterally, posteriorly, and also medially and anteriorly, by considerable longitudinal fibre bundles that do not descend into the medulla oblongata.

The conditions are comparable in the *cerebral peduncle*, into which the aforesaid fibres pass, retaining their relative positions. As determined by the formation of the myelin sheath, the tract is divided into at least four areas of varying importance. I first distinguish an upper area bordering the substantia nigra (*oE* in Fig. 9, Pl. VII) and a lower, lying free in the anterior floor area (*y, p, z*), which is particularly clearly separated from the hemispheres; in the lower the longitudinal fibre bundles come closer together than in the upper where they are often separated from each other by a network of gray matter, etc. For the time being, only the *lower* one is of interest to us. Embryologically it is divided into three sub-sections (longitudinal fibre bundles) of unequal cross section, the *middle* one of which is formed exclusively of the pyramidal fibres (*p* in Fig. 9, Pl. VII). If one imagines the cerebral peduncle cut at right angles to the principal direction of its fibre tracts from the inside to the outside, and into four segments of equal width, then the pyramidal tracts lie predominantly in the *third quarter*. At lower levels, towards the upper margin of the pons, they extend slightly into the second quarter; at the higher ones they limit themselves exactly to the third quarter (*p* in Fig. 9, Pl. VII).

The behavior of the pyramidal tracts in the *internal capsule* may be described in more detail, not only with respect to the outstanding importance of the internal topography of this main traffic route between the psychic area and the periphery, but also because embryology allows explanations of undreamed-of perfection precisely in this part of the cerebrum.

In the internal capsule I distinguish an anterior and posterior segment [or limb], in the first instance merely to facilitate description. The former (*cia*, Fig. 8) lies between the anteromedial surface of the lenticular nucleus and the thalamus. Corresponding to the anterior portion of the latter, the two segments join at an obtuse angle that is open laterally and may be called the "genu of the internal capsule." This genu, as well as the partition of the internal capsule into two limbs produced by it, is particularly noticeable in horizontal sections that have been carried out in the region of the second component of the lenticular nucleus [globus pallidus]. Between the second part on the one hand and the caudate nucleus and thalamus on the other, it is no longer visible. Where then are the pyramidal tracts located?

Insofar as the internal capsule is distinctly divided into two limbs, as indicated earlier, they run upwards in the *posterior* one, and assuming it to be divided into three parts corresponding to the anterior, middle, and posterior *third of the thalamus*, they are in the middle part. They also retain this position at higher levels. In this course, the pyramidal tracts are separated from the tail of the caudate nucleus [posteriorly] by a fibre layer, the elements of which pass from the lateral surface of the thalamus into the corona radiata. However, *laterally* they border (apart from the lowest levels of the internal capsule where a part of the loop of the lenticular nucleus (?) intrudes between them and the first component of the lenticular nucleus [globus pallidus]), directly on the gray substance of the lenticular nucleus, from below upwards touching successively the first [globus pallidus I], second [globus pallidus II], and third parts [putamen] in their most posterior segments.

The *entrance* of the pyramidal tracts into the *centrum semiovale* takes place, counting from before backwards, approximately at the third quarter of the caudate nucleus, close to the upper border of the lenticular nucleus. At the point of entrance its bundles frequently interlace, partly with each other, partly with the heterogeneous fibre bundles that radiate next to them from the internal capsule, so that for the most part one can follow them in the white matter of the hemispheres for only short distances. However, a portion of the pyramidal fibres retains the direction which predominates in the internal capsule; these reach the upper portions of the [pre-]central

convolution, particularly anteriorly, for they run laterally towards the oper-
culum to ½ cm. above the lateral ventricle and subsequently curve medially at the top. My embryological studies have not as yet enabled me to
demarcate precisely the cortical areas that are reached by the fibres of the
pyramidal tracts [see pp. 548–555] . . . . It seems to me beyond question
that the *cortical gray matter* of the areas towards which the pyramidal fibres
turn, contains their *end stations* (in the form of ganglion cells) I
now believe that, based upon my embryological experiments I may now
draw the conclusion that *the lenticular nuclei are in no way very pertinent
to the pyramidal tracts. Nowhere have I seen fibre bundles branch off* from
the tract that I consider to be the continuation of the pyramids and that
passes through the cerebral peduncle and internal capsule, *and proceed to
the lenticular nucleus.* If one considers furthermore that the cross section of
our tract is somewhat larger in the entire area of the internal capsule than
the cross section of the pyramid at the upper end of the medulla oblongata,
then the number of fibres of the capsule does not only correspond to the
total size of the pyramid, but, moreover, there is simply no room within the
pyramid for fibres of different origin in addition to the elements reaching it
from the cerebral white matter. What can be said of the lenticular nuclei is
also valid for the caudate nuclei, the association of which with the pyramids
I earlier declared to be most improbable. *Thus none of the ganglia of the
cerebral peduncle is related to the pyramidal tracts.*

One of the most vital areas in the cerebral hemispheres is the internal capsule,
and Flechsig used his myelogenetic technique to elucidate the arrangement of its
contents. His detailed results appeared in 1881 ("Zur Anatomie und Entwickelungsgeschichte der Leitungsbahnen im Grosshirn des Menschen," *Arch. Anat.
Physiol.,* 1881, pp. 12–75). He examined seven horizontal sections of the capsule,
the levels of which were designated according to their relationship to parts of the
lenticular nucleus, and gave an account of the internal capsule in each. The third
and fourth sections are described in the following selection.

EXCERPT PP. 29–32

3) Section through the *upper half* of the first portion of the lenticular
nucleus [L] above the body of Luys (Fig. 6 [fig. 143]). The internal capsule
is bounded medially by the thalamus instead of by the body of Luys. It is
thereby divided distinctly into *two* large *divisions* [or limbs]: a smaller,
anterior one between the lenticular nucleus and head of the caudate nucleus, and a *posterior* one, located between the lenticular nucleus and the
thalamus. Both limbs meet at an obtuse (almost right) angle; the place
where this occurs might be called the *knee* [genu] *of the internal capsule.*
   a. The bundles of fibres in the *posterior* (principal) *limb* are arranged in

almost their entire length into two approximately parallel layers of which the larger one lies close to the lenticular nucleus ("*external* position"), whereas the other is located partly on the outside, partly within the most external portions of the thalamus ("*internal* position").

α. Only the *external lamina* contains the continuation of the bundle of fibres that ascends from the crus of the peduncle. There can be distinguished in it an anterior, non-myelinated section that lies in almost its entire length close to the first portion of the lenticular nucleus, corresponding to field *c* and partly also to *d* in Fig. 4 [fig. 144], which has a considerably smaller cross section; that is, bundles of fibres that proceed at less than a right angle to the level of the section, than *c* + *d* at lower levels—evidently because a large portion of their fibres, particularly those of *d*, have gone over into the *anterior limb* of the internal capsule. Directly behind the non-myelinated field *c* there are, still within the area of the first part of the lenticular nucleus, a number of fibre bundles that are provided with rudimentary myelin sheaths, and proceed vertically to the plane of the cross section and correspond to *p'* of the lower cuts in size and elementary structure. Lying closely next to them, posteriorly, is the continuation of the *pyramidal tract* [*p*], as a completely separate, medullary column of uniformly developed fibres, of an approximately elliptical cross section. The transversely infiltrating, non-myelinated fibres have been lost and only connective tissue-like septa affect a division into a number of smaller bundles. The pyramidal tract has gone over from the area of the first part of the lenticular nucleus into that of the second (see Fig. 6 [fig. 143, II]). Behind it, on the one hand, between the second [II] and third [III] portions, is the *internal* layer of the capsule that will soon be described; on the other hand, a *new* field *g* is seen (Fig. 6) in which we can distinguish transversely and obliquely cut bundles of fibres at different stages of development. Most of them are *myelinated*, some with fine myelin sheaths that are barely visible, even with strong magnification (similar to *p'*), and some with thicker ones. The former lie close to the pyramidal tract posteriorly, the latter adjacent to the second or third part of the lenticular nucleus. They are later joined by sparse, non-myelinated bundles of fibres, somewhat more numerous in the posterior sections than in the anterior. The myelinated fibres of field *g* have entered the internal capsule between the plane that corresponds to that of section 2 and that under discussion, partly from the thalamus and partly from the subthalamic region; the myelinated ones, which, with regard to their position, might be considered as a continuation of the lateral bundles of the cerebral peduncle (*a*), are so sparse that only a small fraction of them could have advanced to the plane in question. Since, however, non-myelinated bundles of fibres enter field *g* from the thalamus as well as from the lenticular nucleus, and since one may observe at lower levels the direct transition of fibres from *a* into the medullary nucleus of the temporal or occipital lobe, I consider the assumption adequately supported that *in the plane which corresponds to Fig. 6, bundles of fibres from a are no longer in the internal capsule.*

. . . .

β. The *internal lamina* (*f–f'*) of the posterior limb consists of a large number of individual bundles of *myelinated* fibres that are arranged in a long row and cover almost the *entire* outer surface of the thalamus; their cross section is of varying shape and size. The most anterior bundles (*v*) lie close to the lateral lamina of the capsule; they have somewhat thinner fibres than those located more posteriorly, and they lie closer together. Beginning at the area of field *p'*, the row becomes looser and the myelinated fibres appear thicker so that they also differ, particularly from the pyramidal fibres, by a larger content of myelin; the medial lamina moves a little from the lateral one, because a small layer of gray substance that penetrates between them interlaces the inner netlike lamina and, towards the inside, passes over into the gray substance of the thalamus. Towards the rear (*f'*), the inner lamina, extends considerably beyond the internal capsule, insofar as one considers its posterior border to be the posterior edge of the lenticular nucleus. One might be in doubt as to whether the inner lamina, especially the portion which is located posterior to *p'*, may be classed with the internal capsule. Evidently it partly corresponds to the external medullary lamina of the thalamus of other writers; the gray substance that separates it from the outer lamina corresponds to the "lattice layer of the thalamus" [reticular nucleus]. Nevertheless, a direct contact of the outer with the inner lamina is visible also in some parts of the posterior limb, because individual bundles of fibres fill the interstices; and, in addition, I must assume that the bundles of the inner lamina at somewhat higher levels mix, for the most part, with the bundles of the external lamina, so that I have not the slightest scruple about considering the former, too, as belonging to the internal capsule.

A comparison of Figs. 6 and 4 shows that the posterior part of the inner lamina (*f'*) develops at that point at which (Fig. 4 *f'*) the bundles of fibres from the area of the red nucleus of the tegmen and its cover *h* aim [corticorubral tract]. *Therefore one must consider the posterior part of the inner lamina as the direct continuation of bundles of the tegmen of the cerebral peduncles.* I must leave it undecided in how far such fibres are also found in the anterior section of the inner lamina (in front of *f*); a good proportion of the elements of this section derive from the thalamus, so that fibres of different importance mix in the inner lamina. I gain the impression that thalamic fibres predominate in the anterior limb and tegmental fibres in the posterior. Consequently I am calling the latter, in short, the *tegmental radiation*, but, of course, based upon the foregoing I cannot report its total circumference exactly; the most fitting interpretation might be that it lies alongside the pyramidal tract, partly medially and partly laterally (*f–f'*); *parts of field g might also have to be put in with it.*

Because of this the posterior limb of the internal capsule in the plane represented by Fig. 6 consists of two large areas. One contains *large* bundles of fibres related to the cerebral peduncle (*p p' c d* [cortical motor pathways]), while the other (*f f' g*) absorbs the fibres that deploy from the cerebral tegmentum and the *thalamus* [superior and posterior thalamic radiation]. Both areas are probably still separate, because a mixing of the fibre bundles, especially from the peduncle and tegmentum, has not yet taken place.

b. The *anterior* limb of the internal capsule consists very predominantly of non-myelinated bundles that proceed from the area of the genu anteriorly, superiorly, and laterally. With respect to their stage of development, etc., they correspond completely with those of fields *c* and *d* of the posterior limb from which they originate by changing direction [frontopontine tract]. Individual bundles of fibres disappear into the caudate and lenticular nuclei. Some myelinated bundles mix in from the anterior end of the *inner layer* of the posterior limb.

4. Horizontal section *above the inner portion of the lenticular nucleus* [I] just above the union of the internal medullary lamina [of the thalamus] with the internal capsule (Fig. 7 [this is the same as Fig. 8, Pl. VII, in *Archiv der Heilkunde*, 1877, 18. See fig. 82]).

The conditions of stratification, as well as the number of the fields that can be distinguished in the internal capsule, are essentially the same as in cross section 3. The *anterior limb* appears much larger than at lower levels; the non-myelinated bundles, of which it chiefly consists, again originate in the knee area of the internal capsule from the non-myelinated fields of the *posterior limb* with individual bundles also from the anterior part of the thalamus [anterior thalamic radiation]. In the posterior limb the non-myelinated sections *c* and *d* exhibit a further decrease in cross section that is particularly manifested by a decrease in transverse diameter while the longitudinal diameter remains constant. The *pyramidal tract* is distinctly visible as a compact, myelinated tract (of the same basic structure as at lower levels) that lies close to the last part of the second portion of the lenticular nucleus. The field in front of it, *p'*, behaves exactly as *p'* at lower levels. Field *g* behind the pyramidal tract has increased in cross section as well as in bundles of fibres with thicker myelin sheaths; the latter are particularly numerous at the inner level of the third portion of the lenticular nucleus. Numerous medullary bundles flow from the thalamus to the inner lamina, especially from the *lateral* nucleus that is abundant in myelinated fibres. The tegmental radiation has placed itself closer to the outer lamina of the capsule.

CONSTANTIN VON MONAKOW
(See p. 565)

Although Flechsig had effectively disproved the existence of the supposed connections of motor fibres with the basal gray masses, it was clear to many neuroanatomists that the thalamus, at least, made contact with the cerebral cortex. Luys thought that corticothalamic fibres existed, and he even suggested that specific cortical areas were related to specific thalamic nuclei; this, however, remained an unverified hypothesis. It was Gudden's secondary degeneration technique which showed that if a cerebral hemisphere were removed and the thalamus left intact, a decrease in the size of the latter resulted ("Experimentaluntersuchungen über das peripherische und centrale Nervensystem," *Arch. Psychiat. NervKrankh.*, 1870, 2:693–723, see pp. 708–709). One of Gudden's assistants was Constantin von Monakow who spent the first third of his professional life carrying out important neuroanatomical investigations (p. 565). He was inspired by his teacher's observation on corticothalamic pathways and was also influenced by the work of Munk on cortical function, especially that of vision (pp. 528–533).

Monakow's experiments were carried out while he was assistant physician at the St. Pirminsburg Asylum at Pfäfers, near Rogatz. Because of the high mortality rate amongst kittens, and since he was unable to obtain dogs, he used newborn rabbits despite their featureless cerebral surface which meant that his studies lacked precision. The following excerpt is from his report, "Über einige durch Exstirpation circumscripter Hirnrindenregionen bedingte Entwickelungshemmungen des Kaninchengehirns" (*Arch. Psychiat. NervKrankh.*, 1882, 12:141–156), and in it one of his experiments is described. He was able to conclude from it that the lateral geniculate body and the lateral portion of the lateral thalamic nucleus were centers for vision in association with the cortical area removed.

EXCERPT PP. 150–151

II. EXPERIMENT

Rabbit II. (One day old, likewise operated on at the end of March 1880.) The cerebral surface was exposed in the same way as in the previous experiment but only the left occipital region; an area of cerebral cortex was ablated [small circular area indicated on drawing of brain—*a* in Fig. 5 (fig. 145)] This animal also recovered after a few days.

At the end of February 1881 the animal was sacrificed. With the exception of the postoperative scar and an (also relatively) insignificant diminution in size of the cerebral hemisphere which had been operated upon, hardly anything pathological could be demonstrated macroscopically in the freshly removed brain.

In the microscopic investigation of the series of coronal sections that were laid out as in the first rabbit, the following was found:

The lateral layer of the lateral nucleus of the left thalamus was completely retarded in its development (Figs. 5 and 6z [figs. 145 and 147]); the lateral nucleus on the operated side looked exactly as if the lateral part of its vault had been excised obliquely with a sharp knife. The remaining portion of this nucleus was completely normal and showed ganglion cells in all parts as beautifully developed as on the other side. In addition, the lateral geniculate body was atrophic to an extreme degree; almost totally so in the anterior parts, and in the posterior parts it was reduced to the size of a pinpoint. The portion of the internal capsule that corresponds to the two atrophic nuclei was completely absent; the atrophy could be followed beautifully from the section, which began with the atrophic nucleus (middle of the thalamus), posteriorly through the internal capsule and the corona radiata to the excised area [of cortex]. Around the latter, the white matter and the cerebral cortex to some extent also were atrophic. That portion of the tract which originates in the left lateral geniculate body was small compared to that on the right side.

The left anterior quadrigeminal body seemed somewhat flatter than the right, but insignificantly so; furthermore, the left transverse peduncular tract (Gudden [pp. 610–611]) had almost completely disappeared whereas the right one could be seen very nicely.

The right optic nerve, too, seemed smaller than the left, even if insignificantly so.

For the remainder, all the tracts of the brain and the spinal cord were, bilaterally, well developed and normal. In particular, the remaining nuclei of the thalamus, the peduncles, and the medial geniculate body were completely intact.

We found in this experiment very similar results to the preceding ones; extirpation of a circumscribed portion of cerebral cortex—atrophy of certain sub-cortical nuclei. The area upon which we operated coincided rather well with Munk's visual center (Zone A_1, in the dog [see pp. 529–530]), corresponded probably also to area 9 reported by Ferrier [see p. 517] and Fürstner in the rabbit (stimulation of which caused closure of the eye). The actual size of the area ablated has been illustrated exactly in Fig. 2 (*a*) [error for Fig. 5]; the tissue around the damaged area, however, as demonstrated by microscopical examination, atrophied to a considerable extent, so that one may well assume that the larger part of the visual areas had lost its function because of the surgical intervention.

Monakow carried out many more experiments of a similar type in an attempt to relate portions of cerebral cortex to deep nuclei and to correlate them both with function; Seguin (1883) has summarized them briefly. In figure 146 the cortical zones isolated in the rabbit brain are shown. The following is the summary from his second report ("Weitere Mittheilungen über durch Exstirpation circumscripter Hirnrindenregionen bedingte Entwickelungshemmungen des Kaninchengehirns," *Arch. Psychiat. NervKrankh.*, 1882, 12:535–549) which is dated 23 September 1881.

EXCERPT PP. 543–547

If now we briefly summarize the results of our investigations, we have produced atrophy of the following tracts by the ablation of circumscribed areas of cortex:

1. Extirpation of zone A [fig. 146]—atrophy of the pathways belonging to the hemispheres, [that is] of the posterior third of the internal capsule, the lateral geniculate body, the lateral layer of the lateral nucleus of the thalamus, the optic tract and, to a lesser degree, of the transverse peduncular tract, the superior [anterior] quadrigeminal body, and of the optic nerve.

2. Extirpation of zone B—atrophy of the fasciculus of the corona radiata originating in the temporal lobe, of the lowest and most posterior part of the internal capsule, the medial geniculate body, and, to a lesser extent, of the posterior reticular layer [of the thalamus].

3. Extirpation of zone a—atrophy of the dependent fasciculus of the corona radiata, the third fifth of the internal capsule, the lateral [thalamic] nucleus, the lateral part of the [cerebral] peduncle, and to a lesser degree of the laminae originating in the lateral nucleus, the reticular formation, the middle peduncle of the cerebellum, the trapezoid body, and the lateral temporal layer.

4. Extirpation of zone b—atrophy of the dependent fasciculus of the corona radiata, the third fifth of the internal capsule, part of the lateral peduncle, the anterior part of the reticular nucleus, and to a lesser extent, of the posterior reticular nucleus and its continuation in the tegmentum.

5. Extirpation of zone c—atrophy of the dependent hemisphere fasciculus of the anterior nucleus, of the anterior part of the internal capsule, then part of the pyramidal tract (with the claustrum and the substantia nigra), and to a lesser degree of the laminae medullares of the anterior nucleus, as well as of Vicq d'Azyr's bundle.

6. Extirpation of zone d—atrophy of the dependent hemisphere fasciculus of the anterior part of the internal capsule, of tract a, and to a lesser degree also of the anterior reticular nucleus.

7. Extirpation of zones e and f—atrophy of the dependent fasciculus of

the corona radiata, of the most anterior part of the internal capsule, partial atrophy of the pyramidal tract, and of the middle [thalamic] nucleus.

A glance at this sequence of operations suffices to demonstrate that, following the ablation of circumscribed areas of the cerebral cortex, the tracts that depend upon them are isolated and inhibited in their development without regard for their physiological importance. Whether or not the extirpated region serves sensory or motor function, when it has been removed the atrophy progresses in an identical manner and for the most part spreads in two directions. First of all it involves the corresponding nuclei of the subcortical ganglia [thalamus, etc.] and their bundles in the corona radiata. Thus by excision of circumscribed portions of the cerebral cortex leading to the posterior nucleus of the thalamus, which is probably related to basal areas of the cerebral cortex, each nucleus could be made to atrophy on its own. In addition, tracts leading directly [from the cortex] to the periphery, also atrophied. Notable among the latter are the lateral tract of the peduncle, the pyramidal tract and tract a, which depends upon region d, and which atrophied following extirpation of zones *a, b, c, d, e*; furthermore, the hemisphere bundles of the optic tract (Gudden) that project upon zone A. Finally, it should be noted that, apart from the atrophies mentioned, those of a second order also occur; that is, tracts which originate in the atrophied [thalamic] nuclei and proceed into the region of the tegmentum also atrophy. However, these cannot be traced separately for long distances. Thus, for example, upon removal of cortical area *c*, there is atrophy not only of the anterior nucleus but also, to a lesser degree, of the tract of Vicq d'Azyr, as well as of the accompanying laminae medullares; likewise with extirpation of zone A, after atrophy of the fasciculus of the hemisphere, the part of the optic tract that arises from the lateral geniculate body also atrophies.

It can be concluded from all this that individual areas of cerebral cortex are in precise relationship with more than one tract.

If now we try to elucidate the physiological importance of the tracts that have atrophied, it appears to me that the conditions are simplest in the tract that projects on zone A. Undoubtedly it serves psychic vision. In the dog, A, because of its position, corresponds to Munk's zone A [see p. 530]; its extirpation produces visual disturbances, and the result after its excision in newborn animals, as I have pointed out elsewhere, is almost the same as the removal of the eyeball.

. . . .

. . . .

Regarding zone *a*, I have stated in my most recent work that this might serve sensory functions. I believe this assumption to be justified since, when it has been ablated, the part of the internal capsule that perishes is that which, according to Duret's and Veyssière's experiments, when sectioned in the dog, produces hemianesthesia on the opposite side of the body; this is also produced by section of its process, that is the lateral part of the peduncle which, according to Meynert's anatomical investigations, is supposed to serve sensation. But part of the motor area for the hind leg (area 6 of Ferrier and Fürstner) is also in area *a*, and ablation of it also leads to partial atrophy of the lateral nucleus of the thalamus and of the lateral [cerebral] peduncle. We have here a contradiction between Fürstner's results and mine that still awaits resolution. Probably it may be traced to errors in measurement. In any event, zone *b*, upon the extirpation of which the lateral peduncle also partially atrophies, must have similar functions to those of zone *a*. However, nothing definite can be said about it at this time.

. . . .

. . . .

. . . .

Corresponding to the above-mentioned assumptions regarding the character of the individual cortical zones that are connected with the thalamus (*Thal. opt.*), a similar hypothesis might be made for the respective nuclei of the thalamus (*Sehügelkern*). The middle and anterior nuclei would then have to do with motor activity, and the lateral nucleus as well as the reticular layer, with sensation. However, one must not overlook the fact that, even if the connections between individual regions of the cerebral cortex and motion and sensation of the extremities have been ascertained, all the functions of individual regions are as yet very imperfectly known. As long as this is so, one must observe extreme caution before making a direct inference from the cortex to the nuclei of the thalamus, the more so, since, as may be seen from our investigations, more than one tract is related to each zone.

If we now summarize the results of our investigations in a few words, we may establish the following propositions:

1. Following ablation of circumscribed areas of cortex in the newborn rabbit, the tracts that project upon them alone perish, and without regard for their physiological importance.

2. For the most part more than one tract is in exact relation to one cortical area.

3. The individual nuclei of the thalamus, as well as the lateral and medial geniculate bodies are each in precise association with circumscribed areas of the cerebral cortex.

4. The lateral and medial geniculate bodies are structures analogous to the nuclei of the thalamus and ought to be included with them.

JOANNES GREGORIUS DUSSER DE BARENNE   WARREN STURGIS MCCULLOCH
           (6 June 1885—9 June 1940)   (16 November 1898—   )

The methods of tracing the white matter pathways considered thus far have been based on anatomy and embryology, but physiological techniques have also contributed to our knowledge of this part of neuroanatomy. One of the most successful of these has been strychnine neuronography that investigates the course of the intracerebral neuron. It was introduced and named by Dusser de Barenne.

Dusser de Barenne was born at Brielle in The Netherlands and studied medicine at the University of Amsterdam. After having been graduated in 1909, he began studies of the functional analysis of the central nervous system which he continued until his death; his first paper, published in 1910, dealt with the action of strychnine on the central nervous system. He first worked in Amsterdam as a psychiatrist and physiologist and then, after having served as a medical officer in the First World War, held appointments in the departments of physiology and pharmacology at the University of Utrecht. In 1930 he was appointed Sterling Professor of Physiology in Yale University, a post he held for ten years. He is remembered for his work on posture, the effect of strychnine on the cerebral cortex, and for pioneer work in neurochemistry (McC[ulloch], 1940; F[ulton] and G[arol], 1940; Haymaker, 1953, pp. 119–122).

The method of Dusser de Barenne, applied first to the cat's cortex in 1915 (Dusser de Barenne, 1916), was based on the observation that strychnine applied to the living brain will produce electrical activity locally and from all regions to which involved neurons send axons or collaterals. Thus the two ends of a neuron pathway may be delimited accurately, although the intervening course is not revealed. In this way it has been possible to check the anatomists' findings in the living brain and to extend their investigations of white matter pathways, especially as regards non-myelinated fibres which are difficult to follow histologically. When working with Sherrington, Dusser de Barenne applied his technique to the monkey's brain (1924) and thereafter he and his students published extensively on the subject. The following excerpt has been taken from an article of 1939, the year before he died ("Physiological delimitation of neurones in the central nervous system," *Amer. J. Physiol.*, 1939, 127:620–628). It reported four years of experience with a combination of physiological methods that in this instance demonstrated the existence of a direct cortical fillet and of neurons originating in the nuclei cuneatus and gracilis and ending in the globus pallidus.

His collaborator, Warren S. McCulloch, was born at Orange, New Jersey, and received the M.D. degree from Columbia University, New York, in 1927. Like his teacher, he has devoted his life to the elucidation of the functional organization of the central nervous system, especially of the cerebral cortex. He introduced electrical recording into Dusser de Barenne's experiments.

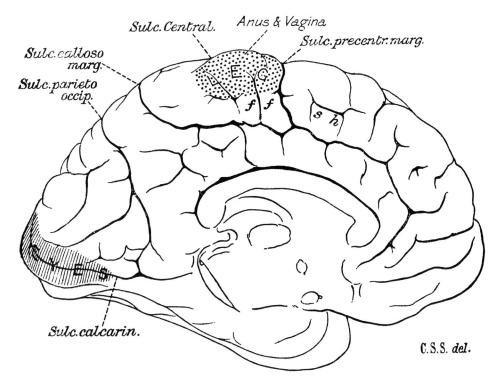

Fig. 129. Grünbaum and Sherrington (1903, p. 154). Left hemisphere, medial surface. See legend to fig. 128.

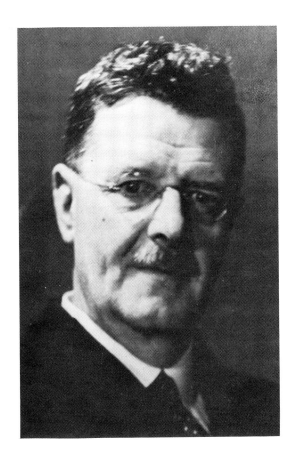

Fig. 130. Gordon Morgan Holmes. Courtesy of Dr. Macdonald Critchley.

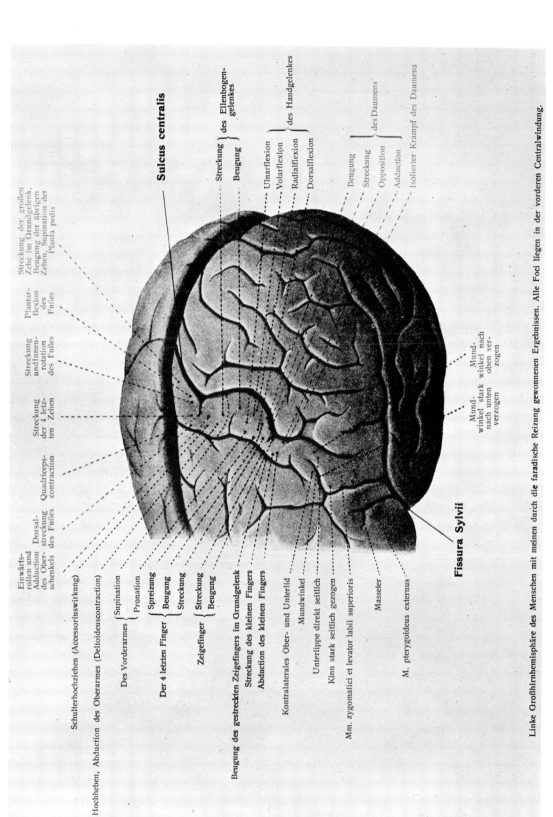

FIG. 131. Krause (1911, p. 185, fig. 66). Human left cerebral hemisphere with foci (all in pre-central gyrus) identified through faradic stimulation.

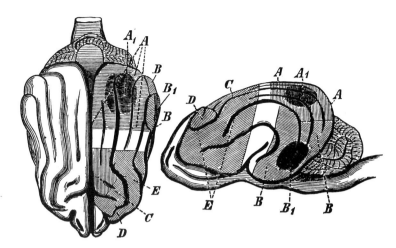

FIG. 132. Munk (1881, p. 29, fig. 1).
Areas: A, visual, B, auditory, C, D, E,
touch. Bilateral removal of A₁ produces psychic blindness; of B₁, psychic
deafness.

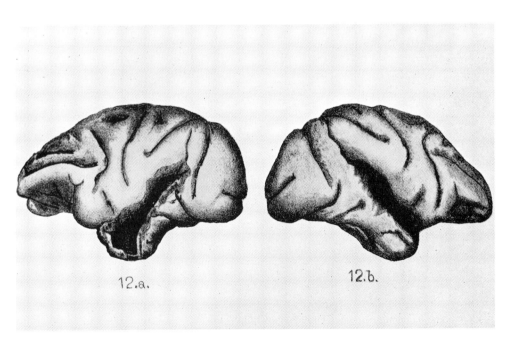

FIG. 133. Brown and Schäfer (1888,
Plate I, figs. 12a–b). Case 12; see text
(p. 542).

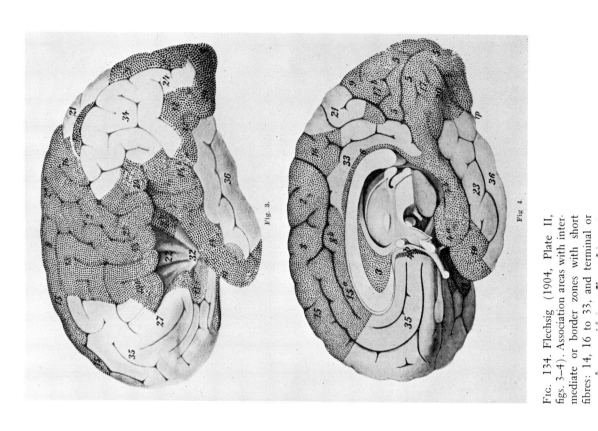

Fig. 134. Flechsig (1904, Plate II, figs. 3–4). Association areas with intermediate or border zones with short fibres: 14, 16 to 33, and terminal or

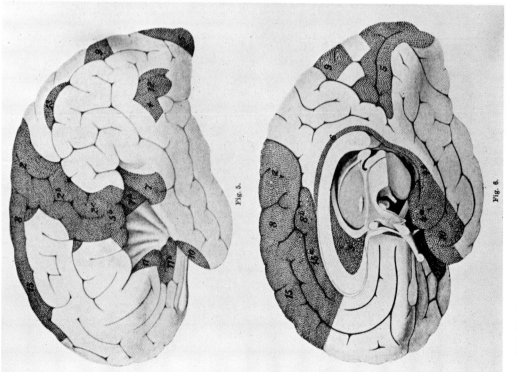

Fig. 135. Flechsig (1904, Plate III, figs. 5–6). Areas with primary, sensory projection fibres: 1, 2, 4 to 8, 15, and areas without these fibres (unknown areas): 3, 9 to 13.

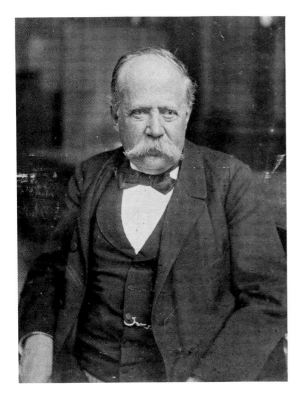

FIG. 136. Friedrich Leopold Goltz and
one of his experimental dogs. Courtesy
of Dr. M. A. B. Brazier.

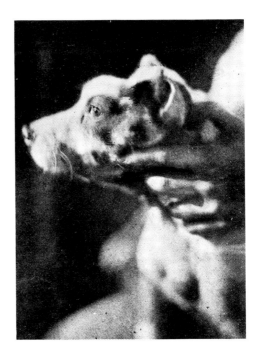

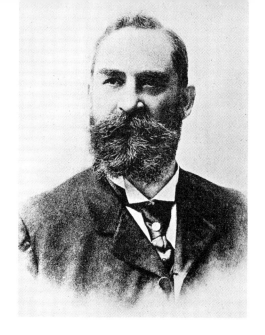

Fig. 137. Constantin von Monakow. By permission of the Wellcome Trustees.

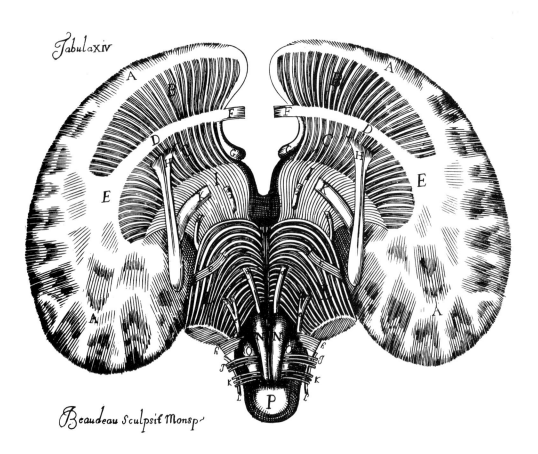

Tabula XIV

Beaudeau sculpsit Monsp

Fig. 138. Vieussens (1684, Plate XIV). Base of brain revealed by scraping: *BB*, lower corpora striata, external and anterior (caudate and lenticular nuclei); *CC*, lower corpora striata, external and posterior (thalami); *DD*, transverse and somewhat oblique tract (*stria terminalis*); *FF*, lowest part of commissure resembling a thick nerve which unites with *DD*, cut and drawn slightly apart (anterior commissure); *L*, pons; *P*, transected medulla oblongata; *N*, pyramid; *O*, olive.

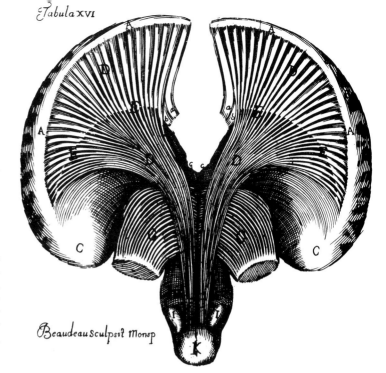

Tabula XVI

Beaudeau sculpsit Monsp

FIG. 139. Vieussens (1684, Plate XVI). Further scraping shows structures deep to those in fig. 138. *DD*, middle corpora striata (internal capsule) continuous with the medullary tracts *FF* (pyramidal tracts); *G*, ? pons; *aa*, commissure resembling a thick nerve (anterior commissure).

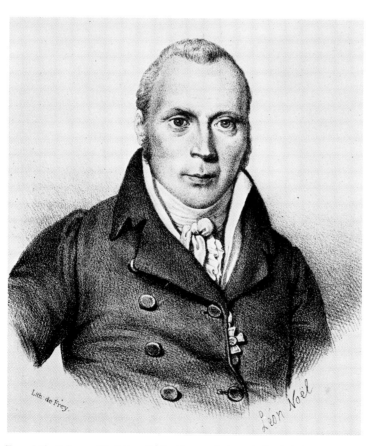

Lith. de Frey.

Léon Noël

FIG. 140. Johann Christian Reil. By permission of the Wellcome Trustees.

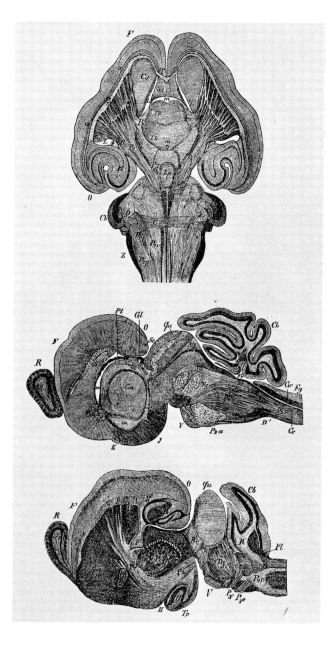

Fig. 141. Meynert (1872, p. 696, figs. 230–232). Horizontal and two sagittal transverse sections of bat's brain. For explanation see text (p. 603).

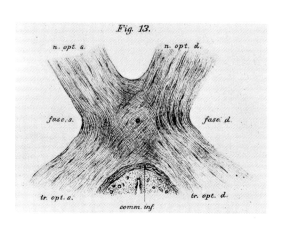

Fig. 142. Gudden (1874, Plate II, fig. 13). Horizontal section through middle of upper half of human chiasma. *Comm. inf.* is the *commissura cerebri inferior,* or posterior commissure of the chiasma.

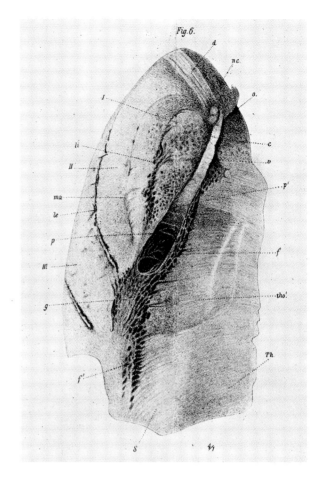

FIG. 143. Flechsig (1881, Plate III, fig. 6). Horizontal section through uppermost division of first part of lenticular nucleus and through lateral nucleus of thalamus. See text (p. 615).

FIG. 144. Flechsig (1881, Plate III, fig. 4). Horizontal section of middle third (lower part) of first portion of lenticular nucleus [I]. For explanation see text (p. 616).

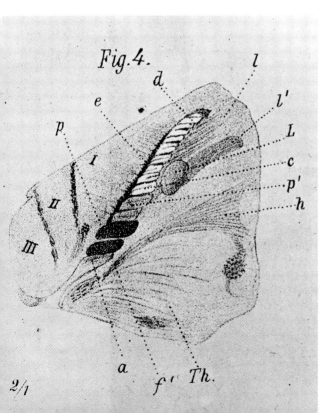

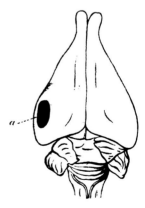

FIG. 145. Monakow (1882, Plate II, fig. 5). Upper surface of brain of rabbit in Expt. II: *a*, area ablated.

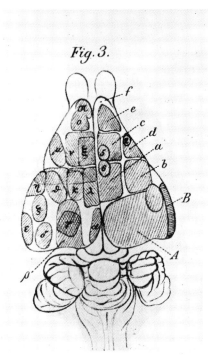

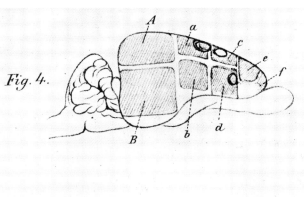

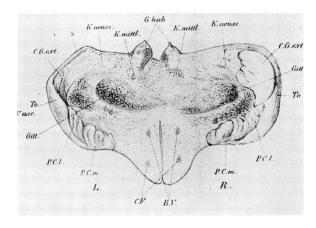

FIG. 146. Monakow (1882, Plate IX, figs. 3–4). Upper (fig. 3) and right lateral (fig. 4) surfaces of rabbit's brain. Fig. 3, ablated areas on left. Zones resulting from investigation on right: A, zone of lateral geniculate body; B, zone of medial geniculate body; a, zone of thalamus; b, zone of reticular nucleus; c, d, e, zones of anterior and medial nucleus; c, e, f, zones of pyramidal tract. See text (p. 621).

FIG. 147. Monakow (1882, Plate II, fig. 6). Section through brain C. G. ext., lateral geniculate body. Gitt. reticular nucleus; z, outermost layer of lateral thalamic nucleus; To, optic tract.

FIG. 148. Vieussens (1684, Plate XII). Coronal section of human cerebellum from behind; g, medullary tracts; h, vessels of choroid plexus; I, superior medullary velum; K, fourth ventricle with choroid plexus, M; superior and N, inferior cerebellar peduncle.

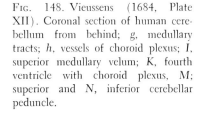

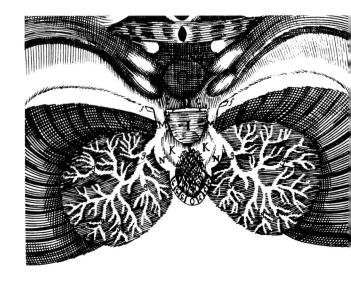

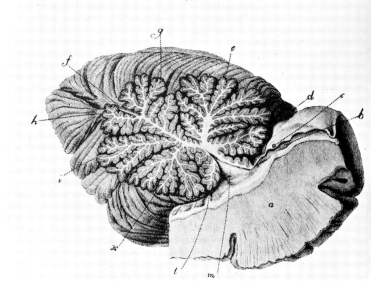

Fig. 149. Reil (1807–1808, Plate III, fig. 1). Midline, sagittal section through vermis: *a*, medulla oblongata and pons; *b*, aqueduct of Sylvius; *c*, superior medullary velum; *d*, central lobe; *e*, complete vertical branch; *f*, cross commissure of posterosuperior lobe between superior and inferior vermis; *g*, four most important branches; *h*, part of horizontal branch that lies below cross commissure of posterior lobes; *i*, pyramid; *k*, uvula; *l*, pyramis; *m*, fourth ventricle.

Fig. 150. Luigi Luciani. By permission, National Library of Medicine.

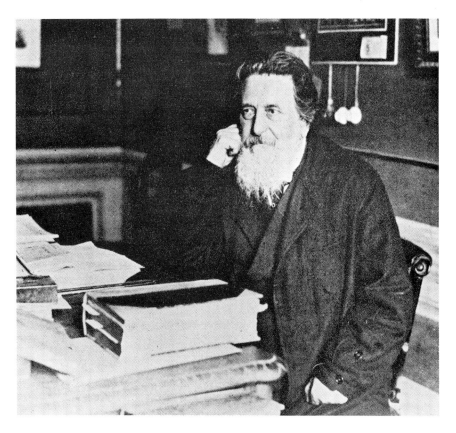

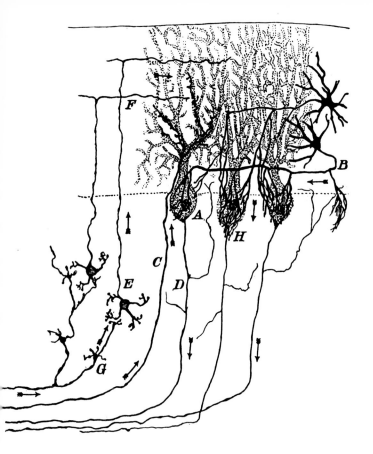

FIG. 151. Ramón y Cajal (1894, p. 459, fig. 5). Connections of Purkyně cells: A surrounded by axon branches; B of star-shaped cells of molecular layer; C, climbing fibres; D, axons of Purkyně cell; E, granular cells ascending axons bifurcate in molecular layer; G, mossy fibres.

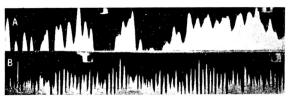

Fig. 1. Cat under chloroform and ether. A, spontaneous potential, waves from cerebral cortex (parietal), about 60 per sec. B, from cerebellar cortex (vermis), about 180 per sec. White marks at top of records give ¼ sec. interval.

FIG. 152. Adrian (1935, fig. 1). See text (p. 701).

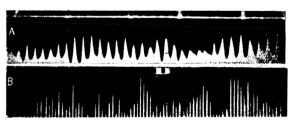

Fig. 2. Rhythmic activity following electrical stimulation. A, cerebrum, waves 30 per sec. B, cerebellum, 190 per sec. (N.B. Recording speed three times as great as in A.) Cat, C. and E.

FIG. 153. Adrian (1935, fig. 2). For explanation see text (p. 701).

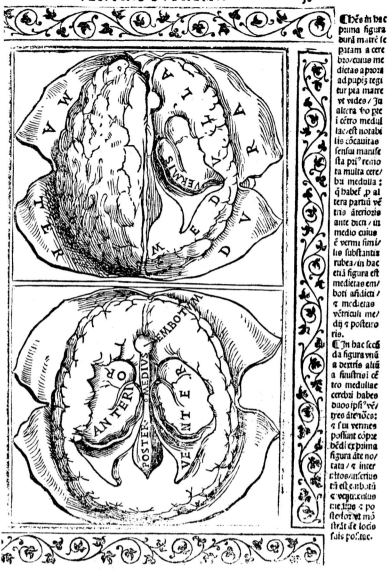

Chẽs in hac prima figura durã matrẽ separatam a cerebro/cuius medietas a priora ad pupi; tegitur pia matre vt vides/ Ju altera vo prei cẽtro medullae/est notabilis cõcauitas sensu manifesta pzi° remota multa cerebri medulla: q̃ habes p altera partuũ vẽtris ãteriozis ante dicti/ in medio cuius ẽ vermi similis subftantia rubea/in hac etiã figura est medietas emboti afidicti/ z medietas vẽtriculi medÿ z posteroris.

Jn hac secũda figura vnũ a dextris aliũ a finiftrisi cẽtro medullae cerebri habes duos ipfi vẽtres ãteriões: z sui vetrtes possunt cõpzebẽdi ex prima figura ãte notata/ z inter ritos/anterius ti est embotũ z vcẽgurculus medius z posterior vt mõstrat de locis suis posttac.

Fig. 154. Berengario da Carpi (1523, p. 56). Lateral ventricles from above. *Embotum* is entrance from third ventricle into iter of Sylvius.

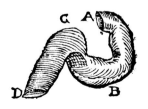

Fig. 155. Wepfer (1658, p. 38). Carotid syphon. For explanation see text (p. 770).

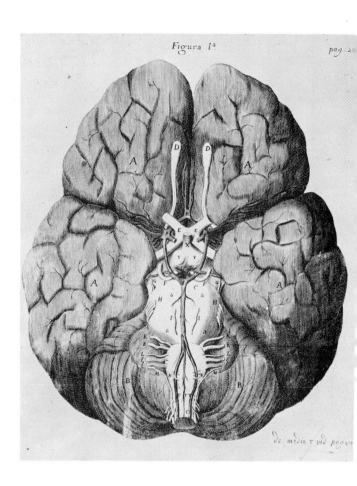

FIG. 156. Willis (1664, Plate Ia).

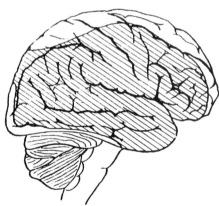

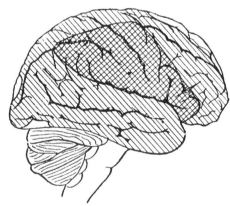

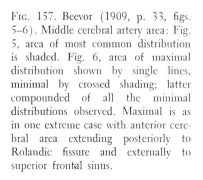

FIG. 157. Beevor (1909, p. 33, figs. 5–6). Middle cerebral artery area: Fig. 5, area of most common distribution is shaded. Fig. 6, area of maximal distribution shown by single lines, minimal by crossed shading; latter compounded of all the minimal distributions observed. Maximal is as in one extreme case with anterior cerebral area extending posteriorly to Rolandic fissure and externally to superior frontal sinus.

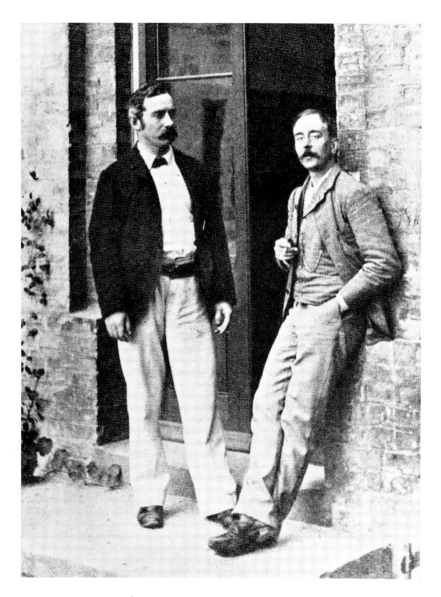

FIG. 158. Charles Smart Roy, left, and
Charles Scott Sherrington in 1893.
With kind permission of Dr. Raymond
Williamson.

EXCERPT PP. 620–622

Heretofore for the delimitation of neurones in the central nervous system (CNS) the only methods available have been anatomical: the Marchi method [pp. 848–850], the Weigert method [pp. 845–848], and the method of retrograde cell degeneration. Although fully recognizing the admirable services these methods have rendered, one should not be blind to their limitations. These methods are time-consuming and require in experimentation sterile operative procedures with a survival of the animal for weeks or even months. These are only small practical disadvantages; heavier weigh the theoretical objections to these methods. We have not in mind here so much the uncertainty often present in the diagnosis of a positive Marchi degeneration, but rather two other objections: 1, the Marchi method does not and can not reveal the actual site of ending of the degenerating myelinated axons, for the last millimeters of these have no myelin sheaths; 2, this method can not help out in the case of non-myelinated neurones. Both objections hold also for the Weigert method, which, furthermore, because it provides a "negative" picture of the degeneration, permits a diagnosis only if the degeneration has occurred in a fairly great number of axons gathered in more or less compact bundles. Similarly the diagnosis of retrograde cell degeneration can only be made if the cells which have atrophied or disappeared were numerous and formed a fairly compact nuclear mass.

For the last four years we have used in this laboratory a combination of physiological methods which has shown itself admirably suitable for the study of problems of "functional organization" in the CNS, namely, the local strychninization of a mass of gray matter in combination with recording of the electrical activity of some other gray matter in the CNS. Strychnine solution applied to a few square millimeters of superficial gray matter, i.e., local strychninization of this mass, results in a typical change in its electrical activity, namely, the appearance of large, rapid voltage fluctuations, "strychnine-spikes." When the local strychninization has been performed somewhere in the sensorimotor cortex these spikes do not remain restricted to the small area strychninized but are also found in other specific areas of this cortex. The distribution of the strychnine-spikes is specific for each strychninized area. The observations that local strychninization of an area *a* (for instance area 6) produces spikes in the electrogram of some other area *b* (for instance area 4), whereas local strychninization of area *b* does *not* produce spikes in the electrogram of area *a* show that this combination of methods reveals *directed* functional relations and, therefore, directed anatomical relations. To correlate these findings with the neuronal structure of the cortex two suppositions are possible: 1, that strychinine acts on the axonal terminations and produces its remote effects by antidromic "firing" of the cell bodies of the neurones whose axonal endings are strychninized; 2, that strychnine acts on the cell bodies (and/or the synapses incrusting these) and produces its remote effects in the direction of the normal conduction in the neurones. That the first of these suppositions is false and the second true follows from the following observations. Local strychninization of the dorsal horn of a spinal segment invariably evokes symptoms of sensory excitation (paresthesiae, hyperesthesia, hyperalgesia) in the corresponding "strychnine-segment zone" and only in this zone. The axonal terminations converging upon the perikarya of the posterior horns of a spinal segment are the endings of neurones originating in many other spinal segments and supraspinal levels. If the strychninization of these axonal terminations "fired" antidromically the cell bodies of the neurones to which they belong, it is impossible to conceive how the sensory symptoms could be projected by the animal into the periphery, into the strychnine-segment zone of the locally strychninized spinal segment and in this zone only. On this supposition the symptoms of sensory excitation should be absent altogether or present in a much larger area of the body, namely, in all portions subserved sensorially by the neurones "fired" antidromically. A second observation which precludes the first supposition is that local strychninization of the posterior horn of a spinal segment does not produce strychnine-spikes in the corresponding posterior root (unpublished experiments). The only alternative left is, therefore, the second supposition mentioned, namely, that the strychnine acts on the cell bodies (and/or the synapses incrusting them) and produces its remote effects in the direction of the normal, i.e., forward, conduction in the reflex arc.

This view is strengthened by the following observations. Local strychninization of a specific area of the sensorimotor cortex, to wit, areas L. or A.4-s, produces strychnine-spikes in the electrogram of the nucleus caudatus, whereas strychninization of this nucleus does not "fire" the cortex. Several neuroanatomists are inclined to admit the existence of cortico-caudate neurones, all deny the existence of caudato-cortical neurones. Local strychninization of the sensorimotor cortex "fires" the sensory thalamic nuclei and local strychninization of these nuclei "fires" the sensorimotor cortex. Here, neuroanatomy recognizes both cortico-thalamic and thalamo-cortical neurones. All available evidence, therefore, points towards the thesis that strychnine acts on the perikarya (and/or the synaptic endings incrusting them), causes these structures to discharge impulses and, by axonal propagation of these impulses, produces strychnine-spikes in those remote, related, portions of gray matter where axons originating in strychninized nerve cells or collaterals of such axons end. If this thesis is accepted, local strychninization with recording of the electrical activity in the course of an acute experiment of a few minutes in the living (narcotized) animal gives the origin and termination of neurones. Thus one obtains physiological delimitation of neurones in the CNS.

Conclusion

The main advances made in the difficult task of elucidating the internal architecture of the cerebral hemispheres and brainstem have depended upon the painstaking pursuit of the white matter fibres. However, only a few of the many intracerebral connections have so far been traced microscopically. The detailed study has taken place almost entirely within the last hundred years and by means of a few relatively simple techniques. However, anatomical and embryological problems still remain and the vast field of function stretches out before the investigator. As has been the case with other organs, the discovery of the form of the cerebral white matter is merely a prelude to the elucidation of function.

CHAPTER XI

THE CEREBELLUM

Introduction

The small brain or cerebellum was mentioned in scientific literature for the first time in the fourth century B.C., in the biological writings of Aristotle. Since then it has been the center of more speculation than almost any other part of the nervous system. It has presented one of the most baffling problems of neuroanatomy and neurophysiology so that precise investigations in the latter field have been possible only relatively recently.

Details of its macroscopic structure did not become available until the end of the eighteenth century, and data concerning its microscopic composition and the various fibre pathways in which it is involved are still being accumulated. The story of cerebellar function is of especial interest because the organ was thought to be in turn the center for motor nerves, the seat of memory, and the controller of involuntary movements such as the cardiac and respiratory, and of sexual activity, before modern physiological investigations began in the first decade of the nineteenth century. Since then other theories have been put forward, and some of these survive today. The cerebellum, however, is still in many respects an enigma to the modern neurophysiologist.

The history of the accumulation of knowledge concerning the cerebellum can best be understood by considering first of all early concepts of form and function, ranging from the statements of Galen in the second century of our era to those of Willis in the mid-seventeenth. Studies of cerebellar anatomy received attention in the eighteenth century, to the complete neglect of function which, however, became of increasing importance in the nineteenth. The latter can be appreciated by considering the work of a few outstanding men who represent a large number of individuals working in the field of cerebellar physiology.

The early and acute experiments of Rolando and Flourens suggested that the organ acted as a whole, and this unitary concept was expanded and supported by Luciani's experiments, by the histological studies of Ramón y Cajal, and by Sherrington's belief that the cerebellum was the center for proprioception. It dominated thought and textbooks from about 1890 to about 1940. Moreover, the expansion of clinical neurology seemed to give important support to the findings in animals.

In retrospect two main themes of cerebellar physiology can be identified in the nineteenth century and traced to the present day: first, the role of the cerebellum in posture and its relationships in particular with vestibular function and tone; second, the localization of function which has now superseded the old unitary concept of Luciani. A third and more recent theme is the investigation of cerebellar electrical potentials. It seems that cerebellar studies will proceed along these three main streams until new or modified concepts arise. There is no adequate history of the anatomy and physiology of the cerebellum, but Dow and Moruzzi (1958) give considerable attention to the latter aspect and have been frequently consulted in regard to the present work. Other sources are Luciani (1891, pp. 247 ff.); Neuburger (1897, pp. 7–38, 311–342); Thomas (1897, pp. 1–40). Fulton (1949, pp. 103–110) and Rawson (1932) provide briefer accounts.

Early Concepts of Form and Function

In the literature of Greco-Roman antiquity available to us there is no description of the cerebellum before that of Galen. It was, however, recognized and differentiated from the cerebrum by Aristotle (p. 8), and Praxagoras (p. 142) referred to it. The Alexandrian anatomists also certainly knew of it, but any description which they may have made has not survived. According to Galen, Herophilus introduced the name *parencephalis*, but Aristotle appears to have used the same word earlier (p. 8). Apparently Erasistratus discussed the cerebellum in man and in animals and, as will be seen below, Galen challenged his conclusions (see also Ch. I, p. 12). On the whole it seems that the Alexandrians regarded the cerebellum and the fourth ventricle as very important structures, but of these beliefs we have no details. Rufus made passing reference to the cerebellum but did not describe it (p. 13). The history of the form and function of the cerebellum as presented here does not, therefore, begin until the time of Galen, the second century A.D.

GALEN

(See p. 14)

Most of the medical writers of antiquity who mentioned the cerebellum contrasted its convolutions with those of the cerebrum. This was the case with Galen who considered it to be the source of motor nerves (p. 149) and even of the spinal cord (p. 630). Moreover, the vermis of the cerebellum was considered to act as a valve in the ventricular system to regulate the flow of animal spirits (p. 631). These were the first suggestions concerning cerebellar function, and although they may not have been original with Galen, they survived for many centuries as part of the

Galenic system of brain function. In the following passage from *The use of parts*, VIII, 11 (Daremberg [1854–1856], I), Galen discussed the problem of nomenclature.

EXCERPT PP. 558–559

Since all the nerves of the body that are distributed from the head to the lower parts must derive either from the *parencephalon* [cerebellum] or from the spinal cord, this ventricle of the cerebellum [fourth ventricle] must be of considerable size to receive the psychic pneuma [animal spirit] elaborated in the anterior [lateral and third] ventricles; it was therefore necessary that there be a channel between them [aqueduct of Sylvius.] Indeed, the ventricle seems large, and the channel that comes from the anterior ventricles and empties there is also very large. This channel alone offers a communication between the parencephalon and the *encephalon* [brain]. Such in fact are the names that Herophilus constantly gives to the one and the other part, above all applying the name of the whole [brain] to the anterior part because of its size.

The encephalon being double, as he said, each of its parts is much larger than the entire parancephalon, but since the anterior part was given the general name, it was not possible to find for the parencephalon a more fitting name than the one it carries. Others, however, do not give it this name but call it *enkranis* [used later to designate "whole content of skull"] and *enkranon*. One must not blame them if, for the sake of clear teaching, they have created a name since in life many things may be designated best in regard to size, power, merit, or value.

In the same work, VIII, 13, Galen dealt with the cerebellum again and made his well-known denouncement of Erasistratus who had been enlightened enough to believe that the gyral pattern of the cerebellum and cerebrum was more complicated in man because of his higher intelligence. Unfortunately, Galen's opinion survived, whereas that of Erasistratus was lost.

EXCERPT P. 563

Having arrived at this point in the discussion one must not leave it without a description of the form of the cerebellum. It does not have great convolutions separated by the pia mater like the cerebrum, but is composed of numerous very small bodies arranged otherwise than in the cerebrum. Indeed, if the psychic pneuma [animal spirit] is contained in all the substance of the brain and not merely in its ventricles, as we have demonstrated elsewhere, one must believe that the origin of the nerves of the entire body is in the cerebellum, that the pneuma is found in very great abundance, and that the intermediate regions that bind the parts are the pathways of this pneuma.

Erasistratus demonstrates very well that the *epenkranis* (as he calls the cerebellum) is of a more varied composition than the cerebrum; but when he claims that the cerebellum, and with it the cerebrum, is more complex in man than in other animals, because these latter do not have an intelligence like that of man, it does not appear to me that he is reasoning correctly, since even asses have a very complicated cerebellum although their imbecile character demands a very simple and unvariegated cerebrum. It is better to believe that intelligence results from the good temperament of the body charged with thinking, whatever this body, and not the variety of its composition. Indeed, it seems to me that it is less the quantity than the quality of the psychic pneuma that is necessary to produce perfection of thought.

The vermis was the only part of the cerebellum to which Galen paid more than passing attention. He described it very briefly and declared that it acted as a valve to regulate the flow of spirit in the aqueduct of Sylvius connecting the third and fourth ventricles. This idea was still current in the seventeenth century. The following passage has been taken from *The use of parts*, VIII, 14 (Daremberg [1854–1856], I, 565–567). There is another account of the vermis on pages 711 to 712. Confusion with authors who used "vermis" to mean the "red worm" or choroid plexus has to be avoided.

EXCERPT PP. 565–567

. . . . there is such a part of the brain itself around the passage [into the fourth ventricle], able both to direct and to regulate the transmission of spirit, but impossible to discover; it is not the pineal, but the process like a worm that is extended through the whole passage. From its shape expert anatomists call it the vermiform process [of the cerebellum].

Such are its position, nature, and its relationship to the neighboring parts . . . . But as well as being variously articulated and appearing to be made up of many parts joined together by thin membranes [pia mater], the vermis also has its distinctive characteristics. Its extremity in the posterior [fourth] ventricle . . . is convex and slender. However, it gradually increases in size and broadens so that its superior surface is equal to the interval between the nates [posterior quadrigeminal bodies]. Because of this it extends along the passage [aqueduct] and obstructs it completely. It surrounds it and thus stretches the membrane attached to the convex parts [anterior medullary velum] posteriorly so that it can open the whole passage as it moves backwards. By wrapping itself up and condensing into itself, it increases in breadth as it decreases in length.

ANDREAS VESALIUS

(See p. 153)

The pre-Vesalian anatomists of the Renaissance had, like Galen, little to say about the cerebellum, although Mondino (p. 22) and Berengario da Carpi mentioned it. The first detailed account of this structure was that of Vesalius, in the *De humani corporis fabrica*, 1543, Bk. VII, Ch. IV) in which he referred only to the external features and made no attempt to discuss its possible function. He did however, refer to the popular belief that the prominence of the bone overlying it, the occiput, was "a measure of the power of memory and intellect." This reflected the ancient idea that memory was located in the fourth ventricle (pp. 464–465) or the cerebellum.

EXCERPT P. 629

THE SITE AND SIZE OF THE CEREBELLUM

The cerebellum is only a tenth or an eleventh the size of the cerebrum. With the origin of the dorsal medulla [spinal cord] it acquires for itself that site in the amplitude of the skull, which is circumscribed by the posterior surface of the projections extending into the cavity of the head for the sake of the auditory organs [petrous temporal bones], and then by two sinuses of the occipital bone that are carved in the cavity of the skull, so that the cerebellum is bounded by the two first sinuses of the dural membrane which we call the right and left mouth (*os* [transverse sinuses]). Nowhere does the cerebellum advance beyond these boundaries which very precisely define its site. In men the cerebellum does not at all extend into the occiput, as perhaps in oxen—which Galen seems only to have used for the study of the brain—so that not even the posterior part of the brain [occipital poles] extends more to the posterior than the cerebellum, and fills what we call the occiput. Indeed, the last and highest part of the human cerebellum scarcely ascends to that point where we can touch the lowest part of the occiput with our fingers [through the foramen magnum]. Nor can any part of the occipital bone that the cerebrum fills be found free of the insertions of muscles, even if anatomists describe the site of the cerebellum as if it stuffed the whole region of that prominence of the occiput, that swelling which the mass of the people consider a measure of the power of memory and talent; the very highest part of the cerebellum extends only to the middle, although some, deluded by oxen and asses or by dreams, have written that the cerebellum ascends from the posterior site of the foramen providing a pathway for the dorsal medulla [foramen magnum] to the part of the lambdoid suture which is joined to the sagittal. Furthermore, the upper part of the cerebellum in men, as in dogs, oxen, and sheep, does not rise up in the shape of a globe, or even more acutely, but is observed to be flat and depressed and by no means prominent in the middle.

SHAPE OF THE CEREBELLUM

And so this site of the skull provided for the cerebellum dictates its confines, shape, and size. For the cerebellum, like its site, is wider than it is long and deep, and in its lower part, and that particularly near its posterior, offers the resemblance of a very widened-out globe; in its middle there is an acute but not very wide impression [vallecula] which it is given by the tuberosity projecting in the form of a very thick line in the occipital bone, that notably increases the strength of that bone to which the dural membrane of the brain is very firmly attached. In the anterior part the cerebellum is extended to the nates of the cerebrum [quadrigeminal bodies]; it is led into a kind of point [lingula of the cerebellum], on all sides accurately fitting the shape of its confines.

EXCERPT P. 631

THE ARRANGEMENT AND APPEARANCE OF THE CONVOLUTIONS OF THE CEREBELLUM

This opinion is supported by reference to the convolutions of the cerebellum which do not penetrate so deeply as those of the cerebrum but are observed to be somewhat more shallow, although numerous and in a somewhat more continuous series. They are shallow because the part to be nourished is smaller and because the cerebellum is more easily penetrated from its deeper convolutions to its ventricle [fourth ventricle]. The convolutions are numerous so that their number may somewhat compensate for the slighter penetration. There are three arrangements of them, much different in appearance from the convolutions of the cerebrum. Because of that impression that the cerebellum receives posteriorly from the tuberosity of the occipital bone, these convolutions appear to be formed in three divisions, right, left, and middle. The right and left divisions [cerebellar hemispheres] have the appearance of two globes placed together, and in the intervening space, that is where the globes do not touch, is the third division of the cerebellum [vermis]; the convolutions [of the latter] resemble a woodworm or a worm such as we find in fresh cheese, since they extend transversely along the length of the cerebellum to form the vermiform process of the brain. In the upper part of the cerebellum, parallel convolutions are extended from the right and left parts; these are also led along the width of the cerebellum and, extended downwards, are, as it were, gathered at that region which adjoins the origin of the dorsal medulla [tonsils]. The convolutions of the right part are extended to that region of the right part adjoining the origin of the dorsal medulla, and those of the left to the like region of its part. These parts of the cerebellum are not separated and disunited from each other but are continuous and constitute a single body, that is, the cerebellum itself.

GALEN ASSIGNED AN INAPPROPRIATE REASON FOR A SINGLE CEREBELLUM

Galen asserted that nature constructed it single and not double like the cerebrum because it would not have been fitting that man have two backs and a like number of dorsal medullae [spinal cords]; as if it would not have been possible that a single dorsal medulla be produced from the cerebrum that had to be divided into two parts, and not a continuous substance, and that therefore it was necessary that the cerebellum be created as a single body so that it might provide a suitable origin for a single dorsal medulla.

COSTANZO VAROLIO
(1543—1575)

When the base of the human brain is inspected, one of its most noticeable features is the pons which is intimately associated with the cerebellum by way of the middle cerebellar peduncles. But so long as the Galenic and Vesalian method of examining the brain *in situ* and from above was practised, an adequate view of the pons could not be achieved. The first anatomist to popularize a method whereby the brain was removed from the skull and dissected from below, was the Italian, Varolio, and he was thus enabled to describe the pons for the first time (for description of his method, see pp. 820–823). This structure, which he and his contemporaries considered to be part of the cerebellum, is still known by his name, the *pons Varolii*.

Varolio was born in Bologna and studied medicine in that city. He was appointed professor of anatomy and surgery there, and after winning a great reputation he went to Rome in 1573 as physician to Pope Gregory XIII—remembered for his revision of the calendar—where Varolio died at the early age of thirty-two. Varolio was renowned as a lithotomist but he was also an outstanding anatomist, and is remembered especially for his work on the brain (see Portal, II, 1770, 26–38; Medici, 1857, pp. 84–98).

Although the pons is now considered to be a part of the brainstem, Varolio's account of it is included here since it is the first detailed description of a cerebellar connection; moreover, in the excerpt below he discussed the cerebellum as well. This appeared in his letter to Hieronymus Mercurialis, *De nervis opticis nonnullisque aliis, praeter communem opinionem in humano capite observatis, epistolae*, (Padua, 1573), a reprint of which was attached to his *Anatomicae . . . libri IIII* (Frankfurt, 1591). He compared the pons appropriately to a bridge spanning a canal and pointed out that the auditory nerve arose from it and therefore from the cerebellum which he considered to be the center for hearing and taste. Galen had also claimed that some of the cranial nerves had their origins in the cerebellum, although this was refuted by some of Varolio's predecessors. Varolio also suggested that the spinal cord had four tracts: two anterior subserving sensation and two posterior for cerebellar functions (cf. Bell, pp. 297–299). The following translation has been made from the 1591 reprint.

EXCERPT PP. 129–130

Furthermore, I have observed one other notable process of the cerebellum which, although it has received notice from no one else, I believe it to be worthy of the greatest consideration as its description will reveal. On each side of the cerebellum near the trunks already described [brainstem] there arises a process which is carried transversely forwards and downwards; by means of this process the cerebellum enfolds the anterior part of the spinal marrow [brainstem] in the same way as the muscles carried to the larynx and that transverse one constituting the third pair of common muscles enfold the beginning of the throat in its posterior part [inferior pharyngeal muscles]. Anyone can observe the site of this transverse process of the cerebellum within the skull near the anterior part of the aperture for the spinal marrow [foramen magnum], for there is a notable transverse depression [clivus] there which provides space for the process. The auditory nerves arise from this process of the cerebellum; hence they do not arise from the cerebrum. Thus certain nerves, such as the auditory, arise only from the cerebellum and not from the cerebrum. Some arise from both, such as the spinal nerves; however, no nerve arises immediately from parts of two origins, but they arise from their own origins either by means of the spinal marrow or by means of the aforesaid transverse process. Observe whether the cerebellum in our head has so slight and obscure a use as the younger anatomists judge, for hitherto we have maintained that the primary origin of the auditory nerve is located there. If it may be permitted to me to name things that I have discovered, since I observe the marrow to be carried under this transverse spinal process in the same way that a flowing channel is carried under a bridge, for the sake of clearer meaning I shall call it a bridge (*pons*) of the cerebellum, as I have been accustomed to call it for a long time, taking the name from that likeness of the process.

Detailed Gross Anatomy

Although in the seventeenth and eighteenth centuries there were no further significant attempts to explain cerebellar function, anatomists began to pay more attention to its anatomical features. Whereas hitherto only the external appearances had been examined with care, its internal structure was now inspected and anatomists were aided by new techniques such as Vieussens' method of boiling the brain in oil and Reil's alcohol fixation process.

At the end of the eighteenth century and the beginning of the nineteenth, interest in the precise structure of the brain was increasing, stimulated to some extent by Gall and Spurzheim. During this period most of the macroscopic features of the cerebellum were described and when the achromatic microscope became available the study of the cerebellum's histological components began. Thus in 1837 the most important cell of the organ was discovered by Purkyně and it is still known today by his name (pp. 55–56).

The history of the anatomy of the cerebellum, although continuous throughout the nineteenth century and up to the present day, will not be taken beyond the work of Reil in 1807 because the contributions to its physiology at this time became of greater importance.

Thomas Willis
(See p. 158)

There were no further important advances in knowledge of the anatomy of the cerebellum until Willis's book on the brain, *Cerebri anatome*, was published in London in 1664. In it he gave a more detailed and reasonably accurate account of the external structure of the cerebellum. This is to be found in Chapter III, entitled "Description of the cerebellum and its processes, and also of the posterior part of the medulla oblongata." Willis was the first to point out, as well as to provide the name for, the three cerebellar peduncles.

EXCERPT PP. 21–23

Below the orbicular prominences [quadrigeminal bodies] *the cerebellum* must next be inspected. Its *shape,* like that of the cerebrum, is somewhat *globular;* indeed, with its *gyri* and *twistings* its *marking* appears uneven; the pia mater covers over the twistings, ridges, and sulci, binds together the peaks, and lines the deep clefts into all of which it extends and deeply inserts plexuses of vessels. Unlike the cerebrum the cerebellum is by no means irregularly variegated by its *gyri* and *convolutions,* but its *folds* are arranged in an orderly series. Its exterior structure appears formed of *thin layers* or *little circles* contiguous to and folded one to another, going about its whole circumference in somewhat parallel positions.

Each region of the cerebellum, that is, *the anterior* and *posterior,* ends in *a vermiform process* [vermis]. At the [superior and inferior] terminations, as if at *two poles*, those *little circles* are *very short*; ascending thence [from the latter] towards the summit, like *an equator*, they gradually widen out like *parallels* on *a sphere*. Outwardly these *little circles* are *cortical* and inwardly *medullary*, and *the marrow* of all of them passes over into two broad *middle markings (meditullia)*; these seem to be the same in *the cerebellum* as *the corpus callosum* in the cerebrum.

. . . .

However, *the cerebellum* itself, whether the aforementioned little protuberances grow on it or are lacking, is found in almost all animals in the same shape and proportion and formed of the same kind of thin layers. Those which have a cerebrum shaped differently from that of man, as *birds* and *fish*, and among quadrupeds, *hares* and *mice*, of which the cerebra lack gyri or convolutions, have the same appearance and a similar arrangement of the folds and composition of the other parts [i.e., the cerebellum]. The reason for *the dissimilarities* in *the cerebrum* and *the similarities* in *the cerebellum* will be given below when we deal with the use of the parts.

Just as the cerebrum has produced *the choroid plexus* within its cavity [ventricle] from various arteries and veins folded together and from very densely interposed little glands, so the cerebellum has similar plexuses of vessels noteworthy because of the very numerous and larger glands than are to be found in the choroid plexus. When the pia mater investing the posterior part of the cerebellum has been separated, *these plexuses* and *accumulations of glands* come readily into view; for there, near the vermiform process [vermis], they creep upwards on either side like two branches; they receive *an artery* on either side from the vertebral artery lying under the base of the medulla oblongata and *the venous ducts*, as they are sent forth from either *lateral sinus*. Later we shall consider the use of this *plexus* and its *glands*.

Meanwhile, now to describe *the site* and *the structures* related to *the cerebellum*; resting on the medulla oblongata it seems to be fixed to its sides through *two* [cerebellar] *peduncles* attached on either side; between *these, the cerebellum above*, and *the trunk of the medulla oblongata below*—since all these ought to be distinguished from one another—there is *a cavity* which is commonly called *the fourth ventricle*.

On either *peduncle* supporting the cerebrum [i.e., brainstem] are found *three* distinct *medullary processes* [cerebellar peduncles]. *The first* of these [superior] issues from the orbicular protuberances and ascends obliquely; *the second* [middle], descending directly from the cerebellum and running across the first, circles around the medulla oblongata; *the third* process [inferior], descending from the rear of the cerebellum, is inserted into the medulla oblongata, and, like an additional cord, augments its trunk. Each of these processes is suitably represented in *the seventh Plate, Q. P. R.* [In

fact only the superior peduncles *Q, Q,* are shown in this illustration of a
sheep's brain which faces p. 130.]

Of equal importance were Willis's speculations on the function of the cerebellum, the first significant contribution to the subject since Galen's work in the
second century A.D. Willis pointed out that the ancients gave no satisfactory
explanations. Some had said that cerebellar and cerebral activity were identical and
others, that the cerebellum was the seat of memory. These Willis refuted and
argued that the cerebellum was, in fact, the seat of involuntary movements, mainly
because of its gyral pattern, because of the origin from it of cranial nerves subserving vital functions, and because its movement in animals affected the heart rate.
But like Varolio, Willis thought that the brainstem was a part of the cerebellum,
and when this is taken into account it appears that his reasoning was not far from
the truth. It can be recalled that cerebellar and brainstem functions were also
confused by Hughlings Jackson, for his so-called cerebellar fits seen in cases of an
expanding cerebellar lesion are now known to result from embarrassment of vital
centers in the brainstem. The following excerpts have been translated from Chapter XV of Willis's *Cerebri anatome* (1664).

EXCERPT PP. 99–102

When some time ago I gave careful and serious consideration to the
function of the cerebellum and revolved in my mind various things concerning it, finally as the result of analogy and much thought about the
matter, I arrived at this (as I believe) true and genuine use of it; that is,
that *the cerebellum is a special fountain of animal spirits that are designed
for certain tasks, wholly distinct from the cerebrum. Imagination, memory,
discourse,* and other superior acts of the animal function are performed
within *the cerebrum* [see pp. 472–473]; furthermore, animal spirits flow
from it into the nervous order [system], by which all *spontaneous movements,* that is, those of which we are conscious and which we direct, are
performed. *The duty of the cerebellum,* however, *seems to be to supply
animal spirits to certain nerves by which involuntary actions take place*
(such as *the heartbeat, normal respiration, concoction of aliment, production of chyme,* and many others); [that is] *those of which we are unaware
or we are unaware of their constant activity.* As often as we undertake
voluntary motion we seem almost aware that the spirits located within us in
the forepart of the head have been aroused to action or influx. But the
spirits inhabiting the cerebellum perform those works of nature silently and
imperceptibly without our notice or concern. Therefore since the cerebrum
has a variety of twistings and, as it were, uncertain meanderings, it is
encompassed by folds and layers disposed in an orderly arrangement; the
animal spirits, according to the rule or manner naturally impressed upon
them, are diffused in the intervening spaces just as in defined orbits and

tracts. Those in the cerebellum, like *an artificial automaton,* seem to have an orderly disposition of that sort within certain compartments and enclosures, so that of their own accord, without a driver to direct and control their movements, they flow out in sequence and in proper and regular order. Therefore, if certain nerves perform some kinds of motions following the instincts and demands of nature, without consultation with the government of the will or desire within the forum of the cerebrum, who may not justly conjecture that the influx of spirits performing these things is derived entirely from the cerebellum? Indeed, for these functions, which ought to be performed without any commotion or disturbance, it seems unsuitable that the spirits should be summoned from the cerebrum where they are continually driven into turbulence by the winds, as it were, of passions and cogitations.

I was led finally to this conjecture regarding the use of the cerebellum by a thread of reasoning to which anatomical study later contributed and clearly confirmed me in my opinion, for in the frequent dissections of the heads of different kinds of animals I made certain observations that seem to put this matter beyond doubt. That is to say, *first* I observed that *the pairs of nerves* which serve the functions normally performed *by instinct of nature* or *by force of passions* rather than *by the judgment of the will* depend so directly from the cerebellum that the influx of animal spirits into their origins seems able to be derived only from there. How the nerves perform only involuntary actions will be stated later; meanwhile we hold in readiness another no less important reason in confirmation of this opinion.

And so *in the second place* we noticed that *the cerebellum* has a *special conformation,* that is, that its mass is composed of folds or little circles in a distinct series, methodically and appropriately disposed at regular intervals (as was said), whence it may be argued that the spirits arising here and flowing outwards are employed in a certain effort limited to one thing. I observed, in addition, that in *whatever animals,* no matter how much they differ in appearance and form, nevertheless *the shape of the cerebellum is always very similar or wholly the same,* but in many *the cerebrum* and *the medulla oblongata* have varying shapes; for as we indicated earlier, there is some difference of these parts in *man* and *quadrupeds,* but between *both of them and fowl and fish* there is a notable difference in those parts. On the other hand, in all these the cerebellum, formed with precisely the same layers or little circles folded alike one to another, is distinguished by the same shape and proportion which is surely indication that in this laboratory the animal spirits are produced in a certain proportion and are dispensed for necessary functions which are performed in the same way in all; these cannot be other than the motions and actions of the viscera and praecordia. As to the other faculties such as *imagination, memory, appetite,* indeed, *local motions* and *sense,* they operate in one way in some animals and in another in others, wherefore the conformation of their cerebrums differs. However, *the motion of the heart* and *respiration* are performed in the same way in whatever ones possess hot blood, that is, by the constant sequence of *systole* and *diastole.* Furthermore, it is necessary to assign another, different function to the cerebellum than is suited to the cerebrum, since where *the folds* and *twistings are lacking to the cerebrum they are constantly to be found in the cerebellum.* In addition to these reasons supplied by anatomy, *pathology* of the human body suggests many others that confirm the aforesaid function of the cerebellum. Very often it happens that cruel and horrid symptoms seize upon the praecordia and the region of the thorax or abdomen, although the morbific cause is in the cerebellum or near it . . . .

1. . . . .

2. From *the blood,* cleared of phlegm in this way and subtilized by a long circulation, a very pure and spiritous liquid is instilled into *the cortical substance* of the cerebellum; this is at once changed into *animal spirits* by the ferment existing there. We have decided that *the spirits are created only in the cortical part of the cerebellum as in the case of the cerebrum;* therefore because this sort of cortex is lacking to *the medulla oblongata and spinal marrow* we believe these latter parts serve only for *the employment* of the animal spirits and not for their production.

3. *The spirits* produced everywhere within *the cortex* or exterior part *of the cerebellum,* where they are immediately prepared for the work of the animal function, are drawn from all *the folds* into *the medullary tracts,* and thence into *two wide middle strips* where they form a welling source or fountain, and there like bubbling waters, with a constant whirling are circulated within, and then run forth [via the peduncles] into the appropriate parts of the nervous system.

RAYMOND DE VIEUSSENS
(*See p. 585*)

Like Willis's book on the anatomy of the brain, the *Neurographia universalis* (Lyons, 1684) of Vieussens was a landmark in seventeenth century neuroanatomy. It contained another important contribution to the anatomy of the cerebellum, but as its author greatly admired Willis, some of the descriptions closely follow those of the *Cerebri anatome.* Like Willis, Vieussens gave an account of the external appearances of the organ, including the anterior (superior) medullary velum that is still occasionally known as the valve of Vieussens; this term reminds us of its supposed function, which was comparable to the activity of the vermis according to Galen (p. 712), to control animal spirit in the aqueduct of Sylvius. In addition, Vieussens studied the internal features of the cerebellum, and he seems to have been the first to record his findings in detail (see p. 581 for Malpighi's brief mention of the resemblance between the cerebellum and the leaf of a tree). Vieussens mentioned, for example, the dentate nucleus ("rhomboid substance or bodies") and the corpus medullare for the first time. The following translation has been made from Book I, Chapter XII, "On the cerebellum," and figure 148 reproduces part of Plate XII which depicts a coronal section through the cerebellum.

EXCERPT PP. 76–79

The cerebellum, like the cerebrum, is composed of two different substances, an ashlike or glandular [gray] substance observed on its whole exterior surface, and a white or medullary one that occupies its interior. When the cerebellum has been stripped of its dura mater and tipped backwards, a somewhat ashen-colored, fairly thick, and soft membrane is revealed that is a prolongation of the pia mater; it is interwoven with a glandular substance not unlike the cerebral cortex. This membrane [Valve of Vieussens], into the front of which a transverse medullary tract is introduced, adheres and is joined to the anterior vermiform process [vermis], to the processes [superior cerebellar peduncles] from the cerebellum to the testes [inferior quadrigeminal bodies], and to the posterior part of the pons Varolii. It can be understood from these things that this membrane lines the anterior [? posterior] part of the cavity of the fourth ventricle and closes off the aqueduct at the rear; hence we assert that it acts like a valve. So it is that after having given consideration to the method of function and the size, we may provide the name of "larger cerebral valve" [Valve of Vieussens or superior (anterior) medullary velum] and so distinguish it from the membranous ligaments within the cavities of the longitudinal [sagittal] and lateral sinuses.

When the cerebellum has been cut into little pieces from the anterior to the posterior, it is seen that its ashen substance is so intermingled with the white that both, mixed together, have the appearance of variegated marble; and at the same time the larger cerebral valve [of Vieussens] and both vermiform processes [the vermis] are clearly revealed [fig. 148]. If the intact cerebellum is cut through the vermiform processes as between twin poles [i.e., superior and inferior extremities of vermis], the white substance of that middle region is observed to be divided into several tracts which spread out everywhere like the branches of trees and are inserted into the cortical substance diffused on all sides. At one and the same time the process from the cerebellum to the testes [the superior cerebellar peduncle], the process from the cerebellum to the spinal marrow [inferior cerebellar peduncle], and the cavity of the fourth ventricle—in which in addition to the larger cerebral valve a choroid plexus is found posteriorly—appear before the eyes. The famous Willis believes this last to differ from the choroid plexuses which rest upon the thalamus [i.e., in the lateral ventricles] because it appears formed from several and larger glands; but we confess that we have never found this different arrangement in the human brain.

Putting aside the larger cerebral valve [superior medullary velum] and the choroid plexus of the cavity of the fourth ventricle, two medullary tracts [in brainstem] are observed in freshly dissected heads by the aid of a microscope or, indeed, without the microscope. They coalesce with certain white fibrils [? striae acousticae] placed transversely on either side which, upon emergence from the medulla oblongata, are separated from one another near their origin. Now the two medullary tracts climb each process from the cerebellum to the spinal marrow [inferior cerebellar peduncle], adhere to them, and then end partly in the soft and partly in the hard branches of the seventh pair of nerves [the auditory and facial cranial nerves respectively]. Furthermore, around the end of the fourth ventricle may be observed as many as three, sometimes four or five, medullary fibrils led out from the cerebellar processes to the spinal marrow, which coalescing on each side form a short, white tract; its lower part is divided into now three, now four fibrils [? striae medullares] which extend into the nerve of the eighth pair [glossopharyngeal, vagus, and accessory]. The upper part, however, communicates some fibrils to the soft branch of the seventh pair of nerves [facial], while the lower serves in the formation of the nerves of the sixth pair [abducens]. From those things said above one can readily deduce reasons for the sympathy between the parts to which the nerves of the sixth, seventh, and eighth pairs contribute.

After the cerebellum has been cut through the vermiform processes so that its deeper parts may come into view and the arrangement of its medullary fibrils may be understood, we cut it again on each side through the middle [horizontally]; then we bend it back partly upwards and partly downwards and note everything in the middle (*meditullium*) of each hemisphere. An ashen or glandular substance [gray matter] is observed which, since it is divided into parts of somewhat rhomboid shape [dentate nucleus], we shall sometimes call the rhomboid substance, sometimes the rhomboid bodies of the cerebellum. Below these rhomboid bodies, all the medullary fibrils of which each cerebellar hemisphere is formed, run together and, joining into a kind of common center, on each side they continue onwards into a medullary or spongy body which we call the medullary center of the cerebellar hemispheres [corpus medullare].

From the aforesaid medullary center of the cerebellar hemispheres six processes [peduncles], that is three on each side formed from the coalescing medullary fibrils, are led forth, and through them the cerebellar medulla communicates with the posterior part of the centrum ovale [of the cerebrum], with the white tracts led forth from the mid-region of the same centrum ovale, and with the spinal cord.

MICHELE VINCENZO GIACINTO MALACARNE
(28 September 1744—4 December 1816)

During the eighteenth century the most outstanding advance in the anatomy of the cerebellum came from the work of the distinguished Italian anatomist and surgeon Malacarne. He made the most detailed examination that had been attempted up to his time and published an account of it in a book that was the first to deal wholly with the cerebellum (*Nuova esposizione della struttura del cervelletto umano*, Turin, 1776). Several of Malacarne's terms such as tonsil, pyramid, lingula, and uvula are still in use today, although like others of their kind they are usually condemned as morphologically meaningless.

Malacarne was born in Saluzzo and was successively professor of anatomy at Acqui, professor of surgery at Turin, professor of surgery and obstetrics at Pavia, and finally professor of the theory and practice of surgery at Padua. He emphasized the importance of comparative anatomy and was recognized for his work on cretinism as well as for many books on anatomy and surgery (see C. G. and V. G. Malacarne, 1819; Castaldi, 1928; Samoggia, 1965).

The following excerpts have been translated from Article I of Malacarne's treatise on the cerebellum and describe the external appearance of that structure. As is often the case with prenineteenth century anatomical works, terminology presents a difficult problem, and although many of Malacarne's descriptions have been identified, some obscurities remain.

EXCERPT PP. 18–25

3. The cerebellum is divided into two *hemispheres*, one on the right, the other on the left; each hemisphere is divided into two *surfaces*, one superior and flat, covered with a *tent* [tentorium cerebelli], the other *inferior*, hemispherical and somewhat irregular, and a little raised in front.

4. Laterally each *hemisphere* describes three-quarters of a circle, and in approaching each other posteriorly they leave a deep and wide *cavity* that I call the *common perpendicular* [posterior cerebellar notch] because in fact it is such, and gives refuge to the occipital falx of the dura mater.

5. In each the hemisphere's two surfaces are separated naturally at the external edge by a sulcus, somewhat wide anteriorly but very narrow poste-

riorly; this on each side is given the name of *horizontal fissure* or *common lateral* [fissure] and each is 14 lines [see p. 41] long.

6. The superior surface is not quite flat, and towards the quadrigeminal bodies it is much elevated and forms a kind of angle upwards and in the center [superior vermis]; anteriorly there is a marked drop to the bottom of a cliff [anterior cerebellar notch]; the same is true posteriorly where the slope is as great, but it is gentle towards the occipital bone.

7. At the lateral side of their anterior part the hemispheres form an angle superiorly, with the margin of the point curving inwards towards the quadrigeminal bodies; I give the name *semilunar* to this *curvature*, which is of 18 or 20 lines but rarely reaching 22.

8. From the center of this curvature to the anterior wall of the *common perpendicular cavity* the medial margins of the same superior surface are united by means of a confused intermingling and irregularity of substance to which I have already given the name of sutures (*raffe*) of the cerebellum [superior vermis].

9. If one examines the inferior surface he finds it divided in two by a wide and deep cavity that rests exactly on the *medulla oblongata*; this already had received the name of *little valley* (*valletta* [= *vallecula cerebelli* = great median fissure of cerebellum]) from the famous Haller; the very raised borders of the *little valley* [walls of vallecula] that are extended somewhat inwards, one towards the other, hide part of its base; they are formed by the medial borders of the hemispheres which are quite separated and do not have *sutures* [cf. no. 8].

10. The whole surface of the cerebellum, especially the superior, has furrows exactly parallel in width; in its side-to-side axis there are very many parallel sulci that descend obliquely, medially, and inferiorly. The inferior surface has semilunar fissures [prepyramidal, postpyramidal, etc.] with anterior and medial branches near to the *little valley* [vallecula], but somewhat distant towards the horizontal fissure; the principal parallel sulci are always shorter and deeper for they are more anterior.

11. Of the sulci, or outlines, the deepest are those that continue to the superior surface through the whole transverse extension of the cerebellum, dividing its hemispheres into *lobes*. A *lobe* therefore is that portion of the cerebellum contained between two very deep sulci.

12. All that portion of each hemisphere contained between two of these very deep sulci [i.e., a lobe] is divided into many subordinate portions by other furrows of lesser depth belonging to the said *lobe*; they are not the same as in the corresponding *lobe* of the other hemisphere; thus, like Heister, I give the name *lobules* to these portions.

13. Then I call *laminated leaflets* [laminae or folia] those other little portions that are separated by shallow sulci because they are part of each

lobule and decorated with now more, now less, layers, and they are noticeable.

14. . . . .

15. . . . .

16. If between one sulcus and another, especially in the sutures, there is raised some *laminated leaflet* not dependent on any of those that form the *lobules* of the hemispheres, that has the name *laminated lingula* [e.g., lingula of superior vermis].

17. Each hemisphere is composed of five lobes; the first is *anterosuperior*, the second, *posterosuperior* [first and second together form our present-day quadrangular lobule], the third, *posteroinferior* [? semilunar lobes], the fourth is called *slender* because rarely does it have a greater thickness than three lines [?]; the last is *biventral* [biventer]. The first two belong to the superior surface of the cerebellum, the last three to the inferior.

18. There is in addition a sixth *lobe* common to both hemispheres, situated between the portion of the sutures [midline] belonging to the anterosuperior lobe [the anterior part of the superior vermis] and the quadrigeminal bodies; it curves inwards with the *ascending portions* of the *arms* of the cerebellum [superior cerebellar peduncles]; it pertains to the superior surface of the cerebellum.

19. In regard to the *common perpendicular cavity* [posterior cerebellar notch] there are seen many bundles of layers, some smooth, others intersected, others more covered, others less, of the cortical substance, which unite the posteroinferior and the posterosuperior lobes of the two hemispheres; these are called *transverse laminated cords* or *commissures* of the cerebellum [tuber of vermis].

20. With the cerebellum reversed and the medulla oblongata raised in order to examine the contents of the *little valley* [vallecula], beginning with the part directly from this, there is seen a thick pyramidal eminence with a base very extended in width although thin; this eminence, because it is all layers, laminated leaflets [folia] and lingulae, I have called the *laminated pyramid* [pyramid or pyramis Malacarnei].

21. Further forwards is seen another long one [eminence], conical, rarely as thick as the little finger [uvula], at the sides of which are seen two thick tangles of layers, and of laminated leaflets [folia] placed as many skeins, one on each side: to these lateral tangles that form the anterior portion of the sides of the *vallecula*, here rather wide, I give the name of *tonsils* of the cerebellum, and to the conical eminence *uvula*, because they much resemble the parts of the same names located in the human fauces.

22. Anterior to the *uvula* is the *laminated tubercle* [nodule of vermis], and at the sides two thin transparent medullary pellicles made in the

manner of a swallow's nest, which are the two true *semilunar valves* of the fourth ventricle [lateral recesses].

23. From the external angle of the free border of the *semilunar valves* the *laminated flakes* [flocculi] are extended by a medullary stem [the peduncle of the flocculus], one on each side, and they come to a point on the neighboring margin of the *pons Varolii* between the *pyramidal eminences* of the medulla oblongata [inferior cerebellar peduncles] and the *tonsils*. The stem or medullary cord [peduncle] from which hang the flocculi in the upside-down cerebellum, remains covered by the roots of the hard portion of the seventh pair [facial nerve] and by those more numerous roots of the eighth pair of nerves [ninth, tenth, and eleventh], and resting against the soft part of the same seventh or auditory cranial nerve.

In the following chapters or articles, Malacarne considered each lobe of the cerebellum in turn. Article IV dealt with the lingula and the lobus centralis, which are both parts of the superior vermis.

EXCERPT PP. 40–42

ART. IV. LOBUS CENTRALIS

54. Although the description of the superior surface of the hemispheres of the cerebellum has been completed, it remains to speak of the *laminated lingula* (16.) that is in the center of the semilunar curvature (7.) [anterior cerebellar notch] and the *central lobe* (18.). The aforesaid lingula is found on the medullary covering [superior (anterior) medullary velum or valve of Vieussens] that descends from the testes [corpora quadrigeminal] and is lost in the [medullary] nucleus of the sutures [vermis]; it is thin, furrowed across so that it has three parallel layers; it is ashlike [in color] on the superior surface, medullary [i.e., white] at the base towards the aforesaid covering [superior medullary velum], and it has a laminated extremity. Ordinarily it has a width of five lines [see p. 41] and a length of six; like a cat's tongue, it is free at its anterior extremity, which is notably higher, and it has a rather wide root concealed under the central lobule. It is not found in all subjects; in some there is only the part corresponding to the superior surface, the inferior combining with the medullary covering (*velo*).

55. The *central lobe* has a very deeply hidden base, and in front of the two quadrilateral lobes [quadrangular lobules] it describes a kind of arc, the convexity of which is posterior and superior. The free border has three projections, two lateral trunks [alae lobuli centralis] and one in the middle [central lobe proper] which gently ascends to a point; among the projections therefore two pronounced curvatures are seen. Both surfaces of this lobe have six sinuous layers along the curves and inclines of the free border. It is thin laterally but often it is somewhat laminated in the middle.

JOHANN CHRISTIAN REIL

(*See p. 593*)

Despite the excellence of Malacarne's description of the cerebellum, it had little immediate effect and it was quite unknown, for example, in Britain. A generation later the German anatomist Reil, making use of his new technique for hardening the brain with alcohol as an aid to dissection (pp. 830–832), published five articles on the cerebellum between 1807 and 1809. His studies were based upon the report of Malacarne, and he freely admitted his reliance upon it. The result was a classic contribution to neuroanatomy and, as Stilling (p. 270, and 1878, III, 352) expressed it, "by means of Reil's work the gross morphology of the cerebellum, which had been established by Malacarne, was placed upon a firm and certain foundation."

Reil's papers on the cerebellum, together with those referred to previously on other parts of the brain (p. 593), appeared in his journal, *Archiv für die Physiologie* (Halle, 1807–1808, 8:1–58, 273–304, 385–426, and 1809, 9:129–135, 485–524). With their excellent copperplate illustrations and detailed legends, these reports were of outstanding significance in the history of knowledge of the cerebellum. Nevertheless, little was known of Reil's work outside the German-reading nations, and even today his contributions to neuroanatomy have not been given sufficient attention. In order to introduce his writings to those who did not read German, Herbert Mayo, a London surgeon and anatomist, published paraphrased translations (1822, 1823) of some of Reil's papers. Unfortunately, the translations were unreliable and were severely criticized by a contemporary commentator on the work of Malacarne and Reil ("Researches," 1824).

The following passages have been translated from Reil's first paper on the cerebellum, "Fragmente über die Bildung des kleinen Gehirns im Menschen" *Arch. Physiol., Halle,* 1807–1808, 8:1–58), which described the vermis and its constituent parts. Reil's comparison of the cerebellum to an electric battery reflected contemporary interest in animal electricity, and his discourse on the developmental aspects of the cerebellum was to be of considerable importance later for understanding the morphological arrangement and functions of the organ. His description of the vermis in animals other than man and his observations on its increased complexity as the scale of animals was ascended, thus taking into account comparative as well as morphological considerations, was the most important up to that time. Little has since been added to it, and in consequence the remainder of the present chapter will deal only with the physiology of the cerebellum.

EXCERPT PP. 26–36

II. THE VERMIS, THE CENTRAL OR TOTAL COMMISSURE PIECE THROUGH WHICH THE TWO HEMISPHERES OF THE CEREBELLUM ARE UNITED

I include in the vermis, or central piece of the two hemispheres of the cerebellum, everything that is contained in a vertical [sagittal] section from the central lobe in the anterior notch [anterior incisure] to the nodule in the posterior notch [posterior incisure], dividing the cerebellum into two completely like parts [fig. 149]. These parts are arranged in the following order: the *anterior* [superior] *medullary velum,* the *superior vermis,* the *simple transverse commissure* of the posterosuperior lobe, the *short, visible, transverse ridges* in the purse-shaped posterior notch [vallecula cerebelli] which lie immediately below that transverse commissure, the *long, hidden, transverse ridges,* the *pyramid,* the *cone* [uvula], and the *little knot* [nodule]; that is, everything belonging to the superior and inferior vermis.

According to the results hitherto obtained from my researches, it seems that two things are essential for a concept of the cerebellum. *First* of all, an apparatus consisting partly of vessels and cortical substance and partly of white matter lying immediately below the cortex closed in from both sides in the shape of a bow, the so-called pons Varolii, just as the circuit of the Voltaic current must be closed. This apparatus always lies outside yet within the confines of the cerebellum and, so to speak, forms its cortex. The vessels and the cortical substance in contact with the white matter may perhaps be the organ that produces activity or the life spirit like electromotor [forces] from a closed circuit. On the other hand, the white matter can be the collector or the area in which the activity collects in the form of disposable excitability. This idea obtains a certain amount of support from a remarkable experiment that I made and which I shall describe hereafter in detail. The cortex and white matter are not continuous but contiguous, and they merely lie on top of one another. I am able to separate them, one from the other, by means of a special manual manoeuvre that destroys the connections between them, as clearly as the auricles of the heart can be separated from their chambers by means of nitric acid. *In the second place,* an apparatus destined for conduction, which is nearer the inside of the cerebellum, forms the roof of the fourth ventricle of the brain and is connected with two conductors: with the cerebral hemispheres by means of two anterior conductors, the superior cerebellar peduncles; and with the spinal cord by means of two posterior conductors, the inferior cerebellar peduncles. The nerves which are undeniably conductors of life activity never come from the cortex or the periphery but all of them invariably come from the inside or medulla; that is, from the part that is more folded and, so to speak, more closely packed [corpus medullare].

The *laminae* [folia] and their *connections* are therefore the essential components of the concept of the cerebellum. They are its primitive qualities and, as it were, the primordial structures. In all solid [i.e., fixed] brains we find this idea, and only this one, expressed; even their structures, which are apparently very heterogeneous, are nothing else but mere modifications of this one concept, if they are dissected without prejudice.

In its most simple form this same shape has been achieved in the *cerebellum of birds* in which it is a pyramidal pile standing erect with double anterior and posterior arrangements of laminae and in its center a narrow, conical, upright cavity out of which arise the peduncles. Here there is as yet nothing but the vermis, and this is a very simple one. The sprouts [i.e., rudimentary structures] and wings, which in more highly evolved animals develop into the hemispheres, are completely missing and are represented only by lateral sprouts that are hardly noticeable.

This simple pile, which in birds represents the whole of the cerebellum, becomes larger and larger in such a way that at its circumference ever new and additional piles are added that in themselves, however, are nothing more than, and in no way different from, the first one. This is the only law according to which the several variations in the function of the cerebellum of higher animals come about. *For it seems that the mere intensity of brain capacity determines the quality and the difference of its function, and again its intensity grows proportionally with its extension and increase in volume in exactly the same way in which the effects of electricity change according to the different degrees of its strength.* The new piles are either separate and only connected by means of the white substance common to them, or they are connected as in an uninterrupted continuum in such a way that cortex and white matter are fused into one. The first I shall call the *sprouts* of the vermis, the latter, the *wings*. In the lower animals there are only a few sprouts, but higher up [the scale] the sprouts around the vermis become more numerous. The vermis extends more laterally, develops wings, and the sprouts disappear in proportion to this increase of wings. The first development of the cerebellum occurs in the anterior and superior region; in the inferior and posterior area, parts of the vermis and the sprouts remain separate. Even in quadrupeds the vermis preponderates in length, breadth, and height; the anterior area has wings already, but few and short ones and on both sides, and in the posterior area all is sprouts, that is, something separated. In proportion as the stages of development continue, the sprouts are changed into wings. They have, so to speak, become part of the wing until in man the hemispheres develop, for in man all sprouts have completely disappeared with the exception of two important flakes [flocculi]. Everything is concentrated into a consolidated organization; the vermis with its wings has become a permanent whole, and in this way a circulation or free community–interchange has been effected which is still interrupted in the sprouts.

. . . .

[DESCRIPTION OF THE VERMIS IN THE HARE, SHEEP, OX, AND HORSE]

The formation of the cerebellum [in animals] begins from the vermis by a multiplication of the primordial structure; the vermis is, as it were, the original pile to which ever-new piles are added in the form of sprouts and wings in proportion to the ascent in the scale of animals. In the quadrupeds, and even in man, this primordial formation is still visible, unobliterated, as in the central lobe. It is true that in man its central piece lacks wings, but it is very broad compared to the wings; the wings are not only very short, but also separated from the central piece by an important sulcus so that it seems to be nothing but an intermediary [stage] between wing and sprout. In proportion as the lobes proceed from the anterior to the posterior notch [incisure], vermis and wings flow together ever more markedly into a continuum and the wings become longer. This is the reason for the pyramidal shape of the cerebellum from the front towards the back; the blunt apex of the pyramid lies in the anterior notch, the base of it is in the part of the posterior lobe of the cerebellum where it is spread most markedly from one corner of the lambdoid suture to the other.

In man the wings form the main part of the cerebellum, that is, its hemispheres. On the superior surface they are a direct continuation of the vermis; on the inferior surface, which, as has been said, is formed later, they are separated from the vermis [on each side] by a deep sulcus and are still somewhat similar to sprouts. It is remarkable that the human cerebellum, which has the most complicated structure of them all, yet expresses most clearly the basic idea and elementary form in its composition. Thus, if one places it erect it is completely similar to the brain of a bird. A simple leaf in the latter, is in man a feathered leaf which is clearly shown in a [sagittal] section of the lobe [fig. 149]. In man leaves surround the white matter as lobes and lobules, and they form a roof under which the peduncles can emerge in all directions, like the feet of a tortoise under its shell.

In proportion as the lateral piles increase in number in the form of sprouts and wings, the vermis becomes smaller and compressed towards the middle. This is most clearly visible in man in whom there are hemispheres. The vermis has remained stationary in all dimensions during the formation of length, breadth, and depth [of the cerebellum]. Anteriorly the horns of a crescent-shaped notch [anterior incisure] protrude, and posteriorly are the [lateral] walls of the purse-shaped notch [vallecula]; the vermis is pushed towards the center in front as well as posteriorly. In the posterior notch and at the cone [uvula] and little knot [nodule] it is scarcely a few lines [see p. 41] broad. In animals it everywhere protrudes over the lateral parts; in man it is on the same level with them on the upper surface and on the lower surface it is remarkably caved in to form the valley [vallecula]. This compression of the vermis from all sides in man is the reason for the modifications in its shape through which it is differentiated from other animal brains. Its organization differs from the hemispheres, but in the quadrupeds it is not different from the structure of the lateral parts [hemispheres]. It is soft in man, in animals hard; the vascular membrane [pia mater] is stronger, more complex, and is provided with more vessels than in the hemispheres. The white matter is far thinner in the vermis than in the hemispheres; thin in the anterior medullary velum and somewhat thicker where the standing and lying branches are united to form the core of the white matter of the vermis [fig. 149]—thicker in the standing than in the lying one—and finally again, very thick in the posterior medullary velum. Anteriorly in the region of the anterior notch it is broadest but becomes narrower towards the posterior notch itself; it is crumpled up into a single leaf in the transverse commissure of the large posterosuperior lobe. It then extends again laterally in the pyramid and finally is again pointed in the uvula and the nodule. On both sides of the superior vermis more or less deep sulci run, in which the substance of the brain is notched and thinned down and the direction of most leaves [folia] between them is changed in such a way that their convexity is turned anteriorly and medially and the arches of the lobules go in exactly the opposite direction. Through the sulci [forming the lateral margins of the vallecula] in which the vessels lie, the lateral branches of the superior vermis are marked exactly, and distinctly differentiated from the boundaries of the lobules. They continue through the vallecula and become deeper in it. Therefore, that is the reason for the protruding midline of the parts that lie in the valley.

What then is the vermis and what is its function? First of all, I make the observation that there is no difference between the superior and inferior vermis, but all parts of the vertical [parasaggital] cross section [fig. 149] are of the same kind as they lie above and below in the center [vermis], between the two hemispheres. This can be seen by merely looking at it. Not all parts of the cross sections have a homogeneous structure and are branched in an analogous way, but they receive deviating formations in the vallecula and posterior incisure through the compression of the hemispheres and the medulla oblongata. In birds the vermis is the only deviating formation; in quadrupeds the main pile; in man, in whom the sprouts and the wings have been fused together into hemispheres, it is partly the same as the lateral parts, that is a *pile*, and partly *total commissure* through which the lateral piles are connected and linked together, that is, the hemispheres superiorly and inferiorly.

Later, in another article, Reil recorded his account of the internal features of the cerebellum ("Untersuchungen über den Bau des kleinen Gehirns im Menschen. Zweyte Fortsetzung über die Organisation der Lappen und Läppchen," *Arch. Physiol., Halle*, 1807–1808, 8:385–426). The following is a translation of a small part of this report.

EXCERPT PP. 404–405

Finally, there follows the *arcuate layer that is made up of coarse fibres.*
This layer is connected mainly with the lateral [middle] peduncles of the
cerebellum and with the anterior [superior] and posterior [inferior] peduncles. With the anterior and posterior peduncles and with the corpus ciliare
[dentate nucleus] it forms the central part [of the cerebellum]. Again, the
lateral peduncles rise posteriorly and laterally [from the pons] in the horizontal fissure, and they spread out in the superior and inferior area of the
bands of the [medullary] nucleus, turning medially towards the vermis
from the horizontal fissure, and being thickest anteriorly and thinnest
posteriorly. The anterior part of these fibres moves on top, over the anterior
peduncles, like a thick bolster, and approaches the superior and inferior
vermis with the part appended to it following. The next fibres run in the
same direction, posteriorly with the medulla [white matter] of the vermis
towards the posterior notch [incisure], and the inner extremities of the
posterior lobe that are present at that place, towards its inside and outside
part; the radiating fibres of this lobe are situated on top of them and at
obtuse angles. If, therefore, a piece of the medullary [nucleus] has remained
on the medullary folia of the posterior lobe, they either finish at the border
or they describe an angle with it in the archlike direction in which the fibres
of the [medullary] nucleus run along the lobes. The dentate nucleus consists of several lobes and can be peeled out of its capsule. Between the
peduncles forming the capsule and the anterior peduncles, the posterior
peduncles squeeze themselves and, together with the lateral peduncles,
cross over the anterior peduncles. The anterior peduncles proceed posteriorly in a straight direction, pierce with delicate bands the lobes of the
dentate nucleus, and border on the anterior [superior] medullary velum and
the [medullary] nucleus of the vermis with which they have the same
anteroposterior direction.

Early Experimental Physiology

Although knowledge of the gross anatomy of the cerebellum was now well
advanced, there was virtually no certain information regarding its function. Willis's
idea that it was the seat of vital functions had received considerable support, partly
from isolated clinical observations on the sequelae of cerebellar trauma. A rival
theory, however, was advanced by Gall and Spurzheim at the beginning of the
nineteenth century; they maintained that the cerebellum controlled sexual function
(F. J. Gall, J. Vimont, and F. J. V. Broussais, 1838). This idea survived for an
astonishingly long time, and William A. Hammond of New York found it neces-

sary to discuss it in 1869, as did Ferrier as late as 1896. No one accepts it today, but the occurrence of genital atrophy with certain forms of cerebellar degeneration has never been adequately explained (Holmes, 1907).

Luigi Rolando

(*See p. 480*)

Meantime a series of experimenters were pursuing a path which would eventually lead to our present-day concept of cerebellar function. Ablation of the cerebellum had been attempted before the nineteenth century but no satisfactory conclusions had been reached. One of the better known experiments was that of Du Verney who in 1673 removed a pigeon's cerebellum, replaced it with flax, and observed the postoperative course (Preston, 1695–1697, p. 461). The first adequate experiments, however, were carried out by Rolando whose studies on a wide variety of animals all showed that by removing portions of the cerebellum, ipsilateral motor activity was impaired. As in his investigations of the cerebral hemispheres (pp. 481–483), so, too, his operative techniques and his observations on the postoperative states of his animals relative to cerebellar investigation were crude. Thus he probably damaged the brainstem as well as the cerebellum in some cases, and the limb phenomena he interpreted as weakness was almost certainly lack of coordination and asthenia (see Fadiga, 1963).

Nevertheless, Rolando was the first clearly to demonstrate the motor nature of the cerebellum's function, and he should be considered as one of the founders of modern cerebellar physiology; he thought, however, that the cerebellum was "the organ controlling locomotion" rather than a regulating influence on motor activity, and this, as Magendie was quick to point out, was his error. He also made the important observation that recovery of function was possible unless the lesion was a severe one, and the observation on the turtle, recorded below, suggested to him that the cerebellum was a reinforcer of voluntary movements. His results were reported in his book, *Saggio sopra la vera struttura del cervello dell'uomo e degl'-animali, e sopra le funzioni del sistema nervoso* (Sassari, 1809); they were translated into French for Magendie in 1823 ("Expériences faites sur le cervelet des mammifères," *J. Physiol. expér. path.*, 1823, *3*:107–111) as part of an article, "Expériences sur les fonctions du système nerveux par le Professeur Rolando" (pp. 95–113), published to refute a charge that Flourens had plagiarized Rolando (see pp. 480–483). They also appeared in Flourens (1824, pp. 293–302). The following passage has been translated from *La vera struttura del cervello*.

EXCERPT PP. 44–49

The structure of the cerebellum, and the important discoveries made by the professor of Padua [Malacarne, see pp. 643–646] regarding the large number of folia of which this organ is composed, prompted me to suspect its true use; I believed that it must serve locomotion, and to confirm my opinion I undertook the following experiments on it.

With a trephine I made a lateral opening at the site of the cerebellum in several pigs and one sheep, and I excised at a stroke as much as I could of this organ; however, scarcely had the lesion been extended beyond the edge of the trephine hole than the animal became hemiplegic and soon died with convulsions and hemorrhage.

It is very difficult to penetrate into the cerebellum of quadrupeds without suddenly depriving them of life, and the animal that I have found most convenient for this experiment has been the kid. Introducing a cutting probe through the trephine opening, I cut the cerebellum of one of these animals in various directions, and after this, as if paralyzed, it could no longer stand on its legs. It lived for twenty-four hours in this condition and died in convulsions. When I examined it, in addition to the aforesaid injuries, I found a quantity of clotted blood in the fourth ventricle, and I believe that this was the main reason for its death and the convulsive spasms. It would be counter to my desire for brevity if I were to report in detail the experiments that I have multiplied in many forms on the cerebellum of a large number of quadrupeds; I shall limit myself for the present to saying that in all of them I have always observed that the lack of movement was proportionate to the larger or smaller injury produced in the cerebellum. Therefore, now totally paralyzed, now half, now only the anterior or posterior limbs remained without movement, according to whether or not this organ, which is of the greatest importance in many functions of the animal economy, was totally or partly destroyed.

OF BIRDS

I trephined the site corresponding to the cerebellum, now laterally, now superiorly, in many fowls, and the movement of the muscles dependent upon the locomotive faculty always disappeared because of the lesion produced. Having made an opening superior to the site of the cerebellum in a chicken, with a suitable instrument I excised approximately half the right side of this organ; the animal was immediately paralyzed and fell on the same side, no longer able to use its right leg in any way or to stand on it. To convince myself the better of this singular phenomenon, I grasped the leg on the injured side, and while it was held in the usual position the chicken supported itself on the other leg and was able to take a few steps; but in a few minutes it could no longer use it, and finally became paralyzed on both sides. I allowed it to live for three days during which time it took no food and hardly drank any water, merely holding its beak immersed in the water.

One must note that despite these lesions in the cerebellum the animal never became drowsy or fell into a stupor; it kept its eyes open and observed all objects; but it was in vain that it attempted to execute any movement through means of the muscles dependent on the locomotive faculty. This is not to deny that from time to time it shook its wings as well as its lower extremities, but these movements seemed to arise solely from the mobility still enjoyed by the muscle fibre or they took place because some considerable piece of the cerebellum remained intact so that it was still able partly to fulfill its function.

When I suddenly lacerated, impaired, or removed this organ, the animal was always completely paralyzed, but if I injured it only slightly, after several hours it regained the faculty of movement.

OF REPTILES AND FISHES

The experiments made on cold-blooded animals were equally conclusive. A turtle in which I resected and raised the cerebellum from the medulla oblongata remained completely paralyzed and lived thus for ten or twelve days without making the slightest movement. Another, after a similar operation, lived for two months, and was very sensitive as usual to the slightest injuries and to the slightest stimulations, but immobile to such a degree that it was unable in any way to remove itself from the spot where it had received the injury. I treated a lizard in the same way and with the same result, but it was more astonishing to see the same effects in two very agile serpents (*coluber natrix*). The organ controlling locomotion not having been well removed in the first and smaller one, it remained paralyzed for two or three hours, unable to move from one place to another; but afterwards it recovered its former ability and escaped. The second one, which was more successfully operated upon, was completely deprived of its faculty of movement; only from time to time was it seen to be agitated by uncertain movements, not directed by instinct, but dependent upon the great mobility of the muscle fibre of these animals; it died after five days.

In order not to leave this experiment untried on fishes, which by their nature die in a short time when kept out of their element, I bound a two-pound *pagello* to a small table, and keeping it thus controlled and immersed I excised almost the whole cerebellum; after I had let it loose it fell as if dead to the bottom of the tub, although it still lived.

I performed the same operation on a catfish (*squalus catulus*) with much greater ease because the bones of its skull are cartilaginous and because it can be kept out of water much longer. It lost its locomotion, and, when it was put back into the water, its movements were vague and uncertain and it could no longer manage to swim.

I observed, as I have already stated, that the injuries made in the cerebellum of several chickens healed very quickly and that they regained their former aptitude for movement. However, I saw this to occur in a more singular way in the first turtle operated on, in which I had only lacerated and divided the aforesaid organ. The animal remained paralyzed for many hours, but then quickly acquired a surprising facility of movement, so that it walked continually with a quadrupled swiftness. I was curious to examine the cerebellum covered only with clotted blood; it seemed to me to be scarred and considerably increased in size. Could it be possible that this animal's cerebellum, having, with the help of a scar, acquired a much greater development, was thus able to contribute to the unusual agility that it enjoyed after the operation?

PIERRE FLOURENS
(*See p. 483*)

Of all the early investigations of cerebellar function, the most famous and the most important were those of the French physiologist Flourens. On the whole, Rolando's experiments had been crude, whereas Flourens not only possessed better techniques but also a better knowledge of the anatomy of the cerebellum.

In the same book in which appeared his ablation experiments on the cerebral hemispheres of animals, considered above (pp. 486–488), Flourens described similar procedures on the cerebellum (*Recherches expérimentales sur les propriétés et les fonctions du système nerveux dans les animaux vertébrés* [Paris, 1824], pp. 36–42, 137–149, 259–262; the last page (p. 262) dealt in detail with the effect of alcohol on the cerebellum). His earliest experiments on the cerebellum were published in *Archs. gén. Méd.*, 1823, 2 (1st ser.):355–356, and his conclusions were succinctly summarized in one of his comments on the work of Rolando included in his book:

> I have shown that all movements persist following ablation of the cerebellum; all that is missing is that they are not regular and coordinated. From this I have been induced to conclude that the *production* and the *coordination* of movements form two classes of essentially distinct phenomena and that they reside in two classes of organs also essentially distinct; to wit, *coordination* in the *cerebellum* and *production* in the *spinal cord* and *medulla oblongata* [p. 297, note 1].

Thus the concept of regulation of motor activity by the cerebellum began with Flourens, "the cerebellum coordinates" (p. x). His idea of coordination was the first step towards our present belief in the cooperation of muscles in movement and in posture, that is, synergia. Like Rolando, Flourens found that sensory, vital, and intellectual functions were not impaired by a cerebellar lesion and that the organ had a great facility for compensation. Moreover, deep lesions produced severe symptoms, whereas extensive but superficial ones did not; this was to be specially important later. However, Flourens did not recognize the weakness associated with a cerebellar deficit nor the release phenomenon. The latter was the work of an Italian contemporary, Michele Foderà (1793–1848) in Magendie's laboratory in Paris, who described the extensor hypertonia following an acute cerebellar lesion in mammals; as Dow and Moruzzi (1958, p. 5) have pointed out, it is an important yet little known contribution.

A report of Flourens' early experiments was read to the Académie Royale des Sciences on 31 March and 27 April 1822 ("Détermination des propriétés du système nerveux, ou recherches physiques sur l'irritabilité et la sensibilité," *J. Physiol. expér. path.*, 1822, 2:372–384; see p. 383). The full article appeared in 1823 (see p. 484), and a report presented by Foderà on 31 December of that same year ("Recherches expérimentales sur le système nerveux," *J. Physiol. expér. path.*, 1823, 3:191–217; the promised continuation was not published, but see *Archs. gén. Méd.*, 1823, 3 (1st ser.):473–474, "A MM. les rédacteurs des Archives"). The following excerpts have been translated from the first edition, 1824, of Flourens' book (see p. 485).

EXCERPT PP. 36–37

EXPERIMENTS TO DETERMINE THE ROLE AND FUNCTIONS
OF THE CEREBELLUM

. . . .

1. I removed the cerebellum from a pigeon slice by slice. During the removal of the first slices, only slight weakness and lack of coordination of movement appeared.

With the middle slices, an almost universal restlessness was manifested although there was no sign of convulsion; the animal performed sudden and disordered movement; it heard and saw.

On the removal of the last slices, the animal, in which the faculty of jumping, flying, walking, and of maintaining an erect posture had become more and more disturbed by the preceding mutilations, lost this faculty altogether.

Placed on its back it was not able to rise. Far from remaining calm and steady as in pigeons deprived of the cerebral lobes [see p. 485], it became vainly and almost continually agitated, but it never moved in a steady and firm manner.

For example, becoming aware of a threatened blow and wishing to avoid it, it made a thousand efforts to do so but without success. When placed on its back, it did not wish to stay there and exhausted itself in vain attempts to get up, but in the end remained in the same position despite its efforts.

Finally, volition, sensation, and perception persisted; the ability to carry out *general movements* also persisted; but the *coordination of these movements* in an orderly and determined manner was lost.

EXCERPT PP. 38–42

4. In a fourth pigeon I removed the upper layers of the cerebellum. When this mutilation was accomplished the animal saw and heard very well; it also kept itself upright, walked, and flew, but in an indecisive and very unsure manner.

I continued my excisions; equilibrium was almost completely lost. The animal had very great difficulty in standing up and could do so only by supporting itself on its wings and tail. When it walked its staggering and unsure steps gave it the appearance of a drunken animal; its wings had to be used to help its legs, and despite this assistance it often fell over and rolled about.

With the removal of the last layers, all semblance of equilibrium, that is all harmony between its efforts, disappeared. Ability to walk, fly, and be stationary were totally abolished; however, I should like you to notice that desire for these movements and tentative efforts to carry them out still persisted.

5. In a fifth pigeon I removed the cerebellum by successive, extremely thin layers so as to follow to the very last detail all the degrees and gradations by which this gradual removal would reduce my pigeon from a state of perfect equilibrium to one of complete abolition of the ability to fly, walk, and stand.

It was a source of astonishment to watch the animal gradually losing its ability to fly, then to walk, and finally to stand, in proportion to its loss of cerebellum.

The ability to keep standing deteriorated little by little before being completely lost. The animal began by being unable to stand firmly on its legs for any length of time; it staggered almost continuously; then its feet could no longer hold it stationary and it was forced to lean on its wings and tail; finally, any stationary and stable position became impossible; the animal made incredible efforts to hold itself in this position but did not succeed.

The ability to walk likewise diminished by degrees. At first the animal maintained a staggering gait very much like the peculiar walk of a drunkard; then it walked only with the help of its wings, and finally it did not know how to walk at all.

By careful excisions one can at will suppress flying only; or suppress flying and walking; or at the same time suppress flying, walking, and the ability to stand. By disposing of the cerebellum, one disposes of all *coordinated movements*, as in disposing of the cerebral lobes one destroys all sensations [pp. 486–487].

The pigeon in which I studied these peculiarities, after the removal of the first layers, evinced only slight weakness and hesitation in its movements.

I should like to note here, in relation to that weakness, that the moment of injury is always the moment when the weakness is most pronounced, and afterwards it decreases more and more until a new mutilation has been made.

With the middle layers, my pigeon saw and heard very well; it had no complaints; its demeanor was gay, its head alert.

Judging by its healthy appearance, certainly no one would have imagined that it was already lacking half its cerebellum; but, on the other hand, its gait was very staggering and agitated; and soon it could not walk any longer except with the help of its wings.

I continued my excisions; the animal lost completely its ability to walk. Its feet would no longer hold it upright, and it could support itself only by leaning upon its knees, its tail, and its wings. Often it tried to fly away or to walk; but these ineffective attempts in several respects resembled the first attempts of young fledglings to fly and walk when they leave the nest.

When it was pushed forwards, it rolled on its head: when pushed backwards, on its tail.

I carried my excisions still further. The animal lost the ability to lean on its knees, tail, and wings. It rolled over itself constantly without being able to hold itself in a fixed position.

Because of this rolling and struggling it became exhausted; and, giving in to fatigue, it then maintained for a moment the position which it had attained by chance: now it rested flat on its stomach, now on its back.

This position on its back, as painful as it must have been, and no matter what efforts it made it could not disengage itself because it no longer knew how.

Otherwise, it saw and heard very well. When resting, the slightest threat, the slightest noise, the least irritation reopened the tumultuous scene of its contortions.

But in the midst of all these so irregular, agitated, and lively contortions, there was not the least sign of convulsions.

6. The results of the excision of the cerebellum varied somewhat according to species.

EXCERPT PP. 138–139

EXPERIMENT IV. ON A SPARROW

I removed the cerebellum carefully in successive layers in a sparrow.

Little by little the animal lost its ability to fly and to walk, while at the same time perfectly preserving vision, hearing, all its senses, and all its intellectual faculties, without ever evidencing the slightest symptom of convulsion.

This small bird offered the most peculiar sight by its tottering, unsure, and queer gait. After it had been for a moment undecided as to how to dart forth, it took three or four steps (sometimes forwards, more often backwards) with an incredible rapidity, and all this ended in a fall or in rolling over.

However, the most curious thing was the manner in which it flew: at one time in the air, it still seemed to roll over, unable to direct itself according to its will, shooting forth in one direction, then turning in another, remaining thus in the air for a moment, fluttering about in indecision and embarrassment and ending by falling down.

This flight completely resembled the walk of a drunkard. Therefore there exists a drunken flight as well as a drunken gait; and, in flying animals, flight is subject to all the influences which affect the gait in walking animals.

EXCERPT PP. 145–146

EXPERIMENT XVI. ON A DOG

In a young but strong dog I injured the cerebellum by deeper and deeper sections. The animal lost more and more its faculty of orderly and regular movement. When I reached the middle region it could walk only with a tottering and weaving step. It retreated when it wanted to advance; when it desired to turn right it turned left instead. Since it made a great effort to move, and could no longer modify this effort, it threw itself forwards impetuously and did not fail to fall or to roll over. If it found an obstacle in its way it could no longer avoid it no matter how hard it tried; it hurled itself right and left; nevertheless it saw and heard very well; when something irritated it, it tried to bite, and, indeed, bit the irritating object if it was able to catch it, but it no longer controlled its movements with sufficient precision to succeed often. It had all its intellectual faculties, all its senses, not a trace of convulsions; it was merely deprived of the ability to command and regulate its movements.

I injured it as far as the final layers of the cerebellum; the animal lost all mobility and all its usual stability.

EXCERPT PP. 148–149

Thus, 1°, in all the animals and at all ages, slight interference with the cerebellum always causes a slight lack of coordination of movement, which always increases with the interference; and the total loss of the cerebellum always causes the total loss of those faculties which regulate movement.

2° However, there remains the very peculiar observation that even with this regularity and with this exact repetition of the phenomena, the movements that have become disorderly because of the cerebellum, always correspond in the different animals to their dominant movements.

In birds that fly much, it is in flight that the disorder mainly appears; in animals that walk, it shows up in the gait; in birds that swim, in their swimming.

There exists therefore a drunken swim and a drunken flight just as there is a drunken gait; and a disturbance in the predominant activity does not prevent its dominating this pattern.

3° Although along with the loss of the cerebellum there is decisive loss of the locomotive faculties, the intellectual and sensory functions remain wholly sound; and, on the other hand, as long as the operation does not exceed the confines of the cerebellum, there is no sign of convulsions.

The faculty exciting convulsions or muscular contractions, the coordinating faculty of these contractions, and the intellectual and sensitive faculties are therefore three classes of functions that are essentially distinct and are located in three orders of nervous organs that are also essentially different.

4° Despite the fact that finally, along with the [ablated] cerebellum, the faculty to command and to coordinate standing and walking is lost, the tendency toward such equilibrium nevertheless continues to exist; and, although all locomotor motions are lost, all movements of [self-] preservation nevertheless always survive. This tendency to a stable and regular equilibrium, these movements of conservation, are therefore not derived from the cerebellum.

The Unitarian Concept of Cerebellar Function

Most of the experimental work on cerebellar function in the nineteenth century was based on ablation procedures which, however, had three main sources of error: (1) differences between animal species were overlooked and findings in lower animals were frequently applied to man, (2) investigators failed to appreciate whether the postoperative states they studied were owing to the activity of the remaining cerebellar tissue or to the rest of the nervous system, (3) there was a lack of histological and gross anatomical controls. As these factors were gradually realized observations became more precise and uniform.

One of the ideas which, in fact, stemmed from Rolando's and Flourens' conclusion that the cerebellum acted as a whole to influence muscle movements, was the unitarian concept of cerebellar function. First of all, the classical work of Luciani

(1891) seemed to substantiate this belief, and support for it was found in the studies of Ramón y Cajal and others on the microscopical appearances of the cerebellum. Sherrington at the turn of the century also concluded that the organ functioned as a whole. It proved to be the predominant concept for several decades.

Luigi Luciani
(23 November 1840—23 June 1919)

The experiments of Rolando and Flourens were repeated and confirmed by many subsequent workers whose interpretations of the results, however, varied. Some like Flourens thought of the cerebellum as an organ that coordinated movements, whereas others considered it to be a center for muscle sense, or for propulsive movements, or for sensation. Another group, following Rolando, concluded that it was a center for the control of muscular energy, and the work of the Italian physiologist Luciani grew out of this idea.

Luciani was born in Ascoli-Piceno and studied medicine at the Universities of Bologna and Naples. After working at the Physiological Institute of the University of Leipzig from 1872 to 1873, he occupied a number of posts in pathology and physiology—at Siena, Florence, and eventually at Rome (1893–1917). His early work was in the field of cardiovascular pathology and physiology, but he is best known for his many neurophysiological investigations. From 1901 to 1911 he published his five-volume textbook of physiology which is a useful source of the history of the subject as well as a brilliant survey of current thought (see Haymaker, 1953, pp. 146–149; Crepax, 1963).

Whereas the experiments of Rolando, Flourens, and subsequent workers were acute, Luciani studied the effects of chronic cerebellar ablations, employing remarkable experimental skill. He was thus the first to discover how a cerebellar deficit could be compensated for by other parts of the nervous system. The new aseptic surgical techniques made these experiments possible and assured the survival of his animals which in most instances were dogs and apes. This was the most significant aspect of his work for at that time the lengthy survival of decerebellated animals was an unusual achievement.

His book, *Il cervelletto. Nuovi studi de fisiologia normale e patologica* (Florence, 1891), was quoted widely, but his analysis of the postoperative states he produced is now judged to have been an oversimplification of very complex phenomena. Unfortunately, his reports were accepted almost universally for more than fifty years and the uncritical perpetuation of his error has in fact hindered progress. His contribution was, nonetheless, an important one for it pointed the way to several modern interpretations, and reference must be made to his main opinions and to his account of cerebellar signs. The cerebellum, according to Luciani, acted as a single functional unit, but he admitted a supervision of the body musculature by the ipsilateral side of the cerebellum.

Luciani helped to begin the modern period of cerebellar physiology. Following Rolando's idea of a diffuse cerebellar influence on all motor activities, Luciani conceived a tonic, facilitating effect upon central structures responsible for the motion of voluntary muscles. The cerebellum acted as a whole, as a single homogeneous organ, and the only distinct anatomical partition of function was its bilaterality; each cerebellar hemisphere governed the bodily musculature of the same side. Its destruction, partial or complete, produced first a transient period of irritation ("dynamic phenomena," or as we would say "release phenomena," owing to the removal of the cerebellar inhibitory influence on muscle tone), second, "deficiency phenomena," and finally a period of compensation. The loss of reinforced movements led to states, later confirmed clinically by Holmes (pp. 677–681), which Luciani termed asthenia, atonia, and astasia (tremors, including titubation and other forms of ataxia); these were the result of a functional influence and there was also a trophic influence. Recovery resulted from compensation by the remaining cerebellar tissue, if any, or by the contralateral cerebral cortex. This division of postoperative phenomena, although not accepted by all, has helped to analyze them. The following translations from Luciani's book of 1891 describe some of these conclusions.

EXCERPT PP. 301–303

One of the great, culminating and truly fundamental facts in respect to this doctrine, confirmed not only by my own investigations but also fully supported by all the better clinical observations and the better experiments conducted by my predecessors, is that extensive and deep ablations, indeed even the total absence of the said organ [cerebellum], produce neither partial nor total *paralysis* of the senses and movements, nor of the sensory, intellectual, and volitional functions that depend upon them.

This fact, together with other related secondary ones (for example, the possibility of long survival in animals deprived of the cerebellum without cessation of any major functions), leads us directly to the assumption that the cerebellum and all its dependencies represent a small, relatively autonomous system that up to a certain point is distinct from the great cerebrospinal system. It is not an intermediate organ introduced along the great pathways of cerebrospinal conduction; it is rather a terminal organ, I should almost say an appendix that by means of special afferent pathways is found to be in relationship—direct or indirect—with the peripheral sense organs and, by means of special efferent pathways, is joined directly with certain masses of gray substance of the cerebrospinal axis, and indirectly with the peripheral apparatus of voluntary movement.

The constant results of our researches have amply demonstrated to us that the cerebellum (like the rest of the central or cerebrospinal nervous system) is histologically and functionally an organ of *bilateral* action, but predominantly *direct* [ipsilateral], contrary to the cerebral hemispheres that also exercise *bilateral* actions but predominantly *crossed* [contralateral] ones. The study of the degenerations following cerebellar hemiextirpation explains to us the reasons for this incontestable fact, common to various classes of vertebrates.

Our experiments lead us to declare that the direct and crossed influence of cerebellar innervation is not limited to the muscles which act in the various forms of standing and moving, but extends to all voluntary muscles; not, however, to the same degree in the different groups of muscles but predominantly to the muscles of the lower or posterior limbs, as well as to the fixed ones of the vertebral column. So far science has been unable to explain this true as well as obscure fact with respect to the anatomicophysiological conditions that determine it.

The manifest result of all our studies is that the middle cerebellar lobe [vermis] does not have in general a greater or different functional importance than the lateral lobes, and that the different cerebellar segments have the same function. In fact the deficiency of the middle lobe can be supplemented in great part, or rather can be *compensated for organically* by the lateral lobes. In general, whatever may be the cerebellar mutilation, symmetrical, asymmetrical, circumscribed, or extensive, the phenomena of deficiency do not differ in their nature or characters, but only in their intensity, extent, and duration, and in their greater or lesser predominance in the muscles of one or other side of the body.

If one desires to remain within the limits of facts acquired up to the present, so long as new, more strongly supported experimental evidence does not lead to modification of our present knowledge, the cerebellum cannot be considered as a collection of centers functionally distinct or different, in the sense that each segment is in very intimate or direct rapport with a specific group of muscles or destined for functions of different kinds. Up to the present we have been led to declare that the cerebellum is an organ functionally homogeneous, that is, an organ in which each segment has the same functions as the whole and is capable of compensating for the deficiencies of others, so long as its normal relationships remain unaltered, either with the afferent pathways by which it receives sensory impressions or with the efferent pathways by which it transmits its influence to the rest of the central system.

What in the cerebellum stimulates the sensory impressions that it receives by way of its afferent pathways? What is the influence that it transmits by its efferent pathways? These are the two principal problems upon the solution of which is based principally the physiological doctrine of the cerebellum.

Hitherto there has been little to say in reply to the first question. It has been well demonstrated that not only the white substance of the cerebellum, that is to say, the peduncular expansions in the depth of the organ, but also the cortical gray substance (at least in certain points not yet exactly determined and probably varying in different species and individuals) *is directly excitable* by electrical, chemical, and mechanical stimuli, in the same way that the same stimuli can excite certain well-known areas in the cerebral cortex. But this fact does not resolve the question. Even if the cerebellar cortex were everywhere shown not to be excitable by artificial, inadequate stimuli, this would not preclude it from reacting to adequate or physiological excitants that are transmitted to it by afferent fibres.

EXCERPT PP. 304–307

Our long, persistent investigations have shown in a clear and consistent manner that cerebellar deficiency is principally characterized by three categories of neuromuscular phenomena, that is, by *asthenic, atonic, astatic* phenomena. It therefore follows logically that the influence which the cerebellum normally exercises upon the rest of the system must occur in *sthenic, tonic,* and *static neuromuscular action,* that is, in a complicated action by which:

a) It increases the *potential energy* that the neuromuscular apparatus has at its disposal (*sthenic action*);

b) the degree of their tone increases during the functional intervals (*tonic function*);

c) the rhythm of the elementary impulses is accelerated during their functional activity and normal fusion and regular continuity of actions occur (*static function*).

Since every *functional* excitant that affects living elements is necessarily associated with a modification in their *nutritive movement,* it is evident that the aforementioned complicated action that the cerebellum transmits by its efferent pathway is intimately associated with a *trophic action,* be it *direct* or *indirect.*

The *direct trophic action* is amply demonstrated by the conspicuous *degeneration* and *sclerosis* that follow ablation of the cerebellum. The *indirect trophic action* is specially disclosed with the slow *muscular* and *cutaneous degeneration* and with the different general and local *dystrophic forms* which are often observed during the course of cerebellar ataxia and constantly with the slower growth and renewal of the tissue elements and with decreased resistance of the animal against the injurious action of external agents through which a healthy animal more readily becomes sick and in general has a relatively brief life.

The trophic influence, transmitted from the cerebellum along its afferent pathways, is by its nature and under normal conditions a *slow, quiet, continuous influence*—insofar as the intensity is variable. Similarly *slow, quiet,* and *continuous* is the *functional* influence (sthenic, tonic, and static) that the cerebellum normally transmits to the other nervous centers.

. . . .

The complex of *irritative phenomena* of cerebellar origin amply confirm what we have deduced from the *deficiency phenomena* [second postablation period] regarding the double influence which the cerebellum normally exercises upon the other nerve centers.

The trophic and the functional influence (asthenic, tonic, and static) most probably represent two sides or different aspects (that is, the internal and external aspects) of one and the same complicated physiological process, the essence of which is unknown to us and of which we know only the effects in their more apparent and appreciable characters.

All this is the logical result, direct as well as indirect, of the sum of our experiments and the critical examination of the phenomena that accompany cerebellar diseases. However, all this is far from hypothetical but is the rational synthesis of the complex of acquired facts which science has elucidated; in other words, it is the total result of experiments and observations concerning the *physiological theory of the cerebellum* without the aid of any hypothesis or speculative element beyond the realm of science.

. . . .

. . . . There is no part of the nervous system in which extirpation, mechanical or simple excision, would not cause ascending and descending degeneration and more or less marked and continuous alterations of general metabolism; in other words, which would not demonstrate that it exercises under normal conditions a *direct trophic action* upon those elements to which its activity is directed and an *indirect trophic action* upon the entire system.

. . . .

It is therefore evident that the *direct* and *indirect trophic action* exercised by the cerebellum, is not a specific characteristic by the activity of which this organ is distinguished in any way from the other centers or segments of the nervous system.

As regards the *functional action* that we have recognized in the cerebellum, at first it seems that it is essentially different from that attributed to the other centers of the system. While in fact the cerebellar deficiencies are expressed with simple *asthenic, atonic, and astatic* phenomena, the deficiencies of the other centers have in consequence true *complete or incomplete sensory and motor paralysis.* But this difference certainly depends upon two facts that we have emphasized as fundamental to the physiology of the cerebellum: on the fact that this organ, with its dependencies, forms a little, relatively independent system, through the lack of which there is no interruption in the pathways of centripetal and centrifugal conduction between the cerebrum and the peripheral sensory and motor apparatus; and on the second fact that the cerebellum does not have its own area of action, that is to say, exclusively reserved to it and to which the influence of the centers of the cerebrospinal axis does not also reach. Precisely for these reasons the cerebellar system, because of the special conditions that control its actions, may be considered as a small *auxiliary* or *reinforcing* system for the large cerebrospinal system.

But even if one admits this, the difference between the functions of the cerebellum and those of the other cerebrospinal centers does not become less distinctive.

We have seen that the *functional activity* under normal conditions develops slowly, quietly, and uninterruptedly, like its *trophic activity*. We have therefore considered these two forms of action as the two different aspects of one and the same process in the cerebellum. On the other hand we know that the most characteristic and best known functions of the cerebrospinal centers occur in violent, interrupted, and, according to the circumstances, changeable manner relative to the special nature of the processes which produce the external *reflex* and *voluntary* actions.

We have also seen that up to now nothing justifies us in the assumption (which has been well established for the cerebrospinal centers) that the functional activity of the cerebellum does not take place in the relative obscurity of the unconscious but has a direct part in any psychic phenomena.

It is therefore evident that the cerebellum plays a less elevated role in the physiological hierarchy of the different foci of activity from which the entire central system results, and that in the slow phylogenetic evolution of the functions, the centers representing the cerebrospinal system have made greater progress, that is to say, have accumulated a greater sum of the hereditary attitudes.

It does not follow from this, however, that the different cerebrospinal centers, in acquiring these new and more elevated attitudes, have lost the older ones. The *trophic* influence that we have seen to have them in common with the cerebellum cannot be associated with a *sthenic, tonic,* and *static* influence perfectly identical with that exercised by the cerebellum, the one and the other form of activity being two different and inseparable aspects of an identical process.

The final conclusion, inevitable from all these considerations, is that the complete physiological activity of the cerebellum is not a *specific* activity *sui generis*; but rather a *common* activity, and therefore *fundamental to the whole nervous system as such*.

SANTIAGO RAMÓN Y CAJAL

(See p. 109)

In his book on the cerebellum Luciani (1891) commented as follows on the contemporary state of knowledge concerning the histological structure of the cerebellum.

EXCERPT P. 311

The knowledge that we possess up to the present of the fine structure of the cerebellum, principally owing to the splendid drawings and detailed descriptions of it furnished by Golgi and his school, is of little value in resolving any physiological problem, much less in illuminating the profound obscurity, or in revealing even in the slightest the mystery that surrounds the innermost process whence cerebellar activity originates. Nevertheless they are of inestimable value since they can provide us with an adequate concept of the relative scarcity of our actual knowledge and of the enormous distance at which, up to now, we find ourselves, from the depth to the height of science that we can vaguely see represented as the ideal of the physiology of the cerebellum.

Although the Purkyně cell of the cerebellum (see pp. 55–56) had been one of the first special nerve cells described (1837), an adequate description of the other cerebellar cortical elements had to await the new techniques and experience of men like Golgi (see p. 91) and Ramón y Cajal. The gradual acceptance of the neuron theory (Chapter II) also made it easier to understand the structure of the cerebellar cortex and, as seen already, the Purkyně cell provided Ramón y Cajal with a vital link in the evidence favoring this doctrine (pp. 110–111).

Ramón y Cajal's findings, together with those of Golgi, showed that the cerebellar cortex, unlike that of the cerebrum, was relatively simple morphologically and that there was a remarkable uniformity throughout its various folia. This was excellent support for Luciani's unitarian concept of cerebellar function, and it partly explains the persistence of his opinion.

A passage from Ramón y Cajal's studies of the histology of the cerebellar cortex has been selected to represent the large amount of work carried out on this subject at the end of the nineteenth century. It has been translated from his Croonian Lecture of 1894 ("La fine structure des centres nerveux," *Proc. R. Soc.*, 1894, 55:444–468) and gives an excellent summary of the microscopic appearances of the cerebellar cortex as they were known at the end of the nineteenth century. Few additions have since been made by light microscopy.

EXCERPT PP. 458–461

Let us see now what are the *neurons and the connections of these neurons in a lamella* [folia] *of the cerebellum* (Fig. 5 [fig. 151]). A transverse section, for example, will show us three concentric layers of neurons.

The first one, or molecular zone, is formed mainly of small, superficial, star-shaped cells. The second, or intermediary one, is made up of Purkyně's cells [pp. 55–56]. The third is the result of an agglomeration of granular cells.

All these elements offer two kinds of relations: intrinsic ones, that is, those established between the cells of three layers; extrinsic connections, that is, those which take place between the neurons of the cerebellum and those belonging to other nerve organs.

Let us examine successively the intrinsic and extrinsic connections. First, the connections of Purkyně's cells with the small, star-shaped elements of the molecular layer. The relations established between these two types of cells constitute the most classic example of pericellular nerve arborizations and the most eloquent factor for transmission by contact, or by contiguity, of nerve activity [see pp. 110–111].

The small star-shaped elements of the molecular layer are flattened in the same way as Purkyně's cells; they possess a protoplasmic, divergent ramification [dendrite] that never extends beyond the thickness of the layer in which they are contained, and a horizontal axis cylinder, the course of which is perpendicular to the longitudinal axis of the cerebellar folia. This axis cylinder extension gives off several descending collaterals and, following a variable course, describes a curve in order to terminate by means of a very rich and varicose arborization, in the region of Purkyně's cells. These terminal arborizations, as well as the collateral descending shoots, branch out repeatedly and constitute a very tight plexus around Purkyně's cells, which ends in a brush point at the inferior part of the body of these cells, at the very place of origin of their axis cylinder. Therefore we have given this arrangement the name of *descending brushes*, but Kölliker, Retzius, and the other authors who have confirmed its existence, prefer the name *terminal baskets*.

Why then not consider these pericellular networks as a means of connection between the star-shaped cells of the molecular layer and Purkyně's cells? And it is very necessary to know that this connection is not an individual one; it is general, which means that each pericellular plexus encloses ramifications coming from several star-shaped cells.

Let us now look at *the relations between the granules and Purkyně's cells*. The granules of the cerebellum [fig. 151, *E*] are small neural elements, the agglomeration of which constitutes almost exclusively the granular layer. They possess three or four short protoplasmic processes [dendrites], adorned at their extremity with a finger-like arborization, and an axis cylinder of extraordinary slenderness. The latter ascends to the molecular zone and there bifurcates at different levels, thus producing a longitudinal fibril which runs parallel to the whole cerebellar folia [fig. 151, *F*]. These interesting fibrils, which we have called *parallel* because they are arranged parallel to the direction of the folia of the cerebellum during their entire passage, are in very close contact with the spinous contours of the protoplasmic branches of Purkyně's cells. As each parallel fibril runs through the entire length of the cerebellar convolution and terminates there in free and rounded endings, it follows that a single granule can act upon a multitude of Purkyně's cells. It is also very probable that each of these latter is subjected to the influence of a considerable number of granular cells.

The *extrinsic relations, or those between the cells of the cerebellum and those of other nerve centers,* have been and still are the most difficult to establish. As Golgi was the first to demonstrate, Purkyně's cells give birth to nerve extensions of the long type, the termination of which has been ignored, and, inversely, axis cylinders coming from other organs, the site of which is still very problematic, terminate in the gray substance of the cerebellum. These are the *mossy* and the *climbing fibres*.

The *mossy* fibres are coarse, myelin tubes that ramify and end in the granular layer where they come into contact with the protoplasmic expansions of these small elements by means of certain outgrowths or collateral eruptions. The terminal branches end in a varicosity or a small ramification in the shape of a rosette.

The *climbing fibres* traverse that layer of granules, skirt Purkyně's cells, and surround the ascending stem and the main protoplasmic branches of these elements in a splendid, terminal, elongated arborization, exactly comparable to that of the motor fibre in muscle bundles.

The conclusion to what we have just reported is that the granular cells and Purkyně's cells can receive nerve impulses from other centers, either by means of mossy fibres, or by climbing fibres; while the small, star-shaped cells of the molecular layer as well as the large star-shaped elements of the granular zone, which belong to the second type of Golgi's cells [p. 94], seem to have no connection with the extrinsic fibres. This has prompted me to name these two latter species of cells as *association corpuscles,* for it seems that their sole role is to unite Purkyně's cells, or the granules, into a dynamic entity, the significance of which is actually obscure.

CHARLES SCOTT SHERRINGTON
(*See p. 238*)

The role of the cerebellum in maintaining the smoothness and effectiveness of muscular movement was emphasized by Sherrington. He conceived of the cerebellum as "the head ganglion of the proprioceptive system" because it regulated the postural tone of muscles or groups of muscles acting as agonists, antagonists, and fixators. It did this by means of the afferent impulses that reached it from proprioceptors in the contracting muscles, in joints, in tendons, and in the vestibular apparatus. It was, in other words, an afferent recipient body, a conclusion supported by Luciani, Jackson, Edinger, and Horsley as well as by Sherrington.

Sherrington thus also supported the unitarian concept of cerebellar function, very vaguely conceived by Rolando but vigorously expressed and supported by Luciani. The first passages below have been taken from Sherrington's contribution to E. A. Schäfer's *Text book of physiology* ([Edinburgh, 1900], Vol. II).

EXCERPT PP. 908–909

The so to say highly technical movements ordered by the cerebral cortex employ comparatively limited aggregates of musculature, e.g., speech employing the muscles of the oral and laryngeal regions, grasp employing the muscles of a single limb. The muscular mechanisms of progression and pose, the innervation of which may, as above suggested, be centred together, perhaps in the thalamencephalon, are of wider spatial distribution, and employ not one side of the trunk but both sides, not one limb but all four. Often they probably involve the musculature of the entire body. It is because of its intimacy of connection with such movements as these that the cerebellum is an organ which justifies Hesiod's ὅσῳ πλέον ἥμισυ παντός. The division into hemispheres and middle lobe is founded merely upon gross anatomy. The organ commonly, probably always, "functions" as a whole. Luciani is right to insist on this, and the reason that it "functions" as a whole seems clearly because it is so largely a piece of mechanism that deals with the innervation, not of this or that piece of musculature, but of the musculature of the body as a whole. The earlier observers, Flourens, Bouilland [*sic*], etc., stated this when they spoke of the cerebellum as an organ of "equilibration."

EXCERPT P. 910

To sum up: the cerebellum is the organ rather of a particular class of reactions than of a particular sense. Its reactions have their sources in the sensifacient organs of various senses, but especially of those pregnant with spatial quality, and in those subserving the "muscular sense," in the widest meaning of that term. It supports the tonus of the majority, perhaps of all, the cranio-spinal motor root cells, of some more than others, e.g., those connected with eye muscles, neck muscles, muscles of the spine. It preponderantly helps to secure co-ordinate innervation of the skeletal musculature, both for maintenance of attitude and for execution of movements. So far as the geotropism and stereotropism of the animal can be "centred" at any one limited field of the central nervous system, that field is cerebellar. It supports habitual posture, and is at least as importantly associated with the movements dependent on the lower cerebral centres (e.g., walking, running), as with those elaborated in connection with the highest (e.g., technical movements).

The main expression of Sherrington's concept of cerebellar function is to be found in his book, *The integrative action of the nervous system* (New Haven, 1906).

EXCERPT PP. 347–349

The cerebellum is the head ganglion of the proprio-ceptive system. If the basis taken for classification of receptors be a physiological one with, as its criterion, the type of reaction which the receptors induce, separate receptive systems may be traced running throughout the whole series of segments composing the total organism. We have seen that such separate receptive systems may be treated as functional unities, extending through the segmental series. In any such system there is evident a tendency for its central nervous mechanisms, that is to say, the components of the central nervous organ which specially accrue to the system in question, to be gathered chiefly where the most important contribution to its receptive paths enters the central nervous system. The receptive system in question has as it were its focus at that place. Thus receptive neurones which can influence respiratory movement enter the central nervous organ at various segments, but the chief respiratory centre lies in the bulb where the receptive neurones from the lung itself make entrance and central connection, the vagal receptors being preponderantly regulative in that function. And we have seen that a proprio-ceptive organ (the labyrinth) in the head segments seems preponderantly regulative in those functions which the proprio-ceptive system subserves. The central neural mechanism belonging to the proprio-ceptive system is preponderantly built up over the central connections of this proprio-ceptive organ (the labyrinth) belonging to the head. Thither converge internuncial paths stretching to this mechanism from the central endings of various proprio-ceptive neurones situate in all the segments of the body. There afferent contributions from the receptors of joints, muscles, ligaments, tendons, viscera, etc., combine with those from the muscular organs of the head and with those of the labyrinthine receptors themselves. A central nervous organ of high complexity results. Its size from animal species to animal species strikingly accords with the range and complexity of the habitual movements of the species; in other words, with the range and complexity of the habitual taxis of the skeletal musculature. This central organ is the cerebellum.

The symptoms produced by its destruction or injury in whole or in part in many ways resemble, therefore, the disturbances produced by injury of the labyrinth itself. It also influences tonus very much as do the simple proprio-ceptive arcs themselves. It is closely connected structurally and functionally with the so-called motor region of the cerebral hemisphere, just as the simpler proprio-ceptive arcs and reflexes are closely associated with the mechanisms of extero-ceptive reactions. Knowledge is not ripe as yet for an adequate definition of the function of the cerebellum. Many authorities have defined it as the centre for the maintenance of the mechanical equilibrium of the body. Others regard it as the organ for co-ordination of volitional movement. Spencer suggested that it was the organ of co-ordination of bodily action in regard to space, the cerebrum he suggested being the organ of co-ordination of bodily action in respect of time. Lewandowski considers it the central organ for the "muscular sense." Luciani, the universally acknowledged authority on the physiology of the cerebellum, describes it as the organ which by unconscious processes exerts a continual reinforcing action on the activity of all other nerve-centres.

It is instructive to note how all these separate pronouncements harmonize with the supposition that the organ is the chief co-ordinative centre or rather group of centres of the reflex system of proprio-ception. The cerebellum may indeed be described as the head-ganglion of the proprio-ceptive system, and the head ganglion here, as in other systems, is the main ganglion.

Clinical Contributions

Accurate and precise experiments on the cerebellum have never been easy to perform because of its location. It is often difficult to expose and the delicate structures in the nearby brainstem are easily damaged. Thus data concerning cerebellar function has had to be collected from all available sources, and one of the most important of these has been clinical observations in man. These have not only supplemented animal experiments which could not be expected to reveal the functioning of the human cerebellum, if only because man stands on two limbs, but they have also confirmed or refuted conclusions derived from them. With the development of neurology in various centers such as Paris, London, Berlin, Vienna, and Philadelphia towards the end of the nineteenth century, new and more precise methods of eliciting and evaluating the clinical manifestations of lesions of the nervous system were perfected. Two of the most important contributions to the elucidation of a cerebellar deficit were those of Babinski of Paris and Holmes of London.

Joseph François Félix Babinski
(See p. 359)

Babinski analyzed with great clarity the clinical manifestations of cerebellar deficit, and several of the terms used to describe them originate from his work. The following passages have been taken from a collection of his writings edited by himself (*Exposé des travaux scientifiques*, Paris, 1913) and include first of all some general remarks. The second passage is an account of one of the signs of cerebellar disorder first described by Babinski as "adiadokokinesia" in 1902 ("Sur le rôle du cervelet dans les actes volitionnels nécessitant une succession rapide de mouvements (diadococinésie)," *Revue neurol.*, 1902, 10:1013–1015).

EXCERPT PP. 134–135

DISORDERS OF THE CEREBELLUM

The anatomic and functional connections that join the cerebellum to the non-acoustic [vestibular] labyrinth explain the close relationship presented by the symptomatology of cerebellar and labyrinthine disorders. This association has been proved, as is known, by Flourens' memorable experiments.

With the exception of the tremor, the scanning speech, difficulty with writing, which by the way have been chiefly studied in multiple sclerosis, and of "cerebellar ataxia," a poorly defined phenomenon, the clinical characteristics attributed in the classic textbooks to cerebellar affections belong also to disturbances of the vestibular apparatus. It is the same with forced attitudes, forced movements, lateral propulsion, the spreading apart of the legs, drunken staggering, vertigo, and nystagmus. Perhaps certain of these disturbances are common even to vestibular lesions, and it is at least unquestionable that in diseases of the cerebellum, their presence or their severity is very often partly owing to involvement of the vestibular nerve or of the nuclei to which it proceeds.

Undoubtedly, these various symptoms are not absolutely identical because their origin is either labyrinthine or cerebellar, but the differences are not sufficiently pronounced so that one may establish a clear and reliable demarcation line between them.

My investigations have led me to discover and to analyze several phenomena which one must rightly consider—while at the same time making some reservations on certain points—as actually belonging to the symptomatology of cerebellar affections. These are: asynergia, adiadokokinesia and cerebellar catalepsy. I am adding to it excessive motions [dysmetria], a sign to the establishment of which I have contributed.

ADIADOKOKINESIA

Adiadokokinesia is the suspension or decrease of the ability to carry out rapidly successive, voluntary movements. It is the very loss of this function which makes us aware of its existence.

A healthy subject is able to carry out a rapid succession of simple movements, such as turning his hand quickly from pronation to supination alternately.

However, in the cerebellar patient, the following may be noted: His muscular strength is intact; he carries out each of the basic movements of pronation and supination as promptly as a normal individual; but he achieves the complete movement, based upon the succession of these two movements, two or three times less rapidly than a healthy subject. The phenomenon becomes particularly obvious if he is made to repeat the same movements many times.

In order to name the function which is thus disturbed, I have proposed a neologism derived from two Greek words, one of which signifies "successive," the other "movement." The word diadokokinesia is a synonym for successive movements, and by extending it, may designate the function which permits the fulfillment of these movements.

Regarding the term "adiadokokinesia" as proposed by Bruns and currently used in the observations, by adding the prefix "a" it expresses the loss or change in this function.

In order to avoid all misunderstanding, I have been careful, from the start, to make it understood that this disturbance should not be considered as actually taking place unless the subject manifests that he is able to execute promptly the basic motions. It is self-evident that an individual who is incapable of carrying out quickly an isolated motion, be it that of pronation or supination, cannot *a fortiori* accomplish a rapid succession of both movements.

Until now, adiadokokinesia has been observed mainly in upper limbs. It is sometimes bilateral, and sometimes unilateral; in the latter case, it depends upon a lesion which involves the same side; this constitutes an important symptom from the diagnostic point of view.

How to explain adiadokokinesia? Here is the interpretation which I have given in my first report on this subject [this exact wording is not to be found in the article of 1902 nor in another article on the subject in the same volume, pp. 470–474]:

"In order to understand adiadokokinesia, it is necessary to analyse diadokokinesia. So that the alternate movements of pronation and supination succeed each other rapidly, it is indispensable that each of these successive motions be well regulated, be not excessive, and that the time lost between the two successive movements be reduced to a minimum. These conditions are realized, thanks to a regulatory action combining the excitomotor action which we are interested in (excitomotor action of reinforcement resulting in a reduction of the duration of time lost between the voluntary stimulus and the end of the contraction). Adiadokokinesia would be the result of a disturbance in this mechanism."

Perhaps it can be said that cerebellar lesions may, without decreasing the muscular energy, induce inertia in a way that would indicate the difficulty of being thrown into action and the impossibility at times of stopping the movement.

In his book of 1913 Babinski also gave original accounts of asynergia, dysmetria, and of "cerebellar catalepsy" which was a disturbance of equilibration. The last, however, was described in 1909 ("Quelques documents relatifs à l'histoire des fonctions de l'appareil cérébelleux et de leurs perturbations," *Revue mens. Méd. interne Thér.*, 1909, 1:113–129).

EXCERPT PP. 123–124

It has been admitted that the cerebellum plays an essential role in equilibration and that cerebellar lesions disturb this function.

This is beyond question, but my observations demand that this concept be further defined, for expressed as it has been until now, it does not hold up against criticism.

The term equilibrium has several connotations. In contemporary speech it means "that a body stands upright without leaning to either side" (Littré).

By using the word in this sense, one may rightly say that a staggering and asynergic cerebellar subject cannot maintain his equilibrium.

But this word has also another meaning: "state of the body maintained at rest under the influence of several forces which counterbalance each other exactly" (Littré). If one understands it in this way, one is justified in saying that a patient stricken with cerebellar catalepsy demonstrates an exaltation of equilibration. Besides, since this patient [whose detailed case study was given in this report] is at the same time asynergic and cataleptic, one is entitled to sustain, according to the point of view one takes, that his equilibratory function is diminished or increased.

This leads me to remark that equilibrium must be looked at from two angles: as the body finds itself in a state of active immobility . . . . or rather that it is in motion, that it changes position.

In the first case equilibrium may be qualified as static and in the second case as kinetic. Moreover, since in the two cases we have seen that the realization of equilibrium requires the intervention of a voluntary act I call these two variations of equilibrium or equilibration volitional. The choice of these expressions can be readily criticized, but we are dealing here merely with a matter of convention and it is sufficient for an understanding.

In the normal state the volitional kinetic equilibrium is realized more easily than the static one. Indeed, it is easier to walk than to stand still without titubation and much more difficult to stand quietly on one leg than to hop on one leg.

. . . .

In cerebellar affections which I am considering particularly here, the volitional kinetic equilibrium may be profoundly disturbed while the volitional static equilibrium is maintained or even increased.

It follows from the foregoing that, on the one hand, the investigators must in the future consider each of these two types of equilibrium separately, and that, on the other hand, the classic reports on disturbances of the equilibrium in cerebellar affections are no longer unimpeachable as far as the volitional kinetic equilibrium is concerned.

GORDON MORGAN HOLMES
(*See p. 537*)

Another outstanding addition to our knowledge of the clinical manifestations of cerebellar dysfunction in man, and thus to our appreciation of the organ's normal function, was a paper published in 1917 by the British neurologist Holmes ("The symptoms of acute cerebellar injuries due to gunshot injuries," *Brain*, 1917, 40:461–535). As with his work on the visual pathways (pp. 537–539), he studied cases of brain damage resulting from World War I, and he also included cases of cerebellar space-occupying lesions. His classic analysis of cerebellar deficit confirmed the experimental findings of Luciani (pp. 662–668) and was aimed at acquiring "an insight into the normal functions and the physiological properties of this organ" (p. 518).

The following excerpts have been taken from Chapter V which deals with atonia, asthenia, and astasia which resulted from injury to the cerebellum, and the remainder of the article considers in turn asynergia, dysmetria, speech defect, nystagmus, etc. Chapter VI contains Holmes's opinions on "functional localisation in the cerebellum," and he concluded as follows:

"But though my observations lend no support to the theory of focal localisation of function in the cerebellar cortex they cannot be accepted as proof that such localisation does not exist" (p. 534). Thus doubt was being cast upon the unitarian concept which at this time was almost universally accepted.

EXCERPT PP. 518–524

The first point which demands attention is the nature of the symptoms already described. Are they to be attributed to destructive or to irritative lesions of the cerebellum? Their constancy, their regularity, their persistence for long periods, and especially their nature, suggest strongly that they are directly due to destruction and that they are consequently negative or defect phenomena. In the case of many of them, as the muscular atonia, this cannot be doubted, and indeed careful observation makes it probable that irritative effects are minimal after gunshot injuries of the cerebellum in man. Those forced movements and attitudes which Luciani has tentatively termed "dynamic phenomena" [pp. 663–665], that occur so commonly after experimental injuries in animals, are very rarely seen in man, or occur at least only as immediate symptoms . . . . It may be consequently safely assumed that the functional disturbances with which we have to deal are produced only by negative or destructive lesions of the cerebellum.

It is worthy of note that, as von Monakow has pointed out, symptoms referable to the effects of shock or diaschisis [pp. 619–623] on other parts of the nervous system are rarely obvious.

Atonia, or diminution of that slight constant tension which is characteristic of healthy muscle, is such a constant and striking feature of all early injuries, and persists for such long periods when the wounds are large, that it is obviously a primary and direct result of the lesion.

The state of the tendon-jerks has been generally taken by clinicians as a measure of tone, and yet it is the rule that even in the toneless limb of a cerebellar patient the knee-jerks and similar reflexes are not abolished, and the excursion of the jerks may be even larger than on the normal side . . . . The presence of the knee-jerk is consequently not an argument against the existence of atonia in cerebellar disease.

But even when septic infection and the effects of increased cerebrospinal pressure can be excluded the knee-jerk and the other tendon reflexes are in some cases depressed, or they may be even for a time absent, on the side of an early and extensive lesion. As far as clinical observations go this seems to be generally associated with an extreme atonicity of the muscles, but their relation is probably not direct. The depression of the reflexes may be due to transient shock or diaschisis as it is [in] an early hemiplegia; but the more probable explanation is that when the muscles are so atonic a tap on the tendon does not produce a sufficient increment of tension in them to be an adequate stimulus. The common observation that a reflex response can be frequently elicited by only one of a series of taps, or when the knee is in a certain position, and that the jerk is then quite brisk, favours the latter hypothesis.

This is probably also the explanation of the failure of the "rebound phenomenon" in the homolateral limbs. The excessive range of the after-movement may be due to absence or too long delay of the voluntary contraction of the antagonistic muscles—the fact that the patient's hand can be flung forcibly into his face shows that prompt voluntary arrest is not possible—but it must be ascribed mainly to failure of the immediate reflex contraction of the antagonists when they are suddenly stretched. The absence of contraction of the hamstring muscles when the knee-jerk is elicited under certain conditions, and the failure of the forearm muscles to contract when they are suddenly elongated by an abrupt jerk of the limb, are similar phenomena; the muscles do not react normally to a sudden putting on stretch.

. . . .

. . . . The study of the knee-jerk by the graphic method shows that the tonic contraction of the quadriceps, which prevents the free and immediate fall of the extended leg under the influence of gravity, is absent or diminished when the homolateral side of the cerebellum is injured; the jerk has then the character of that described by Sherrington when the reflex excitability of postural contraction is low, or when what Langelaan calls plastic tone, that is the slow yielding of the extensor muscles to a continued stress, is absent or diminished.

. . . .

It seems that the various symptoms of atonia described above can be attributed to this loss or diminution of postural contraction or plastic tone; its absence abolishes the normal resistances of the various segments of the limbs to passive movement, leaves the muscles less elastic to sudden stretching, and makes them soft and flabby to palpation.

Clinical experience, therefore, fully confirms the statements of Luciani and other physiologists that atonia is a constant, important, and striking result of acute cerebellar destruction. It diminishes gradually in time, and may, like all the other symptoms, disappear, at least if the lesion is not very extensive . . . .

. . . .

. . . .

The next group of symptoms that claim our attention are those seen in voluntary movement. Certain of them are most easily studied in simple actions against resistance. It has been shown that when a man with a cerebellar lesion attempts to grasp the observer's two hands simultaneously: (1) the power exerted by the affected limb is defective; (2) the initiation and the execution of muscular contractions and relaxations are slower than on the normal side; (3) the grasp is often intermittent and irregularly maintained; and (4) the affected limb tires more quickly than its fellow. These symptoms can be equally well demonstrated in other actions.

Asthenia.—This term, which Luciani has applied to the diminished functional energy of the affected limb, may be conveniently used to describe their lack of normal power in movements that demand its exertion. It differs so definitely from the paralysis and paresis produced by the diseases of the motor system that it is advisable to designate it by a distinct word.

. . . . Asthenia must be consequently regarded as another primary and immediate symptom of cerebellar injury. It is probably pronounced only when the cerebellar nuclei are involved. The abnormal fatiguability of the affected limbs is associated with, and may be regarded as a result of, this asthenia.

Slowness in movement has been noticed by both clinical and experimental observers . . . .

In order to understand its nature it is necessary to study simple actions, and if possible by the aid of the graphic method. It is then seen that the slowness is due both to delay in starting the contraction and to slowness in completing it. Further, careful examination shows that there is usually associated with it a similar delay in commencing and completing the relaxation of the same muscles, which is occasionally even more pronounced . . . . It consequently seems that the cerebellum exerts an influence on the nervous mechanisms, most probably on the spinal, immediately concerned in the execution of voluntary muscular contractions, by virtue of which these react promptly to cerebral impressions.

The cerebellum might be therefore regarded as a motor reinforcing organ, in the sense in which Luciani and others have used this term. It seems, however, probable that it takes no direct part in the processes, whether initiated reflexly or voluntarily, that produce motor effects, and that it does not augment these, but that it "sets," or "tunes," or regulates the activity of certain motor mechanisms, most probably spinal, so that the response to a volitional stimulus is immediate, effective, and proportional to the intensity of the cerebral impulse.

Closely associated with asthenia is the discontinuity and irregularity in the maintenance of muscular contractions. This disturbance can be observed occasionally in voluntary movements and in the contractions of muscles concerned in maintaining posture (static tremor), but it is most easily studied in actions that demand the exertion of power; in these the contractions reach their maximum slowly and intermittently, and while in the normal limb a forcible contraction can be maintained regularly for some time, the grasp or other action which the patient attempts with the affected limb is often discontinuous and irregular, and it is frequently interrupted by sudden relaxations. The outstretched arm if unsupported often, for instance, falls suddenly, and in walking the affected leg frequently gives way under the patient without any apparent cause. The tremor that occurs in maintaining an attitude and in voluntary movement is due to this defect in the regularity and stability of the muscular contractions. Luciani has described this condition as *astasia,* and has attributed it to the imperfect fusion and summation of the single twitch contractions . . . .

Astasia is not, however, such a prominent symptom in most local lesions of the cerebellum in man as it is in animals after experimental destruction, though it varies in degree in different cases. It does not seem to stand in any close relation to the atonia and it is probably not in any way dependent upon it; it is, on the other hand, intimately associated with asthenia. Consequently, in addition to that function by virtue of which it assures that the motor response to a voluntary cerebral impulse shall be immediate and proportional to the impulse, the cerebellum also exerts an influence on the efficiency of this response by determining the complete fusion of the elementary muscle twitches.

Clinical observations consequently confirm Luciani's conclusions that atonia, asthenia, and astasia, the triad of symptoms to which he attributes all the functional disturbances, result from cerebellar lesions.

Modern Approaches

As Dow and Moruzzi (1958) have pointed out, modern research on the physiology of the cerebellum can be divided into three main approaches to the problem:
- *a*) A search for evidence substantiating the equilibratory function of the cerebellum.
- *b*) A search for evidence favoring the theory of functional localization in the cerebellum rather than the unitarian concept.
- *c*) The investigation of cerebellar electrophysiology.

The first two find their roots in the nineteenth century whereas the third is of more recent origin. The pursuit of them will no doubt contribute largely to the solution in the future of some of the major problems concerning cerebellar function.

A. Equilibratory Function

Evidence has accumulated since early in the nineteenth century that the cerebellum plays a role in the maintenance of the body's equilibrium. The subject is, however, of immense complexity, and only in the last few decades has any real advance towards its solution been possible. Three early predecessors of this modern work have been selected below. Magendie's crude experiments of 1824 gave origin to the idea, and Ferrier much later in the century added more precise and detailed experimental evidence for it. Many others have also contributed, in particular A. Stefani ("Contribuzione alla fisiologia del cervelletto," *Atti Accad. Sci. med. nat. Ferrara*, 1877, 12:193–211), but there is no doubt that present-day investigations have developed largely from the pioneer studies of Magnus and his colleagues.

François Magendie
(See p. 299)

It has been claimed by Longet (1842, pp. 743, 749–750) that Pourfour du Petit (p. 265) first described a disturbance of equilibrium following section of the cerebellar peduncles, but this cannot be verified. He did, however, study the effect of cerebellar injury in man and animals (Duckett, 1964) and concluded (1710, p. 20) that "from these experiments it seemed to me that the cerebellum does not produce the spirits for sensation; what kind they are we have not been able to decide with certainty." Peduncle section was, however, carried out by Magendie in 1824 ("Mémoire sur les fonctions de quelques parties du système nerveux," *J. Physiol., Paris*, 1824, 4:399–407), and it provided the first certain evidence of the cerebellum's role in equilibration. He observed that the animal developed skew deviation of the eyes and that it rolled towards the side of the lesion. But like Rolando and Flourens, his techniques were crude and the effects he observed were probably owing to damage of the brainstem vestibular nuclei, for a histological control of the lesions was not, of course, available at that time. Nevertheless, Magendie originated the important idea that the cerebellum might be the center for the nervous mechanism of equilibrium. His original observations were owing to a chance section of the peduncle in a rabbit while trying to cut the fifth cranial nerve.

EXCERPT PP. 400–402

In carrying out this delicate manoeuvre which was entirely new to me, I chanced unwittingly to damage and even to cut transversely one of the two cerebellar peduncles (*crura cerebelli*). Scarcely had I inflicted this accidental injury when I saw the animal turn over quickly on itself and nothing could stop it, or at least nothing could stop it making the necessary efforts to produce this peculiar revolving movement. I placed the animal in several positions, but it rolled incessantly until stopped by a physical object. I thought that this phenomenon would be of short duration but I observed it to continue for more than two hours . . . .

. . . .

[The following day the rotation persisted.] I then made an observation which had escaped me on the previous day. The animal's eyes had lost their alignment and normal movement. They had become fixed in an inverse manner; the one on the side of the lesion was directed downwards and in front and the contralateral one was held upwards and towards the back [skew deviation] . . . . [After eight days] autopsy revealed that I had cut a large part of the cerebellar peduncle corresponding to the side towards which the animal when held had had a tendency to turn.

I took steps to repeat this experiment and cut the same parts in another animal. This I carried out on a second rabbit in which I produced exactly the same phenomena. But as I had cut the left peduncle, the movement of rotation was in the direction from right to left: it may be recalled that it was the reverse in the previous experiment when I had cut the right peduncle.

I verified the correctness of these results on several occasions and I could no longer deny that they were of great importance.

Since the rotary movement was separately caused by section of the cerebellar peduncle, it became very probable that the nerve thread was the transmitting agent of a force which in a healthy animal counterbalances a similar force passing through the other peduncle. It was through the equilibrium of these two forces that the state of standing and even the possibility of rest and of various regular and voluntary movements of the animal resulted.

To verify this conjecture it was necessary to cut both cerebellar peduncles [i.e., bilaterally] in the same animal; then the animal ought not be able to produce any rotatory movement and ought to remain immobile.

Experiment completely confirmed the conjecture I had formed . . . .

DAVID FERRIER

(*See p. 513*)

The modern period of investigations into the equilibratory function began with Ferrier who carried out a series of stimulation experiments on a variety of animals including monkeys and dogs. Although many of his findings have since been shown to be due to faulty experimental techniques, and although he did not envisage a cerebellovestibular connection, his work nevertheless was a pioneer attempt to solve a very complex problem. The following passages have been taken from his book, *The functions of the brain* (London, 1876).

EXCERPT PP. 109–113

The cerebellum would, therefore, seem to be a complex arrangement of individually differentiated centres, which in associated action regulate the various muscular adjustments necessary to maintain equilibrium of the body; each tendency to the displacement of the equilibrium round a horizontal, vertical, or intermediate axis, acting as a stimulus to the special centre which calls into play the antagonistic or compensatory action.

Every form of active muscular exertion must tend to overthrow the balance, and we should therefore expect, on the above hypothesis, that the cerebellum would be developed in proportion to the variety and complexity of the muscular activity of which the animal was capable; a relation which is fully borne out by the facts of comparative anatomy (Owen). We should, further, expect to find that a lesion which annihilates the functional activity of any of the individual cerebellar centres, should manifest itself in a tendency to the overthrow of the balance in the direction naturally opposed by this centre. This also is in accordance with the facts of experiment. We have seen that stimulation of the anterior part of the middle lobe [vermis] excites the muscular combinations which would counteract a tendency to fall forwards. Hence destruction of this part shows itself in a tendency to fall forwards. In this we see both the negative effect caused by the removal of the one centre, and the positive effect exerted by the unopposed and antagonistic centres.

In like manner stimulation of the posterior part of the middle lobe calls into play the muscular adjustments necessary to counteract a backward displacement of the equilibrium, and hence, as we have seen, destruction of this region manifests itself in a tendency to fall backwards.

The lateral lobes of the cerebellum contain centres for complex adjustments against lateral, combined with diagonal and rotatory displacements to the opposite side; and hence, as has been found by experiment, lesions of the lateral lobes exhibit themselves in disturbances of the equilibrium, either laterally, to the side opposite the lesion, or as the resultant of lateral and rotatory displacement in rolling over to the side of lesion. The effects of lesion of the lateral lobes may therefore vary, a fact which may account for some of the discrepancies among the results obtained by different experimenters.

. . . .

. . . .

Hence it is that lesions of the cerebellum, while interfering with the mechanical adjustments against disturbance of the bodily equilibrium, do not cause paralysis of voluntary motion of the muscles which are concerned in these actions. This is an exceedingly important fact which, though disputed by some, seems to be established experimentally beyond all question . . . .

. . . .

In terming the effect of cerebellar lesion a paralysis of reflex adjustment, I do not thereby imply a paralysis of reflex action. This, which would result from [a] spinal lesion, must necessarily coincide with paralysis of voluntary motion, as the path from the hemispheres would thereby be interrupted. What is implied is that the same combinations of muscular action which are co-ordinated in the cerebellum for the maintenance of the equilibrium, are capable of being called into voluntary action by the cerebral hemispheres. Hence, though lesions of the cerebellum destroy the self-adjusting co-ordination of muscular combinations necessary to maintain the equilibrium, they do not cause paralysis of voluntary motion in the same muscles. So, conversely, by removal of the cerebral hemispheres we cause paralysis of voluntary motion, but do not affect the independent mechanism of cerebellar co-ordination. When we make this necessary distinction we are enabled to understand how limited lesions of the cerebellum may produce only transient effects, and how even complete destruction of the cerebellum may ultimately be recovered from.

The disturbance of equilibrium is always most marked immediately after the infliction of injury to the cerebellum. This is to be accounted for by the sudden derangement of the self-adjusting mechanism on which the maintenance of the equilibrium mainly depends. As, however, the animal may supplement the loss of this mechanism by conscious effort, in process of time it acquires the power of voluntary adaptation, and thus is enabled to maintain its equilibrium, though perhaps with a less degree of security than before.

The more extensive the lesion, the greater the disturbance of the mechanism, and the greater the difficulty of effecting through conscious effort all the muscular adjustments necessary to maintain the balance. The disturbances of equilibrium are therefore of a more enduring character, and it is only by a long process of training that volitional acquisition can replace a mechanism essentially independent of consciousness. Even should this point be reached, the constant attention necessary to prevent displacement of the equilibrium would be a heavy strain on the animal's powers, and it would be quite in accordance with this condition, that prolonged or varied muscular effort should cause great apparent exhaustion. . . .

If it were possible to remove both cerebellum and cerebral hemispheres from a pigeon without causing speedy death, it might confidently be predicted that no recovery of the power of equilibration could ever take place.

A similar explanation is applicable to those cases of disease of the cerebellum which have been found to co-exist with little or no disturbance of equilibrium during life. A slowly progressive lesion would be the most favourable condition for the supplementation by conscious effort of a self-adaptative mechanism which is gradually undergoing degeneration. It is questionable, however, whether in man perfect substitution is possible; a want of precision and energy in movement, and a continual tendency to reel or fall being generally observable in cerebellar disease.

RUDOLF MAGNUS

(2 September 1873—25 July 1927)

Babinski's discussion of "cerebellar catalepsy" (pp. 676–677) represented an important clinical contribution to the problem of cerebellar function and equilibration. But the most important experimental attack upon the problem was made by the Dutch physiologist Magnus and his colleagues in Utrecht.

Magnus was born in Braunschweig, Germany, and studied medicine mainly at Heidelberg. Before and after being graduated, he worked in Heidelberg on problems of the cardiovascular, intestinal, and renal systems and in Edinburgh he studied pituitary function. In 1908 he worked with Sherrington in Liverpool on reflexes and in the same year was appointed professor of pharmacology at Utrecht, a position he held until his untimely death eighteen years later. There he carried out his classic experiments on the reflexes of equilibration and the whole question of body posture, as well as studies on choline and the effect of drugs on the nervous system (see Dale, 1930; Fulton, 1927–1928; Haymaker, 1953, pp. 149–152).

Together with his collaborators, such as de Kleijn, whose name today is associated with that of Magnus in the title of the reflexes they first described, he performed fundamental experiments that were the starting point for all modern investigators of this complicated field of body posture and vestibulocerebellar relationships. They studied, in animals, the tonic labyrinthine and neck reflexes and the labyrinthine righting reflexes by which the varying attitudes of the body are assumed in response to the changing needs of the organism and thus they provided basic data for the complex problem of the maintenance of posture. They then observed these reflexes before and after ablations of the cerebellum, cerebrum, brainstem, or cervical spinal cord. On the whole, their negative results appear at first sight to have been disappointing since these reflexes were found to be unchanged, for example, after complete cerebellectomy. However, they prepared the way for the study of posture, muscle tone, labyrinthine cerebellar proprioception fibres and the whole question of the equilibratory functions of the cerebellum. The extensive inquiries that have been carried out since the time of Magnus are, in fact, extensions of his work.

Magnus's first important paper appeared in 1914 ("Welche Teile des Zentralnervensystems müssen für das Zustandekommen der tonischen Hals- und Labyrinthreflexe auf die Körpermuskulatur vorhanden sein," *Pflügers Arch.*, 1914, 159:224–249). The following excerpt is the summary of his results derived from experiments on cats and rabbits.

EXCERPT P. 249

1. The tonic neck and labyrinthine reflexes affecting the muscles of the extremities and the neck can be produced in cats by changing the position of the body as well as by turning the head, and they appear after unilateral section of the eighth cranial nerve. They remain unchanged when the animals are decerebrated, when the entire cerebellum and quadrigeminal bodies are ablated, or when the brainstem is separated at the origin of the eighth cranial nerve by a coronal section.

2. Moreover, if the entry zone of the eighth nerve is removed, the labyrinthine reflexes cease; but the neck reflexes which effect the four limbs and which are produced by turning, bending, lifting, or lowering the head, remain unchanged. The whole of the medulla oblongata can be removed without impairing the neck reflexes. After removing the uppermost cervical segment [of the spinal cord] the neck reflexes are weakened, but after removing the second, they disappear.

The second classic paper on the cerebellum and equilibration was published by Magnus in conjunction with A. de Kleijn ("Über die Unabhängigkeit der Labyrinthreflexe vom Kleinhirn und über die Lage der Zentren für die Labyrinthreflexe im Hirnstamm," *Pflügers Arch.*, 1920, 178:124–178). Their experiments were more precise and better controlled than those of the earlier report but the results were much the same. Although the cerebellum may not be essential for the reflexes Magnus and de Kleijn elicited, nevertheless it still seemed to play an important role in relation to muscle tone and proprioception which were both essential factors in the maintenance of the body's equilibrium and in its variations in posture according to attitude or movement. The presence of a cerebellar control of the brainstem centers of the labyrinthine reflexes was not necessarily rejected by their findings. Magnus and de Kleijn reached the following conclusions which subsequent workers have developed.

EXCERPT PP. 172–173

In the present work, we have proved, on the basis of thorough physiological observations and special anatomical controls, that all the labyrinthine reflexes and reactions we have examined are preserved after the complete removal of the cerebellum, including its nuclei. Also that the centers responsible for them lie in a well-defined local arrangement in the brain-stem, that is, in the medulla oblongata and mid-brain, and that the path-ways serving the labyrinthine reflexes do not run through the cerebellum.

This does not mean, of course, that no stimuli from the labyrinthine can get to the cerebellum in the intact central nervous system, in order to participate in one way or another in this part of the brain, the functions of which are as yet unknown. This [problem] can only be examined when the normal function of the cerebellum has been made more readily accessible to physiological experiment; but at present there is little hope of this, despite the exertions of many researchers.

On the other hand, it is quite possible that the impulses going from the cerebellum to the centers for the labyrinthine reflexes in the brainstem, exert there either a reinforcing or an inhibitory influence on the course of the labyrinthine reflexes. For instance the observations of Bauer and Lei-dler (1911) would speak in favor of this. They have found a considerable reinforcement of the eye-turning reactions after injury to the vermis of the cerebellum.

No possibilities of this kind, however, detract from the final conclusions that the centers for the labyrinthine reflexes are situated outside the cere-bellum and that *therefore the idea that is still very popular, that the cerebellum must be the central apparatus for the labyrinths, must finally be dismissed.*

After reviewing the evidence in favor of a cerebellar control of the labyrinths, they concluded:

Despite these various hints which have been collected above, the belief in a direct functional connection between the labyrinth and the cerebellum is still very widely held. In contrast to this belief, it now appears that the labyrinthine reflexes are independent of the cerebellum [p. 175].

In June 1925 Magnus delivered a Croonian Lecture before the Royal Society in London ("Animal posture," *Proc. R. Soc.*, 1925, 98B:339–353) and in it he reviewed his conclusions regarding the physiology of posture. He ended by pointing out that areas of the brain such as the basal ganglia must also play a part but as yet remained virtually uninvestigated from this point of view. The cerebellum pre-sented no less an enigma.

EXCERPT PP. 352–353

Still worse perhaps is the situation with regard to another very important part of the brain, the *cerebellum*. Experiments have proved that all postural reflexes discussed in this lecture are present and perfectly undisturbed after total extirpation of the cerebellum. Therefore their centres as well as their afferent and efferent tracts are extracerebellar. Through the brilliant investigations of Luciani and others we know that loss of the cerebellum is followed by severe motor and postural disturbances. These symptoms, however, cannot depend on the cerebellum, which has been removed, but are evoked by the rest of the central nervous system, which has been spared. Unfortunately we know not a single function or reflex positively connected with the cerebellum, in such way that it is absent after cerebellar extirpation, and present after ablation of other parts of the brain, as long as the cerebellum remains uninjured. Our evidence of the postural activity of the cerebellum is purely negative. The great advantage during the investigation of the postural functions of bulb and mid-brain was, that we could there deal with positive reflexes (righting and attitudinal) which are present as long as the hind part of the brain-stem is intact. I am convinced that as soon as we succeed in finding positive reflexes connected with the cerebellum, it will be possible to elucidate the mystery of this undoubtedly very important part of the Central Nervous System. Only then can the question of the importance of the different *cortical* centres for posture be raised.

B. Localization

Although Luciani and his supporters believed that the cerebellum acted as a whole and that its several parts did not control individual muscles, the concept of a functional, rather than an anatomical, localization was not necessarily ruled out. The elucidation of this problem forms the second important modern approach to the physiology of the cerebellum. There is now a considerable amount of evidence to show that Luciani's concept is no longer tenable; nor can the cerebellum be considered as an organ solely concerned with proprioception as suggested by Sherrington (pp. 672–673). This part of Luciani's teaching which held the field for so many years and had excellent support from independent sources has therefore been superseded, and it has been shown, mainly by means of comparative anatomical studies, that various parts of the cerebellum control highly integrated functions but not anatomical entities.

John Hughlings Jackson
(*See p. 499*)

One of the earliest references to cerebellar localization was a remark made by Jackson when discussing (pp. 312–318) a paper by A. Hughes Bennett on "Muscular hypertonicity in paralysis" (*Brain*, 1888, 10:288–312). As in the case of his arguments in favor of cerebral cortical localization (see pp. 500–505), he used clinical evidence and theoretical considerations only but no experimental data. The result was a vague but nevertheless important suggestion. It is interesting to note that many of the ideas put forward in this discussion have since been proved to be incorrect. We have selected the one that has survived.

EXCERPT P. 317

. . . . I submit that the cerebrum represents all parts of the body, and that the cerebellum also represents all parts of the body. But the two representations are in inverse order; putting it roughly and neglecting some parts, the cerebral order is, arm, leg, trunk. This is admitted when we say that the "brain is the organ of volition," for the order stated *is* the order of parts as they are most often used voluntarily. The cerebellar order of representation is the opposite—trunk, leg, arm. This is admitted by those who say that the cerebellum is the organ "co-ordinating locomotor movements," for that expression only means an organ where muscles of all parts of the body are represented in certain complex ways. The order of parts getting into play in locomotion, from walking to swift running, is, trunk, leg, arm.

MAX SOLLY LÖWENTHAL   VICTOR ALEXANDER HADDEN HORSLEY
(10 October 1867—8 October 1960)   (14 April 1857—16 July 1916)

While most investigators were confirming the opinion of Luciani that the cerebellum acted as a whole, evidence was also appearing which suggested that the cerebellum, like the cerebrum, possessed a localization of function, although of a quite different nature. Jackson's statement of 1888 (pp. 689–690) had long been forgotten, but in 1897 there were two independent reports which were to be of great significance for this aspect of cerebellar physiology. On 24 May 1895 Löwenthal, a German émigré in Britain, observed that the extensor tonus of decerebrate rigidity could be relaxed by faradic stimulation of the upper surface of the cerebellum. In collaboration with Horsley he investigated this further and together they submitted a paper to the Royal Society on 8 February 1897 and read it on 25 February ("On the relations between the cerebellar and other centres (namely cerebral and spinal) with especial reference to the action of antagonistic muscles (Preliminary account)," *Proc. R. Soc.*, 1897, 61:20–25). One has the impression that this represents mainly Löwenthal's labors. In a later paper (V. Horsley and R. H. Clarke, "The structure and function of the cerebellum examined by a new method," *Brain,* 1908, 31:1–80) Horsley seemed to have forgotten that Löwenthal and he had found the cerebellar cortex responsive to electrical stimuli; he described it as "relatively inexcitable" (p. 71).

Löwenthal was born in Germany and was graduated M.D. from the University of Würzburg in 1892. He went to London in 1894 and spent the rest of his professional career in Britain. At first he worked as a neurophysiologist with Victor Horsley at University College, London, and then was in general practice in Liverpool from 1897 to 1935 when he retired to South Africa where he died. Apart from a small investigation of the spinal cord, he did no further experimental work (see *Brit. med. J.*, 1960, ii:1243–1244, 1606–1607).

Horsley studied medicine at University College, London, and was associated with its medical school and hospital throughout his career. As well as a brilliant neurophysiologist, he was one of the pioneers of neurosurgery and in 1886 became surgeon to the National Hospital in Queen Square, London. His interests in medicine were very wide and included medical politics, the reform of medical education, the social aspects of medicine, and crusades against alcohol and tobacco. He was knighted in 1902 and died of heat exhaustion while on active service in Mesopotamia in World War I (see Paget, 1919; Haymaker, 1953, pp. 429–432).

The following extracts are from the paper of Löwenthal and Horsley; in view of Sherrington's work on decerebrate rigidity (pp. 373–374) they did not extend it beyond a "preliminary account." Using the dog and cat, they studied the responses of the muscles at the elbow to cerebellar and cerebral stimulation.

EXCERPT PP. 20–21

The following is a brief summary of certain results which we have obtained in the investigation of the relations prevailing between the cerebellum and other parts of the nervous system, and which we commenced in consequence of an observation made by one of us (L), on the 24th May, 1895.

This consisted in the observation that when both cerebral hemispheres were removed and, as a result, active extension tonus [decerebrate rigidity] of the limbs was obtained, excitation (faradic) of the upper surface of the cerebellum caused immediate relaxation of such tonus so long as the current was applied, and that on the latter being shut off the tonus was immediately re-established.

As this observation appeared to indicate a distinct relation between the cerebellum and the bulbospinal system of lower centres, it was obviously very important to examine it further, especially as to whether it was a truly central effect or not.

It was soon made clear that the effect was a constant one, provided that the above mentioned tonus was distinctly established, and further that the primary effect of excitation of the cerebellum upon the upper limb in such case was not an active relaxation of the triceps alone, but that there was a marked contraction of the biceps.

Further, this effect, though constant, when tonus is present, was not the character of the muscle changes obtained when the tonus was absent.

It was, therefore, necessary to arrange a large series of experiments to determine a comparison between the changes in the two groups of muscles according as to whether the cortex cerebri, corona radiata, crusta, tegmentum, cerebellum, or cerebellar peduncles were excited either singly or in combination.

After making fifteen experiments in which the contraction of the muscles involved was determined by inspection, passive movement, and palpation only, the movements produced were graphically recorded.

EXCERPT PP. 23–25

G. EXCITATION OF THE CEREBELLUM

Excitation of the cerebellum produced very constant and sharply marked effects according as to whether the "acerebral" tonus [decerebrate rigidity] was present or not, and, further, a notable difference according to the side of the cerebellum excited.

The limits of the excitable region of the cerebellum will not now be discussed, but we may here state that the most excitable area is along the line of junction of the vermis superior with the lateral lobe. (This, it will be noted, is that portion of the cortex of the cerebellum which, in vertical position, is nearest the superior cerebellar peduncle [anterior lobe].)

For the purposes of the present communication excitation of the cerebellum means excitation of this focal area.

(*a*) *Excitation of the Cerebellum when "acerebral" Tonus is established.*—The effect of excitation of the cerebellum when ablation of the cerebral hemispheres has produced general tonic contraction, in extension of the trunk and limb muscles is a striking and *constant* active relaxation so far as the triceps (of the side stimulated) is concerned, and an active contraction of the biceps.

In the absence of graphic record it is impossible to determine precisely what is the nature of this effect on either the biceps or triceps.

We have, however, proved by the graphic method that—

(1) The biceps contracts powerfully;

(2) The triceps actively relaxes, i.e., it does not simply relax by ceasing to contract, but it relaxes so as to lose its normal physiological tonus.

The next step was of course the further investigation whether this phenomenon is unilateral. We have found as the result of twenty-nine experiments that the muscles of the right arm can be influenced by excitation of both halves of the cerebellum, but that the effect is very much greater from excitation of the right half, i.e., the same side. In addition we have excited the two halves of the cerebellum after median division of the organ, and then found that the effect was practically limited to the same side.

This is of course in harmony with the results of ablation of the cerebellar hemispheres obtained by Luciani, Risien Russell, and Ferrier and Turner.

In five experiments it was interesting to find that excitation of the *left* half of the cerebellum, i.e., that of the opposite side, evoked relaxation of the *biceps*. This crossed effect we noticed early in the investigation, and the similarity in the movements of the forelimb in walking was very striking.

The phenomenon of relaxation of the triceps and contraction of the biceps can be obtained also by excitation of the sub-cortical white substance of the cerebellum and of the peduncles in part.

(*b*) *Excitation of the Cerebellum when no "acerebral" Tonus is yet established.*—We have constantly obtained from the cerebellar cortex a tonic *contraction* of either the triceps or biceps, or both together, if the "acerebral" tonus had not appeared.

Sherrington had also made the same discovery independently and reported it in a paper sent to the Royal Society on 15 February 1897 and read on 8 April ("Double (antidrome) conduction in the central nervous system," *Proc. R. Soc.*, 1897, 61:243–246). It is usually said that he referred to cerebellar faradization in a paper read on 21 January 1897 ("On reciprocal innervation of antagonistic muscles. Third note," *Proc. R. Soc.*, 1896–1897, 60:414–417), but there is no direct reference to it there. In any case Löwenthal's observation had been made two years earlier (p. 691). The following is from the paper of 1897.

. . . . Thus, on exciting, especially with electric currents, the mammalian metencephalon (*vermis cerebelli*) and *isthmus rhombencephali*, subsequent to ablation of the parts above, I have seen movements produced in the limbs and trunk, and also inhibitions occur. Thus, in instance of the latter, inhibition of the tonic extensor spasm of the fore and hind limbs combined with contraction of the flexors of knee and elbow, such as is seen under local spinal reflex action . . . . [p. 246].

In a paper on decerebrate rigidity ("Decerebrate rigidity, and reflex coordination of movements," *J. Physiol.*, London, 1898, 22:319–332) he referred again to the phenomenon.

. . . . In the monkey similar inhibition of the decerebrate rigidity can be produced by excitation of the anterior (cerebral) surface of the *cerebellum*, as mentioned in my previous paper. Faradisation of points in a large area extending from near the middle line far out toward the lateral border of the cerebellar surface causes relaxation of the rigid neck and tail muscles, and relaxation of the rigid limbs, especially of the uncrossed side [p. 327].

Sherrington also drew attention to it in another paper ("Experiments in examination of the peripheral distribution of the fibres of the posterior roots of some spinal nerves.—Part II," *Phil. Trans. R. Soc.*, 1898, 190B:45–186; see p. 174) but did not pursue the matter further.

The significance of this finding was not fully appreciated at the time and it had to be rediscovered independently in 1922, again simultaneously in two laboratories (Miller and Banting, 1922; Bremer, 1922). It is now clear that the inhibitory effect produced by excitation of the cortex of the anterior lobe of the cerebellum is of paramount significance and its discovery has been likened to that made by Fritsch and Hitzig (pp. 507–511) with regard to the cerebral cortex. In addition to revealing its existence, Löwenthal, Horsley, and Sherrington demonstrated that an effect could be localized to a definable area of cerebellar cortex. From their work, therefore, more recent attempts to analyze the functional organization of the cerebellum have stemmed and stimulation experiments of the cerebellum began with them.

LOUIS BOLK

(10 December 1866—17 June 1930)

At the beginning of the twentieth century the cerebral cortical map-makers were hard at work and, as it had been shown that a pattern of localized function existed in the cerebral cortex (Chapter IX), it seemed reasonable to argue that a similar arrangement might be found in the cerebellum. A great stimulus to this belief resulted from the work of the Dutch anatomist Bolk who made an extensive comparative study of cerebellar anatomy and on the basis of it speculated concerning cerebellar function and its localization.

Bolk was born at Overschie and studied first at Jus where he qualified as a notary before beginning his medical training. In 1896 he was appointed assistant in anatomy at Utrecht and in 1898, professor *ordinarius*. His numerous studies were in the fields of anatomy, embryology, biology, and anthropology (see Broek, 1931).

In 1906 Bolk published his important work, *Das Cerebellum der Säugethiere* (Haarlem, 1906), and in it he concluded that each coordinated movement of a muscular system was represented in a definable area of cerebellar cortex. The cerebellum was therefore organized on a basis of somatomotor localization and there was a measurable correlation between the development of definite lobules and specific systems of muscles. This ingenious argument was based upon his wide experience of the anatomy and embryology of the animal cerebellum. Thus in all mammals it is formed on the same uniform principles and here Bolk was confirming some of Reil's earlier work (pp. 647–652); there are four growth centers, one anterior and three posterior of which one is medial and two are lateral (pp. 47–49). To cite popular examples, the spider monkey has a prehensile tail, and as its flocculus is elongated, Bolk considered this to be the center for the regulation of tail movements; similarly the long neck of the giraffe was considered to be related to the large lobulus simplex in this animal. Bolk was therefore able to allocate specific portions of the cerebellum to limbs, trunk, head, and neck, and his hypothesis has not been entirely disproved. Moreover, he stimulated many investigations of the problem, including those of Robert Bārāny (1876–1936) of Vienna who showed that the vermis controlled trunk movements, the hemispheres, those of the legs, and the flocculus, the eye movements ("Beziehungen zwischen Bau und Funktion des Kleinhirns, nach Untersuchungen an Menschen," *Wien. klin. Wschr.*, 1912, 25:1737–1739, and "Lokalisation in des Rinde der Kleinhirnhemisphären des Menschen," *ibid.*, pp. 2033–2038).

The following passages have been translated from Bolk's book of 1906 and summarize his main opinions. He first discussed "the structure of the cerebellum in the midline which I have arrived at on the basis of a comparative anatomical investigation" (p. 78).

EXCERPT P. 77

The following is the principal result of my comparative study of the way in which the arbor vitae branches in the median plane and, with this, the formation of lobes by the cerebellum in this plane. With the exception of the cetacea (and according to the work of Ziehen, perhaps of the monotremes [e.g., the duck-billed platypus]) the mammalian cerebella are composed of two lobes, an anterior and a posterior. Almost without exception the former proves to consist of four lobules which, however, in certain forms (anthropomorphs, humans, certain carnivores) cannot always be distinctly differentiated. The latter is composed of three lobules. Two of these are not differentiated in the mammalian orders, and they are probably the least changeable elements of the median posterior lobules; the third lobule is uniform only in the smallest cerebella, but this lobule is precisely the site of important variations. These variations are partly of a progressive character since the originally uniform radiation may branch considerably and the basal branch of this radiation has gained complete independence in all the rather larger cerebella. Consequently, this lobule which was originally uniform, seems to be composed of two sublobules in the majority of mammals. One can therefore imagine ultimately that the posterior lobe, too, is composed of four lobules.

EXCERPT PP. 302–303

I repeat the question: how can one reconcile variability in certain lower cerebellar parts, situated next to others of a more rigid constituency, with the concept of the cerebellum as an organ of homogeneous function in which, as has been asserted by physiologists, one part may be substituted for another. This concept cannot be rejected since Luciani's investigations have proved that a vicarious relationship must exist between areas of the cerebellum, and it must be the duty of experimenters to work out the topographical basis of this physiological principle. It cannot be assumed that defect of functions resulting from extirpation of a given part of the cortex can be gradually restored by any arbitrarily chosen lower part of the cerebellum. In my opinion the ablation of the anterior lobe, for example, cannot be completely nullified by the posterior lobe, and several further such examples could be cited.

If one considers the independent variability of the lower parts of the cerebellum, one almost gains the impression that the cerebellum is a complex of organs, some of them constant, others very variable in their development. It was this phenomenon that became the strongest reason for my assumption that there must be a localization of functions in the cerebellar cortex, and the question arose again and again: why is a lobe so large in one animal and so little developed in another? Originally I favored the opinion that there was a relationship between the massive development of certain lower parts of the muscular system and those of special cerebellar lobules. However, when subsequently applying this postulate, I repeatedly met with contradictions, until I finally found the solution which, in my opinion, partly removes the mystery regarding localization of functions in the cerebellum. For there is no relationship between the lobulization of the cerebellum and the massive degree of development of certain lower parts of the muscular system, but there is one between the lobules and the physiological degree of development of certain muscle areas.

I reached this conclusion ultimately because of a phenomenon that had attracted my attention for some time, but without immediately realizing its importance; that is, that there exists a peculiar correlation between the system of the growth centers in the cerebellum [see p. 694] and the distribution of muscle groups in the body, especially if one compares these in their functional dependence on and independence from each other in the performance of complicated movements.

EXCERPT PP. 306–307

If we now summarize the above we reach the conclusion that one must imagine a number of coordinated centers in the cerebellar cortex, partly paired, partly unpaired. The center for the following group of muscles will be unpaired: muscles of the eye, tongue, mastication, larynx, pharynx, and of facial, cervical, dorsal muscular apparatus, and other muscular apparatus of the trunk. The center for the musculature of the upper and lower extremities will be paired, while, in addition, an unpaired center must be assigned to the musculature of the two extremities. If one compares these physiological deductions with the lobulization of the cerebellum, one is astonished by the agreement between them. If one were now to attempt to illustrate these postulated physiological centers by a schematic presentation, one would demonstrate identical and considerable agreement with the schema of the morphological composition of the cerebellum resulting from my anatomical investigation. Now, if this parallelism between a physiological principle and a morphological phenomenon actually corresponds to a correlation, the necessary consequence must be that, with an increase in the physiological differentiation in one of the mentioned areas of muscles, there is a coordination which occurs simultaneously. I have compared in great detail the morphological differentiation of degree of development of the specific individual muscle groups. Based upon this I have reached the following assumptions regarding the localization of cerebellar functions. *The anterior* [central] *lobe contains the coordination center for the group of muscles of the head* (eyes, tongue, muscles of mastication, facial muscles) *and in addition of the larynx and pharynx; in the lobulus simplex is the coordinating center of the cervical muscles; the upper portion of the lobulus medianus posterior contains the unpaired coordination center for the left and right extremities; in each of the lobuli ansiformis and paramediani is one of the paired centers for the two extremities; and in the remaining part of the cerebellum we find the coordinating centers for the muscles of the trunk.*

Olaf Larsell
(13 March 1886—8 April 1964)

Important as Bolk's work was, to some extent it was speculative and a rigorous experimental analysis of the comparative approach he had used was necessary. This was provided by the American neuroanatomist Larsell and his pupils.

Larsell was born at Rättvik in Sweden and entered the United States in 1891. He studied zoology at Northwestern University, Evanston, Illinois, where he received the Ph.D. degree. Thereafter he held appointments in zoology and anatomy at Northwestern and the Universities of Wisconsin and Oregon. He worked principally in the fields of experimental neurology and neuroanatomy, but his comparative analysis of the cerebellum is his best known study (Jansen, 1965).

His approach was a dynamic, embryological one which has extensively modified the morphological interpretations of the organ and is fundamental to many present-day studies, while its functional terminology is superseding the purely descriptive terminology dating from the eighteenth century (see Malacarne, pp. 643–646).

Larsell's work is represented here because of its considerable influence on the development of cerebellar physiology and because of its contribution to the functional parcellation of the organ.

Larsell's views were summarized in a paper ("The cerebellum. A review and interpretation," *Arch. Neurol. Psychiat.*, 1937, 38:580–607) that he described as "a review of some of the principal facts of the comparative, anatomic, and embryologic development of the cerebellum in relation to the results of experimental anatomic studies of its connections both internally and with other parts of the nervous system . . ." (p. 580).

EXCERPT PP. 605–607

NEOCEREBELLUM AND PALEOCEREBELLUM

The terms paleocerebellum and neocerebellum have a certain value, if it is recognized that there is no real boundary between the regions they designate. As is evident from the preceding description, the lateral parts of the corpus cerebelli in mammals are outgrowths of the medial, or vermian, portion. The pars lateralis of reptiles foreshadows the lateral lobes of the mammalian cerebellum. The anterior lobe of the corpus cerebelli shows the smallest lateral expansion of any major division. This is the oldest part of the corpus cerebelli; yet even here there is some lateral expansion, especially in Bolk's lobulus 4. Hausman stated that a neocerebellar equivalent is provided for each lobule of the vermis except the lingula. Yet the oldest part of the cerebellum phylogenetically, namely, the flocculus, which is connected with the newer vermian nodulus by primitive peduncles and by an ancient commissure, is the most laterally placed developmentally of the cerebellar divisions. It is only by the growth above and around it of other parts of the cerebellum that it has become located relatively near the midplane in larger mammals.

The emphasis on the vermis as a functional entity has been misleading. The vermis is made up of distinct units—some closely related to the ancient vestibular foundation of the cerebellum, others with spinal connections and still others with the newer connections established by the higher centers. Only if the primate cerebellum is taken as the model form, in spite of its greatly hypertrophied ansiform lobule, can the vermis be regarded to some degree as a separate division.

The term neocerebellum is useful, if it is applied in a general way to the region which receives pontile fibres predominantly. The term paleocerebellum should be restricted to the more basal region which receives spinal and vestibular fibers chiefly.

It must be recognized that there are several degrees of newness in the phylogenetic formation of the cerebellum. First appeared the lateral commissure between the acousticolateral areas of the medulla oblongata and then the trigeminal commissura cerebelli between the primary proprioceptive centers. Along each of these commissures there occurred a migration of cells, building a massive corpus cerebelli and a less massive flocculonodular lobe. In land animals the proprioceptive corpus cerebelli became predominant. It soon underwent division into an anterior and a posterior lobe, the latter a new development largely in connection with the growth of the dorsal spinocerebellar tract. This in turn was divided by the fissura secunda into the still newer medial lobe of Elliot Smith and the uvula. The uvula is the more primitive part, as shown by its retention of direct vestibular, as well as spinocerebellar, fibers. Elliot Smith's middle lobe was again subdivided into Ingvar's medial lobe and the pyramis, each with lateral expansions. In the larger mammals the lateral expansions, i.e., the cerebellar hemispheres, become so large as to obscure the medial structures from which they have their origin. It is the medial lobe of Ingvar, with its great lateral development and its connections through the pons with the cerebral cortex, which is the newest major division of the cerebellum, both phylogenetically and functionally.

Phylogenetically, there is basis for division into the archicerebellum, the paleocerebellum and the neocerebellum. The boundaries, especially that between the archicerebellum and the paleocerebellum, cannot be sharply fixed, but in general the archicerebellum should include the flocculonodular lobe and the basis cerebelli, with part of the anterior lobe of the corpus cerebelli and possibly part of the posterior lobe.

The deep nuclei of the cerebellum tell the same story. The fastigial nucleus is the oldest developmentally, corresponding to the nucleus cerebelli of lower vertebrates. Its primitive efferent and afferent connections are retained. It is the nucleus of the first story of the cerebellar superstructure, having to do chiefly with vestibular and muscle sense impulses. The vestibular nuclei are the nuclei primarily of the more purely vestibular flocculonodular "basement." The nucleus interpositus, so far as may be judged from comparative anatomy, has to do chiefly with spinocerebellar stimuli, and possibly others, including those brought by olivocerebellar connections. The nucleus dentatus is the nucleus of the third, or neocerebellar story, so far as the term neocerebellum is justified. It is dominated by corticopontocerebellar impulses. The continuation of fibers from this nucleus to the thalamus, pointed out by Allen, is significant. The connections with distinct parts of the cerebellar cortex demonstrated for these nuclei would seem to indicate that they have different functional values. The tentative conclusions from comparative and experimental anatomic studies, however, must be checked by other methods. The suggestions made in this paper will serve a useful purpose if they point the way for physiologic experiments.

The structural plan of the cerebellum outlined here does not rule out a certain amount of localization of function. Rather, with reference to the primitive distribution of afferent fibers especially, it favors such an interpretation, which is also supported by experimental anatomic evidence. It must be recognized, however, that, in mammals at least, there has developed so much overlapping of fibers from various sources that the primitive pattern is entirely hidden. The two fundamental divisions, namely, the corpus cerebelli and the flocculonodular lobe, receive primarily general proprioceptive and vestibular fibers, respectively. The various tracts which enter the corpus cerebelli of mammals, in addition to trigeminal, spinocerebellar, and possibly tectocerebellar fibers, appear to do so secondarily. Some of these, however, assume a functional importance which appears to transcend that of some of the more direct connections.

From the functional point of view, there are four principal divisions of the cerebellum. These are: (1) the vestibular flocculonodular lobe, having its chief afferent connections with the vestibular nuclei; (2) the vestibular and spinocerebellar anterior lobe, the uvula, and in part the pyramis (spinocerebellar portion), having efferent connections chiefly with the fastigial nucleus and, through the uncinate bundle of Russell, with the vestibular nuclei, the medulla oblongata, and the spinal cord; (3) the lobulus simplex, the pyramis in part, the paraflocculus, and the lobulus ansoparamedianus, connecting with the nucleus interpositus and through it with the nucleus ruber and, possibly, the thalamus, and (4) the medial lobe of Ingvar, connecting with the nucleus dentatus and through it chiefly with the nucleus ruber and the thalamus.

C. Cerebellar Electrophysiology

Edgar Douglas, Lord Adrian
(See p. 224)

One of the more recent advances in cerebellar physiology has been the recording of bioelectric potentials from the cerebellum or related structures. This represents the third and last of the main modern lines of investigation. Early attempts were made by A. Beck and G. Bikeles ("Versuch über die gegenseitige funktionelle Be-einflussung von Gross- und Kleinhirn," *Pflüger Arch.*, 1912, 113:283–295; "Versuche über die sensorische Funktionen des Kleinhirnmittelstücks," *ibid.*, pp. 296–302) with a string galvanometer, but the whole study of cerebellar electrophysiology was inaugurated by Adrian in a paper presented to the Physiological Society on 15 December 1934. ("Discharge frequencies in the cerebral and cerebellar cortex," *J. Physiol.*, London, 1935, 83:32P–33P). He first described the spontaneous electrical activity of the cerebral cortex, and then that of the cerebellum, which he found to be entirely separate.

An entirely different picture is found in records of the potential changes in the exposed cerebellar cortex (vermis or lateral lobes) under anaesthesia or in the decerebrate preparation. There is persistent spontaneous activity consisting of groups of sinusoidal waves at frequencies ranging from 250–150 per sec., and there is no sign of the slower type of oscillation found in the cerebral cortex (Fig. 1 [fig. 152]). In deep chloroform anaesthesia the cerebellar waves often become exceedingly regular, but the rate is still of the order of 150 per sec.

Electrical stimulation of the cerebral and cerebellar cortex reveals the same differences in the frequency of discharge. In the cerebrum stimulation with repeated induction shocks for a few seconds gives a discharge resembling that produced by severe injury. The initial stages are obscured by the stimulus artefact, but the frequency very soon falls to a plateau at 40–50 per sec., and ultimately the discharge changes progressively into a series of large waves which may attain very low frequencies. These resemble the waves due to convulsant drugs, and it can be shown that they spread widely over the cortex.

In the cerebellum electrical stimulation produces a regular series of waves (injury does not), but the whole frequency is still uncertain, but in the later stages of the discharge the waves occur at 250–150 per sec. and cease when the frequency has fallen to 150 per sec. (Fig. 2 [fig. 153]). Here too the waves spread some distance from the stimulated point and are evidently due to a number of neurones pulsating in phase.

The fact that the normal activity of the cerebellar neurones occurs at such high rates suggests that the cerebellum may perhaps exert an inhibitory influence of the Wedensky type on some of the structures innervated by it.

H. W. Magoun   Ray S. Snider

(23 June 1907—   )   (27 January 1911—   )

It must not be implied from the material hitherto presented that there are three wholly independent approaches to the investigation of the cerebellum. Combinations of them are obviously necessary. Sherrington interpreted the abolition of decerebrate rigidity in the monkey by anterior cerebellar lobe stimulation as the consequence of a direct cerebellospinal connection. But this does not exist in mammals, and the effect he observed must have been produced by way of the reticular substance. Attention was first drawn to the role of this structure in the inhibition and facilitation of motor activity by the American anatomist H. W. Magoun in 1944.

Magoun was born in Philadelphia and received the Ph.D. degree from Northwestern University in 1934, where he worked until becoming professor and chairman of the Department of Anatomy in the University of California at Los Angeles in 1950. His department, together with the University's Brain Research Institute, initiated to a very considerable degree through his efforts, has become one of the most active centers of neuroanatomical and neurophysiological research in the world.

Since 1944 there have been widespread investigations into the morphology and function of the reticular substance, and Magoun recently summarized its activities in his book, *The waking brain* (2d ed., 1963).

EXCERPT PP. 187–188

Within the brain, a central transactional core has been identified between the strictly sensory or motor systems of classical neurology. This central reticular mechanism has been found capable of grading the activity of most other parts of the brain. It does this as a reflection of its own internal excitability, in turn a consequence of both afferent and corticifugal neural influences, as well as of the titer of circulating transmitters and hormones which affect and modify reticular activity.

While the functions of this reticular system tend generally to be more widespread than those of the specific systems of the brain, it is proposed to be subdivided into a grosser and more tonically operating component in the lower brain stem, subserving global alterations in excitability, as distinguished from a more cephalic, thalamic component with greater capacities for fractionated, shifting influences upon focal regions of the brain.

Influences of this reticular system which are directed spinalward modify the activities of motor outflows from the cord, in particular those subserving postural control. Reticular influences which are directed forward to the cephalic brain stem and limbic forebrain, affect mechanisms regulating visceral and endocrine functions, as well as innate and emotional behavior.

In its ascending and descending relations with the cerebral cortex, the reticular system is intimately bound up with, and contributes to most categories of, higher nervous activity. It has to do significantly with the initiation and maintenance of wakefulness; with the orienting reflex and focus of attention; with sensory control processes including habituation and external inhibition; with conditional learning; through its functional relations with the hippocampus and temporal cortex, with memory functions; and, through its relations with the midline thalamus and pontile tegmentum, with the management of internal inhibition, as well as light and deep sleep. These manifold and varied capacities of the reticular system suggest that it serves importantly and in the closest conjunction with the cortex in most of the central integrative processes of the brain.

One of the efferent connections of the cerebellum is via the reticular substance, and this appears to have a facilitatory influence on the cerebral cortex. The investigation of this phenomenon has been one of the many contributions to cerebellar physiology made by another American anatomist, Ray S. Snider.

Snider was born in Illinois and in 1937 was graduated Ph.D. from Washington University, St. Louis. Since 1953 he has been a professor of anatomy at the Northwestern University Medical School in Chicago.

Snider and Magoun in 1948 were able through cerebellar stimulation to demonstrate facilitation, and the following is their brief report to the American Physiological Society ("Facilitation produced by cerebellar stimulation," *Fed. Proc.*, 1948, 7:117–118).

In monkeys excitation of (*a*) anterior lobe-lobulus simplex region and (*b*) paramedian lobule-tuber vermis-pyramis region of the cerebellum produced facilitation of reflex activity and of movements evoked from the cerebral cortex. The most pronounced effects were noted when chloralosane anesthesia was used and electrical stimuli of 200–300 cycles per second were applied to the cerebellum from 5–15 seconds before elicitation of the movement. Facilitation occurred following destruction of the superior peduncle suggesting that the cerebellum is exerting its influence through facilitatory centers in the brain stem rather than through the activation of the cerebral mechanism. The distribution of cerebellar facilitatory areas in the monkey is similar to that of the tactile receiving areas and of the area yielding inhibition of movement in the cat. This similarity even extends to the somatotopic representation of body parts for, though overlapping was present, within zone (*a*) movements of the leg were facilitated from points rostral to those for the arm, while within zone (*b*) the reverse was the case.

In a more extensive paper on this topic ("Facilitation produced by cerebellar stimulation," *J. Neurophysiol.*, 1949, 12:335–345) the authors made the following comments.

EXCERPT PP. 342–344

. . . . Thus, not only can inhibitory and excitatory influences result from stimulation of certain areas of the cerebellum but, as shown by the present work, facilitatory influences can be elicited also. Just what this means in terms of total cerebellar function it is difficult to say, but it is interesting to note that all three of these functional manifestations result from the stimulation of two regions of the cerebellum.

The anterior facilitatory area of the cerebellum is located mainly in the ipsilateral lobuli centralis, culmen, and simplex. For maximal effects on leg movements—whether they be reflexly or cortically induced movements—it is necessary to stimulate the anterior folia of this area. On the other hand, if effects upon arm movements are desired, it is necessary to stimulate posteriorly (culmen).

The posterior facilitatory area is located bilaterally in the paramedian lobules and pyramis and, like the anterior area, definite zones exist in which stimulation primarily affects the upper and lower extremity. Although the two zones are not as sharply separated as they are in the anterior lobe, stimulatory effects on the leg are more prominent in the posterior part of the area and those on the arm are more prominent in the anterior part.

. . . .

. . . .

From the standpoint of total cerebellar function a possible explanation of the facilitatory role played by the cerebellum comes when it is realized that tactile, auditory, visual, and proprioceptive impulses, as well as impulses from the cerebrum via the pontine nuclei, come into the cerebellum. This abundance of afferent supply puts into action certain cerebellar mechanisms which, acting through brain stem centers on the spinal cord, can produce facilitation of cortically induced or reflexly induced movement. Certain other areas of the cerebellum, when brought into action, can alter cerebral action. Thus cerebellar influences can be exerted at one or more levels within the nervous system to produce facilitation.

It is not easy to make an appropriate selection from the several very recent and important contributions to the anatomy and physiology of the cerebellum, but the work of Snider has certainly been quite revolutionary (e.g., "Recent contributions to the anatomy and physiology of the cerebellum," *Arch. Neurol. Psychiat.*, 1950, 64:196–219). The following excerpts taken by permission from his article, "The cerebellum" (*Scient. Am.*, 1958, 199:84–90), represent the most recent commentary on the cerebellum.

EXCERPT PP. 85–86

Thus in the first 40 years of this century the cerebellum was established as a center governing the musculature, coordinating both consciously and unconsciously directed action. In engineering parlance, it is the control box in the feedback circuitry of the nervous system. Such a control box does not originate the input of commands to the system, but it is informed of them by the command center; for example, by the setting of a dial. From the sensing instruments at the output end of the system it receives the feedback of data on the output. Comparing output with input, it informs the command centers of the corrections to be made or generates correcting command signals itself. Confident as we are that this is the function of the cerebellum, we are a long way from a complete understanding of how it carries out this function.

EXCERPT PP. 86–90

As in the cerebrum, the various functions of the cerebellum are localized in distinctly defined areas of its cortex. Detection and plotting of the electrical activity of the cortex has made it possible to map these areas. The control of the body's equilibrium, for example, is localized in the extreme front and rear surfaces of the cerebellum. The proprioceptive areas appear as actual maps of the body on the cortex: two distorted homunculi, one face-on and the other in double profile back-to-back . . . .

For a long time it was thought that the plotting of these areas had completed the map of the cerebellar cortex, in line with the notion that the cerebellum was restricted to the management of the body's equilibrium and muscular activity. However, at the Johns Hopkins University in 1942 Averill Stowell and I undertook an investigation which has established that the cerebellum is equally involved in the coordination of the sensations of touch, hearing, and sight.

We worked with animals and, by touching hairs, shining a sharply focused light on the retina or sounding a distinct sound at the ear, we were able to pick up the resulting nerve signals with probes applied to the cerebellar cortex. Interestingly enough, the tactile area coincides with the two proprioceptive areas, while the auditory and visual senses register in a separate overlapping area that lies between them. This arrangement reflects the close association of these two pairs of sensations in behavior: when an animal feels a touch on the leg, for example, its response is to flex the leg; when it hears a sound, it turns to look. In the cerebrum the visual and auditory centers occupy separate areas, and their cellular complexity is many times greater.

Our investigation showed also that the tactile, visual, and auditory centers of the cerebellum are linked to the corresponding centers in the cerebral cortex by the same sort of feedback loop that connects the proprioceptive areas. By stimulating the appropriate areas in the cerebellum directly with electrodes we found we could project the stimulus to the matching areas of the cerebrum, and *vice versa,* and thus lay out the feedback circuits [tactile, visual, proprioceptive, and auditory] . . . . Our studies developed further feedback pathways to the thalamus, the basal ganglia, and the reticular formation of the lower brain stem. This array of feedback loops should stimulate the cerebral servomechanism of any student of cybernetics. In sum, the cerebellar circuitry is an accessory control system imposed upon the basic ascending (sensory) and descending (motor) circuits of the nervous system.

The big question remains: How does the cerebellum play its role? We know that removal of the cerebellum produces severe disturbances in muscular coordination of the animal. On the other hand, it is necessary to remove large areas of the cerebellar cortex in order to produce enduring loss of muscular coordination. How does the nervous system so smoothly absorb so great an insult? Does it mean that the cerebellum acts in such close harmony with some as yet unidentified center that this second center takes over its functions? Or does it mean that the cerebellum has little functional significance? The category of puzzles becomes larger when one considers the cerebellar sensory areas. Few, if any, measurable sensory losses occur when these areas are destroyed.

The electrical characteristics of the cerebellar cortex furnish the principal clues for future investigation. The cerebellum generates electrical waves at the highest frequency in the nervous system. They range from 200 to 400 per second—10 times faster than those of the cerebral cortex. The amplitude of cerebellar discharges, on the other hand, seldom exceeds 200 microvolts; this is a fraction of the operating level of the cerebrum, which runs 10 or more times higher. The cerebellum imposes its peculiar high-frequency, low-amplitude characteristics upon all the impulses that pass through it. Often it seems to "smother" the frequency-amplitude characteristics of impulses originating elsewhere in the nervous system. The characteristic electrical signature of the cerebellum helped us considerably to detect and map the sites at which impulses from its cortex arrive in the cerebrum.

But what purpose is served by this peculiar electrical activity? Modulation of signals is so common and so useful in radio technology that one is tempted to see the cerebellum as the great "modulator" of nervous function. The imposition of high-frequency rhythms on low-frequency impulses would enable appropriate centers to discriminate between impulses modulated by the cerebellum and those not so modulated. This is interesting speculation, but it may not be the mechanism at all. The cerebellum might equally well act as a "band-pass" filter; that is, its fast activity may allow some wave patterns to go through, while blocking or altering others. Another line of speculation argues that wave frequencies have little to do with the case, and holds that the important thing is the total energy added by the cerebellum to the outgoing impulses. Whether these speculations (or any added by the reader) may help to solve the riddles of the cerebellum, only time and more experimentation can tell.

In the meantime we may have to contend with the possibility that the cerebellum is involved in still more diverse aspects of the nervous system. It becomes increasingly evident that if "integration" is a major function of this organ, trips into the realm of mental disease may cross its boundaries more frequently than the guards in sanatariums suspect.

Conclusion

In a chapter entitled "General considerations on the function of the cerebellum" Dow and Moruzzi (1958, p. 373) "admit that we are unable to state precisely how the cerebellum performs its function," but their bibliography of sixty-seven pages testifies to the amount of labor that has been expended in attempts to do so. There seems little doubt, however, that until new technological procedures become available and new points of view are developed, advances will be based very considerably upon the three avenues of experimental approach opened up in the last few decades and upon combinations of them. Nevertheless, the long space of time preceding the very recent historical period saw the accumulation of a vast amount of factual data concerning the anatomy and physiology of the cerebellum, and each of the contributors selected above, together with many more, have helped to make possible recent approaches to new concepts.

CHAPTER XII

THE VENTRICULAR SYSTEM AND CEREBROSPINAL FLUID

Introduction

The cerebrospinal fluid has had a more varied history than any other part of the nervous system. Thus its proposed role in the animal economy has ranged from a humoral excrement contained, according to Galen and his followers, in the ventricles, to that of the seat of man's soul as was suggested by the German anatomist Soemmerring at the end of the eighteenth century. Moreover, its history is one of the lengthiest. As far as recorded anatomical data are concerned, the parts of the nervous system that have the longest history are the meninges, the cerebral convolutions (Chapter VII), and the cerebrospinal fluid. They were all mentioned in the Edwin Smith Surgical Papyrus (pp. 383–384), but in the case of the last two, little is, on the whole, yet known of their function, five millennia later.

The history of the cerebrospinal fluid and its pathways falls naturally into three periods. First, there was the acquisition of anatomical knowledge. In antiquity a good deal was known of the coverings of the brain and of the ventricular system; in fact, these were the best known parts of the nervous system, and during the medieval period the ventricles were frequently the only cerebral structures mentioned (see W. Sudhoff, 1913). Although most of the important anatomical features of the meninges and the ventricular system were known by the seventeenth century, almost nothing had been learned about their contents, the cerebrospinal fluid. The second division or period of this chapter deals therefore with early accounts of the cerebrospinal fluid and the attempts to explain its production and elimination. This period began in the sixteenth century and lasted until the end of the eighteenth when the first reliable account of the fluid, subarachnoid as well as ventricular, was given by Cotugno. Modern investigations of the physiology of the cerebrospinal fluid did not begin, however, until the third decade of the nineteenth century when Magendie began his research on it. Since then attempts to elucidate its functions have been continuous, but it seems likely that this third period has ended very recently and that a fourth, created by the application of radioactive techniques to the problem, has begun.

In respect to the first period, no attempt has been made to continue the history of the meninges beyond Galen's description of them in the second century A.D. Likewise, in our third period only the theories of cerebrospinal fluid production and removal have been illustrated, and those concerning fluid pressure, physical and chemical properties of the fluid, and others have been purposely omitted.

A history of the anatomy of the cerebrospinal fluid is to be found in Woollam (1957) and in Millen and Woollam (1962, pp. 1–24, and *passim*). Christoffel (1944) deals with the work of Magendie and Quincke, and Bing (1954) covers the whole history. There is a review of the literature up to 1842 by Jodin (1842) and up to 1875 by Key and Retzius (1875–1876; see below, pp. 740–744); Bowsher (1960) has made reference to much of the work carried out during the last hundred years. Nevertheless, there is no adequate historical consideration of the whole topic, and most authors have been content to copy earlier writers, with the inevitable transmission of errors.

Early Accounts of the Meninges and Ventricles

Whereas the ancients paid little attention to the solid parts of the nervous system, they had considerable knowledge of the coverings of the brain and spinal cord, and of the ventricular system. In the earlier works available to us, however, these are merely mentioned in passing; thus one of the Hippocratic Writers noted the falx cerebri (*The sacred disease*, VI) and Aristotle spoke of the two meningeal membranes, pia mater and dura mater, as well as of the cavity inside the brain (p. 9). Erasistratus also referred to the meninges and to the lateral, third, and fourth ventricles (p. 12), as did Herophilus (p. 713) and Rufus (p. 13).

Frequent and extensive accounts of the ventricles are to be found in Galen's writings, and the reason for the emphasis laid upon them is presumably owing to the fact that they were considered as storage spaces for the essential animal spirit or psychic pneuma which, according to Erasistratus's original theory, found its way thence into the nerves to execute muscle movement and to subserve sensation (pp. 144–146). In the medieval period and extending as far as the seventeenth century, the localization of psychological functions in the ventricles further indicates the central role they played in the theory of brain function which was universally accepted at this time (pp. 463–469). Mondino in 1316 (pp. 23–25) supported this idea, but Vesalius, like Massa before him (pp. 722–723), attacked it (pp. 714–718) and gave a more detailed account of the ventricles. Aranzi also represents the interest that Renaissance anatomists had in the ventricular system, and his description of it included observations previously omitted.

GALEN
(*See p. 14*)

Galen's account of the ventricular system is the first detailed one we possess. It was of particular importance to him in view of his theory of brain function which called for the ventricles to act as a reservoir for the animal spirit manufactured by the solid parts of the brain, by the choroid plexus, or by the *rete mirabile* (p. 758). The brain was the seat of the soul and also the mediator, by means of the animal spirit, of all bodily motion and sensation. It also took in air through the cribriform plate to be used for olfaction and to help in the formation of the animal spirit. The waste products of brain activity passed out through the sutures if gaseous and through the cribriform plate and pituitary fossa as phlegm if they were fluid.

There are many references in Galen's writings to the brain's meninges—although until the sixteenth century only the pia mater and dura mater were recognized—and to the ventricles. The following passages from his *Use of parts*, VIII, 8–9 (Daremberg [1854–1856], I, 553–554) describe respectively the pia mater and dura mater.

EXCERPT P. 553

Thus the pia mater strengthens the brain at the same time that it covers it, and, furthermore, it also binds together all the vessels that it encloses. It is the same as the chorion in respect to the fetus, and the mesentery. Indeed, both membranes are composed of numerous veins and arteries, situated one next to the other, and of a thin membrane which binds together the intermediate parts. Likewise, the pia mater fastens all the arteries and veins of the brain so that they cannot intersect or intermingle, and so when in motion they cannot deviate from their positions; their base not being very stable, because they rest on such a humid, soft, and almost fluid substance [brain tissue]. That is why the pia mater not only surrounds the brain but also finds its way into its depths, traversing it in all directions, creeping into all its sinuosities, spreading out with the vessels as far as the cavity of the ventricles.

In this regard, I do not know why the majority of anatomists, undoubtedly still very much in the dark, call the part of the pia mater that lines the ventricles, plexus and choroidal fold, and refuse to compare the other parts to the chorion and to designate them in the same way. As for us, we know and we demonstrate that its nature and use are identical to that of the chorion and the mesentery. We say that these latter membranes bind together the arteries and veins, and that the pia mater, in addition to these vessels, also binds together the entire brain.

EXCERPT P. 554

The dura mater is also a covering for the brain, or rather it is not simply a covering but also a protective rampart that prevents the brain from striking against the cranium. As for the pia mater, it is truly an adherent covering of the brain. In fact, the dura mater is separated from it and connected with it only by the vessels that run through it; if nature had not established the pia mater between them, the closeness of the dura mater to the brain would not have been without inconveniences.

In the same work appeared a description of the ventricular system (*Use of parts,* VIII, 10, Daremberg [1854–1856], I, 557–558). Galen explained the reason for two lateral ventricles rather than one and cited the famous case of a head wound penetrating to one of these cavities.

EXCERPT PP. 557–558

Now first we shall consider the ventricles of the brain, the size and position of each of them, their shape, their communications with one another, their number, and then the parts that are superimposed upon or adjacent to them. The two anterior ventricles perform the inspiration, expiration, and exsufflation of the brain. Elsewhere [*The usefulness of breathing,* I, 5] we have demonstrated these facts. We have also demonstrated that they prepare and elaborate for it the psychic pneuma [animal spirit]. Moreover, we have just said [also *Anatomical procedures,* IX, 7] that by their lower [i.e., anterior] parts which communicate with the nostrils, they are at the same time an olfactory organ and a channel for the outflow of superfluities.

It was better that there exist two ventricles rather than a single one, considering that the inferior opening [foramen of Monro] was created double, that all the sense organs are double, that the brain itself is double. This doubling provides still another use of which we shall speak when we come to the sense organs. But the first and most general use of the double organs is that in case one is injured the other may take over its function.

We were witness to an astonishing incident in Smyrna in Ionia; we saw a young man survive an accident, seemingly by the will of God, in which one of the anterior ventricles was injured. It is certain that he would not have survived for a moment if both had been injured simultaneously. Likewise, leaving aside injuries, if some ailment occurs in one ventricle and the other is not harmed, the animal is less affected than it would be if both suffered at the same time. Now if there are two ventricles and both of them have become involved, it is the same as if there were a single one, existing from the beginning, and this single ventricle became diseased. Therefore the presence of a double organ, when it is possible, is a surer guarantee than that of a single organ. But this is not possible in all cases. Thus, the existence of two spines in a single animal was completely impossible; consequently that of two spinal cords; still more, there could not be a double cavity in the cerebellum, for the spinal cord arises from it.

Galen discussed the communication between the third and fourth ventricles in another book, the *Anatomical procedures,* IX, 4–5 (Kühn [1821–1833], II, 728–731). Some have claimed that Galen was not describing the aqueduct of Sylvius, but there seems to be sufficient evidence below to indicate that he was. It was also in this passage that he described the floor of the fourth ventricle, including the *calamus scriptorius* of Herophilus.

EXCERPT PP. 728–731

. . . . When all the parts described here have been properly revealed, you will see the third ventricle between the two first and the fourth in the posterior. For you will observe the passages on which the pineal gland rests, extending to the middle ventricle in such a way that two [ducts] of some size appear in the opening. One stretches back to the cerebellum, and if you extend a probe or spatula through it you will realize that it ends in the posterior ventricle. The other in the bottom of the middle ventricle extends downwards [infundibulum]. However, when the pineal gland has been separated from the surrounding parts and rests intact over the passage, it usually slips down rather than remaining upright as when it was covered with membranes and vessels; usually, too, it slips backwards as it falls.

. . . . The aforesaid passage [aqueduct of Sylvius], which extends from the middle [third] to the posterior [fourth] ventricle and is situated between these nates [inferior quadrigeminal bodies], is covered by a special tunic [? superior medullary velum] of substance like that of the membrane [pia mater] that connects all the vessels of the brain. Therefore, employing care, attempt to remove it from the underlying structures always realizing that it will be torn if you are careless. A certain small part of the brain, which has an outline similar to the shape of the worm found in wood [vermis of cerebellum], lies upon it. Hence the name that anatomists, discovering this vermiform excrescence, gave that body which covers the whole passage. You will see that [the vermis] has two ends, an anterior one that extends towards the pineal gland [superior vermis] and a posterior one that is not yet visible, because the whole posterior part of the brain [occipital lobes] lies above it. Grasping and bending this end [inferior vermis], which is situated near the beginning of the spinal marrow [cord], carry it forwards [posteriorly] until you catch sight of another body which is like a worm [choroid plexus of fourth ventricle]. When this has been found, little by little raise the many things which lie above the bodies so that only those are left which, on each side near the passage [aqueduct of Sylvius], have two ends similar in shape to the aforesaid worms. Here you will see slender bodies that attach the vermiform excrescence to the small parts adjacent to the nates on each side of the brain [superior cerebellar peduncles]. Some anatomists call them tendons. Now when you have completed this part of the anatomy and have investigated in turn each end of the vermiform process [vermis], move the whole body [of the cerebellum] somewhat forwards and somewhat to the rear. I say whole, because a little before I said that the vermis lies over each end of the passage. Then notice how the posterior [fourth] ventricle is exposed when [the vermis] is reflected forwards [posteriorly], and, when it is moved backwards [anteriorly], how most of it is concealed and only that part appears which

Herophilus compared to the groove of a reed pen [calamus scriptorius of floor of fourth ventricle]. It is, in fact, similar, having a groove like a cut in the middle [posterior median sulcus], on either side of which the outer edges rise higher than the middle groove [eminentia facialis] as they do in pens. The pens with which we write are so grooved, particularly in Alexandria where Herophilus lived when he was dissecting; hence it may be gathered that he called it so, influenced by the resemblance.

In a further passage (*Use of parts*, VIII, 11, Daremberg [1854–1856], I, 559) Galen discussed the third ventricle and the aqueduct of Sylvius which connects it with the fourth. According to Herophilus, the latter was the most important cavity in the brain. As Miller and Woollam (1962, p. 8) have pointed out, it is essential to realize that Galen was not dissecting the human brain. Thus in the brain of the ox which he said he used, there is no true third ventricle but instead there are connected passages, owing to the large massa intermedia in this animal. This led to interminable confusion in the sixteenth and seventeenth centuries as well as among modern interpreters.

EXCERPT P. 559

In reality the encephalon [cerebrum] is separated from the parencephalon [cerebellum], as we said before, by the fold of the dura mater [tentorium cerebelli] which, having need of being attached to it, at least at one point, in order to produce the above-mentioned channel [aqueduct of Sylvius] first caused its two ventricles to be brought to the same place. That is, in the opinion of certain anatomists, the fourth ventricle [modern third] of the whole encephalon. It is this which they call the opening of the two ventricles. They pretend that one must not consider it [third ventricle] as a genuine ventricle. Insofar as comprehension is concerned, in my opinion it does not matter whether one regards this cavity as common to the two ventricles or as a third ventricle added to the others.

I should like to describe the common juncture of the anterior ventricles explained by the construction of that channel which attaches them to the parencephalon [cerebellum]. Indeed, this channel, issuing from the [third] ventricle and receiving the pneuma that it encloses, transmits it to the parencephalon. As for the part of the encephalon located above the common cavity [third ventricle], and shaped like the cavity of a hollow sphere, like the roof of a house, it seems to me that there was justification for calling it "vaulted body" [fornix], considering it like those parts of buildings that architects usually call vaults and arches. Those who look upon it as a fourth ventricle pretend that it is the most important one of all in the entire encephalon. Herophilus seemed always to consider as the most important one, not this ventricle but that of the cerebellum [modern fourth].

There is further evidence in another book to suggest that Galen had identified the aqueduct of Sylvius (*Anatomical procedures,* IX, 6; Duckworth, 1962, p. 1); and he explained again how a probe could be passed through it. Elsewhere he described the foramen now known by the name of Monro (p. 712), and his account of excretion from the frontal horns of the ventricles through the cribriform plate into the nose also appeared here (IX, 7, Duckworth, pp. 4–6). This last idea was not disproved until the middle of the seventeenth century (Marx, 1873).

Andreas Vesalius
(See p. 153)

As was the case with so many structures of the body, the first accurate and detailed account of the ventricular system surpassing that of Galen was the work of Vesalius. Admittedly, Leonardo da Vinci had produced a wax cast of the human ventricular system about 1504, but his findings were not known until the nineteenth century (O'Malley and Saunders, 1952, pp. 145–147). Vesalius's description is presented in the following passage (*De corporis humani fabrica* [1543], Bk. VII, Ch. VI). Although he denied the presence of excretory ducts running from the lateral ventricles to the cribiform plate as described by Galen, nevertheless Vesalius accepted the one from the third ventricle to the nasopharynx.

He had already denounced the localization of mental functions in the ventricles (pp. 468–469); he does so again in the following passage, but he had nothing to offer in its place. Elsewhere (pp. 632–633) he also denied that the choroid plexus and vermis were valves for the ventricular system.

EXCERPT PP. 633–636

DESCRIPTION OF THE RIGHT AND LEFT VENTRICLES

The right [lateral] ventricle wholly corresponds to the left in site, shape, size, and all those other things that are ordinarily considered in the structure of the parts; therefore that which is written about each part of the right may be presumed to apply also to the left. Now a ventricle lies extended along almost the whole length of the right side of the brain; its anterior [tip] is as far from the forehead as its posterior is from the occiput, and in those places it is separated from the external surface of the brain as much as the right or exterior side of the ventricle, in the direction of the side of the skull, is distant from the surface of the brain. The medial side of the right ventricle, along the length of the corpus callosum, is very close to the medial side of the left ventricle, and they are separated by only the thin, subtle, little membranous portion of the brain that we call the septum [lucidum]. We have said that it, arisen from the corpus callosum, is continuous and attached along its length to the upper part of the vaulted body [fornix]. Thus the inner sides of the right and left ventricles are only barely separated from one another in that whole area where the septum is extended or through the length of the corpus callosum. But in that part of the brain which is clearly divided, such as that which rests upon the cerebellum [occipital poles] and that which is closest to the frontal bone [frontal poles], there the sides of the ventricles are [in the occipital and frontal lobes] at their greatest distance from one another; for in addition to the cerebral membranes contributing to this separation, also much cerebral substance separates the ventricles. Hence the right lateral side of the right ventricle is led somewhat obliquely, for it moves to the right anteriorly and posteriorly more than in the middle, but the left side is extended more in the middle than at its extremities. The anterior part of the ventricle [frontal horn] is blunt and rounded and it does not seem to me, as all others write, that it ends in a point near the olfactory organs and optic nerves. Nor is any passage extended from the ventricle to this part [as Galen had described] except that one on the inner side which—as I shall soon discuss in greater detail—extends downwards to the third ventricle [foramen of Monro]. The posterior part of the ventricle looking towards the occiput [occipital horn] is also blunt and rounded, but it gradually descends [as the inferior or temporal horn] a little into the substance of the brain towards the slightly compressed forward part until it ends where the olfactory organs and optic nerves take origin, and where the largest branches of the carotid arteries are carried into the brain. If you examine the length of its course, it is longer than half the ventricular length that we said is extended from the occiput to the forehead, and this course is extended under that half length into the substance of the brain, ending in a kind of pointed horn. It does not end in the origins of the optic nerves and olfactory organs by any continuation, but it ends at the base of the brain in one of the convolutions of the brain and receives the largest of the arteries [middle cerebral] seeking the brain with a process of the thin membrane [pia mater] supporting it.

MANY UNTRUE TEACHINGS OF GALEN ARE OMITTED HERE

. . . . The whole surface of the ventricle is smooth and covered with an aqueous humor [cerebrospinal fluid] and sometimes during dissection is observed to be filled with it. The upper part of the ventricle is lacking in all unevenness, as are both walls except that that oblique duct of the ventricle seems to produce a kind of protuberance. A certain sinus [channel between thalamus and caudate nucleus on floor of lateral ventricle] creeping obliquely forwards from the external side of the posterior part of the ventricle to that common cavity of the ventricles [third ventricle] prepared for easier disposal of the pituita, renders the floor of the ventricle uneven. Then that part of the ventricle [inferior horn] that creeps downwards from the posterior part towards the anterior produces an unevenness. For that bending back of the ventricle with that sinus is the reason for a little hillock [thalamus] rising in the anterior and posterior of the floor of the ventricle; this is carried from the right side of the slope to the left towards the common cavity of the ventricles. The floors of the right and left ventricles, which are seen to be continuous with the whole length of the corpus callosum, incline downwards towards the common cavity of both [third ventricle], nor, as in the upper parts and sides, are they separated from one another by any septum.

ACCOUNT OF THE COMMON CAVITY OF THE RIGHT AND LEFT VENTRICLES, OR THIRD VENTRICLE

The common cavity of the ventricles is nothing other than the descent and running together of the lower parts of the right and left ventricles under that body compared by professors of dissection to a tortoise [fornix]. In its lower part this cavity resembles a long valley between two neighboring hills [thalami], or it forms an acute angle longitudinally. In the upper part under the concave part of the tortoise that cavity is seen to be round and smooth . . . .

THE PASSAGES FROM THE THIRD VENTRICLE

One of these passages [infundibular recess] is stretched from the lower part of the third ventricle where it cuts a sharp furrow like a valley along the whole length, then directly downwards to the [pituitary] gland receiving the cerebral pituita. The other passage [aqueduct of Sylvius] which is posterior, not the least part of the third ventricle, extends downwards between [beneath] the testes and nates [quadrigeminal bodies] of the brain and above the beginning of the dorsal marrow [brainstem], posterior to the fourth ventricle. The beginning of this passage appears not exactly round but somewhat triangular, and in its lower part retains its original sharp angularity, but in its upper part near the [pineal] gland the passage, which supervises the division of the vessels seeking the third ventricle of the brain, is observed connected by a transverse line to the sides of that angle and forms two other angles with them. The opening of the passage by which the fourth ventricle looks back under the nates of the brain [inferior quadrigeminal bodies] is of this sort. From the lower angle of the passage where first it begins to be carried under the testes of the brain [superior quadrigeminal bodies], another passage is infrequently led forth which, extended downwards and forwards through the substance of the brain, finally reaches as far as the cup [pituitary fossa] which, as we shall teach, receives the cerebral pituita.

ACCOUNT OF THE FOURTH VENTRICLE

The fourth ventricle, to which the posterior passage of the third ventricle [aqueduct] extends, is formed from the sinuses of the dorsal marrow [brainstem] and the cerebellum, not otherwise than if you were to form a cavity with your two hands, for the whole ventricle is by no means carved into the body of the cerebellum. And so the dorsal marrow [brainstem] goes forth from the cerebrum, where the third ventricle first extends a passage towards the fourth ventricle, and the testes and nates [quadrigeminal bodies] are continued to the origin of the marrow, and leads down that passage of the third ventricle with the origin of the dorsal marrow, so that the upper part of the passage is incised from them, the lower from the dorsal marrow [brainstem]. After that passage has passed the nates [inferior quadrigeminal bodies] the portion of it which seems carved from the dorsal marrow [brainstem] begins to widen and forms a hollow extending almost to that place where the dorsal marrow issues from the calvarium [foramen magnum]. Herophilus very correctly compared this sinus to the hollow of the quill with which we write [calamus scriptorius], because if we compare it to that part of the quill that we dip in the ink, you will notice that the orifice of the pen, where it is still rounded and near the cutoff end, resembles the end of the passage of the third ventricle that spreads out under the nates [inferior quadrigeminal body]. Then you will see that the point with which we write is like the lower part of the cavity producing a kind of pore or narrow passage carved into the dorsal marrow [central canal] where it leaves the skull; but you will see that two angles of the quill, which we cut between the point, and the beginning of the highest part of the cut, as well as the sides of the quill's hollow, are very similar to the sides of the cavity. At the sides of this cavity where those angles are formed [lateral recesses] one on each side, there is one round process of the dorsal marrow to which the cerebellum is attached [inferior cerebellar peduncle] and forms a continuous body with the dorsal marrow. Thus the cavity of the dorsal marrow forms part of the cavity of the fourth ventricle . . . .

THE SEPARATE PARTS OF THE VENTRICLES

In dissection the fourth ventricle is observed to contain nothing except the watery humor [cerebrospinal fluid] that is common to the other ventricles, but not the passage running from the third ventricle into the fourth. The right and left ventricles, in addition to that humor, also contain a plexus which those skilled in dissection compare to the outermost covering of the fetus [choroid plexus]. The common cavity or third ventricle leads down that venous vessel [vein of Galen] which, as we taught in the Third

Book, arises from the fourth [straight] sinus of the dural membrane to form that plexus. Then the anterior part of these ventricles sometimes receives slender venules from that vessel, just as we see very similar ones to adorn the adhering tunic [choroid coat] of the eye. Venules of this sort are readily attached to the surface [wall] of the ventricles, because the substance of the brain is observed to be harder and, so to speak, more callous in the surface [wall] of the ventricles than elsewhere.

. . . .

THE USE OF THE VENTRICLES

I have decided for the present to say nothing about the ventricles other than that they are hollows or cavities in which air, drawn in during inspiration, and vital spirit, transmitted to them by the heart, are altered by the power of the peculiar substance of the brain into animal spirit. Afterwards this is distributed through the nerves to the organs of the senses and of movement, so that by the aid of this spirit and through a construction suited to the functions of such organs they may perform their duty by which the muscles move, the eyes see, the olfactory organs smell, the auditory organs perceive sounds, the tongue recognizes flavors, and, finally, every part to which a nerve is extended recognizes tactile qualities. Hence I do not hesitate to ascribe to the ventricles a share in the production of animal spirit, but I believe nothing ought to be said of the locations of the faculties of the principal soul in the brain—even though they are so assigned by those who today rejoice in the name of theologians, who believe that they may with impunity say what they please. All our contemporaries deny the particular powers of the principal soul to apes, dogs, horses, sheep, oxen, and other animals and, in brief, attribute only to man the faculty of reason, and that, insofar as I am able to understand, equally to all men. Nevertheless in dissection we see that men do not differ from animals by the possession of any special ventricle; not only is the number of ventricles the same, but all other things are very much alike in man and animal except in respect to the mass of the brain and a temperamental urge towards upright conduct.

GIULIO CESARE ARANZI
(*1530—7 April 1589*)

Despite the excellence of Vesalius's account of the ventricular system, he was vague about certain parts of it and the Italian anatomist, Aranzi, made good some of these deficiencies.

Aranzi was born in Bologna where he studied anatomy under Bartolomeo Maggi, and obtained the M.D. degree in 1556. He was eventually appointed professor of anatomy and surgery in the University of Bologna and occupied that position with distinction for thirty-three years. Aranzi is best known for his accounts of the gravid uterus, the fetus, the heart, and the brain, and he made several important discoveries in these and in other organs. He also described the pulmonary circulation (see Portal, 1770–1773, II, 2–27; Fantuzzi, 1781–1794, I, 266–272, IX, 23; Mondella, 1961).

In his book, *De humano foetu liber tertio editus, ac recognitus. Eiusdem anatomicarum observationum liber* . . . (Venice, 1587, Ch. II of the latter work), Aranzi provided an improved description of the temporal or lateral horns of the lateral ventricles, and of the choroid plexus; he also gave the first account of the hippocampus and its relationships with the ventricles. He was the first to give the name "aqueduct" to the passage connecting the third and fourth ventricles which was later named after François de le Boë, Sylvius, 1614–1672 (F. Baker, 1909).

EXCERPT PP. 43–45

CHAPTER I. ON THE VENTRICLES OF THE BRAIN NAMED FROM THE HIPPOCAMPUS

In addition to those sinuses, usually called ventricles, that have been observed in the substance of the brain, in which the wholly pure animal spirit is made from air inspired through the olfactory organ and from vital spirit conveyed through the carotid arteries, I have found two other notable sinuses or cavities hidden and concealed in the deeper parts of the brain. They are not much smaller than the upper sinuses or ventricles, and like them are circumscribed by the membranous and very solid substance of the brain. They lie concealed on either side under the two anterior ventricles and extend forwards like the lower, concealed sleeping quarters of ships. Like the two upper [lateral] ventricles they run together and form the third or common sinus at about the center of the brain [collateral trigone].

CHAPTER II. THE CHOROID PLEXUSES DISTRIBUTED THROUGH THE SAME SINUSES

In that way in which branches of the choroid plexus are distributed into the upper ventricles, so branches of those same plexuses are led around on either side from the third ventricle to each of these [lower] ventricles—in my opinion for the manufacture of animal spirit. These deeply submerged branches are distributed through the [lower] cavities [inferior horns] with such elegant arrangement that the careful observer is readily persuaded that these are true ventricles and not verbal or anatomical figments; for nowhere will you find a plexus of this sort dispersed through the substance of the brain except in the ventricles themselves. When the choroid [plexuses] have issued from the upper ventricles, they unite in the third [ventricle]; with the spirit doubled they communicate at the conarius [pineal body] with a noteworthy vessel approaching from the fourth [straight] sinus of the dural membrane so that with a multiple reticulated plexus of the arteries formed, the spirit runs through all the ventricles, lower as well as upper, and finally there is one confluence and union from the mixture of this elaborated vital spirit and inspired air, and with the concurrence of the brain the animal spirit receives its perfected form. How can anyone consider that the [lower] ventricles are recesses or tunnels of the superior ventricles? but even so they ought not to be overlooked.

CHAPTER III. THE PARTS OF THE BRAIN RESEMBLING A HIPPOCAMPUS

In the floor of those ventricles which face inwardly towards the middle [inferior horns] there appears a raised, partially attached, whitish substance [hippocampal formation] which is extended as an addition from the lower surface. It is continuous with the vaulted body or tortoise [fornix] and is extended lengthwise towards the front [of the brain]; it has an uneven, bent form which resembles the appearance of a hippocampus, that is a sea horse, or rather enfolded on either side by the beginning of the spinal marrow [brainstem] it presents the shape of a white silkworm. We shall discuss its use elsewhere. The small part of it resembling the head is very near to the third ventricle, but the body bent away towards the tail is extended to the anterior. The [lower] ventricles [inferior horns], in distinction to the upper, may be called those of the hippocampus or silkworm. It is also worthy of note that when the choroid plexus has been raised from the base of the ventricles, an astonishingly involved collection of slender vessels is observed, more complicated than in the upper ventricles. It is related to the cavities and other things.

EXCERPT P. 48

CHAPTER VII. THE CAVITY OF THE CEREBELLUM WHICH WE CALL THE CISTERN

At the base of the so-called third ventricles, below the conarium [pineal gland], where the little bodies called *glutia* [superior quadrigeminal bodies] are located, which can be removed with a slight incision, anatomists, as has been seen, place the origin of the fourth ventricle which they have aptly compared to a reed pen [calamus scriptorius]. However, taking other things into consideration, "ventricle" does not seem to be a suitable name for it, and it ought rather to be considered as a channel or aqueduct. It descends from the center of the brain, that is, from what is called the third ventricle, between the cerebellum and the spinal marrow [brainstem] to the occiput, and carries down the confected animal spirit to a cistern or sinus of the brain [fourth ventricle]. Thus in almost the center of the cerebellum, that is, in the most hidden part of it, is situated a cavity, not very far from the base of the head and the aperture of the occiput from which the dorsal marrow slips out [foramen magnum].

Early Accounts of the Cerebrospinal Fluid

Although so much detailed knowledge of the ventricles and brain coverings was known in antiquity, it is astonishing to note that the cerebrospinal fluid was mentioned only vaguely on two or three occasions. It seems likely that the ancient Egyptian commentator of the Edwin Smith Surgical Papyrus was referring to the cerebrospinal fluid when he mentioned the presence of fluid in a penetrating head wound (p. 384). Both a Hippocratic Writer and Galen referred to "humors" in the ventricles, but there is no clear statement discoverable in any of the writings of antiquity. Galen, who must have been aware of the cerebrospinal fluid, was more concerned with the animal spirits and waste products that he believed to be contained in the ventricles.

No doubt Leonardo da Vinci had seen the ventricular fluid in 1504 during his experiments to produce a cast of the ventricular system, but his work remained unknown and therefore had no influence. In his commentary on Mondino's anatomical treatise Berengario da Carpi (1521, fol. 438*v*) discussed the spiritous and fluid superfluities of the ventricles and stated of the latter:

> In my opinion the gross superfluity of the brain ["watery excrement"] can be seen in the majority of heads dissected because some of it is always in the ventricles of the brain . . . . I believe that there is more of this moisture in one body than in another.

Later (fol. 439*r*) he made an analogy between the ventricular fluid and that found in the pericardial sac; in each instance it was "constantly a watery substance." In his *Isagoge* (1523) Berengario published the first perceptual representation of the lateral ventricles (fig. 154).

Following Massa's description in 1536 the cerebrospinal fluid was frequently observed, but until Cotugno's discovery in 1764, only in the ventricles of the brain. It was usually thought to be in some way associated with Galen's ventricular animal spirits or waste products, a belief that persisted tenaciously into the eighteenth century. Many writers thought that it appeared only after death. Although the subarachnoid fluid may have been observed, it could have no significance and the idea of a circulation was impossible so long as the ventricles were considered to be a closed system, as was demanded by the Galenic theory; accordingly, the only exits were by way of the hollow nerves.

Investigators like Willis and Haller suggested that the cerebrospinal fluid was of vascular origin and thought, perhaps correctly, that the site of origin was the choroid plexuses. But the most important advance of this period was made by Cotugno who was the first to describe the fluid surrounding the spinal cord and to suggest that it was in continuity with the ventricular and cerebral subarachnoid fluids. However, his concept of a cerebral and spinal fluid, which is the beginning of its modern physiology, remained in obscurity until rediscovered by Magendie some sixty years later.

NICOLO MASSA
(1485–1569)

The first clear account of the cerebrospinal fluid was given by the Italian anatomist Massa whose importance as a precursor of Vesalius has recently been realized.

Massa was born in Venice and studied medicine at the University of Padua. Thereafter he practised medicine successfully in Venice but found time to carry on anatomical investigations and write an anatomical treatise that included some important contributions to the pre-Vesalian study of the subject; his descriptions of the anterior abdominal muscles, the peritoneum, the prostate, and the olfactory nerves were of especial note. He also wrote on syphilis and its treatment with mercury, and on the plague (see Portal, 1770–1773, I, 350–355; O'Malley, 1964, pp. 122–123, 438–439).

Massa's *Liber introductorius anatomiae* (Venice, 1536) contains his account of the cerebrospinal fluid, but like Vesalius (pp. 714–718), he denied the presence of psychological functions in the ventricles.

EXCERPT FOL. 84v

. . . . Observe the watery superfluity in these cavities, sent there from the other parts of the brain and expurgated through a foramen [imaginary passages, via sphenoid and cribriform plate] from the cavities of the ventricles . . . . It is especially noteworthy that I have always found these cavities full or half-full of the aforementioned, watery superfluity of the rational brain.

EXCERPT FOLS. 85v–86R

. . . . Note that in the middle [third] ventricle no collection of veins or arteries is found; hence there is no power of the mind in it, and it is consonant with reason to place all the powers of the mind in the anterior part of the brain where the spirit is in its vessels, and to say that that middle ventricle is a route carrying the superfluities, like other cavities of this very humid organ . . . . you will see a transit, which is now midway between the anterior brain and the posterior brain which is called the cerebellum, to a cavity descending toward the space [fourth ventricle]. Many unreasonably believe that this space is the posterior ventricle, but if you inspect it carefully you will find also another pathway [aqueduct of Sylvius] proceeding to the posterior brain which, even if it is a small pathway and is found only by the most expert anatomists, nevertheless it is always present and makes transit to the final ventricle.

EXCERPT FOLS. 86R–86V

. . . . you must understand that these ventricles are rather for the collection and expulsion of superfluities than for the diverse operations of the mind, which are performed through different parts, since no veins or arteries are found in the last [fourth] ventricle which proceeds into the posterior cerebellum . . . . You see from these aforesaid ventricles, that is, the anterior, middle, and posterior, nothing primary occurs for the operations of the mind, since there is no spirit in them . . . . but the spirit is in the arteries in the anterior ventricles, in which the spirit in the arteries creates powers of the mind for intrinsic operations. These powers, according to the differences of the grades of the spirit, cause the different operations of the mind. Just as the veins are the proper place for the blood so the arteries are the proper place for the spirit, for the spirit is not found outside the arteries except in the left ventricle of the heart, just as the blood is found outside the veins in the right ventricle.

THOMAS WILLIS
(See p. 158)

By the seventeenth century the gross anatomy of the meninges, the ventricular system, and of the choroid plexuses had been described in considerable detail and further accounts will not be included here. The microscopic appearances were not dealt with until the nineteenth century, and certain special parts of the ventricles such as the foramen of Monro had to await more precise dissection for more complete descriptions (Wilder, 1880; Magendie, 1827*a–c*; Luschka, 1855, and Sharp, 1961).

Meantime the functions of the ventricles and the choroid plexuses and the origin and purpose of the cerebrospinal fluid engaged the attention of investigators. One of the most important was Willis who was the first to suggest a new function for the choroid plexuses. He did not, however, reject entirely the Galenic ideas and still believed, for example, in animal spirit and the excretion of waste products through the infundibulum of the third ventricle. His attempt to explain the activity of the choroid plexuses on a chemical basis was in keeping with his iatrochemical associations. Nevertheless, it is interesting to note how close he was to present-day concepts of cerebrospinal fluid production, albeit in a crude and somewhat fanciful way. The following passages have been translated from Willis's *Cerebri anatome* (London,

1664), Chapters XI and XIV, respectively. They also provide an insight into Willis's general ideas of brain tissue function.

EXCERPT PP. 73–75

With regard to the aforesaid *inwardly remaining faculties*, we may now notice in addition that their more outstanding *operations* are especially and almost solely performed by *the spirits* that have already been *perfected* and highly elaborated. If those *recently-made* or *being-made* spirits are in abundance, they severely obstruct and impede the acts of the animal function; for example, when the subtle fluid is copiously instilled from the vessels everywhere irrigating the cortex of the brain, as the material of the animal spirits, this fluid fills all the pores and passages of the brain and for that period of time blocks off the spirits from their accustomed tracts and pathways of distribution. Therefore, while this very powerful *restoration* of the brain and the spirits is being performed, *sleep* or *the eclipse of the spirits* occurs; *wakefulness* returns when the more subtle part of the fluid has been instilled and refined into very pure animal spirits and the more watery portion resolved into vapor has been partly exhaled, partly absorbed by the venous passages entering the substance of the brain, or has sweated out into the empty spaces lying under the corpus callosum [lateral ventricles]. I hope later to speak more fully about these things. Now to proceed to the remaining matters concerning *the brain,* properly so called, there yet remains the subject of *the ventricles,* but since they are only *an empty space resulting from the folding of the exterior border of the brain,* it does not seem necessary to discuss their function in detail any more than astronomers are accustomed to speak of the empty space contained within the cavity of the universe.

But since there is nothing in nature that has not been destined for some use, certainly we suspect that *this cavity* within the globe of the brain was not established without purpose. *The ancients* so magnified the importance of *this cavity* that they declared it to be the workshop where the animal spirits are created and perform the chief operations of the animal function. On the other hand, *the moderns* consider these places as vile and assert them to be merely sewers for the carrying away of excreted matter. However, the opinion of the ancients can be readily overthrown, because the animal spirits, very subtle and liable to dissipation, do not require so wide and open a space, but rather more narrow passages and little pores such as are produced in the substance of the brain; since this spirit had to be composed in various arrangements and different orders for the different *faculties of the soul,* it must therefore be moved within special tracts and orbits. Furthermore, if one considers exactly the structure of the brain and gives serious thought to the fact that the ventricles are not formed by the primary intention of nature but only secondarily, and result accidentally from the folding of the brain, one will be far from believing that the supreme seat of the soul is fixed there, hemmed in by a very noble *retinue of spirits,* to execute and perform its functions. For it is not at all clear from what kind of material and by what contrivance the animal spirits are created there, nor by what ways of emanation they are sent thence into the other parts of the brain and nervous system. Therefore almost all anatomists of more recent times have given to this more inward chamber of the brain the vile duty of a sewer. Some substance has been added to this belief because in the dead these ventricles are often observed to be filled with water; furthermore, ways seem to lie open from the ventricles for excretion to the infundibulum [infundibular recess] and to *the cribriform plate.* It is observed that wherever *the blood* flows more copiously into some part and irrigates it, there *vapors* or watery *humors* are created from the superfluous serum left in circulation; for the most part they exhale outwards either as *vaporous effluvia* or are returned into the blood through *the veins* or *lymphatic vessels.* But when a copious supply of blood irrigates not only the cortex of the brain, but also the interior medulla [white matter], if *the serous fluid* in the blood is too abundant for its superfluities to be immediately drawn off through the veins or through the lymph ducts (if they are present there), or strained off by the glands, it may slip down into that cave hollowed out within the folding of the brain [ventricles]. In truth, there are many instances plainly indicating that the serous humors are deposited throughout the ventricles of the brain. *Anatomical observations* of men dead from many brain diseases, and especially from soporific diseases, confirm this.

EXCERPT PP. 91–92

From these things thus posited about *the pineal gland,* it will not be difficult also to attribute the use of *the choroid plexus.* There will be little need to refute the common opinion of it according to which it is asserted that the animal spirits supplying the whole brain are created in this plexus; indeed, its vessels instill nothing into the substance of the brain or its appendix [spinal cord] because nowhere are they inserted into it, and it was indicated above that the ventricles of the brain, or the cavity in which the same vessels are suspended, do not at all contain the spirits; this, furthermore, is clearly apparent when in diseases of the brain those ventricles are filled with water and the continuity of the plexus is dissolved by too much moisture, although, meanwhile, the sick are only partly capable of enjoying the animal faculties.

We suppose that this *plexus* serves *a double purpose,* that is, *first,* that the more watery part of the blood destined for the brain may be sent off into its vessels, so that the remaining portion of the fluid in the blood may become more pure and free from excrements for its distillation into spirits, not otherwise than normally occurs in *a chemical distillation;* that is, when a special receptacle is adapted to receive only *the phlegm* and the more pure and subtle spirits are distilled into another more noteworthy receptacle. The more watery blood entering the arterial vessels of this plexus and carried from them into the veins is sent back towards the heart; meanwhile, lest the serum bubbling in these vessels become overfull and hinder the circulation, its superfluities are received for some time by thickly inserted *little glands* [these were in the choroid plexus and may have been the villous processes or cysts] and by *the pineal gland.*

The other and not less noteworthy *use of this plexus* is to conserve the heat arisen from the blood within the complications of the vessels, driven in a kind of circular course and heated as by a hearth within the folding of the brain. Although the pia mater need not insert dense shoots of vessels into *the corpus callosum* and the medullary portion of the brain [white matter], that is given over rather to *the exercise* than to *the generation* of animal spirits, nevertheless, in order that *the heat required for the circulation of the spirits* be constantly maintained there, this *plexus* is suspended in proximity. As the blood collected within the cavities of the sinuses takes the place of *a hot spring* by which the animal spirits are copiously distilled in the outer, cortical part of the brain, so the blood contained within the slender vessels of this plexus seems to fill the place of *a smaller,* more temperate *spring* by which the same spirits may more suitably be circulated in the more inward and medullary substance.

Finally, another reason may be offered as to why *the choroid plexus* is always found within the ventricles or cavity of the brain made from its folding, and with differing configurations; that is, that another kind of commodity may result thence, so that when the vessels of that plexus, carrying too much watery blood, deposit more serum than what the glands are able to receive and contain, that the superfluity may opportunely descend into the underlying cavity as into a sewer. Therefore *the pineal gland,* although located in a more eminent place, yet is always placed near the foramen or duct which lies open towards *the infundibulum* [infundibular process] in every brain.

ALBRECHT VON HALLER

(*See p. 170*)

There were no outstanding additions to knowledge of cerebrospinal fluid production or function until Haller in the middle of the eighteenth century was able to support Willis's opinion with experimental evidence. By the use of injection techniques he argued that the fluid in the cerebral ventricles and on the surface of the brain originated from the arteries. Moreover, since it was taken up by the veins, for the first time the idea of a circulation of cerebrospinal fluid was conceived. Haller used the analogy of similar events in other closed cavities of the body, first set forth by Berengario (p. 764), and he made the first references to the physical properties of the fluid. However, he could not divorce himself entirely from the idea of a gaseous substance in the ventricles; this was a vapor which condensed into a fluid that he termed "water" or "thin humor."

The following passage has been translated from Haller's famous textbook of physiology that was the first of its kind. (*Elementa physiologiae corporis humani*, Vol. IV [Lausanne, 1762], Bk. X, Sec. I, pt. xix.)

EXCERPT PP. 43–45

THE WATER OF THE VENTRICLES

The ceiling of the ventricle, in distinction to the floor, produces a vapor that breathes out from all parts of the membrane lining the ventricle and from the plexuses, as they may be called, and covers all the internal surface of the cavity with a slight moisture. In addition to my own experiments I have, as my witnesses for this, numerous leading anatomists. Since this is a light vapor it does not always collect into water, and is sometimes absent in very fresh, intact cadavers. It has, however, a common relationship with the pericardial fluid and the moisture of the pleural cavity and abdomen.

In the living animal an observable vapor breathes out either from the exterior surface of the brain [subarachnoid space] or from the hollow of the ventricle.

It is clear that the moisture exhales from the arteries, since if a thin liquid is injected into the arteries, it sweats out from all the surface of the ventricles. I have often repeated this experiment.

Also, as I have said, I have often seen a colored, gelatinous impression in the ventricles when I filled the arteries.

The same humor is as clearly drawn into the veins. For if you inject clear or colored water, or glue dissolved in alcohol into the large venous trunks, perspirable humor will sweat from all their surface as clearly as it would be breathed out through the arteries.

There seems little doubt that as in the pericardium, pleura, and other bellows of the human body, so a thin humor constantly exhales from the arteries into the ventricles of the brain, and in the same way is continually drawn back through the veins; this agrees with the examples of all the other cavities in the body.

But as often as the function of the veins becomes weakened, or is weak as is usual in chronic diseases, so often the collected moisture is turned into water and even distends the ventricles of the brain by a notable mass. A great abundance of water has been found in the ventricles of apoplectics, the soporose, phrenetics, convulsives, paralytics, and victims of epidemic fevers; hydrocephalus even more.

I find that 113 *uncias* have been seen in the hydropic cerebrum, and in the ventricles, one, two, three, four, nine, and thirteen *libras*.

For some time after death this exhalation, like other vapors, seems to be generated from the arteries; hence much water is found in the ventricles several hours after death. Even when wiped away it returns in the animal's newly opened brain [excellent evidence for active secretion].

When the ancients found such a quantity they considered it to be pituitous excrement of the cerebrum [i.e., phlegm].

The quality is gelatinous with a diffuse, sour, mineral taste; it gathers into the membranes either by means of spirit of wine or by fire; as a result of other experiments famous men say that perhaps putridity is the cause of such great exhalation. So in the dissected brain of fishes there is distilled an albuminous, coagulable humor, as well as in the hydatids of the brain and in the cellular [areolar] covering of the arachnoid membrane. As often certainly as some experiments produce some coagulable juice, others induce it to evaporate, but more faith ought to be placed in the former. For delay and putridity can render it evaporable but no accident renders it coagulable.

DOMENICO FELICE ANTONIO COTUGNO
(29 January 1736—6 October 1822)

It has been claimed that Valsalva (1666–1723) first recognized the spinal subarachnoid fluid in 1692 (Bilancioni, 1911). He did in fact mention a collection of "humor" around the brainstem ("beginning of the spinal marrow") similar to that found in joints (Morgagni, 1761, p. 180). This, however, was in a dog in which both carotid arteries had been ligated, and even if it had been cerebrospinal fluid it was not spinal, as is usually claimed, and Valsalva made no further reference to it. There is, however, no doubt that Cotugno gave the first adequate description of the spinal subarachnoid cerebrospinal fluid.

Cotugno was born in Ruvo di Puglia in the southeast of Italy. He studied at the University of Naples and then worked there as physician and anatomist until 1766 when he was appointed to the chair of anatomy. At the same time he was the leading Neapolitan physician and was active in the affairs of the University and in public and private charities. He studied the contents of the petrous temporal bone and the acoustic nerve and proposed a theory of hearing which antedated that of Helmholtz by a hundred years. He also wrote on typhus fever and smallpox (see Bianchi, 1928, Viets, 1935).

The book for which Cotugno is justly famous is *De ischiade nervosa commentarius* (Naples, 1764). In it he pointed out that the extracerebral and spinal fluid had not been seen in the past because of the methods of dissecting the nervous system and he described a technique whereby this might be avoided. Like Haller, he suggested that cerebrospinal fluid originated from blood vessels and, most important of all, that the ventricular and spinal fluids were continuous with one another.

A translation of Cotugno's book into English appeared in 1775. Despite this English translation and a further one into German in 1792, little attention was paid to Cotugno's discovery, until Magendie (1827c) resurrected it in 1827 by reprinting the Latin text of paragraphs ix to xvi. The following excerpt has been newly translated from the edition of 1764.

EXCERPT PP. 12–14

. . . . I have always seen the [epidural] space from the dura mater to the walls of the spinal cavity filled with a cellular [areolar] stuffing that is soft, fluid, and fatty . . . . Whatever space exists between the sheath of dura mater and the spinal marrow, it is always *filled* not by the marrow, which is fuller in the living, nor by a vaporous mist, as very eminent men seem to believe of this yet obscure matter, but by *a water* similar to that which is contained around the heart in the pericardium [cf. Berengario, p. 721], or that which fills the ventricular cavities of the brain, the labyrinth of the ear, or, finally, fills the other cavities of the body to which the air has no entry.

x

Not only does this water contained in the tube of dura mater ensheathing the spinal marrow from the occiput to the os sacrum, surround the marrow constantly, but it also abounds in the hollow of the skull and fills all the spaces found between the brain and the encompassing dura mater. Several spaces are always found under the base of the brain, and not rarely a noteworthy space may be found between the remaining circumference of the brain and its embracing dura mater [cistern] . . . . It seems to be a human law that the space around the spinal marrow that is filled with water increases with man's age, for there is almost no space in the fetus in which the dural tube tightly embraces the marrow, especially in the neck; with increase in age the space becomes larger.

xi

Hitherto anatomists have not observed this large collection of water in the spine and around the brain because of the ridiculous method usually employed for the dissection of bodies. When they are about to examine the brain, they usually cut off the head with the neck, and when this has been done, and the tube of dura mater descending through the spine of the neck has been cut through, all the fluid collected around the brain and the spinal marrow is at once lost; thus when the skull is opened, all the spaces between the brain and the dura mater that were once filled with water are found to be empty, and the anatomist is misled by the appearance of empty spaces which perhaps may once have been filled with a now dissipated vapor. There scarcely remains the slightest bit of that water within the cavities of the base of the skull or within the special sheathed space' of the dura mater receiving the nerves from the brain to prove the former existence of the fluid. As a result of this incorrect dissection procedure, when all the fluid collected around the marrow [spinal cord] and brain has flowed out, it is replaced by air which fills those spaces vacated by the fluid. This is the reason why those examining the brain often find little bubbles of air under the arachnoid membrane in the highest part of the brain's sulci. The number is greater or smaller in proportion to the larger or smaller spaces on the convexity of the sulci of the arachnoid and pial membranes of the specimens. There is a very open passage to these spaces from the base of the skull where the arachnoid, descending to the spine, becomes as distant as possible from the pia mater [cisterna magna]; it is through this passage that the cerebral fluid of the sulci readily pours out when the neck has been cut through and permits air immediately to replace the fluid. However, I am never accustomed to find bubbles of air under the arachnoid in those heads which I have carefully opened, still fully joined to the trunk.

EXCERPT PP. 15–17

. . . . Through these [dissection] procedures, performed at different times on about twenty adult male bodies, I was able to draw off easily from the hollow of the spine, four and sometimes even five ounces of water; usually that water is very clear in adults, although sometimes verging slightly to yellowish; however, in fetuses suffocated in difficult birth, little as it was, I always found it an opaque, pale red.

XIII

It may be doubted with considerable probability of truth that this collection of fluid around the brain and spinal marrow is normally to be found in man only after death, and that alive, those spaces are empty or filled with a vaporous mist or a more swollen marrow. For it does not seem likely that an empty space during life will be found filled with a fluid after death; that would oppose the law of nature that states: *There is no space in the body of living things which if it is not filled by air or some solid substance is not filled by a fluid.* Nor, if a vaporous mist were to fill those spaces when man is alive, does it seem that condensed after death it would fill those same spaces with water. Moreover, vivisection of certain animals confirms the presence of a true fluid collected around the brain and spinal marrow, although doubted in a living man. I dissected various fishes either alive or immediately after death, and recently in particular a sea tortoise weighing fifteen pounds. In proportion to the capacity of the skull the mass of its brain was very small so that from the brain to the whole inner circumference of the skull there was a large intervening space; all this space was filled with a large quantity of water which also filled the remaining cavity of the spine and appeared to lie around the marrow itself.* However, I was unable to find this same thing in living dogs and fowl, because their brain and spinal marrow were of such size, living or dead, that they equalled the capacity of the hollows in which they were contained. Even if these animals are not so suitable for proving the presence of a condensed vapor, they do prove, nevertheless, that the brain and spinal marrow do not decrease in size with death. Although there are those who imagine that the spinal marrow is more swollen in life and equals in size the whole surrounding space, they ought to notice that the nerves arising from the spinal marrow run through that space without obstruction in the cadaver, but would then in the living subject be entangled and compressed. Therefore that space found around the spinal marrow is naturally filled with water and in the cadaver is almost without difference from its appearance in the living man.

XIV

It seems astonishing that eminent men who have very carefully examined the fluid in the cavities of the human body have overlooked the very remarkable and, so to speak, chief and abundant collection of fluid in the spine. It seems beyond all possible doubt that the spinal fluid, as well as that which humectifies all the other cavities of the body, constantly oozes from the extremities of the smallest arteries and, finally, is absorbed through very small inhaling veins, so that there is a continual state of renovation. It was I in particular who proved elsewhere by experiment that certain of the inhaling mouths of the dura mater's venules open on its internal surface, once doubted by Abraham Kaavius, grandson of the illustrious Boerhaave. I have no doubt, and recently the famous Haller has given full credence to the belief, that those waters which the cerebellar ventricle receives, whether from the larger ventricles of the cerebrum through the lacuna and the aqueduct of Sylvius, whether from special exhaling arteries, are thereafter mixed with the waters of the spine; the perpendicular position and rather open passage at the hollow of the spine [cistern] are clearly indicative of the flowing down of the fluid into the spine.

* This finding has been used to account for an otherwise inexplicable statement made by Aristotle concerning the presence of an empty space in the occipital portion of the cranial cavity in man. See Clarke and Stannard (1963).

Modern Physiology of the Cerebrospinal Fluid

Magendie's classic accounts of the cerebrospinal fluid in the third decade of the nineteenth century have proved to be the foundation for all subsequent work on its origin, its elimination, its properties, its constituents, and its function. Closer anatomical observations, both gross and microscopic, such as those of Luschka (1855) and Faivre (1853–1854), gave greater clarity to the idea that the fluid circulated and they provided further evidence that the choroid plexuses produced it. The improved injection techniques, introduced for example by Key and Retzius (1875), employed the new products of the German dye industry which were then becoming available; they concluded that the cerebrospinal fluid was removed by way of the arachnoidal villi of Pacchioni, an idea still subscribed to by many but probably incorrect. In the last decade of the nineteenth century the lumbar puncture was introduced and the clinician was thus provided with a new approach to the diagnosis and treatment of diseases of the nervous system. But, interestingly enough, it was not this stimulus which provoked further research into the physiology of the fluid now readily obtainable. The new advances of the second decade of the twentieth century came from the young and virile field of neurosurgery. In his approaches to the central nervous system the surgeon became aware of problems relating to the cerebrospinal fluid that demanded elucidation, and the ease of access to it afforded by his operations in man and in animals was an important factor in this regard. Another significant influence on research into this field has been in the further use of dyes. The investigation of their behavior towards living nervous tissue has led to the concept of the blood–brain barrier and related phenomena.

Thus since the pioneer work of the early decades of the present century, a large mass of data has accumulated, but until quite recently little advance has been made towards universally acceptable theories. Newer techniques employing radioactive materials which, unlike dyestuffs, do not interfere with the dynamics of the cerebrospinal fluid, are now providing information which suggests that some of the long-cherished opinions, such as absorption of the fluid through the Pacchionian villi, may be incorrect.

Only the problems relating to the site of formation and elimination of cerebrospinal fluid can be dealt with here and not the equally important question as to whether fluid production is a process of secretion, transudation, or of both.

François Jean Magendie
(See p. 299)

The opinions of Cotugno, imbedded as they were in a book on sciatica, had little or no immediate effect and nothing of note was added to the knowledge of the cerebrospinal fluid until Magendie began his investigations in 1824. His precise and skillful experiments and perceptive observations once more clarified a confused situation and began a new era of research. Moreover, the term "cerebrospinal fluid" was his.

On 10 January 1825 Magendie read his first paper on the subject to the Académie des Sciences in Paris (Mémoire sur un liquide qui se trouve dans le crâne et le canal vertébral de l'homme et des animaux mammifères, *J. Physiol. exp. path.*, Paris, 1825, 5:27–37). He pointed out that the cerebrospinal fluid was a normal finding in man and mammals. Like Cotugno, he recognized it on the surface of the brain and the spinal cord, and by injection experiments demonstrated a free communication between the two sites and with the ventricular system. It was located "between the pia mater and the internal or cerebrospinal surface of the arachnoid" [p. 37].

Magendie gave full recognition to Cotugno for his prior discovery—in fact he reprinted Cotugno's account of the fluid as an appendix (pp. 83–96) to a paper he read to the Académie on 12 February 1827 ("Troisième et dernière partie du second mémoire sur le liquide qui se trouve dans le crâne et l'épine de l'homme et des animaux vertébrés," *J. Physiol. exp. path.*, Paris, 1827, 7:66–82). This generous action should be taken into account when the notorious priority conflict between himself and Charles Bell concerning the spinal roots (pp. 299–303) is being assessed. The following selection is a summary of Magendie's findings, which included the discovery of the foramen of Magendie in the roof of the fourth ventricle.

EXCERPT PP. 79–80

From facts and experiments reported in the three parts of this Memoir, I have deduced the following conclusions:

1.° The cerebrospinal fluid is one of the natural fluids of the body and henceforth because of its uses it must be given first place in a list of these fluids;

2.° It is indispensable to the free exercise of the functions of the brain and the spinal cord;

3.° It protects these parts from external injuries;

4.° It influences the functions of the brain and the spinal cord by the pressure that it transmits to these parts, by its temperature, and by its chemical nature;

5.° At the base of the fourth ventricle opposite to the calamus scriptorius there is a constant opening which permits an easy communication between the cavities of the brain and the cerebrospinal fluid [foramen of Magendie];

6.° The ventricles are constantly full of this fluid. These cavities can contain two ounces of it without there being any defect of intellectual faculties; beyond that quantity there is a disturbance [of them], ordinarily a paralysis of movement and a more or less considerable decrease of intelligence;

7.° It is extremely likely that from time to time, and particularly with the movements of the brain, there occur a flux and a reflux of the cerebrospinal fluid from the spine into the ventricles and from the ventricles into the spine;

8.° A fluid produced accidentally in the spine soon passes into the cavities of the brain and fills them;

9.° A fluid produced in a ventricle passes without delay into the others and promptly reaches as far as the base of the sacrum;

10.° An accidental fluid which has its source on the surface of the cerebral hemispheres can, in little more than an instant, reach into the cavities of the spine and into those of the brain;

11.° Finally, it is very probable that the natural fluid of the ventricles and that which is found there in diseases have their principal source in the secretion of the vascular membrane which covers the spinal cord.

Magendie described (par. 5 above) the foramen now associated with his name, and in a later paper ("Second mémoire sur le liquide qui se trouve dans le crâne et l'épine de l'homme, et des animaux vertébrés," *J. Physiol. exp. path.*, Paris, 1827, 7:1–29; deuxiéme partie, read before the Académie des Sciences 18 December 1826) he gave more detail.

EXCERPT PP. 21–22

I therefore offer as a *constant anatomical arrangement which is easy to verify, that the fourth ventricle communicates freely with the spinal subarachnoid space*; the communication is established by a *round opening* placed between the two posterior cerebellar arteries [posterior inferior cerebellar], which is *two or three lines* [see p. 41] in diameter. I have often seen it still much bigger; its superior and lateral part is formed by a number of blood vessels of the pia mater which proceed to the cerebellum and to the choroid plexuses of this organ. Laterally and above these vessels this hole is formed by the internal part of the stria terminalis which borders it on the sides, and below the fourth ventricle. Below it is limited by the calamus scriptorius.

. . . .

I propose to call this opening the *entrance of the cavities of the brain*, or if one wishes to preserve the archaic nomenclature, *entrance of the cerebral ventricles*.

In one of his papers (1827b, pp. 80–81) Magendie elaborated a research program to investigate the cerebrospinal fluid as thoroughly as possible and he gathered together the results of it in a paper delivered to the Académie on 16 June 1828 ("Mémoire physiologique sur le cerveau," *J. Physiol. exp. path.*, Paris, 1828, 8:211–229). Fourteen years later he published a book (*Recherches physiologiques et cliniques sur le liquid céphalo-rachidien ou cérébro-spinal* [Paris, 1842]) which contained all his researches on the subject and also included a history of the cerebrospinal fluid by Jodin (pp. 139–161). His attempts to establish the physical and chemical properties of the fluid are also to be found here (pp. 47–52), and they represent the beginning of cerebrospinal fluid analysis which was to provide a useful diagnostic tool later in the century. From his many experiments he concluded that the fluid was formed from the leptomeninges, especially the pia mater, and so was partially correct at least.

The following excerpts have been translated from the 1828 article which contained many observations upon which subsequent research was founded. It also contained a few fanciful beliefs such as the pineal gland's role as a valve for the aqueduct of Sylvius, and Magendie missed no opportunity to provide evidence refuting phrenology. He also made a few remarks that foreshadowed the Monro–Kellie doctrine of the brain (see pp. 788–793).

EXCERPT PP. 214–216

I must begin by giving a name to my fluid; a name is important even in anatomy. I have named it *céphale-spinal* (or *céphale-rachidien* for those whose ears are offended by a hybrid word) because it is found simultaneously in the head and in the spinal cavity. [He had termed it "le liquide céphalo-spinal" in 1827 (above).]

Then I had to ascertain its [cerebrospinal fluid] quantity exactly, and I recognized that in an adult man of medium height enjoying all his mental and physical faculties there are about three ounces of it; women, all things being otherwise equal, have a much larger quantity of it. One sees, then, that that is not one of the advantages that they now have over us. [Intellect was considered to be inversely proportional to volume of fluid.]

In the aged the proportion of cerebrospinal fluid is still greater. It can even increase to as much as six or seven ounces, but it is rare for the intellectual and physical faculties not to be then very weak.

The place that the fluid occupies is worthy of remark. It creates around the brain and the spinal cord a layer of varying thickness according to location; in the neck it is four or five lines [see p. 41] thick; at the lumbar region more than an inch; finally, around the brain it is generally one or two lines and in certain cases and in certain places, nearly an inch.

Are not these facts a powerful objection against a famous system [phrenology] in which nothing less than the recognition of the very small features of the volume and the conformation of the brain by the dimensions and conformation of the cranium is pretended? If there exists, as one can no longer doubt, a layer of fluid between the cranium and the brain, and if this layer may be several lines thick, how is it possible to judge the dimensions of the brain from those of the cranium? And how is it possible to be sure that the protuberances and hollows of the surface of the head correspond to similar details of the configuration of the brain?

. . . .

. . . .

. . . .

. . . .

Thus one of the duties of the cerebrospinal fluid is to replace the brain as often as its total volume is decreased. It has the same use in cases of partial decrease, of which I have been able several times to convince myself, in individuals who, during several years of their lives, had had an arm or a leg *contracted and immobilized*. In this case a fifth or a fourth [part] of a cerebral lobe disappears; a large hollow is formed on the surface of the organ, and this hollow is filled with cerebrospinal fluid so that the cranium is always full.

Remarkable diversity of the means employed by nature! In the chest and abdomen the organs also frequently decrease in volume, but the walls of these cavities are flexible; compressed by the weight of the atmosphere they follow the withdrawal of the organs and emptiness is avoided. In the cranium, on the contrary, the walls being inflexible cannot follow the brain when it loses volume; it is therefore necessary that the cerebrospinal fluid come to occupy the space that the brain abandons.

EXCERPT PP. 221–222

Having acquired the ideas of which I spoke regarding the liquid which surrounds the brain and the spinal cord, I thought that the water which one finds so often in the cerebral cavities could well be the same humor which is found on the surface of the brain. It would follow from this that its presence in the ventricles is a natural condition as the ancient physicians thought, and not at all an effect of disease as is now declared.

One conceives that to confirm this conjecture it would be absolutely necessary that there be an opening for communication between the exterior of the organ and its internal cavities but, however, this opening was not at all known. How could it have escaped the numerous modern investigators of the brain? But as they paid no attention to the cerebrospinal fluid, I did not at all despair, and in fact after some researches made at the conclusion of certain diseases I finally found an opening of two or three lines in diameter, completely hidden by a lobe of the cerebellum and forming a genuine *entrance into the cavities of the brain* [foramen of Magendie].

I had this opening represented very handsomely in wax, and I presented it to the Académie; it is now on display at the Dupont exhibition.

Once this was established it became mechanically necessary that the cerebrospinal fluid enter the cavities of the brain and fill them, for these cavities communicate with one another. I had no difficulty in verifying this deduction on the bodies of individuals dead from accidents that were offered to me; in fact, there is a liquid filling the cerebral cavities and immediately related to the liquid which fills the spine and around the brain.

EXCERPT PP. 223–224

The liquid that fills the cavities is not at rest. On the contrary, it demonstrates a continual agitation through the effects of a sort of flux and reflux that takes place—a remarkable thing—under the influence of respiration. Thus at the moment that we draw air into our chests to breathe, the liquid partly passes out from the cerebral cavities into the spinal canal; on the contrary, at the moment in which we breathe out from the lungs by expiration, the liquid returns into those cavities passing across the conduits mentioned above and particularly running through the *aqueduct* [of Sylvius] which thus carries the liquid in one direction and again in the opposite direction.

The mechanical cause of this flux and reflux of the cerebrospinal fluid is very simple. It results from the alternate swelling of the veins of the spine with blood under the influence of respiration.

HUBERT VON LUSCHKA
(27 July 1820—1 May 1875)

Magendie's description of the midline foramen which provided a communication between the ventricular and subarachnoid fluid was supplemented by Luschka's description of the lateral recesses of the fourth ventricle. This was another important link in the evidence for a circulation of the fluid.

Luschka was born at Constance in Switzerland and studied medicine in Freiburg and Heidelberg. After practising medicine in Meersburg and Constance he was appointed professor *extraordinarius* of anatomy and prosector at Tübingen in 1849 and, following Arnold's departure, became professor *ordinarius* and director of the Anatomical Institute. He held these posts until his early death. He was one of the most outstanding anatomists of the nineteenth century and he studied many parts of the body, adding additional value to his work by considering morbid as well as normal anatomy. His name is associated with the anterior part of the true vocal cord, a tubular structure in the gall bladder wall, the coccygeal gland, cystlike cavities in the urachal canal, the tonsil, and finally the foramina found at the base of the brain (see Langer, 1875; Hirsch, 1884).

Luschka's account of the pathways and production of the cerebrospinal fluid is found in his excellent monograph on the choroid plexuses of the brain (*Die Adergeflechte der menschlichen Gehirnes. Eine Monographie* [Berlin, 1855]). It is noteworthy not only for the detailed and accurate descriptions but also for its elegant illustrations. The following passage describes the foramina of Luschka or lateral recesses.

EXCERPT PP. 27–28

The *outer angle* of the fourth cerebral ventricle [lateral recess] projects very pointedly outwards and forwards. It is bordered 1) by the peduncle of the flocculus and thus also by the lateral end of the inferior medullary velum which forms a thin margin of the peduncle projecting from its mass; 2) by the so-called neck of the cerebellar peduncle to the medulla oblongata [inferior cerebellar peduncle], namely, at the place where the uppermost striae medullares of the floor of the fourth ventricle run laterally.

Not infrequently some of these striae medullares fuse into a thin lamella scarcely a line high, similar to the lingula which is related to the anterior circumference of the lateral end of the peduncle of the flocculus, just as the external end of the inferior medullary velum is related to its posterior circumference; this means that the little peduncle [of the flocculus] has a double margin. The outer angle thus formed proceeds laterally as a channel through which projects the lateral part of the choroid plexus of the fourth cerebral ventricle, while the arachnoid is stretched freely over this area. Therefore, the outer angle puts the fourth ventricle in free communication with the subarachnoid space [foramen of Luschka]. Meanwhile, the gap where pia mater passes over into ependyma is so transferred by the lateral part of the fourth choroid plexus that there remains only a narrow sulcus which, however, is perfectly adequate to allow the liquid, which, with the intact inferior tela choroidea is driven in with the tubulus from below, to appear at that spot under the arachnoid. This anatomical finding is the more important since in many animals, such as the horse, the lower end of the fourth ventricle is found to be completely closed; in this case only the lateral angles of that ventricle could effect a connection between cerebral ventricle and subarachnoid space. As anyone who is familiar with the topics that are now being discussed knows from his own experience, the lateral part of the fourth choroidal plexus already mentioned lies free below the arachnoid membrane at the side of the medulla oblongata. However, that plexus, by proceeding along the free border of the inferior medullary velum, passes along the sulcus that exists in the inferior tela choroidea towards the side of the nodule of the inferior vermiform process, and thus along the necessary openings of the fourth ventricle for free communication with the outside.

Whereas Magendie had thought that the pia mater in particular produced the cerebrospinal fluid, Luschka, in keeping with earlier opinions but with much more accurate and detailed evidence, thought the choroid plexus was the main site of formation. It appeared as a transudate from the blood vessels of the plexuses.

EXCERPT PP. 166–168

In the course of time very differing opinions have been entertained concerning the way in which the fluid is formed in the cerebral ventricles and in the subarachnoid space. Assuming the lining of the ventricles to be a serous membrane, one simply derives the fluid according to an analogy with other serous membranes, or one considers the choroid plexuses to be instruments for secretion. Diemerbrock designated the pituitary body as the most important organ for the secretion of the cerebroventricular fluid. Magendie considered the outer vascular membrane [pia mater] as the anatomical site for the secretion of all the cerebrospinal fluid.

In contrast to the investigations of earlier observers, present-day efforts are focused less upon elucidation of definite secretory organs of the cerebrospinal fluid than upon the manner of its occurrence. From the chemical composition of the cerebrospinal fluid, which has been found to be similar to many dropsical effusions, it was believed that it could be produced as in those instances, by a simple *capillary transudation* through the vessels of the different parts of the pia mater alone, or concomitantly from the ependyma. Based upon this idea, Virchow did not hesitate in the least to call the cerebrospinal fluid *"a physiological type of dropsy."*

This theory of transudation is based upon a very weak foundation insofar as it relies upon chemical analysis, since, on the one hand, no one has as yet succeeded in determining the nature of the organic components of the cerebrospinal fluid, and on the other, the available *evidence* of its composition, as it exists *in life,* must, on the whole, be questioned. The theory that takes into account the hazard to the organism owing to such a creation of its normal constituents that, according to their purpose, should remain qualitatively and quantitatively constant, seems still less tenable. According to this theory one would always be much concerned about becoming the victim of genuine hydrocephalus, since, with the assumption of a simple transudation, what would prevent less transudation into the respective ventricles in accordance with the degree of expansibility of their walls?

In view of these changes to which the cells distributed on the surface of these structures are subjected by the vessels from which the liquid is supposed to be deposited in the ventricles, one is even more justified in doubting such a method of production.

It cannot escape unbiased observation that the *most important* sources for the formation of the cerebrospinal fluid are the choroid plexuses; however, as may be concluded from the metamorphosis of its epithelium, the ependyma and the outer vascular membrane [pia mater] also participate in it.

The process of formation of this fluid agrees completely with the occurrence of substances commonly designated as products of secretion. Different blood elements that have the significance of a blastema, pass through the vessel wall. On the other hand, the degenerated cells of these structures are replaced from this blastema by new ones. On the contrary, certain constituents are absorbed from the older cells so that they can be liberated, following adequate transposition in the cell cavity as elaborated content, partly by way of transudation through the intact wall and partly through complete disintegration of the cell. That part of the fluid transudate which could not help the process of cell formation and nutrition, flows away in order to wash away the product of secretion from the site of its formation, as the latter's vehicle.

Thus it is the metamorphosis of special, formed elements upon which the regularity of formation of the cerebrospinal fluid is based, and which assures the quantity as well as the quality of that fluid which is calculated during a fixed period, as long as general healthy conditions exist.

[ERNST] AXEL [HENRIK] KEY   GUSTAV MAGNUS RETZIUS
(25 October 1832—27 December 1901)   (17 October 1842—21 July 1919)

As well as the problem of how the cerebrospinal fluid was elaborated, an explanation of how it was removed from the system was sought. Willis (pp. 724–726) and Haller (pp. 727–728) had both favored production by arteries and absorption by veins, but although Willis probably thought the site of both was the choroid plexus, no precise data on this was available until the second half of the nineteenth century. The problem of the site of elimination will be discussed here.

The arachnoidal granulations or villi had been seen by Vesalius and others, but the first adequate account of them was made by Antonio Pacchioni (13 June 1665—5 November 1726) of Rome; his name is today associated with the very large villi which are few in number and present only in the adult. In his monograph (*Dissertatio epistolaris de glandulis conglobatis durae meningis humanae, indeque ortis lymphaticis ad piam meningen productis* [Rome, 1705]) he claimed that the villi were lymph-producing glands, and it was a French medical student, Ernest Faivre, at the University of Paris who, in his doctoral thesis, first associated them with the cerebrospinal fluid. In an article ("Observations sur les granulations méningiennes ou glandes de Pacchioni," *Anns. Sci. nat.*, 3d ser. [Zoologie], 1853, 20:321–333) based on his doctoral dissertation he suggested, incorrectly, that the villi were herniations through the dural wall of the sinus owing to the cerebrospinal fluid pressure. He concluded:

> We believe that we have shown that the meningeal granulations are normal structures and that they are intimately connected with the production of the cerebrospinal fluid; it remains for us to seek the functions they carry out in the economy, if, however, they have any.
>
> . . . .
>
> . . . .
>
> . . . .
>
> Rather we believe it necessary to regard the granulations as structures for excretion, for deposition, for elimination, the production of which is normally determined by age.
>
> The blood and cerebrospinal fluid thus get rid of some of the inorganic substances which they contain and which tend to travel incessantly from the inside to the outside of the meninges [pp. 332–333].

Luschka (pp. 737–739) also noted the granulations, but the concept of Faivre was developed by the Swedish anatomists Key and Retzius.

Key was born in Smaland and received his medical qualification from the University of Lund in 1861. He then studied histology with Max Schultze and pathological anatomy with Virchow, in Germany, and for thirty-five years from 1862 he was professor of pathological anatomy in the Caroline Institute, Stockholm, during the last eleven years of which he was rector. He investigated the anatomy of the spleen, the renal circulation, and a variety of pathological states (see Santesson, 1902; Bardeleben, 1902).

G. M. Retzius was born in Stockholm, the son of Anders Adolf Retzius (1796–1860) whose name is associated with the prevesicular space (see Speert, 1958, pp. 116–123). He studied medicine at the Universities of Uppsala, Stockholm, and Lund. In 1871 he was appointed Docent in anatomy at the Caroline Institute in Stockholm, six years later assistant professor in histology, and in 1888, full professor. He retired in 1890 to devote his time to research. His studies in anatomy, biology, and anthropology were widespread but he also published biographies, translations, and other literary writings (see Larsell, 1920; Waldeyer–Hartz, 1919–1920; Haymaker, 1953, pp. 83–86).

Together Key and Retzius published a magnificent work, *Studien in der Anatomie des Nervensystems und des Bindgewebes* (2 vols., Stockholm, 1875–1876), one portion of which (Vol. I, pp. 168–187) was entitled "Die Arachnoidzotten oder die sogenannten Pacchionischen Granulationen." By means of gelatine-dye injections they examined the cerebrospinal fluid pathways and provided the most detailed and elegantly illustrated studies that had so far appeared. They examined in particular the arachnoidal granulations or villi of Pacchioni and proved by their injections that fluid passed through them into the venous system; it now seems, however, that their injection pressure of 60 mm. of Hg. was somewhat high, and their injection mass was unsatisfactory as it contained gelatine. Nevertheless they were the first to implement with extensive evidence the vague suggestion of Faivre and their opinion has been mostly accepted ever since, although very recent evidence suggests that it may be incorrect.

The following excerpts have been translated from the book of Key and Retzius. They had first examined the arachnoidal granulations in detail and then considered their function.

EXCERPT PP. 185–186

The results of the injections described so far refer to the adult human. We have, of course, investigated a significant number of human cadavers in this way. However, we have occupied ourselves not only with the [arachnoidal] villi of the adult, but we have also made injections in the child and even in the newborn. In these we have been able to inject the villi and, with especial beauty, the venous lacunae . . . .

We have also carried out a series of these injection experiments in animals, particularly in the dog and sheep. In these we obtained comparable results . . . . These injections were carried out mainly on animals just dead. But we have also made a series of injection experiments in the living dog (and rabbit). These were to test the [theory of] absorption of the dura upheld by Boehm. We injected either with a syringe or with the method we usually employed, by means of which a small quantity of fluid containing soluble Berlin blue or cinnabar emulsion flowed by itself into the subdural space of the spinal cord. If the animal was not killed by the injection, it was sacrificed after a few hours and the dura carefully exposed and fixed. By means of examination we found blood vessels here and there in the dura filled with the injection fluid. But we never saw this in the tissue of the dural pathways where the vessels could have been injected from the inner surface of this membrane. On the other hand the Pacchionian villi in the lacunae and the sagittal sinus were filled and the injection fluid overflowed freely into these spaces. The finer blood vessels of the dura which were injected were found particularly in the neighborhood of the venous spaces which contained villi. It appears to us from our investigations that the filling of the veins of the dura is not a genuine absorption from its inner layer through specific pathways into the blood vessels, but owing to the injection of the blood vessels by way of the Pacchionian villi.

On the basis of these investigations, what role can be attributed to the Pacchionian villi? Are they only pathological structures or can a physiological function be inferred and what then is the nature of this function? [They are not pathological structures.]

. . . . Their normal occurrence is also demonstrated by their similar existence in animals. The discovery that in general they protrude into the venous spaces, points with certainty to a specific physiological significance. They all arise from the true arachnoidal and subarachnoidal tissue. None of them belongs to the internal surface of the dura (the "arachnoidea parietalis") as Luschka proved, and, in addition, as will be maintained later, none protrudes freely into the subdural spaces of the brain, as he has also asserted.

Since we have in addition demonstrated by means of our injections that fluid under a very low pressure passes through the subarachnoidal villi into the venous spaces from the subdural as well as the subarachnoid space, it is certainly very reasonable to conclude that these arachnoidal villi have a normal physiological function. What then can this function possibly be? Certainly [they are] a communication between the serous spaces, that is the cerebrospinal fluid of the brain, and the blood system. But can two hypotheses be justified? Either the flow of fluid is from the serous to the venous spaces or, in the opposite direction, from venous to serous. Indeed one can imagine even an alternation of these two current directions, according to varying pressure as well as to varying endosmotic conditions in both systems. These two, the *fluid pressure* and *endosmosis*, must be the factors that influence the passage of the fluid from one system to the other. Therefore, we shall first of all consider each in turn.

EXCERPT P. 187

We may well conclude from this, as well as from the other experiments, 1) the positive pressure of the cerebrospinal fluid does not differ very much from that of the blood in the sinus. However, it appears that in general it is slightly higher than the pressure in the sinus, as one might already assume *a priori* when considering the peculiar relations of the venous sinus in question. Yet it must be emphasized here that the experiments on the two pressure values are best carried out in the same animals, in order to establish a valid comparison between them. With our tests therefore only approximately true values are obtained. 2) Furthermore, one finds a fluctuation with respiration; namely, the pressure is slightly less with inspiration than with expiration. In all probability the pressure in the subarachnoid spaces of the brain is approximately the same as in the spinal spaces because of the open circuit connection.

Although the figures resulting from these tests, as stated above, determine only approximately the height of the blood pressure in the sagittal sinus and that of the cerebrospinal fluid in the subarachnoid spaces, it follows, however, that 1) the pressure is positive in both systems; moreover, that 2) it alternates in both in approximately the same degree, and in the same manner, following the various phases of respiration; but that 3) in general it differs very little in the two systems; probably as a rule, however, it appears somewhat lower in the sinus than in the cerebrospinal fluid system. It would follow from this that under normal conditions, according to the difference of pressure in the two systems, a normally weaker filtering out of the cerebrospinal fluid into the sinus occurs by way of the Pacchionian bodies because of the increased pressure of the cerebrospinal fluid (or decreased pressure of the sinus blood); such filtration must take place faster and more abundantly. The balloon-like, stretched shape and the general state of the villi seem indeed very favorable for a flowing out of cerebrospinal fluid towards the sinus.

In addition, we still have to consider the second factor, *endosmosis*. Here we find ideal conditions for its occurrence; on one side there is a fluid of high specific gravity, the thick venous blood, and on the other side a fluid of low specific gravity, the cerebrospinal fluid.

If one now summarizes everything, it seems justifiable to assume that, under normal conditions during life a fluid current is present owing to simple filtration as well as to endosmosis from the subarachnoid spaces (and the subdural space) through the arachnoidal villi into the cerebral venous sinus. With an increased pressure of cerebrospinal fluid, as in our injection experiments, the filtration must take place even faster and more copiously.

This in our opinion adequately illustrates the importance and the physiological significance of the arachnoidal villi.

WALTER EDWARD DANDY
(6 April 1886—19 April 1946)

After the work of Key and Retzius on the cerebrospinal fluid pathways and their suggestion concerning the elimination of the fluid by way of the Pacchionian villi, there were no significant contributions to the subject for nearly forty years. This was partly due to a feeling that the problem had been solved and partly to the absence of new experimental techniques for the examination of the cerebrospinal fluid and its circulation. This is astonishing in view of the fact that the lumbar puncture introduced by H. Quincke and others in 1891 ("Über hydrocephalus," *Verh. Congress. inn. Med.*, Wiesbaden, 1891, 10:321–339) had attracted much attention to the cerebrospinal fluid and its pathways. Meantime aseptic surgery and neurosurgical techniques were developing so that delicate operations on the brains of animals became possible. It was, therefore, the experimental, surgical approach, stimulated by the neurosurgeons' need for more knowledge of the cerebrospinal fluid, that led to the next advances. The leading investigator in this new field was the American neurosurgeon Dandy.

Dandy was born in Sedalia, Missouri, and studied medicine at the Johns Hopkins School of Medicine in Baltimore where he received the M.D. degree in 1910. It was while he was a house officer at the Johns Hopkins Hospital that he carried out his work on the physiology of the cerebrospinal fluid. He later followed Harvey Cushing as professor of neurological surgery in the Johns Hopkins University and was an important pioneer of the surgery of the nervous system. He is especially remembered for his introduction of ventriculography in 1918 (see *J. Neurosurg.*, 1963, 20:450–458) and air encephalography in 1919 (see *J. Neurosurg.*, 1963, 20:531–536) as diagnostic procedures. His remarkable surgical skill, originality, and courage allowed him to invent many important operative techniques (see Fairman, 1946; Campbell, 1951; Haymaker, 1953, pp. 417–420).

Together with a colleague, Kenneth Daniel Blackfan (1883–1941; see Wilson, 1955), Dandy produced an experimental hydrocephalus by blocking the aqueduct of Sylvius, since he had inferred that the cerebrospinal fluid was produced in, but not removed by, the ventricles. Simulating a technique already in use for evaluating renal function, he introduced the inert chemical, phenolsulphonephthalein, into the cerebrospinal fluid as a marker to study the possible routes of absorption that he concluded took place diffusely throughout the subarachnoid space rather than at one site, as, for example, the arachnoidal granulations (pp. 740–744). It seems likely that Dandy was correct in this conclusion although his idea was at first rejected. The following selection has been taken from a paper of 1913 ("An experimental and clinical study of hydrocephalus," *J. Am. Med. Assoc.*, 1913, 61:2216–2217), one of a series of ten.

EXCERPT PP. 2216–2217

Since an internal hydrocephalus can be experimentally produced by occluding the aqueduct of Sylvius, it is evident that absorption of fluid from the ventricles is less rapid than its production. In the studies of the absorption from the ventricles of patients with an internal hydrocephalus due to obstruction in the aqueduct, after the introduction of phenolsulpho-nephthalein in the lateral ventricles, there is excreted in the urine from 0.25 to 1 per cent during a period of two hours; but when it is injected into the subarachnoid space of the same patient there is an excretion of from 35 to 60 per cent in the urine in the same period of time. This demonstrates that the absorption of cerebrospinal fluid takes place almost entirely in the subarachnoid space.

It is evident that the fluid must be absorbed either into the blood or lymph-vessels. When phenolsulphonephthalein or other inert colored solutions are injected into the subarachnoid space, they appear in the lymph of the thoracic and right lymphatic ducts only after an interval of from thirty to fifty minutes, and only a faint trace is present even after two hours, whereas, they appear in the blood in three minutes and in the urine in six minutes and, as mentioned above, from 35 to 60 per cent is excreted in the urine at the end of two hours. These facts indicate that the cerebrospinal fluid passes directly into the blood and that the lymph-vessels are not concerned in its absorption. There are three principal views regarding the manner in which the cerebrospinal fluid passes into the blood: (1) by means of stomata arranged along the venous sinuses; (2) through the pacchionian granulations, and (3) by a general process of osmosis.

When a suspension of fine granules is injected into the subarachnoid space the granules do not pass into the blood except in very minute quantities and after a long interval of time. Consequently the assumption of special openings (stomata) from the subarachnoid space into the venous sinuses seems unlikely. This applies to granules injected into the subarachnoid space under normal conditions of pressure. . . .

That the pacchionian granulations do not play any special rôle in absorption can, we think, also be shown. These granulations are absent in many species of animals, are always variable in number and size and develop principally in adult life. After fine granules are injected into the subarachnoid space, local collections are deposited along the sinuses—especially the superior longitudinal sinus—in the interstices of the fibrous meshwork which forms the walls of the sinuses. These deposits are in all essentials similar to those in the pacchionian granulations. There is always a layer of dura and arachnoid separating these masses of granules from the blood in the veins. This is a much greater mechanical barrier to absorption than is present in the exposed capillaries of the pia-arachnoid.

After the injection of phenolsulphonephthalein into the spinal subarachnoid space (the communication with the cerebral subarachnoid space being closed), there is found to be a quantitative absorption proportionately as great as from the entire subarachnoid space. This shows that the absorption from the spinal subarachnoid space is similar to that from the cerebral. It is obvious, therefore, that cerebrospinal fluid is absorbed by a diffuse process from the entire subarachnoid space and is not restricted to any special locality, as, for instance, the region of the venous sinuses or the pacchionian granulations. From the foregoing observations, absorption from the subarachnoid space appears to be very similar to that from the pleural and peritoneal cavities, though it is somewhat less rapid.

FORMATION OF THE CEREBROSPINAL FLUID

It has long been known that there is an active formation of cerebrospinal fluid as evidenced by the rapidity with which the fluid reforms after it has been withdrawn either by lumbar or ventricular puncture. The endowment of the chorioid plexus with an elaborate blood-supply indicates that it is a structure with a special function. Since the work of Faivre (1854) and Luschka (1855) showing the secretory character of the cells, the chorioid plexuses have been regarded as glands, from which at least part of the cerebrospinal fluid is formed. The discovery of secretory granules by *intra-vitam* staining by Francini, and also by Bibergeil and Levaditi, leaves but little doubt as to the secretory nature of this function.

We have shown that practically no absorption takes place in the ventricles, at least under the pressure from an abnormal accumulation of fluid. Since this is true and since hydocephalus results from an experimental block in the aqueduct of Sylvius, it is evident that the fluid forms in the ventricles. These facts demonstrate an irreciprocal permeability of the fluid-forming structures, and emphasizes the secretory rather than the mechanical formation of the cerebrospinal fluid.

After these preliminary researches Dandy carried out a series of experiments in which he interfered surgically with the ventricles or the choroid plexuses in animals. His results supported his original contentions, and the evidence he presented in 1919 ("Experimental hydrocephalus," *Ann. Surg.*, 1919, 70:129–142) was the strongest single confirmation that the cerebrospinal fluid was produced by the choroid plexuses, probably alone, a view that is today being challenged. The passages below include Dandy's report of a crucial experiment and then his conclusions derived from all his investigations.

EXCERPT PP. 133–134

OCCLUSION OF THE FORAMEN OF MONRO AFTER REMOVAL OF THE CHOROID PLEXUS

The entire choroid plexus of one lateral ventricle can be removed through the same transcortical incision that is made in order to plug the foramen of Monro. If choroid plexectomy is to be done, the incision in the cortex should be even more posteriorly—into the posterior horn of the ventricle—so that the descending horn and the body of the lateral ventricle can be directly illuminated at the same time. The choroid plexus can then be seen through its entire extent. The choroid plexus is picked up with delicate forceps at the foramen of Monro and stripped from its attachment to the velum interpositum as far as the glomus. The tip of the choroid plexus in the descending horn is then picked up and stripped in a similar manner until the glomus is reached. In this way the entire choroid plexus can be removed in one piece. Numerous tiny blood-vessels enter the choroid plexus through its narrow edge of attachment to the ventricular wall. The vessels, however, are quite small, and the slight bleeding can be easily controlled by pledgets of cotton moistened in warm saline solution.

If the entire choroid plexus is removed and the foramen of Monro is blocked at the same time, the ventricle becomes obliterated. A marked contrast is produced by blocking the foramen of Monro on the opposite side without removal of the choroid plexus. Both foramina of Monro being occluded, a collapsed ventricle results on the side from which the choroid plexus has been removed, but the ventricle becomes greatly enlarged on the side in which the choroid plexus is intact. From these experiments *we have the only absolute proof that cerebrospinal fluid is formed from the choroid plexus. Simultaneously it is proven that the ependyma lining the ventricles is not concerned in the production of cerebrospinal fluid.*

EXCERPT PP. 141–142

SUMMARY AND CONCLUSIONS

1. Hydrocephalus has been produced by placing an obstruction in the aqueduct of Sylvius. Dilatation of the third and both lateral ventricles results.

2. One foramen of Monro has been occluded; this is followed by a unilateral hydrocephalus.

3. If the choroid plexus of one lateral ventricle is completely removed at the time the foramen of Monro is occluded, not only does no dilatation occur, but the entire lateral ventricle collapses.

4. This is the only absolute proof that the cerebrospinal fluid is formed from the choroid plexus. At the same time it proves that the ependyma does not secrete cerebrospinal fluid.

5. If the choroid plexus of both lateral ventricles is removed, and an obstruction is placed in the aqueduct of Sylvius, hydrocephalus still results in the third and both lateral ventricles, but at a reduced rate. The fluid forms from the choroid plexus of the third ventricle but cannot escape into the subarachnoid space.

6. Cerebrospinal fluid forms in all the cerebral ventricles. It is absorbed almost entirely in the subarachnoid space. The sole communication between the ventricular system and the subarachnoid space is through the foramina of Luschka and the median foramen of Magendie.

7. The phenolsulphonephthalein test will prove conclusively whether the foramina of Luschka and Magendie are open or closed. Closure of these foramina invariably causes hydrocephalus.

8. Hydrocephalus follows ligation of the vena magna Galeni if the ligature is placed at the origin of this vein. Ligatures beyond or in the sinus rectus have no effect because there is sufficient venous collateral circulation.

9. The communicating type of hydrocephalus has been produced in dogs by a perimesencephalic band of gauze, saturated in an irritant which induces adhesions. This obstruction prevents cerebrospinal fluid from reaching the cerebral subarachnoid space where most of the cerebrospinal

fluid is absorbed. The resultant diminished absorption of fluid results from hydrocephalus.

10. Hydrocephalus follows ligation of the great vein of Galen because of an overproduction of cerebrospinal fluid. In other types of hydrocephalus, both obstructive and communicating, the accumulation of fluid is due to a diminished absorption of cerebrospinal fluid.

EDWIN ELLEN GOLDMANN
(12 November 1863—12 August 1913)

Closely allied to the many investigations being carried out on the formation and elimination of the cerebrospinal fluid was the problem of the barrier between the blood and cerebrospinal fluid systems (see Bakay, 1956, pp. 3–8). In 1885 Paul Ehrlich, the great German chemist, immunologist, and discoverer of chemotherapy, had noted that an acidic dye, coerulein -s[ulphite], injected intravenously stained all organs except those of the nervous system (*Das Sauerstoff-Bedürfnis des Organismus. Eine Farbenanalytische Studie*, Berlin, 1885, pp. 67–72). There was also evidence that whereas certain toxic substances produced cerebral symptoms when introduced directly into the cerebrospinal fluid, they did not do so when placed in the bloodstream. It therefore seemed that an efficient and selective mechanism separated the two systems, recognized today as the "blood–brain barrier." This important concept was largely the work of the German surgeon and biologist Goldmann.

Goldmann was born in Burghersdorp, South Africa, and studied medicine in Breslau, Freiburg, and London. After having been graduated, he studied with Ehrlich, worked on histology and pathological anatomy with Weigert in Frankfurt am Main, and then trained in surgery at Freiburg. He was appointed professor *extraordinarius* of surgery in the University of Freiburg in 1895. Goldmann's research extended into the fields of surgery, physiology, biology, and histology. In particular he examined the effect of vital dyes *intra vitam*, and his work on the liver helped to establish the reticuloendothelial system. He applied his techniques to the functioning of abnormal as well as normal living cells (see Kreuter, 1913; Goldmann, 1913*b*).

Goldmann was the first to carry out a series of experiments that proved the existence of the blood–brain barrier. Using vital dyes, and in particular trypan blue, Goldmann studied the permeability of the barrier. By the intravenous and intrathecal administration of trypan blue he found that the barrier was impermeable to its large molecules, and he concluded that the choroid plexuses were the site of the holdup. The paper reporting his results was presented to the Royal Prussian Academy of Sciences in 1913 just before his death ("Vitalfärbung am Zentralnervensystem. Beitrag zur physico-pathologie des plexus-chorioideus und der Hirnhäute," *Abh. kön-preuss. Akad. Wiss. Berlin*, Phys.-Math. Classe, 1913, Nr. I). In it he referred to chemotherapy of the nervous system which was not, however, to be introduced for thirty years. His suggestion that the cerebrospinal fluid has a nutritive function and that it removes the waste products of nervous tissue metabolism, is today thought to be unlikely (for full abstract and commentary, see Mott, 1913). The following passage summarizing Goldmann's findings and conclusions has been translated from his monograph of 1913.

EXCERPT PP. 54–55

In conclusion, just a word regarding the nature of the cerebrospinal fluid. I shall not enter into detail on the question whether or not it is a lymph fluid, the more so since recently this has been often and thoroughly discussed, above all by Mott, Lewandowsky, Blumenthal, and others. Our experiments have taught us two things. The cerebrospinal fluid receives important metabolic products from the choroid plexus, and these are carried to the nerve substance by the fluid. On the other hand, the plexus is in a position to protect the cerebrospinal fluid, and thus the nerve substance, from the penetration of substances that, by direct entrance into the subarachnoid space, might prove to be extremely toxic to the nerve cells. Furthermore, it has long been known that the cerebrospinal fluid contains *ingredients of the brain substance*; see Reichmann and others. Consequently, Lewandowsky was obviously right when he stated that the cerebrospinal fluid mediates the metabolism of the central nervous system, in that "it carries its nutrients to it, and its waste materials away." From this viewpoint we arrive at an accurate understanding of the very peculiar composition of a fluid that deviates so much from other body fluids, that, in an extremely expedient and perfect manner, makes it possible for the nerve substance to absorb nutritive materials from it and, on the other hand, to excrete waste materials into it. Far be it from me to make the plexus responsible for the *total secretion* of the fluid; however, my experiments do not permit any further doubt that it influences its composition to a large degree and that it supplies it with important ingredients. Every practical attempt to affect the diseases of the central nervous system *chemotherapeutically* will have to rely upon the greater or lesser permeability of the epithelium of the plexus, in case the direct use of effective substances by way of spinal puncture is contraindicated.

Is it therefore astonishing that, as in the *lower vertebrates* (cyclostomata) plexus-like organs can already be distinguished, and that also in the *embryos* of higher vertebrates the choroid plexuses begin their specific function very early? We thus reach the conclusion that the plexus represents an important protective and regulatory mechanism for the central nervous system. If the physiological portal of entry, the choroid plexus, is circumvented and such various substances are brought into direct contact with the nerve elements by way of lumbar puncture, all the doors are opened for the entrance of different substances into the central nervous system.

Lewis Hill Weed
(15 November 1886—21 December 1952)

Considerable evidence had now been assembled to indicate that the cerebrospinal fluid was produced by the choroid plexuses and absorbed by way of the cranial and spinal arachnoideal villi. This opinion is still accepted today by many investigators (Millen and Woollam, 1962, p. 29), and Dandy's work on the choroid plexuses (pp. 747–749), for example, has been widely adopted, although some would claim, uncritically; but whether the fluid is an ultrafiltrate or a secretion has not yet been decided conclusively.

Other theories have been put forward, however, and one of these was elaborated by the American anatomist Weed, who believed that the fluid was produced by diffusion from the meningeal perivascular spaces as well as from the choroid plexuses. Weed was born in Cleveland, Ohio, and attended the Johns Hopkins University Medical School where he received the M.D. degree in 1912. He trained with Harvey Cushing, the neurosurgeon, and was appointed professor of anatomy in the Johns Hopkins University in 1919; he retired in 1950. Weed's anatomical research was principally in the field of experimental neurology, but in later years he devoted much of his time to the administrative aspects of medical science (see Fulton, 1952*b*; Weed, 1953).

In 1914 Weed published a series of papers on the physiology of the cerebrospinal fluid, and the following three excerpts have been taken from one of them, "Studies on cerebro-spinal fluid. No. IV. The dual source of cerebro-spinal fluid" (*J. med. Res.*, 1914, 31:93–117). In it he dealt with the choroid plexuses as the most important source of the fluid and declared that by employing a method of catheterizing the third ventricle, by way of the aqueduct, he could collect cerebrospinal fluid solely from the plexuses.

EXCERPT PP. 98–99

With this method, which permitted the securing of the fluid from the choroid plexuses alone, without admixture by the products of the perivascular system, it has been possible to obtain interesting data regarding the elaboration of the cerebro-spinal fluid . . . .

. . . . We are concerned here chiefly with the method of study and the fact that when the perivascular system is excluded, it is possible to secure fluid from the chambers holding the lateral choroid plexuses—more direct proof apparently than has yet been offered in support of this function of elaboration.

The fluid obtained by the method of ventricular catheterization is, as far as we are able to ascertain, identical microscopically and chemically with normal ventricular fluid. The small quantities obtained, however, render it difficult to make an accurate chemical analysis.

. . . .

The employment of this method of ventricular catheterization affords apparently evidence, of a more direct nature than any heretofore reported, that the choroid plexuses of the cerebral ventricles are the elaborators of the cerebro-spinal fluid. There is no histological evidence that the cells of the lining ventricular ependyma play any part in the formation of this fluid.

On the basis of experiments in which he used Prussian blue reagents, Weed claimed that the second source of the cerebrospinal fluid was the perivascular spaces, and so from the brain substance itself. Some have rejected this opinion on the ground that these spaces are artifacts, but it has not been completely rejected. Likewise some doubt that the fluid removes the products of metabolism.

EXCERPT PP. 102–103

In our opinion these [perivascular] sheaths do carry away the waste products of the nerve cell metabolism, contributing, in part, to the formation of the cerebro-spinal fluid. The fluid, then, obtained by lumbar puncture, represents not only the secretion of the choroid plexuses, but also the fluid waste products of nerve cell activity, poured into the subarachnoid spaces by the perivascular channels . . . . Of course, it may be argued that the fluid waste of nerve cell activity represents the lymph of nervous tissue, just as much as thoracic duct lymph serves as the fluid carrier of waste products of other body tissues. To differentiate these two widely different kinds of lymph seems rather forcing the continued use of the term "lymph" when applied to this fluid content of the perivascular "lymph" spaces.

EXCERPT PP. 108–110

Such evidence indicates that when the experimental cerebro-spinal tension is very high or when an anemia of the nervous system is occasioned, fluid can pass directly into the cerebral capillaries from the subarachnoid space, the pathway being along the perivascular spaces . . . . It seems most likely that actually the flow is from the nerve cell and cerebral capillary toward the subarachnoid space and not from the space toward the capillary.

. . . .

. . . .

This whole accessory fluid system of the cerebro-spinal axis—an intramedullary canalicular system—undoubtedly possesses an active function in maintaining the metabolic exchange and elimination of the nerve cells. Throughout the body in other tissues there is a chief and accessory circulation. For in these other tissues of the body there is in addition to the blood capillary a lymph capillary with the tissue juice or plasma playing the intermediate part in exchange. Nervous tissue lacks entirely the lymphatic system; it would appear that its place is taken by the perineuronal, pericapillary, and perivascular system with its contained fluid, and that this fluid is poured into the subarachnoid space, where it mixes with the fluid from the choroid plexuses.

CONCLUSIONS

1° Cerebro-spinal fluid appears to be derived from two sources: (*a*) The choroid plexuses in the cerebral ventricles; (*b*) the perivascular systems of the nervous tissues.

2° No evidence is afforded by these observations of any absorption of cerebro-spinal fluid into the cerebral capillaries.

3° Under certain pressure conditions an extensive injection of the perivascular system from the subarachnoid spaces can be secured by the ferrocyanide method.

As stated by Bowsher (1961, p. 24) Weed's concept of fluid absorption, although wrong, was accepted, whereas his ideas on its production, which seem to have been mainly correct, were ignored. The following excerpts present these two opinions and also a brief survey of knowledge as it stood in 1922 ("The cerebrospinal fluid," *Physiol. Rev.*, 1922, 2:171–203).

EXCERPT PP. 184–185

In addition to this major venous absorption through arachnoid villi directly into the great dural sinuses, an accessory drainage by way of the lymphatic system was demonstrated. This seemed a much slower, less efficient means of absorption of the fluid, caring for but a small fraction of the total. Such lymphatic absorption was wholly indirect; the fluid reached the true lymphatic vessel only outside of the dura and then by way of perineural spaces.

These anatomical findings, based on a standard of experimentation which approximated the normal, agreed largely with those of Key and Retzius, substituting however for the Pacchionian granulation the normal arachnoid villus . . . .

. . . .

Thus it seems fair to assume that the absorption of the cerebrospinal fluid is a twofold process, being chiefly a rapid drainage into the great dural sinuses, and in a small part a slow indirect escape into the true lymphatic vessels.

EXCERPT P. 177

But even as a working hypothesis, the choroid plexuses must not be considered to be the sole elaborators of the cerebrospinal fluid. Anatomical evidence presented by the writer [Weed, 1914] indicates that the perivascular spaces also pour a certain amount of fluid into the subarachnoid space, where this fluid mixes with the liquid produced in the cerebral ventricles. Such an addition to the cerebrospinal fluid probably accounts for the reported differences between subarachnoid and ventricular fluids on serological and chemical analysis. The ependymal cells lining the cerebral ventricles and the central canal of the spinal cord may also contribute even in the adult a minimal addition to the interaventricular cerebrospinal fluid.

EXCERPT PP. 200–201

. . . . The intracranial vascular and the cerebrospinal fluid pressures have been determined both before and throughout the period of subarachnoid introduction of the foreign solution, so that definite physiological control is afforded. The results indicate that with the increase of osmotic pressure of the blood, due to the intravenous injections of hypertonic solutions, the cerebrospinal fluid is aspirated into the shrinking nervous system, chiefly along the perivascular channels but also through the ependymal lining of the ventricles. Along these channels, under this extraordinary osmotic pull, actual absorption of the fluid into the vessels of the nervous tissue takes place. The findings suggest a reversal, following the injection of the hypertonic solution, of the normal processes; the osmotic pressure of the blood stream, under these conditions, seems to be a determining factor in the absorption of the cerebrospinal fluid. Interpretation of certain of the experimental observations makes it seem likely that diffusion also plays a part in the process.

RÉSUMÉ

. . . .

Our present knowledge of the processes of the cerebrospinal fluid in many respects is inadequate. The conception that this characteristic body-fluid is largely produced by the intraventricular choroid plexuses is based not on any single conclusive piece of evidence but on a mass of suggestive data; when considered from all standpoints, however, the hypothesis seems today well established. The current ideas regarding the circulation of the fluid through cerebral ventricles and subarachnoid space are founded largely on exact anatomical evidence, particularly in regard to the structure of the meninges and the use of these intrameningeal channels as fluid-pathways. And likewise, there are firm and reliable data of an anatomical and physiological nature supporting the contention that the cerebrospinal fluid is absorbed largely into the venous system and to a lesser extent into the lymphatic channels. It is possible now to discard the hypothesis of equality between the cerebrospinal fluid pressure and that of the cerebral veins, and to regard the cerebrospinal fluid as being maintained at an individual, relatively independent pressure at fairly constant levels above that of the sagittal venous sinus. The conceptions of pressure-changes effected by the intravenous injection of solutions of various concentrations are substantiated by dependable observations, but it does not seem as yet justifiable to accept, without further control, the data furnished in regard to similar changes brought about by administration of pharmacological agents and tissue extracts. And the same cautions may be urged in regard to the acceptance of conclusions based on the effects of various agents upon the rate of outflow of the fluid.

Conclusion

Bowsher (1960, p. 7) confessed that "the present state of knowledge on the origin, circulation, and fate of the C.S.F. is still in a state of considerable controversy and doubt." His own work with histo-autoradiographic techniques and that of others, in particular of Davson (1956), have introduced new physiological data that seem to refute some of the studies included above in the third and last period. Although we are at present too close to this recent work to reach a decision, it seems likely that a new analysis of the history of the modern physiology of the cerebrospinal fluid will soon be necessary.

Thus all the lining membranes of the fluid's pathways seem to take part in its absorption and its elaboration; the latter process appears to be partly diffusion and partly active secretion. Specific factors such as the properties of the individual constituents of the fluid, in particular the particle size, are proving to be of vital importance, and it is now clear that the whole problem must be investigated from the point of view of general physiology and of the general laws of hydrodynamics rather than as a local phenomenon obeying local laws.

Despite the fact that the physiology of the cerebrospinal fluid is still in a neonatal state of development, it is nevertheless possible to select a few of the major contributions which, although they may not be entirely correct, are unlikely in the future to be dismissed as wholly insignificant.

CHAPTER XIII

THE CEREBRAL CIRCULATION

Introduction

The history of the cerebral circulation is similar in several respects to that of the cerebrospinal fluid pathways. In both instances the history is a long one, and in Greco-Roman antiquity physicians knew more about the structures involved than about any other parts of the nervous system. The system of brain function introduced by the Alexandrians (pp. 144–146) and elaborated by Galen gave the blood and its contained spirits a vital role to play so that blood vessels and blood flow in the cranial cavity, like the ventricular system and its humors, had to be studied in as much detail as was then possible. However, those who adhered to the Aristotelian theory of cardiac dominance (pp. 7–10) interpreted the cerebral vessels as merely conveyors of blood to be cooled by the otherwise functionless brain. Although considerable anatomical knowledge of arteries, veins, and sinuses was acquired during the Renaissance and in the seventeenth and eighteenth centuries, there was little or no understanding of the physiology of the intracranial circulation of blood before the beginning of the nineteenth century; here, too, a comparison can be made with the history of the cerebrospinal fluid. Of course, a concept of blood circulation in the brain was not possible before Harvey's work on the systemic circulation in the first half of the seventeenth century, but even after the enunciation of his new doctrine no advance was made in this field for about two hundred years.

As late as the nineteenth century little was understood of the function of the cerebral circulation, and apart from the Monro–Kellie Doctrine (1783, 1824), Donders' cranial observation window (1850), and other less important contributions, knowledge of the physiology related to the cerebral circulation did not develop until the last decade of the nineteenth century. Since then much has been learned, but, once more as in the case of the physiology of the cerebrospinal fluid, revolutionary advances appear to have begun only in the last few decades. Today, more so than in the past, the higher incidence of cerebrovascular disease has been an important stimulus.

The history of the cerebral circulation can be considered in two overlapping and, at the same time, parallel lines of development, the first dealing with its anatomy and the second with its physiology. However, the distinction between the anatomy and physiology of any system or organ is a recent and artificial one, and they cannot be separated in the writings of earlier authors. Limitations of space require that only a few of the most significant contributions to knowledge of the cerebral circulation be presented in this chapter, and no reference will be made to the microscopic appearances of cerebral blood vessels or to the anatomy and physiology of the blood vessels of the spinal cord; similarly, little attention will be given to the cerebral veins and sinuses.

There is a survey of the literature on the anatomy of the brain's arteries from the seventeenth to the nineteenth century by Duret (1874, pp. 343–353), and recently Kety (1964), a man who has been responsible for some of the most modern advances in knowledge of the physiology of cerebral blood flow, produced an excellent history of the cerebral circulation.

Anatomy of the Brain's Blood Vessels

From an early time it was known that the brain needed an adequate supply of blood if serious consequences were to be avoided, and those who favored a cephalo-centric system elaborated this belief. The ancient Greeks insisted that the most subtle spirit of the body, the animal spirit, was manufactured in the *rete mirabile* found by Galen and others at the base of the ox's brain and, in consequence, erroneously considered to be present as well in that of man. The concept of the *rete mirabile*, a network of fine arteries fed by the internal carotid arteries, dominated all discussion of cerebral circulation before the seventeenth century. However, in the seventeenth century anatomists like Wepfer and Willis turned their talents to a description of the brain's arteries as a prelude to the important studies carried out by others in the eighteenth. The last quarter of the nineteenth century saw the introduction of injection techniques for determining the distribution of individual vessels, and, more recently, new histological and radiological methods have added to a field of knowledge that is still expanding. The complexity and inaccessibility of the brain's blood vessels have always been a deterrent to progress in understanding of their morphology and their distribution *in vivo*.

GALEN

(See p. 14)

Whereas the Hippocratic physician who mentioned the brain's blood vessels (*The sacred disease*, VI) had little knowledge of them, and Aristotle's information (pp. 7–10) was obtained from animals, the anatomists of Alexandria probably observed their main features directly in man. Unfortunately, none of their writings has survived and we must rely upon later commentators for our knowledge of them. Thus, according to Galen, the term *rete mirabile* was first used by Herophilus, whose name is still occasionally associated with the torcular seemingly described by him for the first time.

As with other aspects of his work, Galen collected the ideas of his predecessors that he considered acceptable, integrated, and extended them. Just as his concept of the ventricular system was of vital importance for his interpretation of the brain's function (pp. 710–714), so the brain's vasculature was equally essential. Thus he considered that the vital spirit in the blood from the heart was changed into animal spirit in the *rete mirabile* and then, as mediator of all the brain's activities, stored in the ventricles. The animal spirit was the working force of the nervous system, and its manufacture and distribution in the blood vessels was of central importance to Galen. Hence, as he often wrote about the ventricular system at the expense of other brain structures, so he made disproportionately frequent reference to the brain's arteries and veins.

The three passages presented below contain in sequence Galen's account of the *rete mirabile* (*Use of parts*, IX, 4; Daremberg [1854–1856], I, 575–578), the vertebral arteries (*Use of parts*, XVI, 11; Daremberg [1854–1856], II, 192–193), and the intracranial distribution of the internal carotid artery (*Use of parts*, XVI, 12; Daremberg [1854–1856], II, 194–195). As in the case of the ventricular system, it is important to remember that Galen was not describing the human brain, and his descriptions must be followed in books on the anatomy of the ox (Sisson and Grossman, 1938) and of the monkey (Hartman and Straus, 1961). The *rete mirabile* occurs in ungulates but not in man. It is interesting to note that Galen recognized the blood vessel anastomoses made possible by the arteries at the base of the brain and by the rich vasculature of the orbit.

EXCERPT PP. 575–578

That plexus called reticular by anatomists, the plexus that embraces the [pituitary] gland itself and extends for a great distance posteriorly, is the most remarkable of the bodies found in this region. Indeed, it extends over almost the whole base of the brain. This network is not simple; one might say [it is] like the many threads of fishermen's nets placed one upon the other. But this naturally occurring net has the special quality that the meshes are so attached to one another that one would find it impossible to remove one of the threads without the others. If one of them is lifted up they are all lifted at the same time because they are all held together and attached to each other. No threads produced by the hand of man can compare with them in delicacy of composition or density of network. Moreover, its formation is no ordinary matter; the largest part of the arteries ascending from the heart to the head [carotid] has been employed by nature for this admirable network. Little branches are given off from these [carotid] arteries to the neck, face, and external parts of the head; all the rest, ascending in a straight line from their source, and mounting towards the head through the thorax and neck, are favorably gathered in that part of the cranium which, pierced with holes [carotid canal], allows them to pass without danger into the interior of the head.

It might perhaps be thought that the dura mater also invests them [immediately] and that it is penetrated in a straight line by the vessels [internal carotid arteries] and that, after all that, it might be believed that these arteries would hasten to reach the brain; but this is not so. Passing into the cranium, they are first divided into a great number of very small and fine branches in the region between the skull and the dura mater. Then travelling, some to the anterior part of the head, some to the posterior, some to the left side, some to the right, and interweaving, they give the impression that they have forgotten their route in the brain. But that is not at all the case. In fact, all these numerous arteries come together again and unite like the roots of a trunk and form another pair of arteries like those that have already given birth to the network; these latter arteries [internal carotid] then penetrate into the brain by holes in the dura mater.

Such is this remarkable arrangement. But why has it been created by nature, which does nothing without purpose? . . . When nature wishes to elaborate something perfectly, she arranges for it to be delayed for a long time [as] in the organs of coction. We have already demonstrated this fact in many places; for the moment, we cite the varicose convolutions [of the epididymis] where she prepares the blood and spirit proper for the production of the sperm; this example will suffice to explain the present case . . . . The animal spirit of the brain demands a much more perfect elaboration than the sperm, so that the reticular plexus has been made more interwoven than the spermatic vessels. We have rightly demonstrated in the *Commentaries* [*On the opinions of Hippocrates and Plato*, VII, 3] that the animal spirit of the brain finds a suitable material of origin in the vital spirit that comes through the arteries [from the heart].

Now we shall repeat an observation made at the beginning of the whole work, namely, that it is not conveniently possible to discover the use of any part if at first one is not perfectly familiar with the function of the whole organ. Thus we demonstrated in the aforesaid *Commentaries* that the rational soul lives in the brain, that we reason by means of this organ, that the largest part of the animal spirit is enclosed there, so that this spirit acquires its special property through the elaboration that it undergoes there.

Let us note here that the structure of the reticular plexus, not less than of other parts of the brain, accords marvellously with our accurate demonstrations. In fact, the brain is entirely interwoven with these arteries that give off various branches; many of them end at the ventricles in the same way as a large number of veins that descend from the upper part of the head [e.g., the sagittal sinus]. Coming from the opposite part [of the brain], they meet the arteries and they distribute themselves like the arteries into all parts of the brain, in the ventricles as well as in the other parts. As in the stomach and intestines, a large number of veins and arteries that discharge bile, pituita, and other analogous humors into the exterior cavity [i.e., the intestinal canal] descend, but retain the blood and vital spirit. So in like fashion the veins discharge their superfluities into the ventricles of the brain, but retain the blood while the arteries principally give off the animal spirit. The arteries, in fact, ascend from the lower parts [of the brain]; the veins, contrarily, descend from above into the brain.

Nature has admirably provided so that the substances that fall from their [venous] orifices traverse the whole brain. In fact, so long as [the animal spirit] is enclosed in the vessels, it circulates with them in all the parts of the body; but once it is discharged, each is directed according to its natural impulse; the light and fine substance rises, the thick and heavy descends . . . . But the arteries of the brain, the direction of which is upwards, always allow the perfectly elaborated spirit to escape into the reticular plexus, whence it is carried by the arteries of the brain in as large quantity as flows into the plexus. In fact, it cannot traverse the arteries of the plexus immediately; it is retained in all their twistings, above, below, at the side, and wandering in all their very numerous and varied circuits so that by taking a long course in the plexus it achieves its elaboration. Once elaborated it immediately falls into the ventricles of the brain, for the spirit must not remain too long in the plexus nor escape still incompletely elaborated.

It is important not only to the ventricles that it be thus, but also it is of great importance to the entire brain. All the parts of the brain in contact with the membrane enveloping the ventricles [choroid membrane; cf. Rufus, p. 13] draw into their vessels the nourishment proper to them.

EXCERPT PP. 192–193

On this occasion the admirable work of nature appears to me analogous to that sometimes executed by artists who carve, bore, and polish their work in such a way as to give it the beauty of perfect finish. In fact, nature, making use of the transverse processes as a rampart for the arteries, could here have caused those which must go to the spinal cord to ascend along these apophyses as far as the head; she did not, however, act in this way and did not content herself with the single protection that we have just indicated, but having hollowed out each process in turn symmetrically and circularly, she formed a passage for these vessels [vertebral arteries] from the succession of holes [foramen transversarium]. According to the way the processes are arranged, one following the other, there exists between the holes only a narrow space through which the nerves issue from the spinal cord. It is also there that a small branch of the artery [radicular] penetrates into the spinal cord. Nature, in fact, here again provided herself with the hole for the nerve to carry the vessels in the spinal canal, and allowed the passage not only of the artery but also of the vein with the artery.

After the vessels that ascend as far as the head [vertebral arteries] have passed the first vertebra, they are divided at their extremity into two branches, of which one is directed internally towards the posterior brain [i.e., cerebellum; cerebrospinal or vertebral artery which unites with its fellow to produce the basilar] while the other [muscular branch] is ramified on the muscles that surround the articulations of the head, attaching themselves to the extremities of the vessels established in the thin membrane [pia mater].

EXCERPT PP. 194–195

In the present book I shall describe briefly the other pair of arteries which from ancient times have been called the carotids; hidden in the depth of the neck, they ascend directly to the head . . . .

The other branch of the carotid artery [internal carotid] which we said is carried rather posteriorly, is also first divided into two considerable parts, but of unequal size; the lesser in volume ascends posteriorly towards the base of the cerebellum [? condyloid artery of ox]; it is received into a large, extensive hole that is found at the lower extremity of the lambdoid suture. The other, coming from the anterior parts by the hole that exists in the petrous bone [carotid canal], ascends to the retiform plexus which is extended, as we said earlier, under almost the whole base of the brain; created by the arteries of which we have just spoken, this plexus presents no slight usefulness; it is doubtful if any other part has so important a function, and this is why nature established it in the most secure of all places . . . . A not insignificant pair of arteries ascends to the brain [anterior choroidal], creating the choroid plexus in the ventricles of the brain and interweaving there with the veins that form the texture of the thin membrane; other small arteries are carried anteriorly and posteriorly, some [posterior cerebral] to the cerebellum and the beginning of the spinal marrow [brainstem], some with the optic nerves that are sent to the orbits of the eyes [ophthalmic]; the extremities of the posterior vessels are united to those that rise through the holes of the cervical vertebrae [vertebral], as I said a little earlier, and the ends of the vessels that go to the eyes are united to those of the face and nose.

Galen's account of the venous sinuses is not easy to follow, but the excerpts below deal first with the *torcular Herophilii* (*Use of parts*, IX, 6; Daremberg [1854–1856], I, 581), and secondly, with the great vein of Galen and other sinuses (*Anatomical procedures*, IX, 3; Kühn [1821–1833], II, 717–718).

EXCERPT P. 581

When these arrangements [of the dura mater] had been made, nature, creating a large number of routes [sinuses] in the dura mater for the passage of the blood, caused veins to go forth from them, some small, some large, some directed upwards towards the diploë of the cranium and the neighboring pericranial membrane, and some downwards towards the underlying pia mater. These veins were not created for a single use, but at one and the same time to nourish, which is the proper and special function of all veins, and to attach all the neighboring bodies to the dura mater.

The folds of the dura mater that direct the blood are united at the top of the head in an empty region, like a reservoir, and therefore ordinarily called the winepress by Herophilus. From there, as from an elevated source, they send branches to all the lower parts.

It would not be possible to calculate the number of streams of blood because it is not possible to count the number of parts that are nourished. There are veins that run even from the central region [of the winepress] into all of the cerebellum, divided and branched like the furrows of a kitchen garden. Others arise from the anterior part that ends at the winepress [straight sinus], and you might say that nature has ingeniously caused a stream of blood to spring forth from the dura mater. For the channels of the dura mater that direct the blood, flow together at the winepress. One of them is directed to the underlying bodies, and nature, no longer entrusting the blood to a single vein, formed a channel [? straight sinus and vein of Galen] for the blood from the parts of the dura mater extending anteriorly, and in the entire course of this channel she gave off numerous branches.

EXCERPT PP. 717–718

After those things that go about the brain [meninges] have been observed, it will then be desirable to dissect the brain itself, beginning with the membrane dividing the anterior part [falx cerebri]. When you have dissected or torn away from this the origins of the veins that extend laterally, beginning with the forward termination, raise it up with your fingers until you reach that large vein [great cerebral] which extends from it and which we have said is carried deeply downwards. Again raising this upwards, give it to someone to hold, and then you yourself loosen it along its length and gently separate with your fingers each part of the brain from the connection of one with the other until you come to that large vein extended there lengthwise [superior or inferior sagittal sinus], and you will immediately recognize its use, for it will be seen to dispatch slender branches to both sides of the brain; then separating that vein from the underlying bodies, cut out the whole of it as far as the torcular, or lifting up whatever extension it may have, lay it on those underlying bodies.

Mondino de' Luzzi

(*See p.* 22)

The form and function of the nervous system as outlined by Galen was everywhere accepted in the medieval period without question or practical verification, and even those who in the fourteenth century carried out human dissection could not divest themselves of Galenic dogmata. Thus Mondino, who dissected the human body, dutifully discovered and described the *rete mirabile*. Like all anatomists before Vesalius, he thought that Galen had described human anatomy, whereas in the case of the brain Galen had, as already mentioned, examined only animals, in particular the ox, in which the *rete* is well developed.

The following brief passage is from the text of Mondino (1316) in Berengario da Carpi's voluminous *Commentaria* (1521).

EXCERPT FOLS. CCCCXLVIIIv–CCCCXLIXr

Continuing, raise the whole brain and then two lower membranes will appear located above the base of the skull, that is, the base and foundation of the brain and of the whole head.

Then lift these two membranes from the bone, and in the middle of the cranial base, in line with the cribriform plate, you will find the *rete mirabile*, woven of a very strong texture, wonderfully doubled and multiplied from very minute arteries finely reticulated, which are the branches of the ascending [internal] carotid arteries. In that network or in the vessels of the network is contained the vital spirit ascending from the heart to the brain so that it may be made into animal spirit; because this spirit is better altered when divided into the minutest form, and because it is especially divided into the minutest parts when it is contained in the smallest and most slender arteries, this *rete* is woven from very small vessels or arteries so that the spirit contained in them may more easily be altered by the brain and tempered and converted into the form of animal spirit, that is, acquire the more perfect form in the ventricles of the brain as the blood does in the ventricles of the heart.

This is one reason why the *rete mirabile* was constructed under the brain as Galen declares [*De juvamentis membrorum*, X, 4].

There is also another reason why this member is worthy of much care and why nature located it in such a very safe place; perhaps nature did this so that the vapors of foods and drinks, condensed by the complexion of the brain and falling downwards, may from time to time cause some obstruction in this *rete mirabile*, and from this obstruction cause sleep. Two pieces of glandular flesh [? pituitary gland] support this *rete*; they were formed primarily for such support, to fill vacuities and to support the two veins ascending to the brain [internal carotid arteries] and the two [? anterior choroidal] arteries ascending to the ventricles of the brain.

GIACOMO BERENGARIO DA CARPI
(c. 1460—c. 1530)

Many Renaissance anatomists, as well as their medieval predecessors such as Mondino, accepted the presence of the *rete mirabile* in man (Belloni, 1958). Thus, for example, Massa (pp. 722–723) referred to the occasional difficulty of seeing it but, nevertheless, accepted its existence in man, declaring:

Nor should anatomists be astonished if sometimes they do not see this *rete*, since sometimes the arteries are lacking in reddish spirit and almost imperceptible. But, if your sight is not defective, by the aid of a candle and a lens you can at least see the processes of very fine arteries like very fine villi . . . . I declare that I have found and dissected that *rete* many times in the presence of others, sometimes so widespread that not even an idiot might deny it; but sometimes I found it so slight that I was unable to remove it [fols. 89*v*–90*r*].

The first person to deny the presence of the *rete mirabile* in the human cranial cavity, although with some reservations, was Berengario da Carpi. A native of the small state of Carpi, Berengario was first trained there in surgery by his father and later, in 1489, was graduated from the University of Bologna. In 1502 he was appointed lecturer in surgery at Bologna, probably owing to the great surgical skill that he had developed. He was also recognized as a notable anatomist and was in fact the most outstanding pre-Vesalian investigator of that field. Although he built up a busy and lucrative medical practice, Berengario found time to publish several books on neurosurgery and anatomy (see Putti, 1937).

Berengario first recorded his doubts regarding the existence of the *rete mirabile* in his *Commentaria cum amplissimis additionibus super anatomia Mundini* (Bologna, 1521). Like Mondino, he took it for granted that Galen's description of the *rete* had been based upon examination of the human head, and thus he could only explain the apparent error by suggesting a defect of observation.

EXCERPT FOL. CCCCLIX*r–v*

Note, reader, that I have worked hard to discover this *rete* and its location; I have dissected more than a hundred heads almost solely for the sake of this *rete* and even now I don't understand it. It is true that posteriorly under the dura mater, at the right and left of the [pituitary] gland beneath the *lacuna* [infundibulum of third ventricle] of Mondino, I often saw and touched something like an intricate network that might be judged to be the *rete mirabile,* and so, too, under the dura mater in the region behind the aperture of the spinal marrow [? foramen magnum], and above the base of the skull towards the occipital bone [clivus] I found a complex as aforesaid; but I do not know whether this is that *rete* or another complex. If there is a *rete mirabile* such as Galen mentions as fact, I believe that the aforesaid complexes are the *rete mirabile,* but since Galen said earlier that the *rete mirabile* is, at least in part, in the substance of the dura mater, I believe that the whole *rete mirabile* could not be seen because the dura mater would be so intricately involved with it that it would not be possible to distinguish one from the other.

However, because Galen says that the *rete mirabile* occupies a large part of the basis cranii, that is forwards, backwards, and to the sides [see p. 758], and because it is not perceptible, I doubt that Galen did otherwise than imagine that a *rete mirabile* is located there. I have careful eyes, hands, and instruments suited to separating the dura mater from the cranium, and I have dissected many heads, as I said above, and did not find such a *rete* except in that place mentioned by me. It is my opinion that if there is a *rete* there in the latter location, it must be concluded that Galen erred, because he says that when the ascending arteries are above the base of the skull, immediately they are divided very minutely and form the *rete;* then he says that from all the branches of the *rete* again two branches of arteries are formed that perforate the dura mater and ascend to the brain. This, however, is not true, because many times I have inserted a little stylus above the dura mater into the aforesaid large ascending branches which are near the optic nerves [internal carotids], and I have found that the stylus penetrates directly downwards through those arteries without any obstacle as far as the base of the skull; and if the aforesaid arteries were so reticulated above the base of the skull and divided very minutely, as Galen says, the stylus would be unable to penetrate downwards through them to the bone because it would find the *rete* to be an obstacle. From that indication I maintain that there is no *rete mirable* there; but I believe that the aforesaid ascending arteries which are divided very minutely in the pia mater are sufficient to refine the vital spirit that, after being refined, passes through the substance of the brain and is distributed there, and from the substance of the brain passes to its ventricles where it is finally distributed. Thus I believe that Galen imagined the *rete mirabile* but never saw it; and I believe that all others after Galen that spoke of the *rete mirabile* did so on the strength of his opinion rather than their own perception of it.

In the following year Berengario produced his *Isagoge breves* (Bologna, 1522) and in it he was more emphatic in denying the existence of the *rete mirabile* in man; by then, too, he had sufficient conviction and courage to state categorically, "I have never seen that net." Although he did not accept the presence of the *rete* in man he was, however, quite willing to accept Galen's general thesis regarding the animal spirit. Thus Berengario suggested that its site or production might, as he declared in the preceding excerpt, be in the vascular pia mater. The following passage has been translated from a section of the *Isagoge breves* entitled "The common opinion regarding the *rete mirabile*."

EXCERPT FOL. 56r–v

Between the dura mater and the base of the skull, in the region of the optic chiasma where the aforementioned colatorium [cribriform plate] exists, two noteworthy arteries [internal carotids] rise up through the base of the skull, one on the right, the other on the left, as was revealed in the chapter on the ascending aorta. It is usually said that immediately above the base of the skull and under the dura mater they form many very minute branches joined into a remarkable network (*rete mirabile*) occupying a large area anteriorly, posteriorly, and laterally; then, that from those many branches there again arise two arteries like the former ones from which the aforesaid minute branches originated, and that these two vessels again become large, ascend with branches [anterior choroidal] above the base of the skull as far as the ventricles of the brain to which they carry the refined spirits of that *rete mirabile*.

Some say that in addition to that network there are two glands supporting it, and that the purpose of that network is to refine the vital spirit, so divided into the most minute particles that it may better be altered for the production of animal spirit; and that perhaps from the vapors arisen from food, then condensed by the brain and imperceptibly fallen back, those very minute branches may more easily be blocked and cause sleep.

I have never seen that network. I believe that nature does not perform through many parts what she can achieve through few, and that she is able to refine this spirit in the very minute branches of the arteries ascending above the dura mater attached to the base of the skull, and continuing through the pia mater as far as the center of the brain. Therefore this network does not exist in that place between the dura mater and the base of the skull; I have given many other reasons for this in the *Commentaria* on Mondino to which for the sake of brevity I refer the readers. Among other reasons I am influenced by sensory experience.

ANDREAS VESALIUS
(*See p. 153*)

Vesalius not only denied the existence of the *rete mirabile* in man much more forcibly than Berengario da Carpi had done earlier, but he was the first to realize that Galen had been describing the brain of the ox and not that of man; in consequence, he was able to explain partly why his more reputable predecessors, and he himself for a time, had subscribed to this erroneous belief. However, Vesalius, like Berengario, recognized the need for a place in which to locate production of the animal spirit and suggested the carotid syphon. His account of the brain's blood vessels is on the whole disappointing, and it does not go beyond that of Galen except in this regard. Moreover, parts of it are confusing because Vesalius occasionally failed to distinguish between artery and vein and believed that they could anastomose.

The first excerpt below has been translated from Book III, Chapter XVIII, of the *Fabrica* (1543) and deals with some of the intracranial branches of the internal carotid, as well as with the *rete mirabile*. The second is from Book VII, Chapter XII, where the *rete* is again discussed.

EXCERPT P. 310

THE FORMATION OF THE PLEXUS IN THE ANTERIOR [LATERAL] VENTRICLES OF THE BRAIN

And so from this [anterior choroidal] artery and the right portion of its branch there is formed in the right ventricle of the brain that plexus which we are aware is called choroeides from the shape of the outermost covering of the fetus, a name that is also often adapted to the thin membrane [pia mater]. In the left ventricle of the brain that plexus is formed from a branch of the left carotid and another part of that branch which, as we wrote earlier, extends from the fourth [straight] sinus to the ventricles of the brain.

GALEN'S RETICULAR PLEXUS

Here I must speak plainly and without any concealment about Galen's reticular plexus [*rete mirabile*], because I have no doubts about the arrangement of the cerebral vessels observed by me; we know that Galen was deceived through dissection of the brain of the ox, not the brain of man, so that he described the vessels of the ox rather than those of man. If you examine the arrangement of the third artery [internal carotid] entering the cranial cavity in man, you will find it as I have now declared; meanwhile you will observe a single branch [formed from] these two which I said run together after they have extended for some distance. If you investigate the artery of the ox and separate the dura mater of its brain at the sides of the gland receiving the brain's pituita, you will find something similar to Galen's reticular plexus; do not be greatly astonished at these contradictory statements as they relate to man and as Galen's description in some degree relates to the ox.

EXCERPT P. 642

How many often unreasonable things have been accepted by Galen's following of physicians and anatomists solely on the word of Galen, easily the most influential professor of anatomy. Among them is that blessed and wonderful reticular plexus which he constantly affirmed in his books. There is nothing of which physicians speak more often, and even though they have never seen it—for there is almost nothing of it in the human body—yet they speak of it on Galen's authority. Indeed, I am now completely astonished at my [former] stupidity and too great trust in the writings of Galen and of other anatomists. Because of my devotion to Galen I never undertook the public dissection of a human head without having available that of a lamb or ox to supply whatever I could not find in the human, and to insure that the spectators not charge me with failure to find that plexus so very familiar by name to all of them. The carotid arteries wholly fail to produce such a reticular plexus as that described by Galen [in his book *On dissection of the veins and arteries*]; much less do the arteries enter the foramen that he described, nor are they wholly taken into that plexus. First, the entire right carotid artery—the arrangement is the same on both sides—seeking to enter the cranial cavity through one foramen, does not enter undivided, as Galen declared, but when it has ascended as far as the base of the skull, it transmits a noteworthy branch [? posterior communicating] to the [jugular] foramen of the sixth cranial nerve [our ninth, tenth, eleventh]. This branch, with a large vein as its consort, empties into the first [lateral] sinus of the dural membrane of the brain. Second, the carotid artery does not have a common foramen with the third pair of nerves [part of our fifth cranial nerve], but the Creator of things used far greater ingenuity than Galen imagined; for he contrived for the larger branch of the carotid artery an oblique foramen [carotid canal] proceeding a long distance through the bone, and through this passage produced what Galen imagined the function of plexus to be, that is, that in the many turnings and twistings of the artery the vital spirit might be thoroughly concocted and its matter made suitable for the preparation of animal spirit. Galen said that when the artery enters the amplitude of the head it is divided into innumerable branches which are so mixed and interwoven that they seem to form a plexus similar to a bunched-up fisher-man's net or a plexus formed from nets piled upon one another. He asserted that this plexus is between the bone and the dural membrane, and that a small portion of the dural membrane extends under the plexus so that it may line the bone. Then, as this plexus is formed from one vessel, or from two if one considers the right joined to the left, so also he declared that the branches of this plexus gradually collect and finally end once more in two vessels, their mass equal to that of those vessels that were said to form the plexus. How far these things are from the truth and how much they demonstrate failure to observe nature will be seen by him who has learned the actual arrangement of that branch of the carotid artery which we said passes through that long passage of the bone into the calvarium. Not to mention other matters, consider how impossible it would be for those vessels to reach the brain as large as when they first reached the skull, since such noteworthy branches are dispersed from the vessels to the dural membrane, to the eyes through the foramina of the second pair of nerves, and to the nasal cavity, before they reach the thin membrane of the brain.

Johann Jakob Wepfer
(23 December 1620—28 January 1695)

Despite the efforts of the Renaissance anatomists, much remained to be learned about the cerebral blood vessels. A very important, but often neglected, contribution was made by the Swiss anatomist Wepfer in his *Observationes anatomicae ex cadaveribus eorum quos sustulit apoplexia* (Schaffhausen, 1658).

Wepfer was born in Schaffhausen and attended the Universities of Basel and Strassburg as well as others in Italy. Graduated from the University of Basel in 1647, he was appointed physician to his native city, and the autopsies he carried out in this capacity provided the material for his book. Later he occupied the post of physician to several German noblemen, and he died while providing medical care for the armies of the Emperor Leopold. His research work was in the fields of pathological and comparative anatomy, and pharmacology (Donley, 1909; Fischer, 1931, 1943; Nigst, 1947).

In his *Observationes* Wepfer not only discussed the pathological findings in four cases of apoplexy, but he also described his observations of the brain's main blood vessels. He was the first to give a detailed account of the internal carotid artery's entrance into the skull and of the so-called carotid syphon. It is of interest that despite the several earlier vigorous denials of Galen's *rete mirabile*, the idea was still under discussion in the middle of the seventeenth century, and Wepfer had to give what was probably the final anatomical proof of its absence in man. The following excerpt deals with Wepfer's observations on the internal carotid artery as it passes through the carotid canal in the base of the skull.

I investigated this course of the artery for two reasons: first, when the dura mater had been torn apart at the sides of the ephippium [sella turcica], I accidentally happened upon it before I had read anything of these matters in [Berengario da] Carpi; for when the dura mater had been divided in the same place, the artery appeared in the form of a vesicle; I thrust a stylus into it there where it pierces the dura mater, and I realized at once that this was an artery, and as carefully as possible I followed it from the sella turcica and pituitary gland as far as the osseous [carotid] canal. Then I followed the carotid artery as far as the styloid process and perceived that here it is curved inwards and extended under the petrous bone through the osseous canal obliquely and anteriorly; and so with as much care and dexterity as possible, with the flesh and membranes removed, I opened the lowest part of the osseous canal for almost the length of an inch (for in almost so much of its length it is hedged on each side by bone), carefully avoiding injury to any artery. When it has slipped out of the canal, it ascends a little towards the posterior [clinoid] process of the sella turcica, then, curved inwards again at the sides of the sella turcica and pituitary gland, it descends; then immediately it ascends again and having become insinuated into and affixed in a deep and conspicuous sinus under the anterior [clinoid] process of the sella turcica, it returns upwards and pierces the dural membrane at the sides of the infundibulum [of the third ventricle]. In the whole of this course it remains intact and undivided, nor have I observed any little branch of significance given off by it to the neighboring parts. How much the course of the internal carotid artery differs here from the Galenic creation of the formerly alleged *rete mirabile*, the unbiased Reader will judge when he has compared both accounts.

Near the end of the osseous canal where the dura mater was cut away and withdrawn on each side, this artery was so twisted above and below in its passage that it resembled the capital Latin letter **S** turned on its back; I have undertaken to make this clear by the addition of an illustration [fig. 155].

It must be noted, however, that in this illustration the surface of the carotid artery is presented somewhat removed from its site, and its sides, normally connected and joined by fibres, are distinct so that its sinuous and twisted course may be better observed. For when its neighboring parts are yet crowded about it, it has the appearance of a bladder at the sides of the sella turcica, and surpassing a nutmeg in size, fills here the whole space under the dura mater.

A. [fig. 155] is the portion of the internal carotid under the sinus of the anterior [clinoid] process of the sella turcica, advancing and about to pierce the dura mater. It is curved inwards because of that same process, but approaching and piercing the dura mater, it ascends again, and having ascended and passed through the dura mater a little, it remains so before it is divided. In some cadavers this anterior process is attached by cartilage to the anterior and superior osseous wall of the sella, so that this arterial portion must traverse the foramen ovale [not the foramen ovale of the cranial base] or, if you prefer, the bony circle, before it reaches that part of the dura mater which it must pierce. I have seen this foramen, or rather this bony semicircle, in several skulls; yet frequently it is absent, perhaps its delicate portion consumed in boiling or for other reasons.

B. is the lowest part of the carotid artery, more swollen and ample than at its exit from the bony canal, and is seen near its entrance to the brain.

C. is the portion of it attached to the posterior [clinoid] process of the sella turcica, where it is bent a little posteriorly, thence about to descend.

D. is the most internal part of the carotid emerging from the osseous duct under the petrous bone, advancing directly for a distance and then ascending to the posterior [clinoid] process.

. . . .

. . . .

Since it has already been shown that in man the *rete mirabile* has no substance but is pure figment, no arteries are derived from it to the dura mater. Many arteries are dispersed through the dura mater; indeed, I have hitherto observed the vessels of the whole dura mater to be only arteries; but not even in brutes do so many arise from the dura mater, as is clearly seen and reason confirms, for what proportion of the innumerable arterial branches of the dura mater [relates] to the *rete mirabile*? How would all the little branches of the *rete mirabile* be able to join together again into one trunk a little before entrance into the brain and equal what it was before its division, as Galen teaches in the *Use of parts* [pp. 758–759] and experience confirms in brutes.

In a later part of his book Wepfer described the various branches of the internal carotid arteries at the base of the brain and also those of the vertebral system. Thus he observed the ramifications of the middle cerebral artery in the sulci and on the gyri of the cerebral hemisphere, but like Vesalius he occasionally confused arteries and veins and considered them to anastomose. The course and distribution of the anterior cerebral, the anterior choroidal, the posterior communicating, the ganglionic or perforating, the posterior cerebral, and the basilar arteries were also dealt with. There is little doubt that the majority of these accounts of 1658 were the best that had appeared up to that time, and some of them were the first.

Wepfer identified most of the basal arteries, and he recognized the connections between the carotid and vertebral systems, but the claim made by Donley (1909, p. 6) and more recently by Nigst (1947, p. 17), Grünthal (1957, p. 101), and Meyer and Hierons (1962) that he described the arterial circle at the base of the brain six years before Willis is not entirely acceptable. After all, Galen had observed this anastomosis (p. 761), and nowhere did Wepfer elaborate on its form or function as did Willis (pp. 776–777). Wepfer did, however, refer to an illustration in Johann Vesling (1598–1649), *Syntagma anatomicum* (Padua, 1647, p. 195, Pl. III, fig. 3), in which the basal arteries were delineated; however, the circle in that illustration is incomplete anteriorly. The following further passage has also been translated from Wepfer's *Observationes*.

EXCERPT PP. 106–114

  As regards the carotid arteries, after issuing intact from the bony canal they advance twisting and incurving to the sides of the sella turcica and pituitary gland where they pierce the dura mater and, still undivided, continue onwards for some distance; but when they have ascended a little above the dural membrane they separate into an anterior and posterior [posterior communicating] branch, but not into an exterior and interior since in the human head no further branch of these arteries is given off to the exterior. When the anterior branch has passed beyond the optic nerve it immediately sends an artery [middle cerebral] to the noteworthy and deep convolutions of the brain there, of notable size, approaching that of a chicken feather; in order that this and the branches and shoots issued from it may be seen more accurately, strip away with your fingers or with a little knife the thin membrane [pia mater] which holds together the outer swellings of the convolutions on the entire surface of the brain and so provides it with a kind of smoothness. In this way that artery and its shoots may be seen within the openings of the convolutions and gyri, in their depths and extending upwards towards the third [sagittal] sinus; for the most part they are free, and they are observed to be firmly attached only through their little shoots interwoven into the pia mater and entering the brain substance. When these shoots have been broken off, they can be lifted and extracted like fibres; I do not hesitate to say that neglect of this stripping off of the membrane was the principal reason why the arteries of the brain were not recognized hitherto and why certain distinguished anatomists dared to write that it was impossible to differentiate between the veins and arteries of the brain. If this method be employed, not only will a clear distinction be discovered between the somewhat larger arteries of the convolutions and the vessels issued from the third [sagittal] sinus—which are veins in form and function—but also their continuity with the vertebral and carotid arteries will be understood. Therefore, from the anterior part of this [middle cerebral] artery branches are given off to all the lateral convolutions—for there is almost no convolution from the depth of which an artery does not creep upwards, so that I believe the convolutions were made in particular for the safe transit of the arteries; these arteries creep through the greatest part of their depth, and as often as they ascend on to a convolution, then they descend into another, neighboring sulcus. While they advance in this way between the convolutions, they give off smaller branches to the thin membrane—for this not only connects the summits of the convolutions, but also binds them together, and everywhere invests their depths—which are partly interwoven into its substance; it is a pleasing sight to see other vessels [veins] of the same size, divided in the same way into small threads but arisen from the third sinus, meet and join these shoots. I have sometimes seen them partly penetrate the pia mater and enter the substance of the brain, not at distant intervals but in many places, and recently in the brain of a septuagenarian cooper who died of tuberculosis. After I had preserved his brain for three days for other purposes, I was able to remove the thin membrane easily, and upon stripping it off I observed many filaments, continuous with the vessels of the thin membrane, entering the substance of the brain; when these had been broken, certain little prickings, as if made by the point of a lancet, as it is called, were brought into view on the surface of the brain.

The closer the arteries, advancing freely within the convolutions, approach the third sinus, the smaller they become because of frequent subdivision; I noticed that they did not at once enter the third sinus, and frequently I saw the extremities of the very small ascending shoots join the minuter descending shoots.

The remaining part of the anterior arterial branch at the base of the brain [anterior cerebral] advances anteriorly more towards the crista galli, and there, where the brain has been divided into two parts, the right branch is joined to the left [anterior communicating artery]; in some instances when a probe was inserted I discovered both branches to be joined; a little later, however, they are again separated and advance merely contiguous to one another to their attachment to the crista galli; in the ox they transmit to the exterior through that little branch. While they thus hasten anteriorly they give off several branches, at one time to the convolutions of the brain's division [i.e., to the medial surfaces] and at another to those facing the forehead [frontal poles]; when these have been subdivided they provide for all those convolutions and in the same way supply little branches to the thin membrane and the brain, as was mentioned earlier.

These two, right and left, branches [anterior cerebral arteries] attached to the crista galli, undertake a contrary route, and there, within the brain's division [longitudinal fissure], directed posteriorly, extend above the corpus callosum; for, in truth, the vessels seen here are arteries, not veins as some believe, inasmuch as they are continuous with the carotid and provided with a thicker covering than the internal veins of the head. These arteries are also free in all this course except where they attach to the neighboring parts through the little branches they give off . . . .

The posterior branch of the carotid artery [posterior communicating] gives off on each side its first branch [anterior choroidal] which enters the ventricles in the base of the brain, where they are fully open, and it enters the sides of the choroid plexus under the border and supplies it with mere filaments and hairlike arteries; but in its whole advance under the border it disperses shoots into the brain, and what remains is communicated to the fourth [straight] sinus and to the convolutions around the fourth sinus.

Then another branch sets forth from that [branch], and advancing behind the crura of the fornix, enters the convolutions there and is carried through them in a varying course like the other arteries; nay more, it transmits little branches on each side to the fourth sinus and to the pineal gland.

After the posterior branch has proceeded about the distance of an inch, it is united with the vertebral artery, again bifurcated [posterior cerebral arteries], and then becomes a continuous duct [basilar artery], as may be recognized if a probe is inserted. From this branch innumerable hairlike arterioles are disseminated on all sides, and the hairlike arterioles are disseminated throughout a little membrane very much like a spider's web, here investing the ivory-colored marrow of the brain; from here a huge number of arterial filaments [central or ganglionic branches] passes into the marrow in the same place [posterior perforating substance] and into the base of the thalami, which you will see clearly if you tear off this very thin membrane, removed without difficulty; for then, with the arterial fibres broken, you will see the many little pricks, as if inflicted with the point of a knife, and the remarkably variegated white surface of the marrow marked with purplish spots of blood. Perhaps some may consider this structure of arteries to be a *rete mirabile* [e.g., the drawing by Vesling, 1647]; however, I believe it ought no more to be called a *rete mirabile* than the pia mater investing the convolutions of the brain, in which arterioles are also everywhere interwoven before they slip into substance of the brain . . . .

As regards the vertebral arteries, they emerge from the nearest foramen, that great orifice through which the spinal marrow descends [foramen magnum]. They advance to the sides of the medulla oblongata, to which they supply many little branches which everywhere enfold the sides; these branches penetrate the marrow in that place otherwise than the distinguished Hoffman believed, for when the marrow has been pressed, not only do bloody points appear, but also the ramifications of the vessels, as I have seen; these are met by little branches of another kind which receive the superfluous blood and carry it to the lateral sinuses, hitherto falsely believed by some to be arteries. When they have almost reached that place where the sixth pair of nerves [ninth, tenth, eleventh cranial nerves] arises, the right and left branches are joined and form a single canal [basilar artery] and remain united along that whole marrowy tract, or the length of this marrowy body formed from four crura and the origins of the spinal marrow [brainstem]; a delineation of this may be seen in the distinguished Vesling's *Syntagma Anatomica* [1647], Ch. 14, Fig. 3, even though in respect to other matters that have been mentioned and those that yet remain to be discussed, he has not shown everything that ought to have been depicted concerning these arteries. These vertebral branches [arteries] join as before into one channel, and then later they send many little branches to the cerebellum, the arrangement of their distribution and communication being the same as of the arteries in the convolutions of the brain, and they end in the deep and posterior part of the cerebellum.

That canal [basilar artery] created a little earlier from the united vertebral arteries, again being divided, sends a noteworthy branch on each side [posterior cerebral arteries] to the anterior part of the cerebellum; it is divided into other branches, it involves almost the whole anterior surface of the cerebellum, and it irrigates the membrane and marrow with a vivifying juice and spirit. After the vertebral arteries have remained united for the length of almost two inches [basilar artery], they are again separated into two branches [posterior cerebral arteries]; from each branch, on whichever side, little branches are given off to the now divided fourth sinus and the choroid plexus [posterior choroidal]. When either branch of the again divided vertebral channel has progressed a little further, it is united to a branch of the posterior carotid [posterior communicating artery], of which mention was made earlier; these joined together into one duct [middle cerebral artery] give off little branches to all the posterior convolutions of the brain in the same way as the noteworthy anterior [cerebral] branch entering a notable convolution, by distributing itself into all the anterior convolutions and providing branchlets for the thin membrane and the brain, is usually distributed.

THOMAS WILLIS
(See p. 158)

Wepfer's work was known and referred to by the English anatomist and physician Thomas Willis (*Cerebri anatome*, London, 1664, p. 7). Willis's own contribution to the investigation of the brain's blood supply was, however, more outstanding. Not only did he describe the arterial anastomosis at the base of the brain and produce a drawing of it [fig. 156], but he also conjectured an explanation for its presence. He considered that it functioned as a collateral system to ensure a constant supply of blood to the brain. Thus he gave observational, pictorial, and experimental evidence, and it is therefore entirely appropriate that his name should be associated with this arterial "circle."

The techniques that Willis employed were novel for his day, since he was one of the first to use injections of colored fluids to help him trace the distribution of the arteries. As was the case throughout his work on the brain's anatomy, Willis studied the vasculature of the animal's brain (*ibid.*, pp. 99–108) as well as that of man, and some of the illustrations in his book depict the animal rather than the human organ; the famous picture of the base of the brain [fig. 156] is said to have been the work of Christopher Wren. The following passage has been translated from the *Cerebri anatome*, Chapter I, entitled "Methods of dissecting the brain or anatomical procedures proposed."

EXCERPT PP. 7–8

One may observe the whole surface of the underlying structure [basal pia mater] covered by plexuses of the vessels like a remarkably variegated network with the appearance of a bushy woodland; the vessels of the brain very aptly represent this *idea* which, however, will be better and more distinctly observed if first you inject a black liquid into the *carotid artery*. Arteries and veins are interwoven into the thin membrane [pia mater]. There are four arteries, that is, *two carotid* and *two vertebral*. The trunks of the cutoff *carotid arteries* appear, ascending on each side of the infundibulum [of the third ventricle], and then on each side they are divided into an anterior [cerebral] and posterior [communicating] branch. *Each pair* moves towards the other [on the opposite side] and they are joined together; furthermore, *the posterior branches* so joined are united with the vertebral branches after they have first been gathered together into one trunk [basilar artery]. The vertebral arteries emerge, first *divided*, from the next-to-last foramen of the cranium, and run along the sides of the medulla oblongata; then *united* at the base of the cranium, they extend through a single canal [basilar artery], as was said, joining with the posterior [communicating] branches of the carotids and are united. From that same place of union a *noteworthy branch* [posterior cerebral] ascends on each side under the edge of the brain, then is carried down upon the crura of the medulla oblongata [cerebral peduncles], and is divided into slender branches like capillaries of which some ascend to the glands located behind the cerebellum [pineal] while the rest form *the arterial part of the choroid plexus*. Before *the anterior branches of the carotids* have been united they give off a noteworthy branch on each side [anterior cerebral arteries] which, creeping upwards like a bordered stream, distinguishes each hemisphere of the brain into, as it were, two provinces; but after the aforesaid branches have been united [by the anterior communicating artery], then withdrawing from one another, they are carried to the anterior part of the brain, and thence bending back between the hemispheres, descend to the corpus callosum. *Before* and *after* all these arteries join one another, they give off branches and shoots on all sides which creep through and, like vine shoots, tightly bind not only the external circumference of this sphere, but also its inner parts and recesses. Such branches of *the carotid* and *vertebral* arteries, as they are found in man, are displayed in *the first Plate* [fig. 156], and in *the second Plate* as in the sheep.

As that *thinner membrane* investing the whole brain and its parts [pia mater] receives *the arteries* ascending, as was said, from a fourfold source, so, too, it is packed throughout with *veins* sent *from the four sinuses*. These vessels meeting together are enfolded with one another, and, through branches derived from both, caused to meet one another; variously twisted together, they constitute almost everywhere retiform plexuses. They are not only exteriorly on the surface, but *wherever,* during dissection, *you are able to separate one part from another without destroying the unity, this sort of plexus of the vessels is to be found.*

The following is Willis's description of the vertebral arterial system, translated from Chapter III of the *Cerebri Anatome*, entitled "A description of the cerebellum and its processes, also of the lower part of the medulla oblongata" [i.e., brainstem].

EXCERPT P. 25

. . . . As for *the vertebral arteries*, they extend from almost the extremity and at the sides of the medulla oblongata, now about to terminate in the spinal cord. As these vessels are more slender than *the carotids*, so they enter the cranium with less preparation, for they are not first spread out into *retiform plexuses*, nor carried by a long, roundabout journey, but each artery passes directly through the cuneiform [sphenoid] bone and joins the medullary trunk on each side. They extend divided for a short distance, but afterwards are united, and extending through a single duct or canal, meet the posterior carotids [posterior communicating arteries]. Thus all the branches meet as at *a crossroads* and are inosculated to one another . . . . In their progress *the vertebrals*, like the *carotids*, give off an innumerable series of shoots [e.g., pontine and cerebellar arteries] which cover over the medulla oblongata, the cerebellum, and all their recesses and cavities, and irrigate everything with a plentiful flow of blood.

Willis was not content only to observe the anatomical arrangement of arteries at the base of the brain, but he also carried out injection experiments to elucidate function. He was thus able to suggest that it served the purpose of a safety device which maintained the brain's blood supply even if one of the carotid arteries were obstructed. A fuller recognition of this mechanism and a more adequate appreciation of its importance in disease of the carotid arteries or the surgical ligation of them has been made possible recently with the introduction of cerebral angiography and with the recognition of the clinical syndromes of carotid or vertebral artery occlusion (Symonds, 1955).

The third excerpt has been translated from Chapter IV, "The parts and some of the contents of the separated skull explained."

EXCERPT PP. 32–33

We have often seen the following sort of experiment repeated. Let *the* [internal] *carotid arteries* be laid bare on either side of the neck so that about a half-inch of their tubes may be brought to view; then let a dyed liquid contained in a large piston [syringe] be injected upwards into the trunk of one side; after one or two injections you will see the colored liquid descend on the other side through the trunk of the opposite artery; indeed, if a very copious injection is made towards the head, the return thence through the artery of the opposite side will go through and below the precordium as far as the lower region of the body. Although little or nothing of that colored liquid is carried through the external or greater jugular veins, when the head has been opened, all the arteries before entrance into the head and the veins accompanying them will be found imbued with the color of the injected liquid. Furthermore, some vestige of that stain will be seen in the vessels that cover over the base of the brain and constitute *the rete mirabile*. The reason that this liquid descends so copiously through *the opposite artery* but not through *the jugular vein*, either the ipsilateral one or the opposite one, is that it would be unable to enter those veins unless the liquid had first passed through the whole brain before entering *the sinus*; but that liquid, so abundantly injected, could not pass so swiftly through the minute vessels covering the brain. Therefore rather than that it be carried to the brain by the violent impulse of the liquid and, flowing abundantly from the injection, threaten the brain with a flood, the arteries, communicating with one another, find a return route for it, even through *the opposite arteries*, before and even after they enter the brain. Here it is impossible sufficiently to admire so provident *a management of the blood within the confines of the brain*, unequalled by any mechanical contrivance. For since the carotid arteries communicate and mutually inosculate with one another in various places, there is a double although contrary benefit: first, by this one and the same arrangement provision is made lest the brain be deprived of its necessary irrigation of blood, and second, lest by the two impetuous flow of the swelling caverns it be overwhelmed. As to the first, lest it happen that one of the carotids perhaps be obstructed, the other may supply the nourishment for both; second, lest the blood rushing in with too full a torrent inundate the hollows and canals of the brain, the flow is checked by a kind of opposite outlet and ordered *to hasten backwards* through the same route of its flow and *to return like an ebbing tide.*

Those *arteries* about to enter the brain are provided with a provision of this sort; nay more, *the venous passages* destined for the return thence of the blood seem also provided with a remarkable artifice. When *the anterior sinuses* [sagittal, etc.] transfer their burden into *the two lateral ones*, which are posterior, these end in *the jugular veins*; it may be observed that those posterior sinuses have carved furrows or cavities which are established on the occiput, and when each sinus, about to enter the jugular vein through its foramen, slips from the cranium, in the exterior part of the calvarium near that foramen a round and *ample cavern* [jugular bulb] is found excavated to increase its capacity and covered by the extremity of each side of the sinus; thus although the blood gushes forth from the head in a torrent it does not burst into the veins with a too rapid and dizzying influx and then besiege the heart itself, because it has here a sufficiently large byway in which the flow may be delayed without any difficulty until a more desirable, open space is granted to its force. Certainly nothing of greater ingenuity can be imagined, or can better demonstrate the providence of the Creator than this suitable disposition of the blood in the brain by its route of reflux in various animals, suited to the necessity of each.

CHARLES EDWARD BEEVOR
(12 June 1854—5 December 1908)

Following the pioneer work of Wepfer (1658) and Willis (1664), anatomists in the seventeenth and eighteenth centuries extended the descriptions of the arteries, veins, and venous sinuses of the cranial cavity. The most notable contributors over the next period were Ruysch (pp. 420–421), who thought that the cerebral cortex was made up only of minute blood vessels, Haller (*Icones anatomicae*, pt. 7 [1754], Pls. I–III), and Vicq d'Azyr (1786, Pls. I–III, VII, VIII, XIX, XXXII–XXXIV). More detailed observations and new discoveries were made during the nineteenth century, a fact reflected in the eponymous nomenclature that is still occasionally employed: the medial striate (recurrent) artery of Heubner (in 1872), the nuclear and striatal arteries of Duret (in 1874), Charcot's artery of cerebral hemorrhage (in 1876–1880), and the anastomotic veins of Trolard (in 1868) and Labbé (in 1879). Such advancements resulted from the use of progressively improved techniques of vascular injection, and the new field of research thus created was dominated by the

French, possibly owing to the Paris school of neurology that flourished in the final quarter of the nineteenth century and thereafter.

As well as following the course of the cerebral blood vessels and observing their variations, workers attacked the important problem of determining the areas of their distribution and drainage in man; this last subject has received attention since the middle of the nineteenth century. In 1872 Heubner published his account of injection experiments of single arteries in thirty human brains, using Berlin blue ("Zur Topographie der Ernährungsgebiete der einzelnen Hirnarterien," *Zbl. med. Wiss.*, 1872, 10:817–821), and in 1874 H. Duret was the first to publish illustrations of arterial distributions ("Recherches anatomiques sur la circulation de l'encéphale," *Archs. Physiol., Paris*, 1874, 1 (2d ser.):60–91, 316–353, 664–693, 919–957). Other investigators also contributed to this new field of research, and one of the most important and influential was the English neurologist Beevor.

Beevor was born in London and qualified in medicine at University College, London, in 1878, whereafter he continued his studies in Germany, Austria, and France. In 1883 he was appointed assistant physician to the National Hospital, Queen Square, and in 1885 was given the same post at the Great Northern Central Hospital. Beevor's work was restricted to neuroanatomy, neurophysiology, and clinical neurology (Brown, 1955, pp. 325–326).

It is now clear that faulty techniques led Heubner and Duret into error. For example, Heubner's method of injecting individual arteries in postmortem material could not reproduce the dynamic state of the living brain. In an attempt to avoid these difficulties, Beevor injected the main cerebral arteries simultaneously with colored, gelatine masses under the same pressure. Unlike his predecessors, furthermore, he based his conclusions on a large number of experiments and so was able to provide important data regarding the arterial territories of the brain.

Beevor's classic paper was submitted to the Royal Society on 8 May 1907 and published in 1908 ("On the distribution of the different arteries supplying the human brain," *Phil. Trans. R. Soc.*, 1908, 200B:1–55). In it he considered each artery and area of distribution in turn and illustrated his results with fourteen colored plates. The following passage is Beevor's account of the distribution of the middle cerebral artery which from the viewpoint of pathology is the most important.

EXCERPT PP. 32–34

The *Middle cerebral artery*, as it winds round the fissura Sylvii, supplies the outer part of the orbital surface, and also the anterior part of the temporal lobe—the extent of its distribution on the inferior surface, and the border line between its area and that of the Posterior cerebral artery, is given under the description of the Posterior cerebral artery. The area supplied by the Middle cerebral artery varies very much in different hemispheres. Its extent superiorly and anteriorly has been given in the account of the anterior cerebral distribution, viz., to the superior frontal sulcus in most cases, and it was there shown that the Anterior cerebral area extends posteriorly in most cases to the anterior half of the gyrus parietalis superior. As the area supplied by the Posterior cerebral artery extends anteriorly to the external parieto-occipital fissure, or, in many brains, along the gyrus parietalis superior, so as to meet the area supplied by the Anterior cerebral artery, the Middle cerebral area in many cases does not reach the middle line. I have found out of 51 cases that the Middle cerebral reached the middle line in 30 cases (fig. 5 [fig. 157]), and did not do so in 21 cases. We have, therefore, every variety between the case of the area supplied by the Middle cerebral reaching the middle line for the distance from the superior praecentral sulcus to the external parieto-occipital fissure, and in the case of the Middle cerebral area not reaching the middle line at all. In rare cases, the Middle cerebral area reaches the middle line just in front of the superior praecentral sulcus, then the upper parts of the two central gyri are supplied by the Anterior cerebral artery, while the superior parietal gyrus is supplied by the Middle cerebral.

. . . .

The extent of the Middle cerebral area posteriorly towards the occiput varies very much in different hemispheres, and I have arranged the varieties in the following table in the order from the most extreme extent in that direction to the least extent. The area was measured in most cases along a horizontal line drawn from the upper end of the Fissura extrema of the Calcarine fissure to the angle of the Parallel sulcus:—

	Cases	Total
To the occipital pole and round to the median surface.. in	1	
To the occipital pole (fig. 6 [fig. 157]) . . . . in	19	
To ¼ or ½ inch anterior to the occipital pole (fig. 5 [fig. 157]) . . . . in	12	32
To the Intraparietal sulcus, posterior end, where it is continued into the anterior occipital sulcus. . . . in	19	19
To the angle formed by the upturned end of the Parallel sulcus. . . . . in	23	
To a point anterior to the angle of Parallel sulcus. . . . in	2	
To a line drawn from the posterior end of the Sylvian fissure to the median line in the middle of the superior parietal gyrus (fig. 6 [fig. 157]) . . . . in	1	26
		77

Dividing the cases into those in which the Middle cerebral area extends to, or within ½ inch of, the occipital pole, in which it reaches to the level of the anterior occipital sulcus from 1 to 1½ inch (2.5–3.8 cm.) from the pole, and in which it reaches to the upturned angle of the parallel sulcus about 2 inches (5 cm.) from the posterior pole, we find that the preponderance is in favour of the occipital pole and ¼–½ inch anterior to it, and then for the angle formed by the parallel sulcus. As will be seen later on, this distribution is of great importance in determining the supply of the optic radiations. The greatest extension of the Middle cerebral area in this direction was to the median surface for the posterior ¼ inch of the Cuneus, and at least was to the Fissure of SYLVIUS.

The extent of the Mid cerebral area downwards varies considerably, and is shown in the accompanying table:—

	Cases
To the middle of the gyrus temporalis inferior (third) (fig. 5)	26
To the lower border of the gyrus temporalis medius (second)	21
To the lower border of the gyrus temporalis inferior (third)	15
To the middle of the gyrus temporalis medius (second)	2
To the fissura Sylvii (fig. 6)	1
	65

It will be seen from the above that in all the cases, except three, the border line between the Middle and Posterior cerebral areas is in the third or inferior temporal gyrus, most frequently at its middle, next at its upper border, and then at its lower border.

Beevor's two important predecessors, Duret and Heubner, had put forward opposing views concerning the anastomoses between brain arteries. Heubner (1874, p. 187) had described an anastomotic network in the pia matter, his *Kanalnetzwerk*, through which all the arteries of a hemisphere could be filled. Duret, however, thought that although some cortical anastomoses may take place, the main basal arteries were nevertheless end arteries. This latter opinion was supported in particular by the German pathologist Julius Cohnheim (1872, pp. 72–78), who argued from the standpoint of pathological studies and stated that since the occlusion of a cerebral artery was invariably followed by tissue ischemia, there could be no anastomoses with neighboring vessels. Each side of the argument had its supporters, but Beevor's findings led him to deny the presence of Heubner's *Kanalnetzwerk* and to agree with Duret that arterioles entering the cortex became end arteries and that the basal and cortical systems were quite distinct and did not anastomose. These ideas were summarized in his presidential address to the Neurological Society on 21 February 1907 ("The cerebral arterial supply," *Brain*, 1908, 30:403–425). It might be added that connections between main arteries at the edges of their territories were, however, admitted.

EXCERPT PP. 413–414

The supply of the centrum ovale is from the medullary arteries of Duret, and the distribution of the arteries corresponds to that of the cortex external to it, so that the line of demarcation between the areas of distribution between any two arteries is quite hard and fast. I can corroborate by experiments Duret's statement that there is no connection between the cortical distribution and that of the basal arteries. I also agree with Duret that there is no anastomotic network [of Heubner] in the pia mater, but that there is an anastomosis between the systems of the three chief arteries at the confines of their areas. This is shown by an experiment which I have made, and which consisted in ligaturing the third cortical branch of the middle cerebral artery, viz., that to the ascending parietal convolution, and then injecting the three chief arteries with separate colours with the same pressure. It was then found that the area supplied by the ligatured branch of the middle cerebral was injected from the anterior cerebral artery at its periphery rather than from the contiguous branches of its own artery, the middle cerebral. It is therefore difficult to understand why, when thrombosis occurs, the circulation in any branch is sufficiently interfered with to produce softening, unless very fine emboli block the capillaries of the cortex. I hold with Duret that the arteries which penetrate and supply the cortex are end arteries, and do not anastomose with their contiguous branches; and I have found that, if the pia mater be carefully removed, or a circular cut be made in it, the subjacent cortex is not injected by the vessels in the surrounding cortex.

RICHARD ARWED PFEIFER
(21 November 1877—15 March 1957)

For about two decades after Beevor's work the occurrence of end arteries in the brain was accepted almost universally, especially by clinicians, and few further investigations of the problem were attempted. Then in the 1920's interest in the brain's blood supply reappeared, and one of those who developed a new technique for examining it, which revolutionized the old concepts, was the German experimental and clinical neurologist Pfeifer. He was able to disprove once and for all the presence in the brain of Cohnheim end arteries.

Pfeifer was born at Brand, Saxony. After having received a Ph.D. degree from the University of Leipzig for studies with Wundt in the field of physiological psychology, he studied medicine at Leipzig and Munich and was graduated M.D. from Leipzig in 1915. Thereafter he studied with Flechsig and in 1924 was appointed professor of psychiatry and neurology, and in 1927 professor of brain research in the University of Leipzig. He founded the Brain Research Institute of the University, and from 1945 to 1952 was provisional director of the psychiatric and neurological clinic. Pfeifer continued Flechsig's myelogenetic technique (pp. 611–619) but his most important work was that on the "Angioarchitektoniks" of the brain (Pfeifer, 1952; Wünscher, 1957).

Using a vital endothelial stain, Pfeifer injected the cerebral vessels of living cats. He was then able to study microscopically, and with benzidine staining, morphological characteristics and distribution of their arteries and veins postmortem. He distinguished artery from vein and could demonstrate many anastomoses of precapillary size between branches of adjacent arteries. He published his first paper on the subject in 1927 and a book in the following year (*Die Angioarchitektonik der Grosshirnrinde*, Berlin, 1928). The following excerpts have been translated from an augmented version of this book (*Grundlegende Untersuchungen für der Angioarchitektonik des menschlichen Gehirns*, Berlin, 1930) with many exquisite illustrations. Pfeifer's work has received much support, and the majority of investigators now believe that there is an endless vascular network, akin to that of Heubner, in the cortex and also in the basal ganglia to which arterioles, capillaries, and venules contribute.

EXCERPT PP. 26–27

The blood vessels of the body as a whole show a vital adaptation of their walls to the hydraulic force of the bloodstream. In this regard Roux has already drawn up laws which are generally valid and which are also essentially true for the circulation in the brain. The brain arteries in particular show a structure and course which are dependent upon hydrodynamic factors. As a consequence of passing [blood] into branches under high pressure, they run in interrupted curves, often spread out over an area. Their branching mostly takes place at nearly a right angle and when the arteries become finer they end in little trees, the branches of which are at a considerable distance from one another. The caliber gradually diminishes according to how much blood has been passed into the branches, and it becomes constantly thinner from the main stem towards the branches. The cone from which larger branches arise has a characteristic shape and it allows the observer to recognize the moulding influence of the bloodstream on the brain to such an extent that one can, in a given case, infer the direction of the bloodstream from the size and the branching angles of the arteries. *Therefore observations of the circulation in the mobile tongue of the frog cannot be used as an analogy for the brain which is an immobile organ.* The individual characteristics of the brain arteries pervade the whole brain with striking homogeneity. There is no division into medullary arteries and cortical arteries in the sense that some supply only the white matter and others only the cortex. We were able to eliminate the basic error which assumes that special medullary vessels issue from the bottom of the gyrus. The point of origin of vessels reaching deep into the white matter can be found on the summit of the convolution as well as on its sides. The course or path of the vessels in the white matter is seen to be not only dependent upon the hydrodynamic factors which are operative in the individual vessel, but it is also influenced by the behavior of other vessels which unite in groups to form stream beds (*Strombetten*). Stout brain arteries are usually flanked on each side by veins when they enter the cortex. Very often, at the junction between cortex and white matter, a transverse distribution of arteries of considerable size takes place. Bifurcation of arteries in the deep layers of the cortex is not rare. *Regarding the proportion of arteries, there can be no doubt that their number in the brain is far smaller than that of the veins.*

EXCERPT PP. 86–88

There is not enough evidence for finding Cohnheim's end arteries in the brain. In Cohnheim's work itself the assumption of end arteries in particular organs was based upon the theory of the origin of the infarct from embolic processes. But despite this there are organs without end arteries in which infarcts occur. An example of this is the intestines. In his work on the consequences of plugging the superior mesenteric artery Litten has given all the essential facts concerning the origin of infarcts in organs which lack end arteries. But one must refuse to accept his new concept of the "functional" end artery. It seems senseless and confusing to assume them, at least in name, in organs in which it has been proved that there are no end arteries. Against Cohnheim's assumption of end arteries in the brain is the observation that a lively exchange takes place between vessels across the midline, despite the bilateral symmetry of the vascular system. Also the conditions for receiving blood flowing through the cerebellum, corpus callosum, and other places in the brain create great difficulties for the recognition of terminal areas. Moreover the cortex and the white matter do not possess separate vascular systems. The general connection of blood vessels in the brain, which can be proved, covers not only the capillaries but also vessels of a larger caliber. There are no "blind" ending vessels in the brain despite the opposite assertion. Duret's opinion that there is a central vein acting as a draining vessel in the medullary center of each convolution cannot be confirmed. Lorente de Nò has confirmed the general vascular arrangement by a completely different technique of investigation. One could also point to Luna who achieved the same result for the brainstem of man with his injection techniques.

EXCERPT PP. 106–108

The characteristic features of the angioarchitechtonics of the cerebral white matter are the "stream beds" which, it is true, in some areas run in the same direction as the [nerve] fibres but otherwise prefer a chief direction towards the ventricle and because of this receive their special topography. The findings in the perfect injection preparation of the cat's brain leave no doubt about this fact. The similarity of the circumstances in man has been shown to be surprisingly close. The "stream beds" cross in many places and cut into the white matter layers as they cross in all directions, and produce the angioarchitectonic boundaries of areas which are just as sharp as in the cortex. Complications appear on account of the introduction of regulatory mechanisms between the derivative and nutritive parts of the circulation of the white matter. While the arteries mainly adopt a ball formation [glomerulus], which can be found irregularly distributed anywhere in the body of the white matter, and which acts as a valve mechanism to slow the blood flow, we find that in the veins there is a direct connection of small vessels with very stout ones, and this is for the same purpose. The connection takes place by means of conical, pointed, blood vessel cones which are stretched out towards each other. The afferent capillary vessels and the capillary venous vessels probably act as a driving mechanism to prevent sluggishness of the blood flow. According to the laws of hydraulics, by which an increase in the diameter of the vessel decreases the blood flow and a diminution increases it, there must necessarily exist a greater measure of regulation for the white matter because in no part of the brain are such great differences in vessel caliber found. In areas where there is a transition from very wide vessels to those of very small caliber, "vessel-strangling-pieces" ("*Gefässdrosselstücke*") are introduced between them as an expression of the purposeful architecture to regulate the circulation and have been described morphologically for the first time. Once the circulation in the cortex and white matter is known, all aspects of the drainage pathways of blood leading to the brain can be surveyed. A considerable portion returns to the surface by way of short-stemmed cortical veins. Another portion is propelled to a distance from its place of entry, sometimes through the pressure gradient in the capillary area, and reappears in large collecting veins which can be found along the brain sinuses. Again, another portion disappears into the vessels of the white matter and is either led back through "sling vessels" ("*Slingengefässe*") or it flows into big veins fed from all sides. Finally, a last portion is conducted along preformed "stream-beds" towards the ventricles in order to join the great vein of Galen together with brainstem vessels. The medulla oblongata has "stream-beds" of a special kind in which masses of parallel blood vessels lie in a paramedian layer. None of the preparations examined gave the impression that the cortex and the white matter possessed separate vascular systems.

EXCERPT P. 136

. . . . After having demonstrated the possibility of showing the exact architectural arrangement of the cat's brain, it now seems to be only a question of time before such investigations will also be made of the human brain. The paucity of the material and the fact that we are restricted to coronal serial sections which show only a few convolutions in the vertical diameter, has limited the present work very considerably from the beginning. Yet this much can be said with certainty, that the angioarchitecture does not follow faithfully and in every detail the cell grouping or the course of the fibres; it possesses its own set of laws which have not yet been investigated in detail. It is true that there are angioarchitectonic forms which reflect, like a mirror, the cytoarchitectonic picture of the same region, but there are also very considerable local structural differences between the two. The criterion for these angioarchitectonics seems to be a different biochemical dignity (*Dignität*) of the nerve cells and the need to provide communicating vascular segments. It is possible that the protoplasmic cell processes [dendrites] and plexuses, which probably have an active metabolism, are decisive factors for the angioarchitectonic picture.

Pfeifer continued his studies on the angioarchitectonic features of the brain tissue and in 1940 published another book in which he attempted to correlate them with cyto- and myeloarchitectonics (*Die angioarchitektonische areale Gliederung der Grosshirnrinde*, Leipzig, 1940).

Conclusion

Recent work by a number of investigators has reaffirmed the presence of intracerebral vascular anastomoses. This conclusion is best summarized by Vander Eecken (1959, p. 139):

Microscopic examination after vascular injection with India ink or by means of the benzidine method showed that the arterial system of the encephalon cannot be regarded as absolutely terminal. On the contrary, everywhere in the brain substance a richly anastomosed network of arterioles is found, fed by perforating branches of the leptomeningeal arteries [i.e., the elements of the Circle of Willis and the anterior, middle, and posterior cerebral arteries] and of the wide, deep arteries [i.e., choroidal and perforating arteries] entering along the base of the skull.

Although end arteries do not exist as morphological entities, the arterioles nevertheless act as such, and so local ischemia follows cerebrovascular occlusion or insufficiency. There are, however, many other factors involved, and as interest in cerebro-vascular physiology and disease grows, further elucidation of them may be expected.

Physiology of the Brain's Blood Vessels

The first section of this chapter contained in its earlier part some speculation on function as well as anatomy. The present section deals only with physiology that is here artificially separated from anatomy. It should properly begin, however, with some consideration of the Galenic concepts of Greco-Roman antiquity, since these ideas survived into the eighteenth century because more satisfactory ones were not forthcoming and because the Harveian revolution of candiovascular physiology was not greatly influential. The Monro–Kellie Doctrine (1783, 1824) was the first important advance of the second period, but further research was only sporadic until the last decades of the nineteenth century. By then physiology was developing rapidly in all its branches, and more knowledge of apparatus and animal experimentation was therefore available. This was of particular importance to investigators of the cerebral circulation who faced the most complicated and difficult part of circulatory research and still do so.

Thus most of the significant advances in the physiology of the brain's circulation have taken place in little more than the last half century, and in consequence are difficult to evaluate accurately. It is clear, nevertheless, that the work of Roy and Sherrington (1891), which indicated that the cerebral vasculature responded to the systemic arterial blood pressure and to inherent stimuli from metabolic products, has been confirmed, although for years it received little or no recognition because of the influence of Hill (1896). A new approach, owing mainly to the studies of Schmidt of Philadelphia and his students, has, in the last twenty years, resulted in a new method of estimating the cerebral blood flow that can be applied to man. Its value seems to be considerable, but judgment of it must be reserved for the present.

ALEXANDER MONRO, SECUNDUS
(See p. 174)

Towards the end of the eighteenth century more and more of the old Galenic beliefs were gradually being abandoned, to be replaced by new concepts, some of which have survived to the present day. One of these revisions, to which Monro gave his attention, concerned the circulation of blood in the cranial cavity. Partly on the basis of anatomical and clinical observations and partly speculatively, he argued that since the brain's bony box is rigid and the brain itself almost in-compressible, the intracranial blood content must be constant. This seems to us to be a reasonable assumption, but when enunciated it was at variance with the universally accepted principle of bleeding for mental disorders and with certain then current ideas on the brain's pathology. Monro discussed the problem in his *Observations on the structure and function of the nervous system* (1783, Ch. I, "Of the circulation of the blood within the head"), where he described the role of the carotid syphon in damping down arterial pressure, noted that the cerebral circulation was greater than that of other parts of the body, examined the structure and uses of the venous sinuses, and finally discussed the intracranial blood volume.

EXCERPT PP. 5–6

For any alternate stop of it [blood returning to the heart], especially when occasioned by the stroke of the corresponding artery, must have had a worse effect on the brain than on other organs; not merely on account of the delicacy of the brain, and the thinness of its veins, but because, being inclosed in a case of bone, the blood must be continually flowing out by the veins, that room may be given to the blood which is entering by the arteries. For, as the substance of the brain, like that of the other solids of our body, is nearly incompressible, the quantity of blood within the head must be the same, or very nearly the same, at all times, whether in health or disease, in life or after death, those cases only expected, in which water or other matter is effused or secreted from the blood-vessels; for in these, a quantity of blood, equal in bulk to the effused matter, will be pressed out of the cranium.

SECT. V

It does not, however, follow from this, that every individual artery or vein within the head is constantly of the same size, or that, at all times, it contains the same quantity of blood, and, of course, that the arteries within the head are immoveable, like metalline tubes, or want pulsation, or are unsusceptible of inflammation. For, whilst the heart is performing its systole, the arteries here, as elsewhere, may be dilating, and, in the meantime, a quantity of blood, equal to that which is dilating them, is passing out of the head by the veins.

During the succeeding period of diastole of the heart and systole of the arteries, the quantity which dilated the arteries of the brain passes into the corresponding veins and sinuses; at the same time, as much passes from the sinuses out of the head, as enters into the head from the contracting trunks of the arteries situated between the heart and the head.

SECT. VI

Neither does it follow, from nearly the same quantity of blood being at all times contained within the head, that opening the arteries or veins on the outside of the head, or in the limbs, can be of no service in the cure of inflammation, apoplexy, and other diseases of the brain. For, although we cannot, by arteriotomy or venesection, lessen much the quantity of the blood within the cranium, we can diminish the force with which it is impelled into it. The great effect of this circumstance needs no other proof than that, in cases of faintness, brought on by inanition, we are relieved by the horizontal posture, and, in cases of plethora, or of inflammation of the brain, we are oppressed by that posture. Nay, the less compressible we suppose the substance of the brain to be, the more readily we understand how the whole of it may be affected by a plethora, or increased momentum of the blood; or a particular part of it injured by an inflammation, or by an extravasation of the blood, or by any other cause of pressure upon its substance.

George Kellie, who elaborated Monro's original idea forty years later, wrote of his teacher as follows (1824, p. 102):

One of my oldest physiological recollections, indeed, is of this doctrine having been inculcated by my illustrious preceptor in anatomy, the second Monro—a doctrine which he used to illustrate by exhibiting a hollow glass ball, filled with water, and desiring his pupils to remark that not a drop of fluid escaped, when inverted with its aperture downwards.

GEORGE KELLIE
(–1829)

Monro had no experimental evidence to support his conclusions regarding the intracranial content, but one of his students, Kellie, was able to supply it. Thus arose the Monro–Kellie Doctrine, as it is still known.

There is little available information about Kellie. He was born at Leith and served as a naval surgeon from 1797; in 1800 he was surgeon to the English prisoners at Valenciennes, and in 1802 he began a surgical apprenticeship in Edinburgh. He was graduated from the University of Edinburgh the following year and appears to have practised medicine in Leith until his sudden death in 1829. He wrote on a variety of experimental and clinical topics such as epilepsy and disorders of the cerebral circulation (see Gurlt, 1931).

Kellie brought forward observations made at autopsies and from animal experiments to establish a concept that, apart from a few modifications, has served ever since as a basis for the interpretation of the physiology of the cranial content. The following passages have been taken from Kellie's article read to the Medico-Chirurgical Society of Edinburgh in 1822 and published two years later ("An account of the appearances observed in the dissection of two or three individuals presumed to have perished in the storm of the 3rd, and whose bodies were discovered in the vicinity of Leith on the morning of the 4th, November 1821; with some reflections on the pathology of the brain," *Trans. med.-chir. Soc. Edin.,* 1824, 1:84–169). In it he reported how he had studied exsanguination in animals, with and without premortem trephination, and had concluded that variation in cerebral blood volume with the skull intact could occur only if "watery effusion," which today we know was cerebrospinal fluid, entered and so maintained the "constant plenitude" of the cranial contents.

EXCERPT PP. 105–107

In our dissections, we do not meet with very striking varieties in the appearances of those [intracranial] vessels: the sinuses of the dura mater, and the veins in general, are found filled, or congested. Even the brains of those who have been largely depleted during life, or who have sunk from inanition, do not appear much voided of their blood. The brains of our apoplectic patients themselves, whom we have, in the course of one or two days, or a few hours perhaps before death, bled to a great extent, with the very purpose of unloading their vessels, are still found congested with blood. In animals bled to death, the brain still retains much of its blood; the vessels on its surface are red, well filled, and sometimes exhibit the appearance even of turgidity and congestion . . . .

. . . .

So far then, these experiments seem to confirm the proposition, that no part of the circulating fluid can be withdrawn from within the cranium, without its place being simultaneously occupied by some equivalent.

EXCERPT PP. 115–116

It is remarkable, I think, that in whatever manner these animals [sheep and dogs] were bled to death, whether from arteries or veins, or both—whether the haemorrhage was rapid or slow—whatever time, in short, was necessary to terminate their life, death did not take place till nearly the same or a proportional quantity of blood was lost . . . .

The summary of these observations, in so far as they apply to our present subject of inquiry, may be thus stated—that though we cannot, by any means of general depletion, entirely or nearly empty the vascular system of the brain, as we can the vessels of the other parts of the body, it is yet possible, by profuse haemorrhagies, to drain it of a sensible portion of its red blood;—that the place of this spoliation seems to be supplied both by extra and intravascular serum, and that watery effusion within the head is a pretty constant concomitant or consequence of great sanguineous depletion.

EXCERPT PP. 124–127

If this be the peculiar condition of the brain, and if the obstacle to the free depletion of its vessels depend mainly on the cerebral system being defended from the weight and pressure of the atmosphere by the solid and unyielding cranium, it seemed probable, that, by removing a portion of the skull, and allowing the atmosphere to gravitate upon the brain, we should succeed in producing a much greater depletion of its vessels by general bloodletting than can be otherwise effected.

To ascertain this point, a portion of the cranium of a dog was removed by the trephine. The dura mater was wounded by the saw, and blood flowed from the surface of the brain. The brain was observed to rise and fall alternately, but so as always to fill the cranium; so that the rise was a sort of protrusion through the opening which had been made. One of the carotid arteries was opened, and in a minute or two afterwards there was an evident gradual sinking of the brain from the margin of the opening. While the blood yet flowed from the carotid, the animal was suspended by the ears, with the view of producing the greatest possible depletion of the vessels of the brain, and allowed to remain in this posture for three hours after death. The brain was sensibly depressed below the cranium, and a space left, which was found capable of containing a tea-spoonful of water. On removing the upper portion of the cranium, the brain appeared of diminished size, or shrunk in its dimensions, so that the membranes, instead of being stretched, seemed loosely extended over it shrivelled-like and unfilled. The membranes and the brain itself were pale and bloodless. No blood was found in any of the sinuses, except at the very terminations of the lateral, at the basis of the cranium. The vessels of the pia mater ramifying between the convolutions of the brain were shrunk, and dwindled to the size of small threads. The choroid plexus was also bloodless, and about a drachm and a half of serum was found effused at the basis of the skull.

. . . .

. . . .

Comparing, then, these with the observations made on animals bled to death by simple haemorrhage, it appears that, when the head is entire, the brain still contains a considerable quantity of blood—when previously perforated, very little: the brain continues to fill the cranium in the one case, and subsides within it in the other.

The same causes which maintain the plenitude of the cranium, and oppose the depletion of the vessels of the brain, may be presumed to present also natural and constant obstacles to the repletion of those vessels; or, as from a consideration of the structure and situation of the brain, it does not appear very conceivable how any portion of its circulating fluid can be withdrawn from within the cranium, without its place being simultaneously occupied by some equivalent; so neither does it seem consistent with the notion of a constant plenitude, that any greater quantity of blood can be forced within the vessels of the brain, without an equivalent compression or displacement.

The first important modification of the Monro–Kellie concept occurred following the work of Magendie on the cerebrospinal fluid (pp. 732–737), and George Burrows (*On disorders of the cerebral circulation* [London, 1846], p. 33) added the new data to the doctrine that he, in fact, opposed: "Regarding this serum [cerebrospinal fluid] as an important element of the contents of the cranium, I admit that the whole contents of the cranium, that is, the brain, the blood, and this serum together, must be at all times nearly a constant quantity." But by the end of the nineteenth century the idea was to some extent discredited and it is only recently that new and more refined techniques have proved it to be substantially correct for the normal, intact, adult cranial cavity. The effect of the doctrine on nineteenth century concepts of intracranial disease is a related topic and seems to have prevailed especially in Britain.

FRANCISCUS CORNELIS DONDERS
(27 May 1818—24 March 1889)

One of the greatest deterrents to the investigation of the brain's vasculature and to further studies of the phenomena revealed by Kellie was the absence of a method of visualizing the blood vessels directly. Admittedly, early investigators such as Haller ("Experimenta ad motum cerebri a reflexu sanguinis natum," Sec. IX of "De motu sanguinis per cor," *Opera minora*, I [Lausanne, 1762], 131–137) had examined the surface blood vessels of the brain in living animals by direct inspection; nevertheless, once the skull and dura were opened an artificial situation was created. What was needed was a technique by which observations could be made under conditions resembling the natural state. Such was the contribution of the Dutch physician Donders.

Donders was born at Tilburg and began the study of medicine in 1835 at the University of Utrecht. He received a medical degree at Leyden, and after having served as a military surgeon and lecturer at the army medical school, was appointed to the faculty of medicine of the University of Utrecht in 1847. In 1863 he was created professor of medicine, a post held until his death. Donders had widespread interests in physiology but he is best known for his classic studies on optical refraction and other aspects of ophthalmology. Together with Graefe of Germany and Bowman of England he helped to establish ophthalmology as a specialty (see Pekelharing, 1919; Donders, 1891, 1963; Colenbrander, 1963).

The obvious necessity for closer study of intracranial blood vessels was a window in the cranium to allow direct observation of them without interference with intracranial dynamics. Donders' paper describing such a cranial window appeared in 1850 ("De bewegingen der hersenen en de veranderingen der vaatvulling van de *pia mater*, ook bij gesloten' onuitzetbaren schedel regtstreeks onderzocht," *Ned. Lancet, The Hague*, 1850, 5 [2d ser.]:521–553; there is an excellent summary of this in *Schmidt's Jb. in-ausländ. ges. Med., Lpz.*, 1851, 69:16–20). Although some of Donders' findings have subsequently been proved incorrect, his invention of the cranial window stimulated considerable research into the problems of the physiology of cerebral circulation, and the principle is still in use today.

The following excerpts have been translated from the original article of 1850, of which the title may be rendered as "The movement of the brain and changes in the filling of the vessels of the pia matter observed directly in the intact, inexpansible skull." Donders was able to measure the caliber of the blood vessels of the pia mater and thus could observe quantitatively their response to the increase or decrease of intracranial blood volume. Thus he observed for the first time the ability of blood vessels in the cranial cavity to vary in size.

EXCERPT P. 542

The conclusion of these investigations is: *in the case of a closed, rigid [inexpansible] skull, no movements of the brain are seen when a part of the skull is replaced by transparent glass. The movements cannot occur in a rigid skull: because the entire space of the brain and spinal cord cavity is continually filled, because therefore the amount of blood cannot noticeably change in a span of time, and because the changes in blood pressure in the vessels, owing to respiration, may be called equal and simultaneous in all arteries and all veins.*

EXCERPT PP. 548–553

The conclusion of these investigations is: *that the forces which bring forth movement in the opened skull will, in the case of the rigid [intact] skull, exert an influence upon the metabolism, the production of heat, and the arterial circulation, and that the functional disturbances, caused by changes in blood pressure, have their origin in the changes to which the metabolism is thereby of necessity subjected.*

IV. THE CHANGES IN THE AMOUNT OF BLOOD IN THE BRAIN CAVITY [CAUSED BY] INCREASED AND DIMINISHED BLOOD PRESSURE

Burrows and Berlin have proved experimentally that the thesis, defended by many, of an invariable amount of blood in the brain, is erroneous; and especially Berlin has clearly shown that blood and cerebrospinal fluid can partly make room for one another, so that with increased blood pressure the amount of blood increases at the expense of the cerebrospinal fluid, or with decreased blood pressure, the latter at the expense of the former. One finds further in his communication a theory which accounts for the facts by demonstrating that with increased blood pressure the physical condition is provided for absorption of nutrient fluid, with decreased blood pressure for its increase. The exceptional situation of the brain and spinal cord in a closed, rigid space will therefore merely impede the blood, but does not abolish it. It could not be decided how much this impediment amounts to, or to what extent and how soon moderate bleeding leads to diminution; increased blood pressure, no matter how it is brought about, leads to increase of blood. In addition, one hears the objection, made by those who themselves do not take the trouble to investigate, that the decision whether the amount of blood is really changed by a raised or lowered blood pressure leads to great difficulty, because it was not possible before the experiment to see the filling with blood, which is after all not the same in all animals. This made me eagerly take the opportunity, offered by the success of my attempt to replace part of the skull by a piece of transparent glass, to investigate directly during life the changes in vascular filling in the pia mater.

Be it observed at once that I found it wholly confirmed that the amount of blood in the brain is modified both by increased and by decreased pressure.

Even with the naked eye it was possible to observe that the redness of the pia mater increased some ten seconds after the respiration had been impeded by closing the nose and mouth. I made use of the microscope for precise observation. A rabbit was loosely tied to a board, and the tube of the microscope was fixed at a suitable height above its head. I employed system 5 of Oberhauser, with an ocular micrometer which yielded a 45-fold magnification. I took the head of the rabbit in my hand and soon learned to place and fix it in such fashion that I could observe the vessels in the pia mater precisely. Already the tying of the animal caused some agitation and thereby sometimes more redness. It was easy to measure and observe a few small vessels if now I brought my hand, with which I moved and held the head to my liking, over the nose and mouth; then ten seconds always sufficed to observe an obvious expansion [of the vessels]. At the same time, it turned out that a greater number of fine vessels became visible than before. The longer the suffocation continued the more this [number] increased. After suffocation had been terminated, more than two minutes passed before the filling with blood was noticeably diminished, and a quarter of an hour later the vascular filling was usually still somewhat greater than before the experiment. But not all vessels were equally expanded. To give an example: two branches, the one 0.04 and the other 0.07 mm. wide, ran parallel to each other over a certain stretch, for a distance of 0.12 mm. With the obstruction to respiration, the larger vessel soon swelled to 0.19, while the thinner not only did not swell, but even seemed to become a little narrower. When the air remained closed off longer so that death from asphyxiation threatened and the animal had to be revived by artificial respiration, both vessels expanded to about the same width, the one to 0.14 and the other to 0.16 mm.; but, what is remarkable, when respiration returned the smaller vessel shrank rapidly again to 0.045 mm. while the larger vessel remained expanded for a long time at 0.13. Probably the one vessel was an artery, the other a vein, but which was the artery, which the vein I could not decide directly. The larger one seemed to divide superiorly, or to penetrate more deeply; the smaller continued uninterrupt-edly up to the superior margin of the hemisphere and seemed therefore to empty into the sagittal sinus. This would suggest that the smaller vessel was a vein, the larger an artery; but observations on another rabbit led me to the opposite conclusion. There I saw veins, recognized with certainty because they emptied into the sagittal sinus, behave just like the larger vessel in the first rabbit, and so I remain somewhat circumspect in my decision, because here I found no arterial branches suitable for observation, and they are always very small anyway.

By hanging the rabbit with its head down, the filling of the vessels likewise increased, as was to be expected.

It is less easy to demonstrate the effect of blood withdrawal upon vascu-lar filling. However, concerning this I have absolutely no doubt left, and if I had wanted to sacrifice the animals for this by letting them bleed to death slowly or rapidly, undoubtedly the phenomenon would have appeared in full force. I preferred to keep them for other observations. The [effect of the] removal of a small amount of blood is not always clearly recognizable. Initially nothing is evident. Many seconds or even minutes must pass until it appears that the surface has become paler, the vessels of the pia mater smaller. A fairly rapid withdrawal of 1½ Dutch lead [approximately 15 gm.], however, caused in the rabbit a very obvious diminution in the blood in these vessels. The diameters of three veins were determined at certain points, as 0.46, 0.41, and 0.18 mm. After the aforementioned withdrawal of blood (13 minutes) they diminished to 0.38, 0.29, and 0.14. Half an hour later the diameters remained sufficiently constant with the exception of the second which had almost returned to its original diameter. [The effect of] *slow* withdrawal of a not-too-large quantity [of blood] is less obvious be-cause everywhere more nutrient fluid becomes absorbed, and the blood volume thus diminishes little or not at all. By contrast, nothing makes its influence more strongly felt than slow withdrawal of a large quantity. Here the original total amount of blood can no longer be restored, and there is ample time to allow an increased exudation of cerebrospinal fluid—a necessary condition as we know for the increase of blood [i.e., of volume of all intracranial contents] in the brain cavity.

Without doubt it has emerged from these conclusions that: *whatever increases blood pressure, and specifically impairs respiration, causes the vascular filling in the pia mater to increase within a short time; that blood withdrawal, if not as immediately as in other parts of the body, also very soon causes the amount of blood in the pia mater to diminish.*

CHARLES SMART ROY   CHARLES SCOTT SHERRINGTON

(27 January 1834—4 October 1897)   (*See p. 238*)

Although the important technique introduced by Donders allowed the observer to follow the changes in the pial blood vessels, a method of measuring the effects of these changes on the intracranial contents in the intact skull was also needed. The first attempt to solve this difficult problem was made by Gustav Gärtner and Julius Wagner in 1887. They measured the outflow from a cerebral sinus to deduce the cerebral circulation and made the important discovery that the systemic arterial blood pressure was one of the main factors of influence. Others, too, were attempting to understand the cerebral circulation, but on the whole such problems received little attention at this time. It can best be represented by the noteworthy contribution of Roy and Sherrington in 1890.

Roy was born at Arbroath in Scotland and received his medical training at the University of Edinburgh. After postgraduate study with Du Bois-Reymond, Virchow, Goltz, and Cohnheim, in 1884 he was appointed to the new chair of pathology in the University of Cambridge. His studies were in the fields of experimental pathology and physiology, especially in problems related to the cardiovascular system. One of his attributes was a mechanical ingenuity and manual dexterity, rivaled only by those of his young collaborator Sherrington (see Roy, 1897*a, b*, Sherrington, 1905).

Roy and Sherrington perfected an ingenious plethysmographic method that recorded variations in the vertical diameter of the dog's brain. A tambour placed over a parasagittal trephine hole was connected with an air-filled system so that changes in intracranial volume were transmitted to a recording pointer. Simultaneous records of systemic arterial and venous pressure were also made. Thus the two experimenters were able to observe graphically the effect on the cerebral volume, and so on the blood flow, of asphyxia, of stimulation of sensory nerves, the vagus, and the medulla oblongata, and of various drugs and chemical substances. This technique, although faulty in several ways, led them to important conclusions, the significance of which was to become apparent only much later. Thus they were able to state that "it must, therefore, be admitted that during asphyxia active expansion of the cerebral vessels takes place in addition to the passive distension which results from the rise of arterial, and in certain instances, of venous pressure" [p. 92]. Moreover, this increase in brain volume with asphyxia appeared earlier than, and therefore independent of, the rise in systemic blood pressure. They could not, however, detect evidence for an intrinsic, vasomotor control of the cerebral arteries that they concluded were under the influence of an inherent cerebral mechanism governed by "chemical products of cerebral metabolism [p. 105]." This observation in particular has been amply verified by recent work.

Unfortunately, the findings of Roy and Sherrington had little effect, for they were soon to be overshadowed by the work of Hill (pp. 801–803). The following excerpts have been taken from their paper dated October 1889 ("On the regulation of the blood supply of the brain," *J. Physiol., London*, 1890, 11:85–108).

EXCERPT PP. 100–106

. . . . One of the most evident of the facts observed by us is that the *blood-supply of the brain varies directly with the blood-pressure in the systemic arteries.*

The higher the arterial pressure, the greater is the amount of blood which passes through the cerebral blood-vessels and *vice versâ*; and, so far as we have been able to learn, this law holds good for all changes in the arterial pressure whatever be their cause. The same may be said regarding the blood-supply of other organs of the body if their connections with the vasomotor centres have been severed; but it applies very much less to the kidney, for example, after complete section of the renal nerves, than it does in the case of the brain. The thinness and extensibility of the walls of the cerebral vessels fit them to undergo much greater variations in calibre as a result of a given rise or fall of the arterial pressure than can be produced in the case of the thicker walled arteries of other organs and tissues.

. . . .

. . . .

. . . .

The vaso-constrictor centres may cause rise of the arterial pressure as a result of nerve impulses reaching them from the periphery of the body by centripetal nerve-fibres, and also as a result of direct excitation of the centres themselves. Let us take the latter case first.

Anaemia of certain parts of the brain may serve as a good example of a natural mode of excitation of the vasomotor centres. Such anaemia may be due to diminution of the arterial pressure, to local obstruction of the blood-vessels or to rise of the extra vascular pressure either locally, from, e.g., tumour-growth, or affecting the whole of the intracranial cavity. In whatever way produced, anaemia of the central nervous system excites the vaso-constrictor nerves with the result that owing to constriction of the vessels of the digestive, urinary and other systems, the arterial blood-pressure rises, causing an increased flow of blood through the cerebro-spinal blood-vessels.

The excitation of the vasomotor centres by anaemia is evidently, then, protective, an increased supply of blood to the central nervous system being obtained by sacrificing the blood-supply of certain other parts of the body whose functional activity can be temporarily diminished or arrested without serious harm to the economy as a whole.

In the excitation of the vasomotor centres by asphyxia the same protective interference with the blood-supply of certain organs is to be met with resulting in an increased flow of blood through the cerebral vessels.

So far as we know, the same explanation holds good for all cases, in which, as a result of interference with the nutrition of the cerebro-spinal axis, excitation of the vaso-constrictor centres takes place. *We conclude, then, that when the vaso-constrictor centres are excited directly in the normal animal, by interference with the nutrition of the brain and spinal cord, the rise of the aortic blood-pressure which results is advantageous to the economy in that it increases the blood-supply of the central nervous system.*

. . . .

. . . .

We conclude then that *the rise of arterial pressure, which may result from certain centripetal nerve-impulses, is of benefit to the economy by increasing the blood-supply of the central nervous system which is called into increased functional activity by the impulses in question,* as well as by aiding the congestion of the part of the body whence the impulses are derived.

We now come to the much discussed question as to whether any centripetal nerves exist which are capable of influencing the blood-vessels of the brain directly, i.e., independently of changes in the general arterial or venous pressure. Our answer to this is, that we have diligently sought for such, and have found no evidence that vasomotor nerves for the brain are to be found outside the cerebro-spinal cavity . . . .

. . . .

. . . .

Are vasomotor nerves for the brain to be found in the medulla or in the spinal cord? We have found no evidence of the existence of such nerves. Direct stimulation of the medulla and cervical cord resulted only, in our observations on the subject, in passive arterial congestion.

Is then the supply of blood to the brain influenced only by changes in the general arterial and venous pressures? Our observations on the effect of various chemical substances on the cerebral circulation shew that the cerebral vessels can undergo *active* changes in calibre. An especially important instance of this is, we think, to be found in the influence on the volume of the brain of comparatively small doses of a free acid introduced into a vein. As we have pointed out, the expansion of the cerebral vessels which is thereby produced, is not due to any passive distension of the cerebral arteries or veins resulting from increase of the arterial and venous pressures. In other words it must be looked upon as being the result of *active* expansion of the blood-vessels of the brain. This active congestion of the brain is too striking a characteristic of the cerebral circulation not to have forced itself strongly upon our attention—the increase of the volume of the brain being great even when only small quantities of acid are injected.

. . . .

. . . .

The experiment, which was made on a dog (A), was arranged so that on the same drum simultaneous tracings were recorded of the arterial pressure in the femoral artery, of the venous pressure in the subclavian vein, and of the volume of the brain. As a part of the preparation for the experiment, an extract of a portion of the brain of another dog (B) had been made in the following way:—some four hours after the animal (B) had been bled to death (the head having in the mean time been kept in an incubator at a temperature of 37 C), the brain was removed, and one of the hemispheres rubbed up in a mortar with about 250 c.c. of warm, normal, neutral salt solution.

The filtrate obtained from the emulsion thus prepared was used for injection into the vascular system of the animal (A) . . . .

. . . . It is evident, then, that in a brain whose blood-supply has been arrested for some little time, there is a substance or there are substances which, when introduced into the circulation, are capable of causing active expansion of the cerebral vessels.

It is, we think, reasonable to suppose, in view of the facts above stated, that the cerebral congestion in this experiment is due to the action on the cerebral blood-vessels of the dog (A), of the products of cerebral metabolism, which had accumulated in the brain of the dog (B) from which the extract had been prepared. These facts seem to us to indicate the existence of an automatic mechanism by which the blood-supply of any part of the cerebral tissue is varied in accordance with the activity of the chemical changes which underlie the functional action of that part. Bearing in mind that strong evidence exists of localisation of function in the brain [see Sherrington, pp. 518–523], we are of opinion that an automatic mechanism, of the kind just referred to, is well fitted to provide for a local variation of the blood-supply in accordance with local variations of the functional activity.

We conclude then, that the chemical products of cerebral metabolism contained in the lymph which bathes the walls of the arterioles of the brain can cause variations of the calibre of the cerebral vessels: that in this re-action the brain possesses an intrinsic mechanism by which its vascular supply can be varied locally in correspondence with local variations of functional activity.

. . . .

There are, then, two more or less distinct mechanisms for controlling the cerebral circulation, viz.—firstly, an intrinsic one by which the blood-supply of various parts of the brain can be varied locally in accordance with local requirements, and secondly, an extrinsic, viz.—the vasomotor nervous system, whose action affects the amount of blood passing through the brain in virtue of the dependence of the latter circulation on the general arterial blood-pressure. Presumably, when the activity of the brain is not great, its blood-supply is regulated mainly by the intrinsic mechanism and without notable interference with the blood-supply of other organs and tissues. When, on the other hand, the cerebral activity is great, or when the circulation of the brain is interfered with, the vasomotor nerves are called into action, the supply of blood to other organs of the body being thereby trenched upon.

There is, however, a third mechanism by which the cerebral circulation can be influenced and the importance of which, we are inclined to think, must be considerable. We refer to the effect on the cerebral vessels of changes of the general venous pressure which, as we have mentioned, may be greater in extent than is usually supposed. The volume of the brain varies with the pressure in the large veins, and it is impossible to overlook the fact that such changes in the pressure of the blood within the cerebral venous capillaries, which have extremely thin walls, must be of importance for the nutritive transudation taking place through those walls.

LEONARD ERSKINE HILL
(*2 June 1866—30 March 1952*)

Occasionally while tracing the development of ideas one must take into account work that retarded rather than contributed to their progress. In these instances experimental findings, which may later be proved erroneous, receive universal acceptance, and examples during the nineteenth century such as Magendie's influence upon the concept of cerebral localization (pp. 682–683) and Luciani's on the physiology of the cerebellum (pp. 662–668) have already been encountered. It can be argued that these episodes were of significance, for they are as much a part of the history of a concept as are the contributions that we today accept as important advancements.

Such was the case with the work of the British physiologist Leonard Hill, later Sir Leonard Erskine Hill (see Douglas, 1952–1953), on the cerebral circulation, the results of which were published in 1896 (*The physiology and pathology of the cerebral circulation. An experimental research*, London, 1896). Hill was principally concerned with disproving results that indicated an intrinsic control of cerebral circulation such as those of Donders and Roy and Sherrington. His experimental techniques were inadequate and faulty, yet he propounded his conclusions with force and authority.

EXCERPT PP. 76–77

(1) No evidence has been found of the existence of cerebral vaso-motor nerves: either by means of stimulation of the vaso-motor centre, or central end of the spinal cord after division of the cord in the upper dorsal region: or by stimulation of the stellate ganglia, and, that is to say, the whole sympathetic supply to the carotid and vertebral arteries.

(2) Evidence is not forthcoming of the existence of any local vaso-motor mechanism.

(3) In every experimental condition the cerebral circulation passively follows the changes in the general arterial and venous pressures. The intracranial or cerebral venous pressure varies directly and absolutely with general venous pressure, but only proportionately with general arterial pressure.

(4) The intracranial pressure is in all physiological conditions the same as the cerebral venous pressure.

(5) The volume of the blood in the brain is in all physiological conditions but slightly variable.

(6) There is no compensatory mechanism by which the intracranial pressure is kept constant. The intracranial pressure or cerebral tension, which in all physiological conditions is circulatory in origin, may vary with the circulatory pressure from zero to 50 mm. Hg. The functions of the brain matter continue in this varying condition of pressure.

(7) In all physiological conditions a rise of arterial pressure accelerates the flow of blood through the brain and a fall slackens it. The cerebral circulation is controlled by the vaso-motor centre acting on the splanchnic area.

(8) There is no evidence of the causation of cerebral anaemia by spasm of the cerebral arterioles.

(9) Arterial hyperaemia of the brain produces no experimental results of

importance. Cerebral venous congestion, on the other hand, is of great pathological significance.

Unfortunately, Hill's opinion that the cerebral circulation passively followed changes in systemic arterial and venous pressure dominated the field for about twenty years and was repeatedly verified. It also had its repercussions in clinical neurology where problems of pathology and therapy were interpreted in the light of it.

HARVEY WILLIAMS CUSHING
(8 April 1869—7 October 1939)

In the growing field of neurosurgery there was an urgent need at the turn of the century for more information regarding intracranial dynamics. It was well known clinically that a rapid increase of intracranial pressure was associated with a high tension pulse and experimentally it could be shown that a rise of blood pressure accompanied artificially induced cerebral compression. The first attempt to explore this phenomenon graphically was made by the American neurosurgeon Harvey Cushing.

Cushing was born in Cleveland, Ohio, and was graduated M.D. from the Harvard Medical School in 1895. After having spent four years in general surgery under the famous William Halsted and a year in Europe (1900–1901), he undertook the development of a neurosurgical clinic at the Johns Hopkins Hospital in Baltimore, Maryland. In 1912 he went to the Harvard University Medical School as professor of surgery whence he retired in 1932. Cushing was the first to devote himself entirely to the surgical problems of the nervous system and became the most outstanding pioneer of this specialty. He trained surgeons from all parts of the world and carried out research on the pituitary, intracranial tumors and many other problems, as well as introducing revolutionary surgical procedures. Cushing had, as well, strong literary and historical interests that were reflected in his biography of Osler (1925), awarded a Pulitzer Prize, his *Biobibliography of Andreas Vesalius* (1943), and many literary and medicohistorical essays. During the years following his retirement from Harvard until his death he held appointment as Sterling Professor of medical history at Yale University and bequeathed his celebrated medicohistorical collection to the Medical Library of that University (Fulton, 1946).

In 1900 Cushing went to Berne to work with the surgeon Theodor Kocher, and there he investigated the interrelation between intracranial tension and systolic blood pressure, mainly in the dog ("Physiologische und anatomische Beobachtungen über den Einfluss von Hirnkompression auf den intracraniellen Kreislauf und über einige hiermit verwandte Erscheinungen," *Mitt. Grenzgeb. Med. Chir.*, 1902, 9:773–808). This paper ended with the statement "Brain compression which produces an intracranial tension far exceeding the normal blood pressure can be the cause of an increase in blood pressure without any other effects" (p. 806). Cushing also published on the subject in English ("Some experimental and clinical observations concerning states of increased intracranial tension," *Amer. J. med. Sci.*, 1902, 124:375–400) and later discussed his results in the light of further clinical experience ("The blood-pressure reaction of acute cerebral compression, illustrated by cases of intracranial hemorrhage," *Amer. J. med. Sci.*, 1903, 125:1017–1044). The following excerpts have been taken from this last paper in which, together with other matters, he pointed out the clinical significance of the relationship between intracranial and systemic pressure. He was especially concerned with correlation of his experimental findings with clinical data in order to devise the most effective therapeutic procedure. A consequence of Cushing's interest in blood pressure was the introduction into the United States of the Riva–Rocci recording instrument (Cushing, 1939, pp. 24–25).

EXCERPT PP. 1018–1019

The experiments above referred to, which for the most part were carried out upon dogs, tended to show, if the interpretation were a correct one, that this rise in blood pressure [which accompanies brain compression] represents a purposeful and not a meaningless reaction. The belief was expressed in a regulatory mechanism which controls the rise, and which, under experimental circumstances at all events, is seemingly so adjusted that the vasomotor centre tends to hold the intravascular pressure (arterial tension) at a level slightly in excess of the external (extravascular) pressure exerted by the compressing force against the arterioles and capillary vessels situated in the medulla. In this way a fatal bulbar anaemia, which otherwise would be the result of an equalization of intracranial and a stationary arterial tension, is warded off. Thus, the high-pressure pulse, which characterizes conditions of intracranial hemorrhage, for example, is easily accounted for, and its measured level of tension may be taken as an indication of the degree of circulatory embarrassment from which the medulla is suffering in consequence of the compressing force. It was pointed out that under these circumstances the continuance of respiration hinged upon the efficiency of the vasomotor mechanism in holding the blood pressure at a certain level. Should the vasomotor centre fail to keep the arterial tension in excess of the experimentally increased intracranial tension, the respiration would immediately cease, owing to the anaemia of the centre governing it. Consequently, as will be emphasized in the discussion of some of the following cases, the sequence of events in case of immoderate intracranial tension is, primarily, exhaustion of the vasomotor mechanism with fall in blood pressure, and, secondarily, failure of respiration in consequence of the ensuing bulbar anaemia.

In the majority of circumstances the vagus centre is likewise stimulated under the effects of compression with the resultant familiar slowing of pulse rate, which, however, does not seem to bear so definite a relation to the degree of increased tension. Aside from the fact of its frequent concomitance the brachycardia does not apparently play any particular part in the reaction under discussion, nor can it be always said that the more advanced the compression the slower will be the pulse rate.

The significance of this vasomotor regulation, should it have been possible to establish it as true for man as well as animals, was fully realized, but, unfortunately, at the time the Mütter lecture was prepared, no opportunity had been offered on clinical cases to satisfactorily corroborate the laboratory findings, much less to put the facts to any practical application.'

The introduction for clinical purposes of a simplified form of the original Riva-Rocci blood-pressure apparatus has enabled us to take observations on arterial tension, and to plot them on charts which simulate in a useful way the invaluable records which in the laboratory may be obtained by taking blood-pressure records directly from an isolated vessel. By employing this apparatus it has been possible to chart graphically the blood-pressure reaction in several cases of intracranial injury, and thus to bring clinical cases in line with the experimentally induced conditions. The results have proven of such interest and the method of observation of such practical value that it is hoped the few cases, which will subsequently be given at some length, may suffice to further illustrate the points which the experimental work has brought out.

EXCERPT PP. 1043–1044

Varying degrees of rapid increased intracranial tension produce corresponding disturbances in the intracranial circulation. To these circulatory disturbances the symptoms of compression are solely due. The condition known as acute cerebral compression may be conveniently subdivided into four stages, dependent upon the degree of circulatory alteration which has been reached. Each of the stages has its own more or less characteristic symptom-complex.

The major or underlying symptoms originate in the centres situated in the medulla, and are only called out when the degree of intracranial tension begins to approach the arterial tension so that anaemia is threatened. A circulatory condition in the medulla which borders upon anaemia has the effect of stimulating the vasomotor centre. Thus, a rise of blood pressure is occasioned which restores the local circulation. The extent of this rise may be taken as an indication of the degree of advancement of the compression. Beyond a certain point, however, this reaction cannot take place. The vasomotor centre under these circumstances fails, and the respiratory efforts cease entirely.

In conjunction with other symptoms, a progressive increase in arterial pressure or a high degree of the same, which has been already reached, or a pressure which exhibits from moment to moment great alterations in level may be taken as a certain indication of the advisability of early operative intervention . . . .

PAUL JENSEN
(*30 October 1868—?*)

A reliable method of measuring the circulation of blood through the brain had been sought ever since the early and crude experiments of Gärtner and Wagner in 1887, but the technical difficulties were immense and at first they were almost insuperable. The first attempts that resulted in a precise figure were made by the German physiologist Jensen, in 1904.

Jensen was born at Stuttgart and studied medicine at Jena, Freiburg im Breisgau, Würzburg, and Berlin. He worked at the Physiological Institute in the University of Breslau and held an appointment as lecturer in physiology at Halle. In 1910 he was created professor *ordinarius* of physiology in the University of Göttingen, and director of the Physiological Institute. He became *emeritus* in 1932. His research was concerned mainly with problems of muscle and circulatory physiology and with biochemistry, evolution, and genetics.

Jensen argued that if he knew the weight of the brain, or part of it, and could measure the amount of blood flowing through it in a given period of time, as well as the blood pressure in the supplying artery, he would be able to calculate the cerebral blood flow. He chose the rabbit for his experiments because unlike other laboratory animals its internal carotid artery is relatively large and it gives off no important branches before it reaches the Circle of Willis. The velocity of the blood in the vessel in the narcotized animal was measured with a Hürthle *stromuhr*. Its territory of distribution was delineated in dead rabbits by the injection of a colored mass, and the area was then dissected free and weighed; Jensen estimated that 23.6 percent of the total brain tissue was supplied by one internal carotid artery (p. 174 of his article; see below).

Unfortunately, this technique, although ingenious, was subject to several errors. Thus the estimation of distribution areas in dead animals was worthless, as those who had investigated the blood supply of individual brain arteries had already discovered. Moreover, Jensen's *stromuhr* was incapable of detecting rapid changes in blood flow. Nevertheless, his experiments marked the beginning of a succession of techniques that are still being employed today.

Jensen's paper, "Über die Blutversorgung des Gehirns" (*Pflügers Arch.*, 1904, 103:171–195), dealt principally with techniques and is thus of little interest now. The final part that detailed his calculations is given below. Cerebral blood flows of

136.4 ccm. per minute for 100 gm. of brain in the rabbit and 138.0 in the dog were much too high.

EXCERPT PP. 194–195

Now we wish to turn to a question arising from the Table [III, which presented his findings in nine experiments]: how much of the internal carotid artery blood is the brain deprived of by its going through the *superior ophthalmic artery?* The second-volume of the latter vessel with an average lumen of 0.08 mm. amounts to about 0.000015 ccm., that is 0.024% of the total second-volume of the internal carotid artery. This small amount can be neglected, for it comes within the limits of error and we can regard the *total second-volume of the internal carotid artery as applying to 2.5 gm. of brain substance.*

From this value we can finally calculate the quantity of blood received *by the whole brain of the rabbit per second, Q,* according to the hypothesis used previously [p. 175; $Q_1:Q_2 = g_1:g_2$ where Q_1 = the flow per second of the basilar artery, Q_2 = the flow per second of the internal carotid artery, g_1 and g_2 = the weights of the respective areas of the brain supplied by these vessels. $Q_2 = 0.0665$ ccm. (Tab. III) and Q replaces Q_1 and represents the total brain flow]:

$$Q : 0.0665 = 10.6 : 2.5$$
$$Q = 0.282 \text{ ccm.}$$

The quantity Q can also be determined in another way, by adding the double second-volume of the internal carotid artery and the second-volume of the basilar artery as has been done in the second of the two procedures mentioned above.

We then obtain:

$$Q = 2 \times 0.0665 \text{ ccm.} + 0.141 \text{ ccm.} = 0.274 \text{ ccm.}$$

For *an average external resistance of the vascular pathways of the whole brain,* we obtained a result by using the first of the two values mentioned above as a figure for Q (= 0.282 ccm.) in the formula already given and for a tube of 1 mm. length and with a lumen of 1.20 mm. [p. 184; $Q = \dfrac{k.h.d^4}{1}$.

Q = second-volume, k = coefficient of viscosity, h = the blood pressure at the beginning of the current pathway, d = the diameter, and 1 = the length of the tube. This is Poiseuille's formula].

If we compare the blood flow of the [rabbit] brain [Tab. III: average of nine experiments = 136.4 ccm. for 100 gm. of brain at 100 mm. of mercury per minute] with the values found by Landergreen and Tigerstedt [1893] and by Tschuewsky [1903] in the dog for other organs, we must place it between the kidneys and the thyroid gland *in order of magnitude of blood supply* in the *dog* and *rabbit*. This scale shows values for organs weighing 100 gm. and with a resulting minute-volume of 100 mm. of mercury:

Hind leg .... 5 ccm.
Skeletal muscle (resting) .... 12 ccm.
Head .... 20 ccm.
Kidney ....100 ccm.
Brain ....136 ccm.
Thyroid ....560 ccm.

Two of my experiments have shown that in the dog the brain occupies the same position [in the table]; their mean is 138.0 ccm. for 100 gm. of brain at 100 mm. of mercury per minute. We may assume, I dare say, that in the human brain the figure is of at least a similar magnitude.

HENRY STONE FORBES   STANLEY COBB
(*27 May 1882—*   )   (*10 December 1887—*   )

The inherent properties of the cerebral blood vessels is the most important aspect of our present-day understanding of the cerebral circulation. Yet Hill's pronouncement that they were like rigid tubes (pp. 802–803) held sway until the 1920's, despite the fact that both earlier evidence, like that of Donders (pp. 794–797) and of Roy and Sherrington (pp. 798–801), and new data, indicated its falsity. The new data, gradually accumulated from the last decade of the nineteenth century onwards, showed that vasomotor nerves did in fact supply the pial and brain tissue vessels and that they could produce vasoconstriction, although less than that seen in other organs; vasodilation was also possible. This knowledge was soon to overthrow the opinion of Hill and led directly to the present-day position.

This new concept of cerebral blood vessels, and thus of the control of cerebral circulation, was the work of many men, but the most active and significant group appeared in Boston in the 1930's. Henry S. Forbes was the most important contributor to the sequence of papers that resulted; in the article cited below his collaborator was Stanley Cobb.

Forbes was born at Milton, Massachusetts, and was graduated in medicine from Harvard University in 1911. Thereafter he held a sequence of appointments in neuropathology and internal medicine, both at Boston and elsewhere. He retired in 1958. He has investigated the effect of the ultraviolet light and heat on protoplasm, carbon monoxide poisoning, asphyxial headache, the cerebrospinal fluid, and the cerebral circulation.

Cobb was born at Brookline, Massachusetts, and also studied medicine at Harvard University where he received the M.D. degree in 1914. He spent his professional career in the fields of neurology, psychiatry, and neuropathology and held many academic positions in Harvard University. He became professor *emeritus* in 1954. His research work has been in the fields of cerebrospinal fluid and cerebral circulation, physiology, epilepsy, language, electroencephalography, and psychosomatic medicine.

In a review of 1938 ("Vasomotor control of cerebral vessels," in *The circulation of the brain and spinal cord, Association for Research in Nervous and Mental Diseases*, Vol. XVIII [Baltimore, 1938], 201–217) Forbes and Cobb first of all surveyed the factors which they thought regulated the cerebral blood flow. They emphasized in particular the unique role the systemic arterial blood pressure and various intrinsic cerebral influences played in this regard; they were, in fact, verifying the work of Donders and of Roy and Sherrington that had been discarded for so many years. This was followed by a brief report of their experiments and a discussion of the results.

EXCERPT PP. 202–204

EXTRACEREBRAL FACTORS

The Systemic Blood Pressure.—This factor appears to dominate all others. The arterial pressure, in turn, depends on complex reflexes from the cardiovascular centers of the central nervous system, the carotid sinuses, and other reflex mechanisms. These reflexes, therefore, play a vital part in controlling the supply of blood to the brain. Other factors contribute to this end: the resistance of arterioles throughout the body, the amount of venous blood returned to the heart, and the state of the heart itself.

CEREBRAL FACTORS

Active Changes in Caliber of Cerebral Arteries.*—Such changes in caliber, due to change in tonus ["tension"—suggested as replacement for "tonus"; personal communication from Forbes] of the arterial walls, may overcome moderate or gradual fluctuations in arterial pressure. Thus, when active changes occur, we usually find arterial constriction following a rise in blood pressure and dilation following a fall. An explanation for this inverse relationship between arterial caliber and intravascular pressure is suggested below in paragraph *c*.

Active changes in caliber result from the following conditions:

a. Direct trauma to vessels' walls.

b. Changes in chemical composition of the arterial blood. Variations in tension of arterial CO_2 are of first importance, for CO_2 strongly dilates all

---

* By the term "active changes in caliber" we mean changes due to alterations in the state of contraction and relaxation of the muscle fibers of the arterial walls (tonus). The fact that the arteries do not behave like inert collapsible tubes (varying in size directly with the internal pressure) indicates that active work is performed by their walls.

cerebral vessels. Many drugs (nitrites, alcohol) and inhaled gases (CO, H_2S) act in a similar fashion.

c. Asphyxia of the tissues due to slow blood flow (termed by Van Slyke "stagnant anoxia"). This condition in the brain may result from general or local causes: low blood pressure, high intracranial pressure or occlusion of vessels supplying the brain. In all of these states we have seen the cerebral arteries dilate. Partial compensation for the slowing of blood flow is thus established. The dilation is probably due to a chemical (asphyxial) effect on the arterial walls, not to a nerve reflex, for it is unaffected by cocaine or by atropine applied locally to the vessels. When the blood pressure rises again, the relaxed walls may dilate still further for a few seconds, but then (while the pressure is still rising) constriction steadily takes place as the asphyxial condition is relieved by the more rapid flow.

d. Regional activity of the brain. There is evidence that active areas of gray matter have a local vasodilation. This may be due to a local increase in CO_2 or other products of active cellular metabolism.

e. Activity of cerebral vasoconstrictor nerves (sympathetic).

f. Activity of cerebral vasodilator nerves (parasympathetic).

These last two conditions have less effect on cerebral blood flow than the chemical conditions mentioned under *b, c,* and *d.*

Passive Changes in Caliber of Cerebral Arteries.—Distension or slight narrowing may occur during abrupt fluctuations of blood pressure. Such changes in caliber are obviously due to mechanical causes. These passive changes in caliber are transient, however, and slight in extent, unless the vessels' walls are in a relaxed state. In that case, a rise in intravascular pressure may cause extreme dilation.

The main object of this paper is to discuss the neural vasomotor mechanism of the brain and to present in some detail the results of recent experimental work. Various methods have been used, both indirect and direct. Each method has its advantages and its drawbacks.

EXCERPT PP. 204–205

In our own laboratory, by use of a cranial window and microscope, we have observed and recorded the changing diameters of vessels in the pia-arachnoid over the parietal cortex. For this work we have used mostly cats, a few dogs, and several monkeys. Our findings, some of them not yet published, may be summarized as follows.

In a large series of experiments, in more than 300 animals, stimulation of the cervical sympathetic nerve has resulted consistently in constriction of arteries in the pia. We have found that the sympathetic fibers responsible for the reaction pass through the middle ear in close association with the carotico-tympanic nerves. The latter serve as pathways for the sympathetic fibers which dilate the pupils. Sympathetic nerve fibers via the stellate ganglion and vertebral nerves exercise no influence, so far as we could determine, on pial arteries of the parietal region.

EXCERPT P. 211

VASODILATION

Evidence of a vasodilator innervation was first obtained in a joint experiment with Penfield conducted in our laboratory [1932]. . . .

The further evidence may be summarized as follows:

Anatomical and histological work by Chorobski and Penfield shows that nerve fibers pass from the facial nerve through the geniculate ganglion and the greater superficial petrosal nerve to the carotid nerve ascending the internal carotid artery.

EXCERPT P. 213

COMMENT

In regard to the functional importance of the cerebral vasomotor mechanism the evidence at hand warrants only a few suggestions. Since it is more effective in some parts of the brain than in others it may aid in diverting the blood from one region to another; it may help arteries to regain their normal caliber, as after extreme dilation, and it may limit undesirable fluctuations and thus aid in maintaining a steady rate of flow through the brain. But there is no evidence from experimental work to show that it can cause the arteries to shut down sufficiently to bring about ischaemia.

SUMMARY

The former confusion regarding regulation of blood flow within the brain and its meninges has been clarified by recent experiments carried on independently in different laboratories. Today there seems to be substantial agreement on several points; that an intracerebral regulation does exist; that in this regulation chemical agents (especially CO_2) play a major part; that cerebral vasoconstrictor nerves are present but that they are only about one-tenth as effective in the pia as the vasoconstrictor nerves are in the skin; that vasoconstrictor nerves are distributed unequally to different parts of the brain. Evidence has been obtained also for the existence of cerebral vasodilator nerves.

With so many regulatory mechanisms one might expect frequent changes in vessel caliber and in blood flow, even under resting conditions. Such changes do not occur normally. The capillaries, at least in the pia, appear to be always open, the arterioles do not change in size appreciably, and the flow is remarkable for its steadiness.

Carl Frederic Schmidt   Seymour Solomon Kety
(29 July 1893—   )   (25 August 1915—   )

Forbes and Cobb and others opened a new chapter in the investigation of the cerebral circulation but had done so by reaffirming earlier views. The work of the Boston group naturally stimulated further studies, and in the late 1940's a considerable amount of experimental evidence was accumulated by a number of investigators. However, it was almost exclusively animal in origin.

Defects of the cranial bones, like deficiencies of the sternum, have always attracted attention because of the access they provide to the underlying organ. Although early experiments making use of a cranial defect have been recorded, the first noteworthy attempt to investigate the cerebral circulation was that of Angelo Mosso, 1881 (see Fischgold, 1963). Mosso's deductions were only partly correct, and a reliable method of measuring the human cerebral circulation did not appear until 1944, when it grew out of the work of the American pharmacologist Schmidt.

Schmidt was born at Lebanon, Pennsylvania, and was graduated M.D. from the University of Pennsylvania in 1918. He has spent most of his career in the University of Pennsylvania School of Medicine in Philadelphia, working in the pharmacological laboratory. His research has been principally in the physiology and pharmacology of respiration and circulation (see Schmidt, 1961).

Schmidt and his pupils, in particular Seymour S. Kety, have been largely responsible for the advances in the physiology of cerebral circulation in the last two decades. In 1943, with P. R. Dumke ("Quantitative measurements of cerebral blood flow in the macacque monkey," *Am. J. Physiol.*, 1943, 138:421–431), Schmidt described the first reliable quantitative measurements of the monkey's cerebral blood flow by means of a bubble flowmeter, and in 1944 he opened the most modern era of investigation with a survey of the field ("The present status of knowledge concerning the intrinsic control of the cerebral circulation and the effects of functional derangements in it," *Fedn. Proc. Fedn. Am. Socs. exp. Biol.*, 1944, 3:131–139) from which the following excerpts have been taken. No account of the techniques then discussed will be given as they are now obsolete.

EXCERPT P. 132

. . . . The blood supply of the brain then becomes a matter of immediate concern, not only because here, as elsewhere in the body, the capacity of the tissue to function is limited by the capacity of its circulation to meet its changing requirements, but for the additional special reason that the brain is unable to contract much of an oxygen debt and therefore is more subject than other tissues to derangement by an insufficient supply of blood. Two major questions then arise: What are the agencies by which the blood supply of the brain, or of its various parts, can be altered either to their advantage or disadvantage? and how would the functional capacity of these structures be affected if their blood supply is either deficient or excessive relative to their requirements?

These questions have been asked and answers to them sought for more than a century, and twenty years ago categorical answers to both of them would have been given without hesitation. The cerebral circulation then was held to be fitted passively to the needs of the brain by adjustments elsewhere in the body, and an intrinsic control over cerebral vessels was regarded as unimportant or non-existent. . . . With these seemingly unequivocal items of experimental evidence as a background, experimenters and clinicians came to hold the opinion that spasms of cerebral vessels, occurring spontaneously or elicited by suitable physical or chemical agencies, would elicit signs of cerebral stimulation and might be responsible for the convulsions produced by disease states or by drugs.

During the past twenty years, however, there has been a gradual accumulation of evidence against both of these older viewpoints. Studies of the cerebral circulation by a number of technics have shown that the cerebral vessels possess considerable capacity for independent control in response to both nervous and chemical agencies; these observations are now so numerous that there is no longer any doubt about the necessity for revising the older idea that the cerebral circulation can be adjusted only passively . . . .

It is scarcely necessary to point out that progress in this as in any other branch of physiology depends on improvement over the methods previously used. In this particular case progress has been impeded by lack of realization of the special anatomical difficulties involved in studies of the cerebral circulation, which appears to indicate that these have not been sufficiently emphasized in the past . . . .

EXCERPT P. 136

The two methods that have been used for quantitative studies of the cerebral circulation in man therefore appear to be fraught with so many uncertainties that the results obtained by them are of limited value until some of the above-mentioned sources of error have been excluded, or at least evaluated. It is unfortunate indeed that now, when data concerning the behavior of the human cerebral circulation are urgently desired, the only thing that can be said is that a considerable amount of fundamental research will have to be done before such data become available. Yet in the past the first step toward real advances in clinical experimentation has often been dissatisfaction with the methods previously utilized, and it is to be hoped that history will repeat itself here.

One of the immediate results of Schmidt's interest and of the encouragement he gave to those working with him, was the introduction by Kety in July 1944 of a method, based on the ability of the brain to absorb nitrous oxide and on the Fick principle for measuring the cerebral blood flow in man ("Quantitative measurement of cerebral blood flow in man," *Meths. med. Res.*, 1948, 1:204–217). Multiple simultaneous samples of arterial blood from the brachial or femoral artery and cerebral venous blood from the superior bulb of the internal jugular vein were taken while the individual was breathing nitrous oxide. The cerebral blood flow could be calculated from the results of the blood analyses, and from it cerebral utilization of oxygen and cerebral vascular resistance computed. Although it seems at the moment that this technique and its more recent modifications are opening a new chapter in the physiology, pharmacology, and pathology of the cerebral circulation, adequate assessment of it cannot yet be made. It can, however, be said that this new approach has stimulated many further studies (see, e.g., Clarke, Jones, Logothetopoulos, 1954).

In 1950 Schmidt summarized in a book the results obtained to date (*The cerebral circulation in health and disease*, Springfield, Ill., 1950), and the following is one of his comments from the introduction to it. His opening remark may seem to be trite, but one of the incomprehensible features of research on the cerebral circulation has been the willingness of investigators to apply results in animals directly to man. This has been especially true in the clinical field and should be recalled before criticizing Aristotle and Galen for a similar practice.

EXCERPT P. 4

. . . . Here it must suffice to point out that the behavior of the cerebral circulation of man in health and disease can be learned only from observations made on man himself, and since the changes to be expected are quantitative, the methods used must be adequately quantitative. Less than five years ago no such methods were available. Since then two have been developed and reported and one of them [that of Kety, applying the Fick principle to cerebral blood flow] has been used sufficiently to indicate that now, for the first time, the clinical physiologist is no longer at a disadvantage in studying the circulation in the human brain. As a matter of fact he is now able to learn more about this, and about its relation to the metabolic functions of the organ supplied, than about any other organ of the body. The change is one of the small profits of the research activities of the war years and is one more example of the benefits to be expected from giving brilliant young men opportunities to develop and test out original ideas.

One thing about the cerebral circulation that has been agreed upon from the start is that it is unique in all essential respects, beginning with the morphological.

Seymour Solomon Kety was born in Philadelphia on 25 August 1915 and was graduated M.D. from the University of Pennsylvania in 1940. He is now Chief, Laboratory of Clinical Sciences, National Institute of Mental Health, Bethesda, Maryland. The following excerpt has been taken from his important paper of 1948; the dye dilution technique referred to in the third paragraph has not been included.

EXCERPT PP. 204–207

Despite its obvious and fundamental importance, information on cerebral blood flow was not placed on a scientific basis until 1943, when Dumke and Schmidt [see p. 812] achieved the first quantitative measurements of cerebral blood flow under conditions approaching the normal. This was soon followed by studies of cerebral metabolism under similar circumstances. These measurements were made on species (rhesus or spider monkeys) whose cerebral circulation resembles that of man in being readily isolated from the extracerebral blood supply of the head. A bubble flow meter interposed in the arterial supply to the brain yielded quantitative values for total cerebral blood flow.

In man so direct a procedure is out of the question, but various methods give indirectly some knowledge of the cerebral circulation in various clinical states. These include observation of the diameter and color of retinal vessels, measurement of cerebral arteriovenous oxygen differences, use of a heated thermocouple introduced into the internal jugular vein and adaptation of the principle of the occlusion plethysmograph to the cranium. The limitations of these methods were discussed in an excellent symposium on cerebral circulation.

Two methods which appear to yield quantitative measurements have been developed: the nitrous oxide method, based on the Fick principle; a dye dilution method, depending on the Stewart principle. These techniques are discussed here in some detail.

1. *Nitrous Oxide Method.*—The brain, unlike the kidney and liver, does not specifically and selectively remove foreign substances from the blood stream, hence the clearance techniques for measuring renal and hepatic blood flows are not applicable. It does, however, absorb by simple solution an inert gas which reaches it by way of the arterial blood, and this phenomenon forms the basis for measurement of cerebral blood flow by the Fick principle. This postulates, in its simplest form, that the quantity of any substance taken up in a given time by an organ from the blood which perfuses it equals the total amount of the substance carried to the organ by arterial inflow less the amount removed by venous drainage during the same time period. For the case of the brain uptake of N_2O, let

$Q_B]u$ = quantity of N_2O taken up by the whole brain in time u measured from the start of inhalation,
$Q_A]u$ = quantity brought to the brain by arterial blood in time u,
$Q_V]u$ = quantity carried away by cerebral venous blood in time u,

A = arterial N_2O concentration,
V = venous N_2O concentration,
TF = total cerebral blood flow/min,

CBF = cerebral blood flow per unit weight of brain/min,
W   = brain weight

From the Fick principle:

$$Q_B]u = Q_A]u - Q_V]u,$$

but since both A and V are variables with respect to time (Fig. 1 [accompanying illustration]),

$$Q_A]u = TF \int_0^u A\,dt$$

and

$$Q_V]u = TF \int_0^u V\,dt,$$

whence

$$Q_B]u = TF \int_0^u (A - V)\,dt$$

or

$$TF = \frac{Q_B]u}{\int_0^u (A - V)\,dt} \tag{1}$$

or, in terms of unit weight of brain,

$$CBF = \frac{Q_B]u/W}{\int_0^u (A - V)\,dt}. \tag{2}$$

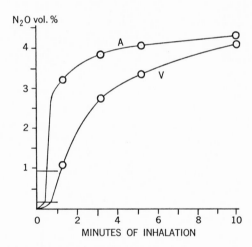

Typical pair of N$_2$O concentration curves for arterial (A) and internal jugular (V) blood.

The quantity $\int_0^u (A - V)\,dt$ is readily obtained from the respective arterial and cerebral venous curves. The numerator, or cerebral concentration of nitrous oxide, is not obtainable directly in man. If the time u is sufficiently long, however, equilibrium will have occurred between brain and blood leaving the brain with respect to nitrous oxide tension. At that time,

$$\frac{Q_B]u}{W} = V\,uS,\tag{3}$$

where S represents a partition coefficient for nitrous oxide between brain and blood $\left(S = \dfrac{\text{solubility of N}_2\text{O/g brain}}{\text{solubility of N}_2\text{O/ml blood}}\right)$. By substituting appropriately and multiplying through by 100, one obtains a value for cerebral blood flow in convenient units:

$$CBF = \frac{100\ V_uS}{\int_0^u (A-V)\,dt}\tag{4}$$

where *CBF* is expressed as ml of blood flow/100 g of brain/min.

Application of this formula to practical measurement of cerebral blood flow, although theoretically valid, necessitates certain assumptions. These were all subjected to experimental evaluation with the following conclusions: (1) Blood from one internal jugular vein at the level of the superior bulb represents mixed cerebral venous blood with only slight contamination by blood of extracerebral origin. (2) After 10 min. of inhalation of a constant tension of nitrous oxide the venous blood is in equilibrium with the brain with respect to nitrous oxide tension. Therefore the value of u in equation (4) may be taken as 10 min. (3) The partition coefficient of nitrous oxide between brain and blood (factor S in equation (4)) equals unity. In addition, simultaneous measurement of cerebral blood flow in monkeys by the nitrous oxide method and the bubble flow meter showed excellent agreement.

Conclusion

Despite a lengthy heritage of almost two millennia regarding knowledge of the cerebral circulation, a clearer understanding of it in man has only recently begun to be possible. Its history is characterized by periods of inactivity during which there was universal acceptance of opinions, such as those of Galen, and more recently of Hill, that were later shown to be quite erroneous. But the greatest deterrent has been the inaccessibility of intracranial blood vessels and the need to examine them in the living state. Thus, despite a rich accumulation of anatomical knowledge in earlier periods, function could not be adequately investigated until the techniques of physiology had advanced to the point where adequate experimental procedures could be devised. The most important recent source of knowledge has resulted from the perfection of a method applicable to man. The whole field of the pharmacology as well as the physiology of the brain's circulation now stretches before the investigators whose techniques will no doubt increase in precision as new physical methods are applied to them. Already it is evident that the cerebral blood flow is amazingly complex and that the factors affecting it are many (Wells, 1960). Moreover, these studies are closely linked with the overall function of the nervous system in health and in disease, and a solution of the many problems related to the cerebral circulation will contribute enormously to an eventual understanding of the fundamental mechanisms of man's nervous system.

NEUROANATOMICAL TECHNIQUES

Introduction

The history of knowledge of the brain is also the history of the techniques that have been employed to elucidate its structures, both gross and microscopic. Some have already been discussed, but in addition, a few of the more important and classic methods used in the past, and in some instances still employed, are represented below by excerpts from the writings of their discoverers or popularizers. In all but three cases—Blum, Marchi, and Weigert—excerpts from the works of these investigators have been included above so that the following selections supplement what has already been presented. The examination of the morphology of the brain is a vast field, and only a very small part of it can be represented here. It is best considered under the following headings: 1) Dissection techniques; 2) Fixation and preservation; 3) Coloring agents; 4) Tract tracing techniques.

Dissection Techniques

The ways in which anatomists have dissected the brain have determined their knowledge, and these methods have had a long and interesting history. The records at present available begin with the techniques used by Galen who described them in his *Anatomical procedures* from which excerpts have already been presented. Some of these techniques were used by Vesalius who, however, also employed the method of slicing horizontally through the brain *in situ*, and observations revealed in this way have likewise been presented above. Although the Vesalian procedure was an easy one to perform, it created difficulties for understanding of the relationships of the various parts of the brain; nevertheless, it was still being used to some extent by Vicq d'Azyr (pp. 590–593) at the end of the eighteenth century.

The method of Costanzo Varolio (pp. 820–823) was revolutionary inasmuch as he examined the brain from the base upwards after it had been removed from the cranial cavity with the attached eyes and cranial nerves. This method was further exploited in the seventeenth century by Willis (pp. 582–585) and by Vieussens (p.

588) who emphasized the importance of tracing white matter fibres, originally mentioned by Willis and by Steno (pp. 584–585).* In addition, Steno proposed a research protocol and in so doing demonstrated remarkable foresight. Gall and Spurzheim also traced fibres macroscopically, and their general influence on brain anatomy is now admitted to have been an important one.

In addition to examination of the adult, human brain, investigation of this organ in animals and in the human fetus also provided significant information. Tiedemann in 1816 was not the first to insist on a comparative and embryological approach to brain anatomy, but his influence was considerable, especially in respect to the cerebral convolutions (pp. 827–829).

The gross techniques of brain dissection used by students today remain based upon the work of these and other pioneers.† No revolutionary additions have been made since the beginning of the nineteenth century, although special techniques have been evolved such as the injection of the cerebrospinal fluid pathways (Chapter XII) and of the intracranial blood vessels (Chapter XIII). For a general history of macroscopic anatomical preparation, see Faller (1948).

VAROLIO

(See p. 634)

Until the time of Costanzo Varolio (1543–1575) there was only one method of examining the brain, that described by Galen (Kühn, 1821–1833, II, 707–713; Duckworth, 1962, pp. 10–17), also used in part by Vesalius (1543, pp. 650–658; also see Eriksson, 1959, pp. 218–221). The brain was dissected *in situ* by means of a series of horizontal slices beginning at the upmost part of the cerebral hemispheres.

Varolio, however, proposed starting from the base of the removed brain, and one of the immediate results of this new approach was his description of the pons Varolii (see pp. 634–635). The new method also used later by Willis, was described by Varolio in *De nervis opticis nonnullisque aliis, praeter communem opinionem in humano capite observatis, epistolae* (Padua, 1573). The following excerpt has been translated from the reprint of 1591.

EXCERPT PP. 140–144

. . . . You are aware of the usual manner of dissecting the head—that used by the ancients as well as the moderns—which begins with its upper part. First, the upper part of the calvarium is cut off and removed, and then, as you are well aware, the membranes and substance of the brain as far as the ventricles and the rest of the parts. However, I, considering most organs of the brain to be near the base of the head, and the brain by its

* The problem imposed by the term "fibre" must be kept continually in mind (p. 29).

† The dissection techniques of Reil and Stilling have been dealt with in the sections concerned with their fixation methods (respectively p. 830, and p. 833).

weight, especially in the dead, to compress them between itself and the calvarium, judged this usual method of dissection to cause many difficulties; therefore I usually begin the dissection from the opposite part of the head, that is, from the base of the brain. If one proceeds in this way, each of its organs may be observed as completely as desirable, but as this method of dissection is unusual so also it is very difficult.

First, I remove all the bones of the head from the underlying dural membrane of the brain in such a way that the brain is left with the eyes attached, as well as all the pairs of [cranial] nerves and a portion of the spinal marrow [cord]; all these things, I say, remain enveloped by the aforesaid dural membrane. Then I invert the brain so that the base is uppermost and remove the dural membrane from the base of the brain, but leave those parts of it that are around the nerves lest they be ruptured; when the membrane has been removed, the base of the brain is exposed as Vesalius delineated it immediately after the first chapter of his fourth book. Then I turn to that first membrane which I said binds the spinal marrow to the brain in its anterior part; grasping it with a hook I cut it lightly with forceps and remove it from the underlying parts. I said forceps because the parts now being dissected are so soft, yielding, and fragile that they cannot like muscles be separated directly from one another with a curved scalpel.

When the membrane has been removed, it will be seen at once that the spinal marrow [brainstem] does not take origin thence where it was first attached, but ascends further upwards and anteriorly and is reflected from its origin in such a way that the membrane contains not only the marrow adhering to the brain but also that reflected. Indeed, that part of the brain at its base is reflected a little posteriorly towards the spinal marrow, and in its middle there is a concavity called the infundibulum [of the third ventricle], of which there is a foramen in the middle of that membrane now removed. With that membrane removed, there appears under it a plexus of vessels crossing one another which anyone may, if he wishes, call the *rete mirabile*. Then I remove all those vessels, whereupon the reflection of the spinal marrow anteriorly and its progress upwards is revealed more clearly; but if the membrane of this sort is also removed posteriorly from the underlying spinal marrow—some may perhaps believe such removal fruitless or impossible—a series of swelling transverse fibres is uncovered, different from the straight fibres of the spinal marrow. This is the process of the cerebellum that I call the bridge (*pons*), from which the auditory nerve is clearly seen to depend [pp. 634–635]. When these things have been observed, I grasp the thin membrane of the brain [pia mater] in that place usually attributed to the origin of the optic nerves and remove some portion of it, but carefully so that the nerve will not be injured. With the removal of the membrane the brain begins to appear there not as continuous to itself but only contiguous, and I follow this division towards the middle of the head around the spinal marrow [brainstem]. I carefully draw the brain attaching to that marrow somewhat outwards until I find the optic nerves hidden in that space known to all from their conjunction [optic chiasma], rounded on each side and separated from all the surrounding parts; they are carried to the posterior as far as the site mentioned earlier, and in that hidden space they determine for themselves their own limits just as they do in the part long known to everyone. Hence if a probe be inserted between them and the parts to which they attach, they may be elevated without violence from the underlying parts as far as the place whence we said they first originate.

While these things are being done, at the same time the primary origin of the spinal marrow will be observed. Where the second pair of nerves [oculomotor] are usually considered to arise, I cut a small portion of the brain, extending as far as that site from which I said it takes origin. Furthermore, with the left hand I grasp the middle prominence of the brain and draw it lightly upwards; then with forceps I cut the angle formed between the said prominence and the anterior; because of that incision and upward drawing those prominences are easily separated from one another, inasmuch as they are mutually contiguous but not continuous as perhaps all anatomists hitherto believed. Then the olfactory organ is observed in this space, attaching to the superior part of the brain and, as I said, progressing as far as the extreme sides of the brain. These things having been seen in this way, I remove the eyes and divide the conjunction of the optic nerves [optic chiasm], drawing each one to its side. Then I cut the pons of the cerebellum, and the spinal marrow near the head's division into two parts [i.e., at the upper midbrain], preserving each portion on each side; then I remove the cerebellum completely, but first observing the processes [peduncles] that it transmits to the spinal marrow. And so the brain has been disposed of in this way, and turned so that its base is downwards, and its parts separated from one another [i.e., separating the two hemispheres], I observe the whole corpus callosum, its true size and construction, which I mentioned above.

Again turning the base upwards, I grasp the other part of the spinal marrow and draw it lightly to the side; then in the lowest part on each side a fissure appears extended slightly curved along the length of the head, of which the middle of the base of the brain forms the exterior. When these fissures have been seen, from the other extremity I cut the cerebrum anteriorly, almost at its extremity. Then I undertake another incision posteriorly, and thereafter I divide the brain in the same way from the lowest aforesaid fissure through the whole middle prominence so that the incisions are of this shape; in consequence the notable size and shape of the ventricles, which I mentioned above, appears, and the root of the spinal marrow [basal ganglia] is observed, which is where the anterior cavity [lateral ventricle] is reflected to the middle [third ventricle]; around that root in the cavity of the ventricle there is a plexus called retiform [choroid] so that it is near the fissures by which I said the ventricles are expurgated into the common space called the third ventricle, and at the same time the primary origin of the optic nerve can be properly seen from that site of the spinal marrow [thalamus] that looks back to the internal cavity of the ventricle.

NICOLAS STENO
(1 January 1638—25 November 1686)

In 1665 the Danish anatomist Nicolas Steno (see Scherz, 1958) read a paper in Paris (*Discours de Monsieur Stenon sur l'anatomie du cerveau* [Paris, 1669]) before a group of scholars that were shortly to form the Académie Royale des Sciences. Essentially it was a critical review of current concepts of brain anatomy and function, but, as well, it denounced the ideas of men such as Descartes. Steno also made several constructive suggestions concerning the examination of the brain, and in fact he outlined a whole program of research that included studies in comparative and morbid anatomy, embryology, physiology, experimental neurology, and neuropharmacology. These are some of the basic methods of modern investigations of the brain, and it is a great pity that Steno was never able to put into practice the very remarkable suggestions his genius produced.

EXCERPT PP. 7–8

If, as I have just said, the substance of the brain is little known to us, the true manner of dissecting it is not any better known. I do not speak of those who cut the brain into slices; it has been recognized for a long time that this does not provide any anatomical elucidation. The other [method of] dissection in which the gyri are unfolded is a little more artistic, but it only shows us the outside of what we are interested in and even that quite imperfectly.

The third, which adds to the development of the gyri, a separation of the gray body [cortex] from the white substance, goes a little further; it does not penetrate, however, beyond the surface of the medulla.

Various combinations of these three methods of dissection have been used, and various types of longitudinal and transverse sections can be added.

As for me, I hold that the true [method of] dissection would be to follow the nerve threads through the substance of the brain in order to see where they go and where they end. It is true that this method is full of difficulties so that I do not know if one may dare to hope that it could be completed without very special preparations. The substance [of the brain] is so soft and the fibres so delicate that they can scarcely be touched without breaking them. Thus, since anatomy has not yet arrived at such degree of perfection that it is able to carry out the proper dissection of the brain, let us not flatter ourselves any longer, and rather admit our sincere ignorance so that we do not deceive ourselves first and others later, by promising to show them the real structure.

EXCERPT PP. 46–51

It is not enough to be attentive at all times; it is necessary to add changes in the methods of dissection that are so many proofs of the truth of your performance, and that can equally satisfy you yourself and convince others.

. . . . The principal reason why many anatomists have persisted in their error and why they have failed to go further than the ancients in their dissections has been because they believe that everything has already been adequately observed and nothing further remains for the moderns; and, as they have held the ancient rules of dissecting as inviolable laws, they have done nothing all their lives but demonstrate the same parts by the same method; whereas anatomy should not be submitted to any rule and it should vary as many times as the times we begin to dissect . . . .

. . . . .

. . . .

. . . .

After a true and very accurate plan of the parts of the brain has been made, and the errors as well as their causes discovered, and a decision made upon the true method of demonstrating the parts, using all the necessary precautions, it is also necessary to try to express what has been seen by accurate and faithful figures; for it is better not to have them at all than to have them false or imperfect.

EXCERPT PP. 53–57

What I have said up to now is but the least part of what I believe must be done to acquire knowledge of the brain; for it is necessary to dissect and examine as many heads as there are different kinds of animals and different conditions in each species. In the fetus of animals one sees how the brain is formed, and that which could never be seen in the healthy and intact brain will be seen in the brain that has been altered by some disease.

In living animals all those things are to be considered that can cause some change in the actions of the brain, whether it come from the outside, like liquors, wounds, or medicines; or whether the causes be internal, as in diseases, of which medicine counts a large number. There is also another reason for working on the brains of animals, and this is that we can treat them as we please. Trephining can be carried out as well as all other surgical operations in order to learn how to perform them; why not perform these same operations to see if the brain has any movement and if on applying certain drugs to the dura mater, to the brain substance, or to the ventricles any special effects can be detected?

Various tests might also be made without opening the skull, by applying different drugs from the outside, by mixing others with foods, by making injections into the vessels, to learn in this way what disturbs the animals' actions and what is most suitable for their recovery when they are disordered.

The brain is different in different species of animals, which is a new reason for examining them all; the brain of the bird and of the fish are quite different from that of man; and in animals that approach us most closely I have not seen one in which I have not found some quite manifest difference.

. . . .

. . . .

We have seen so far, gentlemen, the inadequacy of the systems of the brain, the defects of the method that has been followed for dissection and understanding, and the infinity of researches that must be carried out on man and on animals, and that under all the different conditions under which it is necessary to examine the small amount of light we find in the writings of those who have preceded us. All those considerations which need to be taken into account in working on such delicate parts must undeceive those who hold to what they find in the books of the ancients. We shall be always in miserable ignorance if we are contented with the little light that they have made for us; if the men most suited to undertake research do not unite their work, their industry, and their studies in order to arrive at some knowledge of the truth, which ought to be the principal goal of those who reason and who study in good faith.

FRANZ JOSEPH GALL   JOHANN CASPAR SPURZHEIM
(*See p.* 392)

Although Gall and Spurzheim won notoriety because of their system of phrenology, nevertheless they stimulated considerable interest in the gross anatomy of the brain, and for Gall this was the primary purpose of his studies. Their technique was mainly an extension of that introduced by Varolio and by Vieussens (p. 819). It not only revealed certain structures for the first time and displayed known structures more clearly, but it also provoked bitter controversy that was itself a useful stimulus to brain dissection. Thus John Gordon (1817) published an entire book attacking their technique and unjustifiably denouncing Gall and Spurzheim as plagiarists.

A description of their method of dissection appeared in several of the writings of Gall and Spurzheim, but the following excerpts have been translated from the first volume of their great work, *Anatomie et physiologie du système nerveux en général, et du cerveau en particulier* (Paris, 1810). It is of interest that they did not use the microscope. Like Bichat, the famed investigator of tissues, they believed that they could not trust it and declared that a knowledge of the microscopic constituents of the nerve fibre, whether globules or other structures, "gives no hint as to how their function may be ascertained" (p. xix).

EXCERPT PP. XVIII–XIX

Perhaps it is thought that we have contrived all sorts of procedures and instruments to see things in the brain that our predecessors in anatomy were unable to see. But with the exception of some experiments by which we have sought to make evident the fibre structure of the white matter of the brain and the fibre layers of the convolutions for those who do not wish to see them, we have only an ordinary dissecting case that contains merely scissors, forceps, a tube, several scalpels, a hammer, a saw for the skull, and cutting pincers.

All our skill or all our dexterity consists not in cutting but in following the nerve threads by scraping without damaging their surface. We have entirely given up the use of the microscope. Besides the fact that these lenses too often become spectacles through which each one sees what he wants to see, the mass of the brain does not seem to be suitable for this kind of research . . . . Thus we have preferred to report from observation with the naked eye, especially as the fibre structure is readily seen when our method is followed.

EXCERPT P. 174

The obvious outcome of these considerations is that every method that prevents the discovery of the parts that gradually bring the brain to perfection, that cuts the organs before their completion, or that begins with the mutilation of the perfect organs by slicing and cutting them from above downwards, etc., is contrary to nature and to the purpose of cerebral organization. What can be said of contemporary professors of anatomy [e.g., Vicq d'Azyr] who, despite our indisputable principles, continue to defend this wretched method of Vesalius? What can be said of those who although publicly admitting the disadvantages of that method continue to use it? Perhaps they wish faithfully to imitate their predecessors and, like them, not employ improvements until they have been recognized for fifty years.

If one follows our method and begins by examining each part at its primary source, it is not difficult to follow its course and direction by scraping, to recognize the successive reinforcements, the addition of new parts and their natural connections and, finally, to approach the laws of brain organization. Vieussens was indebted, for most of the discoveries he made in the brain, to the care he used in scraping the fibres along their length.

Despite all that we have published about our method and our principles, nothing has been grasped except that we begin the dissection of the brain from below, whereas, since the time of Vesalius, all schools have followed the custom of beginning this operation from above. Because Varolio, Vieussens, Monro, Vicq d'Azyr, and several other anatomists have made their cuts from below or at the base, and because our opponents know the principles of these anatomists hardly better than our own, they have pretended that our method was nothing but that of Varolio and of Vieussens. It matters little to science who may have been the first to introduce a better way of observing. However, our answer to the report of the commissioners of the Institute [*Recherches sur le système nerveux en général . . . mémoire,* Paris] contains considerable detail regarding the various methods of dissecting the brain, and in it we have proved by the history of anatomy and by passages from the authors cited, how far they were from our principles and our method. Besides, it is only too well known that before us the application of physiological and philosophical views to the anatomy of the brain were almost completely neglected, perhaps from ignorance, perhaps from timidity.

When we occupy ourselves with examining at what point the skull is the expression of the form of the brain, it will be realized how important it is for the physiologist to know accurately the position of each part of the brain; and as our anatomical designs must likewise be consulted for the physiology as well, we have, as far as possible, represented the brain in its natural position in the skull.

FRIEDRICH TIEDEMANN

(*See p. 395*)

Willis, Steno, Haller, and others emphasized the need to examine the brains of animals, and Steno also included the growing brain in his research protocol. Nevertheless, even at the beginning of the nineteenth century little comparative or embryologico-anatomical data had been amassed. At this time Tiedemann, as well as other anatomists, stimulated inquiries into both these fields by means of his widely popular book on the development of the human fetal brain (*Anatomie und Bildungsgeschichte des Gehirns im Foetus des Menschen*, Nuremberg, 1816). The following passages have been translated from the introduction.

EXCERPT PP. 2–4

In my opinion the only two paths that can lead to a knowledge of the structure of the brain, but that are still infrequently used, are those of comparative anatomy and the anatomy of the fetus; for this labyrinth they are like Ariadne's thread. Comparative anatomy shows us the origin and the gradual formation and progression of the nervous system and brain from the lower and simply fashioned animals up to man. In the formation of no other system of organs does such a perfect gradation from a simple to a complex structure take place as in the case of the brain and nervous system. So, with the structure of the brain and nervous system there is found a distinct basic type through the whole scale of animals. Through a consideration of the increasing complexity and development of the animal brain we shall be in a firm position to understand and to interpret the very complicated structure of the human brain in its confluences and in its organic connections.

Although the importance of comparative anatomy in anatomical investigations of the brain's structure has been recognized by modern dissectors of the brain, nevertheless more is made of the idea than of the reality. If we examine the new work of Gall on the brain and nervous system, we find the idea expressed everywhere that the structure of the nervous system and of the brain must be followed from the lower animals upwards to the higher animals and so to man. But what in reality has Gall done? He has described and portrayed nothing more of the animals' nervous system than the nerves of the caterpillar, the brain and spinal cord of a hen and of a few mammals, and this itself in part faulty. If conclusions are to be reached from such scanty and fragmentary investigations of the brain and nervous system, the object of the investigation is merely [to produce] more confusion than clarity. All such fragmentary investigations are to be considered only as the building materials of an edifice which, if they are used as elements towards general conclusions on brain structure, only lead to new errors and false steps. No inference concerning an anatomical or physiological subject is accurate if it is not fully set off with sagacity based on facts and observations.

As we must arrive at a knowledge of the gradual formation and composition of the brain by way of investigation of the nervous system and of the brain of the animal, so we also need a comparative psychology in order to understand the significance and action of parts of the brain. That is to say, the manifestations and appearances of the brain and soul action of animals from the lower to the higher up to man must be observed and followed, and, finally, a comparison must be made of these with the structure of the brain. By means of a comparison of soul action and the brain structure of various animals, we shall attain a knowledge of the function of individual parts of the brain, a knowledge that we still wholly lack and that we can acquire in no other way than in that one indicated. Hitherto it has been believed that we can observe the soul action of animals of the same species to increase as we perceive greater complexity and development in the structure of the brain and nervous system. Moreover, we find the sensory nerves and their places of origin in the brain of the animal so much larger, as the sense organs become progressively developed and larger, etc. It is to be considered as a truth that an intimate connection and a close relation exists between the soul action of the animal and the structure of the parts of the brain.

In this way it is at least possible to attain knowledge of the function of the parts of the brain even if the reason, the last argument and the why of these appearances, remains unknown . . . . Thus I repeat that the structure of the brain and the function or action of its parts may possibly be uncovered by means of anatomy, physiology, or psychology but by no means the reason and final argument themselves. This is my belief.

. . . .

Another part of the anatomy and physiology of the brain that is almost entirely neglected is the origin and embryology of the brain in the embryo and fetus. There is a law, established by the discerning Harvey and more recently very adequately proved by German anatomists and physiologists, that the human and animal embryo do not appear in a perfect and diminutive form [of the adult], but that they start in an elementary form, that they gradually pass through lowly stages of formation, and that they finally reach a higher stage of development. Why, I wonder, should not a similar process take place in the structure of the brain of the embryo and fetus from a simple to a complicated formation, and why should not this give an explanation regarding the fashioning and formation of the brain that, in its perfect state, is so complicated? In order that I may answer these questions I have for some years been occupied with the structure of the brain in the embryo and fetus and now make known the results of my investigations in this work, because it allows many explanations of the structure of the brain that seem to me to be not unimportant [see pp. 395–397 for embryology of cerebral gyri].

Fixation and Preservation of Nervous Tissue

No matter how refined the techniques of dissection became, examination of the brain and spinal cord was bound to be difficult and confusing in the absence of any means of hardening and preserving them. Yet this was the situation up to the first decade of the nineteenth century. Earlier investigators may occasionally have used hardening and preserving techniques such as soaking in wine or freezing but they never referred to them. As noted already (p. 820), the appearance of some of the early illustrations of the brain such as the famous one in Willis's book (1664, fig. 156) suggests that some method of hardening was used, and it is known that Vieussens employed boiling in oil for this purpose and that Malpighi boiled his specimens in water.

Reil's method of preparing the brain by soaking it in alcohol was, however, the first to be used widely and it was thus a milestone in the history of the anatomy of the brain. As various chemicals became available in the nineteenth century, other agents were employed, and Hannover and Stilling used chromic acid to fix and preserve the brain and spinal cord respectively. This, too, was an important stimulus, and at the end of the century Blum introduced formaldehyde which is still the most commonly used substance for fixing nervous tissue.

Johann Christian Reil
(See p. 593)

Reil's use of alcohol to preserve and harden the brain was an important landmark in the history of neuroanatomy. By its use he was able to make many contributions to the knowledge of the brain's gross anatomy (pp. 593–598, 647–652, and 830–832). The paper containing the description of his methods is entitled "Untersuchungen über den Bau des grossen Gehirns im Menschen . . . Vierte Fortsetzung VIII" (*Arch. Physiol., Halle,* 1809, 9:136–146).

EXCERPT PP. 137–142

The chief merit of my work lies in the preparation of the brain for dissection and the method of dissecting. For the art of dissecting the brain is so important that it is equivalent to a knowledge of the brain's organization, so that both must be discovered simultaneously and at one stroke. Hence my care in the description of my preparations, procedures, and method of dissection, so that anyone may duplicate what I have discovered.

We shall never be successful in puzzling out the complicated web of the brain so long as we hack blindly into it and, as Vicq d'Azyr did, slice it in all directions. Initially, I made numerous random cuts, but when I dissected next, was unable to repeat what I had previously laid bare by chance. Today I am in a position to determine with absolute certainty those cuts that must be made in the cerebrum as well as in the cerebellum in order to observe certain organizations. I have submitted an idea for the dissection of the brain and I have fortunately been able to show the path so that everybody can now walk in this direction and easily fill in the deficiencies. The method leads to the discovery of the parts, and an acquaintance with them in turn leads to the perfection of a procedure by which they can be best presented. For if one knows exactly the course and direction of the [lateral] lemniscus, of the anterior [superior] cerebellar peduncles, of the commissures, etc., it is not going to be difficult for us to consider a method and with its help to exhibit them to the greatest advantage. Gall's method is inadequate. Without being prepared, the brain is too pulpy and fluid and therefore cannot be dissected in continuity. It may also have certain structures that are not sufficiently prominent in themselves and, like the muscular apparatus of the crystalline lens, can only be made visible by appropriate means. However, this subject, too, has not been exhausted; certainly there are still other suitable procedures for dissecting and better means of preparation that have to be elucidated. Alcohol compresses [dehydrates] nervous tissue with such force that the brain loses a quarter of its volume and thereafter cannot be easily separated again. The simultaneous or subsequent use of potash, although decreasing the disadvantage of the compression [dehydration], does not completely prevent it. If the cerebral fibres, like the nerve fibres, were partitioned by a neurilemmal sheath, another far from negligible obstacle to the dissection of the brain would arise. In the preparation of nerves, I dissolved the cell substance [? areolar tissue] with nitric and hydrochloric acid, of which only the latter succeeded in breaking up the nerve fibres, whereas the former compressed them into cords. However, the brain's substance is too voluminous, so that the acids have difficulty in penetrating; nitric acid renders it so brittle that it cannot be displayed, and hydrochloric acid, according to my experience to date, does not affect the brain in the same way as it does the nerves. In addition, the nerve fibres that have been separated by hydrochloric acid are so fluid that they cannot be touched. Therefore it could only be applied partly to small pieces of brain, and partly to those parts in which the fibres are parallel in position.

Among those methods that I have tried in the dissection of the brain, I have found the following to prove useful: 1) The brain is fixed in alcohol for several days, and then placed in a solution of carbonate of potash or of pure potash for several days; after it has become softened in the potash it is again fixed in alcohol. This method has the advantage that the brain tissue can be separated more readily and the difference between the gray and white matter becomes visible again, after it had been more or less lost in the process of hardening with alcohol. The gray matter takes on a blackish-gray color because of the potash and turns out to be slippery and gelatinous in consistency. 2) Pure potash or carbonate of potash is immediately added to the alcohol in which the brain is to be fixed. 3) It is placed in alcohol in which ammonia has been dissolved. Both methods yield good specimens and may perhaps be preferred to the first one because they decrease the severe compression of pure alcohol. 4) Finally, I started to prepare for examination the superficial parts of the brain on the fourth, sixth, and eighth days immediately following fixation in alcohol and proceeded with the dissection of the deeper parts as they gradually became harder. This last method seemed to me almost the best and might perhaps be even more successful if one were to add some potash or ammonia to the alcohol at the start. In this initial preparation the parts are revealed more beautifully, they are tougher and firmer, and the alcohol penetrates better into the deeply situated parts because they are exposed earlier. The membranes in particular hinder the penetration of the alcohol. It would therefore be very advantageous if they could be partially or totally separated from the fresh brain at the start. However, sometimes even small brains that have been left for years in alcohol lose their membranes very nicely.

There are probably still other methods that might be wholly superior to mine, such as the use of sublimate or sulphuretted potash solutions, the addition of dyes to the potash and ammonia solutions, the acceleration of fixation by heat, the dissection of the brain under water after it has been well softened in potash solutions, etc., with none of which I have so far experimented.

If one has first become acquainted with the general connections of the brain, one can fix it in small portions and dissect it later.

As instruments for dissection I used my fingers, the handle of a scalpel, a styloid-like instrument, a narrow, ivory disc, rounded at the tip, and a small ivory knife with a straight blade and a bent, rounded, and medium sharp back. One must bend apart as firmly as possible the parts that one wants to separate and dissect with the tool, not the part that one wants to demonstrate but the part that covers it.

I have not the slightest doubt that with the gradual perfection of the methods of preparation and dissection of the brain, the point will be reached when it can be dissected with the same ease as that with which one dissects any other part.

Adolph Hannover
(See p. 59)

The discovery of chromic acid as an agent to harden nervous tissue was made by Hannover in 1840. The following passages have been translated from "Die Chromsäure, ein vorzügliches Mittel beim mikroscopischen Untersuchungen" (*Arch. Anat. Physiol.*, 1840, pp. 549–558).

EXCERPT PP. 549–550

. . . . I tested other media with just as little success until I finally discovered in chromic acid the liquid in which not only outer form and inner structure [of the specimen] are perfectly preserved, but also that which sets it to such a degree that one can prepare the finest sections without their elements being disordered. Even the various color shades, for example, those of the brain and the spinal cord, are still visible after months of preservation; indeed, the yellowish stain in transparent and very delicate objects is distinguished to advantage. I have the honor of listing some of the matters in which I employed this excellent medium.

EXCERPT P. 555

Chromic acid was extremely useful in the exploration of the stratiform arrangements in the cerebrum and the spinal cord, because I could cut them with a very sharp knife into the thinnest slices and thus follow piece by piece [serial section]. However, the disadvantage here is that the harder the cerebrum has become, the less transparent is the section, and in these investigations one must be extremely careful, employing only light pressure, and covering with only a small glass plate; nevertheless, one can make the thinnest sections. But if the hardening is less, the sections are less successful and cannot be made so thin; in these instances slight pressure will help. It is best to avoid extremes in the hardening; one soon learns to achieve this by carrying out tests.

Benedikt Stilling
(See p. 270)

One of the most detailed and precise examinations of the spinal cord carried out in the nineteenth century was that of Benedikt Stilling, and some of his references to the technique he employed have already been cited (pp. 270–275). In January

1842 he first cut sections from the frozen cord and then developed a technique for making serial sections in various but specific directions, such as transverse, longitudinal, and oblique, through the organ. By his method and careful study of the material produced, Stilling laid the foundation for the modern anatomical study of the spinal cord, medulla oblongata, and pons. Rolando (pp. 653–656) had previously made thin slices of nervous tissue, but Stilling was able to reconstruct organs by means of his series of sections. The following selections have been translated from *Untersuchungen über die Textur des Rückenmarks* (Leipzig, 1842), written by Stilling in collaboration with J. Wollach.

EXCERPT P. 17

Although I now recognized the different directions of the fibres in individual parts of the spinal cord, I lacked a precise survey of the entire course of the fibres in general and of the spinal cord as an entity. I therefore undertook an exploration of very thin sections through the entire thickness of this organ. In a calf's spinal cord, moderately frozen, I first succeeded in obtaining a very thin section, that is an exceedingly thin slice of the entire thickness of the spinal cord, and I put it under the microscope between two sheets of glass, being very careful to compress it only very slightly. With a magnification of 15 (Ocular No. C, lens No. 1) at first glance I saw here the admirable structure of the spinal cord of which up to now I had only a faint idea. I now saw clearly and demonstrably the transition, connection, and the relations of the fibres of both substances of the spinal cord.

Stilling also cut longitudinal sections of the cord, and the following account illustrates his method of doing so in a fresh specimen (*Untersuchungen über den Bau und die Verrichtungen des Gehirns*, Jena, 1846).

EXCERPT P. 10

From the white lateral tracts of a fresh, human spinal cord or of a calf one takes a slice as thin as possible by making a longitudinal cut parallel to the long axis of the spinal cord, carefully compresses it between two glass plates or in a compressorium so that it is transparent and suitable for microscopic examination. With fifteen times magnification and transmitted light one can distinguish primary fibres, well known from earlier investigations, of the same dimensions as in the hardened spinal cord. The dark contours and light masses of the contents of the primary fibres, as well as the light interstices between the individual fibres, yield a beautiful picture which on the whole appears silver-gray under the microscope. The fibres do not all lie in the same direction; however, most of them lie lengthwise, parallel to one another; the many fibres that lie in other directions must be considered as being shifted from their natural position. When cutting off the section with a knife many fibres become dislocated, and this dislocation is further increased by the compression.

The following are Stilling's comments on transverse sections of fresh material, from the same book of 1846.

EXCERPT P. 10

It is impossible to make as fine transverse sections from fresh as from hardened spinal cord. Therefore, the appearance of a cross section of the former is quite different under the microscope from a similar one of the latter. For example, a transverse section from the fresh spinal cord of a calf, carefully compressed between two glass plates or in a compressorium, appears under the microscope with fifteen magnifications as a dark gray (with strong compression, light gray or silver gray) mass, that looks completely disorderly; with more careful examination it shows itself to be composed (in the white lateral, posterior, and anterior tracts) of fragments of primary fibres which, shorter or longer depending upon the thinness of the section, lie together in the most variable directions. Imbedded between them is an excessively large mass of those spherical masses of the nerve content (mentioned with the longitudinal sections) that made this confusion still more complete, in such a way that one cannot make a sure judgment from the microscopic examination of only such a preparation for the evaluation of the stratification of the fibres in the spinal cord. A similar result is noted in oblique sections of fresh spinal cord.

After pursuing his studies of the spinal cord with very intense industry for seventeen years, in 1859 Stilling published his huge book, *Neue Untersuchungen über den Bau des Rückenmarks* (Cassel, 1859). In it he included detailed instructions for the preparation and examination of the spinal cord, presented in such detail as to allow the selection of only a small portion of his practical advice, and the following excerpt (from Bk. I, "Über die Methode der anatomischen Untersuchung des Rückenmarks im Allgemeinen wie im Besondern") contains a few general comments and then Stilling's account of his method of fixing the cord, the basic principles of which are still in use today.

EXCERPT P. 1029

The anatomical investigation of the spinal cord is for the purpose of providing us with knowledge of its form, area, and gross parts, visible with the naked eye, as well, mainly, as an insight, as exact as possible, into its most subtle structure; that is, a knowledge of the most diverse elements of the spinal cord, its anatomical and material properties and their mutual relations with regard to form, situation, connection, origin, cause, and ending. But it is only possible to obtain this knowledge by mechanically isolating the different parts of the spinal cord and by investigating them with the help of the microscope.

EXCERPT PP. 1030–1031

From what I have said already, the anatomical techniques can be divided into two main divisions, that is, 1) the preparation of the spinal cord for anatomical investigation; 2) the investigation of the prepared parts of the cord with the help of the microscope. The preparation of the spinal cord itself is divided into the following subdivisions: *a*) into that of hardening the cord; *b*) into the cutting up of the cord into fine segments. The staining of the cord must be regarded as part of the first division. In addition, a part of the second is, in certain rare cases, the further division of the fine segments by teasing them with needles under the microscope in order to isolate mechanically individual elements, as well as in even rarer cases, treating the segments with different chemical reagents in order to make individual portions of the tissue of the relevant segments more clearly visible. Moreover, as it is important to conserve the prepared segments of the spinal cord for longer and repeated investigation, one has to add to the points of the anatomical-preparation technique already mentioned, a further one. That is, the most suitable method for storing the fine sections for microscopical examination. All these more mechanical manipulations and methods are, however, only the preparations for the actual research which, as mentioned before, consists of the appropriate microscopical investigation of the relevant objects.

EXCERPT PP. 1032–1033

. . . . The prepared cord with its coverings is lowered into a strong, glass cylinder that is filled with chromic acid solution (the preparation of which will be noted below) and which is 3 to 4 feet in length and 1½ to 2½ inches in diameter, so that the lower end of the cord is put in first with a stone tied to it. Because of its own weight, but more because of that of the stone, it gradually enters the cylinder so deeply that finally even the top end of the cord is drawn into the cylinder below the fluid level. Then two small, firm, wooden sticks are put through two thread loops that were drawn through the uppermost end pieces of the dura mater. These sticks are placed parallel to each other across the top of the cylinder in such a way that now the cord, suspended on the two wooden sticks, floats freely in the fluid of the long, glass cylinder but is kept under a certain tension and straight by the weight of the suspended stone.

The fluid in the cylinder can be distilled water or ordinary, fresh, cold well water to which has been added a small quantity of crystalline chromic acid, dissolved beforehand by shaking in such a way that the color of the fluid is light wine yellow. It is not important whether there is more or less acid, but as a start, 10 grains in one pound of water [is enough].

The spinal cord is left quietly in this way in the cylinder for 24 hours in a cool and shady spot. During this time it is noticed that the dura mater, and in part the arachnoid, nerve roots, etc., mostly stand out from the cord, and that the chromic acid solution has free access to the subarachnoid spaces and to the spinal cord. On each of the following 5 to 8 days fresh quantities of crystalline chromic acid are added to the fluid so that on the second day about 20 grains of acid are added to one pound of water, and in the end the solution will contain about one ounce of acid for each pound of water. But there is no need for anxiety concerning the exact relation of acid to water. As soon as the solution has taken on an intensive dark wine yellow color I do not add any more fresh acid. Now the cord remains in the cylinder quietly and undisturbed for 14 to 20 days. After the end of this period, the cord is lifted out of the cylinder a little and by pressing on the medulla oblongata one attempts to discover whether it feels like wax. If this is the case, the hardening can be regarded as completed. But if the mass of the cord can be indented by finger pressure so that one is convinced that the center of the cord is softer than the periphery, the cord must be left in the fluid for another 8 to 14 days until it has reached a degree of uniform hardness in all its inner and outer layers as far as can be judged from finger pressure.

When this has come about, the cord is taken out of the chromic acid solution and put on the table. The attached stone is removed as well as the thread loops and the cord is put into a suitable vessel containing the purest rectified spirit (97%) so that it can be used either straightaway or after a shorter or longer time and investigated, that is, divided into small segments or in other ways for different purposes. It is either all put in or it is cut into individual larger or smaller pieces according to the intended purpose of the investigation. It is true that the spinal cord can remain even longer in the chromic acid solution, for as long as several months without becoming unsuitable for investigation, but this is less advisable as will be remarked below.

FERDINAND BLUM
(3 October 1865—)

Ferdinand Blum was the first to suggest that formaldehyde should be used as a tissue fixative and preservative. It has been the commonest substance so employed ever since, and it is especially useful for nervous tissue. The following excerpt has been translated from Blum's paper announcing his discovery, "Der Formaldehyd als Härtungsmittel" (Z. *wiss. Mikrosk.*, 1893, 10:314–315). For the early history of its use in neurology, see Fish (1895).

EXCERPT PP. 314–315

As I demonstrated recently ["Der Formaldehyd als Antisepticum," *Münch. med. Wschr.*, 1893, 40:601–602], formaldehyde in aqueous solution has the remarkable quality of killing micro-organisms with excellent certainty, not only in concentrated solution but also when extremely diluted. This slow, sure disinfection seems to be based upon a peculiar transformation of the organic matter, during which process the tissues—the constituents of which will remain wholly undiscussed at this point—change from their semisolid aggregate state to an essentially more resistant, hardened state.

I first made this observation on my own fingers which, while handling formaldehyde, acquired a completely hardened epidermis; I then noticed that a cut-up anthrax mouse that had lain overnight in a formaldehyde solution, after such a short time, felt like an alcohol preparation; and I became certain of the above-stated thesis concerning the effect of formaldehyde when, according to plan, I put pieces of tissue into the solution. A formaldehyde solution diluted ten times hardens even large pieces of tissue such as liver, kidneys, gastric mucous membrane, brain, etc. (definitely faster than alcohol!), in the shortest time. At the same time the macroscopic structure of the tissue remains better preserved than when hardened in alcohol: for example, the white and gray substance in the hardened brain, the central vein and its periphery in the acini of the liver contrast markedly with one another; however, noticeable shrinkage does not occur.

With microscopic examination that was carried out following dehydration and celloidin imbedding in stained preparations, the tissue of liver, kidney and gastric wall appeared well preserved and receptive to hematoxylin as well as to anilin dyes, particularly to Weigert's fibrin and micro-organism stains. Micro-organisms retained their specific stainable properties even when they had been pretreated for days with formaldehyde.

The investigations with formaldehyde as a hardening medium for the brain and spinal cord will be continued by courtesy of Professor Weigert, and for the other organs by myself. I have reported the present observations to the dye works, formerly Meister, Lucius and Brüning at Hoechst/Main, which provided me with the formaldehyde for investigation, for their use; the firm will market the concentrated formaldehyde under the name of "Formol."

The Use of Coloring Agents in Neurohistology

Increasingly refined methods of gross dissection aided by techniques of fixation could give only a limited amount of information, and further elucidation was to depend upon the microscopic examination of nervous tissue. But this, too, was limited until ways of coloring the nerve elements could be discovered. The early microscopists who used the new compound, achromatic machine (pp. 29–30) made fundamental discoveries without the help of this refinement, but the development of neurohistology from the second half of the nineteenth century onwards has been determined by the exploitation of coloring agents that were themselves dependent upon the development of the dyestuffs industry, mainly in Germany.

As Baker (1945) pointed out, the history of this subject must consider non-vital dyeing, vital coloring of preexistent structures, histochemical color tests, impregnation with opaque substances, coloring by phagocytosis, and injection of colored substances. For further relevant contributions to the history of staining, see Lewis (1942); Hintzsche (1943); Conn (1946 and 1948).

Of the various methods of subjecting tissues to coloring agents the works of the authors presented below illustrate three: non-vital dyeing by Gerlach's use of carmine, Weigert's method for myelin, and Nissl's nerve cell stain; histochemical color tests by Marchi's method for myelin; and impregnation with opaque substances by Golgi's silver stain. Vital staining has already been referred to in the work of Ehrlich on the staining of the nervous tissue with methylene blue (pp. 97–99) and in that of Goldmann who investigated the blood-brain barrier with vital dyes (pp. 749–751), especially trypan blue. Likewise, there was Ruysch's method of injecting colored substances into blood vessels in the study of the cerebral cortex (pp. 420–421), and Pfeifer's microtechnique of examining blood vessels (pp. 783–787) belongs partly to this group. In addition, Malpighi had used ink to outline the "glands" that he discovered in the cerebral cortex (p. 418), although not as a stain, and other authors mentioned in Chapter II, such as Ranvier, Held, and Ramón y Cajal, referred to the use of coloring agents as a means of identifying the morphological characteristics of the neuron; Ranvier (pp. 78–81) used both a silver impregnation method and a non-vital dye, picrocarminate, to demonstrate the "constriction ring" of the myelinated nerve fibre that still bears his name.

Joseph von Gerlach
(*See p. 88*)

Joseph von Gerlach was responsible for the widespread use of carmine as a non-vital dye substance in the microscopic investigation of animal tissues. He was by no means the first to use it as a dye, for its properties with regard to botanical material had been discovered a century before. He did, however, introduce it as a means of dyeing animal material (see Baker, 1945, pp. 9–10; Conn, 1948, pp. 15–17, 25–26, 29). The following excerpt has been translated from Gerlach's book, *Mikroscopische Studien aus dem Gebiete der menschlichen Morphologie* (Erlangen, 1858), and describes his chance discovery of carmine as a coloring agent of nervous tissue.

EXCERPT PP. 1–3

Four years ago while exploring the walls of injected blood vessels, I became aware that nuclei take up the dye [ammonium carminate] avidly, and thus behave differently from the cells [cytoplasm] and intercellular substances.

Although the cells absorb dye, too, they do so much more slowly and in smaller quantity than do the nuclei. The intercellular substance is almost indifferent to the dye, and even after prolonged exposure scarcely takes on a visible strain. The easiest way to be convinced of this is to place fine sections of hyaline cartilage in a solution of ammonium carminate. By the way, the same results are obtained with this dye by treating epithelial and connective tissue cells and smooth and striated muscles.

Some time ago I had the idea of applying this behavior of elementary living structures towards staining to the investigation of the central nervous system. I placed especially fine sections of the brain and spinal cord, that had been fixed in potassium bichromate, in a somewhat concentrated solution of ammonium carminate, left it standing for 10 to 15 minutes, washed it for several hours in water that was changed frequently, then added acetic acid, and, following this, absolute alcohol to remove the water, and preserved it with Canada balsam. With this procedure I obtained rather pretty specimens of nerve cells with markedly red nuclei, lighter stained cells and their processes, and barely stained ground mass. These were particularly instructive for the visualization of the topographic distribution of nerve cells in the central [nervous system] organs, since, as a result of staining the cells and their processes, the structures which mattered here most became much more strikingly obvious. Sections of the spinal cord that I have also shown to my Würzburg colleagues, Kölliker and H. Mueller, looked especially good; by the way, I must confess that these did not yield any additional information and they agreed completely with the illustrations of the spinal cord that Stilling published only recently [see pp. 270–275].

It was chance which now revealed to me a method for using the pigment which achieves much more than the one just described. In a cup that had not been thoroughly rinsed, a residuum of dye remained, and I poured water over this so that the liquid was of a weak, rosy-red color. In this solution I left a section of a cerebellar convolution overnight. On account of the infinitesimally small quantity of dye and its enormous dilution, I did not expect any staining at all; however, the following morning I was extremely surprised when I discovered the sections changed in this way: the hue of the white medullary mass [white matter] that continued into the convolutions was hardly changed to the naked eye; however, this was followed by the deep red (infinitely redder than the rosy colored liquid), stained, internal layer of the gray matter that was joined to the outer layer of a somewhat weaker red color. Microscopic examination now revealed at once that I had a specimen before me that promised something quite different from the ones prepared according to the former method. Granules and cells were stained intensively red, and the equally pigmented processes of the latter more massive, long, and branching than I had ever seen before in any cell of the central organ. This observation showed me at the same time that we were not dealing here with simple diffusion or soaking; for the solution in which the section had been placed was so little stained that it was completely impossible to differentiate it from ordinary water under the microscope, and yet, the cells and granules resting in it had been colored intensively, whereas the finely granular ground substance and the tissue-containing nerve fibres had not undergone any change from the dye.

. . . . the stain that had been absorbed by the cells and the granules of the central nervous system could not be washed out with water. I kept stained specimens for four weeks in water, renewed it every second day, but not a trace of color change could be noted [in the water], while the specimens themselves did not become discolored.

The procedure which I used in my research was as follows: with a razor blade I cut extremely fine sections from the cerebellum of an eight-year-old girl and of an adult male that had been left standing for four weeks in a solution of potassium bichromate of a wine yellow color. These sections were placed in water to which 2 to 3 drops of a concentrated solution of ammonium carminate per ounce of water were added. The sections remained in this solution for 2 to 3 days and were then further examined, partly in the same state and partly teased out with needles.

Camillo Golgi

(*See p. 91*)

As in the instance of Gerlach, so Golgi was not the first to use the type of coloring technique for which he is famous. Ranvier, for example, had used silver impregnation of nerve fibres a few years earlier (p. 79). But working under very primitive conditions Golgi perfected a comparable but vastly improved method that consisted of impregnation of the nerve cell and its processes with silver nitrate after exposure to potassium dichromate. His discovery was one of the most significant in the history of the neuron because for the first time it allowed the observer to see all parts of the structure and to realize the exceeding complexity of nervous tissue.

By skillfully exploiting his new techinque Golgi evolved the theory that a network connected all neurons. At the same time the Spanish neurohistologist Ramón y Cajal, using the same technique and modifications of it, took issue with Golgi, maintaining that the neurons were in contiguity, not in continuity. So began the famous net versus neuron controversy that was to last for several decades (pp. 87–138). For his contributions to the morphology of the neuron, made possible by his staining method, in 1906 Golgi shared a Nobel Prize for physiology and medicine with his adversary, Ramón y Cajal.

The following passage has been translated from an early account of the method "Sulla fina struttura dei bulbi olfattoria," *Riv. sper. Freniatria Med. legal.*, 1875, 1:66–78; it also appeared in Golgi's *Opera omnia*, I, "Istologia normale 1870–1883" [Milan, 1903], pp. 113–132, and the pagination given below is from this latter source). Although subsequently several modifications were made in details of the technique, the basic principles remained the same as those Golgi followed in his classic work reported in 1883 (pp. 92–96). A later and more detailed account appeared in English in *Alienist and Neurologist*, 1886, 7:126–134.

EXCERPT PP. 127–131

METHOD

In regard to the methods employed in this anatomical study, I shall say that I undertook all those that might give better results in the study of the central nervous system, ranging from that very simple one of ordinary section of either fresh material or after its slight hardening with the bichromate, to the method discovered by me, based on the combined action of bichromate and silver nitrate, as well also as trials with the other modern methods using gold chloride or osmic acid.

Since among all these methods the one that gave the best results was mine (by which one can, by means of controlled variations, obtain black staining of only cells, nerve fibres, or connective elements, and also at the same time staining of one part of the one or of the other elements), hence in this note I wish to limit my reference very briefly to certain necessary conditions regarding its use. Permit me to advise, however, that I do not find myself as yet in a position to explain with precision all the necessary procedures for the best results. These are still partly fortuitous.

Essentially the method followed by me is the result of two different procedures, that is, 1. Hardening of the specimens with bichromate of potassium and of ammonia. 2. Immersion of the specimens in a solution of silver nitrate.

The best solution for the hardening is that prepared according to Müller's formula (Bichromate of potassium, gm. 2, sodium sulphate, gm. 1); but it is convenient to increase the amount of bichromate by degrees daily for 8 days, reaching finally 3½—4 gm. The results are better in proportion to the greater freshness of the specimens to be studied; so that it is desirable to place in the bichromate some detached [olfactory] bulbs of animals just killed. The bulbs of considerable size, such as those of the dog, ox, etc., must previously have been cut into bits so that there may be uniform action of the bichromate on the parenchyma. Because the special reaction on the elements is verified by their passage through the silver solution, the duration of immersion necessary to obtain a suitable hardness or to reduce the specimen to the most suitable condition, varies not only according to the differing concentration of the hardening liquid, but otherwise, and much more, according to the surrounding temperature. In cold surroundings a longer immersion is required and the opposite in hot, and the variations in this matter can be very great. For example, the reaction that can be obtained during the hot season after 30 to 40 days of immersion in the bichromate, during the cold season often does not succeed until after 3, 4, or even more months. Thus it is that one cannot stabilize a precise norm and that good results, as I said, arise partly from chance.

The more difficult, and also the more important part, of my method is consequently the determination of the time at which one ought to proceed to the second step, that is to say, to the removal of the specimens from the bichromate solution to that of the silver nitrate. The lack of precise directions must be supplemented by frequent tests; in addition, the following few data are also of value.

In the cold season the tests ought to be made only after 3 months of immersion in the bichromate, and repeated every 10 days. With the gradual change from the cold to the hot season one must proportionately anticipate the tests and shorten the period of repetition, so that in the hotter season one can commence the tests of the reaction with the silver salt after 30 to 40 days, repeating them at intervals of 4 or 5 days.

As to the rule of sequence of the different actions on the cells, nerve fibres, and connective elements, etc., I must equally declare that I have not yet succeeded in determining with certainty why under the same conditions, at least in appearance, I have often obtained very different results. Yet I can assert that the rule for the more frequent success of the reaction on the different elements is the following: 1.° bundles of nerve fibres that form the most superficial layer of the bulbs that some of the [olfactory] glomeruli penetrate; 2.° large nerve cells arranged in regular series at the internal border of the gray layer; 3.° bundles of nerve fibres of the white matter layer; almost at the same time or a little after, the little pyramidal cells located in the remaining spaces between the bundles of the nerve fibres of this same layer; 4.° connective elements and blood vessels. These, almost as a rule, are also partly stained in the preceding periods, together with the cells and the nerve fibres, as they prevail now in one, now in the other layer; but their more complete, extensive, and elegant staining is always accomplished after a long period of hardening; 5.° as an indefinite rule, the large, solitary nerve cells disseminated in the internal, middle layer are stained sometimes with the connective elements, sometimes with the nerve fibres.

I believe it is almost unnecessary to note that these different phases of the reaction proceed in a rapid or slow manner according to the surrounding temperature and to the time intervals indicated when I spoke of the duration of the immersion of the specimens in the bichromate; therefore it is understood that in accordance with the sequence of the phases almost as many gradations and transitions are encountered as there are gradations of passage from the lowest to the highest temperature of our climate. Again it is readily understood that seldom will one be able to identify a distinct sequence of the different phases, since in fact there is a gradual passage from one to the other; not seldom it happens otherwise, that as a result of the uneven action of the bichromate the reaction of a given series of elements occurs in one part of the specimen, while that of another series occurs in another part.

Ordinarily I use a solution of silver nitrate in the proportion of 1:100. Weaker solutions also give equally good results; for example, either 0.50 or 0.75 per hundred, but the solutions have to be renewed after 12, 15, or 20 hours, and the various specimens have to be immersed so much longer in a proportionately smaller quantity of liquid. The necessity of renewing the solution is indicated by the yellowish color that it acquires.

As to the duration of the immersion of the specimens in the solution of silver nitrate, it is not important to set a rigorous period of time, since it can be prolonged through weeks and months without harmful effects; still, it will be useful to note that the reaction with the silver nitrate also occurs somewhat more rapidly in warm surroundings than in cold. In general, if a few hours are enough for traces of the reaction to become manifest in the more superficial layers of the specimen, it will extend to all the specimen in about 24 hours in the summer and 48 hours or more in the winter. The minimum immersion will consequently be the number of hours that I have indicated; but, as I said, it can be prolonged for weeks or months, so much the more so as the specimens in the same nitrate solution preserve a special consistency. In any event, to preserve them for years it is desirable to keep the specimens in alcohol.

For microscopic examination the sections are placed in damar varnish [resin from the Dámmara species of conifer] or in Canada balsam after they have been dehydrated through the use of absolute alcohol and have been rendered transparent with creosote.

Time and light continually spoil the microscopic prepartions obtained with my method; hence for the purpose of making demonstrations it is desirable always to keep some macroscopic bits in alcohol, from which one can in a short time obtain new microscopic preparations. Minute care and especially the very careful extraction of water from the single sections with alcohol at 46° R and storing away from the influence of light can much retard the spoilage, so much so that after several years the preparations are still usable; but then some spoiling, at least diffuse yellowing, will appear.

As a last observation in respect to my method, I wish to say that experience has demonstrated to me that with artificial raising of the surrounding temperature in which the specimens are located, the period of immersion in the bichromate, normally so long, can be reduced; but as yet I am not in a position to furnish precise data since I have not had an opportunity to make such experiments with the necessary rigor.

Carl Weigert

(19 March 1845—4 August 1904)

Carl Weigert of Frankfurt am Main (see Rieder, 1906; Haymaker, 1953, pp. 222–225; Freund and Berg, 1963–1964, II, 463–473) was an outstanding pathologist who invented several staining techniques. The one to be described here stained the myelin sheath and was first reported in 1882 ("Über eine neue Untersuchungs-methode des Centralnervensystems," *Z. med. Wiss.*, 1882, 20:753–757, 772–774). It has been one of the most widely used microscopical stains for the eaxmination of nervous tissue.

EXCERPT PP. 754–757

Concerning the preparation of objects to be stained according to this method, I was able thus far to use only those that had been fixed in the usual manner for at least eight weeks in Müller's solution [hardening agent containing potassium bichromate 2 gms., sodium sulphate 1 gm., distilled water 100 ml., introduced in 1859 by Heinrich Müller 1820–1864]. Although it may be only temporary, this method, which is limited to specimens treated for a long time with potassium bichromate, has its advantages and disadvantages. The advantage is that organs already available and mostly treated with Müller's solution may also be used for the new method. Indeed, even sections not yet green and subsequently hardened in alcohol readily lend themselves to the staining technique described; this is a decided advantage in the preparation of sections. However, the disadvantage is that I have so far not found any other method of fixation which would be more quickly effective and yet facilitate the new staining process. Simple fixation in alcohol and, indeed, even in chromic acid, for example, does not suffice.

I cannot say whether a differential staining of pieces *in toto* is possible, but I am inclined to doubt it, *a priori*; so far, I have stained only sections themselves. Duval's collodion method [introduced in 1878 and replaced by the celloidin technique of Schiefferdecker in 1882] to which Schiefferdecker recently drew attention, should be highly recommended for this purpose. Also the collodion need not be extracted, since (provided one does not employ the method of double staining that will be discussed below) it remains unstained and can hardly be seen. Because the nerve roots might be cut and lost, it is advisable not to remove the area of collodion that surrounds the sections. To accomplish this one must employ a method which makes the subsequent application of balsam possible and yet neither dissolves the collodion nor makes it sticky as oil of cloves does. Such a medium is xylol. Although it is very sensitive to water residues in the sections, one may, as we shall see, carry through the dehydration as far as necessary despite it and in a sufficiently short time.

It should be noted that the ordinary oil of cloves treatment yields very good preparations.

As concerns the staining process itself, the sections, which must not be more than 0.025 mm. thick, are first placed in an aqueous saturated solution of acid fuchsin (beaker i) for at least one hour. (It may be left in this solution much longer, for overstaining will not occur even after days.) . . . . This acid fuchsin is the sodium salt of rosanilinesulfonic acid, that is the rosaniline in which one H is substituted by SO_3H. The staining principle is an acid, in contrast to the ordinary fuchsin which is a base. Both dyes, acid fuchsin and [ordinary] fuchsin, are histologically completely different tinctures . . . . Above all, the acid fuchsin is not a means for "staining nuclei" as are the "basic" dyes (in Ehrlich's sense) of the group of the rosaniline derivatives (for instance, fuchsin) or that of the pararosaniline (i.e., methyl violet). Only under very special circumstances can one accomplish the differential nuclear staining; with the ordinary method of staining with coal tar dyes (washing in alcohol, etc.) the tincture becomes more diffused, however. With good carmine, nigrosin, or other aniline blue preparations, sections of the central nervous system then take on a great similarity.

However, if after the diffusely adhering dye substances have been rinsed off into a large beaker (beaker ii) filled with water, and the section is placed in an alcoholic potash solution (beaker iii), the picture changes very strikingly. For the present purpose the alcoholic solution is prepared as follows: one gram of caustic potash is placed in 100 cc. of absolute alcohol. One waits 24 hours until whatever is soluble is dissolved. Of this alkaline parent liquid, which is kept on hand, one takes 10 cc. for each 100 cc. alcohol and washes the sections in this solution. This washing procedure is the most important step and must be stopped exactly at the right moment. It can be seen that when the sections have been spread upon a spatula and put into the alcoholic solution of potash, a red cloud rises immediately. The section is now agitated with a needle and, as soon as the first sign of gray matter appears, the section is lifted with the spatula and placed in a large beaker (beaker iv) filled with clean water (it need not be distilled water; however, the first one, beaker iii in which the sections have been rinsed, cannot be used for this purpose because it is too red). This water must not contain any trace of acid since otherwise the differentiation disappears again; however, a small amount of alkali (for instance, a few drops of the parent liquid that have adhered to the spatula) are not detrimental. The section floats of course on the surface. It is submerged carefully and rinsed until it no longer gives off a red cloud. It is now placed in a fresh beaker (beaker v) of clean water (the one used first will always be slightly red) and inspected [to see] whether the gray portions of the sections are now lighter than the white ones. If this is the case and the section is still red at this time, the procedure may be considered successful and complete. If the section is too pale, it has to be restained; if the gray matter is not differentiated by a lighter color, the section must be briefly returned to the weak alcoholic potash solution and must again be rinsed with water in beakers iv and v. Since the new staining of the sections takes up more time than repeated treatment with potash alcohol, it is better to leave it in the solution for too short rather than for too long a period.

These procedures are repeated until sufficient differentiation is achieved, [which is] something one learns to evaluate quickly since the gray matter is always a good yardstick. By the way, aqueous potash solutions do not produce this differentiation.

Now, all that remains to be done is to dehydrate the sections, for which I used alcohol saturated with sodium chloride. It seemed to me that the red dyes were retained better in this solution than in ordinary alcohol. If one then wishes to use xylol instead of oil of cloves as an intermediate fluid for the balsam, two different beakers with alcohol are required (beakers vi and vii), since the former will have too much water adhering to the section to permit saturation with xylol. However, a few moments only suffice to complete the thorough dehydration.

Despite the many beakers which are necessary in this procedure, the staining is not at all complicated. All that is required is scrupulous accuracy and cleanliness.

In sections that have been prepared as described above, only nerve fibres, in a manner soon to be discussed, are stained bright red (the red blood corpuscles more purplish red). The nerve cells, the intermediate substances especially in sclerosis, the pia [mater], etc., all vary in staining, from a very pale appearance to an exquisitely bluish hue according to the duration of the rinsing process with potash alcohol. However, if one wishes to accentuate the bluish color and wants to make the nuclei stand out sharply blue, one can do this without employing a new stain, by placing the sections from beaker v into one with hydrochloric acid (1:5 water), then rinsing in water, dehydrating in alcohol, etc. It is absolutely necessary here that not a trace of the diffuse stains remain in the sections, since this would interfere with the differentiation.

VITTORIO MARCHI
(1851–1908)

Vittorio Marchi (see Haymaker, 1953, pp. 61–63) and Giovanni Algeri discovered that the products of Wallerian degeneration in the myelin sheath of a nerve fibre (pp. 71–74) could be stained by a simple technique involving a chromic salt and osmic acid. Thus in the presence of diseased fibres, as in Türck's work (pp. 851–853), or of experimentally induced nerve decay, as in Gudden's method (pp. 854–857), and in cortical ablation experiments, the investigator could by Marchi's technique trace individual fibres by means of the degenerated myelin stained black; it works best on about the twelfth day of degeneration. Its mode of action is still obscure, but it has nevertheless been responsible for many important advances in neuroanatomy by elucidating myelinated nerve fibre pathways. The following account of the method has been translated from a paper by Marchi and Algeri entitled "Sulle degenerazioni discendenti consecutive a lesioni sperimentale in diverse zone della corteccia cerebrale" (*Riv. sper. Freniatria Med. legal.*, 1885, 11:492–494, 1886, 12:208–252). There have been several modifications of the technique, especially by Davenport and Swank in 1934, and a later description of it by the inventor himself, "On the minute structures of the corpora striata and the thalami optici" (*Alien. Neurol.,* 1888, 9:1–23).

EXCERPT PP. 226–227

The method of investigation employed in our researches on degenerations following the afore-described [cortical] ablations, differs somewhat from those hitherto employed. The usual staining with carmine, hematoxylin, aniline dyes, etc., although on the one hand it places all the more conspicuous, sclerosed parts in relief, on the other, it allows some small but extremely important parts, constituting the principal object of our researches, to escape the eye of the observer. Therefore, although we have not disregarded the aforesaid methods of staining, nevertheless we have been served here by the valuable reaction of osmic acid in combination with bichromate of potassium. We used the following mixture: osmic acid in a 1 percent solution, one part, Müller's fluid [see p. 846], two parts. The whole specimens were placed first in only Müller's liquid for a week or two; then we reduced them to the size of about a half centimetre and placed them in the aforesaid mixture; in brief, after 5 days they were ready for our examination. We noted at once that there should not be more than 3 or 4 specimens in an appropriate quantity of liquid so that they could be well penetrated by the osmic acid. The reaction of the osmic acid in union with the bichromate of potassium has for its effect to stain intensely in black the myelin that has just separated out in the altered [i.e., degenerated] fibres; it is worth saying that in these circumstances the myelin has the property of reducing the osmic acid; meanwhile by degrees the normal fibres acquire an ashen color, so much so that it is possible to distinguish clearly their [myelin] covering and the axis cylinder; that is to say, it can no longer be recognized in the degenerated fibres. It must be noted that this reaction serves remarkably well for rather recent material, about a month old, so long as the altered myelin of the fibres has not been completely reabsorbed, while in old degenerations in which the nerve tissue is replaced by connective tissue (neuroglia), the osmic acid does not serve, and the other staining substances are used instead. If the nerve fibres exposed to degeneration are seen in transverse section, they are revealed as completely black in their center, and only very rarely does the axis cylinder come into view; the sheath of Schwann is clearly distinguished; the normal fibres that are found mixed with the degenerated fibres preserve their structure completely. On studying the fibres through dilaceration, with the same treatment it is revealed that at brief intervals in their length there are collections of small drops of myelin perfectly stained in black; some are small, others larger, elongated, or rounded, and they are between the sheath of Schwann and the axis cylinder. This appearance that the degenerated nerve fibre assumes with the aforesaid treatment is in fact not met with in the healthy fibres; therefore, in a part of the cerebrospinal axis where there may be an area of degeneration, one can count the fibres, so conspicuous are they because of their black stain.

Franz Nissl
(See p. 81)

First Gerlach's carmine preparation and then Golgi's chrome-silver technique and Ehrlich's vital staining (pp. 97–99) permitted a closer examination of the nerve cell body, but it was Franz Nissl who perfected a method of staining that revealed its more intimate structure. He insisted that this gave information concerning only the morphology of the cell's contents and that, contrary to the assertions of other investigators, its chemical characteristics could not necessarily be assessed by it. The following description of his technique has been translated from Nissl's article, "Über die sogenannten Granula der Nervenzellen" (*Neurol. Zbl.*, 1894, 13:676–685, 781–789, 810–814) that contains his description of the granules that now bear his name. Part of this article has been included in Chapter II.

EXCERPT PP. 785–786 (FOOTNOTE 2)

My methylene blue method is, in its improved state, as follows: Careful hardening in 96° alcohol of blocks [of tissue] approx. 1 to 1.2 ccm. in size. These are cut without imbedding, subsequent to fixing the block on cork with gum arabic, after Weigert's method. The [microtome] blade is moistened with 96° alcohol and the sections, which are always less than $\frac{1}{100}$ mm. thick, are stored in 96° alcohol. The sections are stained in the staining solution which is heated with a spirit lamp until a large number of audibly exploding air bubbles rise. The temperature now reached is 65–70° C. The section is then washed out in aniline oil alcohol until no more heavy clouds of stain develop. Then the differentiated section is placed upon the slide where it is dried with filter paper. Following this procedure, it is completely covered with oil of cajeput and the oil then dried off with filter paper. A few drops of benzine remove all superfluous [oil] from the section which is now enclosed in benzine colophonium. Since it is essential that the enclosed mass render diffusion of the stain impossible, the section, which is covered with benzine colophonium, is passed through a spirit burner whereupon it ignites. If the flame is extinguished at once, this procedure may be repeated without ill effects until there are no vapors of benzine present, i.e., until the mixture will no longer ignite immediately. However, owing to the fact that the benzine has been mostly removed from the compound, it has lost its finely liquid, collective state and from this point on the diffusion of stains has become impossible. Although danger of scorching the cells exists, it is not important since it can be avoided with some skill. By the way, I suggest that everyone should scorch cells deliberately once so that one can correctly assess the extremely characteristic artificial products that are thereby produced, so that mistakes can be avoided. The staining solution is as follows:

Methylene blue B patent	3.75
Venetian soap	1.75
Distilled water or soft well water	1000.0

I am indebted to a suggestion by Dr. G. Frank (Bacteriology Laboratory of Fresenius, Wiesbaden) for the addition of Venetian soap. The differential solution consists of 10 vol. aniline oil to 90 vol. 96° alcohol. The aniline oil should be as water-clear as possible and like that delivered to me by the Hoechster Farbwerke upon request. I order oil of cajeput from the pharmacy; benzine colophonium is prepared by dissolving ordinary, commercial colophonium [common resin or rosin] in benzine. The superficial clear layer which forms after 24 hours of standing is poured off. Through the process of evaporation of the benzine, thicker or thinner preparations are obtained at will.

Tract Tracing Techniques

The presence of the myelin sheath that surrounds certain nerve fibres has proved a vital factor in tracing the pathways adopted by bundles of these fibres. Its characteristic behavior during development and the reverse, degeneration, has formed the basis of several important techniques. Thus the degeneration first described in 1850 by Waller (pp. 70–74) was used by Türck to trace spinal cord tracts, and by Gudden to follow the intracerebral connections of sense organs, the cerebral cortex, and of certain brain nuclei. Flechsig's technique, on the other hand, was to investigate the growth of myelin in the central nervous system and to use this as a means of identifying specific parts of its white matter.

LUDWIG TÜRCK
(See p. 284)

Türck's most important neuroanatomical contribution was his demonstration that Wallerian degeneration of the spinal cord tract (pp. 284–287) resulting, for example, from compression of the cord (pp. 852–853) corresponded to the direction in which the tract conducted, and his tracing of the tracts on the basis of this finding. Türck's work was based upon pathological studies and it was of the greatest importance to knowledge of the anatomy of the cord. It led him to identify distinctly six spinal cord tracts, one of which formerly carried his name (*Hülsen-Vorderstrangbahn*, i.e., anterior corticospinal tract), and to formulate his concept of system disease of the spinal cord. The following excerpt has been translated from "Über sekundäre Erkrankung einzelner Rüchenmarkstränge und ihrer Fortsetzungen zum Gehirne" (*Z. kais. kön. Ges. Ärzte Wien*, 1853, 9 [ii]:289–317), a paper read on the 9 June 1853. Türck's first contribution to the subject had appeared in 1849 (*ibid.*, 1849, 1:173–176).

EXCERPT PP. 309–311

The *compressed portion of the spinal cord* acted as follows: With intensive, continuous compression at a certain level, caused mostly by an exudate on the dura mater owing to vertebral caries, the entire cross section of the spinal cord was uniformly and intensively diseased; the most severe pressure had occurred in this area. At the same site, in the cases of milder compression, there was a marked prevalence of involvement noticeable in the lateral tracts; the anterior and posterior ones behaved similarly. In the higher region, the involvement of the anterior tract decreased rapidly until, in [cases of] vertebral caries and almost always still within the confines of the exudate of the dura mater, it disappeared completely, whereas the disease of the posterior tract persisted as complete; when the compression was significant the disease became intensive.

Below the level of most severe compression the disease of the posterior tract decreased successively and disappeared completely when that of the anterior tract persisted, mostly still within the extent of the exudate of the dura mater.

In all the cases cited above, in the entire extent of secondary disease of the posterior and lateral tracts, the degeneration always extended upwards to one or several sites of insertion [spinal levels] beyond the compressing exudate or secondary material. In the same manner the disease of the entire lateral and anterior tracts, in the six cases cited, later extended further down than the exudate; therefore, the total disease of these tracts cannot very well be considered as a direct result of the compression that sometimes presses more upon the anterior and sometimes more upon the posterior surface of the spinal cord, since, under the various conditions of compression, the same tracts were always affected in the same manner above, and others again below the most severe compression. From the discussion so far, it therefore follows necessarily that certain tracts (the posterior ones) can become diseased secondarily centripetally, others (the anterior ones) centrifugally only, and still others (the lateral ones) in both directions.

The concept is that individual tracts of the spinal cord in certain old cerebral lesions or with continuous compression of an area of the spinal cord no longer receive any impulses in a centrifugal or centripetal direction. They degenerate as a result of the long-disrupted conduction. This secondary disease (spoken of in the sense of nerve conduction in the respective tract) must therefore always occur in front of the lesion of the cerebrum or the spinal cord, or, what amounts to the same thing. It seems quite evident and the only plausible explanation for this disease that the tracts of the spinal cord conduct in the direction in which they are secondarily affected. However, more recently we have made observations that indicate that this subject cannot yet be considered a closed issue.

These observations are as follows:

a) the limitation of the secondary disease at a greater distance from the area of compression of the spinal cord to exposed portions of such cords, which in a lesser distance from the compressed site are diseased in their entire circumference, has already been discussed here in detail;

b) the complete lack of secondary disease in several cases that we observed in chronic, partial diseases of the white substance of the spinal cord which even resulted occasionally in complete disappearance of the nerve fibres;

c) the behavior of the spinal cord in individuals who had suffered amputation a long time previously. In two such cases that I examined, in one an amputation of the thigh had been carried out almost two years previously, and in the second case (amputation of the upper arm in the vicinity of the elbow joint) more than two years before. The spinal cord above and below the origin of the respective nerve plexus, the medulla oblongata, the pons, as well as the brain in some sections, were completely normal when examined microscopically. The nerve roots of the lowest three cervical segments as well as the first thoracic nerve were significantly atrophied in the second case . . . .

These observations demonstrate that conduction interrupted in a considerable number of nerve fibres, does not suffice to cause secondary disease of the spinal cord. It shows that there are still factors involved that we have missed entirely. . . .

Frequently, one could demonstrate at the area of compression of the spinal cord, as well as in the secondarily diseased tracts above and below, a very striking difference in the intensity of the formation of granular cells [compound granular corpuscles] on the two sides, which, undoubtedly, and often distinctly demonstrable, depended upon the uneven compression; it was accompanied by a difference in the paralytic phenomena on the two sides. As definitively as one can often establish the age of a primary cerebral lesion, so little is it possible of course to determine in any case of successively continuing compression of the spinal cord, how long this specific degree of compression existed in order to produce granular cells.

Bernhard Aloys von Gudden
(See p. 606)

Gudden's contribution to experimental neurology was a technique for producing secondary atrophy of central brain structures by the removal of a peripheral sense organ or cranial nerve in a neonatal animal. Gudden attacked all nuclear parts of certain cerebral pathways, as, for example, in the experiment for the ablation of the anterior quadrigeminal body described below, and in his work on the thalamocortical pathways that was continued by his student Monakow (pp. 619–623). The underlying principle was to remove nerve cells and either to trace their degenerated axons (Wallerian degeneration) or to observe their absence and thus to trace the pathway of the white matter. The following excerpts have been translated from Gudden's paper, "Experimentaluntersuchungen über das peripherische und centrale Nervensystem" (*Arch. Psychiat. NervKrankh.*, 1870, 2:693–723). He first of all dealt with general technical matters and then with his experiments; the report of the thirteenth experiment is included below.

EXCERPT PP. 693–697

The method that was used in the following investigations is new insofar as young animals have been subjected to it purposely. The younger the animal the more rewarding and striking are the results. Operations were performed in rabbits, and generally, for the most part in those that were no more than one or two days old. In addition, a small series of experiments concerning the optic nerves was conducted in pigeons, twelve to eighteen hours after they had been hatched.

Contributing essentially towards facilitating the operations and in part also promoting their objectives are:

1) in general, a limited development of the sense of pain,
2) the lack of hair,
3) the greater coagulability of the blood,
4) the extraordinary rate of growth.

1) With regard to pain sense, the fifth nerve, which with the olfactory nerve is the leader during the suckling period, constitutes an exception to some extent. It nevertheless demonstrates by its yet relatively weak response that this sensation is still limited . . . . As a result of this dulled sensation the small animals offer little resistance to the scalpel and scissors and can therefore be handled more easily. Every day of delay is a lost one since it causes increased pain as well as defensive movements.

2) As is known, the young rabbits are born naked . . . . The advantage of the nakedness is, moreover, that the skin does not require any further

preparation, that a clean incision can be made, and that it can be easily sutured again.

3) One must not underestimate the surgeon's relief because of the rapidity of blood coagulation. Even if larger vessels have to be cut, coagulation always sets in rapidly and spontaneously. This is of particular importance for such surgical operations, for example, as the removal of portions of the brain when a vessel ligature is almost impossible, and, even if possible, would be extremely damaging since some of the ligatures would have to be left behind.

4) However, the most essential advantage of surgery in newly born animals is the almost unbelievably rapid and perfect healing of the wounds by first intention, unaccompanied by disturbing secondary complications . . . .

It is good practice to mark the operated animals by making a small incision in the ear. They are kept alive for six to eight weeks; if one should desire, even longer (until they reach adulthood), which may be indicated in some cases; they are then sacrificed, for which I recommend a subcutaneous injection of hydrocyanic acid.

. . . .

. . . .

. . . .

The results of the experiments performed are constant and leave nothing to be desired in this respect. The macroscopic results and those that are obtained with minimal magnification of sections rendered transparent, are reported. I have no doubt that everyone who, from his own experience, is quite familiar with those not too rare difficulties and mishaps in the Rolando-Stilling method of cutting [pp. 271–275], will doubly appreciate the definite progress that has been made in decreasing these difficulties by the experimental preparation of the specimens. The actual microscopic exploration still offers special obstacles. To overcome these completely may not be possible until methods have been devised by which we may recognize the composition and mutual connection of the finest components of the central nervous organs more definitively and with more certainty than has so far been the case.

EXCERPT PP. 718–720

EXPERIMENT XIII

Removal of one of the anterior quadrigeminal bodies in the rabbit. The operation, when performed well, is very elegant. Holding the scalpel in a slanting position (to avoid injury of the dura mater) one separates the lambdoid suture, inserts a fine scissors' blade into the separated suture, as far away as possible from the midline of the skull (in order to provide sufficient space for the use of the forceps that are to be used later), carefully advances it between bone and hard cerebral meninges [dura mater], and cuts through the parietal bone to the coronary suture on both sides. When this operation was successful there was scarcely a drop of blood lost. The bone cover prepared in this way is broken off at the coronary suture, whereupon the quadrigeminal bodies are completely exposed. One then applies a pair of fine, curved forceps as deeply as possible, to the anterior body and, with one manoeuvre, simultaneously lifting the instrument so that the incision does not penetrate into the body too far beyond the nerve cell layer, one pinches it off and then removes it. Even if the first attempt with this operation is not completely successful and is accompanied by considerable bleeding, the removal of the anterior body can be carried out without difficulty, provided that one moves swiftly and uses the very instant when, while the skull cap is being raised, the blood is aspirated into the cavity. The injury to the brain is always followed by considerable loss of blood and this is even less avoidable since, of the sinuses of the dura mater originally kept intact, the sagittal sinus at least cannot be protected when the anterior body is being pinched off. However, little attention is paid to this and the skull cap is immediately shut again; the exuding blood is dabbed a few times with a small linen cloth, the skin wound sutured, and the animal returned to its nest. The surgery is easily tolerated. It is obvious, by the way, for anyone who, especially after working with sliced specimens, is familiar with the stratification and the extension of the superficial nerve cell layer of the anterior body, which alone is to be considered, that the latter is not completely removed by the procedure suggested. However, this limits the success of the operation by degree only. A partial extirpation is actually to be preferred to a total one, because of its convincing demonstration. The latter, conditioned by the stratification of its parts, could not be carried out in isolation, that is, without removing deeper lying layers along with it. However, the more perfect the excision was (always provided that no other parts were also removed, which can be verified from the sections; and, should it have been the case, these animals eventually would have to be sacrificed), the more was the impairment of visual function of the associated eye. Yet this is actually more of a conclusion than a true observation since, as anyone who is going to repeat these tests will soon become convinced, there exist considerable difficulties regarding a correct assessment of the degree of visual impairment. The most reliable measure of the latter position of head and ears (compare with statements made in experiment viii) usually tends to be present by inference only. Examination of the pupils also has its drawbacks. In this connection one must be particularly aware of the fact that the reaction of the pupils towards changes in light is, under normal conditions, a gradually progressive one only. In order to discount the disturbing effect of this peculiarity as much as possible, I carry out my experiments in a dark room into which a cone of light falls through a narrow opening. The eyes are directed uniformly and not too slowly from the dark across the light, with the result that the pupil that is associated with the injured anterior quadrigeminal body becomes larger with light and narrower with darkness than the pupil of the other eye. If one then carries out an autopsy one notices an optic nerve which is more or less retarded in its development. The tractus peduncularis transversus [see pp. 609–611] is also less developed. However, and so far I cannot explain this, at least in some specimens it is not developed to the degree that I had expected.

Paul Flechsig

(*See p. 277*)

Flechsig studied the developing rather than the degenerating myelin. Thus his method is known as myelogenesis and depends upon the fact that myelinization of nerve fibres in different cerebral pathways reaches maturity at different times. A chronological sequence that served to differentiate some of the innumerable cerebral and spinal tracts was therefore made available and its use has proved an important technique in the discrimination between cerebral cortical areas (pp. 447–457) as well as white matter in the cord (pp. 287–290) and brain (pp. 611–619). The following description of the method has been translated from Flechsig's book, *Die Leitungsbahnen im Gehirn und Rückenmark des Menschen auf Grund entwicklungsgeschichtlicher Untersuchungen* (Leipzig, 1876).

EXCERPT PP. 255–256

With the investigation of the local course of the formation of the myelin sheath, a path has been broken that has contributed to the knowledge of the organization of the central nervous system that would have been hardly possible to ravel with former research methods. We discovered that the human fetus was a particularly suitable subject for the revelation of the arrangement, course, and structure of the nerve fibre substance within the central [nervous system] organs. This seems to be the place to reemphasize the basic merits of this exploratory method that is preferable to those that have already been used for similar purposes.

In brief, they are as follows: during certain periods of fetal life *fibres, which in the adult are of uniform constituency and differ very little* [from one another], *can be distinguished from each other in a very striking manner.* This is because some of them already have a complete *myelin sheath*, whereas others still exhibit their *naked axis cylinders.* Thus we are in a position, especially in the case of the compact white matter, to follow for a considerable distance fibres and fibre bundles that later on, owing to the uniformity of their components, become masked in their course. Furthermore, while, owing to the different progress in their development, individual fibre bundles stand out, we become aware of their separate existence, and we are directly challenged to explore them more precisely in relation to their course, their ending, etc. At the same time there exists an additional important motive in that the differentiation of the central mass of fibres exhibits in general a systematic character and that at times certain *fibre systems are morphologically sharply characterized by their total size, in contrast to other fibres with which they are in contact and which surround them.* We find now a whole system equipped with medullary sheaths proceeding between bundles of non-medullated fibres (for instance, the posterior, longitudinal bundles in the medulla oblongata, and in the region of the pons in specimens approximately 25–28 cm. long), now a non-medullary system between the universally medullated (the pyramidal tracts in the fetus which are from 34–49 cm. long). Thus in the human embryo we have become familiar with an object, in which also virtually different systems, in the adult morphologically little or not at all differentiated, are characterized by specific structure and thus recognizable in their course and extent.

Considering the direct information that can be gained by following the procedure mentioned above, we obtain in addition information of certain *laws of the local course* of fibre development, especially, as well, of the development of the myelin sheaths, that, as far as we regard them as commonly valid, may serve as a basis for *general guiding points of view* for the anatomical study of the central organ and can lead us directly to noteworthy conclusions.

BIBLIOGRAPHY

ABERCROMBIE, M.
1961. "Ross Granville Harrison, 1870–1959," *Biogr. Mem. Fellows R. Soc.*, 7:111–126.

ACKERKNECHT, E. H.
1953. *Rudolf Virchow. Doctor. Statesman. Anthropologist.* Madison, University of Wisconsin Press.
1956. *Franz Joseph Gall, inventor of phrenology, and his collections.* Translated by C. St. Leon. Madison, Dept. of History of Medicine, University of Wisconsin Medical School.

ADAM, C.
1910. *Vie et oeuvres de Descartes. Étude historique.* Paris, Cerf.
1937. *Descartes; sa vie et son oeuvre.* Paris, Boivin.

ADELMANN, H. B.
1966. *Marcello Malpighi and the evolution of embryology.* Ithaca, N.Y., Cornell University Press. 5 vols.

ADRIAN, E. D.
1913–1914. "The all-or-none principle in nerve," *J. Physiol., London,* 47:460–474.
1926. "The impulses produced by sensory nerve endings—Part I," *J. Physiol., London,* 61:49–72.
1932. *The mechanism of nervous action. Electrical studies of the neurone.* Philadelphia, University of Pennsylvania Press.
1935. "Discharge frequencies in the cerebral and cerebellar cortex," *J. Physiol., London,* 83:32P–33P.
1947. *The physical background of perception.* Oxford, Clarendon Press.
1955. "Sir Henry Dale's contributions to physiology," *Br. med. J.,* i:1355–1356.
1965. "Alexander Forbes," *Nature,* 206:1095–1096.

ADRIAN, E. D., and ZOTTERMANN, Y.
1926. "Impulses from a single sensory end-organ," *J. Physiol., London,* 61:viii.

AFNAN, S. M.
1958. *Avicenna. His life and works.* London, Allen & Unwin.

ALDINI, G.
1792. "Memorie sull'elettricità animale," *G. fis.-med. L. Brugnatelli,* 1 (ii):146–187, 241–270, 287–290.
1803. *An account of the late improvement in galvanism,* [etc.]. London, Cuthell and Martin, & Murray.

859

ALIX, E.
1868. "Notice sur les travaux anthropologiques de Gratiolet," *Mém. Soc. Anthrop. Paris*, 3:lxxi–cii.

AMACHER, M. P.
1964. "Thomas Laycock, I. M. Sechenov, and the reflex arc concept," *Bull. Hist. Med.*, 38:168–183.

ANDREOLI, A.
1961. *Zur geschichtlichen Entwicklung der Neuronentheorie.* Basel, Schwabe.

ANTON, G.
1914. "Nachruf auf E. Hitzig," *Arch. Psychiat. NervKrankh.*, 54:1–7.
1930. "Theodor Meynert. Seine Person, sein Wirken und sein Werk," *J. Psychol. Neurol., Lpz.*, 40:256–281.

ARANZI, G. C.
1587. *De humano foetu liber tertio editus, ac recognitus. Eiusdem anatomicarum observationum liber.* . . . Venice, Brechtanus.

ARETAEUS THE CAPPADOCIAN
1856. *The extant works of Aretaeus the Cappadocian,* edited and translated by Francis Adams. London, Sydenham Society.

ARISTOTLE
1910. *Historia animalium,* [translated] by D'Arcy Wentworth Thompson. Oxford, Clarendon Press.
1911. *De partibus animalium,* translated by William Ogle. Oxford, Clarendon Press.
1912. *De motu animalium. De incessu animalium,* [translated] by A. S. L. Farquharson. Oxford, Clarendon Press.

ARNETT, L. D.
1904. "The soul—a study of past and present beliefs," *Am. J. Psychol.*, 15:121–200, 347–382.

ASRATYAN, E. A.
1953. *I. P. Pavlov. His life and work.* Moscow, Foreign Languages Publishing House.

ATTI, G.
1847. *Notizie edite ed inedite della vita e delle opere di Marcello Malpighi* . . . *raccolte da G. Atti.* Bologna, Volpe.

AUBURTIN, S. A. E.
1861a. "Sur la forme de la cavité crânienne d'un Totonaque, avec réflexions sur la signification du volume de l'encéphale," *Bull. Soc. Anthrop. Paris*, 2:66–67.
1861b. "Reprise de la discussion sur la forme et le volume du cerveau," *Bull. Soc. Anthrop. Paris*, 2:209–220.

AUSTRIAN, C. R.
1943. "Lewellys Franklin Barker," *Bull. Johns Hopkins Hosp.*, 73:401–404.

AVICENNA
1930. Gruner, O. C. *A treatise on the Canon of Medicine of Avicenna incorporating a translation of the first book.* London, Luzac.
1952. Rahman, F. *Avicenna's psychology. An English translation of Kitāb al-Najāb, Book III, Chapter VI, with historical-philosophical notes and textual improvements on the Cairo edition.* London, Oxford University Press.

BABINSKI, J. F. F.
1896. "Sur le réflexe cutané plantaire dans certaines affections organiques du système nerveux central," *C. r. Séanc. Soc. Biol.*, 3:207–208.
1898. "Du phénomène des orteils et de sa valeur sémiologique," *Sem. méd.*,

18:321–322; partial English translation in Fulton and Keller (1932, pp. 3–6).

1902. "Sur le rôle du cervelet dans les actes volitionnels nécessitant une succession rapide de mouvements (diadococinésie)," *Revue neurol.*, 10:1013–1015.

1903. "De l'abduction des orteils," *Revue neurol.*, 11:728–729.

1909. "Quelques documents relatifs à l'histoire des fonctions de l'appareil cérébelleux et de leurs perturbations," *Revue mens. Méd. interne Thér.*, 1:113–129.

1913. *Exposé des travaux scientifiques*. Paris, Masson.

BABKIN, B. P.

1950. *Pavlov. A biography*. Chicago, University of Chicago Press.

BAILEY, P., and BONIN, G. VON

1951. *The isocortex in man*. Urbana, University of Illinois Press.

BAILLARGER, J. G. F.

1840. "Recherches sur la structure de la couche corticale des circonvolutions du cerveau," *Mém. Acad. roy. Méd. Paris*, 8:149–183; English translation in Bonin (1960, pp. 22–48).

BAILLET, A.

1691. *La vie de M. Descartes*. Paris, Dezallier.

BAKAY, L.

1956. *The blood-brain barrier with special regard to the use of radioactive isotopes*. Springfield, Ill., Thomas.

BAKER, F.

1909. "The two Sylviuses. An historical study," *Bull. Johns Hopkins Hosp.*, 20:329–339.

BAKER, J. R.

1945. *The discovery of the uses of colouring agents in biological micro-technique*. London, Williams & Norgate.

1948–1953. "The cell-theory: a restatement, history and critique," *Q. Jl. microsc. Sci.*, 89:103–125; 90:87–108; 93:157–190; 94:407–440.

BÁRÁNY, R.

1912a. "Beziehungen zwischen Bau und Funktion des Kleinhirns, nach Untersuchungen an Menschen," *Wien. klin. Wschr.*, 25:1737–1739.

1912b. "Lokalisation in des Rinde der Kleinhirnhemisphären des Menschen," *Wien. klin. Wschr.*, 25:2033–2038.

BARD, P., and RIOCH, D. McK.

1937. "A study of four cats deprived of neocortex and additional portions of the forebrain," *Bull. Johns Hopkins Hosp.*, 60:65–147.

BARDELEBEN, K. VON

1902. "Nekrolog Axel Key," *Dt. med. Wschr.*, 28:87.

BARKER, L. F.

1897a. "The phrenology of Gall and Flechsig's doctrine of association centres in the cerebrum," *Bull. Johns Hopkins Hosp.*, 8:7–14.

1897b. "The sense-areas and the association centres in the brain as described by Flechsig," *J. nerv. ment. Dis.*, 24:325–356.

1899. *The nervous system and its constituent neurones*. New York, Appleton.

1942. *Time and the physician. The autobiography of Lewellys F. Barker*. New York, Putnam.

BARTHOLIN, C.

1641. *Institutiones anatomicae*. Leiden, Hack.

BARTHOLOW, R.
  1874. "Experimental investigations into the functions of the human brain," *Am. J. med. Sci.*, 67:305–313.
BASTHOLM, E.
  1950. *The history of muscle physiology.* Copenhagen, Munksgaard.
BAUMANN, E. D.
  1937. "Praxagoras von Kos," *Janus*, 41:167–185.
BAYLE, A. L. J., and THILLAYE, A. J.
  1855. *Biographie médicale par ordre chronologique.* Paris, Delahaye. 2 vols.
BAYLISS, W. M.
  1919. "Keith Lucas 1879–1916," *Proc. R. Soc.*, 90B:xxxi–xlii.
  1920. "Ludimar Hermann, 1838–1914," *Proc. R. Soc.*, 91B:xxxviii–xl.
BEACH, F. A., HEBB, D. O., MORGAN, C. T., and NISSEN, H. W.
  1960. *The neurospychology of Lashley.* New York, McGraw-Hill.
BEARE, J. I.
  1906. *Greek theories of elementary cognition from Alcmaeon to Aristotle.* Oxford, Clarendon Press.
BECK, A., and BIKELES, G.
  1912a. "Versuch über die gegenseitige funktionelle Be-einflussung von Gross- und Kleinhirn," *Pflügers Arch.*, 113:283–295.
  1912b. "Versuche über die sensorische Funktionen des Kleinhirnmittelstücks," *Pflügers Arch.*, 113:296–302.
BÉCLARD, P. A.
  1823. *Eléments d'anatomie générale.* Paris, Béchet Jeune.
BEEVOR, C. E.
  1908. "The cerebral arterial supply," *Brain*, 30:403–425.
  1908. "On the distribution of the different arteries supplying the human brain," *Phil. Trans. R. Soc.*, 200B:1–55.
BEHREND, C. M.
  1957. "Fedor Krause und die Anfänge der Neurochirurgie in Deutschland," *Dt. med. Wschr.*, 82:519–520.
BELL, C.
  1811. *Idea of a new anatomy of the brain submitted for the observations of his friends.* [London, Strahan and Preston]; reprinted *J. Anat. Physiol.*, 1869, 3:147–182; *Med. Class.*, 1936, 1:105–120; Gordon-Taylor and Walls (1958, pp. 218–231).
  1823. "Second paper on the nerves of the orbit," *Phil. Trans. R. Soc.*, 113 (i):289–307.
  1870. *Letters of Sir Charles Bell, K.H., F.R.S.L. & E. Selected from his correspondence with his brother George Joseph Bell.* London, Murray.
BELLINGERI, C. F.
  1834. "Elogio storico del Professore Luigi Rolando," *Memorie r. Accad. Sci. Torino*, 37:153–193.
BELLONI, L.
  1958. " 'Rete mirabile' (Introduzione storica)," pp. 3–17, *Pathophysiologia diencephalica. Symposium internazionale, Milano, Maggio 1956.* Vienna, Springer.
  1963a. *Per la storia della neurologia italiana. Atti del simposio internazionale di storia della neurologia. Varenna—30. VIII. / 1. IX. 1961 editi da Luigi Belloni.* Milan, Istituto di Storia della Medicina, Università degli Studi.
  1963b. "L'opera nevrologica di Domenico Cotugno," in Belloni (1963a, pp. 51–66).

BENASSI, E.
1963. "Ipotesi elettropatogenetiche e proposte elettroterapiche nell'opera di Luigi Galvani," in Belloni (1963a, pp. 131–138).

BENCE JONES, H.
1852. *On animal electricity: being an abstract of the discoveries of Emil du Bois-Reymond.* London, Churchill.

BENEDIKT, M.
1895. "Wladimir Alexewitsch Betz," *Wien. med. Wschr.*, 45:cols. 33–37.
1906. *Aus meinem Leben.* Vienna, Konegan.

BENNETT, A. H.
1888. "Muscular hypertonicity in paralysis," *Brain*, 10:288–312.

BERENGARIO DA CARPI, G.
1521. *Commentaria cum amplissimis additionibus super anatomia Mundini una cum textu ejusdem in pristinum et verum nitorem redacto.* Bologna, Benedictis.
1522. *Isagoge breves.* Bologna, Hectoris.

BERG, A.
1942. "Die Lehre von der Faser als Form- und Funktionselement des Organismus," *Virchows Arch. path. Anat. Physiol.*, 309:333–460.

BERLIN, R.
1858. *Beitrag zur Strukturlehre der Grosshirnwindungen.* Erlangen, Junge. Inaugural dissertation.

BERLUCCHI, C., and TRASCHI, G.
1963. "Bartolomeo Panizza," in Belloni (1963a, pp. 149–163)

BERNARD, C.
1840–1849. [On P. Flourens], *Recl. Discours Acad. française*, pp. 21–36.
1857. *Leçons sur les effets des substances toxiques et médicamenteuses.* Paris, Baillière et Fils.
1865. *Introduction à l'étude de la médecine expérimentale.* Paris, Baillière.
1881. *L'oeuvre de Claude Bernard.* Paris, Baillière.

BERNSTEIN, J.
1902. "Untersuchungen zur Thermodynamik der biolektrischen Ströme," *Pflügers Arch.*, 92:521–562.

BETZ, V. A.
1874. "Anatomischer Nachweis zweier Gehirncentra," *Zbl. med. Wiss.*, 12:578–580, 595–599.
1881. "Über die feinere Struktur der Grosshirnrinde des Menschen," *Zbl. med. Wiss.*, 19:193–195, 209–213, 231–234; French translation: "Quelques mots sur la structure de l'écorce cérébral," *Revue Anthrop.*, 4 (2d ser.):427–438; partial English translation in Bailey and Bonin (1951, pp. 2–5).

BIANCHI, L.
1895. "The functions of the frontal lobes [translated from the original MS by A. de Watteville]," *Brain*, 18:497–522.
1920. *La meccanica del cervello e la funzione dei lobi frontali.* Turin, Fratelli Bocca.
1922. *The mechanisms of the brain and the function of the frontal lobes,* translated by J. H. Macdonald. Edinburgh, Livingstone.
1923. "Domenico Cotugno," *Rif. med.*, 39:1–14.

BILANCIONI, G.
1911. "Valsalva, scrittore del liquido cefalo-rachidiano," *Policlinico*, 18:1047–1048.

Bing, R.
1954. "Medicohistorisches über den Liquor cerebrospinalis," *Schweiz. med. Wschr.*, 84:181–183, 204–207.

Blasius, W.
1964. "Die Bestimmung der Leitungsgeschwindigkeit im Nerven durch Hermann v. Helmholtz am Beginn der naturwissenschaftlichen Aera der Neurophysiologie," in Rothschuh (1964*a*, pp. 71–84).

Blum, F.
1893. "Der Formaldehyd als Härtungsmittel," *Z. wiss. Mikrosk.*, 10:314–315.

Bogaert, L. van
1961. "L'Institut Korbinian Brodmann à Tübingen (Allemagne)," *Wld. Neurol.*, 2:846–848.

Bolk, L.
1906. *Das Cerebellum der Säugethiere.* Haarlem, Bohn.

Bonin, G. von
1950. *Essay on the cerebral cortex.* Springfield, Ill., Thomas.
1960. *Some papers on the cerebral cortex.* Springfield, Ill., Thomas.

Bonin, G. von, and Bailey, P.
1947. *The neo-cortex of Macaca mullatta.* Urbana, University of Illinois Press.

Borelli, G. A.
1680–1681. *De motu animalium.* Rome, Bernabò. 2 vols.

Boring, E. G.
1942. *Sensation and perception in the history of experimental psychology.* New York, Appleton-Century.
1960. "Lashley and cortical integration," in Beach *et al.* (1960, pp. xi–xvi).

Boruttau, H.
1914. "Ludimar Hermann," *Dt. med. Wschr.*, 40:1529.
1922. *Emil du Bois-Reymond.* Vienna, Rikola.

Bouillaud, J.-B.
1825. "Recherches cliniques propres à démontrer que la perte de la parole correspond à la lésion des lobules antérieurs du cerveau, et à confirmer l'opinion de M. Gall, sur le siège de l'organe du langage articulé," *Archs. gén. Méd.*, 8:25–45.

Bowditch, H. P.
1871. "Über die Eigentumlichkeiten der Reizbarkheit welche die Muskelfasern des Herzen zeigen," *Ber. sächs. Akad. Wiss.*, Math.-nat. Klasse, 23:652–689.

Bowsher, D.
1960. *Cerebrospinal fluid dynamics in health and disease.* Springfield, Ill., Thomas.
1961. *Introduction to neuroanatomy.* Springfield, Ill., Thomas.

Brazier, M. A. B.
1959*a*. "The historical development of neurophysiology," pp. 1–58, *Handbook of physiology*, I, Washington, D.C., American Physiological Society.
1959*b*. "The evolution of concepts relating to the electrical activity of the nervous system," pp. 191–222, *The history and philosophy of knowledge of the brain and its functions.* Oxford, Blackwell.
1963. "Felice Fontana," in Belloni (1963*a*, pp. 107–116).

Bremer, F.
1922. "Contribution à l'étude de la physiologie du cervelet et la fonction inhibitrice du palée-cérébellum," *Archs. int. Physiol.*, 19:189–226.

BROADBENT, W.
1903. "Hughlings Jackson as pioneer in nervous physiology and pathology," *Brain*, 26:305–382.

BROCA, P.-P.
1861*a*. "Sur le volume et la forme du cerveau suivant les individus et suivant les races," *Bull. Soc. Anthrop. Paris*, 2:139–204.

1861*b*. "Perte de la parole, ramollissement chronique et destruction partielle du lobe antérieur gauche du cerveau," *Bull. Soc. Anthrop. Paris*, 2:235–238, 301–321.

1861*c*. "Remarques sur le siège de la faculté du langage articulé; suivies d'une observation d'aphémie (perte de la parole)," *Bull. Soc. anat. Paris*, 36:330–357; complete English translation in Bonin (1960, pp. 49–72).

1863. "Localisation des fonctions cérébrales.—Siège du langage articulé," *Bull. Soc. Anthrop. Paris*, 4:200–202.

1865. "Éloge funèbre de Pierre Gratiolet," *Mém. Soc. Anthrop. Paris*, 2:cxii–cxviii.

BRODMANN, K.
1903*a*. "Beiträge zur histologischen Lokalisation der Grosshirnrinde. I. Mitteilung: die Regio rolandica," *J. Psychol. Neurol., Lpz.*, 2:79–107.

1903*b*. "Beiträge zur histologischen Lokalisation der Grosshirnrinde. II. Mitteilung: Der Calcarinatypus," *J. Psychol. Neurol., Lpz.*, 2:133–159.

1908. "Beiträge zur histologischen Lokalisation der Grosshirnrinde. VI. Mitteilung: Die Cortexgliederung des Menschen," *J. Psychol. Neurol., Lpz.*, 10:231–246.

1909. *Vergleichende Lokalisationslehre der Grosshirnrinde in ihren Prinzipien dargestellt auf Grund des Zellenbaues.* Leipzig, J. A. Barth; English translation of Ch. IX, "Versuch einer physiologischen Cortexorganologie," of which excerpts have been included in Ch. IX of the present work, in Bonin (1960, pp. 200–230).

BROEK, A. J. P. V. D.
1931. "Louis Bolk," *Morph. Jb.*, 65:497–516.

BROUSSAIS, F. J. V.
1838. *On the functions of the cerebellum*, translated by G. Combe. Edinburgh, Maclachlan and Stewart.

BROWN, G. H.
1955. "Albert Sidney Frankau Leyton [Grünbaum]," in *Lives of the Fellows of the Royal College of Physicians of London, 1826–1925* [*Munk's Roll*, Vol. IV]. London, by the College.

BROWN, S. M.
1892. "On hereditary ataxy," *Brain*, 15:250–268.

BROWN, S. M., II.
1928. "Dr. Sanger Brown," *J. nerv. ment. Dis.*, 67:643–644.

BROWN, T. G.
1947. "Sherrington the man," *Br. med. J.*, ii:810–812.

BROWN-SÉQUARD, C.-E.
1849. "De la transmission des impressions sensitives par la moelle épinière," *C. r. Séanc. Soc. Biol.*, 1:192–194.

1850. "Mémoire sur la transmission des impressions sensitives dans la moelle épinière," *C. r. hebd. Séanc. Acad. Sci., Paris*, 31:700–701.

1889. Recherches cliniques et expérimentales sur les entrecroisements des conducteurs servant aux mouvements volontaires," *Archs. Physiol. norm. path.*, 21:219–245.

BRUETSCH, W. L.
1960. "In memoriam. Oskar Vogt, M.D., 1870–1959," *Am. J. Psychiat.*, 116:958–960.

BUESS, H.
1964. "Vom Beitrag der schweizer Ärzte zur Geschichte der Neuronentheorie," in Rothschuh (1964*a*, pp. 186–210).

BURDACH, E.
1837. *Beitrag zur mikroskopischer Anatomie der Nerven.* Königsberg, Bornträger.

BURN, J. H.
1955. "Sir Henry Dale's contribution to therapeutics," *Br. med. J.*, i:1357–1359.

BURROWS, G.
1846. *On disorders of the cerebral circulation.* London, Longman.

C., J. R.
1880. "Paul Broca of Paris," *Edin. med. J.*, 26:186–192.

CAMERON, G. R.
1955. "Rudolf Albert Kölliker (1817–1905)," *Ann. Sci.*, 11:167–172.

CAMPBELL, A. W.
1903. "Histological studies on cerebral localisation," *Proc. R. Soc.*, 72:488–492.
1905. *Histological studies on the localisation of cerebral function.* Cambridge, University Press.
1938. [Obituary notice], *Med. J. Aust.*, i:181–185.

CAMPBELL, E.
1951. "Walter E. Dandy—surgeon, 1886–1946," *J. Neurosurg.*, 8:249–262.

CANGUILHEM, G.
1955. *La formation du concept de réflexe aux XVIIe et XVIIIe siècles.* Paris, Presses Universitaires.
1964. "Le concept de réflexe au XIXe siècle," in Rothschuh (1964*a*, pp. 157–167).

CANNON, D. F.
1949. *Explorer of the human brain. The life of Santiago Ramón y Cajal (1852–1934).* New York, Schuman.

CANNON, W. B.
1934. "The story of the development of our ideas of chemical mediation of nerve impulses," *Am. J. med. Sci.*, 188:145–159.

CAPPARONI, P.
1939. "Domenico Mistichelli e la sua scoperta della decussatio pyramidum," *Atti Accad. stor. arte san.*, 5:261–275.

CARDINI, M.
1927. *La vita e l'opera di Marcello Malpighi.* Rome, Pozzi.

CARMICHAEL, L.
1927. "Robert Whytt: a contribution to the history of physiological psychology," *Psychol. Rev.*, 34:387–394.
1959. "Karl Spencer Lashley, experimental psychologist," *Science*, 129:1410–1412.

CARRON DU VILLARDS, C.-J.-F.
1830. "Notice necrologique sur le Professeur Rolando," *Bull. Soc. anat. Paris*, 5:195–205.

CASTALDI, L.
1928. "Un manoscritto di Vincenzo Malacarne saluzzese sull'anatomia delle meningi," *Riv. Stor. Sci. med. nat.*, 19:62–73.

CAUSEY, G.
  1960. *The cell of Schwann*. Edinburgh, Livingstone.
CERLETTI, V.
  1959. "Erinnerungen an Franz Nissl," *Münch. med. Wschr.*, 101:2368–2371.
CESALPINO, A.
  1588. *Tractationum philosophicarum tomus unus . . . . Quaestionum peripateticarum libri* V. Geneva, Vignon.
CHAPMAN, L. F., and WOLF, H. G.
  1961. "The human brain—one organ or many?" *Arch. Neurol.*, 5:463–471.
CHARPENTIER, A.
  1934. *Un grand médecin. J. Babinski 1857–1932*. Paris, Bernouard.
CHRISTOFFEL, H.
  1944. "Zur Geschichte der Liquorforschung," *Schweiz. med. Wschr.*, 74:339–342.
CLARKE, E.
  1963. "Aristotelian concepts of the form and function of the brain," *Bull. Hist. Med.*, 37:1–14.
CLARKE, E., JONES, N. C. H., and LOGOTHETOPOULOS, J.
  1954. "The action of tolazoline hydrochloride on cerebral blood flow in cerebral thrombosis," *Lancet*, ii:567–570.
CLARKE, E., and STANNARD, J.
  1963. "Aristotle on the anatomy of the brain," *J. Hist. Med.*, 18:130–148.
COBB, S.
  1960. "A salute from neurologists," in Beach *et al.* (1960, pp. xvii–xx).
COFFMAN, B. R.
  1934. "Bibliographical material for the study of Haller's literary work," *Philolog. Q.*, 13:333–339.
COHEN OF BIRKENHEAD, LORD
  1958. *Sherrington: physiologist, philosopher and poet*. Liverpool, University Press.
COHEN, M. R., and DRABKIN, I. E.
  1948. *A source book in Greek science*. New York, McGraw-Hill.
COHNHEIM, J.
  1872. *Untersuchungen über die embolischen Processe*. Berlin, Hirschwald.
COLE, F. J.
  1937. "Leeuwenhoek's zoological researches," *Ann. Sci.*, 2:1–46, 185–235.
COLENBRANDER, M. C.
  1963. "Franciscus Cornelis Donders and his time," *Opusc. selecta Neerl. Arte med.*, XIX, ix–xv.
COLLANDER, R.
  1933. "Ernst Overton. Ein Nachruf," *Protoplasma*, 20:228–231.
CONEL, J. LeR.
  1953. "Contribution of S. Ramón y Cajal to the knowledge of the anatomy of the cerebral cortex," *New Engl. J. Med.*, 248:541–543.
CONN, H. J.
  1946. "Development of histological staining," Ciba Symp. Summit, N.J., 7:270–300.
  1948. *The history of staining*. Geneva, N.Y., Biotech Publications.
CORNFORD. See PLATO
COTUGNO, D. F. A.
  1764. *De ischiade nervosa commentarius*. Naples, Fratres Simonii.
  1775. *A treatise on the nervous sciatica, or nervous hip gout, by Dominicus Cotun-*

nius [probably translated by Henry Crantz] London, Wilkie; a part of this translation appears in Viets (1935, pp. 715–720); also see Magendie (1827*c*).

CRANEFIELD, P. F.

1957. "Charles E. Morgan's *Electro-physiology and therapeutics*: an unknown English version of du Bois-Reymond's *Thierische Elektricität*," *Bull. Hist. Med.*, 31:172–181.

CREPAX, P.

1963. "The first Italian contributions to the study of cerebellar functions and the work of Luigi Luciani. Part II," in Belloni (1963*a*, pp. 225–236).

CUNNINGHAM, D. J.

1890. "On cerebral anatomy," *Br. med. J.*, ii:277–283.

CUSHING, H. W.

1902. "Physiologische und anatomische Beobachtungen über den Einfluss von Hirnkompression auf den intracraniellen Kreislauf und über einige hiermit verwandte Erscheinungen," *Mitt. Grenzgeb. Med. Chir.*, 9:773–808.

1902. "Some experimental and clinical observations concerning states of increased intracranial tension," *Amer. J. med. Sci.*, 124:375–400.

1903. "The blood-pressure reaction of acute cerebral compression, illustrated by cases of intracranial hemorrhage," *Amer. J. med Sci.*, 125:1017–1044.

1939. A *bibliography of the writings of Harvey Cushing.* Springfield, Ill., Thomas.

DA FANO, C.

1926. "Camillo Golgi, 1843–1926," *J. Path. Bact.*, 29:500–514.

DALE, H. H.

1914*a*. "The occurrence in ergot and action of acetyl-choline (Preliminary communication)," *J. Physiol.*, London, 48:iii–iv.

1914*b*. "The action of certain esters and ethers of choline, and their relation to muscarine," *J. Pharmac. exp. Ther.*, 6:147–190.

1930. "In memoriam Rudolf Magnus (1873–1927)," *Stanford Univ. Publs.*, Med. Sci., 2:241–247.

1937–1938. "Du Bois-Reymond and chemical transmission," *J. Physiol.*, London, 91:4P.

1938*a*. "Acetylcholine as a chemical transmitter of the effects of nerve impulses. I. History of ideas and evidence . . . ," *J. Mt. Sinae Hosp.*, 4:401–415.

1938*b*. "Acetylcholine as a chemical transmitter of the effects of nerve impulses. II. Chemical transmission at ganglionic synapses and voluntary motor nerve endings. Some general considerations," *J. Mt. Sinae Hosp.*, 4:416–429.

1954. "The beginning and the prospects of neurohumoral transmission," pp. 7–13, of "Symposium on neurohumoral transmission," *Pharmac. Rev.*, 6:1–131.

1958. "Autobiographical sketch," *Perspect. Biol. Med.*, 1:125–137.

1961. "Thomas Renton Elliott 1877–1961," *Biogr. Mem. Fellows R. Soc.*, 7:53–74.

1962. "Otto Loewi 1873–1961," *Biogr. Mem. Fellows R. Soc.*, 8:67–89.

1963. "Some fifty years in British medical science," in Ingle (1963, pp. 1–13).

1965. "Some recent extensions of the chemical transmission of the effects of nerve impulses," *Nobel lectures physiology or medicine 1922–1941.* Amsterdam, Elsevier Publishing Co., pp. 402–413.

DALLY, E.

1884. "Éloge de Paul Broca," *Bull. Soc. Anthrop. Paris*, 7 (3d ser.):921–956.

DANDY, W. E.

1919. "Experimental hydrocephalus," *Ann. Surg.*, 70:129–142.

1928. "Removal of right cerebral hemisphere for certain tumors with hemiplegia," *J. Am. Med. Assoc.*, 90:823–825.

DANDY, W. E., and BLACKFAN, K. D.

1913. "An experimental and clinical study of hydrocephalus," *J. Am. Med. Assoc.*, 61:2216–2217.

1854–1856. DAREMBERG. See GALEN.

DAVIS, H.

1965. "Alexander Forbes, 1882–1965," *J. Neurophysiol.*, 28:986–988.

DAVSON, H.

1956. *Physiology of the ocular and cerebrospinal fluid.* London, Churchill.

DAWSON, P. M.

1928. "The life and work of Ernst Heinrich Weber," *Phi Beta Phi Q.*, 25:86–116.

DEITERS, O. F. K.

1865. *Untersuchungen über Gehirn und Rückenmark des Menschen und der Säugethiere.* Braunschweig, Vieweg und Sohn.

DEJEANT, H. J.

1930. *La vie et l'œuvre de Bouillaud.* Paris. Thesis.

DELLA TORRE, G. M.

1776. *Nuove osservazioni microscopiche.* Naples.

DENNIS, W.

1948. *Readings in psychology.* New York, Appleton-Century-Crofts.

DESCARTES, R.

1637. *Discours de la methode pour bien conduire sa raison, & chercher la verité dans les sciences. Plus la dioptriques. . . .* Leiden, Maire. Reprinted in the *Oeuvres* (1956–1957, VI, 1–228).

1647. *Les meditations metaphysiques . . . et les objections . . . .* Traduites par Mr. C. L. R. Paris, Camusat et le Petit. The third edition of 1673 has been reprinted in the *Oeuvres* (1956–1957, IX, 1–245; English translation of Descartes' replies to the "quatrièmes objections" in E. S. Haldane and G. R. T. Ross, *The philosophical works of Descartes*, Cambridge, University Press, II, 1912, 96–122.

1649. *Les passions de l'ame.* [Amsterdam, Elsevier]. Reprinted in the *Oeuvres* (1956–1957, XI, 301–497; English translation of those parts pertinent to the present work in Haldane and Ross, *loc. cit.*, I, 329–427, and selections in N. K. Smith, *Descartes' philosophical writings*, London, Macmillan, 1952, pp. 283–312.

1662. *De homine.* Leiden, Moyardus and Leffen.

1664. *L'homme.* Paris, Angot. Reprinted in the *Oeuvres* (1956–1957, XI, 119–209).

1956–1957. *Oeuvres de Descartes publiées par C. Adam & P. Tannery.* Paris, Vrin. 13 vols.

DEWHURST, K.

1964a. "The murder of Dr. von Gudden," *Practitioner*, 193:220–227.

1964b. *Thomas Willis as a physician.* Los Angeles, William Andrews Clark Memorial Library.

DEZEIMERIS, J. E.

1828–1839. *Dictionnaire historique de la médecine ancienne et moderne.* Paris, Béchet Jeune. 4 vols.

DIBNER, B.

1952. *Galvani-Volta. A controversy that led to the discovery of useful electricity.* Norwalk, Connecticut, Burndy Library.

DIELS, H.
   1964. *Die Fragmente der Vorsokratiker,* I. Zürich, Weidmann.
DIEPGEN, P.
   1927. *Zweie grosse Naturforscher des 19. Jahrhunderts.* Leipzig, Barth.
   1960. *Unvollendete; vom Leben und Wirken frühverstorbener Forscher und Ärzte
       aus anderthalb Jahrhunderten.* Stuttgart, Thieme.
DIXON, W. E.
   1907. "On the mode of action of drugs," *Med. Mag., London,* 16:454–457.
DOBELL, C.
   1932. *Antony van Leeuwenhoek and his "little animals."* London, Staples Press.
DOBSON, J. F.
   1925. "Herophilus of Alexandria," *Proc. R. Soc. Med.,* 20:19–32.
   1927. "Erasistratus," *Proc. R. Soc. Med.,* 20:825–832.
DODDS, W. J.
   1878. "On the localisation of the functions of the brain: being an historical and
       critical analysis of the question," *J. Anat. Physiol.,* 12:340–363, 454–494,
       636–660.
DOMANSKI, B.
   1900. "Die Psychologie des Nemesius," *Beitr. Gesch. Phil. Mittelalt.,* III, pt. 1.
DONDERS, F. C.
   1850. "De Bewegingen der hersenen en de veranderingen der vaatvulling van de *pia
       mater,* ook bij gesloten' onuitzetbaren schedel regtstreeks onderzocht," *Ned.
       Lancet, The Hague,* 5 (2d ser.):521–553.
   1891. "In memoriam F. C. D.," *Proc. R. Soc.,* 49:vii–xxiv.
   1963. "Address by Professor F. C. Donders," *Opusc. selecta Neerl. Arte med.,* XIX,
       270–293.
DONLEY, J. E.
   1909. "John James Wepfer, a renaissance student of apoplexy," *Bull. Johns Hopkins
       Hosp.,* 20:1–19.
DOUGLAS, C. G.
   1952–1953. "Leonard Erskine Hill 1866–1952," *Obit. Not. Fellows R. Soc.,*
       8:431–443.
DOW, R. S.
   1940. "Thomas Willis (1621–1675) as a comparative neurologist," *Ann. med. Hist.,*
       2 (3d ser.):181–194.
DOW, R. S. and MORUZZI, G.
   1958. *The physiology and pathology of the cerebellum.* Minneapolis, University of
       Minnesota Press.
DUBOIS, F.
   1806. "Recherches historiques sur les dernières années de Louis et de Vicq d'Azyr,"
       Gaz. hebd. Méd. Chir., 3:625–629, 641–650, 657–669, 689–698.
DU BOIS-REYMOND, E.
   1843. "Vorläufiger Abriss einer Untersuchung über den sogenannten Froschström
       und über die elektromotorischen Fische," [Poggendorffs] *Annln. Phys.,*
       58:1–30.
   1848–1884. *Untersuchungen über thierische Elektricität.* Berlin, Reimer. 2 vols. in 3.
   1853. *On Signor Carlo Matteucci's letter to H. Bence Jones.* London, Churchill.
DUCKETT, S.
   1964. "Étude de la fonction cérébelleuse par François Pourfour du Petit (1710),"
       Encéphale, 53:291–297.

1962. Duckworth. See Galen.

Dufresne, A.-J.-L.-M.

1906. *Notes sur la vie et les oeuvres de Vicq d'Azyr (1748–1794).* Bordeaux. Thesis.

Duret, H.

1874. "Recherches anatomiques sur la circulation de l'encéphale," *Archs. Physiol., Paris,* 1 (2d ser.):60–91, 316–353, 664–693, 919–957.

Dusser De Barenne, J. G.

1916. "Experimental researches on sensory localization in the cerebral cortex," *Quart. J. exper. Physiol.,* 9:355–390.

1924. "Experimental researches on sensory localization in the cerebral cortex of the monkey (Macacus)," *Proc. R. Soc.,* 96B:272–291.

Dusser De Barenne, J. G., and McCulloch, W. S.

1939. "Physiological delimitation of neurones in the central nervous system," *Am. J. Physiol.,* 127:620–628.

Earles, M. P.

1960. "The experimental investigation of viper venom by Felice Fontana (1730–1805)," *Ann. Sci.,* 16:255–268.

Ebbecke, U.

1951. *Johannes Müller . . . .* [with a reprint of] *Über die phantastischen Gesichtserscheinungen.* Hannover, Seefeld.

Eccles, J. C.

1957. *The physiology of nerve cells.* London, Oxford University Press.

1964. *The physiology of synapses.* Berlin, Springer.

1965. "The synapse," *Scient. Am.,* 212:56–66.

Ecker, A.

1869. *Die Hirnwindung des Menschen nach eigenen Untersuchungen insbesondere über die Entwicklung derselben beim Fötus.* Braunschweig, Vieweg.

1873. *On the convolutions of the human brain,* translated by J. C. Galton. London, Smith, Elder.

Eckhard, C.

1849. "Über Reflexbewegungen der vier letzten Nervenpaare des Frosches. I. Abhandlung," *Z. rationelle Med., Heidelberg,* 7:281–310.

1881. "Beiträge zur Geschichte der Experimentalphysiologie des Nervensystems. Geschichte der Entwickelung der Lehre von den Reflexerscheinungen," *Beitr. Anat. Physiol, Giessen,* 9:29–192.

Economo, C. von, and Koskinas, G. N.

1925. *Die Cytoarchitektonik der Hirnrinde des erwachsenen Menschen.* Vienna, Springer.

1929. *The cytoarchitectonics of the human cerebral cortex* [abbreviated English translation by S. Parker]. London, Oxford University Press.

1930. *The EDWIN SMITH surgical papyrus. Published in facsimile and hieroglyphic transliteration with translation and commentary by James Henry Breasted,* I. Chicago, University of Chicago Press.

Ehlers, E.

1906. "Albert von Kölliker. Zum Gedächtnis," *Z. wiss. Zool.,* 84:i–xxvi.

Ehrenberg, C. G.

1833. "Nothwendigkeit einer feineren mechanischen Zerlegung des Gehirns und der Nerven vor der chemischen, dargestellt aus Beobachtungen von C. G. Ehrenberg," [Poggendorffs] *Annln. Phys.,* 28:449–473.

1838. *Die Infusionsthierchen als volkommene Organismen.* Leipzig, Voss.

EHRLICH, P.

    1885. *Das Sauerstoff-Bedürfnis des Organismus. Eine Farbenanalytische Studie.* Berlin, Hirschwald.

    1886. "Über die Methylenblaureaction der lebenden Nervensubstanz," *Dt. med. Wschr.*, 12:49–52.

ELLIOT, H.

    1917. *Herbert Spencer.* London, Constable.

ELLIOTT, T. R.

    1904. "On the action of adrenalin (Preliminary communication)," *J. Physiol., London,* 31:xx–xxi.

    1905. "The action of adrenalin," *J. Physiol., London,* 32:401–467.

    1961a. Obituary notice. *Br. med. J.,* i:752–754.

    1961b. Obituary notice. *Lancet,* i:567–568.

ERB, W. H.

    1875. "Über Sehnenreflexe bei Gesunden und bei Rückenmarkskranken," *Arch. Psychiat. NervKrankh.,* 5:792–802.

ERIKSSON, R.

    1959. *Andreas Vesalius' first public anatomy at Bologna 1540. An eyewitness report by Baldasar Hessler.* Uppsala, Almqvist and Wiksells.

ERLANGER, J.

    1964. "A physiologist reminisces," *Annual Review of physiology,* Palo Alto, California, XXVI, 1–14.

ERLANGER, J., and GASSER, H. S.

    1924. "The compound nature of the action current of nerve as disclosed by the cathode ray oscillograph," *Am. J. Physiol.,* 70:624–666.

EWALD, J. R.

    1903. "Friedrich Goltz," *Pflügers Arch.,* 94:1–64.

FADIGA, E.

    1963. "The first Italian contributions to the study of cerebellar functions and the work of Luigi Luciani. I. Researches accomplished before Luciani," in Belloni (1963, pp. 203–223).

FAIRMAN, D.

    1946. "Evolution of neurosurgery through Walter E. Dandy's work," *Surgery,* 19:581–604.

FAIVRE, E.

    1853. "Observations sur les granulations méningiennes ou glandes de Pacchioni," *Anns. Sci. nat.,* 3d ser. (Zoologie), 20:321–333.

FALLER, A.

    1948. *Die Entwicklung der Makroskopischanatomischen Präparierkunst von Galen bis zur Neuzeit, Acta Anat.,* Suppl. VII.

FANTUZZI, G.

    1781–1794. *Notizie degli scrittori Bolognesi.* Bologna, S. Tommaso d'Aquino. 9 vols.

FARRAR, C. B.

    1954. "I remember Nissl," *Am. J. Psychiat.,* 110:621–624.

FEARING, F.

    1928. "The history of the experimental study of the knee-jerk," *Am. J. Psychol.,* 40:92–111.

    1929. "René Descartes. A study in the history of theories of reflex action," *Psychol. Review,* 36:375–388.

1930. *Reflex action. A study in the history of physiological psychology.* Baltimore, Williams & Wilkins.

FERRIER, D.

1873. "Experimental researches in cerebral physiology and pathology," *West Riding Lun. Asyl. med. Rep.,* 3:30–96.

1876. *The functions of the brain.* London, Smith, Elder.

1878. *The localisation of cerebral disease.* London, Smith, Elder.

1890. *The Croonian Lectures on cerebral localisation.* London, Smith, Elder.

FICK, R.

1921. "Gedächtnisrede auf Wilhelm von Waldeyer-Hartz nebst einem Verzeichnis seiner Schriften," *Sber. k. preuss. Akad. Wiss. Berlin,* 33:508–546.

FIELD, G. C.

1930. *Plato and his contemporaries. A study in fourth century life and thought.* London, Methuen.

FINLAYSON, J.

1893. "Herophilus & Erasistratus: a bibliographical demonstration," *Glasgow med. J.,* 39:321–352.

FISCHER, H.

1931. *Johann Jakob Wepfer 1620–1695. Ein Beitrag zur Geschichte des 17. Jahrhunderts.* Zürich, Rudolf.

1943. *Briefe Johann Jakob Wepfers (1620–1695) an seinen Sohn Johann Conrad (1657–1711) studiosus medicinae zu Basel und Leyden.* Aarau, Sauerländer.

FISCHGOLD, H.

1963. "D'Angelo Mosso à Hans Berger. Comment est née l'electro-encéphalographie," in Belloni (1963*a*, pp. 237–254).

FISH, P. A.

1895. "The use of formalin in neurology," *Proc. Amer. microsp. Soc.,* 17:319–330.

FLECHSIG, P.

1876. *Die Leitungsbahnen im Gehirn und Rückenmark des Menschen auf Grund entwicklungsgeschichtlicher Untersuchungen.* Leipzig, Engelmann.

1877–1878. "Über 'Systemerkrankungen' im Rückenmark," *Arch. Heilk.,* 18:101–141, 289–343, 461–483, 19:52–90, 441–447.

1881. "Zur Anatomie und Entwickelungsgeschichte der Leitungsbahnen im Grosshirn des Menschen," *Arch. Anat. Physiol.* (Anat. Abt.), pp. 12–75.

1900. "Les centres de projection et d'association du cerveau humain," *XIIIe Congrès International de Médecine* (Sect. Neurologie), Paris, pp. 115–121.

1901. "Developmental (myelogenetic) localisation of the cerebral cortex in the human subject," *Lancet,* ii:1027–1029.

1904. "Einige Bemerkungen über die Untersuchungsmethoden der Grosshirnrinde, insbesondere des Menschen," *Ber. Verh. k. sächs. Ges. Wiss. Leipz.,* Math.-Phys. Klasse, 56:50–104, 177–248.

1920. *Anatomie des menschlichen Gehirns und Rückenmarks auf myelogenetischer Grundlage,* I. Leipzig, Thieme.

1927. *Meine myelogenetische Hirnlehre mit biographischer Einleitung.* Berlin, Springer.

FLINT, A., JR.

1868. "Considérations historiques sur les propriétés des racines rachidiens," *J. Anat. Physiol., Paris,* 5:520–538, 577–592.

FLORIAN, J.
1932. "The early history of the cell theory," *Nature*, 130:634–635.

FLORKIN, M.
1960. *Naissance et déviation de la théorie cellulaire dans l'oeuvre de Théodore Schwann.* Paris & Liège, Hermann.

FLOURENS, P.
1822. "Détermination des propriétés du système nerveux, ou recherches physiques sur l'irritabilité et la sensibilité," *J. Physiol. expér. path.*, 2:372–384.
1823. "Recherches physiques sur les propriétés et les fonctions du système nerveux dans les animaux vertébrés," *Archs. gén. Méd.*, 2:321–370.
1824. *Recherches expérimentales sur les propriétés et les fonctions du système nerveux dans les animaux vertébrés.* Paris, Crevot. Parts of this work are presented in English by Bonin (1960, pp. 3–21); and Fulton (1966, pp. 286–288).
1843. *Examen de la phrenologie.* Paris, Paulin.
1862. "Éloge historique de Frédéric Tiedemann," *Recueils des éloges historiques.* Paris, Garnier Frères, pp. 251–295.

FODERÀ, M.
1823. "Recherches expérimentales sur le système nerveux," *J. Physiol. expér. path.*, 3:191–217.

FOERSTER, O.
1933. "The dermatomes of man," *Brain*, 56:1–39.
1936. "Motorische Felder und Bahnen," in Bumke and Foerster, *Handbuch der Neurologie*, VI, Berlin, Springer, 1–357.

FONTANA, F.
1767. *Ricerche fisiche sopra il veleno della vipera.* Lucca, Giusti.
1781. *Traité sur le vénin de la vipère.* Florence. 2 vols.
1784. "Lettre de M. l'Abbé Fontana a M. Gibelin, à Aix en Provence, datée de Florence du 10 Juillet, 1782," *J. de Physique*, 24:417–421.
1787. *Abhandlungen über das Vipergift.* Berlin, Himburg.
1795. *Treatise on the venom of the viper*, translated by J. Skinner. 2d ed. London, Cuthell. 2 vols.

FORBES, A.
1915. "Electrical studies in mammalian reflexes. I. The flexion reflex," *Am. J. Physiol.*, 37:118–176.
1939. "Problems of synaptic function," *J. Neurophysiol.*, 11:465–472.

FORBES, A., CAMPBELL, C. J., and WILLIAMS, H. B.
1924. "Electrical records of afferent nerve impulses from muscular receptors," *Am. J. Physiol.*, 69:283–303.

FORBES, H. S., and COBB, S.
1938. "Vasomotor control of cerebral vessels," in *The circulation of the brain and spinal cord*, Association for Research in Nervous and Mental Diseases, XVIII, Baltimore, Williams & Wilkins, 201–217.

FOREL, A. H.
1887. "Einige hirnanatomische Betrachtungen und Ergebnisse," *Arch. Psychiat. NervKrankh.*, 18:162–198.
1935. *Rückblick auf mein Leben. Mit einem Nachwort von O. L. Forel.* Zürich, Europa.
1937. *Out of my life and work.* New York, Norton.

Fossati, J.-A.-L.
  1858. "François-Joseph Gall," *Nouvelle biographie générale,* XIX, Paris, Firmin Didot frères, cols. 271–284.

Foster, M.
  1897. *A text-book of physiology,* Pt. III. London, Macmillan.
  1899. *Claude Bernard.* London, Unwin.
  1901. *Lectures on the history of physiology during the sixteenth, seventeenth and eighteenth centuries.* Cambridge, University Press.

Fredericq, H.
  1962. "In memoriam. Otto Loewi (1873–1961)," *Archs. int. Pharmacodyn. Thér.,* 137:1–5.

Freeman, K.
  1959. *The pre-Socratic philosophers,* 2d ed. Oxford, Blackwell.

Freund, H., and Berg, A.
  1963–1964. *Geschichte der Mikroskopie; Leben und Werk grosser Forscher.* Frankfurt am Main, Umschau. 2 vols.

Fulton, J. F.
  1927–1928. "Rudolf Magnus 1872–1927," *Boston med. surg. J.,* 197:323–324.
  1932. *The sign of Babinski. A study of the evolution of cortical dominance in primates.* Springfield, Ill., Thomas.
  1933. "Joseph François Félix Babinski 1857–1932," *Archs. Neurol. Psychiat., Chicago,* 29:168–174.
  1937. "A note on Francesco Gennari and the early history of cytoarchitectural studies of the cerebral cortex," *Bull. Hist. Med.,* 5:895–913.
  1938a. "Alfred Walter Campbell, M.D., Ch.M., 1868–1937," *Archs. Neurol. Psychiat., Chicago,* 40:566–568.
  1938b. "Cytoarchitecture of the gorilla brain," *Science,* 88:426–427.
  1946. *Harvey Cushing. A biography.* Springfield, Ill., Thomas.
  1947. "Sherrington's impact on neurophysiology," *Br. med. J.,* ii:807–810.
  1949a. *Physiology of the nervous system.* 3d ed. New York, Oxford University Press.
  1949b. *Functional localization in the frontal lobes and cerebellum.* Oxford, Clarendon Press.
  1951. "Jules Baillarger and his discovery of the six layers of the cerebral cortex," *Gesnerus,* 8:85–91.
  1952a. "Sir Charles Scott Sherrington, O.M. (1857–1952)," *J. Neurophysiol.,* 15:167–190.
  1952b. "Lewis Hill Weed 1886–1952," *Yale J. Biol. Med.,* 25:215–217.
  1966. *Selected readings in the history of physiology.* 2d ed. Springfield, Ill., Thomas.

Fulton, J. F., and Cushing, H.
  1936. "A bibliographical study of the Galvani and Aldini writings on animal electricity," *Ann. Sci.,* 1:239–268.

Fulton, J. F., and Garol, R. W.
  1940. "Joannes Gregorius Dusser de Barenne 1885–1940," *J. Neurophysiol.,* 3:283–292.

Fuortes, M. G. F.
  1959. "Revue historique," *Archs. ital. Biol.,* 97:276–277.

Gaizo, M. Del
  1904. "Il 'De motu animalium' di G. A. Borelli studiato in rapporto del 'De motu cordis et sanguinis' di G. Harvey," *Atti r. Accad. med.-chir. Napoli,* 67:195–227.

1908. "Giovanni Alfonso Borelli e la sua opera De motu animalium: discorso," *Atti r. Accad. med.-chir. Napoli*, 62 (n.s.):147–169.

1909. "L'oeuvre scientifique de J. A. Borelli, étudiée dans rapports avec l'école hollandaise," *Janus*, 14:506–511.

GALEN

1821–1833. *Opera omnia. Editionem curavit C. G. Kühn*. Leipzig, Cnobloch. 20 vols. in 22.

1854–1856. *Oeuvres anatomiques, physiologiques et médicales . . . traduites sur les textes imprimés et manuscrits . . . par C. Daremberg*. Paris, Baillière. 2 vols.

1916. *Galen on the natural faculties with an English translation by A. J. Brock*. London, Heinemann.

1956. *Galen on anatomical procedures . . . Translation of the surviving books with introduction and notes by C. Singer*. London, Oxford University Press.

1962. *Galen on anatomical procedures. The later books. A translation by the late W. L. H. Duckworth, edited by M. C. Lyons and B. Towers*. Cambridge, University Press.

GALL, F. J., and SPURZHEIM, J. C.

1809. *Recherches sur le système nerveux en général, et sur celui du cerveau en particulier . . . .* Paris, Schoell and Nicolle. English translation: "Report on a memoir of Drs. Gall and Spurzheim relative to the anatomy of the brain," *Edin. med. surg. J.*, 1809, 5:36–66.

1810–1819. *Anatomie et physiologie du système nerveux en général, et du cerveau en particulier . . . .* Paris, Schoell *et al.* 4 vols. and atlas.

GALVANI, L.

1791*a*. "De viribus electricitatis in motu musculari commentarius. Pars prima," *Bononien. Sci. Art. Instit. Acad.*, 7:363–418.

1791*b*. The same. Bologna, Ex typographia Instituti Scientiarum.

1953*a*. *A translation of Luigi Galvani's De viribus electricitatis in motu musculari commentarius, by R. M. Green*. Cambridge, Mass., Licht.

1953*b*. *Commentary on the effects of electricity on muscular motion, translated . . . by M. G. Foley, with notes and a critical introduction by I. B. Cohen . . . and a bibliography of the editions and translations . . . by J. F. Fulton and M. E. Stanton*. Norwalk, Conn., Burndy Library.

1937. *Memorie ed esperimenti inediti di Luigi Galvini*. Bologna, Capelli.

GALVANI, L., and ALDINI, G.

1794. *Dell'uso e dell'attività dell'arco conduttore nelle contrazioni dei muscoli* [with supplement]. Bologna, Aquino.

GARRISON, F. H.

1935. "Felice Fontana. A forgotten physiologist of the Trentino," *Bull. N.Y. Acad. Med.*, 2:117–122.

GARTNER, G., and WAGNER, J.

1887. "Über den Hirnkreislauf vorläüfige Mittheilung," *Wien. med. Wschr.*, 37: cols. 601–603, 640–642.

GASSER, H. S.

1955. "Sir Henry Dale, his influence on science," *Br. med. J.*, i:1359–1361.

1963*a*. Obituary notice, *Br. med. J.*, i:1482–1483.

1963*b*. Obituary notice, *Lancet*, i:1167–1168.

1964. "Mammalian nerve fibers," *Nobel lectures physiology or medicine 1942–1962*. Amsterdam—London—New York, Elsevier Publishing Co., pp. 34–47.

GASSER, H. S., and ERLANGER, J.
    1922. "A study of the action currents of nerve with the cathode ray oscillograph," *Am. J. Physiol.*, 62:496–524.
GAULT, R. H.
    1904. "A sketch of the history of reflex action in the latter half of the nineteenth century," *Am. J. Physiol.*, 15:526–568.
GENNARI, F.
    1782. *De peculiari structura cerebri nonnullisque ejus morbis*. Parma, Ex regio typographeo.
GENTY, M.
    1935. "Paul Broca (1824–1880)," *Biog. méd.*, 9:209–274.
GEOFFROY, J.
    1878. *L'anatomie et la physiologie d'Aristote*. Paris.
GEORGE, J. D.
    1837–1838. "Contribution to the history of the nervous system," *London med. Gaz.*, 2:40–47, 93–96; with accompanying editorial comment and correspondence provoked, pp. 72–73, 128, 160, 248–249, 252–254.
GERLACH, J. VON
    1858. *Mikroscopische Studien aus dem Gebiete der menschlichen Morphologie*. Erlangen, Enke.
    1872a. "Über die Structur der grauern Substanz des menschlichen Grosshirns. Vorläufige Mittheilung," *Zbl. med. Wiss.*, 10:273–275.
    1872b. "Von dem Rückenmark," in Stricker (1869–1872, II, 665–693); English translation, "The spinal cord," in Stricker (1870–1873, pp. 327–366).
GERTLER-SAMUEL, R.
    1965. *Augustus Volney Waller (1816–1870) als Experimentalforscher*. Zürich, Juris. (Zürcher medizingeschichte Abhandlungen, N. R. Nr. 25.)
GLEES, PAUL
    1955. *Neuroglia, morphology and functions*. Oxford, Blackwell.
    1961. *Experimental neurology*. Oxford, Clarendon Press.
GLISSON, F.
    1654. *Anatomia hepatis*. London, Pullein.
    1672. *Tractatus de natura substantiae energetica*. London, Brome & Hooke.
    1677. *Tractatus de ventriculo et intestinis*. London, Brome.
GOLDMANN, E. E.
    1913a. "Vitalfärbung am Zentralnervensystem. Beitrag zur physico-pathologie des plexus-chorioideus und der Hirnhäute," *Abh. kön.-preuss. Akad. Wiss. Berlin*, Phys.-Math. Classe, Nr. 1.
    1913b. Obituary notice, *Br. med. J.*, ii:893–894.
GOLGI, C.
    1875. "Sulla fina struttura dei bulbi olfattoria," *Riv. sper. Freniatria Med. legal.*, 1:66–78.
    1883–1884. "Recherches sur l'histologie des centres nerveux," *Archs. ital. Biol.*, 3:285–317, 4:92–123.
    1886. "Professor Golgi's method of black coloring of the central nervous organs," *Alien. Neurol.*, 7:127–131.
    1903. "Sulla fina struttura dei bulbi olfattoria," *Opera omnia*, Milan, Hoepli, I, 113–132.
    1908. "La doctrine du neurone," *Les Prix Nobel en 1906*, Stockholm, P. A. Norstedt & Söner.

GOLTZ, F. L.

1881a. *Gesammelte Abhandlungen.* Bonn.

1881b. [Report on Goltz's decerebrate dogs], *Trans. International Medical Congress, London, 2–9 August, 1881.* London, Kolckmann, I, 218–243.

1888. "Über die Verrichtungen des Grosshirns," *Pflügers Arch.,* 42:419–467; English translation in Bonin (1960, pp. 118–158).

1892. "Der Hund ohne Grosshirn. Siebente Abhandlung über die Verrichtungen des Grosshirns," *Pflügers Arch.,* 51:570–614.

GOODSPEED, A. W.

1902. "Contributions of Helmholtz to physical science," *J. Am. Med. Assoc.,* 38 (i):552–566.

GORDON, J.

1817. *Observations on the structure of the brain comprising an estimate of the claims of Drs. Gall and Spurzheim to discovery in the anatomy of that organ.* Edinburgh, Blackwood.

GORDON-TAYLOR, G., and WALLS, E. W.

1958. *Sir Charles Bell. His life and times.* Edinburgh, Livingstone.

GRANDEAU, L.

1865. *Pierre Gratiolet.* Paris, Hetzel.

GRANIT, R.

1965. *Charles Scott Sherrington.* London, Nelson.

GRAPOW, H.

1954. *Grundriss der Medizin der alten Ägypter, I. Anatomie und physiologie.* Berlin, Akademie-Verlag.

GRASHLEY, H.

1886. "Bernhard von Gudden," *Arch. Psychiat. NervKrankh.,* 17:i–xxix.

1887. "Nachtrag zum Nekrolog auf Bernhard von Gudden," *Arch. Psychiat. NervKrankh.,* 18:898–910.

GRATIOLET, L. P.

1854. *Mémoires sur les plis cérébraux de l'homme et des primates.* Paris, Bertrand.

1857. *Anatomie comparée du système nerveux,* II. Paris, Baillière.

1861. "Sur la forme de la cavité crânienne d'un Totonaque, avec réflexions sur la signification du volume de l'encéphale," *Bull. Soc. Anthrop. Paris,* 2:66–71.

GROTE, L. R.

1925. *Die Medizin der Gegenwart in Selbstdarstellungen,* V. Leipzig, Meiner.

GRÜNBAUM, A. S. F., see LEYTON, A. S. F.

GRUNDFEST, H.

1963. "The different careers of Gustav Fritsch (1838–1927)," *J. Hist. Med.,* 18:125–129.

GRUNER. See AVICENNA (1930)

GUDDEN, B. VON

1870a. "Über einen bisher nicht beschriebenen Nervenfasernstrang im Gehirne der Säugethiere und des Menschen," *Arch. Psychiat. NervKrankh.,* 2:364–366.

1870b. "Experimentaluntersuchungen über das peripherische und centrale Nervensystem," *Arch. Psychiat. NervKrankh.,* 2:693–723.

1874. "Über die Kreuzung der Fasern im Chiasma nervorum opticorum," *Albrecht v. Graefes Arch. Ophthal.,* 20 (ii):249–268.

1881. "Über den Tractus peduncularis transversus," *Arch. Psychiat. NervKrankh.,* 11:415–423.

GURLT, E.
   1931. "George Kellie," *Biographisches Lexikon der hervorragenden Ärzte*, 2d ed., Berlin, Urban & Schwarzenberg, III, 498.

GUTHRIE, W. K. C.
   1962. *A history of Greek philosophy*, I. Cambridge, University Press.

HABERLING, W.
   1924. *Johannes Müller. Das Leben des rheinischen Naturforschers.* Leipzig, Akademische Verlags. gesellschaft M. B. H.

HAHN, L.
   1882. "Otto-Friedrich Carl Deiters," *Dictionnaire encyclopédique des sciences médicales.* Paris, Masson, 1st ser., XXVI, 276.

HALDANE, E. S.
   1913. "The life of Descartes," *Q. Rev.*, 219:48–65.

HALES, S.
   1733. *Statical essays, containing haemastaticks*, II. London, Innys, Manby, & Woodward.

HALE-WHITE, W.
   1935. *Great doctors of the nineteenth century.* London, Arnold.

HALL, C.
   1861. *Memoirs of Marshall Hall, by his widow.* London, Bentley.

HALL, M.
   1826. "On the nervous circle which connects the voluntary muscles with the brain," *Phil. Trans. R. Soc.*, 116 (ii):163–173.
   1833. "On the reflex function of the medulla oblongata and medulla spinalis," *Phil. Trans. R. Soc.*, 123:635–665.
   1837. "On the reflex function of the spinal marrow; by Prof. Müller," *London Edin. philos. Mag. J. Sci.*, 10 (i):51–57, 124–129, 187–193.
   1850. *Synopsis of the diastaltic nervous system.* London, Mallett.

HALL, W. S.
   1902. "The contributions of Helmholtz to physiology and pyschology," *J. Am. Med. Assoc.*, 38 (i):558–561.

HALLER, A. VON
   1753. "De partibus corporis humani sensibilibus et irritabilibus," *Comment. Soc. Reg. Sci. Göttingen.*, 2:114–158.
   1755. *Dissertation sur les parties irritables et sensibles des animaux. Par M. de Haller.* Traduite par Tissot. Lausanne, Bosquet.
   1755. *A dissertation on the sensible and irritable parts of animals by M. A. Haller, M.D.* London, J. Nourse. [Translated from the French by an unidentified translator].
   1936. *A dissertation on the sensible and irritable parts of animals* . . . [London, J. Nourse, 1755]. Introduction by Owsei Temkin. Baltimore, Johns Hopkins Press.
   1743–1756. *Icones anatomicae* . . . . Göttingen, Vandenhoeck. 8 pts. in 1 vol.
   1762. *Opera minora*, I, Lausanne, F. Grasset, 131–137.
   1762. *Elementa physiologiae corporis humani*, IV. Lausanne, Grasset.
   1774. *Bibliotheca anatomica*, I. Zürich, Orell, Gessner, Fuessli.

HALSTEAD, W. C.
   1947. *Brain and intelligence. Quantitative study of the frontal lobes.* Chicago, University of Chicago Press.

HAMMARBERG, C.
1893. *Studier öfver idiotiens klinik och patologi jämte undersökningar af hjärnbarkens normala anatomi.* Uppsala, Almqvist & Wiksells. German translation by W. Berger. Uppsala, Berling, 1895.

HAMMOND, W. A.
1869. "The physiology and pathology of the cerebellum," *Q. J. psychol. Med. and med. Jurisprud.,* April.

HANNOVER, A.
1840. "Die Chromsäure, ein vorzügliches Mittel beim mikroscopischen Untersuchungen," *Arch. Anat. Physiol.,* pp. 549–558.

HANSTEIN, J.
1877. *Christian Gottfried Ehrenberg. Ein Tagwerk auf dem Felde der Naturforschung des neunzehnten Jahrhunderts.* Bonn, Marcus.

HARRISON, R. G.
1907. "Observations on the living developing nerve fiber," *Anat. Rec.,* 1:116–118.
1908. "Embryonic transplantation and development of the nervous system," *Anat. Rec.,* 2:385–410.

HARTMAN, C. G., and STRAUS, W. L., Jr.
1961. *The anatomy of the rhesus monkey (Macaca mulatta).* New York, Hafner.

HASSLER, R.
1962. "Die Entwicklung der Architektonik seit Brodmann und ihre Bedeutung für die moderne Hirnforschung," *Dt. med. Wschr.,* 87:1180–1185.

HAYMAKER, W.
1951. "Cécile and Oskar Vogt on the occasion of her 75th and his 80th birthday," *Neurology,* 1:179–204.
1953. *The founders of neurology: one hundred and thirty-three biographical sketches prepared for the fourth International Neurological Congress in Paris by eighty-four authors.* Springfield, Ill., Thomas.

HAZEN, A. T.
1939. "Johnson's life of Frederick Ruysch," *Bull. Hist. Med.,* 7:324–334.

HEAD, H., and CAMPBELL, A. W.
1900. "The pathology of herpes zoster and its bearing on sensory localisation," *Brain,* 23:353–523.

HEIDEL, W. A.
1941. *Hippocratic medicine. Its spirit and methods.* New York, Columbia University Press.

HELD, H.
1897*a.* "Beiträge zur Structur der Nervenzellen und ihrer Fortsätze. Zweite Abhandlung," *Arch. Anat. Physiol.* (Anat. Abt.), pp. 204–294.
1897*b.* "Beiträge zur Structur der Nervenzellen und ihrer Fortsätze. Dritte Abhandlung," *Arch. Anat. Physiol.,* Anat. Abt. Suppl. Bd., pp. 273–312.

HELMHOLTZ, H. VON
1842. *De fabrica systematis nervosi evertebratorum.* Berlin, Inaugural dissertation.
1850. "Vorläufiger Bericht über die Fortpflanzungsgeschwindigkeit der Nervenreizung," *Arch. Anat. Physiol.* (Anat. Abt., Supplement-Bd.), pp. 71–73; translation in Dennis (1948, pp. 197–198).
1852. "Messungen über Fortpflanzungsgeschwindigkeit der Reizung in den Nerven, zweite Reihe," *Arch. Anat. Physiol.,* pp. 199–216.

HEMMETER, J. C.
1908. "Albrecht von Haller: scientific, literary and poetical activity," *Bull. Johns Hopkins Hosp.*, 19:65–74.

HENSCHEN, S. E.
1893. "On the visual path and centre," *Brain*, 16:170–180.
1924. "On the value of the discovery of the visual centre. A review and a personal apology," *Scand. scient. Rev.*, 3:10–63.

HERMANN, L.
1863. *Grundriss der Physiologie des Menschen*. Berlin, Hirschwald.
1870. *Grundriss der Physiologie des Menschen*. 3d ed. Berlin, Hirschwald.
1874. *Grundriss der Physiologie des Menschen*. 5th ed. Berlin, Hirschwald. English translation: *Elements of human physiology*, translated by A. Gamgee. London, Smith, Elder, 1875.
1905. *Lehrbuch der Physiologie*. 13th ed. Berlin, Hirschwald.
1884. "Über sogenannte secundärelektromotorische Erscheinungen an Muskeln und Nerven," *Pflügers Arch.*, 33:103–168.

HERRICK, J. B.
1940. "Jean-Baptiste Bouillaud and his contribution to cardiology," *Bull. Soc. med. Hist. Chicago*, 5:230–246.

HEUBNER, J. B. O.
1872. "Zur Topographie der Ernährungsgebiete der einzelnen Hirnarterien," *Zbl. med. Wiss.*, 10:817–821.
1874. *Die luetische Erkrankung der Hirnarterien*. Leipzig, Vogel.

HIERONS, R., and MEYER, A.
1962. "Some priority questions arising from Thomas Willis' work on the brain," *Proc. R. Soc. Med.*, 55:287–292.
1964. "Willis' place in the history of muscle physiology," *Proc. R. Soc. Med.*, 57:687–692.

HILL, L. E.
1896. *The physiology and pathology of the cerebral circulation. An experimental research*. London, Churchill.
1932–1935. "Sir Edward Albert Sharpey-Schäfer 1850–1935," *Obit. Not. Fell. R. Soc. London*, 1:401–407.

HINTZSCHE, E.
1943. "Die Entwicklung der histologischen Färbetechnik," *Ciba-Z.*, 8:3074–3109.
1953. *Gabriel Gustav Valentin (1810–1883). Versuch einer Bio- und Bibliographie.* Bern, P. Haupt. (Berner Beiträge zur Geschichte der Medizin und der Naturwissenschaften, Nr. 12.)
1963. *Zellen und Gewebe in G. Valentin's "Histiogenia comparata" von 1835 und 1838.* Bern, Haupt. (Berner Beiträge zur Geschichte der Medizin und der Naturwissenschafte, Nr. 20.)

HIPPOCRATES
1839–1861. *Oeuvres complètes d'Hippocrate, traduction nouvelle par É. Littré.* Paris, Baillière. 10 vols.
1849. *The genuine works of Hippocrates. Translated from the Greek by Francis Adams.* London, Sydenham Society. 2 vols.

HIRSCH, A.
1884. "Hubert Luschka," *Allgemeine deutsche Biographie*, XIX. Leipzig, Duncker & Humblot, cols. 653–655.

HIS, W.
1887. "Zur Geschichte des menschlichen Rückenmarkes und der Nervenwurzeln," *Abh. k. säch. Ges. Wiss.*, Math.-Phys. Classe, 13:477–514.
1888. "Über die embryonale Entwickelung der Nervenbahnen," *Anat. Anz.*, 3:499–506.
1894. "Über mechanische Grundvorgänge thierische Formenbildung," *Arch. Anat. Physiol.*, pp. 1–80; summation by His of his life's work, pp. 35–41, 51.

HIS, W., Jr.
1931. *Wilhelm His der Anatom. Ein Lebensbild.* Berlin, Urban & Schwarzenberg.

HITZIG, E., and FRITSCH, G. T.
1870. "Über die elektrische Erregbarkeit des Grosshirns," *Arch. Anat. Physiol.*, pp. 300–332; English translation in Bonin (1960, pp. 73–96); and H. Wilkins, "Neurosurgical classics XII," *J. Neurosurg.*, 1963, 20:904–916.

HODGE, C. F.
1890. "A sketch of the history of reflex action," *Am. J. Psychol.*, 3:149–167.

HODGKIN, A. L.
1964. *The conduction of the nervous impulse.* Liverpool, University Press.

HODGKIN, T., and LISTER, J. J.
1827. "Notice of some microscopic observations of the blood and animal tissues," *Phil. Mag.*, ii:130–138.

HOFF, H. E.
1936a. "Galvani and the pre-Galvanian electrophysiologists," *Ann. Sci.*, 1:157–172.
1936b. "Vagal stimulation before the Webers," *Ann. med. Hist.*, 8:138–144.
1940. "The history of vagal inhibition," *Bull. Hist. Med.*, 8:461–496.
1942. "The history of the refractory period. A neglected contribution of Felice Fontana," *Yale J. Biol. Med.*, 14:635–672.
1959. "A classic of microscopy: an early, if not the first, observation on the fluidity of the axoplasm, micromanipulation, and the use of the cover-slip," *Bull. Hist. Med.*, 33:375–379.

HOFF, H. E., and GEDDES, C. A.
1957. "The rheotome and its pre-history," *Bull. Hist. Med.*, 31:212–234, 327–347.
1960. "Ballistics and the instrumentation of physiology: the velocity of the projectile and of the nerve impulse," *J. Hist. Med.*, 15:133–146.

HOFF, H. E., and KELLAWAY, P.
1952. "The early history of the reflex," *J. Hist. Med.*, 7:211–249.

HOFFMEIER, H. K.
1963. "Christian Gottfried Ehrenberg (1795–1876)," *Z. ärztl. Fortbild.*, 52:740–741.

HOLLAND, J. W.
1904. "Memoir of Roberts Bartholow," *Trans. Stud. Coll. Physns. Philad.*, 26 (3d ser.):43–52.

HOLMES, G. M.
1907. "A form of familial degeneration of the cerebellum," *Brain*, 30:466–489.
1917. "The symptoms of acute cerebellar injuries due to gunshot injuries," *Brain*, 40:461–535.
1919. "Lecture I—The cortical localization of vision," *Br. med. J.*, ii:193–199.
1966a. Obituary notice: "Gordon Morgan Holmes," *Lancet*, i:101.
1966b. Obituary notice: "Sir Gordon Morgan Holmes," *Br. med. J.*, i:111–112.

HOLMES, G. M., and MAY, W. P.
1909. "On the exact origin of the pyramidal tracts in man and in other animals," *Brain*, 32:1–43.

HOLMSTEDT, B., and LILJESTRAND, G.
1963. *Readings in pharmacology*. New York, Macmillan.

HOPF, A.
1962. "Cécile Vogt," *J. Hirnforsch.*, 5:245–248.

HOPSTOCK, H.
1921. "Leonardo as an anatomist," *Studies in the history and method of science*, edited by C. Singer, II, Oxford, Clarendon Press, 151–191.

HORSLEY, V. A. H., and CLARKE, R. H.
1908. "The structure and function of the cerebellum examined by a new method," *Brain*, 31:1–80.

HUARD, P.
1960. "Panorama de Paul Broca (1824–1880)," *Bull. Soc. Anthrop. Paris*, 1 (11th ser.):277–291.
1961. "Paul Broca (1824–1880)," *Rev. Hist. Sci.*, 14:47–86.

HUBER, J. J.
1741. *De medulla spinali speciatim de nervis ab ea provenientibus commentatio cum adjunctis iconibus*. Göttingen, Vanderhoeck.

HUGHES, A.
1959. *A history of cytology*. New York, Abelard-Schuman.

HUNT, J.
1868–1869. "On the localisation of the functions of the brain with special reference to the faculty of language," *Anthrop. Rev.*, 6:329–345, 7:100–116, 201–204.

HUSCHKE, E.
1854. *Schädel, Hirn und Seele des Menschen und der Thiere nach Alter, Geschlecht und Raçe*. Jena, Mauke.

HUSEMANN, T.
1931. "Johann Jacob Huber," *Biographisches Lexikon der Hervorragenden Ärzte aller Zeiten und Völker*. Berlin, Urban & Schwarzenberg, III, 320.

HUTCHINSON, J.
1911. "The late Dr. Hughlings Jackson," *Br. med. J.*, ii:1551–1554.

INGLE, D. J.
1963. *A dozen doctors. Autobiographical sketches*. Chicago, University of Chicago Press.

INGVAR, S.
1931. "Salomon Eberhard Henschen. In memoriam," *Acta med. scand.*, 74:325–333.

IRELAND, W. W.
1898. "Flechsig on the localisation of mental processes in the brain," *J. ment. Sci.*, 44:1–17.

IRSAY, STEPHEN D'
1930. *Albrecht Haller. Eine Studie zur Geistesgeschichte der Aufklärung*. Leipzig, Thieme. (Arbeiten des Institut für Geschichte der Medizin an der Universität. Leipzig, Bd. I.)

ISCHLONDSKY, N.
1958. "The life and activity of I. M. Sechenov," *J. nerv. ment. Dis.*, 126:367–391.

JACKSON, J. H.
1864. "Loss of speech," *Clin. Lect. Rep. Med. Surg. Staff London Hosp.*, 1:388–471.

1870. "A study of convulsions," *Trans. St. Andrews med. Grad. Assoc.*, 3. Published as separate monograph, London, Odell and Ives, 1870; reprinted in *Selected writings*, 1931, I, 8–36.

1873. "On the anatomical and physiological localisation of movement in the brain," *Lancet*, i:84–85, 162–164, 232–234 [no continuation as promised]. Reprinted with an article by W. Gowers: *Clinical and physiological researches on the nervous system, No. 1.* London, Churchill, 1875.

1911*a*. Obituary notice. *Br. med. J.*, ii:950–954.

1911*b*. Obituary notice. *Lancet*, ii:1103–1107.

1931. *Selected writings of John Hughlings Jackson*, edited by J. Taylor. London, Hodder and Stoughton. 2 vols.

JAEGER, W. W.
1914. *Nemesius von Emesa. Quellenforschungen zum Neuplatonismus und seinen Anfängen bei Poseidonios.* Berlin, Weidmann.

1934. *Aristotle. Fundamentals of the history of his development*, translated by R. Robinson. London, Oxford University Press.

JANSEN, J.
1965. "Komparativ anatomi - komparativ - neurologi," *Tidsskr. norske Laegeforen*, 85:87–92.

JEFFERSON, G.
1949. "René Descartes on the localisation of the soul," *Irish J. med. Sci.*, 6th ser., no. 285, pp. 692–706.

JEITTELES, A. L.
1858. "Wer ist der Begründer der Lehre von den Reflex Bewegungen?" *Vjschr. prakt. Heilk.*, 4:50–72.

JENSEN, P.
1904. Über die Blutversorgung des Gehirns," *Pflügers Arch.*, 103:171–195.

JODIN, J.-N.
1842. "Recherches historiques sur le liquide céphalo-rachidien," in Magendie (1842, pp. 139–161).

JOHN, H. J.
1959. *Jan Evangelista Purkyně, Czech scientist and patriot.* Philadelphia, American Philosophical Society.

JOHNSSON, J. W. S.
1915. "Adolph Hannover," *Mitt. Gesch. Med. Naturw. Tech.*, 14:109–111.

JOLLY, J.
1923. "Louis Ranvier (1835–1922)," *Archs. Anat. microsc.*, 19:l–lxxii.

JOURDAN, A. J. L.
1820–1825. *Dictionnaire des sciences médicales. Biographie médicale.* Paris, Panckoucke. 7 vols.

KAPPERS, A., HUBER, G. C., and CROSBY, E. C.
1936. *The comparative anatomy of the nervous system of vertebrates including man.* New York, Macmillan. 2 vols.

KAYSERLING, A.
1901. "Die Medizin Alcmaeons von Kroton (um 520 n. chr.)," *Z. klin. Med.*, 43:171–179.

KEEGAN, J. J., and GARRETT, F. D.
1948. "The segmental distribution of the cutaneous nerves of the limbs of man," *Anat. Rec.*, 102:409–437.

KEELE, K. D.
1957. *Anatomies of pain*. Oxford, Blackwell.

KEHRER, F. A.
1905. "Zu Erinnerung an Konrad Eckhard," *Münch. med. Wschr.*, 52:1296–1297.

KELLAWAY, P.
1946. "The part played by electric fish in the early history of bio-electricity and electrotherapy," *Bull. Hist. Med.*, 20:112–137.

KELLETT, C. E.
1942. "The life and works of Raymond de Vieussens," *Ann. Med. Hist.*, 4 (3d ser.):31–54.

KELLIE, G.
1824. "An account of the appearances observed in the dissection of two or three individuals presumed to have perished in the storm of the 3rd, and whose bodies were discovered in the vicinity of Leith on the morning of the 4th, November 1821; with some reflections on the pathology of the brain. Part I," *Trans. med.-chir. Soc. Edin.*, 1:84–124; "Reflections on the pathology of the brain. Part II," *ibid.*, 125–169.

KENNEDY, R.
1897–1898. "Degeneration and regeneration of nerves. An historical review," *Proc. phil. Soc. Glasgow*, 29:193–229.

KETY, S. S.
1948. "Quantitative measurement of cerebral blood flow in man," *Meth. med. Res.*, 1:204–217.
1964. "The cerebral circulation," *Circulation of the blood—men and ideas*, edited by A. P. Fishman and D. W. Richards. New York, Oxford University Press, pp. 703–742.

KEY, E. A. H., and RETZIUS, G. M.
1875–1876. *Studien in der Anatomie des Nervensystems und des Bindgewebes*. Stockholm, Norstedt & Söner. 2 vols.

KING, L. S.
1954. "Plato's concepts of medicine," *J. Hist. Med.*, 9:38–48.

KIRCHHOFF, T.
1921. *Deutsche Irrenärzte*, I. Berlin, Springer.

KISCH, B.
1954. *Forgotten leaders in modern medicine*. Philadelphia, American Philosophical Society.

KLEIJN, A. de, and MAGNUS, R.
1920. "Über die Unabhängigkeit der Labyrinthreflexe vom Kleinhirn und über die Lage der Zentren für die Labyrinthreflexe im Hirnstamm," *Pflügers Arch. f. Physiol.*, 178:124–178.

KLEIN, E.
1883–1884. "Report on the parts destroyed on the left side of the brain of the dog operated on by Prof. Goltz," *J. Physiol.*, London, 4:310–315.

KLOTZ, O.
1936. "Albrecht von Haller (1708–77)," *Ann. Med. Hist.*, 8 (n.s.):10–26.

KLÜVER, H.
1936. "An analysis of the effects of the removal of the occipital lobes in monkeys," *J. Psychol.*, 2:49–61.

KNAPP, H.
1902. "A few personal recollections of Helmholtz," *J. Am. Med. Assoc.*, 38 (i):557–558.

KOELLIKER, R. A. VON
1849. "Neurologische Bemerkungen," *Z. wiss. Zool.*, 1:135–163.
1850–1854. *Mikroskopische Anatomie.* Leipzig, Englemann, 3 vols.
1852. *Handbuch der Gewebelehre des Menschen.* Leipzig, Englemann.
1853. *Manual of human histology*, translated by G. Busk and T. Huxley. London, Sydenham Society. 2 vols.
1856. "Physiologische Untersuchungen über die Wirkung einiger Gifte," *Virchows Arch. path. Anat. Physiol.*, 10:1–77.
1896. "Vom Nervensysteme," in *Handbuch der Gewebelehre des Menschen.* 6th ed. Leipzig, Englemann, II, 1–874.
1899. *Erinnerungen aus meinem Leben.* Leipzig, Englemann.

KOENIGSBERGER, L.
1902–1903. *Hermann von Helmholtz.* Braunschweig, Vieweg. 3 vols.
1906. Compressed English version by F. A. Welby: *Hermann von Helmholtz.* Oxford, Clarendon Press.

KOLLE, K.
1956–1963. *Grosse Nervenärzte; Lebensbilder.* Stuttgart, Thieme. 3 vols.

KONING, P. DE
1903. *Trois traités d'anatomie arabes.* Leiden, Brill.

KONORSKI, J.
1948. *Conditional reflexes and neuron organisation*, translated by S. Garry. Cambridge, University Press.

KOSHTOYANTS, K.
1962. "I. M. Sechenov (1829–1905)," in I. M. Sechenov, *Selected physiological and psychological works.* London, Central Books.

KRAUSE, F.
1908–1911. *Chirurgie des Gehirns und Rückenmarkes nach eigenen Erfahrungen.* Berlin, Urban & Schwarzenberg. 2 vols.
1910 ff. *Surgery of the brain and spinal cord based on personal experiences.* London, H. K. Lewis. 3 vols. Vol. I translated by H. A. Haubold; Vols. II–III, "English adaptation by M. Thorek."

KRAUSE, F., and SCHUM, H.
1931. *Die epileptischen Erkrankungen.* Stuttgart, F. Enke. (Vol. 49, pt. 1, of *Neue Deutsche Chirurgie*, edited by H. Küttner.)

KREUTER, A.
1913. "Edwin E. Goldmann. Ein Nachruf," *Münch. med. Wschr.*, 60:2735–2736.

KRUGER, L.
1963. "François Pourfour du Petit 1664–1741," *Expl. Neurol.*, 7:ii–v.

KRUTA, V.
1949. *Georgius Procháska 1749–1820. Professor of anatomy, physiology and opthalmology at the Universities of Prague and Vienna.* Brno.
1962a. *Jan Evangelista Purkyně.* Prague, State Medical Publishing House.
1962b. "The physiologist George Procháska (1749–1820) and the reflex theory," *Epilepsia*, 3 (4th ser.):446–456.
1964. *K počátkům vědecké dráhy J. E. Purkyně.* Brno, Lékářská Fakulta University J. E. Purkyně.

KRYNAUW, R. A.
1950. "Infantile hemiplegia treated by removing one cerebral hemisphere," *J. Neurol. Neurosurg. Psychiat.*, 13:243–267.

KUDLIEN, F.
1964. "Mondinos Standort innerhalb der Entwicklung der Anatomie," *Med. Mschr.*, 5:210–214.

KÜHN. See GALEN

KÜHNE, W.
1862. *Über die peripherischen Endorgane der motorischen Nerven.* Leipzig, Engelmann.
1869. "Nerv und Muskelfaser," in Stricker (1869–1872, I, 147–169); English translation: "The mode of termination of nerve fibre in muscle," in Stricker (1870–1873, I, 202–234).
1888. "On the origin and the causation of vital movement (Über die Enstehung der vitalen Bewegung)," *Proc. R. Soc.*, 44:427–447.

KUSSMAUL, A.
1879. *Dr. Benedict Stilling. Gedächtnissrede.* Strassburg, Trübner.

LANGER, C.
1875. "Hubert von Luschka," *Wien. med. Wschr.*, 25:322–323.

LANGLEY, J. N.
1883–1884. "Report on the parts destroyed on the right side of the brain of the dog operated upon by Prof. Goltz," *J. Physiol.*, London, 4:286–309.
1916–1917. "Captain Keith Lucas, F.R.S.," *Nature*, 98:109.

LANGLEY, J. N., and GRÜNBAUM [LEYTON], A. S.
1890. "On the degeneration resulting from removal of the cerebral cortex and corpora striata in the dog," *J. Physiol.*, London, 11:606–624.

LANGLEY, J. N., and SHERRINGTON, C. S.
1884–1885. "Secondary degeneration of nerve tracts following removal of the cortex of the cerebrum in the dog," *J. Physiol.*, London, 5:49–65.

LARSELL, O.
1920. "Gustav Retzius, 1842–1919," *Scient. Mon.*, 10:559–569.
1937. "The cerebellum. A review and interpretation," *Arch. Neurol. Psychiat.*, 38:580–607.

LASHLEY, K. S.
1933. "Integrative functions of the cerebral cortex," *Physiol. Rev.*, 13:1–42; reprinted in Beach *et al.* (1960, pp. 217–255).
1937. "Functional determinants of cerebral localization," *Arch. Neurol. Psychiat.*, 38:371–387.
1950. "In search of the engram," *Symposia of the Society for Experimental Biology, No. IV, Physiological mechanisms in animal behavior.* Cambridge, University Press. Reprinted in Beach *et al.* (1960, pp. 454–482).
1958. Obituary notice. *Br. med. J.*, ii:694–695.

LASHLEY, K. S., and CLARK, G.
1946. "The cytoarchitecture of the cerebral cortex of Ateles: a critical examination of architectonic studies," *J. comp. Neurol.*, 85:223–305.

LASSEK, A. M.
1954. *The pyramidal tract. Its status in medicine.* Springfield, Ill., Thomas.

LAUTOUR, A.-M.
1948. "Auburtin," *Dictionnaire de biographie française*, IV, Paris, 1948, col. 300.

LAYCOCK, T.

1845. "On the reflex function of the brain," *Br. foreign med. Rev.*, 19:298–311.

LE BOË, FRANCISCUS DE (Sylvius)

1681. *Opera medica.* Geneva, Tournes.

LEEUWENHOEK, ANTONY VAN

1674. "More observations from Mr. Leewenhook, in a letter of Sept. 7, 1674. sent to the Publisher," *Phil. Trans. R. Soc.*, 9:178–182.

1675. "Microscopical observations of Mr. Leewenhoeck, concerning the optic nerve . . . ," *Phil. Trans. R. Soc.*, 10:378–380.

1677. "Mr. Leewenhoeks letter written to the publisher from Delff the 14th of May 1677, concerning observations by him made of the carneous fibres of a muscle, and the cortical and medullar part of the brain," *Phil. Trans. R. Soc.*, 12:899–895 [905].

1685. "An abstract of a letter of Mr. Anthony Leewenhoek, Fellow of the Society; concerning the parts of the brain of severall animals . . . ," *Phil. Trans. R. Soc.*, 15:883–895.

1693. "An extract of a letter from Mr. Anthony van Leeuwenhoek, to the R. S. containing his observations of the . . . optic nerves . . . ," *Phil. Trans. R. Soc.*, 17:949–960.

1719. *Epistolae physiologicae super compluribus naturae arcanis.* Delft, Beman.

1722. "De structura cerebri diversorum animalium: etc." in *Opera omnia, seu arcana naturae*, I, Leiden Langerak, pp. 29–41. This is the full Latin version of the English abstract cited immediately above.

1807. *Antony van Leeuwenhoek.* The selected works by Samuel Hoole. London, Philanthropic Society. Vol. II, 303–306, contains an inaccurate and incomplete translation of the letter of 2 March 1717.

LEGALLOIS, C. J. J. C.

1812. *Expériences sur le principe de la vie, notamment sur celui des mouvements du coeur, et sur la siége de ce principe.* Paris, D'Hautel.

1813. *Experiments on the principle of life, and particularly on the principle of the motions of the heart, and on the seat of this principle*, translated by N. C. and J. G. Nancrede. Philadelphia, Thomas.

1814–1815. "Notice biographique sur M. Legallois," *Bull. Fac. Soc. Méd., Paris*, 4:105–109.

1830. "Notice sur l'auteur," in *Oeuvres de C^{ar} Legallois*, edited by M. Pariset, I, Paris, Le Rouge, 1–11.

LENZ, G.

1924. "Erwiderung auf die Arbeit Henschens: 40 jähriger Kampf um das Sehzentrum und seine Bedeutung für die Hirnforschung," *Z. ges. Neurol. Psychiat.*, 90:628–637.

LESKY, E.

1964. "Ludwig Türck (1810–1868), Neuroanatom und Neurophysiologe," in Roth-schuh (1964a, pp. 121–133).

LEURET, F.

1839. *Anatomie comparée du système nerveux considéré dans ses rapports avec l'intelligence.* Paris, Baillière.

LEVY-VALENSI, J.

1933. *La médecine et les médecins français au XVIIe siècle.* Paris, Baillière.

LEWES, G. H.
 1860. *The physiology of common life*. Edinburgh, Blackwood. 2 vols.
 1864. *Aristotle: a chapter from the history of science*. London, Smith, Elder.
LEWIS, A.
 1958. "J. C. Reil's concepts of brain function," in *The history and philosophy of knowledge of the brain and its functions*, Oxford, Blackwell, pp. 154–166.
 1965. "J. C. Reil: innovator and battler," *J. Hist. behavior. Sci.*, 1:178–190.
LEWIS, F. T.
 1942. "The introduction of biological stains: employment of saffron by Vieussens and Leeuwenhoek," *Anat. Rec.*, 83:229–253.
LEWIS, W. B.
 1878. "On the comparative structure of the cortex cerebri," *Brain*, 1:79–96.
 1929*a*. Obituary notice. *Br. med. J.*, ii:833–834.
 1929*b*. Obituary notice. *Lancet*, ii:954–955.
LEWIS, W. B., and CLARKE, H.
 1878. "The cortical lamination of the motor area of the brain," *Proc. R. Soc.*, 27:38–49.
LEYTON (GRÜNBAUM), A. S. F.
 1921*a*. Obituary notice. *Br. med. J.*, ii:579.
 1921*b*. Obituary notice. *Lancet*, ii:825–826.
LEYTON (GRÜNBAUM), A. S. F., and SHERRINGTON, C. S.
 1902. "Observations on the physiology of the cerebral cortex of some of the higher apes (Preliminary communication)," *Proc. R. Soc.*, 69:206–209.
 1903. "Observations on the physiology of the cerebral cortex of the anthropoid apes," *Proc. R. Soc.*, 72:152–155.
 1917. "Observations on the excitable cortex of the chimpanzee, orang-utan, and gorilla," *Q. Jl. exp. Physiol.*, 11:135–222. Partial reprint in Sherrington (1939, pp. 396–439) and complete in Bonin (1960, pp. 283–396).
LIDDELL, E. G. T.
 1960. *The discovery of reflexes*. Oxford, Clarendon Press.
 1839–1861. LITTRÉ. See HIPPOCRATES
LIVINGSTON, R. B.
 1947. "Hermann von Helmholtz and the conservation of energy. A centenary note," *Stanford med. Bull.*, 5:182–184.
LOEB, J.
 1884. "Die Sehstörungen nach Vorletzungen der Grosshirnrinde," *Pflügers Arch.*, 34:67–172.
LÖWENTHAL, M. S.
 1960. Obituary notice. *Br. med. J.*, ii:1243–1244, 1606–1607.
LÖWENTHAL, M. S., and HORSLEY, V. A. H.
 1897. "On the relations between the cerebellar and other centres (namely cerebral and spinal) with special reference to the action of antagonistic muscles (Preliminary account)," *Proc. R. Soc.*, 61:20–25.
LOEWI, O.
 1921. "Über humorale Übertragbarkeit der Herznervenwirkung. I. Mitteilung," *Pflügers Arch.*, 189:239–242.
 1922. "Über humorale Übertragbarkeit der Herznervenwirkung. II. Mitteilung," *Pflügers Arch.*, 193:201–213.

1926. "Über humorale Übertragbarkeit der Herznervenwirkung. X. Mitteilung. Über das Schicksal des Vagusstoffs," *Pflügers Arch.*, 214:678–688.

1935. "The Ferrier Lecture on problems connected with the principle of humoral transmission of nervous impulses," *Proc. R. Soc.*, 118B:299–316.

1954. "Introduction," pp. 1–6, of "Symposium on neurohumoral transmission," *Pharmac. Rev.*, 6:1–131.

1955. "Salute to Henry Hallett Dale," *Br. med. J.*, i:1356–1357.

1961. "An autobiographical sketch," *Perspect. Biol. Med.*, 4:3–25.

1963. "The excitement of a life in science," in Ingle (1963, pp. 109–131).

LONES, T. E.

1912. *Aristotle's researches in natural science.* London, West & Newman.

LONGET, F. A.

1841. *Recherches expérimentales et pathologiques sur les propriétés et les fonctions des faisceaux de la moelle épinière et des racines des nerfs rachidiens.* Paris, Bechet Jeune & Labé.

1842. *Anatomie et physiologie du système nerveux de l'homme,* I. Paris, Fortin, Masson.

LORD, J. R.

1928. "Leonardo Bianchi," *J. ment. Sci.*, 74:381–385.

LORENTE DE NÓ, R.

1949. "Architectonics and structure of the cerebral cortex," in Fulton (1949a, pp. 288–330).

LUCAS, K.

1909. "The 'all or none' contraction of the amphibian skeletal muscle fibre," *J. Physiol., London*, 38:113–133.

1912. "The process of excitation in nerves and muscles," *Proc. R. Soc.*, 85B:495–524.

1917. *The conduction of the nervous impulse.* London, Longmans, Green.

LUCIANI, L.

1891. *Il cervelletto.* Florence, Successori Le Monnier.

LUCIANI, L., and SEPPILLI, L.

1885. *Le localizzazioni funzionali del cervello.* Naples, Vallardi.

LUDWIG, C.

1878. *Rede zum Gedächtniss an Ernst Heinrich Weber.* Leipzig, Veit.

LUNDSGAARD-HANSEN-FISCHER, S.

1959. *Verzeichnis der gedruckten Schriften Albrecht von Hallers.* Bern, Haupt. (Berner Beiträge zur Geschichte der Medizin und der Naturwissenschaften, Nr. 18.)

LUSCHKA, H. VON

1855. *Die Adergeflechte der menschlichen Gehirnes. Eine Monographie.* Berlin, Reimer.

MACCALLUM, W. G.

1905. "Marcello Malpighi. 1628–1694," *Bull. Johns Hopkins Hosp.*, 16:275–284.

MAGENDIE, F. J.

1822a. "Expériences sur les fonctions des racines des nerfs rachidiens," *J. Physiol. exp. path., Paris*, 2:276–279; English translation in A. Walker (1839, pp. 87–91).

1822b. "Expériences sur les fonctions des racines des nerfs qui naissent de la moelle épinière," *J. Physiol. exp. path., Paris*, 2:366–371; English translation in A. Walker (1839, pp. 92–101).

1823. "Sur le siège du mouvement et du sentiment dans la moelle épinière," *J. Physiol. exp. path., Paris*, 3:153–157.

1824. "Mémoire sur les fonctions de quelques parties du système nerveux," *J. Physiol. exp. path.*, Paris, 4:399–407.

1825. "Mémoire sur un liquide qui se trouve dans le crâne et le canal vertébral de l'homme et des animaux mammifères," *J. Physiol. exp. path.*, Paris, 5:27–37.

1827*a*. "Second mémoire sur le liquide qui se trouve dans le crâne et l'épine de l'homme, et des animaux vertébrés," *J. Physiol. exp. path.*, Paris, 7:1–29.

1827*b*. "Troisième et dernière partie du second mémoire sur le liquide qui se trouve dans le crâne et l'épine de l'homme et des animaux vertébrés," *J. Physiol. exp. path.*, Paris, 7:66–82.

1827*c*. "Extrait de la dissertation de Cotugno *De ischiade nervosa*," *J. Physiol. exp. path.*, Paris, 7:83–96. Contains the Latin text of pars ix–xvi.

1828. "Mémoire physiologique sur le cerveau," *J. Physiol. exp. path.*, Paris, 8:211–229.

1842. *Recherches physiologiques et cliniques sur le liquide cephalo-rachidien ou cérébro-spinal.* Paris, Méquignon-Marvis.

MAGNUS, R.

1914. "Welche Teile des Zentralnervensystems müssen für das Zustandekommen der tonischen Hals- und Labyrinthreflexe auf die Körpermuskulatur vorhanden sein," *Pflügers Arch.*, 159:224–249.

1925. "Animal posture," *Proc. R. Soc.*, 98B:339–353.

MAGOUN, H. W.

1944. "Bulbar inhibition and facilitation of motor activity," *Science*, 100:549–550.

1963. *The waking brain.* 2d ed. Springfield, Ill., Thomas.

MAHAFFY, J. P.

1880. *Descartes.* Edinburgh, Blackwood.

MAJOR, R. H.

1932. "Raymond Vieussens and his treatise on the heart," *Ann. med. Hist.*, 4 (n.s.):147–154.

MALACARNE, C. G., and MALACARNE, V. G.

1819. *Memorie storiche intorno alla vita e alle opere di Michele Vincenzo Giacinto Malacarne da Saluzzo, anatomico e chirurgo.* Padua, Tip. del Seminario.

MALACARNE, M. V. G.

1776. *Nuova esposizione della struttura del cervelletto umano.* Turin, Briolo. Reprinted in Malacarne's *Encefalotomia nuova universale*, Turin, Briolo, 1780, pt. 3, pp. 17–129, under the title "Notizie generali intorno a tutte le parti che entrano nella composizione del cervelletto umano."

MALL, F. P.

1905. "Wilhelm His, his relations to institutions of learning," *Am. J. Anat.*, 4:139–161.

MALPIGHI, M.

1665. "De cerebro epistola," pp. 1–46 of *Tetras anatomicarum epistolarum de lingua et cerebro.* Bologna, Benati. There is a partial English translation in Gordon (1817).

1666. *De viscerum structura exercitatio anatomica.* Bologna, Montius.

MARCHAND, J. F., and HOFF, H. E.

1955. "Translation of Felice Fontana: the law of irritability," *J. Hist. Med.*, 10:197–206, 302–326, 339–420.

MARCHI, V.

1888. "On the minute structures of the corpora striata and the thalami optici," *Alien. Neurol.*, 9:1–23.

MARCHI, V., and ALGERI, G.
1885–1886. "Sulle degenerazioni discendenti consecutive a lesioni sperimentale in diverse zone delle corteccia cerebrale," *Riv. sper. Freniatria Med. legal.,* 11:492–494, 12:208–252.

MARIE, P.
1906. "Revision de la question de l'aphasie; l'aphasie de 1861 à 1866; essai critique historique sur la genèse de la doctrine de Broca," *Sem. méd.,* 26:241–247, 493–500, 565–571.

MARION, H.
1882. "François Glisson," *Rev. phil.,* 14:121–155.

MARQUANDT, M.
1949. *Paul Ehrlich.* London, Heinemann.

MARSHALL, C.
1936. "The functions of the pyramidal tracts," *Q. Rev. Biol.,* 11:35–56.

MARX, K. F. H.
1838. *Herophilus: ein Beitrag zur Geschichte der Medicin.* Karlsruh, Marx.
1873. *Konrad Victor Schneider und die Katarrhe.* Göttingen, Dieterich.

MASSA, N.
1536. *Liber introductorius anatomiae, sive dissectionis corporis humani, nunc primum ab ipso auctore in lucem aeditus.* Venice, Bindonus & Pasinus.

MATTEUCCI, C.
1838. "Sur le courant électrique ou propre de la grenouille," *Bibl. univ. Genève,* 7:156–168.
1840. *Essai sur les phénomènes électriques des animaux.* Paris, Carillian, Goeury & Dalmont.
1842*a.* "Deuxième mémoire sur la courant électrique propre de la grenouille et sur celui des animaux á sang froid," *Annls. Chim. Phys.,* 6 (3d ser.):301–339.
1842*b.* "Sur un phénomène physiologique produit par les muscles en contraction," *Annls. Chim Phys.,* 6 (3d ser.):339–343.
1844. *Traité des phénomènes électro-physiologiques des animaux.* Paris, Fortin, Masson.
1847. *Lectures on the physical phenomena of living beings,* translated by J. Pereira. London, Longman, Brown, Green, & Longman.

MAYO, H.
1822–1823. *Anatomical and physiological commentaries.* No. 1, August 1822; no. 2, July 1823. London, Underwood.

McCULLOCH, W. S.
1940. "Joannes Gregorius Dusser de Barenne (1885–1940)," *Yale J. Biol. Med.,* 12:743–746.

McGILL UNIVERSITY. THE NEUROLOGICAL INSTITUTE
1936. *Neurological biographies and addresses.* London.

McINTYRE, A. R.
1947. *Curare. Its history, nature and clinical use.* Chicago, University of Chicago Press.

McKEAG, A. J.
1902. *The sensation of pain and the theory of specific sense energies.* Boston, Ginn.

MEDICI, M.
1845. *Elogio di Luigi Galvani.* Bologna, Volpe.
1857. *Compendio storico della scuola anatomica di Bologna.* Bologna, Volpe & Sassi.

MEIER, F. X.
1937. *Über den Versuch Borellis, die Physiologie der Bewegung mit Hilfe der Mechanik zu beschreiben.* Munich, Hohenhaus. Inaugural dissertation.

MERCIER, C.
1912. "The late Dr. Hughlings Jackson," *Br. med. J.,* i:85–86.

MEYER, A., and HIERONS, R.
1962. "Observations on the history of the 'Circle of Willis,'" *Med. Hist.,* 6:119–130.
1965. "On Thomas Willis's concepts of neurophysiology: Part II," *Med. Hist.,* 9:142–155.

MEYER, G. H.
1843. "Glisson's Irritabilitäts– und Sensibilitätslehre," *Arch. ges. Med.,* 5:1–17.

MEYNERT, T.
1867–1868. "Der Bau der Gross-Hirnrinde und seine örtlichen Verschiedenheiten, nebst einem pathologisch-anatomischen Corollarium," *Vjschr. Psychiat.,* Vienna, 1:77–93, 198–217, 2:88–113.
1872. "Vom Gehirne der Säugethiere," in Stricker (1869–1872, II, 694–808); English translation, "The brain of mammals," in Stricker (1870–1873, II, 367–537); also in *A manual of histology,* New York, Wood, 1872, pp. 650–766.
1884. *Psychiatrie: Klinik der Erkrankungen des Vordeshirns . . . . Erste Hälfte.* Vienna, Braumüller.
1885. *Psychiatry. A clinical treatise on diseases of the fore brain . . . . Part I,* translated by B. Sachs. New York, Putnam.

MILLEN, J. W., and WOOLLAM, D. H. M.
1962. *The anatomy of the cerebrospinal fluid.* London, Oxford University Press.

MILLER, F. R., and BANTING, F. G.
1922. "Observations on cerebellar stimulations," *Brain,* 45:104–112.

MINKOWSKI, M.
1911. "Zur Physiologie der Sehsphäre," *Pflügers Arch.,* 141:171–327.
1931. "Constantin von Monakow 1853–1930," *Schweiz. Arch. Neurol. Psychiat.,* 27:1–63.

MISTICHELLI, D.
1709. *Trattato dell'apoplessia.* Rome, Rossi.

M'KENDRICK, J. G.
1899. *Hermann Ludwig Ferdinand von Helmholtz.* London, Unwin.

MOELI, C.
1890. *Zur Erinnerung an Carl Westphal.* Berlin, Hirschwald.

MONAKOW, C. VON
1870. "Über einen bisher nicht beschriebenen Nervenfaserstrang," *Arch. Psychiat. NervKrankh.,* 2:364–366.
1882a. "Über einige durch Exstirpation circumscripter Hirnrindenregionen bedingte Entwickelungshemmungen des Kaninchengehirns," *Arch. Psychiat. NervKrankh.,* 12:141–156.
1882b. "Weitere Mittheilungen über durch Exstirpation circumscripter Hirnrindenregionen bedingte Entwickelungshemmungen des Kaninchengehirns," *Arch. Psychiat. NervKrankh.,* 12:535–549.
1911. "Lokalisation der Hirnfunktionen," *J. Neurol. Psychiat.,* 17:185–200; full English translation in Bonin (1960, pp. 231–250).

1914. *Die Lokalisation im Grosshirn und der Abbau der Funktion durch kortikale Herde.* Wiesbaden, Bergmann.

MONDELLA, F.

1961. "Giulio Cesare Aranzio," *Dizionario biografico degli Italiani,* Rome, Istituto della Enciclopedia Italiana, III, 720–721.

MONDINO

1925. *The Fasciculo de medicina* Venice 1493, with an introduction by C. Singer, pt. 1. Florence, Lier.

1930. *Mondino de' Liucci anatomia,* edited by L. Sighinolfi. Bologna, Cappelli.

MONRO, A., PRIMUS

1746. *The anatomy of the human bones and nerves [etc.].* 4th ed. Edinburgh, Hamilton & Balfour.

1758. *The same.* 6th ed. Edinburgh, Hamilton & Balfour.

1781. *The works of Alexander Monro M.D.* Edinburgh, Elliot.

MONRO, A., SECUNDUS

1779. [Untitled communication on the nerve fibre], *Med. phil. Comment. Soc. in Edinburgh,* 6 (i):111–113.

1783. *Observations on the structure and functions of the nervous system.* Edinburgh, Creech & Johnson.

MOORE, N.

1949. "Francis Glisson, M.D.," *Dictionary of National Biography,* London, Oxford University Press, VII, 1316–1317.

MOREAU, J. L.

1805. "Discours sur la vie et les ouvrages de Vicq d'Azyr," pp. 1–88 in *Oeuvres de Vicq d'Azyr,* Paris, Duprat-Duverger.

MORGAGNI, G. B.

1761. *De sedibus et causis morborum,* I. Venice, Remondiniana.

MORUZZI, G.

1955. "Luigi Luciani," *Scientia med. ital.* [English edition], 3:381–389.

1963. "The electrophysiological work of Carlo Matteucci," in Belloni (1963, pp. 139–147).

1964. "L'opera elettrofisiologica di Carlo Matteucci," *Physis,* 6:101–140.

MOSSO, A.

1881. *Über den Kreislauf im menschlichen Gehirn.* Leipzig, Veit.

MOTT, F. W.

1894. "The sensory motor functions of the central convolutions of the cerebral cortex," *J. Physiol., London,* 15:464–487.

1913. "The late Professor Edwin Goldmann's investigations of the central nervous system by vital staining," *Br. med. J.,* ii:871–873.

MÜLLER, J.

1826. *Zur vergleichenden Physiologie des Gesichtssinnes des Menschen und der Thiere.* Leipzig, Cnobloch.

1831. "Bestätigung des Bell'schen Lehrsatzes, dass die doppelten Wurzeln der Rückenmarksnerven verschiedene Functionen haben, durch neue und entscheidende Experimente," *Notiz. Gebiete Nat.-Heilk, Erfurt,* 30:cols. 113–117. There is an extended French version: "Nouvelles expériences sur l'effet que produit l'irritation mécanique et galvanique sur les racines des nerfs spinaux," *Annls. Sci. nat.,* Paris, 1831, 23:95–112.

1835. *Handbuch der Physiologie des Menschen für Vorlesungen,* I. 2d ed. Coblenz, Hölscher.

1838. *Elements of physiology*, translated by W. Baly, Vol. I. London, Taylor & Walton. This translation has been severely criticized for incompleteness and inaccuracy.

MÜNZER, F. T.
1939. "The discovery of the *cell of Schwann* in 1839," *Q. Rev. Biol.*, 14:387–407.

MUNK, H.
1877. "Zur Physiologie der Grosshirnrinde," *Berl. klin. Wschr.*, 14:505–506.

1881. *Über die Functionen der Grosshirnrinde. Gesammelte Mittheilungen aus den Jahre 1877–80*. Berlin, Hirschwald. The third *Mittheilung*, pp. 28–53, appears in English translation in Bonin (1960, pp. 97–117).

1890. "Of the visual area of the cerebral cortex, and its relation to eye movements [trans. F. W. Mott]," *Brain*, 13:45–67.

MUNK, W.
1878. *The roll of the Royal College of Physicians of London*. 2d ed. London, by the College. 3 vols.

NACHMANSOHN, D.
1959. *Chemical and molecular basis of nerve activity*. New York, Academic Press.

NAGEOTTE, J.
1922. "Louis-Antoine Ranvier," *C. r. Soc. Biol.*, Paris, 86:1144–1152.

NATHAN, P. W., and SMITH, M. C.
1955. "The Babinski response. A review and new observations," *J. Neurol. Neurosurg. Psychiat.*, 18:250–259.

NEMESIUS OF EMESA
1955. *The nature of man*, in *Cyril of Jerusalem and Nemesius of Emesa*, translated and edited by W. Telfer. Philadelphia, Westminster Press. There is an unreliable seventeenth century English translation: *The character of man*. London, Crofts, 1657.

NEUBURGER, M.
1897. *Die historische Entwicklung der experimentellen Gehirn und Rückenmarksphysiologie vor Flourens*. Stuttgart, Enke.

1910. "Ludwig Türck als Neurologe," *Jb. Psychiat. Neurol.*, 31:1–21.

1913. *Johann Christian Reil*. Stuttgart, Enke.

NIELSEN, J. M.
1936. *Agnosia apraxia aphasia. Their value in cerebral localization*. 2d ed. New York, Hoeber.

1963. "The myelogenetic studies of Paul Flechsig," *Bull. Los Angeles Neurol. Soc.*, 28:127–134.

NIESCHLAG, E.
1965. "Otto Deiters (1834–1863)," *Med. Welt*, no. 4, pp. 222–226.

NIGST, H.
1947. *Das anatomische Werk Johann Jakob Wepfers*. Aarau, Sauerländer.

NISSL, F.
1894. "Über die sogenannten Granula der Nervenzellen," *Neurol. Zbl.*, 13:676–685, 781–789, 810–814.

1895. "Bernhard von Gudden's hirnanatomische Experimentaluntersuchungen zusammengefasst dargestellt," *Allg. Z. Psychiat.*, 51:527–549.

NOBILI, L.
1825. "Über einen neuen Galvanometer," *J. Chem. Phys.*, Nuremberg, 45:249–254.

OLMSTED, J. M. D.
1939. *Claude Bernard, physiologist*. London, Cassell.

1943. "The aftermath of Charles Bell's famous 'Idea,'" *Bull. Hist. Med.*, 14:341–351.

1944. *François Magendie.* New York, Schuman.

1946. *Charles-Édouard Brown-Séquard. A nineteenth century neurologist and endocrinologist.* Baltimore, Johns Hopkins University Press.

1952. *Claude Bernard and the experimental method in medicine.* New York, Schuman.

1953. "Pierre Flourens," in *Science, medicine and history. Essays . . . in honour of Charles Singer.* London, Oxford University Press, II, 290–302.

O'Malley, C. D.

1964. *Andreas Vesalius of Brussels 1514–1564.* Berkeley, University of California Press.

O'Malley, C. D., and Saunders, J. B. DeC. M.

1952. *Leonardo da Vinci on the human body.* New York, Schuman.

Oppenheimer, J. M.

1966. "Ross Harrison's contribution to experimental embryology," *Bull. Hist. Med.*, 40:525–543.

Ortlob, F.

1694. *Nova anatomia ratiociniis illustrata.* Württemberg, Kühn.

Osterhout, W. J. V.

1931. "Physiological studies of single plant cells," *Biol. Rev.*, 6:369–411.

Osterhout, W. J. V., and Hill, S. E.

1929–1930. "Salt-bridges and negative variations," *J. gen. Physiol.*, 13:547–552.

Overton, E.

1902a. "Beiträge zur allgemeinen Muskel- und Nervenphysiologie," *Pflügers Arch.*, 92:115–280.

1902b. "Beiträge zur allgemeinen Muskel- und Nervenphysiologie, II. Mittheilung. Über der Unentbehrlichkeit von Natrium- (oder Lithium-) Ionen für den Contractionsact des Muskels," *Pflügers Arch.*, 92:346–386.

Owen, R.

1835. "On the anatomy of the cheetah, Felis Jubata, Schreb," *Trans. Zool. Soc. London,* 1:129–136.

1842. "Lectures on the anatomy and physiology of the nervous system," *Med. Times, London,* 7:1, 35, 75–76, 101.

1868. *On the anatomy of vertebrates,* III. London, Longman, Green.

1894. *The life of Richard Owen.* London, Murray. 2 vols.

Pacchioni, A.

1705. *Dissertatio epistolaris de glandulis conglobatis durae meningis humanae, indeque ortis lymphaticis ad piam meningen productis.* Rome. In the present work reference has been made to the *Opera*, Rome, Pagliarini, 1741, in which the "Epistola de inventione glandularum et lymphaticorum durae matris . . ." is to be found on pp. 123–134.

Pagel, J.

1901. "Hermann Munk," *Biographisches Lexikon hervorragender Ärzte des neunzehnten Jahrhunderts.* Berlin, Urban & Schwarzenberg, cols. 1177–1178.

1895. "Gabriel Gustav Valentin," *Allgemeine deutsche Biographie*, Leipzig, Dunker & Humblot, XXXIX, 463–464.

Pagel, W.

1958. "Mediaeval and renaissance contributions to knowledge of the brain and its functions," pp. 95–114 in *The History and philosophy of the brain and its functions*. Oxford, Blackwell.

PAGET, S.
1919. *Sir Victor Horsley. A study of his life and work*. London, Constable.

PANIZZA, B.
1855. "Osservazioni sul nervo ottico," *G. I. r. Ist. Lombardo Sci. Lett. Arti Biblioteca ital.*, 7:237–252.

PAOLETTI, I.
1963. "La scoperta, sulla struttura della corteccia cerebrale, di Francesco Gennari (1752–1797) anatomico parmense: la stria del Gennari," *Minerva Med.*, 54:1574–1580.

PAVLOV, I. P.
1907. [Untitled Nobel Oration], in *Les prix Nobel en 1904*. Stockholm, Norstedt & Söner.
1913. "The investigation of the higher nervous functions," *Br. med. J.*, ii:973–978.
1928–1941. Lectures on conditioned reflexes, translated by W. H. Gantt. London, Lawrence. 2 vols.

PEKELHARING, C. A.
1919. "Franciscus Cornelis Donders," *Janus*, 24:57–76.

PELOUZE, T. J., and BERNARD, C.
1850. "Recherches sur le curare," *C. r. Acad. Sci., Paris*, 31:533–537.

PENFIELD, W.
1947. "Some observations on the cerebral cortex in man," *Proc. R. Soc.*, 134B:329–347.

PENFIELD, W., and BOLDREY, E.
1937. "Somatic motor and sensory representation in the cerebral cortex of man as studied by electrical stimulation," *Brain*, 60:389–443.

PETELLA, J. B.
1901. "La décourverte du centre visuel cortical revendiquée par un anatomiste italien," *Janus*, 6:629–635.

PETROV, B. D.
1954. *The role of Russian scientists in medicine*. Moscow, State Medical Literature Publishing House.

PFAFF, C. H.
1795. *Über thierische Elektricität und Reizbarkeit. Ein Beytrag zu den neuesten Entdeckungen über diese Gegenstände*. Leipzig, Crusius.

PFEIFER, R. A.
1928. *Die angioarchitektonik der Grosshirnrinde*. Berlin, Springer.
1930a. *Grundlegende Untersuchungen für die Angioarchitektonik des menschlichen Gehirns*. Berlin, Springer.
1930b. "Nekrolog. Paul Flechsig. Sein Leben und sein Wirken," *Schweiz. Arch. Neurol. Psychiat.*, 26:258–264.
1940. *Die angioarchitektonische areale Gliederung der Grosshirnrinde*. Leipzig, Thieme.
1952. "Professor Dr. phil. et med. Richard Arwed Pfeifer zum 75. Geburtstag am 21. 11. 1952," *Psychiat. Neurol. med. Psychol.*, 4:349.

PFLÜGER, E. F. N.
1859. *Untersuchungen über die Physiologie des Electrotonus*. Berlin, Hirschwald.

PICCOLOMINI, A.
1586. *Anatomicae praelectiones explicantes mirificam corporis humani fabricam.*
Rome, Bonfadinus.

PIERRO, F.
1965. *Arcangelo Piccolomini Ferrarese (1525–1586) e la sua importanza nell'anatomia postvesaliana.* Ferrara, Università degli Studi. (Quaderni di storia della scienza e della medicina vi.)

PIZZOLI, U.
1897. *Marcello Malpighi e l'opera sua. Scritti varii di G. Atti [et al.] raccolti da U. Pizzoli.* Milan, Vallardi.

PLATO
1892. *The dialogues of Plato,* translated by B. Jowett, II. 3d ed. Oxford, Clarendon Press.
1937. *Plato's cosmology. The Timaeus,* translated with a running commentary by F. M. Cornford. London, Routledege & Kegan Paul.

PLATT, W. B.
1896. "Johannes Müller, a university teacher," *Bull. Johns Hopkins Hosp.,* 7:16–18.

PORTAL, A.
1770–1773. *Histoire de l'anatomie et de la chirurgie.* Paris, Didot, 6 vols. in 7.

POURFOUR DU PETIT, F.
1710. *Lettres d'un medecin des hôpitaux du roy a un autre medecin de ses amis.* Namur, Albert.

POWER, D'A.
1950. "Augustus Volney Waller," *Dictionary of National Biography,* London, Oxford University Press, XX, 579–580.

PRAXAGORAS
1958. *The fragments of Praxagoras of Cos and his school,* collected, edited, and translated by F. Steckerl. Leiden, Brill.

PRESTON, C.
1695–1697. "An account of a child born alive without a brain, and his observables in it on dissection," *Phil. Trans. R. Soc.,* 19:457–467.

PROCHÁSKA, J.
1784. *Adnotationum academicarum. Fasciculus tertius.* Prague, Gerle. There is a partial English translation in Unzer (1851, pp. 429 ff.).

PUPILLI, G. C., and FADIGA, E.
1963. "The origins of electrophysiology," *J. Wld. Hist.,* 8:547–589.

PURKYNĚ, J. E.
1838. *Bericht über die Versammlung deutscher Naturforscher und Ärzte in Prag im September, 1837.* Prague. Pt. 3, sec. 5, A. Anatomisch-physiologische Verhandlungen, pp. 177–180. This report of the paper read by Purkyně on 23 September 1837 has been reprinted in his *Opera selecta,* Prague, pp. 111–114.

PURKYNĚ SOCIETY
1937. *In memoriam: Joh. Ev. Purkyně 1787–1937.* Prague, Purkyně Society.

QUINCKE, H.
1891. "Über hydrocephalus," *Verh. Congress. inn. Med., Wiesbaden,* 10:321–339; there is an English translation in *J. Neurosurg.,* 1965, 32:294–304.

RAMÓN Y CAJAL, S.
1888a. "Estructura de los centros nerviosos de los aves," *Rev. trimest. Histol. norm. patol.,* 1:305–315.
1888b. "Estructura del cerebelo," *Gac. méd. Catalana,* 11:449–457.

1891. "Sur la structure de l'écorce cérébrale de quelques mammifères," *Cellule*, 7:123–176.

1894. "La fine structure des centres nerveux," *Proc. R. Soc.*, 55:444–468.

1908. "Structure et connexions des neurones," *Les Prix Nobel en 1906*. Stockholm, Norstedt & Söner, pp. 1–25, separate pagination.

1909–1911. *Histologie du système nerveux de l'homme et des vertébrés*, translated by L. Azoulay. Paris, Maloine. 2 vols.

1913–1914. *Estudios sobre la degeneración y regeneración del sistema nervioso*. Madrid. 2 vols.

1928. *Degeneration and regeneration of the nervous system*, translated by R. M. May. London, H. Milford. 2 vols.

1923. *Recuerdos de mi vida*. 3d ed. Pueyo.

1937. *Recollections of my life*, translated by E. H. Craigie and J. Cano. Philadelphia, American Philosophical Society.

1933. "Neuronismo o reticularismo? Las pruebas objectivas de la unidad anatómica, de las celulas nerviosas," *Archos. Neurobiol.*, 13:217–291, 579–646. Reprint: *Neuronismo o reticularismo?* Madrid, Instituto Ramón y Cajal, 1952. There is a German version: "Die Neuronenlehre," in O. Bumke and O. Foerster, *Handbuch der Neurologie*, Vol. I, "Anatomie," Berlin, Springer, 1935, 887–994; English translation: *Neuron theory or reticular theory. Objective evidence of the anatomical unity of nerve cells*, translated by M. U. Purkiss and C. A. Fox, Madrid, Instituto Ramón y Cajal, 1954.

1955. *Studies on the cerebral cortex [limbic structures]*, translated by L. M. Kraft. London, Lloyd-Luke.

1959. *Degeneration and regeneration of the nervous system*, translated by R. M. May. New York, Hafner. 2 vols.

RAND, C. W.
1953. "The role of the astrocyte in the formation of cerebral scars with an introduction to Cajal's contribution to our knowledge of neuroglia," *Bull. Los Angeles Neurol. Soc.*, 17:57–70.

RANDAL, B. A.
1902. "The debt of otology to Helmholtz," *J. Am. Med. Assoc.*, 38 (i):561–562.

RANDALL, J. H., Jr.
1960. *Aristotle*. New York, Columbia University Press.

RANKE, J.
1887. "Alexander Ecker," *Arch. Anthrop.*, 17:i–vi.

RANVIER, L.-A.
1871. "Contributions à l'histologie et à la physiologie des nerfs periphériques," *C. r. hebd. Acad. Sci., Paris*, 73:1168–1171.

1872. "Recherches sur l'histologie et la physiologie des nerfs," *Archs. Physiol. norm. path.*, 4:129–149.

RASMUSSEN, A. T.
1947. *Some trends in neuroanatomy*. Dubuque, Iowa, Brown.

RAWSON, N. R.
1932. "The story of the cerebellum," *Canadian Med. Assoc. J.*, 26:220–225.

REIL, J. C.
1795. "Über den Bau des Hirns und der Nerven," [Gren's] *Neues J. Phys., Lpz.*, 1:96–114; reprinted in Reil (1817, pp. 113–132) with the title extended by the phrase "In einem Schreiben an Gren."

1807–1808*a*. "Fragmente über die Bildung des kleinen Gehirns im Menschen," *Arch. Physiol., Halle*, 8:1–58.

1807–1808*b*. "Untersuchungen über den Bau des kleinen Gehirns im Menschen. Zweyte Fortsetzung, über die Organisation der Lappen und Läppchen," *Arch. Physiol., Halle*, 8:385–426.

1809*a*. "Untersuchungen über den Bau des grossen Gehirns im Menschen . . . . Vierte Fortsetzung VIII," *Arch. Physiol., Halle*, 9:136–146.

1809*b*. "Das Hirnschenkel-System oder die Hirnschenkel-Organisation im grossen Gehirn," *Arch. Physiol., Halle*, 9:147–171; condensed version in Neuburger (1913, pp. 85–86).

1809*c*. "Das Balken-System oder die Balken-Organisation im grossen Gehirn," *Arch. Physiol., Halle*, 9:172–195.

1809*d*. "Die sylvische Grube," *Arch. Physiol., Halle*, 9:195–208.

1817. *Kleine Schriften*. Halle, Curt.

1960. "Johann Christian Reil," *Nova Acta Leopoldina*, 22 (n.s.):no. 144; papers by H.-H. Eulner, J.-H. Scharf, K. Ponitz, W. Piechocki.

Reisch, G.

1503. *Margarita philosophica*. Freiburg im Breisgau, Schott.

Remak, R.

1836. "Verläufige Mittheilung mikroscopischer Beobachtungen über den innern Bau der Cerebrospinalnerven und über die Entwicklung ihrer Formelemente," *Arch. Anat. Physiol.*, pp. 145–161.

1837. Weitere mikroscopische Beobachtungen über die Primitivfasern des Nervensystems der Wirbelthiere," [Froriep's] *Neue Notizen*, 3: cols. 35–40.

1838. *Observationes anatomicae et microscopicae de systematis nervosi structura*. Berlin, Reimer.

1841. "Anatomische Beobachtungen über das Gehirn, das Rückenmark und die Nervenwurzeln," *Arch. Anat. Physiol.*, pp. 506–522.

1844. "Neurologische Erläuterungen," *Arch. Anat. Physiol.*, pp. 463–472.

1824. "Researches of Malacarne and Reil—present state of cerebral anatomy," *Edin. med. surg. J.*, 21:98–141.

Révész, B.

1917. *Geschichte des Seelenbegriffes und der Seelenlokalisation*. Stuttgart, Enke.

Rieder, R.

1906. *Carl Weigert und seine Bedeutung für die medizinische Wissenschaft unserer Zeit. Ein biographische Skizze*. Berlin, Springer.

Riese, W.

1959. *A history of neurology*. New York, MD Publications.

Riese, W., and Arrington, G. E.

1963. "The history of Johannes Müller's doctrine of the specific energies of the senses: original and later versions," *Bull. Hist. Med.*, 37:179–183.

Riese, W., and Hoff, E. C.

1950–1951. "A history of the doctrine of cerebral localization," *J. Hist. Med.*, 5:50–71, 6:439–470.

Ritchie, A. D.

1947. "Sherrington as a philosopher," *Br. med. J.*, ii:812–813.

Ritti, A.

1892. "Éloge de J. Baillarger," *Annls. méd.-psychol.*, 16:5–58.

Robertson, W. F.

1899. "Normal and pathological histology of the nerve-cell," *Brain*, 22:203–327.

ROLANDO, L.

1809. *Saggio sopra la vera struttura del cervello dell'uomo e degl'animali, e sopra le funzioni del sistema nervoso.* Sassari, Stampa Privileg. Annotated French translation by Flourens: "Expériences sur les fonctions du système nerveux," *J. Physiol. expér. path.,* 1823, 3:95–113.

1831. "Della struttura degli emisferi cerebrali," *Mem. r. Accad. Sci. Torino,* 35:103–146.

ROLLESTON, J. D.

1930–1931. "Jean-Baptiste Bouillaud (1796–1881). A pioneer in cardiology and neurology," *Proc. R. Soc. Med.,* 24:1253–1262.

ROOK, A.

1964. *The origins and growth of biology.* London, Penguin.

ROSIN, H.

1894. "Entgegnung auf Nissl's Bemerkungen: Über Rosin's neue Färbemethode des gesammten Nervensystems und dessen Bemerkungen über Ganglienzellen," *Neurol. Zbl.,* 13:210–214.

ROSS, W. D.

1923. *Aristotle. A complete exposition of his works and thought.* London, Methuen.

ROTHMANN, M.

1909. "Hermann Munk zum 70. Geburtstag," *Dt. med. Wschr.,* 35:258–259.

1912. "Hermann Munk," *Neurol. Zbl.,* 31:1343–1344.

ROTHSCHUH, K. E.

1958. "Vom spiritus animalis zum Nervenaktionsstrom," *Ciba Z.,* 8:2951–2980.

1963. "Die neurophysiologischen Beiträge von Galvani und Volta," in Belloni, (1963a, pp. 117–130).

1964a. *Von Boerhaave bis Berger. Die Entwicklung der kontinentalen Physiologie im 18. und 19. Jahrhundert mit besonderer Berücksichtigung der Neurophysiologie,* edited by K. E. Rothschuh. Stuttgart, Fischer.

1964b. "Emil du Bois-Reymond (1818–1896) und die Elektrophysiologie der Nerven," in Rothschuh (1964a, pp. 85–105).

ROY, C. S., and SHERRINGTON, C. S.

1890. "On the regulation of the blood supply of the brain," *J. Physiol., London,* 11:85–108.

1897a. "Charles Smart Roy, M.S. Cantab., M.D. Edin., F.R.S.," *Lancet,* ii:954.

1897b. "Obituary. Charles Smart Roy, M.A., M.D., F.R.S.," *Br. med. J.,* ii:1031–1032.

RUDOLPH, G.

1959. "Albrecht von Haller (1708–1777)," *Annls. Univ. sarav.,* 2. Medizin, 7:273–289.

1964. "Hallers Lehre von der Irritabilität und Sensibilität," in Rothschuh (1964a, pp. 14–34).

RÜDINGER

1881. "Emil Huschke," *Allgemeine Deutsche Biographie,* Leipzig, Duncker & Humblot, XIII, 449–451.

RUFUS OE EPHESUS

1879. *Oeuvres de Rufus d'Ephèse,* translated by C. Daremberg and C. E. Ruelle. Paris, Imprimerie Nationale. 2 vols.

RUYSCH, F.

1737–1744. *Opera omnia anatomico-medico-chirurgica,* I–III. Amsterdam, Jansson-Waesberg.

SABIN, F. R.
  1905. "On Flechsig's investigation of the brain," *Bull. Johns Hopkins Hosp.*, 16:45–49.
SACHS, B.
  1910. "Raymond de Vieussens. Noted neuro-anatomist and physician of the XVIIth century," *Proc. Charaka Club*, 3:99–105.
SAINT-GERMAIN, B. DE
  1869. *Descartes considéré comme physiologiste et comme médecin.* Paris, Masson.
SALOMONSEN, C. J.
  1915. *Adolph Hannovers liv og virken særligt i ungdomsaarene.* Tilskueren.
SAMOGGIA, L.
  1965. "I rapporti fra Francesco Aglietti e Vincenzo Malacarne in una lettera inedita del 1789," *Pag. Stor. Med.*, 9:54–68.
SANTESSON, C. G.
  1902. "Axel Key," *Münch. med. Wschr.*, 49:242–243.
SARTON, G.
  1954. *Galen of Pergamon.* Lawrence, Kansas, University of Kansas Press.
SCARFF, J. E.
  1940. "Primary cortical centers for movements of upper and lower limbs in man. Observations based on electrical stimulation," *Arch. Neurol. Psychiat.*, 44:243–299.
SCHÄFER, E. A. See SHARPEY-SCHÄFER, E. A.
SCHERZ, G.
  1958. *Nicolas Steno and his Indice.* Copenhagen, Munksgaard.
SCHIERBEEK, A.
  1959. *Measuring the invisible world. The life and works of Antoni van Leeuwenhoek, F.R.S.* New York, Abelard-Schuman.
SCHILLER, F.
  1965. "The rise of the 'enteroid processes' in the 19th century: some landmarks in cerebral nomenclature," *Bull. Hist. Med.*, 39:326–338.
SCHMIDT, C. F.
  1944. "The present status of knowledge concerning the intrinsic control of the cerebral circulation and the effects of functional derangements in it," *Fedn. Proc.* 3:131–139.
  1950. *The cerebral circulation in health and disease.* Springfield, Ill., Thomas.
  1961. "Pharmacology in a changing world," *Ann. Rev. Physiol.*, 23:1–13.
SCHMIDT, C. F., and DUMKE, P. R.
  1943. "Quantitative measurements of cerebral blood flow in the macacque monkey," *Am. J. Physiol.*, 138:421–431.
SCHOEPS, C. G.
  1827. "Über die Verrichtungen verschiedener Theile des Nervensystems," *Arch. Anat. Physiol.*, pp. 368–416.
SCHUBERT, G. H. VON
  1877. *Die Geschichte der Seele.* 6th ed. Stuttgart, Cotta.
SCHULTZE, F.
  1922. "Wilhelm Erb," *Dt. Z. NervHeilk.*, 73:i–xviii.
SCHUMACHER, J.
  1963. *Antike Medizin.* 2d ed. Berlin, de Gruyter.

Schwann, T.
  1839. *Mikroskopische Untersuchungen über die Übereinstimmung in der Struktur und dem Wachsthum der Thiere und Pflanzen*. Berlin, Reimer.
  1847. *Microscopical researches*, translated by H. Smith. London, Sydenham Society.
Sechenov, I. M.
  1863. *Physiologische Studien über die Hemmungsmechanismen für die Reflexthätigkeit des Rückenmarkes im Gehirne des Frosches*. Berlin, Hirschwald. Reprinted in Sechenov (1935, pp. 153–176).
  1935. *Selected works*. Moscow, State Publishing House.
  1962. *Selected physiological and psychological works*. Moscow, Foreign Languages Publishing House.
  1965. *Autobiographical notes*. Washington, D.C., American Institute of Biological Sciences.
Seguin, E. C.
  1883. "Gudden's atrophy method: and a summary of its results," *Arch. Med., New York*, 10:126–145, 235–270.
Seller, W.
  1864. "Memoir of the life and writings of Robert Whytt, M.D. Professor of Medicine in the University of Edinburgh from 1747 to 1766," *Trans. R. Soc. Edin.*, 23:99–131.
Semelaigne, R.
  1930. *Les pionniers de la psychiatrie française avant et après Pinel*, I. Paris, Baillière.
Sharp, J. A.
  1961. "Alexander Monro Secundus and the interventricular foramen," *Med. Hist.*, 5:83–89.
Sharpey-Schäfer, E. A.
  1900. *Text book of physiology*, II. Edinburgh, Pentland.
  1935a. Obituary notice. *Br. med. J.*, i:740–742.
  1935b. Obituary notice. *Lancet*, i:843–845.
Sharpey-Schäfer, E. A., and Brown, S. M.
  1888. "An investigation into the functions of the occipital and temporal lobes of the monkey's brain," *Phil. Trans. R. Soc.*, 179B:303–327.
Shaternikov, M. N.
  1935. "The life of I. M. Sechenov," in Sechenov (1935, pp. vii–xxxvi).
Shedlovsky, T.
  1964. "W. J. V. Osterhout, 1871–1964," *Rockefeller Inst. Rev.*, 2:11–13.
Sherrington, C. S.
  1892. "Notes on the arrangement of some motor fibres in the lumbo-sacral plexus," *J. Physiol., London*, 13:621–772.
  1894. "Experiments in examination of the peripheral distribution of the fibres of the posterior roots of some spinal nerves," *Phil. Trans. R. Soc.*, 184B:641–763.
  1897a. "Cataleptoid reflexes in the monkey," *Lancet*, i:373–374.
  1897b. "On reciprocal innervation of antagonistic muscles. Third note," *Proc. R. Soc.*, 60:414–417.
  1897c. "Double (antidrome) conduction in the central nervous system," *Proc. R. Soc.*, 61:243–246.
  1898a. "Experiments in examination of the peripheral distribution of the fibres of the posterior roots of some spinal nerves—Part II," *Phil. Trans. R. Soc.*, 190B:45–186.

1898*b*. "Decerebrate rigidity, and reflex coordination of movements," *J. Physiol., London,* 22:319–332.

1899. "On the spinal animal," *Med.-chir. Trans.,* 82:449–477.

1905*a*. "C. S. Roy. 1854–1897," *Proc. R. Soc.,* 75:131–136.

1905*b*. "Correlation of reflexes and the principle of the common path," *Rep. Br. Ass. Advmt. Sci.,* 74th meeting, trans. Sec. I.—Physiology, pp. 728–741.

1906. *The integrative action of the nervous system.* New Haven, Yale University Press.

1925. *The assaying of Brabantius and other verse.* London, Oxford University Press.

1928. "Sir David Ferrier, 1843–1928," *Proc. R. Soc.,* 103B:viii–xvi.

1935. "Santiago Ramón y Cajal 1852–1934," *Obit. Not. R. Soc.,* no. 4, pp. 425–441.

1939. *Selected writings of Sir Charles Sherrington,* edited by D. Denny-Brown. London, Hamilton.

1952*a*. Obituary notice. *Br. med. J.,* i:606–609.

1952*b*. Obituary notice. *Lancet,* i:569–571.

SHERRINGTON, C. S., CREED, R. S., DENNY-BROWN, D. E., ECCLES, J. C., and LIDDELL, E. G. T.

1932. *Reflex activity of the spinal cord.* London, Oxford University Press.

SIEMERLING, E.

1890*a*. "Carl Westphal. Nekrolog," *Arch. Psychiat. NervKrankh.,* 21:I–XXII.

1890*b*. "Carl Westphal," *J. ment. Sci.,* 36:312–313.

SIGERIST, H. E.

1961. *A history of medicine,* II. New York, Oxford University Press.

SINGER, A.

1937. *Der Begriff der Irritabilität bei Glisson und bei Haller,* Munich, Kallmünz & Lassleben. Inaugural dissertation.

SINGER, C.

1925. *The evolution of anatomy.* London, Kegan Paul, Trench, Trubner.

1956. See GALEN

SISSON, S., and GROSSMAN, J. D.

1953. *The anatomy of the domestic animals.* Philadelphia, Saunders.

SNIDER, R. S.

1950. "Recent contributions to the anatomy and physiology of the cerebellum," *Arch. Neurol. Psychiat.,* 64:196–219.

1958. "The cerebellum," *Scient. American,* 199:84–90.

SNIDER, R. S., and MAGOUN, H. W.

1948. "Facilitation produced by cerebellar stimulation," *Fedn. Proc.,* 7:117–118.

1949. "Facilitation produced by cerebellar stimulation," *J. Neurophysiol.,* 12:335–345.

SOBOTTA, J.

1922. "Zum Andenken an Wilhelm von Waldeyer-Hartz," *Anat. Anz.,* 56:1–53.

SOEMMERRING, S. T.

1788. *Vom Hirn und Rückenmark.* Mainz, Winkopp.

SOLMSEN, F.

1961. "Greek Philosophy and the discovery of the nerves," *Mus. Helvet., Basel,* 18:150–167, 169–197.

SOUQUES, A.

1938. "Descartes et l'anatomo-physiologie du système nerveux," *Rev. neurol.,* 70:221–245.

SPEERT, H.
  1958. *Obstetric and gynecologic milestones.* New York, Macmillan.
SPENCER, H.
  1855. *The principles of psychology.* London, Longman, Brown, Green, & Longman.
  1904. *An autobiography.* London, Williams & Norgate. 2 vols.
SPILLMAN, R.
  1941. "Félix Vicq d'Azyr and Benjamin Franklin," *J. nerv. ment. Dis.,* 94:428–444.
SPURZHEIM, J. C.
  1817. *Examination of the objections made in Britain against the doctrines of Gall and Spurzheim.* Edinburgh, Macredie, Skelly, & Muckersy.
STECKERL. See PRAXAGORAS
STEFANI, A.
  1877. "Contribuzione alla fisiologia del cervelletto," *Atti Accad. Sci. med. nat. Ferrara,* 12:193–211.
STENO, N.
  1669. *Discours de Monsieur Stenon sur l'anatomie du cerveau.* Paris, Ninville.
  1950. *A dissertation on the anatomy of the brain,* with a preface and notes by E. Gotfredsen. Copenhagen, Busck.
  1965. *Nicolaus Steno's lecture on the anatomy of the brain,* introduction by G. Scherz. Copenhagen, Busck.
STEUDEL, J.
  1964. "Johannes Müller und die Neurophysiologie," in Rothschuh (1964a, pp. 62–70).
STEWART, T. G.
  1928. "Sir David Ferrier," *J. ment. Sci.,* 74:375–380.
STIEDA, L.
  1899. "Geschichte der Entwicklung der Lehre von den Nervenzellen und Nervenfasern während des 19. Jahrhunderts. I. Teil: von Sömmerring bis Deiters," pp. 79–196 in *Festschrift zur 70. Geburtstag von Carl v. Kupffer.* Jena, Fischer.
STIEVE, H.
  1936. "Hans Held zu seinem siebzigsten Geburtstage am 8. August 1936," Z. *mikrosk.-anat. Forsch.,* 40:1–28.
STILLING, B.
  1842a. *Untersuchungen über die Functionen Rückenmarks und der Nerven.* Leipzig, Wigand.
  1842b. *Untersuchungen über die Textur des Rückenmarks.* Leipzig, Wigand.
  1846. *Untersuchungen über den Bau und die Verrichtungen des Gehirns. I. Über den Bau des Hirnknotens der den Varoli'schen Brücke.* Jena, Mauke.
  1859. *Neue Untersuchungen über den Bau des Rückenmarks.* Cassel, Hotop.
  1878. *Neue Untersuchungen über den Bau des kleinen Gehirns des Menschen.* Cassel, Fischer. 3 vols. and atlas.
  1910. [Centenary note]. *Lancet,* i:1152–1153.
STIRLING, W.
  1881. "Historical references to the structure of nerve fibres," *J. Anat. Physiol.,* 15:446–447.
  1896–1897. "The last of a brilliant quartette of physiologists—E. du Bois-Reymond," *Med. Chron., London,* 7 (n.s.):241–250.

STOOKEY, B.

1954. "A note on the early history of cerebral localization," *Bull. N.Y. Acad. Med.*, 30:559–578.

1963. "Jean-Baptiste Bouillaud and Ernest Auburtin. Early studies on cerebral localization and the speech center," *J. Am. Med. Assoc.*, 184:1024–1029.

STRAUSS, L.

1910. "Zum 100. Geburtstag Dr. Benedikt Stilling. (22. Februar 1910)," *Münch. med. Wschr.*, 57:699–700.

STRICKER, S.

1869–1872. *Handbuch der Lehre von den Geweben des Menschen und der Thiere.* Leipzig, Engelmann. 2 vols.

1870–1873. *Manual of human and comparative histology*, translated by H. Power. London, New Sydenham Society. 3 vols.

STUDNIČKA, F. K.

1927–1928. "Joh. Ev. Purkinjes und seiner Schule Verdienste und die Entdeckung der thierschen Zellen und um die Aufstellung der Zellentheorie," *Anat. Anz.*, 64:140–144.

1931–1932. "Aus der Vorgeschichte der Zellentheorie. H. Milne Edwards, H. Dutrochet, F. Raspail, J. E. Purkinje," *Anat. Anz.*, 73:390–416.

1936. "Joh. Ev. Purkinjes histologisches Arbeiten," *Anat. Anz.*, 82:41–66.

SUDHOFF, W.

1913. "Lehre von dem Hirnventrikeln in textlicher und graphischer Tradition des Altertums und Mittelalters," *Arch. Gesch. Med.*, 7:149–205; also published separately: Leipzig.

SYLVIUS. See LE BOË, F. DE

SYMONDS, C. P.

1955. "The circle of Willis," *Br. med. J.*, i:119–124.

TAYLOR, A. E.

1956. *Plato. The man and his work.* New York, Meridian Books.

TAYLOR, J.

1912. "John Hughlings Jackson," *Dictionary of National Biography*, Supplement, 1901–111, London, Oxford University Press, pp. 356–358.

TEMKIN, O.

1946. "The philosophical background of Magendie's physiology," *Bull. Hist. Med.*, 20:10–35.

1947. "Gall and his phrenological movement," *Bull. Hist. Med.*, 21:275–321.

1964. "The classical roots of Glisson's doctrine of irritability," *Bull. Hist. Med.*, 38:297–328.

THEOPHRASTUS

1866. *Opera quae supersunt omnia, edita* Fridericus Wimmer. Paris, Firmin-Didot.

THESLEFF, S.

1964. "Ernest Overtons forskargärning," *Nordisk Med.*, 71:549–553.

THOMAS, A.

1897. *Le cervelet.* Paris, G. Steinheil. With the exception of pp. 1–40, this work appears in English translation as *Cerebellar functions.* New York, Journal of Nervous and Mental Diseases, 1912.

THOMAS, H. M.

1910. "Decussation of the pyramids—an historical inquiry," *Bull. Johns Hopkins Hosp.*, 21:304–311.

THOMAS, K. B.
1964. *Curare. Its history and usage.* London, Pitman.

THORNDIKE, L.
1943. *A history of magic and experimental science,* I. New York, Columbia University Press.

TIEDEMANN, F.
1816. *Anatomie und Bildungsgeschichte des Gehirns im Fœtus des Menschen.* Nuremberg, Steinischen Buchhandlung.
1823. *Anatomie du cerveau,* traduite par A. J. L. Jourdan. Paris, Baillière.
1826. *The anatomy of the fœtal brain,* [translated from the French edition of 1823 by W. Bennet]. Edinburgh, Carfrae.
1821. *Icones cerebri simiarum.* Heidelberg, Mohr & Winter.

TRELAT, U.
1857. "Notice sur François Leuret," in Leuret, *Anatomie comparée,* 2d ed., Paris, Baillière, I, xiii–xxxii.

TREVIRANUS, G. R.
1816. *Vermischte Schriften. Anatomischen und physiologischen Inhalts,* I. Göttingen, Röwer.

TSCHERMAK, A. V.
1919. "Julius Bernstein's Lebensarbeit. Zugleich ein Beitrag zur Geschichte der neueren Biophysik," *Pflügers Arch.,* 174:1–89. Contains a bibliography of Bernstein's writings.

TÜRCK, L.
1852. "Über sekundäre Erkrankung einzelner Rückenmarkstränge und ihrer Fortsetzungen zum Gehirne," *Z. kais. kön. Ges. Ärzte Wien,* 8 (ii):511–534.
1853. "Über sekundäre Erkrankung einzelner Rückenmarkstränge und ihrer Fortsetzungen zum Gehirne," *Z. kais. kön. Ges. Ärzte Wien,* 9 (ii):289–317.
1856. "Vorläufige Ergebnisse von Experimental-Untersuchungen zur Ermittelung der Haut-Sensibilitätsbezirke der einzelnen Rückenmarksnervenpaare," *Sber. kaisl. Akad. Wiss., Wien, Math.-nat. Kl.,* 21:586–589.
1869. "Über die Haut-Sensibilitätsbezirke der einzelnen Rückenmarksnervenpaare," *Denkschr. kaisl. Akad. Wiss., Wien, Math.-nat. Kl.,* 29:299–326.
1910. "Ludwig Türck's gesammelte neurologische Schriften," *Jb. Psychiat. Neurol.,* 31:23–194.

TURNER, A. L.
1919. *Sir William Turner, K.C.B., F.R.S.* Edinburgh, Blackwood.

TURNER, W.
1866. *The convolutions of the human cerebrum topographically considered.* Edinburgh, Maclachlan & Stewart.

UNZER, J. A.
1771. *Erste Grunde einer Physiologie der eigentlichen thierischen Natur thierischer Körper.* Leipzig, Weidermanns, Erben & Reich.
1851. *The principles of physiology, by John Augustus Unzer; and a dissertation on the functions of the nervous system by George Prochǎska,* translated by T. Laycock. London, Sydenham Society.

VALENTIN, G. G.
1836. "Über den Verlauf und die letzten Ende der Nerven," *Nova Acta phys.-med. Acad. caes. Leopold.-Carol. Nat. Curiosorum, Breslau,* 18 (i):51–240.

VANDER EECKEN, H. M.
    1959. *The anastomoses between the leptomeningeal arteries of the brain.* Springfield, Ill., Thomas.

VAROLIO, C.
    1573. *De nervis opticis nonnullisque aliis praeter communem opinionem in humano capite observatis epistolae.* Padua, Meitti. Edition used in Varolio, *Anatomicae . . . libri IIII.* Frankfurt, Wechel & Fischer, 1591.

VERGA, A.
    1869. *Sulla vita e sugli scritti di Bartolomeo Panizza.* Milan, Bernadoni.

VERVORN, M.
    1913. *Irritability.* New Haven, Yale University Press.

VESALIUS, A.
    1543. *De humani corporis fabrica libri septem.* Basel, Oporinus. There is a translation of Bk. VII by C. Singer, *Vesalius on the human brain,* London, Oxford University Press, 1952. It must, however, be used with some caution since it is based partly on the edition of 1555.

VESLING, J.
    1647. *Syntagma anatomicum.* Padua, Frambotti.

VICQ D'AZYR, F.
    1784. "Recherches sur la structure du cerveau, du cervelet, de la moelle elongée, de la moelle épinière; et sur l'origine des nerfs de l'homme et des animaux," *Hist. Acad. roy. Sci.*, 1781, pp. 495–622.
    1786. *Traité d'anatomie et de physiologie.* Paris, Didot l'Aine.

VIETS, H. R.
    1935. "Domenico Cotugno: his description of the cerebrospinal fluid," *Bull. Hist. Med.*, 3:701–738.
    1938. "West Riding, 1871–1876," *Bull. Hist. Med.*, 6:477–487.

VIETS, H. R., and GARRISON, F. H.
    1940. "Purkinje's original description of the pear-shaped cells in the cerebellum," *Bull. Hist. Med.*, 8:1397–1398.

VIEUSSENS, R. DE
    1684. *Neurographia universalis.* Lyons, Certe.

VIRCHOW, R.
    1846. "Über das granulirte Ansehen der Wanderungen der Gehirnventrikel," *Allg. Z. Psychiat., Berlin*, 3:242–250.
    1854. "Über eine im Gehirn und Rückenmark des Menschen aufgefundene Substanz mit der chemischen Reaction der Cellulose," *Arch. path. Anat. Physiol.*, 6:135–138; English translation: "On a substance presenting the chemical reaction of cellulose found in the brain and spinal cord of man," *Q. J. microscop. Sci.*, 2:101–108.
    1856. *Gesammelte Abhandlungen zur wissenschaftlichen Medizin.* Frankfurt am Main, Meidinger & Sohn.
    1867. "Zur pathologischen Anatomie des Gehirns. I. Congenitale Encephalitis und Myelitis," *Virchows Arch. path. Anat. Physiol.*, 38:129–142.

VOGT, O., and VOGT, C.
    1903. "Zur anatomischen Gliederung des Cortex cerebri," *J. Psychol. Neurol.*, 2:160–180.
    1919. "Allgemeinere Ergebnisse unserer Hirnforschung," *J. Psychol. Neurol.*, 25:273–462.

VOIT, C.
1900. "Nachruf Willy Kühne gewidmet," *Z. Biol.*, 40:I–VIII.

VOLKMANN, A. W.
1842. "Von dem Baue und den Verrichtungen der Kopfnerven des Frosches," *Arch. Anat. Physiol.*, pp. 367–377.

VOLPRECHT, A.
1895. *Die physiologischen Anschauungen des Aristoteles.* Greifswald, Abel. Inaugural dissertation.

WALDEYER-HARTZ, H. W. G. VON
1891. "Über einige neuere Forschungen im Gebiete der Anatomie des Centralnerven-systems," *Dt. med. Wschr.*, 17:1213–1218, 1244–1246, 1267–1269, 1287–1289, 1331–1332, 1352–1356.
1919–1920. "Gustaf Retzius," *Anat. Anz.*, 52:261–268.
1920. *Lebenserinnerungen.* Bonn, Cohn.

WALKER, A.
1839. *Documents and dates of modern discoveries in the nervous system.* London, Churchill.

WALKER, A. E.
1951. *A history of neurological surgery.* Baltimore, Williams & Wilkins.
1957a. "Stimulation and ablation: their role in the history of cerebral physiology," *J. Neurophysiol.*, 20:435–449.
1957b. "The development of the concept of cerebral localization in the nineteenth century," *Bull. Hist. Med.*, 31:99–121.

WALKER, W. C.
1937. "Animal electricity before Galvani," *Ann. Sci.*, 2:84–113.

WALLER, A. D.
1905. "Emil du Bois-Reymond, 1818–1896," *Proc. R. Soc.*, 75:124–127.

WALLER, A. V.
1850. "Experiments on the section of the glossopharyngeal and hypoglossal nerves of the frog, and observations of the alterations produced thereby in the structure of their primitive fibres," *Phil. Trans. R. Soc.*, 140 (i):423–429.
1852a. "Examen des altérations qui ont lieu dans les filets d'origine du nerf pneumo-gastrique et des nerfs rachidiens, par suite de la section de ces nerfs au-dessus de leurs ganglions," *C. r. hebd. Acad. Sci., Paris*, 34:842–847.
1852b. "Septième mémoire sur le système nerveux," *C. r. hebd. Acad. Sci., Paris*, 35:301–306.
1852c. "Huitième mémoire sur le système nerveux," *C. r. hebd. Acad. Sci., Paris*, 35:561–564.

WALSH, J.
1774. "Of torpedos found on the coast of England," *Phil. Trans. R. Soc.*, 64 (ii):464–473.

WALSHE, F. M. R.
1956. "The Babinski plantar response, its forms and its physiological and pathological significance," *Brain*, 79:529–556.
1958. "Karl S. Lashley," *Neurology*, 8:870.

WARTENBERG, R.
1945. *The examination of reflexes.* Chicago, Year Book Publishers.
1947. "The Babinski reflex after fifty years," *J. Am. Med. Assoc.*, 133:763–767.

1951. "Babinski reflex and Marie-Foix flexor withdrawal reflex," *Arch. Neurol. Psychiat.*, 65:713–716.

WASER, M.

1933. *Begegnung am Abend, ein Vermächtnis.* Stuttgart, Deutsche Verlagsanstalt.

WATERMANN, R.

1960a. *Theodor Schwann, Leben und Werk.* Düsseldorf, Schwann.

1960b. "Theodor Schwanns Beitrag zur Neurologie," *Dt. Z. NervHeilk.*, 181:309–330.

WEAVER, T. A.

1937. "Anatomical relations of the commissures of Meynert and Gudden in the cat," *J. comp. Neurol.*, 66:333–342.

WEBER, E. H., and WEBER, E. F. W.

1846. "Muskelbewegung," in Wagner, *Handwörterbuch der Physiologie mit Rücksicht auf physiologische Pathologie*, Braunschweig, Vieweg, Vol. III, pt. 2, pp. 1–122.

WEED, L. H.

1914. "Studies on cerebro-spinal fluid. No. IV. The dual source of cerebro-spinal fluid," *J. med. Res.*, 31:93–117.

1922. "The cerebrospinal fluid," *Physiol. Rev.*, 2:171–203.

1953. "Lewis Hill Weed," *J. Am. Med. Assoc.*, 151:400.

WEIGERT, C.

1882. "Über eine neue Untersuchungsmethode des Centralnervensystems," *Z. med. Wiss.*, 20:753–757, 772–774.

WELDON, W. F. R.

1898. "Albert von Kölliker," *Nature*, 58:1–4.

WELLS, C. E.

1960. "The cerebral circulation. The clinical significance of current concepts," *Arch. Neurol.*, 3:319–331.

WEPFER, J. J.

1658. *Observationes anatomicae ex cadaveribus eorum quos sustulit apoplexia.* Schaffhausen, Sutur.

WESTPHAL, K. F. O.

1875. "Über einige Bewegungs-Erscheinungen an gelähmten Gliedern," *Arch. Psychiat. NervKrankh.*, 5:803–834.

WHYTT, R.

1751. *An essay on the vital and other involuntary motions of animals.* Edinburgh, Hamilton, Balfour & Neill.

1765. *Observations on the nature, causes, and cure of those disorders which have been commonly called nervous hypochondriac, or hysteric, to which are prefixed some remarks on the sympathy of the nerves.* Edinburgh, Becket, Hondt, & Balfour.

1768. *The works of Robert Whytt, M.D. published by his son.* Edinburgh, Becket, Hondt & Balfour.

WICKENS, G. M.

1952. *Avicenna: scientist and philosopher.* London, Luzac.

WIEBERG, J.

1914. "The anatomy of the brain in the works of Galen . . ." *Janus*, 19:17–32.

WILDER, B. G.

1880. "The foramina of Monro: some questions of anatomical history," *Boston med. surg. J.*, 103:152–154.

WILLIS, T.
  1664. *Cerebri anatome.* London, Martyn & Allestry. English translation in Willis (1684).
  1670. "De motu musculari," pp. 69–107 in *Affectionum quae dicuntur hystericae & hypochondriacae.* London, Allestry. English translation of *De motu musculari* in Willis (1684).
  1672. *De anima brutorum.* London, Davis. English translation in Willis (1684).
  1684. *Dr. Willis's practice of physick . . . new translated by S. Pordage.* London, Dring.

WILSON, J. L.
  1955. "Kenneth D. Blackfan (1883–1941)," *J. Pediat.,* 47:261–267.

WILSON, L. G.
  1955–1956. *The works of Giovanni Alfonso Borelli on muscular movements in animals.* Unpublished dissertation, University of London.

WINKLER, C.
  1923. "Die Bedeutung der Arbeit Constantin von Monakow's für die Wissenschaft," *Schweiz. Arch. Neurol. Psychiat.,* 13:11–24.

WOLLENBERG, R.
  1908. "Eduard Hitzig," *Arch. Psychiat. NervKrankh.,* 43:III–XV.

WOOD, C. A.
  1902. "Hermann von Helmholtz—the invention of the ophthalmoscope," *J. Am. Med. Assoc.,* 38 (i):552–557.

WOOLLAM, C. H. M.
  1957. "The historical significance of the cerebrospinal fluid," *Med. Hist.,* 1:91–114.

WRIGHT-ST. CLAIR, R. E.
  1964. *Doctors Monro. A medical saga.* London, Wellcome Historical Medical Library.

WUNSCHER, W.
  1957. "In memoriam Richard Arwed Pfeifer," *Psychiat. Neurol. med. Psychol.,* 9:131–132.

YOUNG, J. Z.
  1935. "Structure of the nerve fibres in Sepia," *J. Physiol., London,* 83:27*p*–28*p*.
  1945. "The history of the shape of a nerve fibre," pp. 41–94, *Essays on growth and form presented to D'Arcy Wentworth Thompson,* edited by W. E. Le Gros Clark and P. B. Medawar. Oxford, Clarendon Press.

ZANOBIO, B.
  1959. "Le osservazioni microscopiche di Felice Fontana sulla struttura dei nervi," *Physis,* 1:307–320.

INDEX

Volume II

Principles and Practice of
EMERGENCY MEDICINE

Edited by

GEORGE R. SCHWARTZ, M.D.

Director of Emergency Medicine
University of New Mexico Medical Center;
Associate Professor of Community,
Family and Emergency Medicine
University of New Mexico School of Medicine
Albuquerque, New Mexico

Formerly, Director, Northeastern Emergency
Medical Services (a multi-hospital group);
Clinical Assistant Professor of Emergency Medicine
The Medical College of Pennsylvania
Philadelphia, Pennsylvania

PETER SAFAR, M.D., Dr. h.c.

Distinguished Service Professor
Resuscitation Research Institute
University of Pittsburgh; Past Chairman
Department of Anesthesiology/Critical Care Medicine
University of Pittsburgh
School of Medicine

JOHN H. STONE, M.D.

Professor of Medicine (Cardiology) and
Director, Emergency Medicine Residency
Grady Memorial Hospital/
Emory University School of Medicine, Atlanta, Georgia

PATRICK B. STOREY, M.D.

Professor of Medicine and Associate Dean
University of Pennsylvania School of Medicine, Philadelphia, Pennsylvania

DAVID K. WAGNER, M.D.

Professor of Surgery and Emergency Medicine
Associate Professor of Pediatrics
The Medical College of Pennsylvania, Philadelphia, Pennsylvania

1978

W. B. SAUNDERS COMPANY
Philadelphia, London, Toronto

W. B. Saunders Company: West Washington Square
Philadelphia, PA 19105

1 St. Anne's Road
Eastbourne, East Sussex BN21 3UN, England

1 Goldthorne Avenue
Toronto, Ontario M8Z 5T9, Canada

Library of Congress Cataloging in Publication Data

Main entry under title:

Principles and practice of emergency medicine.

Includes index.

1. Medical emergencies.   I. Schwartz, George R.
II. Title: Emergency medicine. [DNLM: 1. Emergencies.
2. Emergency medicine.   3. Critical care.
WB105 P957]

RC86.7.P74   616'.025   75–25277

ISBN 0–7216–8031–3 (v.-1)

Principles and Practice of Emergency Medicine

Volume I   ISBN   0-7216-8031-3
Volume II   ISBN   0-7216-8033-X
Set   ISBN   0-7216-8034-8

Last digit is the print number: 9   8   7   6   5   4   3   2   1